S0-BZD-433

Disability Evaluation

Disability Evaluation

second edition

Stephen L. Demeter, M.D., M.P.H.
Staff Physician
Verde Valley Medical Center
Cottonwood, Arizona
Former Professor and Head of Pulmonary and Critical Care Medicine
Northeastern Ohio Universities College of Medicine
Rootstown, Ohio,
Immediate Past President
American Academy of Disability Evaluating Physicians
Chicago, Illinois

Gunnar B.J. Andersson, M.D., Ph.D.
Professor and Chair
Department of Orthopedic Surgery
Vice Dean, Surgical Sciences and Services
Rush University,
Senior Attending
Vice President of Medical Affairs
President, Medical Staff
Rush-Presbyterian-St. Luke's Medical Center
Chicago, Illinois

MOSBY
An Affiliate of Elsevier Science

American Medical Association
Physicians dedicated to the health of America

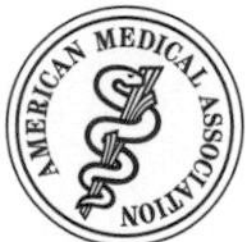

MOSBY
An Affiliate of Elsevier Science

11830 Westline Industrial Drive
St Louis, Missouri 63146

DISABILITY EVALUATION ISBN 0–323–00959–X

Notice

Medicine is an ever-changing field. Standard safety precautions must be followed, but as new research and clinical experience broaden our knowledge, changes in treatment and drug therapy may become necessary or appropriate. Readers are advised to check the product information currently provided by the manufacturer of each drug to be administered to verify the recommended dose, the method and duration of administration, and contraindications. It is the responsibility of the treating physician, relying on experience and knowledge of the patient, to determine dosages and the best treatment for each individual patient. Neither the Publisher nor the editor assume any liability for any injury and/or damage to persons or property arising from this publication.

THE PUBLISHER

First Edition 1996

Library of Congress Cataloging-in-Publication Data

Disability evaluation / [edited by] Stephen L. Demeter, Gunnar B. J. Andersson.—2nd ed.
p. ; cm.
Includes bibliographical references and index.
ISBN 0–323–00959–X
1. Disability evaluation. I. Demeter, Stephen L. II. Andersson, Gunnar.
[DNLM: 1. Disability Evaluation. W 925 D611 2003]
RC963.4 .D56 2003
616.07'5—dc21 2002037858

EXPO/MVY

Printed in the United States of America

Last digit is the print number: 9 8 7 6 5 4 3 2 1

This book is dedicated to all people who have struggled with physical or emotional disabilities in their lifetime. Their perseverance is an inspiration to us all. Their ability to overcome their difficulties is a reflection of God's mercy. Their willingness to take on the battles needed to overcome their restrictions, though, is a measure of their spirit and a reflection of some of the best qualities of man.

This book is also dedicated to my wife, Baze. Without her love and support, I would only be a shadow.

It is also dedicated to my parents, Steve and Arline Demeter who have always had my love, but have also earned my deepest respect.

Lastly, again with apologies to the Society of Jesus, "Ad Dei gloriam majorum."

STEPHEN L. DEMETER

To my wife, Kerstin, for her never-ending support and encouragement.

GUNNAR B.J. ANDERSSON

Contributors

Harvey L. Alpern, M.D.
Assistant Clinical Professor of Medicine, University of California at Los Angeles; Attending, Cedars-Sinai Medical Center, Los Angeles, California
Cardiac Impairment; Cardiac Disability

Gunnar B.J. Andersson, M.D., Ph.D.
Professor and Chairman, Department of Orthopedic Surgery, Vice Dean, Surgical Sciences and Services, Rush University, Senior Attending, Vice President of Medical Affairs, and President, Medical Staff, Rush-Presbyterian-St. Luke's Medical Center, Chicago, Illinois
Joint Systems: Thoracic and Lumbosacral Spine; Orthopedic Disability: The Spine

Arnold A. Angelici, Jr., M.D.
Assistant Clinical Professor of Community Health (Aerospace Medicine), Wright State University, Dayton, Ohio
Disability under the Federal Aviation Administration

Thomas J. Armstrong, Ph.D.
Professor, Center for Ergonomics, Department of Industrial Operations Engineering, University of Michigan, Ann Arbor, Michigan
Cumulative Trauma

Gerald M. Aronoff, M.D., F.A.A.D.E.P., D.A.B.P.M.
Assistant Clinical Professor, Tufts Medical School, Boston, Massachusetts; Chairman, Department of Pain Medicine, Presbyterian Hospital, Charlotte, North Carolina
Evaluating and Rating Impairment Caused by Pain

Charles G. Atkins, J.D.
Adjunct Professor of Law, University of Cincinnati College of Law, Cincinnati, Ohio
Legal Issues of Off-Work

Christopher T. Bajzer, M.D., F.A.C.C.
Associate Director, Carotid & Peripheral Intervention, The Cleveland Clinic Foundation, Cleveland, Ohio
Cardiac Diagnostic Techniques

Peter S. Barth, Ph.D.
Professor of Economics, University of Connecticut, Storrs, Connecticut
Economic Costs of Disability

Christopher Bell, J.D.
Jackson and Lewis Law Firm, Minneapolis, Minnesota
Overview of the Americans With Disabilities Act and the Family and Medical Leave Act

Thomas W. Bevan, Esq.
Bevan and Associates LPA, Inc., Northfield, Ohio
State Workers' Compensation Programs

Don B. Chaffin, Ph.D.
The G. Lawton and Louise G. Johnson Professor, Department of Industrial and Operations Engineering and Biomedical Engineering, and Professor, Department of Environmental and Industrial Health, University of Michigan, Ann Arbor, Michigan
Ergonomic Basis for Job-related Strength Testing

Daniel J. Clauw, M.D.
Professor of Medicine, and Director, Center for Advancement of Clinical Research, University of Michigan, Ann Arbor, Michigan
Functional Somatic Syndromes

Brian S. Cohen, M.D.
Center for Advanced Orthopedics and Sports Medicine, Chillicothe, Ohio
Joint Systems: Shoulder and Elbow

Mark S. Cohen, M.D.
Associate Professor and Director of Orthopedic Education, Rush Medical College; Director of Hand and Elbow Program, Department of Orthopedic Surgery, Rush-Presbyterian-St. Luke's Medical Center, Chicago, Illinois.
Joint Systems: Hand and Wrist

August Colenbrander, M.D.
Director Emeritus, Low Vision Services, Department of Ophthalmology, California Pacific Medical Center;

Affiliate Senior Scientist, Smith-Kettlewell Eye Research Institute, San Francisco, California
Visual Impairment

Alan L. Colledge, M.D.
Associate Professor and Adjunct Clinical Faculty, Department of Family and Preventive Medicine, University of Utah Sciences Center, Salt Lake City; Staff Physician, Utah Valley Hospital, Provo, Utah
Introduction to Fitness for Duty

Geraldine T. Demeter, M.A.
Office Manager, Editorial Assistant to Stephen L. Demeter, M.D., M.P.H., Sedona, Arizona
The Generic Functional Capacity Assessment

Stephen L. Demeter, M.D., M.P.H.
Staff Physician, Verde Valley Medical Center, Cottonwood, Arizona; Former Professor and Head of Pulmonary and Critical Care Medicine, Northeastern Ohio Universities College of Medicine, Rootstown, Ohio; Immediate Past President, American Academy of Disability Evaluating Physicians, Chicago, Illinois
Introduction to Disability and Impairment; The Historical Development of Disability Programs in the United States; Contrasting the Standard, Impairment, and Disability Examination; The Impairment-Oriented Evaluation and Report; Pulmonary Diagnostic Techniques; Pulmonary Impairment; Peripheral Vascular Impairment; Endocrinological Impairment; Impairment Evaluation in Functional Somatic Syndromes; The Disability Evaluation and Report; The Generic Functional Capacity Assessment; Pulmonary Disability; Peripheral Vascular Disability; Biostatistics and Epidemiology: A Review of Topics Found in this Book; How to Fill Out Disability and Return-to-Work Forms

Anthony J. Dorto, M.D.
Past President, American Academy of Disability Evaluating Physicians, Chicago, Illinois; West Gables Rehabilitation Hospital, Miami; Attending Physiatrist, Disability Assessment Center, P.A., Miami, Florida
Department of Labor Guidelines for Job Categorization

Byron A. Eliashof, M.D.
Clinical Professor, John A. Burns School of Medicine, University of Hawaii; Honorary Staff, Queens Medical Center, Honolulu, Hawaii
Psychological Impairment

Eugene P. Frenkel, M.D.
Professor of Medicine and Radiology, Patsy R. & Raymond D. Nasher Distinguished Chair in Cancer Research, University of Texas Southwestern Medical School; Attending Physician, Zale-Lipshy University, and Parkland Memorial Hospital, Dallas, Texas
Hematologic and Oncologic Impairment

John W. Frymoyer, M.D., M.S.
Retired Professor and Chair Emeritus, Department of Orthopedics and Rehabilitation, University of Vermont Medical School, Burlington, Vermont
Joint Systems: Thoracic and Lumbosacral Spine

Steven R. Garfin, M.D.
Professor and Chair, Department of Orthopaedics, University of California, San Diego, University of California, San Diego, Medical Center, and Veterans Administration Hospital, San Diego, California
Joint Systems: Cervical Spine

Elizabeth Genovese, M.D., M.B.A.
Clinical Assistant Professor of Medicine – Associated Faculty, University of Pennsylvania School of Medicine, Philadelphia; Medical Director, IMX Medical Management Services, Bala Cynwyd, Pennsylvania
Causality

Tee L. Guidotti, M.D., M.P.H.
Professor and Chair, Department of Environmental and Occupational Health, and Professor of Health Policy and Epidemiology, School of Public Health and Health Sciences, Professor and Director, Division of Occupational Medicine and Toxicology, and Professor of Pulmonary Medicine, Department of Medicine, School of Medicine and Health Sciences, The George Washington University Medical Center, Washington, D.C.; Adjunct Professor, Department of Public Health Sciences, University of Alberta Faculty of Medicine, Edmonton, Alberta, Canada
Evidence-Based Medical Dispute Resolution

Scott Haldeman, D.C., M.D., Ph.D., F.R.C.P.(C)
Clinical Professor, Department of Neurology, University of California, Irvine, Irvine, California
Neurological Diagnostic Techniques

James E. Hansen, M.D., F.A.C.P., F.C.C.P.
Professor of Medicine, Department of Medicine, UCLA School of Medicine, Los Angeles; Professor of Medicine, Division of Respiratory and Criticial Care Physiology and Medicine, Los Angeles County Harbor UCLA Medical Center, Torrance, California
The Integrated Cardiopulmonary Exercise Stress Test

Robert H. Haralson III, M.D., M.B.A.
Associate Clinical Professor, University of Tennessee Center for the Health Sciences; Medical Director, Southeastern Orthopaedics, Knoxville, Tennessee
Orthopedic Disability: The Joints

Natalie P. Hartenbaum, M.D., M.P.H.
Adjunct Assistant Professor, Department of Emergency Medicine, Hospital of the University of Pennsylvania, Philadelphia; Chief Medical Officer, OccuMedix, Inc., Dresher, Pennsylvania
Fitness to Work for Commercial Drivers

Richard J. Herzog, M.D.
Professor of Radiology, Weill Medical College of Cornell University; Chief, Division of Teleradiology, Hospital for Special Surgery, New York, New York
The Role of Radiologic Imaging in the Orthopedic Impairment Evaluation

Edward B. Holmes, M.D., M.P.H.
Assistant Professor – Occupational Medicine, and Occupational Medicine Clinic Director, University Hospital, University of Utah Health Sciences Center, Salt Lake City, Utah
Introduction to Fitness for Duty

George B. Holmes, Jr., M.D., M.P.H.
Assistant Professor, Department of Orthopaedic Surgery, Rush Medical College; Attending Orthopaedic Surgery, Rush-Presbyterian-St. Luke's Medical Center, Chicago, Illinois
Joint Systems: Foot and Ankle

Susan J. Isernhagen, P.T.
Founder, Isernhagen Work Systems, Duluth, Minnesota
Work Hardening

Richard E. Johns, Jr., M.D., M.S.P.H.
Professor, Adjunct Faculty, Department of Family and Preventive Medicine, University of Utah Health Sciences Center, Salt Lake City, Utah; Fellow, ACOEM and AADEP, and CIME – ABIME, Chicago, Illinois
Introduction to Fitness for Duty

Barbara Judy, R.N., M.A.
Americans with Disabilities Act/504 Compliance Director, West Virginia University, Morgantown, West Virginia
Overview of the Americans With Disabilities Act and the Family and Medical Leave Act; Resource Lists

David M. Kalainov, M.D.
Assistant Professor of Clinical Orthopaedic Surgery, Department of Orthopaedic Surgery, Northwestern University Feinberg School of Medicine; Active Staff, Northwestern Memorial Hospital, Department of Orthopaedic Surgery, Chicago, Illinois
Joint Systems: Hand and Wrist

Choll W. Kim, M.D., Ph.D.
Assistant Professor, Department of Orthopaedics, University of California, San Diego; Assistant Professor and Staff Orthopaedic Surgeon, Department of Orthopaedics, Veterans Administration Hospital and University of California Medical Center, San Diego, California
Joint Systems: Cervical Spine

Jeffrey D. Klein, M.D.
Instructor in Orthopaedic Surgery, Attending Spine Surgeon, Hospital for Joint Diseases, New York University School of Medicine, New York, New York
Joint Systems: Cervical Spine

Edwin H. Klimek, M.D., F.R.C.P.C., F.A.A.D.E.P.
Consultant Neurologist, Department of Medicine, Niagara Health System, St. Catharines, Ontario, Canada; Director, American Academy of Disability Evaluating Physicians, Chicago, Illinois
Central Nervous System Impairment; Central Nervous System Disability

J. Bruce Kneeland, M.D.
Professor of Radiology, Hospital of the University of Pennsylvania, Philadelphia, Pennsylvania
The Role of Radiologic Imaging in the Orthopedic Impairment Evaluation

Randall D. Lea, M.D.
Clinical Assistant Professor of Orthopaedic Surgery, Tulane University, New Orleans; Orthopaedic Surgeon, Center of Orthopaedic Care & Evaluative Medicine, Baton Rouge, Louisiana
Joint Systems: Knee and Hip

Barry S. Levinson, M.D.
Associate Professor, University of Texas Southwestern Medical Center; Chief of Hematology – Oncology, Dallas Veterans Administration Medical Center, Dallas, Texas
Hematologic and Oncologic Impairment

Richard P. Levy, M.D.
Adjunct Professor of Medicine, Dartmouth Medical School, Hanover, New Hampshire; Research Professor of Internal Medicine, Northeastern Ohio Universities College of Medicine, Rootstown, Ohio; Attending Endocrinologist, Dartmouth Hitchcock Medical Center, Lebanon; Staff Endocrinologist, Cheshire Medical Center, Dartmouth-Hitchcock, Keene, New Hampshire
Endocrinological Disability

James V. Luck, Jr., M.D.
Professor and Executive Vice Chairman, Department of Orthopaedic Surgery, University of California, Los Angeles/Orthopaedic Hospital, University of California, Los Angeles; President, Chief Executive

Officer, and Medical Director, Orthopaedic Hospital, Los Angeles, California
Joint Systems: Knee and Hip

Alvin Markovitz, M.D., F.A.C.P., F.A.C.O.E.M., F.A.A.D.E.P.
Associate Professor of Medicine, University of Southern California School of Medicine, Los Angeles; Medical Staff – Chairman of Medical Education, St. John's Hospital and Medical Center, Santa Monica; Medical Staff, Santa Monica-University of California, Los Angeles Medical Center, Santa Monica; Medical Staff, Los Angeles County-University of Southern California Medical Center, Los Angeles, California
Hematological and Oncological Disability

Leonard N. Matheson, Ph.D.
Associate Professor, Occupational Therapy, and Neurology, Washington University School of Medicine; Director, Occupational Performance Center, Rehabilitation Institute of St. Louis, St. Louis, Missouri
The Functional Capacity Evaluation

Tom G. Mayer, M.D.
Clinical Professor, Department of Orthopedic Surgery, University of Texas Southwestern Medical Center; Medical Director, PRIDE and PRIDE Research Foundation, Dallas, Texas
Range of Motion Evaluation

John D. McLellan, Jr., A.B., J.D.
Formerly Attorney, Alexandria, Virginia, Director of the Federal Employees Compensation Program, and United States Department of Labor
The Historical Development of Disability Programs in the United States; Federal Workers' Compensation Programs

James R. McPherson, M.D., M.Sc., F.A.C.P.
Emeritus Professor of Medicine, Mayo Medical School, Rochester, Minnesota
Gastrointestinal Impairment; Gastrointestinal Disability

Stanley R. Mohler, M.D., M.A.
Professor and Vice Chair, and Director of Aerospace Medicine, Department of Community Health, Wright State University School of Medicine; Courtesy Staff, Family Practice, Good Samaritan Hospital, Dayton, Ohio
Disability under the Federal Aviation Administration

Kenneth D. Nibali, J.D.
Associate Commissioner for Disability, Social Security Administration, Baltimore, Maryland
Social Security Disability Programs

Inder Perkash, M.D., M.S., F.R.C.S. (Edin), F.A.C.S.
Professor of Urology, Physical Medicine and Rehabilitation, and Paralyzed Veterans of America Professor of Spinal Cord Injury, Stanford University School of Medicine, Palo Alto; Chief, Spinal Cord Injury Service, Stanford University, Stanford, Veterans Affairs Palo Alto Health Care System, Palo Alto, California
Genitourinary Impairment

Lawrence P. Postol, J.D.
Seyfarth, Shaw, Fairweather and Geraldson, Washington, DC
The Medical—Legal Interface

David C. Randolph, M.D., M.P.H.
Department of Occupational and Environmental Medicine, University of Cincinnati, Cincinnati, Ohio; President, The American Academy of Disability Evaluating Physicians, Chicago, Illinois
The Historical Development of Disability Programs in the United States

Anthony A. Romeo, M.D.
Associate Professor, Department of Orthopedic Surgery, Rush Medical College; Attending Surgeon, Orthopedic Surgery, Rush-Presbyterian-St. Luke's Medical Center, Chicago, Illinois
Joint Systems: Shoulder and Elbow

Robert T. Sataloff, M.D., D.M.A.
Professor of Otolaryngology – Head and Neck Surgery, Thomas Jefferson Medical College; Chairman, Department of Otolaryngology – Head and Neck Surgery, Graduate Hospital, Philadelphia, Pennsylvania
Otolaryngological (ENT) Impairment

Brian Schulman, M.D., C.I.M.E.
Occupational Psychiatry, Bethesda, Maryland
Evaluating and Rating Impairment Caused by Stress

Karl D. Schwarze, M.D., M.S.
Associate Professor of Clinical Internal Medicine, Division of Nephrology, Northeastern Ohio Universities College of Medicine, Rootstown; Director of the Acute Hemodialysis Unit, Akron General Medical Center, Akron, Ohio
Renal Disability

Lynn C. Slaby, J.D.
Judge, 9th District Court of Appeals – Akron; Graduate of the University of Akron, Akron, Ohio
The Physician as a Witness

Jon Streltzer, M.D.
Professor of Psychiatry, John A. Burns School of Medicine, University of Hawaii, Honolulu, Hawaii
Psychological Impairment

Rand S. Swenson, D.C., M.D., Ph.D.
Associate Professor of Medicine (Neurology) and Anatomy, Dartmouth Medical School, Hanover; Staff Physician, Dartmouth-Hitchcock Medical Center, Lebanon, New Hampshire
Neurological Diagnostic Techniques

James B. Talmage, M.D.
Medical Director, Occupational Health Center, Cookeville Regional Medical Center, Cookeville, Tennessee
Resource Personnel Used in a Disability Evaluation; Can Joe Work?

James S. Taylor, M.D.
Head, Section of Industrial Dermatology, The Cleveland Clinic Foundation, Cleveland, Ohio
Dermatological Impairment; Dermatological Disability

Marc T. Taylor, M.D.
Clinical Assistant Professor of Surgery, Division of Plastic Surgery, University of Texas at San Antonio Health Science Center; Past President, American Academy of Visability Evaluating Physicians; President, Bexar County Medical Society, San Antonio, Texas
Peripheral Nervous System Impairment; Peripheral Nervous System Disability

Moshe S. Torem, M.D.
Professor, Department of Psychiatry, Northeastern Ohio Universities College of Medicine, Rootstown; Medical Director, The Center for Mind-Body Medicine, Akron General Health and Wellness Center, Akron, Ohio
Psychiatric Diagnostic Techniques; Psychiatric Disability

Ronald J. Washington, M.D., F.A.A.D.E.P.
Former Clinical Instructor of Internal Medicine, University of Texas, Southwestern Medical Center, Dallas, Texas
The Impairment-Oriented Evaluation and Report; The Disability Evaluation and Report

Karlman Wasserman, M.D., Ph.D.
Professor of Medicine, Department of Medicine, UCLA School of Medicine, Los Angeles; Professor of Medicine, Division of Respiratory and Critical Care Physiology and Medicine, Los Angeles County Harbor UCLA Medical Center, Torrance, California
The Integrated Cardiopulmonary Exercise Stress Test

John M. Williams, D.Ed.
President, Dr. John M. Williams & Associates, Health and Rehabilitation Consultants, Pompano Beach, Florida
The Role of the Vocational Rehabilitationist

Lee C. Woods, M.D.
Private Practice, Whittier, California
Joint Systems: Foot and Ankle

Dennis J. Wright, M.D.
Assistant Professor of Surgery, Northeastern Ohio Universities College of Medicine, Rootstown, Ohio
Peripheral Vascular Impairment; Peripheral Vascular Disability

Preface

This second edition of *Disability Evaluation* has been written for three reasons: to update and expand the introductory section, to make the second section follow the newest edition of the Guides, and to add a third section on disability and return-to-work issues.

The introductory material has been expanded to include chapters on causality and evidence-based medicine. These chapters should provide a firmer basis for the legal aspects of disability medicine, a specialty which bridges the medical-legal interface more commonly than any other branch of medicine other than the forensic disciplines such as forensic psychiatry or pathology. However, unlike these disciplines, disability medicine is a branch of medicine that will be used by most physicians who take care of patients. Clinicians frequently face issues such as filling out the forms sent to them by the Social Security Administration for their patients; they treat injuries and provide activity restrictions for their patients; and they write return-to-work prescriptions for these patients. Unfortunately, there is a paucity of published materials that teach physicians how to accomplish these and other tasks covered under the blanket term, "disability medicine." It is certainly not a topic discussed in medical school or taught during residency or fellowship programs.

As recently as last year, I received a consult in my office for the express intent of filling out Social Security forms for the patient of a fellow practitioner. When I told him what the SSA needed from him and what the forms were intended for, it was if the sun rose in his eyes and he finally understood what this part of disability medicine covered. For this reason, the chapter on Social Security was changed to make it more of an instructional chapter for the practicing physician. In a similar vein, the remaining chapters in the introductory section were rewritten to allow the practicing physician to better understand the "system" in which they work and interface.

In 2001, the American Medical Association published the fifth edition of the AMA Guides. One of the express purposes of the first edition of this book was to provide the background material for the Guides so that the impairment-evaluating physician would be able to understand why the Guides did things in the manner that it did. As mentioned in the preface of the first edition, "these rating systems, many times, take the appearance of 'cookbooks.'" The Guides is an excellent example of this concept, although the fifth edition was rewritten to provide some explanation of the methods behind the evaluating process found in this new edition. However, it still does not explain much of the medical concepts underlying the details of its methods or conclusions. This book, co-published by the AMA, provides those explanations. The same remarks can be made for the other rating systems that physicians may use for an impairment evaluation such as the Social Security system, the various state workers' compensation systems, the Veteran's Administration system, and others. Material is found in the book that addresses each of these systems although not in the same detail as for the AMA Guides. However, and more importantly, the concepts developed in this book will allow the impairment-evaluating physician to understand these systems better and to produce a better examination and report.

A new, third section covers the topic of return-to-work issues. As noted above, these are areas which practicing physicians need to have familiarity with, will use frequently, and are generally poorly knowledgeable about. Most primary care physicians should find this material of great utility in their practices. It is approached from two perspectives—a medical and a legal. The medical/scientific background material necessary for performing this aspect of disability medicine are provided. The legal implications are discussed. Using this part of the text, the physician should be able to provide a better service to their patients and avoid legal liability.

One issue that is usually not discussed when reading articles on the subjects of impairment rating or disability and return-to-work issues, is the almost total lack of scientific research underlying most of this material. Much of what was written in this book is taken from mainstream medicine and then extrapolated into the impairment or disability concepts. There have been frequent calls for scientific research on the topics of impairment medicine and disability medicine. Considering the financial impact of this branch of medicine, it is curious that so little valid research has been performed. This preface makes another plea to the medical and legal community to fund and perform this research. Many of the chapters in this book make note of this need and offer recommendations for future lines of study.

Finally I will give my personal reasons for undertaking the second edition of this book. It has been a labor of love, one that starts with the love that I have for an organization of which I am a "Founding Fellow"—the American Academy of Disability Evaluating Physicians. This is and continues to be an emerging discipline under the broad umbrella of medicine and I feel privileged to be a part of on ongoing, growing, and new branch of medical science.

I would like to make many of the same acknowledgements found in the first edition. My love and respect for my parents, Steve and Arline, grows with the years. My love for my children likewise continues to increase. My attempt at an American haiku will be repeated as my love, respect, and admiration for my wife deepens.

I would also like to acknowledge the contributions of individuals who have assisted me with this book including my secretaries Darlene Guillard and Cindy Campbell and the librarians at Akron General Medical Center, especially Judy Knight, MLS. I would also like to pay respect to my mentor and friend of the last 25 years, Dr. Edward Cordasco, an exemplary physician, teacher, and human being.

Lastly, I would like to acknowledge my brother-in-law, George Sampas who didn't really do a darn thing for this project but who told me that he never had his name mentioned in a book and that he felt that his life would be successful if only it were. Marrying my sister should have been sufficient for that.

Stephen L. Demeter, MD, MPH

Contents

PART I
INTRODUCTION

PART II
IMPAIRMENT

PART I

Introduction

CHAPTER

1

Introduction to Disability and Impairment*

STEPHEN L. DEMETER, MD, MPH

This book is intended as a reference source for impairment or disability-oriented evaluations, protocols, and techniques. The first edition of this book was organized into three broad categories: introductory chapters, impairment evaluation chapters (which explained and extended the material published in the fourth edition of the AMA Guides[5]), and reference/resource chapters. This edition of the book significantly differs from the first edition in two major areas.

In the impairment section of the book (Part II), the chapters continue to expand on the principles outlined in the fifth edition of the AMA Guides.[3] As can be expected, there has been an evolution in the impairment ratings found in the Guides.

In 1956, the Board of Trustees of the AMA created the ad hoc Committee on Medical Rating of Physical Impairment. Its charge was to develop a series of practical guides for rating physical impairment due to organic diseases. The scope of the Committee's work was broadened and its name was changed to the Committee on Rating of Mental and Physical Impairment. The Committee published a series of 13 separate papers in the Journal of the American Medical Association between 1958 and 1970. These papers were published as a single volume in 1971. A republication occurred in 1977.[4]

In 1981, the AMA's Council on Scientific Affairs undertook a review of the Guides and established an advisory panel to determine the need for revising the published criteria. At their direction, 12 expert panels were established to update the Guides. The second edition was published in 1984.[1] Further revision yielded the third edition in 1988,[6] the third revised edition in 1990,[2] and the fourth edition in 1993.[5] Ratings for various diseases and medical conditions have been constantly revised as greater experience has been acquired and as medical science has progressed culminating in the current edition.

The fifth edition[3] has continued this tradition of reworking the material found in prior editions. Application of the fifth edition, as well as differences between the fourth and fifth editions of the AMA Guides are discussed thoroughly in the AMA Guides companion, Masters the AMA Guides.[10] The second edition of *Disability Evaluation* reviews, expands, and explains the material found in the fifth edition.

A new section in this book addresses disability evaluation. To the beginner, the distinction between impairment and disability appears to be trivial, yet it is important and the two concepts are distinct.

One important issue concerning a disability evaluation that is not covered in this book is the timing of return to work after an acute injury, illness, or surgical procedure. These issues are beyond the scope of this book and have been addressed in other published texts.[7,8] These sources are recommended for those issues. This edition addresses how to certify that an individual is ready to return to work, how to fill out the forms or to prepare a report, when and how to place restrictions on the examinee's ability to return to the work setting, whether job changes are necessary, and whether accommodations are needed.

As in the previous edition, certain concepts are crucial to the understanding of an impairment or a disability evaluation. These concepts are adherence to rigid definitions of impairment and disability, ability to communicate effectively, and knowledge and awareness of one's role in the process.

*Parts of this chapter were previously published in the First Edition. George Smith, MD, MPH, and Gunnar Andersson, MD, PhD contributed to that chapter.

Need for Precise Definitions

A disability could be defined as an inability or altered ability to accomplish a given task successfully. Such a definition would ill suit the purposes of this book and would not help to distinguish what is being evaluated during the disability process. The goal is not to define and describe all the limitations that nature has imposed on each individual. In an impairment evaluation, the evaluator is charged with defining and measuring an individual's health status with regard to that individual's prior health status. In a disability evaluation, the clinician is interested solely in those deficiencies that are important for specific tasks, especially in the workplace. Further, the investigator is not interested in all the deviations in capability that serve to segregate an individual's place in the workplace; only those created owing to an alteration of prior capabilities caused by a departure from an individual's "normal" state of health. For example, the issue of why an individual cannot be a championship marathon runner or a concert pianist is not addressed. However, why an individual can no longer be a marathon runner or a concert pianist is important. To measure, define, and rate those causes (the impairment evaluation) is the goal. After measuring and defining those causes, in the second instance, the individual's capabilities to accomplish certain activities such as running a marathon or playing the piano at a professional level (the disability evaluation) are described.

Disability (or non-ability) arises out of an individual's inability to perform a task successfully because of an insufficiency in one or more areas of functional capability: physical function, mental function, agility, dexterity, coordination, strength, endurance, knowledge, skill, intellectual ability, or experience. Disability is not necessarily related to any health impairment or medical condition, although a medical condition or impairment may cause or contribute to disability. (For example, a 5-year-old cannot teach a college course on calculus; neither can a 50-year-old college professor who had a brain injury limiting his awareness of time and place.) Disability requires a conceptual definition; it is "the gap between what a person *can* do and what the person *needs*, or *wants* to do."[9(p3)] A medical condition may limit the individual's capacity for physical or mental activity, thus creating the disability, or it may lead to restrictions placed on the individual's activities to prevent future harm.

Both impairment and disability may be temporary or permanent depending on the capacity of the medical condition to resolve, the degree of resolution, and the care that the individual receives toward that resolution. In addition, there are degrees of resolution, or degrees of impairment and disability, which are termed partial or complete. A partial or complete impairment refers to the degree of deviation from normality. Partial impairment refers to a medical condition that prevents to some degree, but not totally, a normal bodily function. Complete impairment refers to the total loss of that bodily function (which may be physiologic, anatomic, or biochemical, for example). Partial disability refers to the ability to perform some, but not all, the required tasks of a job; complete disability means that the individual can perform none of those tasks.

Both impairment and disability can be measured. In measuring impairment, the evaluator must be aware of the normal functions or expectations for that part of the body being measured. Physicians possess this ability owing to their education and experience. The foundation of arriving at a diagnosis in clinical medicine is the assessment of deviations from normality. However, there is a large gap between a skilled and eminent diagnostician and an impairment evaluator. This gap is created by the direction in which the examiner proceeds after cataloging those deviations. The clinician uses the deviations as the basis for a diagnosis and a therapeutic regimen. The impairment evaluator applies them to a set of artificial expectations that usually culminate in a financial settlement. The disability evaluator, on the other hand, must weigh the medical impairment, the demands of the occupation, and how these two interact. The disability evaluator addresses issues such as whether the job can be modified to fit the individual's abilities or whether the worker can be retrained or rehabilitated so that he or she can perform that job or a different job.

Confusion occurs when dealing with the distinctions between impairment and disability, as noted previously. That confusion is heightened when dealing with the language of laws, regulations, or policies and procedures, which ordinarily confuse the two concepts, making no distinction between them and using them interchangeably, and also speaking of the consequences of disability rather than accurately defining the disabled state.

The fifth edition of the Guides and its Masters companion, offers examples of various definitions of both impairment and disability from several sources.[3,10] Many other examples exist and could be cited. Common to all these definitions is an underlying need to define impairment and disability in an operational sense to fulfill the needs of the organization that developed it. These definitional differences are most marked between private industry (e.g., insurance companies) and governmental agencies.

For the purposes of this book, an impairment is defined as deviation of an anatomic structure, physiologic function, intellectual capability, or emotional status from that which the individual possessed prior to an alteration in those structures or functions or from that expected from population norms. A disability is defined as a medical impairment that prevents an individual from performing specified intellectual, creative, adaptive, social, or physical functions. Disability is the inability to complete a specific task successfully that the individual was previously capable of completing or one that most members of a society are capable of completing owing to a medical or psychological deviation from prior health status or from the status expected of most members of a society.

A handicap relies on the concept of disability. A person with a medical impairment may or may not be disabled (for example, a paraplegic may be a successful business person but not a professional basketball player). If an assistive device allows a medically impaired individual to perform a specified task successfully that he or she would not have been capable of performing (either totally or partially) without the use of that assistive device, then a handicap exists. A handicap also exists if the task circumstances can be modified so that the medically impaired individual can perform the task without the use of personal assistive devices. For example, if a company only purchases desks that one stands behind as opposed to sitting at, then the individual with an above the knee amputation who can successfully accomplish his or her job tasks with various accommodations to allow him or her to use that desk is considered handicapped. He or she is medically impaired but not disabled because he or she is capable of performing the specified tasks while using that desk. However, that capability is created by using a personal assistive device (such as an artificial leg) or by modifying the task circumstances (for example, a special desk with a chair purchased solely for this one individual). Thus a person with a medical impairment may or may not have a disability. The coexistence of a handicap, by definition, mitigates the impact of the impairment and alters the disability.

Role Awareness

Physicians, in their traditional role in medicine, are decision makers. They are so accustomed to this concept that this role does not enter into their conscious awareness. They stand at the top of a flow of information, taking, assimilating, organizing, and using that information when making decisions about or giving recommendations to their patients. In circumstances where their role at the pinnacle of this information flow is impeded or circumvented, they feel threatened, uncomfortable, and even angry. Yet this is the norm in impairment and disability evaluations.

In a standard medical evaluation, or in the course of the normal practice of medicine, input from a variety of sources flows upward, stopping at the decision maker—the physician. The following situation provides an example (Fig. 1–1 graphically conveys the following concept, with the internist at the top of the decision making pyramid). An internist is caring for an elderly man in a hospital. The patient enters with signs of dementia and is found to have sepsis caused by pneumonia. The flow of information is upward and comes from a variety of sources, including the pathology department (chemistries, hematology, microbiology), the radiology department, other physicians (consultants such as infectious disease or pulmonary specialists), the respiratory therapy department (oxygen analyses, pulmonary hygiene recommendations), a social worker (for family interactions regarding resuscitation decisions and posthospital placement or care), nurses, and others. The internist may have an emotional reaction if a medical professional who was one of the components of the information flow decided to become a decision maker. For example, if the radiologist wrote in the report that "the patient has lobar pneumonia, most likely pneumococcal, and should receive 4 million units of penicillin every 4 hours intravenously, 5 liters of oxygen by nasal cannula, an aerosol with a sympathomimetic every 4 hours, and a stat consult to the pastoral care department," the internist may feel usurped.

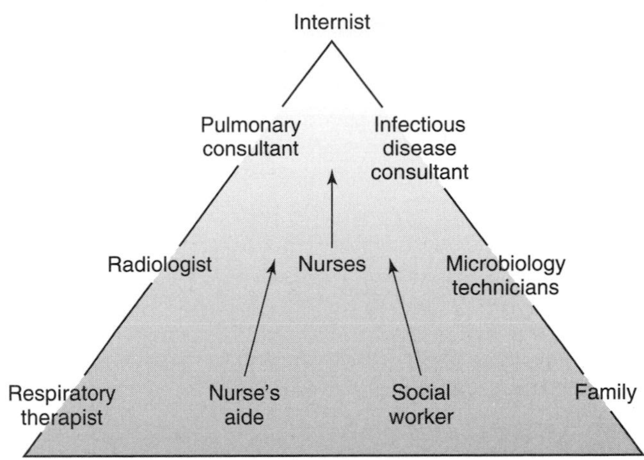

Figure 1–1. An example of the upward flow of information to the internist caring for a hospitalized patient with pneumonia, dementia, and sepsis. Other sides of this pyramid would have other sources of input (see example in text).

The anger and frustration that the internist would feel in the example caused by the usurption of his or her role as the decision maker by someone lower in the information flow is understandable. In impairment and disability examinations, physicians frequently develop these feelings of anger and frustration for the same reason—they feel that they are being bypassed in their role as the decision maker. The point that physicians rarely understand is that they are being bypassed because they are no longer the decision maker. Someone else is. That someone might be an attorney, an insurance administrator, a workers' compensation examiner, a nurse, an administrative law judge, or others. As seen in Figure 1–2, during the course of a person's impairment or disability evaluation, the physician occupies a lower position

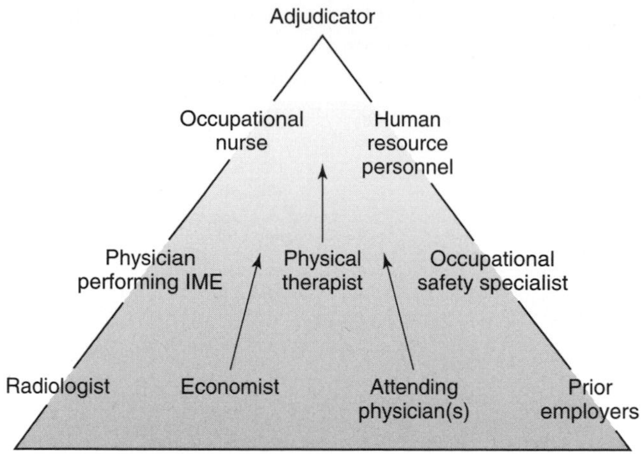

Figure 1–2. An example of the upward flow of information to a workers' compensation adjudicator for a claimant with a work-related crush injury of an arm. Other sides of the pyramid would have other sources of input: for example, social workers, vocational rehabilitationists, psychologists, and others.

in the information flow, which leads to the decision maker. The physician is responsible for providing medical information regarding impairment or disability to the decision maker. That is his or her sole responsibility unless further input is requested. Unless requested, further information is neither desired nor appreciated.

Cognitive assimilation of this positional shift (or role awareness) is vital for the physician. Otherwise, anger and frustration ensue—not only for the physician, but also for the decision maker who occupies the pinnacle of the information flow and who cannot understand why physicians seem so hard to work with.

Communication

In communication, a thought or idea is expressed by the sender and delivered to a receiver. For that thought or idea to be properly interpreted by the receiver, both sender and receiver must have a common frame of reference and speak the same language. In relation to impairment and disability evaluations, physicians and nonmedical personnel must be able to communicate about medical problems and limitations using a common language.

Communication can be thought of as the bridging of an idea from one person to another. There is a sender and a receiver. Because a person cannot read another person's mind, this bridging is done by language—either oral or nonoral. For the sender to communicate effectively with the receiver, they must have a common language and share a common reference and background (for example, no matter how patiently and simply an astrophysicist explains celestial mechanics, a 5-year-old will never understand the subject because of a lack of common reference and background).

Physicians are trained to assemble and analyze medical information, communicating with each other within a framework of established medical diagnostic criteria and generally accepted medical principles and practice. They use highly technical and specialized medical language to communicate with each other and with other health care professionals. When communicating with nonmedical users of medical information, they must speak in nontechnical terms. The information that flows each way across this information interface must be understandable, supportable, reasonable, and useful to each party. All parties who work in the impairment and disability arenas depend on each other for the system to work efficiently and properly. The same applies to nonmedical professionals. All professions, not just medicine, utilize highly specialized language. In order to obtain useful information, the nonmedical professional must ask the medical professional questions that the medical professional can understand. Figure 1–3 illustrates the dynamics of this type of communication.

As seen in Figure 1–3, the bridge between these technical languages is "plain English." The first and foremost rule that should apply in all communication between professionals with different professions is never to assume that the other professional understands what is meant by a technical term.

BRIDGE BETWEEN TECHNICAL LANGUAGES		
MEDICAL LANGUAGE This language is spoken by the physician, physical therapist, nurse, and others.	PLAIN ENGLISH	NON-MEDICAL LANGUAGE This language may be the language of lawyers, human resource personnel, insurance administrators, and others.

Figure 1–3. Bridge between technical languages.

The Report

Physicians must become more than casually acquainted with the specific provisions and procedures of the employment and workers' compensation laws and regulations in the states where they practice, the Social Security Act, the Americans with Disabilities Act, the Family and Medical Leave Act, and the regulations published by the federal agencies administering these statutes. By becoming knowledgeable regarding these matters, physicians will be able to assess the requests and reasons for an impairment or disability-oriented medical evaluation; ask appropriate questions of the requestor; understand the needs of the requestor; and provide a report that is complete, accurate, supportable, and responsive to the stated needs. The user of the medical information must also understand the technical medical statements the physician uses in formulating conclusions and recommendations and know when to ask for clarification if the physician relies more on medical jargon than on plain English.

By the same token, those on the nonmedical side of impairment and disability management must understand the role, functions, thought processes, and limitations of the physician so that they can formulate questions and have realistic expectations regarding the evaluation's outcome. The request for an impairment or disability-oriented medical evaluation must explain enough regarding the evaluation's objectives for the physician to assess those objectives, translate them into a medical evaluation protocol appropriate for that system, and provide a responsive report.

In the end, the report is the final product of the impairment or disability evaluation. Chapters 11 and 43 discuss the report more fully. Communication is the vital element in a successful report. The purpose of this book is to provide the necessary concepts to both physician and nonphysician readers to allow that communication to take place.

References

1. American Medical Association: Guides to the Evaluation of Permanent Impairment, 2nd ed. Chicago, American Medical Association, 1984.
2. American Medical Association: Guides to the Evaluation of Permanent Impairment, 3rd ed, rev. Chicago, American Medical Association, 1990.
3. Cocchiarella L, Andersson GBJ (eds): Guides to the Evaluation of Permanent Impairment, 5th ed. Chicago, American Medical Association, 2001.
4. Committee on Rating of Mental and Physical Impairment: Guides to the Evaluation of Permanent Impairment. Chicago, American Medical Association, 1977.
5. Doege TC, Houston TP: Guides to the Evaluation of Permanent Impairment, 4th ed. Chicago, American Medical Association, 1993.
6. Engelberg AL: Guides to the Evaluation of Permanent Impairment, 3rd ed. Chicago, American Medical Association, 1988.
7. Reed P: The Medical Disability Advisor: Workplace Guidelines for Disability Duration, 4th ed. Denver, Reed Groups, 2001.
8. Work Loss Data Institute: Official Disability Guidelines, 2001, 6th ed. Corpus Christi, Work Loss Data Institute, 2000.
9. Demeter SL, Andersson GBJ, Smith GM: Disability Evaluation. Mosby, Philadelphia and the American Medical Association, Chicago, 1996.
10. Cocchiarella L, Lord SJ Master the AMA Guides Fifth: A Medical and Legal Transition to the Guides to the Evaluation of Permanent Impairment, Fifth Edition. First Edition. Chicago, American Medical Association, 2001.

CHAPTER

2

The Historical Development of Disability Programs in the United States*

DAVID C. RANDOLPH, MD, MPH ■ STEPHEN L. DEMETER, MD, MPH ■ JOHN D. McLELLAN, JR., JD

As long as humankind has existed there has inevitably been impairment and disability. The life-giving processes of gestation and birth themselves can result in physical and mental incapacities that impede an individual's full, normal function. Natural disasters such as earthquakes and hurricanes cause injuries and impairment, as do accidents of all kinds and in all situations. Accidents can occur at home, at work, while on vacation, or while using transportation. Violent aggression, from single-encounter assaults or ethnic conflicts or full-scale wars, can also create disability. The process of life and aging itself guarantees that if one lives long enough, impairment of some sort will occur.

Throughout history, disability and impairment have been unwanted human conditions; therefore, they have been the subject of miraculous recoveries (Jesus healing the lame and the blind) or caused ostracism and even punishment (disabled and impaired persons in concentration camps were the first to be exterminated in Nazi Germany). Between the extremes of miraculous cures and extermination, from ancient to modern times, impairment and disability have been addressed through religious and secular charity. It is only in modern times that they have been accorded legal status. Unlike other human conditions that have been accorded legal status, such as poverty, gender, childhood, old age, and race, disability has challenged and continues to challenge definitive categorical boundaries. All over the world, governments and adjudicating bodies struggle to determine who is disabled. The definitions of disability expand and contract more along political and ideological lines than according to any clear physical determinations.

ATTITUDINAL BASES OF DISABILITY PROGRAMS

For many years, social scientists have been searching for ways to distinguish mankind from the animal world. Purported factors have included the development of language and the use of tools. However, research has made it clear that animals use communication skills for a variety of purposes and some of these forms of communication are verbal in nature. Similarly, the use of primitive forms of tools has been observed in some animals, such as monkeys, which put sticks into the ground to pull insects from their burrows, or otters, which use stones to break oyster shells. In fact, most intellectual and reasoning skills that humans possess can be seen as a continuum from lesser to more advanced creatures. The development of religion and superstition may represent such an advance that divides humankind from other animals. Perhaps another difference lies in the way that humans treat other members of their own species. Humans show a true dichotomy in their concept of the worth of another human being. At times, life seems worthless, or even less. Witness concepts such as ethnic cleansing, which is the purposeful destruction or annihilation of human life for the most trivial of reasons. The attitude toward the sick, injured, malformed, and disabled represents another departure. Just as humans can be calloused and sink to incredible depths in their attitude toward others, they can rise to great heights in their attitude toward individuals who are less fortunate.

Anthropologists and archeologists have tried to understand the functions of many of the objects that

*This chapter contains parts of Chapter 2, "History of Disability As a Legal Construct," by Judith Goodwin Greenwood, and Chapter 6, "Workers' Compensation," by Donald Elisburg, published in the previous edition.

primitive man used. Particularly intriguing is the evidence pointing to the development of religious belief, including cave paintings and stylized earth mothers. Just as intriguing are the burial chambers of primitive man. Some of the skeletons that have been retrieved show evidence of disease and injury. For a primitive man to have had, for example, a broken leg and to have been buried with evidence that that fracture had healed many years before that person's death gives credence to the concept that primitive man had some respect for individuals in their community that went beyond their ability to hunt, gather food, or protect the community. Their community supported these individuals until they had time to heal. In some instances, they were also supported well after that event since their ability to be of practical use to the community was limited by their physical deformities. Thus they either had some alternative use to the community or the development of a compassionate society had begun to emerge.

The development of American culture is a reflection, in part, of the historical and attitudinal development of individuals living in the Mediterranean Basin region.

ANCIENT EGYPT

> Do not laugh at a blind one and do not mark a dwarf. Do not harm a dumb one and do not mark a man who is in the hand of God and do not be wrathful to him when he falls (Amenemope, ca. 1200 B.C.)

The majority of our understanding of ancient Egyptian culture comes from hieroglyphs. Imhotep, an ancient Egyptian physician (circa 2600 B.C.), was commemorated as one who "lets the needy become well," indicating ancient homage to medical treatment of the poor.

The hieroglyphs depicted individuals with varying degrees of disabilities including morbid obesity, traumatic amputations, hernias, and others.[1] Individuals with congenital dwarfism were highly respected and were chosen to look after the wardrobe and jewelry of kings and noblemen. The hieroglyphs also show individuals with spinal deformities believed to be indicative of tuberculosis. The hieroglyphs indicate that these afflicted individuals were able to attain high functions in that society, illustrating that such disabilities did not necessarily result in loss of social stature. There are even notations that dwarfs received special honors and were carried on altars, indicating their elevated role in society.

Pictorial representations show the extremely long fingers and toes of a priest of the sixth dynasty (Meren-Ra-Nefer) (circa 2000 B.C.) that were prominent enough to suggest the possibility of inherited disease.[1] The Pharaoh Akhenaten was depicted in hieroglyphs as having "feminine breasts, filled out hips, sunken stomach and an egg-head."[1] Other hieroglyphs depict individuals with other physical afflictions including muscular dystrophy and thyroid problems. Even the Egyptian gods were not immune to physical disability: Horus (head physician in the house of Ra) was missing one eye (according to legend, he lost the eye in battle).

As seen by the quotation at the beginning of this section, Egyptian culture encouraged understanding and acceptance of those with mental and physical afflictions.

THE BIBLE

There are multiple references to physical and mental disabilities in the Bible. In the book of Leviticus (chapter 21:16) the following statement is found: "[if one has] any blemish let him not approach to offer the bread of his God." This restriction was also extended to "a blind man or a lame man or he that hath a flat nose . . . or a man that is broken footed or broken handed, with a crooked back, or a dwarf, or he that hath a blemish in his eye, or be scurvy or scabbed or hath his bones broken."

The status of the disabled in this society was diminished for individuals who were legally "unclean." They were capable of participating in various religious observances, but could not function as priests or make sacrifices. They were not welcome in sacred areas.[2]

In general terms, disabilities were judged as "impurities disqualifying their bearers from active participation in the cult." A regulation reflecting the attitude of Essene Judaism found in the Qumran shows that individuals with disabilities were denied the opportunity of participating in combat or communal meals:

> In no man lame, blind or crippled, or having an incurable defect of the flesh or afflicted by an impurity of the flesh, none of these shall accompany them to battle . . . Every person afflicted by these impurities unsuited to occupy a place in the midst of the congregation and every person stricken in his flesh, paralyzed in the feet or hands, lame, or blind, or deaf, or mute, or stricken in his flesh with a defect visible to the eye . . . let not these persons enter to take a place among the congregation of men of repute. If one among them has something to say to the counsel of sanctity he will be questioned apart, but this person shall not enter into the midst of the congregation for he is afflicted.[3]

Leprosy was also identified by the Old Testament as a disabling condition resulting in the need for social exclusion. According to Leviticus, priests would function essentially as dermatologists and determine whether leprosy was in fact present. If so, the sufferer was physically excluded. This exclusion was based on legal grounds according to Levitican regulation. The restrictions are also found in Job (2:7–8), where lepers were excluded even during times of mourning. These restrictions, or quarantines, were in place many thousands of years before the understanding of germs and infectious diseases and the quarantines, as noted, extended not only to (possible) transmissible diseases but also to physical deformities.

Intriguing in its complexity is a passage from Exodus (21–28) dealing with reparations for disability. This passage describes the responsibility of an owner of an ox that has caused a disabling injury or death of a man or a woman, boy or girl, or male or female slave. The passage further outlines various penalties to be extracted from the owner depending on the owner's knowledge of the habits of the ox or whether the owner had any liability with respect to the ox's behavior. One cannot help but draw a comparison between these passages and present-day social liability associated with workers' compensation and civil litigation.[3]

The New Testament is replete with references to a major change in attitudes toward the poor, sick, and disabled. There is a discontinuation of the "connection between disability and individual fault."[3] The attitude in the New Testament is one of integration of those individuals who had been thrust from society. The altered attitudes of the New Testament resulted in a "destabilization"[3] of the social system. Traditional concepts were reversed by the teachings in the New Testament, which Jesus, by his teaching, "suspends the ancestral prohibition" against the sick and disabled.[3] Jesus, in fact, was noted to express affection for the disabled and the ill, stating that they are closer to God and are cited as "examples of faith and grace."[3] The direction of the New Testament was toward acceptance of individuals previously cast out by social norms.

ANCIENT GREECE AND ROME

The writings of Hippocrates give direction for the treatment of various diseases and afflictions, both of a physical and mental nature.[4] Epilepsy was described as a medical condition and not the work of the gods or demons. This rational approach found in the Hippocratic writings covered an array of medical afflictions. It announced a cultural shift toward understanding these afflictions and attempting to deal with them. Nevertheless, malformed infants (including those with a club foot or webbed hands) were left to die.[5] The method of dealing with these deformed infants was to place them in a hole or drown them. This was not considered execution, but rather "returning them to the gods." They were not killed; they were sacrificed.[5] These deformed infants were considered to be harmful to society and the decision to eliminate them was made by a council of wise men representing the state. Early Roman law stipulated that this decision would be made by the head of the family in the presence of five neighbors.[5] However, this decision to expose deformed infants was not extended to older individuals with other problems such as blindness, deafness, or emotional problems.

Cicero indicated that blind and deaf people could have rewarding special characteristics noting their ability to compensate for their abnormalities. He stated that their afflictions might allow them to enjoy "pleasures of the dark and of silence."[6] Tuberculosis and mental afflictions were considered illnesses, specifically different from various congenital malformations. Nevertheless, Plato indicated that "the insane should not appear in the city, but each of them shall be kept in the home by those close to him."[7]

Greek literature contains references to other disabilities. Oedipus was described as having some type of disability. The essence of the actual disability is unclear but it was of a physical nature. The survival of Oedipus, despite his disability, may reflect an accepting attitude toward such afflictions. The Greek God Hephaestus was born lame and deformed, causing his father, Zeus, to expel him from Olympus. Hephaestus later surfaces in the Iliad as a master of metals and other objects of magic and later as the lord of fire. He is identified in the Iliad as a craftsman with artistic powers, in part owing to his deformities.

These stories address cultural attitudes of Greco–Roman society toward the sick and disabled. They show a rejection of birth defects but a tolerance, to some degree, of individuals with deformities and disabilities, and that these individuals can contribute to society despite their physical limitations.

MIDDLE AGES

The next millennium was not characterized by any particular event with respect to the science of medicine or the attitude toward the sick or disabled. During this time, the Catholic church was the primary social agency. Life was divided between urban and agrarian societies. In the small villages, the care of the sick and injured was performed on a local level.

At the end of the Middle Ages, with a shift from a local to a more regional economy, craft guilds in Europe began to provide funds to members who were sick or injured. At the onset of the Industrial Revolution, major population shifts were seen, with people moving from their farms to the cities where a higher wage for their work could be found. Major changes in social systems ensued. The forces behind these changes included a loss of identification with the land, greater mobility, increased population densities, and a greater exposure to workplace hazards.

THE ENGLISH POOR LAW DEVELOPMENT

The English Poor Law of 1601 was passed in response to the decline of feudalism and community bonds that existed for the protection of all, not only against outsiders seeking to acquire property or to wreak revenge, but for the protection of individuals with special needs: children, the elderly, and the infirm and impaired. Within the feudal system, charity from community members took care of deserving people with special needs. The new economic system, however, brought with it a new class of people: unemployed wanderers or vagrants who turned to begging or charity together with people with special needs, such as orphans, the blind, and the physically defective. These two categories—vagrants and the infirm or persons with special needs—could overlap, as some disabled persons may have been intermittent workers who moved from job to job as their conditions permitted.

The English Poor Law of 1601 was a culmination of earlier laws in the sixteenth century that initially provided voluntary funds for those unable to work. When those funds proved insufficient, compulsory contributions were sought within towns and parishes. With these compulsory contributions it became necessary to clearly identify those persons in need who would qualify for assistance. Thus, local government replaced religious charity. Whereas the codified Old Poor Law (as the Poor Law of 1601 came to be known) was national legislation, the parish remained the administrative unit. The law was enforced by both local justices and church wardens who assessed and collected a household contribution (or tax) and determined the distribution of funds among the needy.

The question of legitimacy for poor relief was paramount. As Deborah Stone has observed:

> The phenomenon of vagrancy was virtually an obsession with social theorists and law makers all over Europe in the sixteenth, seventeenth, and eighteenth centuries. It is unlikely, therefore, that the specific causal theories elaborated for the English case tell the whole story. (Enclosure or conversion of public grazing land to private property was probably the one phenomenon unique to England, at least in scope.) Bad harvests, currency debasement, price inflation, and the conclusion of wars may have temporarily exacerbated an existing situation, but the problem was clearly fundamental and pervasive. And whatever its actual magnitude in terms of actual numbers of vagrants, it was serious enough to command enormous intellectual, economic, and political effort.[2(p30)]

To control the vagrancy problem and provide for persons in need, English policy makers in the early seventeenth century with the Old Poor Law and again in the nineteenth century with the New Poor Law made work ability and locality predominant issues. Workhouses were set up for those poor persons who were able to work. Poor children and orphans were apprenticed to craftsmen. "Settlement Laws" restricted movement of the poor between parishes, but also gave parishes the power to remove young family members from "families overburdened with children" and to send orphans to apprenticeships.

The issue of work ability and need for some relief for the poor came to a head with the New Poor Law of 1834, which stated the "principle of least eligility" wherein a poor person's economic situation had to be below that of an independent laborer of the least means in order to qualify for a workhouse. Need for assistance outside of or beyond a workhouse (then referred to as "outdoor relief") was based on inability to work according to various categories: the sick, the insane, the "defective" (blind, deaf, and dumb; then, later, "lame" and "deformed"), the aged and infirm, and children. All except children became part of the developing concept of sanctioned disability and were classified as unable to work.

Thus categorization and means testing became an essential part of English welfare policy from the seventeenth century onward. The concept of need was drawn ever more stringently into opposition with work ability. Certification of legitimacy for assistance became the imperative in separating the ablebodied from those who were poor because of some specified condition of physical or mental impairment that prevented work.

With regard to the ablebodied, the New Poor Law restrained labor mobility either by forcing lower-class laborers to accept low wages to avoid the workhouse or by confining poor ablebodied persons of "least eligibility" to workhouses, often under harsh conditions.

THE GERMAN INVALIDITY AND PENSION LAW OF 1889

In Germany, as in England, taking care of the needs of those persons who were unable to take care of themselves fell to the church when society was primarily agrarian. As industry developed in the German states in the mid-1800s, the Catholic church, which was not affiliated with the states as was the Protestant church, became particularly active in charitable work helping individuals displaced by the emerging economic order. As industry was developing, Otto von Bismarck ascended to political power, first as prime minister to King Fredrick William IV of Prussia, then as chancellor to William, who became emperor of a unified Germany under the name of Wilhelm I. The unification of the separate German states was consummately forged by Bismarck.

Chancellor Otto von Bismarck, a conservative, determined that social insurance was the way to instill patriotism and loyalty to the new German state as well as to quell political activism in the rival Social Democratic party. In contrast to the English Poor Laws, the German social legislation of the 1880s was not a codification of earlier laws directed at controlling vagrancy and the needs of the poor, but part of a planned and concentrated effort of state-sponsored social welfare that was concerned with social hierarchy and labor mobility. As noted previously, the shift in Europe from a feudal and community resource-based economy to a wage-based manufacturing economy required governments to focus on the work ability of its citizens. Three laws comprised Bismarck's approach.

In 1883, national health insurance was introduced for a large segment of workers. In 1884, after three draft laws, a plan to compensate workers for lost wages when injured on the job was enacted with costs paid fully by employers. (Bismarck had to give up his idea of a federal contribution owing to opposition from other conservatives.) In 1898, when addressing work disability, the government decided that disability was a function of lost earning capacity and job opportunity, and not, as narrowly interpreted in the English Poor Laws, a categorical incapacity to work.

The concept of disability as a function of lost earning capacity allowed the German state to promote regional job mobility for persons with skills needed in the economy of other localities, while protecting individuals who already held jobs requiring similar education and experience. The interest of the nation-state was to provide comparable jobs for displaced workers or to provide disability pensions. Whereas acceptable alternative job options for educated, clerical (white collar) workers were relatively narrow, the available job market for manual (blue collar) workers was considerably broader. Thus, as German law developed, white-collar workers were considered separately from blue-collar workers. Earning capacity again determined the difference: white-collar workers had to demonstrate a loss of half their earning capacity to qualify for a disability pension, whereas blue-collar workers had to demonstrate a two-thirds loss of earning capacity. The concept of disability was clearly and carefully tied to both occupational and social structure and was used to preserve a person's sense of security within the social system.

An analytic observation was made by Deborah Stone, who has studied and written in detail on disability as a special status for public assistance:

> Disability in German policy, as in English policy, serves to demonstrate the boundaries between the work and need system, but the boundaries are defined very differently. In Poor Law policy the purpose of the categories was to help people in the work-based system as long as possible so as not to lose their productivity. Disability was thus defined very narrowly, and restricted (originally) to a small set of recognizable conditions that permanently incapacitated a person or totally incapacitated him or her temporarily. The Poor Law concept allowed people out of the work-based system and into the need-based system only when they were absolutely devoid of productive ability. In German social insurance, the effect of the category was to preserve very fine distinctions in the internal occupational hierarchy. The German definition of disability thus let people out of the work-based system when keeping them in would disrupt the social hierarchy.[2(pp66–67)]

Two very different philosophies of welfare are evident. Prior to 1870, Germany had been a loose confederation of separate principalities until Prussia with Bismarck at the helm exerted leadership in a drive toward unification and industrialization. Thus in the German system, social insurance was instituted as a material benefit given by the state to its citizens, and the cost of providing the insurance was viewed as a political expediency to maintain their loyalty if an appropriate work status could not be maintained.

On the other hand, in England, where the events of history allowed a slower shift from an agrarian to an industrialized, mercantilist economy, any "out-door relief" or direct government subsidy was seen as a drain on resources that could otherwise have gone to productive development. Stone notes that in late eighteenth century England, Jeremy Bentham, the philosopher–industrialist, proposed that the blind could indeed knit and suggested that children "would be harnessed to a seesaw apparatus designed to pump water as a by-product of their play."[2] Productivity of any kind, not social status and earning capacity, was the issue.

Both systems provided the basics for current American laws and attitudes toward disability and social relief.

WORKERS' COMPENSATION IN THE UNITED STATES

The first legal recognition of disability in the United States developed out of the tremendous industrial expansion that started after the Civil War and extended into the early twentieth century. Injuries and fatalities related to work were very common and accepted as inevitable. There were spectacular catastrophes, including the death of 362 miners in a mining explosion in West Virginia in 1907 and 164 women in New York in the Triangle Shirtwaist fire in 1911.[8] Whether there was death or injury, the only recourse employees or their families had was to bring a tort action against the employers in court to claim damages.

Employers, however, had three common law defenses, known as the "unholy trinity," that were difficult to overcome: assumption of risk (employees supposedly knew the risks of the job before accepting employment), the fellow-servant rule (co-worker negligence), and contributory negligence by the employee. Nevertheless, as traumatic work-related injuries and fatalities mounted in the early twentieth century, judges allowed more and more cases to be brought to trial, and more and more frequently juries were holding employers culpable and determining monetary awards. Still, many injured employees and their families did not have the resources to go to trial; consequently, many employees and their families were left destitute. There was a growth of social concern for a remedy to the poverty caused by work-related injuries and fatalities. At the same time, employers were increasingly faced with the uncertainty of potential liability for injuries and the unpredictability of jury awards if a lawsuit was brought.

The plight of workers in the United States at the end of the 19th century has been well documented. As noted, injured workers and their survivors, for the most part, had no right to compensation when their injuries or deaths were work-related. Relief, if any, was through the common-law tort system of personal injury action. As plaintiffs, workers were subject to defenses including contributory negligence, fellow-servant rules, and assumption of risk. Few workers could overcome these hurdles and recoveries were few and small.

Otto Bettmann described those times in vivid terms:

> "Aside from the steel mills the railroad industry was the most lethal to its workers, killing in 1890 one railroader for every 306 employed and injuring one for every 30 employed. Out of a work force of 749,301 this amounted to a yearly total of 2451 deaths, which rose in 1900 to 2675 killed and 41,142 injured. It should be noted that these casualty lists cover only railroaders in the line duty: civilian casualties in train collisions and level-crossing accidents were another matter. The *New York Evening Post* concluded that the deaths caused by American railroads between June 1898 and 1900 and were about equal to British Army losses in the three-year Boer War.
>
> ". . . In the high-risk job category the circus stuntman and test pilot today enjoy greater life assurance than did the brakeman of yesterday, whose work called for precarious leaps between bucking freight cars at the command of the locomotive's whistle. In icy weather it often became a macabre dance of death. Also subject to sudden death—albeit to a lesser degree-were the train couplers, whose omnipresent hazard was loss of hands and fingers in the primitive link-and-pin devices. It took an act of law in 1893 to force the railroads to replace these man-traps.
>
> ". . . Industry's cavalier attitude to safety had a predictable effect on lower-echelon bosses. One rail-road-yard superintendent refused to roof a loading platform, even though in the cold his men had contracted rheumatism and asthma. His observation: "Men are cheaper than shingles . . . There's a dozen waiting when one drops out."
>
> ". . . Whether a worker was mutilated by a buzz saw, crushed by a beam, interred in a mine, or fell down a shaft, it was always "his own bad luck." The courts as a rule sided with the employer; in any event, few accident victims or their kin had the money to bring suit. Companies disclaimed responsibility, refused to install protective apparatus, and paid no compensation. Their only concession to human life was to pay for burying the dead!"[36(pp 70–71)]

FEDERAL EMPLOYERS LIABILITY ACT

The Federal Employers Liability Act (FELA) was enacted amidst a general outcry by railroad workers and others for protective legislation. Congress, in its first venture into the realm of worker disability, enacted the initial FELA in 1906 and the present version of FELA in 1908. It was an effort to provide workers with some ability to obtain injury compensation through the courts by modifying the negligence standards and eliminating or modifying certain of the railroads' defenses such as contributory negligence, the fellow-servant rule, and the assumption of risk. In a major change, contributory negligence gave way to comparative negligence. The significance is that, under FELA's comparative negligence test, injured workers are not denied compensation if they contributed to the fault for the accident. Rather, their compensation can be reduced according to the percentage of the fault that was theirs. Furthermore, FELA provides that if the railroad violated a safety standard, any degree of fault by injured workers is disregarded in determining compensation.[9–11]

The FELA was amended at various times to provide more liberal interpretations, and changes in 1939 eliminated any remaining doctrine of assumption of risk. The basic FELA statute was used in 1920 when Congress enacted the Jones Act to provide similar protection for seamen. Clearly, the two statutes were designed to cover workers where Congress saw a national industry—i.e., railroads, and maritime on the navigable waters—over which the federal government had exclusive control.[10,12,13]

In practice, the FELA is the product of decades of judicial interpretation. The Supreme Court has ruled on its effect numerous times and, in the context of a fault-based system, has determined that the required proof of negligence by the railroad is extremely liberal (only a "scintilla" of negligence is needed). The coverage of the Act to workers is also extremely broad (for example, occupational illnesses are fully covered).[9–11]

The FELA and Jones Act can be characterized as workers' compensation systems in that the railroads and ship owners have developed extensive claims filing procedures, investigations, and examinations to handle the vast bulk of claims under these laws. A review of a typical FELA or Jones Act file would contain essentially the same information about the injured worker's medical and economic circumstances as in the typical state or federal workers' compensation file.

Participants have developed guidelines for economics and impairment. In a typical FELA case, the injured worker will file a claim that will be processed through the system as though it were a workers' compensation claim. In cases of dispute, the injured worker will seek counsel and proceed through an elaborate system of administrative process within the railroad personnel or claims department, both before and after a proceeding is filed in court. The cases are brought under extremely liberal venue with an option of federal or state courts and the right to a jury trial. Perhaps the most distinguishing feature of the FELA is the ability to have a jury determine whether there was negligence by the parties and for the jury to determine the extent of the damages. Also, by statute, the FELA does not have a schedule of awards, nor a formula for determining benefit levels.[9–11,14]

FEDERAL EMPLOYEES' COMPENSATION PROGRAM

The United States Congress, 25 years before the enactment of a federal workers' compensation law, showed an interest in protecting injured employees by finding ways of maintaining their pay during disability caused by job injury. In 1882, a program was enacted to continue the pay of federal workers in "hazardous occupations" who sustained injury. "Hazardous occupations" was defined to include primarily workers in life-saving situations (Coast Guard and occupations on the navigable waters). Full salary for up to 2 years was provided but no medical benefits were given. In the event of death in such employment, the worker's family would receive the worker's pay for 2 years.

Later, but before the turn of the century, Congress authorized the Postmaster General to continue the salary of postal employees during the period of disability caused by injury on the job.

Then, in 1908, Congress passed what is often referred to as the first workers' compensation law for federal employees. This law, again, was for only those employees in hazardous occupations, but the expanded definition included about 25% of federal employees. Compensation was paid for job injury disability. In essence, the compensation was a continuation of the full pay of the employee for the first year and then 50% pay for the second year.

This law, although an improvement over the past minimal attempts, still left the great majority of federal workers without protection against loss of wages because of injuries. Congress quickly corrected this coverage gap by passing the Federal Employees' Compensation Act in 1916 to provide a workers' compensation program for its own employees.[15] Because the doctrine of sovereign immunity protected the federal government from lawsuits, the federal system never was required to replace an existing tort system. Basically, Congress provided full coverage to all employees in a system that was much less adversarial than that which developed under the FELA and the state-based no-fault systems. As a self-insurer, the federal government was not obliged to set up a system that functioned with private carriers or insurance funds. In addition, from the enactment of the statute, Congress made the administrative decision final with no appeals to the courts.

All federal employees were covered except, initially, for federal officers. Compensation for wage loss was originally provided at 66⅔% of the injured or killed workers' pay. At the same time compensable wages were set at $100, meaning that, at the beginning, no injured worker received more than $66.67 a week in compensation. For the first time, reasonable medical care was provided in addition to the income maintenance compensation payments. Injuries covered then, as today, were personal injuries, which includes not only traumatic injuries but also what we today refer to as occupational disease and illness.

The federal employees' compensation program was run initially by an independent U.S. Employees' Compensation Commission composed of three commissioners who also administered the Longshore and Harbor Workers Compensation Act passed in 1927. In 1946, these functions were placed in the new Bureau of Employees' Compensation (BEC) in the recently formed Federal Security Agency. In 1950, BEC was placed in the Department of Labor. BEC was abolished in 1974 and its functions placed in the new Office of Workers' Compensation Programs in the U.S. Department of Labor.[16]

The issue confronting the federal government and the protection of some 2 million federal employees has been one of tinkering with the administrative process and the need for Congress to increase the benefit schedule periodically.

In the 1970s Congress improved the FECA by making it conform to the recommendations of the National Commission on State Workmen's Compensation Laws. In addition, a growing backlog of cases convinced Congress to provide an experiment permitting the government to continue an injured worker's pay while the case was being processed. This innovative approach presented difficulties in administration in the 1970s, particularly as the caseload continued to grow substantially.[12,17]

DEVELOPMENT OF THE STATE-BASED WORKERS' COMPENSATION SYSTEM

About the same time that Congress began to struggle with the FELA, there was activity in the states to provide a disability compensation system that would be a no-fault approach modeled on the social experiments in Germany and Great Britain in the 1880s and 1890s.

Credit is generally given to Bismarck for the enactment of the first workers' compensation system in the 1880s in Germany. Other historians have traced the first such systems in Europe to the 1830s. In America, the historical product of the industrial revolution was the desire to eliminate the country's terrible cost in human lives during its rise as an industrial power.[18]

A political consensus grew for finding a clear and certain remedy to the problem. State after state, beginning with Wisconsin in 1911, mandated an employer-financed insurance program. At first the program was limited to the most hazardous occupations, and it compensated workers and their families for lost wages resulting from work-related injury or death. Workers lost their right to sue the employer for damages, but gained assurance of a certain level of wage replacement benefits and coverage of medical expenses, if they were injured. Employers accepted limited liability for all work-related injuries and deaths. Within this original "no-fault" system, injured workers were considered to be victims of inevitable industrial accidents and, as conceived in Germany, society or the state had an obligation to offer some limited form of wage-based social insurance. Unlike the German form, however, there was initially little or no concern within state workers' compensation programs for using insurance benefits as a way to maintain social hierarchy and labor mobility. Like the original English Poor Law, prevention of poverty, not disability and its social management, was the driving concern for the development of workers' compensation programs in the United States.

By 1920, 42 of the 48 states and the District of Columbia had workers' compensation laws in place. The state-by-state process of legislating workers' compensation laws has been called the "most dramatic event in the twentieth century history of American civil justice."[19] For 25 years after its inception, workers' compensation was the only social disability income program in the United States.

The glory was short-lived, however. The 1920s saw a workers' compensation system in relative decline compared to the aspirations of reformers and early proponents of the system. Programs became dominated by disputes over whether certain injuries were work-related and over the exact extent of disability or impairment and the corresponding amount of benefits. Also, politically appointed administrators who lacked appropriate legal expertise and objectivity in labor–management relations contributed to the developing adversarial climate. The basic concept of workers' compensation as a self-contained program for the provision of wage replacement benefits and for the adjudication of disputes between employers and employees regarding those benefits became fixed. By the mid-1930s, when the debate heated up over wider disability coverage through Social Security, workers' compensation was not considered a model program because leading reformers saw little distinction between occupational disability and non-occupational impairment. They also expressed skepticism over the quality of medical care that was provided for the injured worker by the large number of company doctors.

Interestingly, the state-by-state approach was not achieved easily. It was not until 1949 that Mississippi finally enacted a workers' compensation statute. Even today, not all workers are protected by a workers' compensation scheme. In a number of states, agricultural and small-employer exemptions, along with those provided in Federal programs, still leave large numbers of workers without protection and force them to go to the courts similar to the situation found a century ago. It is also note-worthy that in three states—Texas, South Carolina, and New Jersey—workers' compensation is not even compulsory (see Chapter 5).[20]

Thus, although a comprehensive scheme of workers' compensation has been enacted in very state, the process has taken more than 90 years and is still not complete. It is also true, that although the concept of workers' compensation was to provide adequate and uniform benefits, the achievement of that result has been painful, difficult, inconsistent, and elusive.

From the inception of the state systems, there has been a struggle to provide adequate benefits and to maintain these benefits in line with increases in wages and costs of care. For example, most state laws provide for a benefit level of 66⅔% of the workers' wages. However, the imposition of caps on total benefits has frequently resulted in many workers of average or higher wages receiving less than 50% of their salary, and in some states the caps are so low that, even at the maximum, benefits are at poverty levels.[21] Additionally, the early state laws did not provide uniform coverage of all occupations and many state laws did not adequately cover occupational diseases.

RAILROAD WORKERS, SEAMEN AND LONGSHORE AND HARBOR WORKERS

Neither railroad workers nor seamen have had the protection of the type of coverage for work injuries afforded by state and federal workers' compensation laws. They have, however, been provided coverage under the Federal Employers' Liability Act, 45 U.S. Code Annotated §§51–60, which extended and enhanced their common-law rights to proceed in court against their employer to obtain damages for job injuries (see above).

Railroad Workers

As discussed previously, workers on the railroads in the late 1800s found themselves in a very hazardous occupation with little hope for an adequate recovery in their common law court actions aimed at getting money from their railroad employers to pay the medical expenses and to compensate for their loss of earnings due to their work injuries. These victims of the hazardous employment environment found their quest for damages constantly defeated in the courts by the use by the railroads of the available common-law defenses of contributory negligence, negligence of a fellow servant, and assumption of risk. If the railroad could show that in some way the injury was caused in part by the employee's own negligence or the negligence of one of the employee's fellow workers or that the employee voluntarily assumed the risk of the (hazardous) job, then the claim for damages would not succeed, leaving the employee's family to shoulder the burden of this injury and wage loss as best they could.

Congress, in 1908, let it be known clearly that the railroads should shoulder a greater share of the cost of railroad employee injuries by passing the Federal Employers' Liability Act.[22] This law provided specifically that the railroads would be liable in damages to its workers who suffered work injuries and effectively modified or did away with the common-law defenses that were the impediments to successful recoveries.[23]

Seamen[24]

Seamen (crew members[25]), although never having experienced the advantages of a workers' compensation law, have been held by tradition or general admiralty or maritime law, perhaps going back to the Middle Ages, to be entitled to income maintenance during a period of illness or disability. This entitlement was termed "maintenance and cure." This concept was accepted by U.S. courts as part of the general maritime law of the United States. In cases where a seaman became sick or suffered injury while in service of his ship, the vessel and her owner were found liable for maintenance and cure in addition to liability to the seaman for an indemnity (damages) for injuries received by the seaman as a result of the unseaworthiness of the ship and her appliances. The seaman, however, could not recover damages or indemnity for injuries sustained through the negligence of the master or a member of the crew.[26]

The maritime tradition and general maritime law requiring maintenance and cure of the vessel and her owner was placed into an international convention in 1936 (Shipowners' Liability Convention), which was then made applicable in the United States by a Presidential Proclamation signed by President Franklin D. Roosevelt on September 29, 1939 (54 Stat 1693). The Convention provisions pertinent to a shipowner's maintenance and cure as thus officially adopted into U.S. law provide, in part, that medical care and maintenance at the expense of the shipowner comprises the following: medical treatment and the supply of proper and sufficient medicines and therapeutic appliances, and board and lodging, shall be provided. The shipowner shall be liable to defray the expense of medical care and maintenance until the sick or injured person has been cured, or until the sickness or incapacity has been declared of a permanent character. Where the sickness or injury results in incapacity for work, the shipowner shall be held liable to pay full wages as long as the sick or injured person remains on board, and if the sick or injured person has dependents, to pay wages in whole or in part as prescribed by national laws or regulations from the time when the worker is landed until the worker has been cured or the sickness or incapacity has been declared of a permanent character.[27]

Subsequently, Congress passed the Jones Act,[28] which extended to seamen (crew members) the same privileges that railroad workers had obtained through the passage of FELA.[29] In fact, FELA was specifically extended by the Jones Act to seamen to give seamen the right to sue for damages when suffering injury due to the negligence of the master or a member of the crew. This act gives to seamen or their personal representatives a right of action against the employer for negligence. The remedy is the same as that of railroad workers under FELA, and the common-law defenses are similarly modified.

LONGSHORE AND HARBOR WORKERS'

The Longshore and Harbor Workers' Compensation Act (LSA)[30] was passed by Congress in 1927 to provide injury protection to workers performing duties on the navigable waters of the United States, excluding seamen. It was made necessary because the U.S. Supreme Court had ruled earlier that a state could not apply its workers compensation law to protect workers working on the navigable waters of the United States because, the court held, this was the exclusive jurisdiction of the United States (federal government).[31]

The LSA is a workers' compensation law covering workers on or adjacent to the navigable waters of the United States. Persons covered include any person engaged in maritime employment, including any longshore worker or person engaged in longshoring operations and any harbor worker, including those engaged in ship repair, shipbuilding, and shipbreaking activities on the navigable waters of the United States or adjoining pier and dock areas. The law does not cover a master or member of a crew of any vessel.

The LSA has been extended to cover some other groups of workers not covered by other workers' compensation laws, such as employees engaged in certain operations conducted on the Outer Continental Shelf of the United States; civilian employees of nonappropriated fund instrumentalities (Post-Exchanges [PXs], Officers' Clubs) of the Armed Forces; employees outside the United States on U.S. Defense Bases; and employees outside the United States carrying out "public work contracts" or other U.S.-funded contracts.

MILITARY VETERANS

Similar to seamen, the Armed Forces have had a long tradition of caring for their sick and wounded. Congress responded to the needs of its veterans of the Revolutionary War and the War of 1812. The present laws covering veterans and administered by the Department of Veterans Affairs (VA) and are reviewed in Chapter 4.

BLACK LUNG BENEFITS ACT

As previously stated, the federal government's role, with the exception of covering railroad workers and seamen, has largely been to provide compensation systems to those workers not otherwise eligible for state protections.

One significant exception to this approach was the black lung legislation. In the 1960s the public and Congress became aware of a serious problem with respect to coal miners and the failure of existing state workers' compensation laws to cover the occupational disease of coal workers' pneumoconiosis or "black lung." Partly as a result of the definition of this disease, and partly as a result of statute of limitations on discovery of this long-latent disease, hundreds of thousands of afflicted miners had no program of compensation.

Congress reacted by providing a series of programs to create a compensation program for coal miners with this illness. Initially a federal payment program, the Black Lung Benefit program was extended in the 1970s to coal mine operators, first on a responsible operator basis, and then to a coal industry-funded program. Because of its extensive application, a number of railroad workers may also be eligible for benefits under this statute. This became an extremely costly and controversial program because of the enormous number of claims, a congressionally mandated liberal eligibility program, and administrative difficulties made this an extremely costly and controversial program. This program provided massive relief to thousands of coal workers and their families who had no other source of benefits or medical care.[12]

SOCIAL SECURITY DISABILITY

The two-decade Social Security debate over wider disability coverage, lasting into the 1950s, was not about whether entitlement to benefits was appropriate, but about the definition of disability and how disability was to be determined. At that time, disability clauses in private insurance carrier life insurance policies usually defined disability as being "wholly" and "totally" incapable of working. However, the courts generally interpreted these statements with some leniency, taking the position that a person need not be totally helpless.[2(p74)] For a variety of reasons, including judicial interpretation, poor underwriting practices, and industry competition, the commercial insurance carriers experienced significant losses in disability coverage and their experience increased the skepticism and fears of conservatives about adding disability coverage into the Social Security program.

The liberals, however, pursued a strategy of incrementalism. Social Security historian Martha Derthick observes that "incremental change in whatever institutional setting has less potential for generating conflict than change that involves innovation in principle."[32(p314)] Thus disability insurance through Social Security came about in a gradual process. The first step was taken in 1954 when disabled persons were exempted from making Social Security contributions but still remained eligible for an old-age pension at age 65. Disability was then defined as the "inability to engage in any substantial gainful activity because of any medically determinable physical or mental impairment that can be expected to be of long, continued, and indefinite duration."[33(p1)]

In 1956, the law was amended to provide disability benefits to individuals between the ages of 50 and 65 who, because of disability, were unable to work according to the above definition. In 1958, the law was amended so that monthly benefits were payable to dependents of disabled workers. In 1960, the age 50 limitation for eligibility was removed, and in 1965, the duration of disability was changed to what it remains today: disability needs to have lasted, or be expected to last, for a continuous period of not less than 12 months.[34] In 1972, benefits were substantially increased, and Medicare benefits were made available to beneficiaries who received disability benefits for 2 years or longer. Over this nearly 2-decade period, not only did Congressional amendments to the Social Security Act liberalize the rules and regulations for determining disability, but liberal judicial interpretations resulted in the disability program taking on "some of the features of an unemployment compensation program."[35(p36)] This meant that there must be a lack of readily available employment opportunities for an individual, along with a physical or mental impairment. A theoretical ability to engage in substantial gainful activity of any kind, anywhere, was deemed by the courts insufficient to disprove disability.

Through all the incremental developments of this federal disability program, however, physical or mental impairment, along with its measurement, has remained the anchor of the decision making. Impairment and its measurement provided political expediency for the proponents of the Social Security Disability Insurance program because it allowed them to present disability as a relatively narrow and measurable concept to skeptical conservatives. Although presenting disability as synonymous with impairment may have been the path of least resistance to win over support initially, it has led to confusion of the entire disability construct, which is an amalgam of a number of factors, with impairment being only one (see Chapter 6).

SUMMARY

This chapter has attempted to trace the development of the current U.S. laws and regulations concerning its various disability systems starting with a brief review of the attitude toward the disabled found in the history of Western civilization. The way Americans approach their sick and disabled has been influenced by their Judeo–Christian heritage. America's laws reflect that heritage and the laws promulgated in Western Europe over the past few centuries. Our current Social Security laws have many of their bases in the attitudes that shaped the first English Poor Laws. Current workers' compensation, likewise, owes its origins to Bismarck's political maneuverings. Through its various and varied programs, America has covered its disabled workers with protection for loss of income through many different mechanisms.

References

1. Stetter C: The Secret Medicine of the Faros. Chicago, Quintessence Publishing, 1993.
2. Stone DA: The Disabled State. Philidelphia, Temple University Press, 1984.
3. Stiker HJ: A History of Disability (William Sayres Translater). University of Michigan Press, East Lansing, MI, 1999.
4. Edelstein L: Temkin, Temkin (ed): In: Ancient Medicine. Baltimore, Johns Hopkins University Press, 1987.
5. Delcourt M: Stérilité, Mystérieuse. Naissance Maléfique Dans l'Antiquité. Liéege, Classique, 1938.
6. Cicero: Tusculanes. Book 5, 38.
7. Plato: The Laws. 11:10, 1079.
8. Speiler E: Perpetuating risk: Workers' compensation: The persistence of occupational injuries. Houston Law Review 3:119–264, 1994.
9. Cost Containment & Reform Activity Report, vol 1, issue 3, July 1991, and vol. 1, issue 4, September 1991. Boca Raton, National Council on Compensation Insurance.
10. Havens AL, Anderson AA: The Federal Employers' Liability Act: A compensation system in urgent need of reform. Federal Bar Journal 34: 1987.
11. Victor RA (ed): Challenges for the 1990s. No. WC-90–3. Cambridge, Mass, Workers' Compensation Research Institute, 1990.
12. DeCarlo DT, Minkowitz M: Workers' Compensation Insurance and Law Practice: The Next Generation. Fort Washington, Pa, LRP Publications.
13. Elkind AB: Should the Federal Employers' Liability Act be Abolished? Chicago, Forum, American Bar Association, Tort and Insurance Section, 1981.
14. Federal Employers' Liability Act. U.S. House of Representatives, Committee on Energy and Commerce, Subcommittee of Transportation and Hazardous Materials, 101st Congress, November 1, 1989.
15. Title 5 U.S. Code, Part 8100.
16. See Nordlund WJ: A History of the Federal Employees' Compensation Act. Washington, DC, U.S. Department of Labor, Employment Standards Administration, Office of Workers' Compensation Programs, 1992.
17. Nordlund WJ (ed): Proceedings of a Conference Celebrating the 75th Anniversary of the Federal Employees' Compensation Act, sponsored by U.S. Department of Labor and Rutgers University, July 1992.
18. Rosenblum M (ed): Compendium on Workers Compensation. Washington, DC, The National Commission on State Workmen's Compensation Laws, Government Printing Office.
19. Darling-Hammond L, Kneisner TJ: The Law and Economics of Workers' Compensation. Santa Monica, Rand Publications, 1980.
20. California Workers' Compensation Institute Bulletin, No. 91–12. San Francisco, California Workers' Compensation Institute, 1991.
21. 1994 Workers' Compensation and Unemployment Insurance Laws. AFL-CIO Publication No. R-36–0394–15, Washington, DC, AFL-CIO, 1994.
22. For FELA, see generally Title 45, U.S. Code Annotated, West Publishing, §§51–60, for background, history, text, and pertinent court cases.
23. FELA provided in part that railroads (common carriers) in interstate or foreign commerce are "liable in damages to any person suffering injury while he (or she) is employed by such carrier . . . for such injury or death resulting in whole or in part from the negligence of any of the officers, agents, or employees of such carrier, or by reason of any defect or insufficiency due to its negligence, in its cars, engines, appliances, machinery, track, roadbed, works, boats, wharves, or other equipment" (45 U.S.C.A., §51); that ". . . the fact that the employee may have been guilty of contributory negligence shall not bar recovery, but damages shall be diminished by the jury in proportion to the amount of negligence attributed to such employee: (but there is no contributory negligence in any case) where the violation by such common carrier of any statute enacted for the safety of employees contributed to the injury or death of such employee" (45 U.S.C.A., §53); and that ". . . such employee shall not be held to have assumed the risks of his employment in any case where such injury or death resulted . . . from the negligence of . . . (railroad employees, or where there was a violation of a safety statute by the railroad)" (45 U.S.C.A., §54).
24. For background and history generally In: Larson A, Larson R, (eds) see 46 U.S.C.A., §688, Notes.
25. "There seem to be no significant distinction between the concepts of 'seaman' and 'crew member.' " Workmen's compensation. Matthew Bender, 1994; §90, citing *Gahagan Constr. Corp. v Armao*, 165 F.2d 301.
26. Pate v Standard Dredging Corp., 193 F.2d 498.

27. See generally Annotation, Supreme Court's Views as to a Seaman's Right, Under Maritime Law, to Maintenance and Cure; Allan L. Schwartz, J.D.; 43 L. Ed. 2d 912, Lawyers Cooperative Publishing 1993; and Norris, The Law of Seamen, 3rd ed, as quoted therein.
28. The Jones Act is in actuality the Merchant Marine Act, 41 Stat. 1007 (1920), 46 U.S.C., §688 (1952).
29. See data on railroad workers: FELA, 45 U.S.C.A., §51.
30. Longshore & Harbor Workers' Compensation Act (LSA), 33 U.S. Code, Chap. 18, §§ 901–950. The regulations applying to this Longshore Program are found at 20 CFR, Parts 701–704.
31. Southern Pacific v Jensen, 244 U.S. 205 (1917).
32. Derthick M: Poicymaking for Social Security. Washington, DC, Brookings Institution, 1977.
33. Social Security Amendments: P.L. 761, Title 1, Section 215(i), Par. 3, Washington, DC, 1954.
34. Social Security Amendments: P.L. 89–97, Title 3, Washington, DC, 1964.
35. Rockman S: Judicial Review of Benefit Determination in the Social Security and Veterans Administration. Report to the Committee on Grants and Benefits. Washington, DC, Administrative Conference of the United States, 1970.
36. Bettmann O: The Good Old Days—They were terrible! New York, Random House, 1974.

CHAPTER

3

Economic Costs of Disability

PETER S. BARTH, PhD

The purpose of this chapter is to explore a set of issues relating to the economics of disability, focusing in particular on the costs imposed by disability. Like a number of other social sciences, economics has extended its reach into subjects that are customarily the domain of others. Consequently, serious studies that examine "the economics of ..." extend into many fields that traditionally have not been exposed to economic analysis. Because the economics of disability have begun to receive attention only within the past few years, the field must be considered as formative and incomplete.

Before the costs of disability can be estimated, some acceptable definition of disability is needed. Unfortunately, this is no simple issue. Chapter 1 described the concepts of impairment and disability from a medical and legal perspective. This chapter will address disability from an economic standpoint. The concept of disability changes with each perspective. As seen in Chapter 1, no universal definition of disability exists. However disability is defined, the definition should be such that it can be measured as a step in assessing its economic costs. Once a working definition of disability has been constructed, the next step is to determine the appropriate method of calculating costs.

An analogy can be drawn here with the development of the concept of poverty at the outset of the Great Society. The decision was made early to create a measurable definition of poverty. This enabled the Johnson administration to accomplish several goals. First, the definition established that the extent of the problem was substantial, justifying a War on Poverty. Second, the measurements that followed the definition identified the sociodemographic characteristics of the poor (i.e., by defining "poverty," target groups could be established). Third, a precise definition allowed for measurement to be made of the changes in the number of poor people that occurred as economic conditions changed and as policies were implemented. That same definition is used today to establish eligibility for certain public entitlement programs (e.g., programs are available for persons with income levels at or below 150% of the poverty threshold).

Sources of Disability Measures

Multiple sources of data on disability exist. Significant differences exist in the definitions used. As such, resulting counts can be expected to yield inconsistent outcomes. One such source of data on the number of disabled people is from the Survey of Income and Program Participation (SIPP), a panel study.[6][AU2] According to the SIPP, a person is considered disabled if he or she has difficulty performing certain functions (seeing, hearing, talking, walking, climbing stairs, lifting, or carrying), has difficulty performing activities of daily living, or has difficulty with certain social roles. A person who is unable to perform one or more activities, who uses an assistive device, or who needs assistance from another person to perform basic activities is considered severely disabled. In contrast, the Current Population Survey (CPS) defines disability in terms of ability to work.[1,6,40] Therefore, some persons considered to have a limitation in the SIPP survey would not be included in the CPS survey if they have never been employed.

Another source of data is the National Health Interview Survey (NHIS), which has been carried out continuously since 1957. It consists of a representative sample of the civilian, non-institutionalized population.[1,6] Approximately 120,000 individuals are included in each sample survey. Persons are asked if an impairment or health problem prevents or limits their activities and whether that condition is chronic (lasting 3 months or more). Respondents are classified according to the degree of activity limitation. Persons with limitations that are not in their major activity are considered to have the least severe limitations. Those with the most severe limitations are unable to carry out their major activity. The concept of major activity is defined according to one's age, so that for children it is attending school, for those aged 18 to 69 it includes working or keeping house, and for those aged 70 and older it is living independently. Each of these concepts (i.e., chronic condition, limits, major activity, and age cutoffs) can be subject to some second-guessing.[9] Further, that the NHIS is based on self-reporting is of some concern. However, the concepts permit measurement, and the degree of stability in the approach permits comparisons to be made over time.

It is difficult to quarrel with the report that concluded that disability statistics are "a patchwork of data that reflect the complexity of the concept of disability" or that "it is clear that the number of persons with disabilities depends on the definition of disability."[40]

The NHIS data suggest that in 1995, 14.7% of the population was limited in activity owing to a chronic condition.[50] A total of 10.1% of the population was limited in a major activity owing to chronic conditions. Additionally, about 2 million disabled persons reside in institutional facilities. Disability rates as defined are higher for male, black, low-income, and older individuals.

By contrast, the SIPP panel study found 20.6% of the total population (53.9 million) to have a disability. It also found that 9.9% of the total population (26.0 million) had a "severe" disability.[6] Among persons aged 15 to 64, the rate of any disability was 18.7% and the rate of severe disability was 8.7%. In contrast, the CPS in March 1996 found that 10.1% of the civilian, non-institutionalized population aged 16 to 64 had a work disability.[49] The study reported that 6.5% of those aged 16 to 64 were severely disabled. Clearly, serious differences exist in the estimates of the number or rate of disabled persons. The point is that any estimates of the costs of disability depend directly on the estimated incidence in the population, which in turn depends on the definitions and concepts used. Cost estimates are also sensitive to the characteristics of those persons who are disabled. If disability is concentrated among low wage earners, as appears to be the case, the impact on costs will be less. The CPS finds that disability is more likely to be found in persons with less education and in minorities, and is slightly higher among women. Back disabilities are the leading cause of work disability.[6,35,47]

Although the need for measurement imposes some constraints on the way that disability is defined, this definition need not be synonymous with the medical and legal definitions. The economic impact of impairment or disability depends on several factors, including one's occupation, the state of the labor market, and a person's willingness and ability to make an occupational shift.[5,33,39] Further, with changes in any of these factors, disability could disappear or reappear while the individual's health status remains stable.

Conceptualizing Costs

Estimating the costs of disability requires establishing both the number of disabled people and the average cost of disability. This exercise can be carried out for reasons that extend beyond any academic challenge. Estimates that appear to demonstrate a high cost of disability might suggest a significant public policy burden. Estimates that seem low would provide less justification for new and expanded programs to curtail disability through workplace safety or to assist impaired workers. This is not to impugn the motives of those carrying out such studies. Rather, it is to explain the substantial degree of interest that greets each new set of cost estimates.

Researchers who attempt to estimate the costs of disability or of particular illnesses or conditions have used one of two approaches. One approach, the prevalence method, relies on cumulating the costs incurred, however conceived, of all the persons with a condition in a given year. In this calculation, the time of onset of the condition is of no concern. What matters is that the condition exists in that year. Alternatively, one could calculate the lifetime costs incurred by those who first develop a condition in the current year. The second approach, the incidence method, derives the present value of lifetime costs by summing the current cost and the discounted value of all future costs. Both approaches, although they are conceptually and calculation-wise quite different, attempt to determine the costs of a specific health condition.

Although economists may measure costs in different ways, in broad terms they conceive of them in the same manner. Typically, an economist asks how much output, or product, is expended or is foregone owing to the presence of disability. A foregone output, for example, is the partial or total loss of a disabled person's work-connected earnings. A number of studies of disability costs are limited to this set of losses only. Another foregone output is the partial or total loss of earnings from family and household members owing to their inability to earn because of the time devoted to caring for the disabled person. Losses attributable to foregone earnings or output are described by some as the indirect costs of disability. The more direct costs of disability include the medical, hospital, pharmaceutical, attendant, equipment, and refurbishing expenses needed to care for the impaired or ill individual.[42] Note that the sources of the funding for this last category are not relevant under this operational concept of disability.

Providing these services and products means that real resources are being expended, regardless of whom the ultimate payers are. The indirect costs together with the direct costs are the total costs of disability.

Where perfectly functioning labor markets are assumed to exist, economists can comfortably argue that workers' earnings perfectly reflect their productivity. This allows one to measure the value of any output foregone by the degree to which a worker sustains reduced earnings. Although such perfection may exist at best in the long run and at worst in textbooks only, this conventional treatment seems more appropriate than other methods. Typically, where impairment leads to unemployment, reduced hours of work, or a lower level of wages, the cost is evaluated based on the overall earnings decline, as a proxy for the lost output to society. This conceptualization stems from the economist's traditional framework that considers full, or near to full, employment as the norm. However, Drummond et al have noted the difficulty of valuing lost production due to disability in the presence of unemployed labor.[15] The very low unemployment rates in the United States in recent years have rendered this criticism of the conventional assumption somewhat less compelling.

Disability is likely to result in reduced productivity at times even without any decline in earnings. Although such a situation is not likely to occur in businesses that seek to survive over the long run, such temporary phenomena are possible. For example, other employees may pitch in and assist a worker with a problem that reduces his or her productivity. This may involve stepping up their own work effort (which means no overall loss of productivity has occurred) or it may mean that they aid in covering up any shortfall in a coworker's normal output (here a loss of productivity does occur). Reductions in output without any consequences in earnings may also represent poor monitoring by the managers of employee performance. In either case, an underestimate of the costs of disability seems likely where the measure is loss of earnings, yet employees continue to receive their pre-disability earnings despite operating at reduced levels of productivity. There are no global estimates of the costs of such hidden productivity losses.

As an example of the hidden productivity loss concept, a study by Greenberg et al of major depression, bipolar disorder, and dysthymia places their overall economic costs to society at $36.2 billion annually (excluding the costs attributable to death by suicide).[25] The authors assume that the reduced productivity of continuing employees with these conditions yields a 20% reduction in worker output, resulting in an economic cost of $12.1 billion. This figure exceeds the costs of work days actually lost, and is about equal to the estimated annual costs of hospitalization, outpatient care, and drugs associated with these illnesses. The study is notable for two reasons. First, it attempts to place a dollar value on the hidden or obscured cost that is associated with certain illnesses and disabilities. Second, this valuation helps to contribute to a very high overall estimate for a single set of conditions, suggesting that the work of Chirikos or Hill may substantially undervalue the costs of disability. In a later study, Greenberg et al ascribe 88% of the indirect costs of anxiety disorders to lost productivity while at work.[23] The remaining loss (12%) is due to actual absenteeism.

Persons not familiar with the foregone earnings method of calculating costs should note some of its other characteristics. First, because younger and older persons are generally not members of the labor force, the costs of their disability tend to be lower, as their disability does not result in any direct diminution of output. Some critics of the foregone earnings approach view this as a significant shortcoming. That aside, if others are forced to reduce their working time in order to assist such persons, their output would fall as gauged by their reduced earnings (foregone output).

Second, disability for young persons can result in direct reductions in future output. One could estimate, therefore, the lifetime direct costs of a disabled person by calculating the reduced or lost earnings in future years. All future losses must be subjected to some time rate of discount, leading to lower cost estimates for younger disabled persons. If many of the disabled are quite young, the incidence method would show a higher social cost than would the prevalence approach.

Third, it is likely that some household members may feel compelled to enter the workforce as a result of the loss of earnings of another member of that household who has become disabled. In such cases it is not appropriate to parallel the treatment given to household members who have reduced their working time to assist the disabled person. That is, one should not reduce the estimated costs of disability because a family member's earnings have increased. Clearly, the earnings increase in that case has come at the expense of either time lost from household duties or from time previously at leisure, both of which have real value.

To estimate the costs of health care treatment and rehabilitation, it is necessary to add all expenditures made on behalf of the disabled person (regardless of who pays the bill) and subtract those expenditures that would have been made for conditions other than those pertaining to the disability.

It should be apparent that efforts to carry out these calculations involve employing a variety of assumptions. Clearly, overall estimates may be quite sensitive to the assumptions selected. Assumptions aside, the underlying data tend to be fragmented and not entirely consistent, suggesting that these estimates must be approached with caution.

Until recently, most economists used foregone output exclusively as a measure of the cost of illness or disability. Indeed, this method is still employed regularly by many and it is the approach used in the courts to assess damages in actions for personal injury or death. However, an alternative method favored by some academic economists is growing in use. With this methodology, based on contingent valuation, the value of avoiding a disability or a life-threatening condition can be established, either by assessing behavior or by asking people to evaluate their preferences. As a result, individuals need not be producers or potential producers in order for a disabling condition to be costly. Nor would this measure exclude the costs of preventing disability in a calculation of the costs of disability. In certain cases it has been shown that the foregone earnings approach at best serves as a lower bound on the estimate based on contingent valuation.[4,32]

An interesting variant of the contingent valuation approach to measuring costs of disability employs the concept of the quality-adjusted life year (QALY).[14,19] This approach seeks to establish a common unit of measurement for both the quality and quantity of life. In this method, individuals are asked to rate different states of health based on their preferences and aversions to various health outcomes using a scale ranging from zero (death) to one (unimpaired health). The result is an index of utility or satisfaction. Levels of QALY or changes therein can be aggregated. Using this methodology, one will find that the value of an added year of life is positive but lower where the person is left in poorer health. However, it would also be affected positively where individual health is improving for many individuals. The QALY will increase, also, as it may be easier to function with disease today than in the past.

Proponents of the foregone earnings approach argue that it provides more consistent and readily measured values. Experience and familiarity in using and applying it may explain why the courts have continued to rely on it. However, critics of the approach attack its use on more than theoretical grounds. Glied, for example, demonstrates that the foregone earnings approach lacks accuracy and that it yields outcomes that are highly sensitive to the data applied.[21] Further, there is still substantial room for differences in selecting the rate of time preference (discount rate) to employ.[34]

Estimates of Costs

An excellent analysis by Chirikos, using the prevalence approach, places the aggregate costs of disability in 1980 at $177 billion, about 6.5% of gross domestic product.[7,8] The methodology he employed parallels the description above. He acknowledges that his estimates could be adjusted if more data were available. Because his assumptions appear to be consistently cautious, his estimate can be regarded as a reasonable lower bound of disability costs that year.

Using a set of techniques that are similar to those used by Chirikos, but employing an alternative data set, using different assumptions, and limiting the group to those aged 18 to 64, Hill reports the direct costs of disability in 1984 to be $145 billion.[29] Although the Chirikos estimate of the direct costs in lost time and earnings for the disabled was for 1980, adjusting that estimate for the subsequent 33% growth in the consumer price index would place his estimate in 1984 dollars at about $91 billion. Clearly, the differences between the Chirikos and Hill estimates highlight the margins of approximation that exist even when highly competent researchers undertake this type of effort. More recent estimates place the costs nearer to $300 billion.[6]

Chirikos found that 51% of the costs of disability derive from the medical care and other goods and services provided to the disabled. About 39% of the overall total stems from the lost earnings (foregone output) of the disabled, and about 10% from the labor market losses of household members of persons with disabilities. About 65% of the labor market losses were for men.

Chirikos[7,8] acknowledges that he ignores those who sustained no earnings loss because of expenditures made to overcome the consequences of an existing impairment. Moreover, there is no estimate of the costs of pain and suffering, yet these are real costs that courts and juries are regularly called upon to evaluate. That they are difficult to assess in the aggregate suggests that a wise course is simply to note their existence without seeking to attach some precise value. Indeed, the difficulty is magnified when one recognizes that the suffering may extend to household members of the person disabled and that courts do award damages, for example, for loss of consortium to those affected by another person's disability.

Because pain and suffering are so difficult to evaluate, and because there are economic incentives to embellish or to diminish their scope, it is understandable that substantial suspicion surrounds claims for damages that they cause. One way to measure the value of pain and suffering is to calculate the amount that one would spend to avoid incurring them. Although this is an indirect approach, it can be measured. The bottom line is that pain and suffering substantially contribute to the costs that individuals, and thereby society, incur owing to disability, and excluding them leads to an underestimation of the aggregate economic impact of disability.[4]

A variant of the Chirikos methodology is employed by Haveman et al in estimating the "loss of earning capabilities" attributable to disability.[28] They define this loss to be the difference between potential earnings capacity and actual earnings capacity. Among other considerations, the authors take into account part-time work (by both disabled and nondisabled workers) and wage effects. They conclude that the cost of disability in the

United States for the working age population in 1984 is in the range of about 5 to 10% of potential earning capacity ($131 to 285 billion in terms of 1988 dollars). Haveman et al report that this represents a slight decline over time owing to a reduction in the number of persons with limitations. The lost earning capacity itself of persons with limitations did not decline.

Several other, more recent global estimates of the costs of disability exist. Hoffman et al estimate the costs of chronic conditions, not disability per se, to be $659 billion in 1987, with 64% as direct costs and 36% ($234 billion) as indirect costs.[30] A more recent study by Brandt and Pope uses NHIS and CPS data to calculate the loss due to the effects of reduced labor force participation rates and wages, adjusting for skill and experience of the disabled, and arrives at earnings loss in the range of $93 to 111 billion in 1994.[6]

Several estimates of losses apply only to industrial injuries or illnesses.[3] Rossman et al estimated the loss of earnings due to work injuries only (excluding fatalities and injuries with less than 3 days of lost time) at $21.5 billion in 1989.[43] These are the costs of work injuries only in that year and include both direct and indirect costs.

In recent years, cost estimates have tended to be less global. A variety of studies have focused on disability costs associated with specific conditions. A number of them examine the health care costs and the foregone earnings or labor force participation of persons with anxiety or mental disorders.[16,18,22–24,38] A Surgeon General's report finds that mental health impairments in 1996 resulted in $69 billion in direct costs and $79 billion more in indirect costs (of which $12 billion was due to mortality costs).[52] Schizophrenia alone accounted for $53 billion in indirect costs. Yelin examined the costs associated with musculoskeletal conditions.[55] In an even more disaggregated approach to a cluster of conditions, the economic costs of cardiovascular diseases in California have been estimated.[20]

A recent study used the National Comorbidity Survey to evaluate the labor market effects of psychiatric disorders.[18] It found that persons with recently occurring disorders experienced lower employment rates of 11 percentage points for male and female workers, that the disorders resulted in reduced hours of employment for male workers, and that earnings declined for male workers by 13% and for female workers by 18%. On-the-job productivity decline was given as the reason for the decline in earnings.

Who Pays for Disability?

Although economists typically measure an item's cost in terms of the real resources used or foregone by it, the public view of costs is often quite different. Noneconomists usually focus on expended resources or the calculation of the costs of health care and rehabilitation, where actual dollars are exchanged for specific services and products. In this case, the two measures of costs are essentially the same.

Transfer payments, a major source of dollars spent, are not considered economic costs although noneconomists often treat them as such. A transfer payment is a payment from one agent to another that is not a payment for a product or a service currently rendered. Insurance benefits, both private and social, are transfers when money is paid out. Payments by government to those with perceived economic needs are also transfer payments. Welfare recipients may be needy as a consequence of disability, but these benefit payments are not the economic costs of disability. Instead, one household has money transferred to it to spend, resulting in someone else having less available for that purpose; for example, a taxpayer. Because one person's gain is balanced against someone else's loss, no real resources are lost to society. That economists do not consider transfer payments as economic costs does not diminish the interest in the dollar payments due to disability.

Tracking the extent of these transfer payments is no simple matter. One study estimated that there are 129 separate programs, administered by 14 different federal agencies, providing $175 billion per year in assistance to the disabled.[6] Note that this estimate does not include privately funded programs. The Commissioner of the US Equal Employment Opportunities Commission has testified that in fiscal year 1987, "one dollar in every 12 that the Federal Government spent was a direct payment to a disabled person or to a disability program [about $85 billion]. What had started out as a minor cost has escalated into a major drain on our economy."[11]

Two of the major programs providing cash benefits to the disabled are Social Security Disability Insurance (SSDI) and Supplemental Security Income (SSI). The latter is a welfare program targeted primarily at the blind and the disabled. In 1999, cash benefits for SSDI recipients were $51.3 billion (of which $46.5 billion were to workers, the balance to their survivors or dependents), up 107% from the level of 1990.[45,46] (This does not include any expenditures for Medicare benefits, vocational rehabilitation, or training services.) Over the period, the consumer price index rose by more than 31%.[17] SSI benefits for the blind and disabled exceeded $25 billion. Cash benefits under workers' compensation programs were $41.7 billion in 1998, up 21.5% from 1989; that is, the growth rate was below that of the consumer price index.[37] Thus, in constant dollar terms, cash benefits actually declined over the period for this program. Moreover, benefits should be understood to have fallen even more, considering that employment was also growing over this period by approximately 12%.[46]

Trupin et al estimate that 50% of the medical costs of all disabled people are paid for from public funds.[48] Of all such medical expenditures, 30% are from the Medicare program, 10% from Medicaid, and the balance from other programs including veteran's health benefits and community mental health centers.

Both workers' compensation and SSDI are economic mainstays of disabled workers and their families. The goal of either program is to replace the earnings lost for covered workers who meet certain eligibility criteria. Yet neither program seeks to replace the full earnings loss due to disability; as a consequence, the disabled shoulder some of the financial burden of disability inevitably. Most workers' compensation programs aim to replace two-thirds of lost gross earnings. All programs have initial waiting periods that are uncompensated, and all have statutory caps on weekly compensation benefits. Permanent disability benefits are very rarely compensable for a lifetime and few states provide any cost-of-living adjustments for long-term benefits. Not infrequently, workers must also pay for the costs of litigating for the benefits they receive.

SSDI benefits are payable only after a 5-month waiting period, have ceilings on benefits, and provide health care benefits only 24 months after cash benefits begin. Offsets exist in order to limit any stacking of benefits under this program with workers' compensation. Offsets under private disability insurance programs also typically limit any stacking of those benefits with either worker's compensation or SSDI.

Benefits under workers' compensation, SSDI, and private disability insurance are usually linked by formula to an employee's pre-disability earnings. Yet with the partial exception of health care benefits and Social Security old age retirement benefits, a work disability will substantially jeopardize an employee's supplemental benefits. Totally disabled workers do not have health care for themselves or their families provided by workers' compensation (except for the disabling condition of the employee) and all other supplemental benefits of the employment can cease. Recipients of SSDI are able to gain eligibility eventually for Medicare, and the Social Security old age benefits are not reduced owing to prior disability. However, other supplemental benefits, such as privately funded retirement contributions, cease. It seems clear that a sizeable gap exists between losses incurred by the disabled and the transfer payments typically provided. The gap is especially large in the case of persons who lose time from work while disabled, and particularly where a full job loss results from the condition.

Changing Incidence of Disability

The economic costs of disability are a product of the incidence of disability and average cost per disabled person. Differences in survey methodologies and definitions mean that a simple conclusion regarding the incidence rate of disablement in the population is perilous. The changing age composition of the population becomes a significant element in evaluating any changes in incidence rates over a long-term period. A changing political climate along with varying incentives available to claimants renders interyear comparisons of successful applications for SSDI and SSI (for blindness and disability) poor indicators of changing disability rates. Several excellent studies of the changing incidence rates of disability can be found in Chirikos,[7] Crimmins et al,[12,13] Colvez and Blanchet,[10] Haveman and Wolfe,[26,27] Kaye et al,[31] Wolfe and Haveman,[53] Yelin and Katz,[57] and Ycas.[54]

Ycas, in 1991, stated that "overall work disability rates have not changed a great deal over time. They probably rose in the mid-70s and since may have tended to decline. All this variation is vastly smaller than one would expect from the doubling and halving of disability benefit award rates."[54] A work disability is a health condition that has lasted 6 months or more and limits the kind or amount of work that one can do at a job or business. The release of the 1990 decennial census findings confirmed Ycas's conclusion. In 1990, 12.8 million persons aged 16 to 64 had a work disability.[42] Of these, 6.6 million, more than half, were defined as severely disabled (i.e., unable to perform work of any type). Nationally, the rates of severe and nonsevere work disability decreased by 3.9% and 4.7%, respectively, from 1980 to 1990, and the incidence of work disability declined from 85.2 to 81.5 per 1000 persons.[42] This has subsequently been reversed. In 1999, the Census Bureau found that 17.0 million persons in the 16 to 64 age range were work disabled, a rate of 97 per 1000. Of these, 68% were categorized as severely work disabled.[51]

Kaye et al rely on data from the NHIS to conclude that by 1994 disability rates had "risen markedly."[31] Yelin and Katz warn that disability rates are sensitive to the economic environment.[57] This would seem to be in line with rising disability rates by 1994, as Kaye et al have found, but hardly with the data for 1999, a year with one of the lowest rates of unemployment experienced in the past 5 decades.

Although disputes continue over the incidence of disability, there is little doubt that utilization of the SSDI and SSI programs has grown substantially. From 1990 to 1999, the number of worker beneficiaries in the SSDI program increased from 3.0 million to 4.9 million—approximately 63%.[46] In 1980, the number of such recipients was 1.5 million. Strikingly, the average age of male and female recipients has fallen by 7.2 and 7.7 years, respectively, over the previous 20 years.[40] Thus, persons are entering these programs at considerably younger ages than before. Participation in the SSI program, with about 3.7 million persons receiving welfare benefits who are blind or disabled, has also grown more rapidly than the labor force or working age population. However, upward trends in SSDI and SSI participation may reflect more on the administration of these programs than on the actual number of disabled persons.

Summary

One cannot estimate the costs of disability without a definition of disability that is measurable. Economists are generally in agreement that the costs of disability represent the resources used plus those not used owing to the presence of an impairment. This is consistent with the manner in which economic costs are generally calculated. Changing labor market conditions can profoundly affect the calculations of costs.

In a society that is increasingly sensitive to considerations of cost-effectiveness, measures of costs of disability take on considerable importance. The public's interest in the costs of disability is likely centered on the direct expenditures made on behalf of the disabled by government, and perhaps by others. Relatively little interest appears to exist in the matter of the economic burden of disability that is borne by the individual.

References

1. Adams PF, Benson V: Current estimates from the National Health Interview Survey, National Center for Health Statistics. Vital Health Stat 10:181, 1991.
2. American Medical Association: Guides to the Evaluation of Permanent Impairment, 3rd ed, rev. Chicago, American Medical Association, 1990.
3. Andreoni D: The Cost of Occupational Accidents and Diseases. Geneva, International Labour Office, 1986.
4. Berger M, Blomquist G, Kenkel D, Tolley G: Framework for valuing health risks. In Tolley G, Kenkel D, Fabian R (eds): Valuing Health for Policy: An Economic Approach. Chicago, University of Chicago Press, 1994, pp 23–41.
5. Berkowitz M, Hill MA: Disability and the labor market: an overview. In Berkowitz M, Hill MA (eds): Disability and the Labor Market: Economic Problems, Policies and Programs. Ithaca, NY, ILR Press, 1986.
6. Brandt EN Jr, Pope AM (eds): Enabling America: Assessing the Role of Rehabilitation Science and Engineering. Washington, DC, National Academy Press, 1997.
7. Chirikos TN: Accounting for the historical rise in work disability prevalence. Milbank Q 64:271–301, 1986.
8. Chirikos TN: Aggregate economic losses from disability in the United States: Preliminary assay. Milbank Q 67(Suppl. 2, Part 1):59–91, 1989.
9. Chirikos TN, Nestel G: Economic determinants and consequences of self-reported work disability. J Health Econ 3:117–136, 1984.
10. Colvez A, Blanchet M: Disability trends in the U.S. population 1966–1977: Analysis of repeated causes. Am J Public Health 71:464–471, 1981.
11. Committee on Education and Labor, U.S. House of Representatives, 101st Congress: Legislative History of Public Law 101–336: Americans with Disabilities Act (Vol. 2). Washington, DC, U.S. Government Printing Office, 1990.
12. Crimmins E, Reynolds S, Saito Y: Trends in health and ability to work among the older working-age population. J Gerontol B 54:S31–40, 1999.
13. Crimmins E, Saito Y, Reynolds S: Further evidence on recent trends in the prevalence and incidence of disability among older Americans from two sources: the LSOA and the NHIS. J Gerontol B 52:S59–71, 1997.
14. Cutler D, Richardson E: Measuring the health of the U.S. population. In Brookings Papers on Economic Activity: Microeconomics. Washington, DC, Brookings Institution, 1997, pp 217–282.
15. Drummond M, Ludbrook A, Lowsin K, Steele A: Studies in Economic Appraisal of Health Care. Oxford, Oxford University Press, 1986.
16. DuPont R, Rice D, Miller S, et al: Economic costs of anxiety disorders. Anxiety 2:167–172, 1996.
17. Economic Report of the President. Washington, DC, U.S. Government Printing Office, 1999.
18. Ettner S, Frank R, Kessler R: The impact of psychiatric disorders on labor market outcomes. Industrial and Labor Relations Review 51:64–81, 1997.
19. Fabian R: The QALY approach. In Tolley G, Kenkel D, Fabian R (eds): Valuing Health for Policy: An Economic Approach. Chicago, University of Chicago Press, 1994, pp 118–136.
20. Fox P, Gazzaniga J, Karter A, Max W: The economic costs of cardiovascular disease in California, 1991: Implications for public health policy. J Public Health Policy 17:442–459, 1996.
21. Glied S: Estimating the indirect cost of illness: An estimate of the foregone earnings approach. Am J Public Health 86:1723–1728, 1996.
22. Greenberg P, Finkelstein S, Berndt A: Economic consequences of illness in the workplace. Sloan Management Review 36:26–38, 1995.
23. Greenberg P, Sisitsky T, Kessler R, et al: The economic burden of anxiety disorders in the 1990s. J Clin Psychiatry 60:427–435, 1999.
24. Greenberg PE, et al: Depression: a neglected major illness. J Clin Psychiatry 54:419–426, 1993.
25. Greenberg PE, et al: The economic burden of depression in 1990. J Clin Psychiatry 54:405–418, 1993.
26. Haveman RH, Wolfe B: The decline in male labor force participation [comment]. J Political Economy 92:532–549, 1984.
27. Haveman RH, Wolfe B: The Disabled from 1962 to 1984: Trends in Number, Composition and Well Being (Special Report No. 44). Madison, Wisc, Institute for Research on Poverty, 1987.
28. Haveman R, Wolfe B, Buron L, Hill S: The loss of earnings capability from disability/health limitations: Toward a new social indicator. Review of Income and Wealth 41:289–308, 1995.
29. Hill MA: The economics of disability. In Thompson-Hoffman S, Storck IF (eds): Disability in the U.S.: A Portrait from National Data. New York, Springer, 1991.
30. Hoffman C, Rice D, Sung H: Persons with chronic conditions: Their prevalence and costs. JAMA 276:1473–1479, 1996.
31. Kaye HS, Laplante MP, Carlson D, Wenger B: Trends in Disability Rates in the US, 1970–1994. San Francisco, Disability Statistics Center, UCSF, 1996.
32. Kenkel D: Cost of illness approach. In Tolley G, Kenkel D, Fabian R (eds): Valuing Health for Policy: An Economic Approach. Chicago, University of Chicago Press, 1994, pp 42–71.
33. Leonard JS: Disability policy and the return to work. In Weaver CL (ed): Disability and Work: Incentives, Rights, and Opportunities. Washington, DC, AEI Press, 1991.
34. Lipscomb J, Weinstein M, Torrance G: Time preference. In Gold M, Russell L, Siegel J, Weinstein M (eds): Cost Effectiveness in Health and Medicine. Oxford, Oxford University Press, 1996, pp 214–246.

35. Loprest P, Rupp K, Sandell S: Gender disabilities and employment in the health and retirement study. J Hum Resources 30(Suppl.):S293–318, 1995.
36. Manton K, et al: Chronic disability trends in the elderly U.S. population. Proc Natl Acad Sci U S A 94:2593–2598, 1997.
37. National Academy of Social Insurance: Workers' Compensation: Benefits, Coverage and Costs, 1997–98, New Estimates. Washington, DC, 2000.
38. O'Neill DM, Bertullo D: Work and earnings losses due to mental illness: Perspectives from three national surveys. Administration and Policy in Mental Health 25:505–523, 1998.
39. Parsons DO: Measuring and deciding disability. In Weaver CL (ed): Disability and Work: Incentives, Rights, and Opportunities. Washington, DC, AEI Press, 1991.
40. Pope AM, Tarlov AR: Disability in America: Toward a National Agenda for Prevention. Washington, DC, National Academy Press, 1991.
41. Prevalence of Work Disability in the United States—1990. MMWR Morb Mortal Wkly Rep 42:757–772, 1993.
42. Rice DP, et al: The economic cost of illness: a replication and update. Health Care Financing Rev 7:61–80, 1985.
43. Rossman S, Miller R, Douglass J: The Costs of Occupational Traumatic and Cumulative Injuries. Washington, DC, The Urban Institute, 1991.
44. Rupp K, Stapleton D: Determinants of the growth in the Social Security Administration's disability programs: An overview. Soc Secur Bull 58:43–70, 1995.
45. Soc Secur Bull 56(4), 1993.
46. Soc Secur Bull (Annual Statistical Supplement), 2000.
47. Storck IF, Thompson-Hoffman S: Demographic characteristics of the disabled population. In Thompson-Hoffman S, Storck IF (eds): Disability in the United States: a Portrait from National Data. New York, Springer, 1991.
48. Trupin L, Rice D, Max W: Medical Expenditures for People with Disabilities in the US, 1987 (Disability Statistics Report No. 5). National Institute for Disability and Rehabilitation Research, 1996.
49. U.S. Bureau of the Census: Census Brief, Economics and Statistics Administration (CENBR/97-5). U.S. Bureau of the Census, 1997.
50. U.S. Bureau of the Census: Current Estimate from the National Health Interview Survey, Vital and Health Statistics (Series 10, No. 199). U.S. Bureau of the Census, 1995.
51. U.S. Bureau of the Census: Selected Characteristics of Persons 16–74, 1999: Available at www.census.gov.hhes/www/disable.
52. U.S. Department of Health and Human Services: Mental Health: A Report of the Surgeon General. U.S. Department of Health and Human Services, 1999.
53. Wolfe BF, Haveman R: Trends in the prevalence of work disability from 1962 to 1984 and their correlates. Milbank Q 68:53–80, 1990.
54. Ycas M: Trends in the incidence and prevalence of work disability. In Thompson-Hoffman S, Storck IF (eds): Disability in the United States: A Portrait From National Data. New York, Springer, 1991.
55. Yelin E: The economic and social and psychological impact of musculoskeletal conditions. Arthritis Rheum 38:1351–1362, 1995.
56. Yelin EH: Disability and the Displaced Worker. New Brunswick, NJ, Rutgers University Press, 1992.
57. Yelin EH, Katz PP: Labor force trends of persons with and without disabilities. Monthly Labor Review 117:36–42, 1994.

CHAPTER

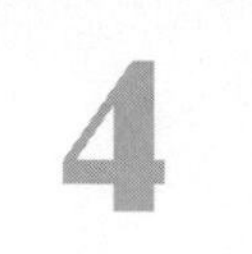

Federal Workers' Compensation Programs

JOHN D. McLELLAN, JR., AB, JD

This chapter discusses disability systems that have been established by Congress to meet the needs of specific groups not generally covered under state workers' compensation or other disability laws. Two of these systems are workers' compensation programs providing the full range of workers' compensation benefits to federal employees (the Federal Employees' Compensation Program) and longshore and harbor workers (the Longshore and Harbor Workers' Compensation Program). Another workers' compensation system, the Black Lung Program, was established solely to provide disability benefits to qualified coal miners with a disabling black lung medical condition due to their employment in or around coal mines. For further information on workers' compensation programs in general, see Chapter 5.

Also discussed are the disability benefits provided by the Department of Veterans Affairs to many military veterans and their families. Attention is given to how nonworkers' compensation law and the Federal Employers' Liability Act work to assist railroad employees and seamen (crew members) in obtaining disability damages from their employers, and other disability benefits available to these two groups.

The discussion herein is meant to acquaint the reader with the identified programs. It does not intend to be a detailed guide on processing individual claims through the different systems. For up-to-date information on claims processing the reader should contact the agency administering the program or the sources listed in this chapter. For those who need readily available up-to-date information on any of these programs administered by a federal agency, such information is easily obtained by accessing the Internet Web site of the program. If, for instance, a physician needs to know the medical/disability rating procedures and policies of one of these federal programs, the procedures and policies may be obtained through a visit to the Web site of the agency administering the program using the address given in this chapter under the programs covered. For the historical developments of these programs, see Chapter 2.

FEDERAL EMPLOYEES' COMPENSATION PROGRAM

The Federal Employees' Compensation Act (FECA) is the workers' compensation law covering federal civilian employees and their dependents. FECA emphasis is on providing continuing income maintenance payments during periods of wage loss caused by disability due to a work injury sustained "while in the performance of duty" (lump sum awards or settlements are not available[1]). In addition, FECA provides full medical care for such injury and, in the event of injury-related death, benefits to survivors. FECA claims are received, adjudicated, and paid by the federal government.[2]

Definitions and Eligibility[3]

The FECA covers civilian employees of the federal government, including the Postal Service. Certain other individuals may be covered under defined circumstances. For instance, state and local government law enforcement officers (not employees of the federal government) who are injured while assisting in the enforcement of criminal laws of the United States may be entitled to FEC benefits to supplement, but not replace, state workers' compensation benefits.

As stated previously, the emphasis in the FEC program is to provide regular income maintenance payments (compensation) to federal employees who sustain loss of earnings or decreases in wage earning capacity due to disability resulting from personal injury sustained while in the performance of duty. The payments continue for the duration of such disability. There is no overall maximum number of weeks or monetary amount that limits payments. When the employee qualifies for government retirement, the disabled employee may elect (revocable) to continue on FEC or to take government retirement. FEC payments would continue until such time as the employee is found to have no further disability—no further wage loss or loss of earnings or earning capacity—owing to the effects of the accepted injury. Lump sum payments to injured workers to settle the government's liability to make continuing payments for disability are not available because the FEC is intended as a wage loss program with the benefits being paid on a continuing periodic basis during the continuance of disability.[4]

Disability is the incapacity, because of employment injury, to earn the wages the employee was receiving at the time of injury.[5]

Injury or *personal injury* is a wound or condition of the body induced by accident or trauma, including disease or illness, proximately caused by the employment for which benefits are provided under the Act. Injuries or deaths specifically not covered are those caused by willful misconduct of the employee; those caused by the employee's intention to bring about the injury or death of the employee or another; and those proximately caused by alcohol intoxication or illegal drug use of the injured employee. Note that the definition of injury is straightforward in the sense that neither unusual effort on the part of the employee nor exposure to unusual employment conditions must be shown to establish a covered injury.

Although OWCP (Office of Workers' Compensation Programs) has specified forms for medical reports, the use of the forms is not required if the physician's report containing all the above information is submitted in narrative form on the physician's letterhead stationery and signed by the physician.

If the report being submitted is in support of a claim for a schedule loss or award (see following discussion on schedule award), the physician's medical report must contain accurate measurements of the function of the organ or member, in accordance with the most recent AMA Edition of the Guides to the Evaluation of Permanent Impairment. These measurements may include the actual degree of loss of active or passive motion or deformity; the amount of atrophy; the decrease, if any, in strength; the disturbance of sensation; and pain due to nerve impairment.[6]

The employee must advise the treating physician of the employing agency's willingness to accommodate where possible the employee's work limitations and restrictions and return to work when the employing agency offers duties within the limitations and restrictions warranted by the medical condition.

Compensation: Monetary Benefits for Disability

When a covered employee sustains a traumatic injury, the employee is entitled to receive full pay (regular paycheck) during the period of injury-caused disability for up to 45 calendar days. The continuation of pay (COP) payments are taxed as is the regular pay.[7] After 45 days, the still-disabled employee would be entitled to appropriate compensation.[8]

Compensation and disability compensation are money payments made under FECA to compensate an injured worker for the disability (lost wages) or permanent impairment (schedule award) sustained as a result of a traumatic injury or occupational disease or illness. For traumatic injuries, compensation would be paid for disability after the 45-day COP period. For occupational disease or illness, compensation would begin at the earliest eligible date following pay loss (3-day waiting period).

The amount of the compensation paid (weekly compensation rate, total disability, and schedule awards) is computed at 75% (for workers who are married or have dependents) or 66⅔% (for those who are not married and have no dependents) of the workers' pay rate on the date of injury. The compensation rate for partial disability (injury-related loss of earnings or earning capacity) is based on 75% or 66⅔% of the difference between the pay rate on the date of injury and the lower earnings or earning capacity after the injury.

Schedule awards are provided for permanent impairment of certain specified members or parts of the body (the head and back are not included) after maximum medical improvement has been achieved. These awards are paid for a specified number of weeks based on the extent of impairment as determined using the current AMA Guides and are paid regardless of whether there is any disability (injury-related loss of earnings).[9] Following is an illustration of this point and the different disabilities described previously.

Johnny Fed falls at work during his normal working hours and breaks his leg. It is considered an injury while in the performance of duty, and he is found entitled to FEC benefits. The injury prevents him from doing his job as a Navy shipyard worker. He is placed on COP for the temporary total disability (total loss of earnings) caused by this traumatic injury. He is entitled to COP for up to 45 calendar days of medically supported disability.

After the 45 days he is entitled to receive compensation for total disability or partial disability depending on whether he continues with total or partial injury-related disability (loss of earnings). When maximum medical improvement has been reached and it appears that Johnny Fed will have a permanent impairment in his injured leg, the treating physician will be asked to supply an opinion as to the extent of the injury-caused impairment based on the current AMA Guides.

If it is found that a 25% permanent impairment remains in the injured leg, Johnny will be entitled to receive 72 weeks of compensation (288 weeks is statutorily provided for 100% loss of use or impairment of a leg; 25% of 288 weeks is 72 weeks). If he has returned to work, he will still be entitled to these payments. If he continues to be disabled, Johnny's total or partial disability compensation will stop while he is paid the 72 weeks' compensation.

If, at the end of the 72 weeks he is still disabled, constituting a total or partial loss of wages or earning capacity owing to the effects of his injury (he cannot go up and down ladders in the shipyard), he could be put back on disability compensation for the duration of his disability. His employing government agency (the Navy) has a responsibility to place Johnny in employment suited to his capabilities and qualifications, and Johnny has a responsibility to accept this suitable employment. If the Navy succeeds in returning him to employment in which he suffers no wage loss compared to his earnings at the time of injury, his compensation for wage loss (total or partial disability) will cease. It also would cease if he returned to employment elsewhere (government or private employment) with no wage loss. If he returned to employment but at lower wages, he would be entitled to compensation for partial disability based on the difference between what he was paid at the time of the injury and what he receives in his current job.

If Johnny Fed had suffered an injury to his leg after climbing ladders over more than 1 day (not a specific incident in 1 day but caused by his climbing ladders over more than 1 day), his injury would have been classified as an occupational disease or illness, not a traumatic injury. He would not be entitled to COP (traumatic injuries only) but would receive compensation for his disability (wage loss) during the duration of that injury-related total or partial disability. His entitlement to schedule awards would be the same as for a traumatic injury.[10]

Role of Physicians in Litigation

The role of the physician in regard to litigation is to provide a clear, thorough, and detailed report concerning the facts of the accident (history) and the medical results of the accident on the individual. Most FECA cases are decided based on documents mailed to the FEC concerning the injury. A good detailed medical report (see also Chapter 12) will usually lead to a prompt decision on the claim and little delay in the disabled employee's receiving appropriate compensation. Inadequate medical reports can lead to questions, confusion, delays, and ultimately litigation. Under FECA, hearings are provided for, and physicians may be asked to testify, especially when the medical issue cannot be readily resolved. On the whole, however, under FECA, good medical reports submitted by the treating or examining physician can result in little or no need for the doctor to be called to a hearing to testify.

Administering Agency[2]

The OWCP, Employment Standards Administration (ESA), Department of Labor (DOL) administers the FEC program. The official OWCP Web page is found at www.dol.gov/esa/owcp_org.htm. In that Web page, clicking on the link entitled "Division of Federal Employees' Compensation" or "FEC" provides up-to-date information on the program, including newly revised regulations. The parts of the regulations cited in the references are available there.

LONGSHORE AND HARBOR WORKERS' COMPENSATION ACT

The Longshore and Harbor Workers' Compensation Act (LSA) is a workers' compensation law covering workers on or adjacent to the navigable waters of the United States. Persons covered include any person engaged in maritime employment, including any longshore worker or person engaged in longshoring operations, and any harbor worker, including those engaged in ship repair, shipbuilding, and ship-breaking activities upon the navigable waters of the United States or adjoining pier and dock areas. The law does not cover a master or member of a crew of any vessel. (Seamen are discussed later in this chapter.)

The LSA has been extended to cover some other groups of workers not covered by other workers' compensation laws, such as employees engaged in certain operations conducted on the Outer Continental Shelf of the United States; civilian employees of nonappropriated fund instrumentalities (Post-Exchanges [PXs], Officers' Clubs) of the Armed Forces; employees outside the United States on US defense bases; and employees outside the United States carrying out "public work contracts" or other United States-funded contracts.

The LSA is similar to many state workers' compensation laws that provide wage loss and schedule loss benefits for injuries arising out of and in the course of employment. Full medical care is also provided, as are death benefits for survivors of a work-injury death. Lump sum awards or settlements are available. The benefits are paid by the employers themselves (as authorized self-insurers) or through employer-obtained insurance.

The LSA program provides for income maintenance (compensation) payments for disability resulting from a covered injury. The LSA program uses the AMA Guides as its rating source.

Injuries that can be shown to have occurred on the job while the employee was in the performance of duty are generally covered without question. Specifically not included are injuries caused solely by intoxication of the employee or by the willful intention of the employee to injure or kill him- or herself or another. There are specific presumptions written into the LSA; it is presumed, in the absence of substantial evidence to the contrary, that the claim comes within the provisions of the Act, that sufficient notice has been given, and that the injury was not occasioned by the intoxication of the injured employee or the willful intention of the employee to injure or kill him- or herself or another.

Medical Examinations and Rules[11]

The worker may select a physician (not limited to MDs) of his or her choice. Full medical care is provided by the law and is to be paid by the employer or the employer's insurance carrier. There is no overall maximum as to the total amount that may be paid, but the OWCP office having jurisdiction may use a local fee schedule such as a local state workers' compensation fee schedule to determine whether the individual medical charges are reasonable.

Physicians asked to treat these patients receive Form LS-1 which is completed by the employer and authorizes treatment. The back side of that form is to be used by the treating physician as the initial medical report, and the report is to be received by the employer within 10 days.

Physicians asked to examine or evaluate workers for disability should give sufficient medical information in the physician's report so that the OWCP claims official can make a determination whether the injury-related medical condition precludes the worker from returning to his or her usual work or some other type of employment, or is unable to perform any work. In evaluating the worker for a schedule loss (permanent impairment) it would seem best for the physician to use the AMA Guides. The ultimate decision as to extent of impairment and disability is made by the OWCP claims official. That official is to consider other factors in addition to the medical evaluation reports in arriving at his or her decision. For an example of the type of medical report most helpful in these workers' compensation cases, see the Medical Report section in the previous FEC discussion. See also Chapter 12.

The LSA Medical Rules can be found on the LSA page via the OWCP Web page (see previous discussion) by choosing LS Regulations following the procedure described. The LSA Medical Rules can be found by selecting 20 CFR Part 702, Subpart D—Medical and Supervision. A shortcut is to access the OALJ (Office of Administrative Law Judges) Law Library at www.oalj.dov.gov and select Regulations, Tittle 20, Part 702, Subpart D—Medical Care.

Compensation Program

Typically, the totally disabled injured worker would receive compensation based on two-thirds of the worker's weekly pay at the time of the injury. This compensation would continue during the medically supported total disability. If the worker has a partial loss of earnings or is otherwise considered partially disabled, the worker will be paid two-thirds of his or her actual or computed loss of earnings.[12] The maximum weekly compensation rate is 200% of the current national average weekly wage as determined each year by the Secretary of Labor.

If the injury is to a member (e.g., arm, hand, leg, foot), when maximum medical improvement is reached the compensation for time loss will stop (if it has not stopped sooner because the employee could or did return to work) and the worker will be evaluated for scheduled loss (extent of permanent impairment). The AMA Guides may be used in this evaluation, but the law or regulations do not require its use except in hearing-loss cases and for an occupational illness of a retired worker.

Compensation for serious disfigurement of the face, head, or neck or of other normally exposed areas likely to handicap the employee in securing or maintaining employment is provided to a maximum of $7,500.

Once the schedule loss is paid, the worker is not entitled to additional compensation for wage loss. Workers who have a back or head injury disability would not normally be entitled to a scheduled award but are entitled to continued compensation based on two-thirds of the loss of earnings.

Note that the benefits for occupational disease are the same as for injury except where the disease becomes manifest after the employee retires. In such a case compensation is paid for impairment rather than wage replacement and therefore paid as a permanent partial disability benefit as determined in accordance with the AMA Guides.[13]

Role of Physicians in Litigation

The role of physicians in regard to litigation under the LSA is as stated in the FECA section. The physician needs to provide clear, thorough, and detailed reports (see Chapter 12) concerning the facts of the accident and the medical results on the injured individual. A thorough, good, clear report will, in most situations, lead to a much quicker resolution of any issues and the lessening of any litigation. Generally, there is more litigation of issues under the LSA than under the FECA. Under the LSA, insurance representatives and attorneys generally participate in hearings and physicians may be expected to be called to testify and be cross examined.

Administering Agency

The OWCP, Employment Standards Administration, US Department of Labor administers the LSA program through offices located in many of the port cities of the United States.

The LSA Web page is available by accessing the OWCP Web page at www.dol.gov/esa/owcp_org.htm and selecting the Division of Longshore and Harbor Workers' Compensation. For the LSA Regulations and other LSA documents you may go directly to the OALJ Law Library without going through OWCP: www.oalj.dol.gov/.

The OWCP's responsibility in administrating the LSA differs from that of administrating the FECA. In the FEC program, the OWCP receives, adjudicates, and pays the disability benefits. The LSA requires the Longshore employer to obtain reports of injury, decide on benefits due, and pay those benefits. The OWCP's job is to monitor the response of employers to the LSA requirements for providing benefits and medical care. It also furnishes the mechanism to resolve disputes.[14]

BLACK LUNG BENEFITS FOR COAL MINERS AND THEIR FAMILIES[15]

Definitions and Eligibility

BL (black lung) benefits are provided to miners who are disabled owing to pneumoconiosis (black lung) and to certain survivors of miners who died owing to or while totally or partially disabled by pneumoconiosis under the authority of Title IV of the Federal Coal Mine Health and Safety Act of 1969, as amended.[17] An applicant or claimant for benefits therefore must establish that the definition of miner has been met and that the miner has a prescribed disability owing to the defined pneumoconiosis (black lung).

A miner is defined as "any person who works or has worked in or around a coal mine or coal preparation facility in the extraction, preparation, or transportation of coal, and any person who works or has worked in coal mine construction or maintenance in or around a coal mine or coal preparation facility."[18]

Total disability in a miner is considered "if the ... pneumoconiosis ... prevents or prevented the miner: (1) from performing his or her usual coal mine work; and (2) from engaging in gainful employment in the immediate area of his or her residence requiring the skills or abilities comparable to those of any employment he or she previously engaged with some regularity over a substantial period of time."[19]

Pneumoconiosis is a chronic dust disease of the lung and its sequelae, including respiratory and pulmonary impairments, arising out of coal mine employment. For the purposes of this definition, a disease "arising out of coal mine employment" includes any chronic pulmonary disease resulting in respiratory or pulmonary impairment significantly related to, or substantially aggravated by, dust exposure in coal mine employment. The definition includes coal workers' pneumoconiosis, anthracosilicosis, anthracosis, anthrosilicosis, massive pulmonary fibrosis, progressive massive fibrosis, silicosis, or silicotuberculosis, arising out of coal mine employment.[20]

Medical Examination and Rules[21]

In filing an initial claim with an office of the DCMWC (Division of Coal Mine Workers' Compensation), the claimant will be referred by letter to a medical specialist who will be asked to perform the designated testing and examinations necessary to put together the medical documentation needed by DCMWC to determine whether the diagnosis of pneumoconiosis has been established. The cost of this examination, including travel costs, is paid by DCMWC and is not to be paid by the claimant. The claimant may request that DCMWC authorize this medical evaluation through a qualified physician of the claimant's choice.

The DCMWC letter to the evaluating medical specialist will typically ask for one or more of the following: chest x-ray (single view, posteroanterior only); pulmonary function tests; arterial blood gas study (as specifically defined); and physical examination.

More information can be accessed at the Black Lung Web page (see previous) by clicking on "Black Lung Regulations (CFR)" and on the Regulations page, "CFR 20 Parts 700–799," by clicking on "Part 718—Standards for ... Disability ... ," which leads to a detailed presentation of the medical aspects of the Black Lung Program.

Compensation Program

As noted, there are income maintenance benefits payable to those covered by this program. The amount of the benefits and how they are determined is spelled out in the Regulations, Part 725, Subpart G—Payment of Benefits, particularly Part 725.520. More information is available from the BL Regulation Web page, as shown previously, by selecting "Part 725, Subpart G—Payment of Benefits."

Role of Physicians in Litigation

The role of the physician in regard to litigation is the same as noted under FEC and LSA. The physician needs to provide clear, thorough, and detailed medical reports (see previous [BL] Medical Examination and Rules and Chapter 12). Hearings are provided for under the BL program so there is the possibility of doctors being asked to testify and be cross examined. Providing good written reports may lessen the hassle the physician could experience in the litigation process.[22]

Administering Agency

The Department of Labor, through the Division of Coal Mine Workers' Compensation (DCMWC) of the OWCP, administers the Black Lung Program (BL) through offices located in coal-producing areas of the United States. Social Security Offices are authorized by DCMWC to receive black lung claims and to forward them to DCMWC for processing and adjudication.

The DCMWC (BL) Web page may be accessed through the OWCP Web page—www.dol.gov/esa/owcp_org.htm. —by clicking on "Division of Coal Mine Workers' Compensation." The helpful materials available through that page include the BL Act and the BL Regulations.

Some black lung benefit claimants may be required to process their claims through the state workers' compensation system where their coal mine employment was located when such system has been found adequate by the Secretary of Labor. The BL Web page can provide help on this issue.

BENEFITS FOR VETERANS AND THEIR FAMILIES[23]

Definitions and Eligibility[24]

To receive benefits the person applying must establish basic eligibility as a veteran or the dependent or survivor of a veteran. Once this is established the person must meet the entitlement requirements for the specific benefits applied for. A very general overview of some of the qualifying requirements is given in the following. More specific and detailed entitlement information is available at local VA offices.

A veteran is a person who served in the active military, naval, or air service, and who was discharged or released under conditions that were not dishonorable. Although "undesirable" or "bad conduct discharge" from a Special Court Martial may disqualify benefit entitlement, it seems clear that a bad conduct discharge from a General Court Martial or a dishonorable discharge definitely will bar benefits.

Active military, naval, or air service includes active duty, any period of active duty for training during which the individual was disabled or died of disease or injury incurred or aggravated in the line of duty, and any period of inactive duty training during which the individual was disabled or died of disease or injury incurred or aggravated in the line of duty.

A showing of service during wartime is necessary to qualify for some benefits such as pensions. Specific periods were defined from the Civil War and Indian wars through the present time. Length of service may determine entitlement to and extent of some benefits, but length of service rules do not apply to service-connected disability compensation benefits.

"Willful misconduct" is a statutory bar to benefits. For instance, disabilities resulting from a person's willful misconduct are not compensable; drug addiction and primary alcoholism are considered misconduct, but hepatitis, cirrhosis of the liver, and AIDS are not considered willful misconduct.

Medical Examinations and Rules[25]

The rules and procedures for conducting medical examinations for the purpose of determining compensable disability are provided in the detailed "Schedule for Rating Disabilities" found in Part 4, Title 38 of the Code of Federal Regulations (CFR). Direct Internet access to that schedule can be found at http://www.access.gpo.gov/nara/cfr via the Code of Federal Regulations page; after clicking on "Retrieve CFR sections by citation ... ," the CFR—Retrieve CFR by citation page provides boxes to be filled in as follows: revision year = most recent available, title = 38, CFR part = 4, section = (blank), subpart = B, type of file = text. For the application of this schedule, accurate and fully descriptive medical examinations are required, with emphasis on the limitation of activity imposed by the disabling condition.[26]

> This ... schedule is primarily a guide in the evaluation of disability resulting from all types of diseases and injuries encountered as a result of or incidental to military service. The percentage ratings represent as far as can practicably be determined the average impairment in earning capacity resulting from such diseases and injuries and their residual conditions in civil occupations. Generally, the degrees of disability specified are considered adequate to compensate for considerable loss of working time from exacerbations or illnesses proportionate to the severity of the several grades of disability.[26]

It is essential that the evaluating physician have knowledge of what is required. Therefore, the physician requested by a veteran to examine him or her and provide such an evaluation needs an up-to-date copy of the VA's *Physician's Guide*, or at least a copy or computer printout of the latest update of the chapter that covers the condition the physician is evaluating. The physician can obtain this document from a local VA service officer. As noted previously, the Guide is also found in

Title 38, Part 4 of the Code of Federal Regulations, which is available from the Government Printing Office and through the Internet (see previous). Local public or legal libraries may also be able to obtain a copy.

Compensation and Pension Programs[25]

Service-Connected Disability Compensation

This program provides compensation for disabilities incurred in or aggravated during a period of military service. This could be a battlefield injury or a football injury incurred during active service. For a disability to be service connected it should be shown that it is directly related to the service (this could be done through military medical records showing that the condition was diagnosed during military service), it was aggravated during service (a condition prior to that military service became worse during military service), or a statutory presumption applies. For instance, the condition was manifested—not necessarily diagnosed—within 1 year of discharge (one year rule) for chronic diseases, including arteriosclerosis and arthritis (defined conditions), and certain other diseases including tropical diseases such as cholera, dysentery, malaria, or filariasis; or at any time for diseases specific to prisoners of war such as beriberi, psychosis, any anxiety state, dysthymic disorder, or depressive neurosis. A service-connected disability also could be a condition secondarily related to a service-connected condition (i.e., proximately caused by or linked to a service-connected condition) or an injury that occurred in a VA medical facility.

Determining service-connected disability benefits involves arriving at the appropriate percentage of covered disability by fixing (determining) the diagnosis (see codes and rating schedule),[27] fixing (determining) the symptoms (will affect the degree of disability), and then comparing them against the VA Schedule for Rating Disabilities.[25] The percentage of (covered) disability thus obtained is intended to reflect the average impairment of earnings capacity, but the result does not necessarily meet this goal. Good medical documentation and support on the veteran's part will make the case here. In a case where there are multiple disabilities, percentages are not added arithmetically, but by the use of the Table of Combined Disabilities. Percentages are set in increments of 10, but may be zero.

With the above-determined percentage rating, the level of benefit payments is fixed by statute. Special or increased monthly compensation in special need cases may be available (above the 100% amount).

Increased compensation is payable when disability rated at less than 100% (sole cause) results in unemployability. A veteran unable to secure or follow a substantially gainful occupation as a result of service-connected disabilities generally only may be paid at the 100% rate. To qualify, the veteran's disability status must be either one disability rated at 60% or more or two or more disabilities, one of which is rated at least at 40%, and sufficient additional disability to bring the combined rating to 70% or more; or if the above percentages are not met, in rare cases the Director of Compensation and Pension Service may allow a claim. Evidence must be submitted to establish unemployability. This includes statements of employers and vocational rehabilitation evaluations. Marginal employment up to national poverty level may not bar unemployability benefit. The VA Form 21-8940 is used.

Non-Service-Connected Disability Pension

VA pension benefits were designed to supplement the income of disabled veterans who, because they gave up career opportunities to serve their country during a time of war, were unable to advance their careers or accumulate enough resources to support themselves adequately after they became disabled. Need and permanent and total disability are crucial factors.

There are three pension programs: Improved (effective January 1, 1979), Section 306 (effective July 1, 1960 to December 31, 1978), and Old Law (before July 1, 1960). Most VA pensioners have the Improved pension. Under this plan the maximum benefit level is reduced by the recipient's (all family) income on a dollar-for-dollar basis for the monthly pension. If the family income exceeds the specified limit, the pension may be totally offset. There may be some offset in the other two plans also. "Countable income" for VA pension purposes does not include Supplemental Security Income payments or welfare benefits.

There are several basic eligibility criteria for a pension. The veteran must be discharged under conditions other than dishonorable; have wartime service of 90 days; have disabilities that are permanent (i.e., impairment is reasonably certain to continue throughout the life of the disabled person) and total (i.e., 100% under the Schedule for Rating Disabilities) (total disability may be assigned with a less-than-total schedular rating under certain defined conditions); have limited countable income and net worth that does not provide adequate maintenance; and the disability must not be due to the willful misconduct of the veteran.

There may be an Increased or Special Monthly Pension for persons with special needs.

Detailed information on what is required to meet the VA eligibility criteria is available from the local VA office.[27]

Role of Physicians in Litigation

The role of the physician in regard to litigation under the VA programs is as stated in the FEC, LSA, and BL programs (see previous). Physicians need to provide clear, thorough, and detailed reports. See (VA) Medical Reports and Rules and Chapter 12. The VA relies heavily on the documentation submitted in the cases. A good medical report will do much to move a case forward without involving the physician in protracted litigation or hassles.

Administrating Agency

The Department of Veterans Affairs (DVA) administers the VA benefit program through regional offices located throughout the United States. The DVA Web page is available at http://www.va.gov/. Clicking on "Health Benefits & Services" and/or "Compensation & Pension Benefits" will lead to up-to-date information on VA benefits.

RAILROAD WORKERS AND SEAMEN

Neither railroad workers nor seamen have had the protection of the type of coverage for work injuries afforded by state and federal workers' compensation laws. They have, however, been provided coverage under the Federal Employers' Liability Act, 45 US Code Annotated §§51–60, which extended and enhanced their common-law rights to proceed in court against (sue) their employer to obtain damages for job injuries.

Present-day Protection for Railroad Workers (FELA)

The FELA provides the basis for work injury damages, payable to injured railroad workers and their families, and is enforceable in court. Although there is no workers' compensation law covering these workers, there is a program providing a form of income maintenance during periods of short-term sickness and unemployment, whether job related or not. This program, funded by railroad employers, is administered by the Railroad Retirement Board (RRB), an independent agency of the federal government (Web page: http://www.rrb.gov).

A railroad employee injured in railroad employment and disabled for work can claim and receive the sickness and unemployment benefits to which the employee may be entitled while pursuing an action for damages under the FELA. However, a railroad employee may be entitled to reimbursement, from any monies received under FELA, for some or all benefits paid by the RRB. Long-term disability is covered under the railroad workers' disability retirement program, also administered by the RRB.

Present-day Protection for Seamen (Jones Act)

Although seamen (crew members) have no protection under a workers' compensation law as such, an injured seaman has three potential causes of action (enforceable in court) against an employer: the right to recover maintenance and cure to which he is entitled irrespective of negligence or fault, unless the injury was brought about by his own willful misbehavior; the right, under general maritime law, to recover indemnity for injury caused by the unseaworthiness of the vessel; and the right, under the Jones Act (46 USCS @ 688), to recover indemnity for a personal injury suffered in the course of his employment and due to the negligence of the shipowner.[28]

References

1. Title 20, Code of Federal Regulations 10.422, 1999.
2. 20 CFR, Part 10, contains the regulations concerning the administration of the FECA.
3. For a valuable guide to the FECA see Graham H: Federal Employees' Compensation Act: Practice Guide. New York, WEST Group.
4. 20 CFR, Section 10.422.
5. 20 CFR, Section 10.5, for definitions.
6. 20 CFR, 10.333.
7. 20 CFR, 10.205–10.224, for COP.
8. 20 CFR, 10.400–10.541, for compensation generally.
9. 20 CFR, 10.404, for schedule awards.
10. 20 CFR, Part 10, generally.
11. 20 CFR, Section 702.401–702.441.
12. A worker with an injury-caused permanent impairment of the back may be entitled to compensation for permanent partial disability and loss of earning capacity even if he or she returns to work with no actual loss of earnings. See Travelers v McLellan, 288 F.2d 250 (1961).
13. See the LS Regulations in general, 20 CFR, Part 702.
14. For a good short practical guide to the Longshore Act and its application, see Sevel BJ: Introduction to the Longshore and Harbor Workers' Compensation Act. In: Maryland Workers' Compensation Manual. Baltimore, MICPEL, 2001.
15. Federal Coal Mine Health & Safety Act of 1969, Subchapter IV, as amended. This subchapter may be cited as the "Black Lung Benefits Act." 30 U.S.C., §§901–945; Regulations: 20 CFR, §§718–727.
16. For more on the background and history, see Larson A, Larson LK: Larson's Workmens' Compensation Law Treatise. New York, Matthew Bender, §§41.90–41.98 (the 11-volume version).
17. 20 CFR, §718.1.
18. See 20 CFR, §725.202, for more detailed information.
19. 20 CFR, §718.204. Total disability.
20. 20 CFR, §718.201.
21. 20 CFR, Part 718 contains the standards for determining coal miners' total disability or death due to pneumoconiosis.
22. Title 5 U.S. Code, Part 8100.
23. Department of Veterans Affairs, DVA (VA) Benefits. The basic law, Title 38 U.S. Code, §1–End. The regulations, 38 CFR, §0–End. An excellent reference is the Veterans Benefits Manual (VBM), Stichman, Abrams and Addlestone, and the National Veterans Legal Services Program (NVLSP) (LEXIS Law). The VBM, written in nonlegal style, has proved very helpful in dealing with this complex subject.
24. Refer to the Veterans Benefit Manual (VBM) (see reference 23), especially Chapter 3.
25. VBM (see reference 23), Part I.
26. 38 CFR, Part 4.1
27. VBM (see reference 29), Chapter 5, generally.
28. Norris, The Law of Seamen, 3rd ed, @ 557, as quoted in 43 L. Ed. 2d 912.

CHAPTER

5

State Workers' Compensation Programs

THOMAS W. BEVAN, ESQ

Workers' compensation rests on the principle that employers that enjoy the economic benefits of business should ultimately bear the costs of injuries and death that are incident to the manufacture, preparation, and distribution of goods and services. The cost of compensating employees for injuries is treated as a cost of doing business without consideration of whether the injury was someone's fault or from an unavoidable circumstance. In theory, the employer initially absorbs the cost of work injuries, and ultimately passes it down the stream of commerce through the prices of its products or services until it is spread among the consuming public.

Workers' compensation attempts to accommodate the rights and duties of employers and employees. Each party relinquishes certain common-law rights and duties in exchange for new statutory rights and duties.

Before Workers' Compensation

Prior to the enactment of workers' compensation laws, workers relied on common law—based recovery for work-related injuries. The common law—based recovery, however, required a finding of fault or negligence on the part of the employer. The injured worker had to hire a lawyer and had the burden of proving a work-related injury and that the employer's negligence was the cause of the injury. The employer, in turn, had much greater resources to hire lawyers and defend injured workers' lawsuits.

Furthermore, common law allowed employers to assert three very strong common-law defenses: doctrine of contributory negligence, fellow-servant rule, and assumption of the risk.

Common law recovery for injured workers was particularly problematic in the 19th and early 20th centuries, when access to attorneys and the civil justice system was more difficult than it is today (see also Chapter 2).

Modern Workers' Compensation Law

Workers' compensation differs from the conventional common-law liability in two important respects: fault on the part of either employers or employees is made irrelevant and compensation is made payable according to a prescribed and limited scheme. All modern workers' compensation statutes accept these two foundational premises no matter how markedly they may differ in other particulars.

Workers' compensation represents a compromise in which both employers and employees surrender certain advantages in order to gain others deemed to be more important. Employers give up the immunity that would otherwise apply in cases where they were not at fault, and employees surrender their formal right to full damages in the few incidents where they could recover under common law and accept a more modest assured benefits for all injuries, diseases, and deaths. The importance of the compromise cannot be overemphasized, and various workers' compensation statutes vary greatly with reference to the proper point of balance. For the employer, the cost of industrial injuries and deaths must be predictable and fixable in an amount that would not disrupt the production and sale of goods and services. Thus, reasonable predictability and moderate costs are necessary from the employer's economic viewpoint. On the other hand, compensation levels must be high enough to provide adequate income to replace lost earnings of injured workers and to create an incentive for employers to adopt injury prevention measures. Otherwise, employers would be tempted to take the risk of paying workers' compensation claims rather than making more costs and expenditures to avoid injuries.

The administration of workers' compensation systems varies greatly from state to state. In most jurisdictions, administration responsibility and authority are vested in a special state agency. A few states, however, still rely on substantial court involvement in the administration of workers' compensation laws.

Court administration of workers' compensation is generally considered inferior to agency administration. Courts are not equipped to handle all aspects of worker's compensation administration effectively. For example, the court system is usually too slow and expensive to meet the primary goals of a worker's compensation program: to provide an injured worker with his or her benefits in a timely and cost-effective manner.

In contested claims, states that utilize an administrative agency to adjudicate disputed worker's compensation claims generally employ informal and expeditious procedures that avoid the sometimes technical and cumbersome procedures that govern civil litigation. These agencies commonly employ referees or hearing officers who are highly skilled in workers' compensation law and medicine to adjudicate claims. The obvious purpose is to facilitate prompt, inexpensive, and fair resolution to claims.

Occupational Injuries

What constitutes a work-related injury is frequently disputed in workers' compensation claims. Work-related injuries are often defined as injuries sustained "in the course of" and "arising out of" the worker's employment. These common tests are used to insure that a worker's injuries are properly charged to the employment.

The "in the course of" test involves when and where the injury occurred. What was the employee doing at the time of the injury? Did the employer have control over the employee at the time of injury? Did the employment subject the worker to some special hazard?

Injuries that occur at a fixed work site during a worker's normal scheduled working hours are always "in the course of" employment. Generally, injuries incurred while traveling to or from a fixed work site are not compensable. Furthermore, injuries incurred when a worker leaves a fixed work site for a lunch break are not compensable. Injuries incurred in an employer-owned or controlled parking lot of a fixed work site are generally compensable.

A fixed work site that creates a "special hazard" may be the basis for finding that an injury was sustained "in the course of" employment. The special hazard rule has been extended to apply in cases where the off-premises site of the injury is on the only route that employees can traverse to reach the employer's premises. The Ohio Supreme Court awarded compensation to an employee who sustained fatal injuries while crossing railroad tracks adjacent to the plant's only entrance.

Non-fixed or semi-fixed work sites create much greater controversy. Such employment may include outside salespeople, truck drivers, lawyers traveling from an office to court, or physicians traveling from one hospital to another. Generally, injuries that occur while employees are actively performing assigned work when and where they are supposed to do it are always "in the course of" employment. Disputes often arise when social relations and work get mixed. The question whether social activities are part of the job often arises in sales work and compensation is frequently awarded.

After entering into the course of employment, an employee can deviate from the employment by undertaking a personal activity. Such deviations from the course of employment may remove the employee from the course of employment. For example, the lawyer who leaves court and, prior to returning to the office, makes a personal trip home, has removed him- or herself from the course of employment. Voluntary intoxication that renders an employee incapable of performing the work constitutes a departure from the course of employment.

Once the "in the course of" test is satisfied, the "arising out of" test is often undisputed. A broken leg injury sustained by a worker who falls 15 feet off a ladder while working clearly arises out of employment. By contrast, some injuries are plainly not the responsibility of the employer; for example, an injury caused by a genetic deficiency. As always, however, there is a wide gray area of dispute.

The worker who suffers an epileptic seizure and fractures his or her jaw when he or she lands on the floor probably has not sustained an injury arising out of employment. If, however, the worker suffered the seizure while on an elevated scaffold and the fall causes him or her to fracture his or her leg, he or she has most likely sustained an injury arising out of employment.

The natural deterioration of a body part often is not considered arising out employment. Preexisting conditions that are aggravated or accelerated by a work-related injury, however, are often compensable.

Occupational Diseases

All states afford workers compensation coverage for occupational diseases. Some do it by separate statutes. Some incorporate occupational disease provisions into their workers' compensation law by expanding the definition of injury.

In earlier years, some of the laws restricted occupational disease compensation to a specified list or schedule of diseases named in the statute. These diseases included those most commonly associated with the industry in which the worker suffered the exposure. An example of a list of such diseases includes anthrax, lead poisoning, tenosynovities, silicosis, and coal miner's pneumoconiosis (Ohio Revised Code Section 4123.68). Over time, many states retained a schedule of diseases but added a general clause affording coverage for any occupational disease.

There is a belief that occupational diseases pose special challenges for the workers' compensation system. The number of potential occupational disease claims is large. The 1972 President's Report on Occupational Safety and Health, a controversial but frequently cited report, estimates that 100,000 workers die each year from occupational diseases and an additional 390,000 workers contract some form of work-related illness. In another article reviewing occupational disease studies, it was estimated that 817,000 to 907,400 new cases of occupational illness occurred and 46,900 to 73,700 deaths resulted from occupational diseases in the United States in 1992.[1] The workplace is thought to be responsible for 6% to 10% of cancer cases, 5% to 10% of coronary heart disease cases, 5% to 10% of cerebrovascular disease cases and 10% of chronic obstructive pulmonary disease cases in the United States.[2]

Many workers' compensation statutes define occupational disease to exclude ordinary diseases of life. Others include only those diseases caused by conditions "characteristic of and peculiar to" employment. The courts will often compare the level of risk created by the work environment with that existing outside the job. If a worker contracts a cold from a fellow worker, he or she is not entitled to compensation because all employment creates a like risk. The worker who contracts lung cancer owing to asbestos exposure, however, is entitled to compensation because not all employment creates such a risk.

Benefits

The first form of benefits common to all workers' compensation systems is medical. Theoretically, a claimant may seek treatment consistent with his or her allowed condition for the life of the claim. Practically speaking, there are many administrative hurdles that must be negotiated before the requested treatment will be authorized and paid for.

Many state-run programs have recently begun using managed care organizations to oversee claims. In this type of system, all requests for treatment are routed to the managed care organization, where they are analyzed, and a recommendation is then made to the state agency as to whether the request of the claimant should be granted. In these systems any decision can be appealed, and the issue will then pass to a hearing officer or referee for review.

Great care should be taken by the worker to become familiar with the rules and regulations in a managed care system. Many of these systems contain provisions that require a claimant who disagrees with a decision to first file an objection to the decision of the managed care organization directly with the organization. Only after all alternative dispute resolution measures have been exhausted will the claim be referred back to the state administrative agency for adjudication. The number one fault of these systems is the imposition of delay in the claimant gaining necessary and often time-sensitive treatment.

The second category of benefits are disability benefits. These benefits are often referred to as income, disability, indemnity, or wage loss benefits. These benefits are most commonly calculated as a percentage of the worker's average weekly wage, often subject to a specified dollar limit. In Ohio, for example, temporary total disability is compensated at the rate of 72% of the worker's full or average weekly wage, but no more than $541 for a 1998 injury (Ohio Revised Code Section 4123.56). The maximum weekly benefit differs widely among the states. For example, in 1998, a totally disabled worker in Alaska could receive as much as $700 per week (Alaska stat. Sec. 23.30.175), whereas in Georgia the maximum was $325 (Ga. Code ANN. Sec. 34–9–261). The most common categories of disability benefits are temporary total disability, permanent total disability, and permanent partial disability.

The vast majority of claims for work injuries involve a temporary total disability rendering the injured employee unable to work for a limited period of time. Temporary total disability benefits are normally payable until the worker is capable of returning to his or her former position of employment or until the worker's disability has become permanent. Permanency is sometimes also referred to as "maximum medical improvement." Maximum medical improvement or permanency denotes a condition that will, with reasonable probability, continue for an indefinite period of time without any indication of recovery therefrom. Despite accounting for the greatest number of claims, only 18% to 19% of the total cost of disability payments is for temporary total disability.[2]

Permanently and totally disabled employees are unable to undertake any substantial work and are not expected ever to do so. Some states limit permanent total benefits by amount or duration. Many states, however, pay permanent and total disability benefits for the duration of the disability or life. Claims of permanent total disability are fewer in number, but greater in average costs. Although only two or three of 1000 worker's compensation claims involve permanent total disability, these claims account for 9% of all disability benefits paid under the various worker's compensation systems.[3]

The most common category of disability benefits is permanent partial disability. More dollars are paid out for permanent partial disability than for any other category of disability. In fact, 65% of all disability benefits paid to injured workers are for permanent partial disabilities.[2,3] This class of cases involves employees who are permanently impaired in some manner but are able to perform some other fairly substantial type of work.

Permanent partial disability benefits are often broken down into two categories: scheduled and nonscheduled loss. Scheduled losses provide for specific amounts of benefits paid for particular injuries such as loss of an eye, loss of hearing, loss of an arm, or loss of a leg. The amount of benefits payable for loss of a specific body part may vary greatly from state to state.

Nonscheduled permanent partial disability compensation is usually measured in terms of impaired earning capacity, simple physical impairment, or a combination of the two. Under the impaired earning approach, the injured worker must prove a physical impairment and that such impairment has caused an actual wage loss or a loss of earning potential. As stated by the Michigan Supreme Court, the impaired earning approach adapts readily to the widely varied circumstances of given cases. The lawyer who lost a little finger will receive little or nothing; the concert pianist with the same injury will be entitled to benefits until reasonable alternative employment is made available (Sobotka v Chrysler Corporation, 447 Mich. 1, 523 N.W.2d 454, 459 [Mich. 1994]).

Most states have recognized the American Medical Association's Guidelines to the Evaluation of Permanent Impairment as authoritative in the calculation of actual physical impairment for purposes.[4] In 1972, The Report of a National Commission of State Workman Compensation Laws recommended that states use the AMA Guides as a source of standardized and medically justified criteria for measuring physical impairment. The actual amount of compensation paid for permanent partial disability varies greatly from state to state (see Tables 5–1 through 5–5). These guidelines contain recommended examination techniques and tables for interpreting the results. The guidelines are currently in their fifth revision.

Whereas workers' compensation represents a substitute for tort remedies, it must also provide benefits to the surviving spouse and dependents of a worker who dies as a result of a work-related accident. These benefits are paid subject to the rules governing disability benefits. Payments to a dependent child, until the child reaches the age of majority, are provided in most states and often can be extended to age 25 if the child is a full-time student. Payments to the surviving spouse are usually made for the lifetime of the spouse if he or she does not remarry. Most statutes terminate a surviving spouse's death benefits in the event of remarriage. Frequently, however, a lump sum payment of a prescribed period of benefits is paid upon remarriage.

Rehabilitation benefits are somewhat new. These benefits have grown out of the desire to get an injured worker back to work as soon as possible. Although each

TABLE 5–1

Scheduled Loss of Member

State	Arm at Shoulder	Hand	Leg at Hip	Foot	Eye
Alabama	48,840	37,400	44,000	30,580	27,280
Alaska					
Arizona	84,006	70,113	70,113	55,896	42,003
Arkansas	59,010	44,398	51,704	36,811	29,505
California					
Colorado	59,379	29,689	59,379	29,689	39,681
Connecticut	195,936	158,256	149,464	118,064	147,580
Delaware	102,777	90,444	102,777	65,777	82,222
District of Columbia	260,463	203,696	240,428	171,138	133,571
Florida					
Georgia	73,125	52,000	73,125	43,875	48,750
Hawaii	161,928	126,636	149,472	106,395	83,040
Idaho	75,240	67,716	50,160	35,112	43,890
Illinois	258,840	163,932	237,270	133,734	138,048
Indiana	53,500	39,500	46,500	32,500	32,500
Iowa	218,000	165,680	191,840	130,800	122,080
Kansas	82,350	54,900	73,200	45,750	43,920
Kentucky					
Louisiana	73,400	55,050	64,225	45,875	36,700
Maine	118,629	94,815	94,815	72,442	71,442
Maryland	180,800	150,516	180,800	150,516	150,516
Massachusetts	30,096	23,797	27,296	20,297	27,296
Michigan	156,020	124,700	124,700	93,960	93,960
Minnesota					
Mississippi	58,572	43,929	51,251	36,608	29,286
Missouri	68,377	51,578	61,009	44,210	44,262
Montana					
Nebraska	105,300	81,900	100,620	70,200	58,500
Nevada					
New Hampshire	176,400	158,760	117,600	82,320	70,560
New Jersey	130,680	79,380	124,740	66,240	50,400
New Mexico	78,410	49,006	78,410	45,086	50,967
New York	124,800	97,600	115,200	82,000	64,000
North Carolina	134,400	112,000	112,000	80,640	67,200
North Dakota	104,250	83,400	97,578	62,550	62,550
Ohio	127,575	99,225	113,400	85,050	70,875
Oklahoma	53,250	42,600	53,250	42,600	42,600
Oregon	87,168	68,100	68,100	61,290	45,400
Pennsylvania	241,080	208,740	241,080	147,000	161,700
Rhode Island	28,080	21,960	28,080	18,450	14,400
South Carolina	106,363	89,442	94,277	67,686	67,686
South Dakota	84,600	61,200	65,280	51,000	61,200
Tennessee	103,000	77,250	103,000	64,375	51,500
Texas	73,200	54,900	73,200	45,750	36,600
Utah	60,775	54,600	40,625	28,600	39,000
Vermont	156,305	127,225	156,305	127,225	90,875
Virginia	106,800	80,100	93,450	66,750	53,400
Washington					
West Virginia					
Wisconsin	92,000	73,600	92,000	46,000	50,600
Wyoming	46,500	37,820	41,850	31,000	29,140

Values are in dollars.

TABLE 5–2

Permanent Total Disability

State	Percentage of Worker's Wage	Maximum Weekly Rate, $	Maximum Period
Alabama	66 2/3	493.00	Duration of disability
Alaska	80% of worker's spendable earnings	700.00	Duration of disability
Arizona	66 2/3	323.10	Life or duration of disability
Arkansas	66 2/3	375.00	Duration of disability
California	66 2/3	490.00	Life
Colorado	66 2/3	519.61	Life
Connecticut	75% of worker's spendable earnings	764.00	Duration of disability
Delaware	66 2/3	411.11	Duration of disability
District of Columbia	66 2/3 or 80% of spendable earnings	834.82	Duration of disability
Florida	66 2/3	522.00	Duration of disability
Georgia	66 2/3	325.00	Duration of disability
Hawaii	66 2/3	519.00	Duration of disability
Idaho	67	410.40 for first 52 weeks; thereafter 273.60	52 weeks, thereafter 60% of SAWW for duration of disability
Illinois	66 2/3	468.00	Life
Indiana	66 2/3	468.00	500 weeks
Iowa	80% of worker's spendable earnings	947.00	Duration of disability
Kansas	66 2/3	366.00	Duration of disability
Kentucky	66 2/3	487.20	Duration of disability
Louisiana	66 2/3	367.00	Duration of disability
Maine	80% of worker's spendable earnings	441.00	Duration of disability
Maryland	66 2/3	602.00	Duration of disability
Massachusetts	66 2/3	699.91	Duration of disability
Michigan	80% of worker's spendable earnings	580.00	Duration of disability
Minnesota	66 2/3	615.00	Until age 67
Mississippi	66 2/3	292.86	450 weeks
Missouri	66 2/3	562.67	Duration of disability
Montana	66 2/3	411.00	Duration of disability
Nebraska	66 2/3	468.00	Duration of disability
Nevada	66 2/3	532.63	Life
New Hampshire	60	840	Duration of disability
New Jersey	70	539	450 weeks; in some cases benefits are payable for life
New Mexico	66 2/3	392.05	Lifetime
New York	66 2/3	400	Duration of disability
North Carolina	66 2/3	560	Duration of disability
North Dakota	66 2/3	417	Duration of disability
Ohio	66 2/3	567	Life
Oklahoma	70	426	Duration of disability
Oregon	66 2/3	576.64	Duration of disability
Pennsylvania	66 2/3	588	Duration of disability
Rhode Island	75% of worker's spendable earnings	65.00	Duration of disability
South Carolina	66 2/3	483.47	500 weeks
South Dakota	66 2/3	408	Duration of disability
Tennessee	66 2/3	515	400 weeks
Texas	75	523	Life for injuries listed in statute as consituting PTD; otherwise 401 weeks
Utah	66 2/3	414	312 weeks or life if claimant cannot be rehabilitated
Vermont	66 2/3	727	Duration of disability with a minimum of 330 weeks
Virginia	66 2/3	534	Duration of disability
Washington	60–75	692.70	Life
West Virginia	66 2/3	466.11	Life
Wisconsin	66 2/3	538	Life
Wyoming		310	344 weeks; benefits may be extended by the district court

SAWW, statewide average weekly wage

TABLE 5–3

Workers' Compensation Insurance

State	State Fund Insurance	Private Insurance	Employer Self Insurance	Group Employer Self Insurance
Alabama	No	Yes	Yes	Yes
Alaska	No	Yes	Yes	No
Arizona	Optional	Yes	Yes	Yes
Arkansas	No	Yes	Yes	Yes
California	Optional	Yes	Yes	No
Colorado	Optional	Yes	Yes	Yes
Connecticut	No	Yes	Yes	Yes
Delaware	No	Yes	Yes	No
District of Columbia	No	Yes	Yes	No
Florida	No	Yes	Yes	Yes
Georgia	No	Yes	Yes	Yes
Hawaii	Optional	Yes	Yes	Yes
Idaho	Optional	Yes	Yes	No
Illinois	No	Yes	Yes	Yes
Indiana	No	Yes	Yes	No
Iowa	No	Yes	Yes	Yes
Kansas	No	Yes	Yes	Yes
Kentucky	Optional	Yes	Yes	Yes
Louisiana	Optional	Yes	Yes	Yes
Maine	Optional	Yes	Yes	Yes
Maryland	Optional	Yes	Yes	Yes
Massachusetts	No	Yes	Yes	Yes
Michigan	Optional	Yes	Yes	Yes
Minnesota	Optional	Yes	Yes	Yes
Mississippi	No	Yes	Yes	Yes
Missouri	Optional	Yes	Yes	Yes
Montana	Optional	Yes	Yes	Yes
Nebraska	No	Yes	Yes	No
Nevada	Exclusive	No	Yes	No
New Hampshire	No	Yes	Yes	Yes
New Jersey	No	Yes	Yes	No
New Mexico	Optional	Yes	Yes	Yes
New York	Optional	Yes	Yes	Yes
North Carolina	No	Yes	Yes	Yes
North Dakota	Exclusive	No	No	No
Ohio	Exclusive	No	Yes	No
Oklahoma	Optional	Yes	Yes	Yes
Oregon	Optional	Yes	Yes	Yes
Pennsylvania	Optional	Yes	Yes	Yes
Rhode Island	Optional	Yes	Yes	Yes
South Carolina	No	Yes	Yes	Yes
South Dakota	No	Yes	Yes	Yes
Tennessee	No	Yes	Yes	Yes
Texas	Optional	Yes	Yes	No
Utah	Optional	Yes	Yes	No
Vermont	No	Yes	Yes	No
Virginia	No	Yes	Yes	Yes
Washington	Exclusive	No	Yes	Yes
West Virginia	Exclusive	No	Yes	No
Wisconsin	No	Yes	Yes	No
Wyoming	Exclusive	No	No	No

Most states mandate that all employers have workers' compensation insurance. There is great variability, however, in the manner in which an employer may obtain workers' compensation insurance. Most states allow large employers to be self-insured for workers' compensation. In such instances, the employer will set up a workers' compensation department and act as an insurance company. Some states allow for smaller employers to form a self-insured group. These groups will have an administrating company that processes the claims and pays the benefits. Most states also allow for private insurance carriers to provide workers' compensation insurance. Some states have created a state workers' compensation insurance fund that acts in the same manner as a private insurance company. In some instances, these state insurance funds are exclusive and in other instances the state funds compete with private insurance companies.

state's benefits vary, they most commonly include vocational rehabilitation, retraining, and counseling. Often, these programs are offered though other state agencies and, as such, an agreement must be entered into among the claimant, rehabilitation agency, and workers' compensation agency to insure that the costs associated with the plan will be absorbed by the employee's claim. Many states also impose an obligation upon the injured worker to accept certain rehabilitation services as a condition on the continued receipt of full compensation benefits.

Settlements and compromises make up the smallest portion of benefits available to claimants. Many states allow for the final settlement of a claim. Of these states, most require that the amount of the settlement be agreed on and authorized by the state agency. Lump sum settlements are not very popular because they are thought to conflict with the benevolent purposes of workers' compensation.

TABLE 5-4

Temporary Total Disability

State	Percentage of Worker's Wage	Maximum Weekly Rate, $	Maximum Period
Alabama	66 2/3	493.00	Duration of disability
Alaska	80% of worker's spendable earnings	700.00	Duration of disability until date of medical stability
Arizona	66 2/3	323.10	Duration of disability
Arkansas	66 2/3	375.00	450 weeks
California	66 2/3	490.00	Duration of disability
Colorado	66 2/3	519.61	Duration of disability
Connecticut	75% of worker's spendable earnings	764.00	Duration of disability
Delaware	66 2/3	411.11	Duration of disability
District of Columbia	66 2/3 or 80% of spendable earnings	834.82	Duration of disability
Florida	66 2/3	522.00	104 weeks
Georgia	66 2/3	325.00	400 weeks
Hawaii	66 2/3	519.00	Duration of disability
Idaho	67	410.40 for first 52 weeks; thereafter 273.60	52 weeks, thereafter 60% of statewide average weekly wage for duration of disability
Illinois	66 2/3	862.80	Duration of disability
Indiana	66 2/3	468.00	500 weeks
Iowa	80% of worker's spendable earnings	947.00	Duration of disability
Kansas	66 2/3	366.00	Duration of disability
Kentucky	66 2/3	487.20	Duration of disability
Louisiana	66 2/3	367.00	Duration of disability
Maine	80% of worker's after-tax earnings	441.00	Duration of disability
Maryland	66 2/3	602.00	Duration of disability
Massachusetts	60	699.91	156 weeks
Michigan	80% of worker's spendable earnings	580.00	Duration of disability
Minnesota	66 2/3	615.00	104 weeks or 90 days after maximum medical improvement
Mississippi	66 2/3	292.86	450 weeks
Missouri	66 2/3	562.67	400 weeks
Montana	66 2/3	411.00	Duration of disability or until worker is released to preinjury job or similar employment
Nebraska	66 2/3	468.00	Duration of disability
Nevada	66 2/3	532.63	Duration of disability
New Hampshire	60	840	Duration of disability
New Jersey	70	539	400 weeks
New Mexico	66 2/3	392.05	Lifetime
New York	66 2/3	400	Duration of disability
North Carolina	66 2/3	560	Duration of disability
North Dakota	66 2/3	417	Duration of disability or until claimant is age 65 and eligible for Social Security retirement benefits
Ohio	66 2/3	567	Duration of disability or until claimant reaches maximum medical improvement
Oklahoma	70	426	156 weeks
Oregon	66 2/3	576.64	Duration of disability
Pennsylvania	66 2/3	588	90 days
Rhode Island	75% of worker's spendable earnings	544	Duration of disability
South Carolina	66 2/3	483.47	500 weeks
South Dakota	66 2/3	408	Duration of disability
Tennessee	66 2/3	515	400 weeks
Texas	70% of worker's spendable earnings	523	104 weeks or upon reaching maximum medical improvement
Utah	66 2/3	487	312 weeks
Vermont	66 2/3	727	Duration of disability
Virginia	66 2/3	534	500 weeks
Washington	60–75	692.70	Duration of disability
West Virginia	70	466.11	208 weeks
Wisconsin	66 2/3	538	Duration of disability
Wyoming	66 2/3	465	Duration of disability

TABLE 5-5

Methods of Physician Selection Provided by Workers' Compensation Statutes

Employee Free Choice	Selection From List Prepared by State Agency	Selection From List Maintained by Employer	Employer Selects Physician	Employer Selects/ May be Changed by State Agency	Employer Selects/ Employee has Free Choice After Specified Period of Time
Alaska	District of Columbia	Georgia	Alabama	Arkansas	California
Arizona	New York	Tennessee	Florida	Colorado	Maine
Connecticut		Virginia	Idaho		Michigan
Delaware			Indiana		New Mexico
Hawaii			Iowa		Pennsylvania
Illinois			Kansas		
Kentucky			Missouri		
Louisiana			New Jersey		
Maryland			North Carolina		
Massachusetts			South Carolina		
Minnesota			Utah		
Mississippi			Vermont		
Montana					
Nebraska					
Nevada					
New Hampshire					
North Dakota					
Ohio					
Oklahoma					
Oregon					
Rhode Island					
South Dakota					
Texas					
Washington					
West Virginia					
Wisconsin					
Wyoming					

References

1. Paul J, et al: Occupational injury and illness in the United States. Arch Intern Med 267: 1157–1562, 1997.
2. Worral, Appel: Some benefit issues in workers' compensation. In: Worral, Appel (eds): Workers' Compensation Benefits 4. 1985.
3. Worral, Appel: Some benefit issues in worker's compensation. In: Worral, Appel (eds): Workers' Compensation Benefits 5. 1985.
4. Cocchiarella L, Andersson GBJ (eds): Guides to the Evaluation of Permanent Impairment, 5th ed. Chicago, American Medical Association, 2001.

CHAPTER

6

Social Security Disability Programs

KENNETH D. NIBALI, JD

Medical professionals play a variety of roles in the Social Security Administration (SSA)'s disability programs. Each year, the SSA processes over 2 million new disability applications as well as hundreds of thousands of appeals and reviews of the continuing entitlement of its beneficiaries (Table 6–1). Program physicians, psychologists, and certain other medical professionals, called medical consultants and psychological consultants, are involved in most of these determinations. Instead of examining claimants and beneficiaries, however, they must rely on reports and copies of records from treatment sources and other medical professionals, as well as other information from lay sources. For this reason, detailed, well-explained reports from physicians, psychologists, and other health care workers who have treated and examined claimants and beneficiaries are critical to SSA's ability to make timely, accurate, and fair decisions.

Physicians, psychologists, and other medical professionals play other roles as well. This chapter describes these roles and the importance of the medical professional throughout the benefit application process and provides an overview of the various kinds of disability benefits available from SSA and the process for applying for benefits. This information will help readers understand the enormously complex disability benefits programs and, in turn, be better able to help patients and clients who may be in need of the benefits SSA can provide. Box 6–1 shows some incorrect beliefs about SSA's disability programs.

SUMMARY OF THE PROGRAMS

The Social Security Act provides cash benefits to individuals with disabling physical and mental disorders under two major programs: Social Security Disability Insurance (SSDI) and Supplemental Security Income (SSI). Often, receipt of disability benefits also provides access to health care.

Claimants file with SSA at a field office in their community or by calling SSA's toll-free number. Once an application is taken, the case goes to a state agency, where medical and lay personnel review the available evidence and make the initial determination of disability for SSA. These state agencies, generically called Disability Determination Services (DDSs), are fully

TABLE 6–1

Social Security Disability Benefit Data—December 2001

Disabled SSDI beneficiaries	6 million
Total benefits paid	$52.3 billion
Average disabled worker benefit	$787
Disabled SSI beneficiaries	5.2 million, including about 880,000 children
Total benefits paid	$24.2 billion (federal SSI payments)
Average benefit	$411 (adults), $464 (children)

SSDI, Social Security Disability Insurance; SSI, Supplemental Security Income funded by SSA. They make their determinations using SSA regulations and instructions.

If claimants disagree with their initial disability determination, they can appeal their cases—first, to a DDS reconsideration, then to an SSA administrative law judge. If they are still dissatisfied, they have the right to further appeal to the SSA Appeals Council and eventually to the federal courts.

There are several kinds of disability benefits:

1. SSDI comprises a number of disability benefits for workers and their dependents. Entitlement is based on contributions to the Social Security trust funds through Federal Insurance Contribution Act (FICA) taxes.[1] Individuals who qualify for SSDI benefits are entitled to receive medical benefits from the federal Medicare program after they have been entitled to benefits for 24 months. SSDI benefits include the following:
   a. Disability insurance benefits.[2] These are cash benefits paid to workers who have not reached retirement age,[3] who are disabled as defined in the Act, and who meet other requirements for entitlement described later in this chapter.
   b. Widow's and widower's insurance benefits based on disability. Disabled widows or widowers of workers may receive benefits if they are at least 50 years old.[4] In general, the disability must have started before the worker died or within 7 years after the worker's death. However, disability may begin later for widows and widowers who received certain types of Social Security benefits in the past. Surviving divorced spouses with disabilities may also qualify for this disability benefit.
   c. Child's insurance benefits based on disability. An unmarried, disabled child of a worker who has died, retired, or is receiving disability insurance benefits may receive this benefit. In general, the individual must be unmarried and 18 years old or older to qualify. The individual must have been continuously disabled since before age 22.

   There are also benefits for nondisabled spouses and children of SSDI recipients. To receive a benefit, the spouse must be age 62 or or older, or

BOX 6–1 Incorrect Beliefs About SSA's Disability Programs

Myth #1:	People who have never worked and who have not paid Social Security taxes cannot get disability benefits.
Fact:	There are disability benefits for disabled widows or widowers and disabled children of workers who were covered by Social Security. SSA also provides a benefit called Supplemental Security Income (SSI) to adults and children with disabling physical and mental disorders. SSI is not based on Social Security taxes but eligible individuals must have limited income and resources.
Myth #2:	It is important that I provide a certification to SSA that my patient or client is disabled.
Fact:	SSA must make the decision whether your patient or client is disabled. Medical information and certain opinions you provide may be the crucial evidence in SSA's decision, but you do not make the decision. Therefore, although SSA will consider your opinion that your patient is "disabled" or "unable to work," it is more helpful if you provide medical records and your opinions about your patient's symptoms and ability to function.
Myth #3:	Once I have given information about my patient or client to SSA, I will not hear from them again.
Fact:	SSA often has to recontact treatment sources for clarification of their reports or additional information. SSA realizes that this is an imposition on your time—it also slows the processing of the case. Sometimes it is necessary, however. To minimize recontacts, provide the most thorough information you can, including an explanation of any opinions you have offered.
Myth #4:	People qualify for SSA disability benefits if they can no longer do their last job.
Fact:	The definition of disability in the Social Security law is very strict. A person must not only be unable to do past work but also any other kind of work that exists in the national economy considering the medical condition and the patient's age, education, and work experience.
Myth #5:	Claimants who do not have impairments that meet or equal listings are generally denied.
Fact:	About 40% of individuals who qualify do so at Step 5 of sequential evaluation.
Myth #6:	Most people who get benefits from SSA were denied when they first applied and had to go through a long appeal.
Fact:	About two thirds of the people who get benefits from SSA were allowed at the first stage of the process. It is true, however, that most people who apply are denied: only 35% to 40% of people who apply are found disabled at the first stage of the process.

be caring for a child of the worker who is under age 16 or who is disabled and also receiving benefits. To receive child's benefits, a child of a disabled worker need only be under age 18, or be under age 19 and a full-time student.

2. SSI benefits are paid to aged (age 65 and older), blind, or disabled individuals who have limited means. Individuals under age 65, including children (individuals under age 18), must be blind or disabled to qualify for benefits.[5] SSI benefits are funded from general revenues, not the Social Security trust funds, and individuals may qualify regardless of whether they have worked. SSI is not an entitlement program like SSDI, but an eligibility program. Individuals who qualify for SSI may receive medical benefits from their state Medicaid programs.

In most states, SSI payments consist of a federal benefit and a supplementary benefit added by the state. The basic federal benefit rate for an individual in 2002 is $545 per month. State supplements vary from state to state and may also vary to reflect different living arrangements; for example, the state supplement may be higher if the person lives alone than it would be if the person lived with someone else. Also, as noted later in this chapter, benefits are often reduced to reflect other income.

People who have paid FICA taxes and who have limited means may qualify for SSDI and a partial SSI payment. Over a third of current SSI beneficiaries also qualify for SSDI benefits.

THE ROLE OF THE MEDICAL PROFESSIONAL

Medical professionals play three major roles in the SSA disability programs:

1. As sources of medical evidence and medical opinions, they provide the evidence that is the foundation of SSA's disability decisions. Most often, medical professionals provide SSA with copies of their treatment records or prepare reports based on their treatment. But in many cases, SSA will also purchase examinations from medical sources on a consultative basis in order to complete the evidence.
2. As medical and psychological consultants in the DDSs and other offices that make disability determinations for SSA, they are decision-makers and expert consultants to decision-makers.
3. As independent medical experts at the hearings and appeals levels of SSA's appeals process, they provide advice and assistance to SSA's federal administrative law judges and Appeals Council.

Providers of Medical Evidence

Each person who files a claim for disability benefits must submit medical and other evidence to support the claim. As explained later in this chapter, SSA will help the person get the evidence he or she needs, and will often make requests for this information on behalf of the person. The faster the information is provided, the faster a decision regarding benefits can be made.

The Act and SSA's regulations require that a person's disability must result from a medically determinable impairment that must be shown by medical evidence. Medical evidence means clinical signs, laboratory findings, and the individual's complaints of symptoms. To establish the existence of a medically determinable impairment, the medical evidence must come from a physician or a licensed psychologist, although there are exceptions for certain kinds of impairments specified in SSA's rules. Collectively, these sources are called "acceptable medical sources" in SSA's regulations.

Once the existence of a medically determinable impairment is established, evidence from other health care professionals, as well as lay sources, can provide crucial information about the severity of the individual's medical impairments. SSA may use this evidence to establish whether the medical impairment meets the standard of disability in the Act. For example, in SSI child cases, educational personnel and school records are two of the best sources of evidence about how a school-age child is functioning, and whether there have been changes in the child's functioning. In this example, SSA asks school professionals to provide information about academic performance, school psychologist evaluations, attendance, behavior, testing, therapeutic interventions, use of special services, individual educational programs, and other assessments that provide information about the child's ability to perform age-appropriate activities.

SSA's rules give preference to information from treating sources. SSA has a unique definition of this term. A treating source is not merely someone who has provided the claimant with treatment. Rather, under SSA's regulations, a treating source is a claimant's own physician, psychologist, or other person who is an acceptable medical source, who has provided the claimant with medical treatment or evaluation, and who has had an ongoing treatment relationship with the claimant. SSA recognizes that because of this relationship treating sources are usually the best sources of medical evidence about the nature and severity of their patients' impairments. SSA rules provide that treating sources are likely to be the medical professionals most able to provide a detailed, longitudinal picture of their patients' impairments. Based on their knowledge of their patients, they may also provide a perspective that cannot be obtained from objective medical findings alone or from reports of single examinations or brief hospitalizations.

SSA will also obtain reports and copies of existing medical evidence from medical sources that are not technically treating sources under SSA's rules. These sources include hospitals and other medical institutions and individual medical providers who may have examined the claimant on a consultative basis in the past.

Neither treating sources nor any other sources of information decide whether their patients are disabled for SSA. The determination of disability is legally SSA's responsibility. Therefore, although SSA will consider notes to the effect that "My patient is disabled" or "My patient is unable to work," this kind of opinion is insufficient for SSA purposes. However, it is impossible to overstate the importance to SSA of detailed medical evidence from treating sources. In most cases, treating source medical evidence is all that SSA needs to make its decision.

Consultative Examinations

If the evidence from a claimant's own medical sources is insufficient for a determination (for example, it does not provide information about one of the claimant's alleged impairments or information about the claimant's ability to do work-related activities), the DDS may purchase one or more independent medical examinations, which SSA calls consultative examinations. SSA regulations provide that treating sources are the preferred sources for such evaluations if they are willing and able to provide the examinations that SSA needs. In most cases, SSA obtains these examinations from independent specialists who have agreed to perform them for the DDSs following SSA rules and accepting fees set by each state. Consultative examinations are performed by physicians, psychologists, or, in certain circumstances, other health care professionals. All sources must be currently licensed, certified, or otherwise qualified in their states and have the training and experience to perform the types of examinations and tests SSA requests.

The states maintain lists of consultative examiners, but are always in need of additional sources. Throughout the year, professional relations officers who work for the states are available to provide information about how medical professionals can become consultants. More information about qualifying as a consultative examination provider is available from SSA's Web site (see the sources at the end of this chapter) and from the local DDS. SSA and the states often exhibit at professional conferences and meetings, where medical professionals can ask questions and obtain written information.

Medical Reports

SSA rules prescribe a list of basic elements of "complete" medical reports. Most of these elements are familiar to all health care professionals: medical history, the results of physical and mental status examinations, laboratory findings (including the results of psychological testing), diagnoses, treatment and response (including adverse effects), and prognosis. This information may be provided in formal reports written about patients for their SSA claims, on special forms provided by the DDSs or claimant representatives, in copies of documents from the patient's chart,[6] or in any combination of these (e.g., a formal report with photocopies of laboratory studies or hospital discharge summaries). To the extent possible, the medical documentation should paint a picture of the claimant's condition and functioning over time so that the DDS can determine the onset and duration of the impairment and make judgments about expected duration and severity.

Dysfunction is a crucial focus of SSA's disability evaluations, but medical records from treatment sources often deal largely with diagnosis and medical management and do not provide information about functional capabilities that are relevant to SSA's determination. Although physicians and other providers might make mental notes about such observations as gross muscle function, muscle strength, the ability to grasp, pinch, and manipulate, and the ability to follow instructions, tolerate work stresses, and work with other people, these kinds of observations are often not in copies from the individual's chart.

Therefore, SSA will also ask for what it calls a medical source statement. SSA uses this term to describe a medical source's opinion about what the claimant can do despite his or her physical or mental impairments. For adult claimants, this opinion will be in terms of work-related activities. In the physical realm, this would include activities such as sitting, standing, walking, lifting, carrying, manipulating, seeing, hearing, speaking, and traveling, and consideration of environmental factors, such as the ability to tolerate dust, extremes of temperature, or noise. In the mental realm, abilities such as understanding, carrying out, and remembering instructions and responding appropriately to supervision, coworkers, and work pressures are considered. For child claimants, the opinion is requested in terms of age-appropriate functioning, and may be expressed in formal terms, such as developmental quotients or years of development, or in more descriptive terms, such as descriptions of activities of daily living. Areas to consider include, but are not limited to, learning, motor functioning, self-care activities, communicating (including hearing, language, and speech), social functioning, and executive functioning. In all cases, medical sources are asked to make judgments about the individual's ability to perform the functions on a maximal or sustained basis. Also helpful are professional estimates of duration of any limitations or restrictions, such as whether they will be lifelong and progressive, of shorter duration, or episodic.

When the DDSs request information from medical sources, they always provide guidelines for report content. Many DDSs provide forms that medical sources may complete or follow as guides in writing their reports or to help determine whether the records they are submitting are sufficient for SSA purposes. The DDS will always ask for a medical source statement and provide guidance for its content. In some cases, the request will include a convenient form that guides the completion of the opinion; in others, there will be an explanation of the kind of medical source statement the DDS needs in the letter the DDS sends. In either case, an essential element is a brief narrative explanation of the reasons for any opinions provided.

Explanations are especially important when a claimant's limitations or abilities are not self-evident from the objective medical findings, as is often the case when claimants are limited primarily by their symptoms, such as pain, fatigue, or anxiety. SSA rules require that in such cases adjudicators must determine the credibility of a claimant's complaints and allegations regarding limitations in functioning. SSA will base this finding on all the evidence in the record, including the objective medical findings and more subjective information tending to support or refute a claimant's statements. Therefore, the better a medical source can explain the reasons for an opinion regarding limitations and abilities, the more likely SSA will be able to accept the opinion.

WHY SSA RECONTACTS MEDICAL SOURCES

For a variety of reasons, SSA may have to ask for additional information from a source who has already submitted a report. For example:

- The evidence may not be complete enough for a decision under SSA's rules, and SSA believes that the medical source may have additional information that may be sufficient to complete the case.
- SSA may need clarification of the medical source's findings or an opinion. This is especially common when there appears to be a conflict between the reported medical findings and an opinion that is not explained by the report or that SSA cannot resolve with other evidence in the claimant's record.
- SSA often obtains other evidence from other sources. When this evidence is, or appears to be, inconsistent with a medical source's report, SSA may have to resolve the conflict and may recontact a medical source for clarification or more information.
- SSA may need updated medical information in cases that are under appeal. An administrative law judge or a claimant's attorney (or other representative) may ask a DDS to obtain this additional information.

In all these cases, a medical or psychological consultant or lay examiner at the DDS will write or telephone the medical source and ask for the necessary information. SSA and the DDSs are keenly aware that this is an imposition on the medical sources' time and try to keep these contacts to a minimum. However, they are necessary both legally and to ensure the fairest and fastest decisions for claimants. As suggested previously, the more complete the initial report, the less likely the need for recontact.

PROGRAM MEDICAL PROFESSIONALS

Psychologists and physicians of virtually all specialties review claims for disability benefits in the DDSs, in SSA regional offices and at the national level. Some of these positions are full-time employment; others are on a part-time consulting basis.

Under the Act, DDSs are generally responsible for collecting medical and other evidence regarding disability and for making the initial determinations whether the claimant is disabled or blind under SSA. In most cases, a team composed of a medical or psychological consultant and a lay specialist, called a disability examiner, reviews all the evidence in the record and determines eligibility. SSA has been testing, and intends to implement, a process in which disability examiners are given enhanced authority to make disability determinations in many cases, with physicians, psychologists, and other medical professionals serving as true "consultants" on difficult and complex cases. As noted, the disability determination is generally made based on a review of the written evidence.

At the federal level, SSA employs physicians, psychologists, and other medical professionals in its 10 regional offices and at SSA headquarters in Baltimore, Maryland. Most of these individuals perform quality review functions and help provide guidance to the DDSs. A number of consultants work for a special federal DDS located in the Baltimore headquarters in the same capacity as medical and psychological consultants in the state DDSs. A small number of medical officers employed at the national headquarters help develop SSA policy and provide national policy guidance.

SSA and the DDSs also employ health care professionals who are not physicians or licensed psychologists, such as speech/language pathologists. For further information, see the sources at the end of this chapter.

OFFICE OF HEARINGS AND APPEALS—MEDICAL EXPERTS

Medical experts are physicians and mental health professionals who provide impartial expert opinion at Administrative Law Judge (ALJ) hearings either by testifying at a hearing or by responding in writing to questions posed by the ALJ, although live testimony at a hearing is preferred. Claimants and their representatives also have the opportunity to question the medical experts.

The main reason ALJs call upon medical experts is to gain information that will help evaluate the medical evidence in a case. Medical experts testify about issues such as the meaning of technical medical evidence, treatment (such as the usual dosage and effect of particular drugs), the onset of medical impairments, and whether a given impairment meets or equals the criteria of a listing in SSA's Listing of Impairments. (See following explanation of the disability process.) Medical experts do not make disability decisions, and ALJs are not required to accept their testimony. Their testimony is opinion evidence that the ALJ considers along with all the other evidence.

Medical experts do not examine claimants. In fact, when an individual who is on the Office of Hearings and Appeals' roster of medical experts has treated or examined a given claimant, he or she is precluded from testifying as a medical expert in that case.

SSA hearings and appeals regional offices maintain rosters of individuals who have agreed to be medical experts.

DEFINITION OF DISABILITY AND SSA'S DECISION PROCESS FOR ADULTS

The Act is divided into sections called "titles." Title II of the Act includes the SSDI programs, Title XVI of the Act is for SSI. For adults (including persons claiming child's insurance benefits based on disability under Title II), disability is defined in the Act under both Title II and Title XVI as the "inability to engage in any substantial gainful activity by reason of any medically determinable physical or mental impairment which can be expected to result in death or which has lasted or can be expected to last for a continuous period of not less than 12 months."[7]

The Act also states that an adult:

> . . . shall be determined to be under a disability only if his physical or mental impairment or impairments are of such severity that he is not only unable to do his previous work but cannot, considering his age, education, and work experience, engage in any other kind of substantial gainful work which exists in the national economy, regardless of whether such work exists in the immediate area in which he lives, or whether a specific job vacancy exists for him, or whether he would be hired if he applied for work.

Therefore, the statutory definition of disability is fundamentally functional, based on a person's physical and mental ability to do work. It should also be evident that the statutory definition is very strict. It does not provide for partial disability payments as other disability programs do. It does not provide payments to people simply because they are unable to do their customary work and it does not provide for short-term disability payments. In most cases, an individual must be unable to work for at least 12 months, and the great majority of individuals who qualify are disabled for much longer than that. The 12-month rule and its alternative, "expected to result in death," are called the "duration requirement."

The provisions in the Act for considering age, education, and work experience mitigate somewhat the severity of the definition for many individuals. For example, individuals who are older generally do not need to be as functionally limited to qualify as do individuals who are younger.

To implement the statutory definition, SSA regulations provide a five-step algorithm, called the sequential evaluation process,[8] which tracks the various requirements in the statutory definition (Fig. 6–1). The steps are followed in order until a decision can be made. If a decision can be made at a given step, the process stops. The steps are as follows:

1. Is the individual engaging in substantial gainful activity? For individuals alleging disability, substan-

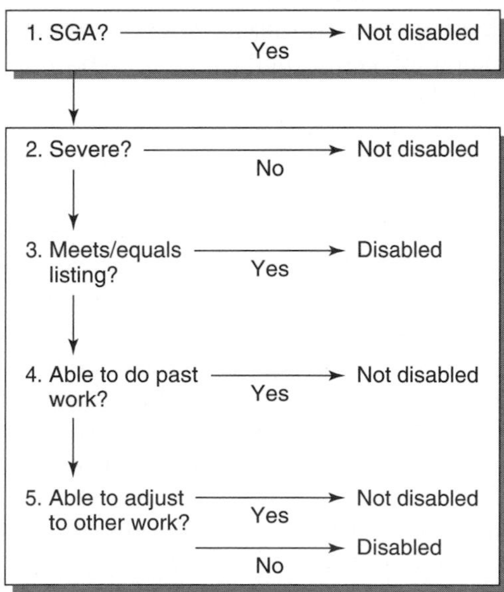

Figure 6–1. Sequential evaluation process for adults (Social Security Disability Insurance and Supplemental Security Income).

tial gainful activity is generally defined as earnings of at least $780 per month in 2002,[9] although there are alternative criteria that consider the value of work in which the earnings may be lower. Also, SSA may not consider all of a person's earnings if the earnings are subsidized because of a disability or if the person has impairment-related work expenses.

If the individual is working and the work is substantial gainful activity, he or she is not disabled. Otherwise, the evaluation proceeds to step 2 of the sequence.

2. Does the individual have an impairment or combination of impairments that is "severe"? At this step of the process, SSA determines whether an individual has a medically determinable physical or mental impairment and whether it affects the individual's ability to do work-related functions.

In SSA parlance, the term impairment means any medical condition, regardless of whether the condition actually impairs the individual's functioning; in fact, it is not always necessary to establish a precise diagnosis. The Act and SSA's regulations provide that the medically determinable impairment "must result from anatomical, physiological, or psychological abnormalities which can be shown by medically acceptable clinical and laboratory diagnostic techniques." Therefore, a physical or mental impairment must be shown by medical evidence consisting of clinical signs, symptoms, and laboratory findings.[10] SSA's rules recognize that symptoms (e.g., pain, fatigue) often play a crucial role in limiting an individual's ability to function and, hence, in determining whether the individual is disabled. However, the Act and SSA regulations provide that an individual may not be found disabled based on symptoms alone; there must always be some objective medical information to support the finding.

The term "severe" is a term of art in SSA's regulations. Under SSA's rules, an impairment or combination of impairments is "severe" if it significantly limits an individual's physical or mental abilities to do basic work activities. An impairment that is not severe is a slight abnormality (or a combination of slight abnormalities) that has no more than a minimal effect on the ability to do basic work activities. Therefore, step 2 of the sequential evaluation process is a screening step. It excludes (screens out) from the programs individuals whose impairments or combinations of impairments are so minor that they cannot be the basis for a finding of disability.

Most individuals who apply for disability benefits have severe impairments. However, if an individual does not have an impairment or combination of impairments that is severe, he or she is not disabled. If the individual has an impairment or combination of impairments that is severe, the evaluation proceeds to step 3 of the sequence.

3. Does the individual's impairment meet or equal the severity of a listing? The Listing of Impairments includes impairments with specific medical and functional criteria that are so serious that SSA presumes that an individual who satisfies the criteria is disabled. Like step 2, step 3 is also a screening step. Unlike step 2, it includes (screens in) individuals whose impairments or combinations of impairments are so significant that SSA does not have to consider other factors to decide that they are disabled.

The listings are published in SSA's regulations.[11] When a person has an impairment or a combination of impairments that meets or medically equals the severity of a listing and meets the duration requirement, the person is disabled based on medical factors alone; i.e., without considering the vocational factors of age, education, and work experience.

The listings are divided into two large sections. Part A contains the listings for people who are at least 18 years old, although occasionally SSA may use listings in Part A for people who are younger than 18 in appropriate circumstances. Part B contains the listings for people who are under 18. The Part B listings are not used to evaluate disability for people who are age 18 or older.

Each part of the listings is divided into sections called "body systems." The body systems include traditional body systems, such as cardiovascular and musculoskeletal, as well as body systems that SSA has created for its convenience. These body systems categorize impairments by their primary manifestations, such as mental disorders.

Each body system contains a preface with instructions and guidance about how to evaluate the impairments included in the body system and how to interpret particular listings. After the preface, the second part of the body system comprises the listings themselves; i.e., the rules that establish disability at this step of the sequence. Each listing consists of one or more sets of medical criteria or a combination of medical and functional criteria. A person's impairment meets the requirements of a listing when it matches exactly the criteria of a listing and meets the duration requirement.

Under the Act and SSA's regulations, individuals may establish disability based on any medical impairment or combination of impairments of sufficient severity. Because no set of listings could include all possible disabling impairments or combinations of impairments, SSA's regulations also provide for a showing of "medical equivalence" to the severity of a listing. An impairment (or a combination of impairments) is medically equivalent to a listing when it does not meet the criteria of any listing but is equal in severity and duration to a listed impairment. When the medical findings are sufficiently severe, medical equivalence applies to types of impairments that are not included in the listings, impairments that are included but do not meet exactly the criteria of a listing, and combinations of impairments, no one of which meets or medically equals the criteria of a listing but that in combination are of equivalent severity to a listing.

A common misconception about SSA's rules is that, to be found disabled, individuals must show impairments that meet or medically equal listings. Although the majority of disabled individuals qualify under the listings, well over a third of individuals who are found disabled qualify at step 5 of the sequence.

When an individual's impairment(s) does not meet or medically equal a listing, the evaluation proceeds to step 4.

4. Does the individual have the ability to perform any past relevant work? To reach this step, SSA has determined that the individual is not engaging in substantial gainful activity and has a severe impairment, but that the impairment does not meet or medically equal the severity of a listing. At this step, SSA assesses the individual's residual functional capacity and decides whether the individual is able to do work he or she has done in the past.

   Residual functional capacity (RFC) is what the individual can still do despite limitations imposed by his or her physical and mental impairments. The RFC assessment considers only functional limitations and restrictions that result from an individual's medically determinable impairment(s), including the impact of any related symptoms. Therefore, age is not a consideration in assessing RFC. However, SSA considers age in determining whether an individual can make an adjustment to other work if the analysis proceeds to step 5.

   Ordinarily, RFC is an assessment of an individual's ability to do sustained work-related physical and mental activities in a work setting on a regular and continuing basis. A "regular and continuing basis" means 8 hours a day, for 5 days a week, or an equivalent work schedule. However, past relevant work may have been part-time work, so in some cases SSA may assess an individual's RFC for fewer hours or fewer days of work per week. Therefore, when SSA asks treating and other medical sources for their opinions about how an individual is able to function despite his or her impairment(s)—the medical source statement already described—it asks for opinions about the length of time and sustainability of performance as well as maximal ability.

   SSA does not ask treatment sources to determine their patients' RFC. The RFC assessment is an administrative finding of fact that is legally reserved to SSA. However, SSA considers opinions from treating sources about their patient's abilities and limitations to be very important evidence for making its findings.

   In deciding whether the individual can do past relevant work, SSA does not necessarily count all work an individual has done. In general, the work must have been performed within the past 15 years and must meet other technical requirements set out in SSA's rules. However, SSA does consider past work both in the way the individual actually performed it and in the way it is generally performed in the national economy if that is different.

   If the individual still has the ability to perform past relevant work, he or she is not disabled. If not, the evaluation proceeds to step 5 of the sequence.

5. Does the individual's impairment(s) prevent him or her from performing other work that exists in the national economy? At this step, SSA again uses the RFC assessment made at step 4. SSA considers this RFC assessment together with the vocational factors of age education, and work experience to determine whether the individual has the ability to make an adjustment to work other than work he or she has done in the past. If the individual is unable to do so, and if the duration requirement is met, the individual is disabled. If not, he or she is not disabled.

   The determination whether an individual is able to make an adjustment to other work is very complex, involving extensive rules and guidelines set out in SSA's regulations and rulings. Considering the interaction of the individual's RFC, age, education, and any relevant work experience, including any skills the individual may have that may be useful in other work, SSA must establish whether there are jobs that exist in significant numbers in the national economy that the individual is able to do. The regulations include tables (often referred to as grid rules) that present various combinations of facts regarding physical RFC, age, education, and work experience, with conclusions for each combination of facts establishing whether the individual is disabled. When the facts of a case match the facts of a rule, the rule directs a decision.[12] When the facts of a case do not match all the facts of a rule, as is frequently the case, the rules are used as a "framework" for decision-making. SSA may also make use of various vocational resources, including vocational experts who testify at ALJ hearings and vocational publications that provide information about the physical and mental requirements of various occupations and the numbers of jobs within local regions and throughout the nation.

There are also special disability rules for individuals who have worked many years at arduous, unskilled labor, and for older individuals who have no relevant work history and limited education or who are unable to communicate in English. Detailed discussions of these and the other vocational rules would be too extensive for the present chapter. However, the Act specifies that the finding regarding disability must not consider whether a job exists in the immediate area in which the person lives, whether a specific job vacancy exists, or whether the person would be hired. The only consideration is whether the person has the capability to do the work. Again, this determination is made by SSA.

DEFINITION OF DISABILITY AND SSA'S DECISION PROCESS FOR CHILDREN CLAIMING DISABILITY BENEFITS UNDER SSI

The SSI program for children has undergone extensive changes since 1990. When the SSI law became effective on January 1, 1974, the Act's provision for childhood disability indicated only that a child would be disabled if he or she had an impairment that was of "comparable severity" to an impairment that would disable an adult. Because the vocational concepts of "past relevant work" and "ability to adjust to other work" considering age, education, and work experience are generally not applicable to children, SSA's rules originally provided that a child would be found disabled only if his or her impairment(s) met or medically equaled the requirements of a listing. If a child did not have an impairment that met or medically equaled a listing, the claim was denied.

In 1990, the Supreme Court ruled in *Sullivan v Zebley*[13] that this "listings-only" approach used to decide children's SSI claims did not carry out the "comparable severity" standard in the Act. The decision ordered SSA to develop another step in the evaluation process for children, analogous to the vocational rules used for adults, that would consider a child's ability or inability to function in a manner similar to children of the same age.

In response to the Supreme Court's decision, SSA made many changes to its rules for evaluating disability in children. Most importantly, SSA developed an expanded definition of comparable severity, a new method of determining equivalence to listings based on functional limitations (called Functional Equivalence), and a process known as the Individualized Functional Assessment (IFA). The last of these provided a step beyond the listings step at which children could establish disability.[14]

Between 1990 and 1996, the number of children eligible for SSI benefits increased from approximately 310,000 to more than 965,000. Although some people have assumed that this dramatic increase was an outcome of the change in the rules resulting from *Zebley*, the facts are more complicated and there were actually several causes. For example, provisions of SSI legislation enacted by Congress in 1989 required SSA to make outreach efforts to locate children who could qualify for SSI. In 1990, SSA published updated and expanded listings for evaluating mental disorders in children. Also, in addition to the new rules that resulted from *Zebley*, the *Zebley* court order required SSA to readjudicate several hundred thousand class member cases and to engage in heightened outreach. Finally, there was an increase in the number of children living below the poverty line and, hence, an increase in the number of children with disabling physical and mental disorders who could qualify. However, it is true that about one-third of all eligible children were found eligible based on the IFA. In addition, there were anecdotal reports of parents coaching children to qualify for benefits, although studies by SSA, the Office of the Inspector General, and the General Accounting Office did not find any evidence of widespread fraud or abuse.

Nevertheless, on August 22, 1996, the Personal Responsibility and Work Opportunity Reconciliation Act of 1996, the "welfare reform law,"[15] established a new definition of disability specifically for children in the Act. This is the law under which SSA has decided childhood SSI cases since August 22, 1996.

The current statutory definition provides that an individual under age 18:

> . . . shall be considered disabled . . . if that individual has a medically determinable physical or mental impairment, which results in marked and severe functional limitations, and which can be expected to result in death or which has lasted or can be expected to last for a continuous period of not less than 12 months.[16]

Among other provisions affecting children and families, the 1996 law also directed SSA to discontinue the use of the IFA and to redetermine the eligibility of children who were receiving SSI based on an IFA as well as some other children. About 101,000 children, out of approximately 965,000 children who received SSI at the time of the change in the law in 1996, lost eligibility for monthly benefits as a result of those changes. However, a 1997 amendment to the law ensures continuing Medicaid eligibility for children who lost eligibility for SSI because of those changes.[17]

Based on the change in the Act, SSA regulations[18] provide that the term "marked and severe functional limitations" means listing-level severity; i.e., that the impairment or combination of impairments must meet, medically equal, or functionally equal the severity of the listings. Although this is a return to a listing-level standard, it is in fact somewhat broader than the pre-*Zebley* standard because it includes the post-*Zebley* policy of functional equivalence, itself broadened somewhat to better recognize physical impairments.

Therefore, for children, SSI provides a three-step sequential evaluation process (Fig. 6–2).

The first two steps of the process are essentially the same as in adult claims. Although it is very unusual for a child to be engaging in substantial gainful activity, it is possible, especially for older children. The term "severe" for children is defined in SSA's regulations in terms of functioning appropriate to the child's age instead of work activities. Likewise, children meet and medically equal listings in the same manner as adults.

The policy of functional equivalence, which applies only to children, is based on the premise that it is the functional limitations of a child that make the child disabled, regardless of the particular medical cause. For example, a child who uses a wheelchair is disabled because of an inability, or seriously limited ability, to walk, regardless of its cause.

Under current regulations,[19] SSA determines functional equivalence by considering a child's functioning in broad areas of functioning called "domains." There are six domains: Acquiring and using information; Attending and completing tasks; Interacting and relating with others; Moving about and manipulating objects; Caring for yourself; and Health and physical well-being. The regulations provide detailed descriptions of the domains of functioning in terms appropriate to five age groups from birth to age 18.

Using this method, a child's impairment functionally equals a listing if the child has "marked" limitations in two domains or "extreme" limitations in one. The terms "marked" and "extreme" are terms of art defined in SSA's regulations in terms related to age-appropriate development and functioning.

Under the provisions of the 1996 law, when a child who is receiving SSI disability benefits attains age 18, SSA is required to redetermine eligibility using the rules for adults.

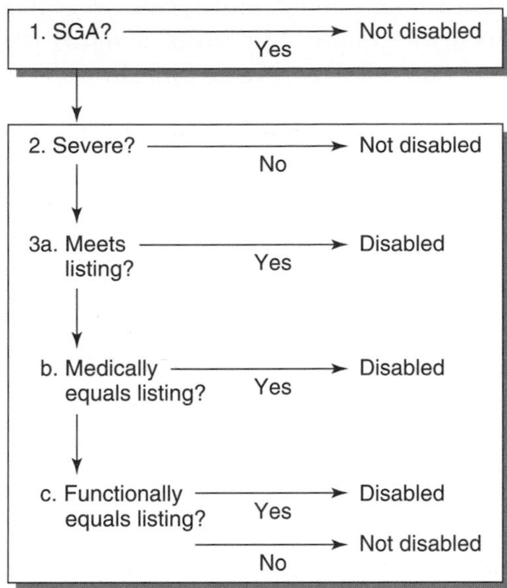

Figure 6–2. Sequential evaluation process for children (Supplemental Security Income).

DEFINITION OF BLINDNESS

Under the Act, the SSI program consider blindness as a separate entity from disability. Both the SSDI and the SSI programs define statutory blindness as central visual acuity of 20/200 or less in the better eye with the use of a correcting lens or a limitation in the field of vision of the better eye so that the widest diameter of the visual field subtends an angle no greater than 20 degrees. There are also a number of special rules for individuals who are blind, and there are differences between the SSDI and SSI programs that are too extensive for discussion in the present chapter.

NONDISABILITY CRITERIA

In addition to the disability requirements, both the SSDI and SSI programs include nondisability criteria. Both programs require a formal application for benefits. It is important that individuals file their applications as soon as they believe they may qualify because the date of filing may affect the benefits they can receive. SSI benefit payments cannot begin until the month after the month in which the application is filed; SSDI applications may be retroactive for as many as 12 months before the date of filing. An individual may file an application even if he or she does not yet have all the information that SSA requires. This information can be obtained after the application is filed. In many cases, SSA will help the individual obtain the information, or even obtain it for the individual.

Disability Insurance Benefits

To qualify for Disability Insurance benefits, a worker (an employee or a self-employed person) must have worked both long enough and recently enough under Social Security to have fully insured status (status for retirement benefits) and a special disability insured status.

By working and paying FICA taxes on levels of earnings prescribed in SSA's regulations, workers earn up to a maximum of four work credits, sometimes called quarters of coverage, per year. To show that they have worked long enough (i.e., have fully insured status), workers must have earned a specified number of credits based on their age when their disability began. There is a maximum of 40 credits to establish fully insured status, and a minimum of six for the youngest workers. For fully insured status, it does not matter when the credits were earned, only whether there is a sufficient number.

To show that they have worked recently enough to qualify for disability insurance benefits (i.e. have disability insured status), fully insured workers must have earned a specific number of work credits in a set period immediately before they became disabled. This also depends on the workers' age when they became disabled. Workers of any age qualify if they have earned 20 credits in the 40 quarters (10 years) ending with the time they became disabled; workers who are at least 31 years old must meet this requirement.

Younger workers may qualify with fewer work credits earned in fewer than 10 years based on their age when their disability began. The minimum, for workers who have not attained age 24, is six credits in the 3 years (12 quarters) ending with the time they became disabled.

In most cases, when an individual's application is approved, he or she will be paid benefits beginning with the sixth full month after the date disability began. The preceding 5 months are called a "waiting period." The waiting period is prescribed by the Act. Depending on when the disability began, benefits may be paid for as many as 12 months before the month of the application.

Supplemental Security Income

There is no work or insured status requirement to establish eligibility for SSI. Individuals must only show that they have limited income and resources. The limits on income and resources are specified in the Act.

"Income" may be either earned (e.g., from part-time work) or unearned (e.g., SSDI benefits, benefit payments from another agency, or in-kind support, such as room and board, provided by someone else). When an individual with a disability is married, SSA "deems" part of the income of his or her spouse to the individual. Likewise, part of the income of parents is deemed to a child with a disability. The Act and SSA regulations include complex rules for disregarding or reducing the amount of income SSA counts against the limit or deems to an individual. Individuals with limited income should never try to determine for themselves whether they qualify, but should always file an application and let SSA make this determination.

"Resources" are cash or other liquid assets (e.g., a savings account) and property that an individual owns that could be converted to cash. As with income, the Act and SSA regulations include provisions for deeming a spouse's resources to a disabled individual or a parent's resources to a disabled child, but also include provisions for disregarding some resources. For example, SSA generally does not count a person's home as a resource if it is the person's principal residence.

Because SSI is a program based on need, there is no waiting period as in SSDI. However, there is no provision for payment of benefits prior to the time of the application. The earliest month for which a benefit can be paid is the month after the month of the application.

For both the SSDI and SSI programs there are many other rules regarding other nondisability issues, such as proof of age, establishing work credits, relationship, residency, and dependency, that are not covered in this chapter. This information is readily available from SSA offices and the other sources cited at the end of this chapter.

THE ADMINISTRATIVE REVIEW PROCESS

Application

Most initial disability claims are processed through a network of approximately 1300 Social Security field offices and 54 DDSs. SSA field offices take applications and information from claimants that the DDSs need so that they can obtain evidence and decide the claims (Fig. 6–3). Field office employees also make determinations about the nondisability aspects of claims, including whether individuals who are working at the time of application are engaging in substantial gainful activity.

When individuals are dissatisfied with any aspect of their determinations, they may appeal, first within the agency and ultimately to federal courts. At every stage in the process beginning with the application, claimants have the right to attorney or nonattorney representation and to review the evidence SSA and the DDS have gathered for their claims.

Social Security Field Office

An SSA field office representative takes the application for disability benefits in person, by telephone, or by mail. During the application process, SSA will obtain a formal application, at least one disability interview form,

Administrative Review Process— Initial Applications		
1. Application (Field Office) and initial determination (DDS)	⟶	Initial determination
↓ Claimant dissatisfied		
2. Reconsideration (DDS)	⟶	Reconsideration determination
↓ Claimant dissatisfied		
3. Request for hearing (ALJ)	⟶	ALJ hearing decision
↓ Claimant dissatisfied		
4. Request for review by Appeals Council	⟶	Appeals Council action or decision
↓ Claimant dissatisfied		
5. Civil action (Federal District Court, U.S. Court of Appeals, U.S. Supreme Court)	⟶	Decision, dismissal, remand

Figure 6–3. Adminstrative review process—initial applications.

and a number of authorizations for release of medical and other information. SSA will ask the claimant for information about his or her impairment(s), symptoms, and functional limitations. The claimant will also be asked for the names and addresses of medical and other sources, identifying information (such as clinic numbers) for those sources, dates of treatment (which need not be exact), school information for child claimants, work history, the physical and mental requirements of any past work, and other information that relates to the alleged disability. The claimant will also be asked for information about age, relationships, income, and other information relating to the nondisability requirements of his or her claim(s).

Claimants may submit medical and other information at the time of their applications, but are not required to do so. The field offices obtain signed authorizations from claimants for the release of medical and other information. The DDSs use these authorizations to request medical and other evidence for the claimants to complete the claims.

The SSA field office verifies nonmedical eligibility requirements. If the claimant is working at the time of the application, the field office will determine whether the work is substantial gainful activity. If necessary, the field office will help the claimant obtain evidence related to any nondisability issue within its jurisdiction. In many cases, the field office will request and obtain this information for claimants if the claimants do not already have it. The field office may also help claimants obtain medical or lay evidence to support allegations of disability, but in most cases this will be left to the DDS so as not to delay processing of the claims. When the field office verifies that the nonmedical eligibility criteria are met, the case is forwarded to the DDS.

State Disability Determination Services

As already noted, the DDS is responsible for collecting medical and other evidence regarding disability and for making the determination whether the claimant is disabled or blind under the law. The DDS is authorized to pay for this evidence; each state sets the fees it will pay. After the DDS makes its determination, it sends a notice to the claimant explaining the determination and the claimant's appeal rights. The DDS also determines whether the claimant is a candidate for vocational rehabilitation (VR). If so, a referral to the state VR agency is made.

When a claimant is dissatisfied with an initial determination, he or she may appeal. Claimants appeal most often when the DDS has found that they are not disabled. However, appeals are taken for other reasons, such as to dispute the date on which the DDS found that disability began. Some claimants even appeal determinations that are wholly favorable to them. Most often in these cases, they dispute the basis for the favorable decision, such as when SSA finds that a claimant who has alleged a physical disability is disabled because of a mental disorder. Many claimants are not aware that SSA's decisions are confidential. SSA does not share information about its decisions without the individuals' authorization.

DDS Reconsideration

If a claimant wishes to appeal an initial determination, he or she may file a request for reconsideration at the SSA field office within 60 days of receiving the notice of initial determination. Failure to file the appeal within 60 days of the letter without good cause results in dismissal of the request for reconsideration, an action that cannot be appealed. Therefore, it is critical that individuals who may wish to appeal their determinations file their requests as soon as possible after receipt of the determination notice. As with initial applications, claimants need not have all necessary information before they request reconsideration. This information may be gathered later, and SSA and the DDS will help.

The determination process is the same for reconsideration as for initial determinations. However, a team of DDS staff different from the team that made the initial determination makes the reconsidered determination.

Hearing Office

Claimants who are dissatisfied with their reconsideration determinations may request a hearing before a federal ALJ in SSA's Office of Hearings and Appeals within 60 days of receiving the reconsideration decision. (As at the reconsideration level, an appeal may be filed later than 60 days after the notice of reconsideration if the claimant has good cause for such late filing. Otherwise, the request will be dismissed.) There are over 1000 ALJs holding hearings in 140 hearing offices throughout the country. ALJs also travel to over 300 additional sites to reduce claimant and representative travel to the hearing when there are long distances involved.

Generally, claimants appear at a scheduled hearing where they can orally present their case to the ALJ. The hearing is usually the first opportunity claimants have to speak to the person who makes the decision in their case. However, at a claimant's request the ALJ will make a decision without a hearing based only on the documentary record, although SSA does not encourage this choice. In some cases, ALJs will make decisions favorable to claimants before holding a hearing based solely on their review of the documentary record; ALJs are not permitted to make unfavorable decisions in this way for claimants who have asked for a hearing.

ALJ hearings are formal proceedings but are run in an informal manner. A taped record is made of the proceeding, but there are no strict rules of evidence and claimants are allowed to speak freely about their medical conditions. ALJs are often said to serve three functions. They are required to be impartial decision-makers, but are also required to represent the interests of the claimant and the interests of SSA. Claimants do not need representation at ALJ hearings, but about 80% of claimants choose to be represented by an attorney or a nonattorney representative.

The ALJ considers the case *de novo*; i.e., as though it is a new claim and without ruling on the correctness of the previous determinations made by the DDS. The ALJ can, and often will, develop additional evidence from the claimant's medical and other sources and through consultative examinations. When an ALJ needs such evidence, he or she will usually ask the DDS to obtain it, although ALJs sometimes write directly to medical sources and also have subpoena power. The claimant's attorney or other representative will often provide additional evidence as well, and may ask a claimant's medical and other sources to prepare reports.

As already noted, the ALJ may also call for testimony at the hearing from expert witnesses: a physician or psychologist, called a medical expert, or a vocational specialist, called a vocational expert, or both. The claimant has the right to question these witnesses, and also has the right to present his or her own witnesses. These witnesses may be experts, but need not be. They may be family members, friends, or other individuals who can testify about the claimant's disability.

Appeals Council

A claimant who is dissatisfied with the ALJ's decision may request review of the decision by the Appeals Council. As with the previous appeals, this appeal must be filed within 60 days of receipt of the decision, or the claimant must show good cause for late filing.

The Appeals Council, based in Falls Church, Virginia, functions differently from the first three levels. The most significant difference is that the Appeals Council's review is not *de novo*. Rather, the Appeals Council reviews the ALJ's decision to determine whether it was supported by substantial evidence, a legal standard of review, and to determine whether there was an error of law or an abuse of discretion. The Appeals Council will also consider new evidence, but only in limited circumstances; the evidence must relate to the period on or before the ALJ's decision.

If the Appeals Council grants the request for review, it has several options. In most cases in which review is granted, the Appeals Council vacates the ALJ's decision and remands the claim to the ALJ who made the decision with instructions to take additional actions, hold a new hearing, and issue a new decision. In some cases, the Appeals Council may obtain evidence on its own and issue its own decision, which may or may not be favorable to the claimant. The Appeals Council may also dismiss the request for review for various reasons.

The Appeals Council may also review on its own motion an ALJ's decision that has not been appealed by a claimant. The Appeals Council reviews only a small number of decisions on its own motion (fewer than 10,000 in 2001). The decisions reviewed are generally ones that are favorable to claimants. The reason for choosing these favorable decisions is to provide some balance in the review of ALJ decisions. Virtually all claims that are appealed to the Appeals Council ask the

Appeals Council to review ALJ decisions that were unfavorable to claimants. Therefore, the own-motion reviews are almost the only favorable decisions the Appeals Council reviews. Cases for own-motion reviews are selected based on fact-based profiles. The Appeals Council does not select particular ALJs for review.

In the vast majority of cases, the Appeals Council considers only the evidence in the documentary record, the taped testimony from the ALJ hearing, and any briefs, letters, or additional evidence submitted in connection with the request for review. However, unlike the ALJ hearing, there are limits, set out in SSA's regulations, on new evidence that the Appeals Council will consider. On very rare occasions, the Appeals Council may hold a hearing, but only if it decides that a case raises an important question of law or policy or that oral argument would help it to reach a proper decision.

If the Appeals Council denies or dismisses the request for review, the ALJ's decision becomes the final decision of the Commissioner of Social Security. If the Appeals Council grants review and issues a decision, its decision becomes the final decision of the Commissioner. A claimant's recourse after these actions is outside of the agency, in the federal courts.

Federal Courts

A claimant who is dissatisfied with the action of the Appeals Council may, within 60 days of the date of receipt of the notice of action, file an appeal in federal district court. Federal court review is limited by statute to whether SSA's decision was supported by substantial evidence.

Also, unlike the previous levels, SSA may itself appeal a federal court's decision if it is dissatisfied with the decision. If the claimant or SSA is dissatisfied with the decision of the District Court, either may appeal to a United States Court of Appeals (also called a circuit court) and, ultimately, to the United States Supreme Court.

CONTINUING DISABILITY REVIEWS

So far, we have discussed the process for initial applicants. However, SSA also regularly reviews the continuing entitlement and eligibility of individuals who are already receiving disability benefits. In general, benefits continue for as long as a person is disabled. But the Act mandates that SSA periodically reexamine the cases of all beneficiaries to see if they are still disabled—even beneficiaries whose disabilities are clearly permanent. These reexaminations are called continuing disability reviews.[20]

For many individuals, SSA asks only that they complete a brief form, which is mailed back to SSA at no cost to the individuals, to confirm their continuing disability status. Based on a beneficiary's answers on the form, SSA decides whether a more formal medical review is required. For many others, SSA conducts a formal medical review to confirm whether they are still disabled. SSA notifies these individuals by mail that their claims will be reviewed and they are asked to come to the local SSA field office to provide information.

At that point, an SSA field office representative will ask the beneficiary if his or her impairment has improved and obtain information about the claimant's current conditions, similar to the information obtained when the individual first applied. This includes information about treatment and medical evaluations the beneficiary has received since originally qualifying or since the last review. If the beneficiary has new medical impairments that were not present at the last review, the SSA representative will take detailed information about those conditions as well.

As in initial claims, the field office will then forward the case to the DDS for development of evidence and a determination. The process for developing evidence (including the purchase of consultative examinations) is the same as for initial claims. Likewise, a team comprising a physician or psychologist and a disability examiner will make the determination.

However, the standards for deciding whether disability continues are somewhat different from the initial standards for establishing disability. The Act and SSA regulations provide that, in general, a beneficiary's disability must be found to continue unless the evidence establishes that the impairment that was the basis for the finding of disability has medically improved and the individual is not currently disabled considering all current impairments. Even if there has been medical improvement, the improvement must be of a certain degree (called medical improvement related to the ability to work). Even if there has been medical improvement related to the ability to work, benefits will continue if the individual is nevertheless currently disabled, considering all current impairments and, if necessary, the vocational factors of age, education, and work experience. There is a separate sequential evaluation process specifically for continuing disability reviews.[21]

The Act provides a number of exceptions to a showing of medical improvement that may result in the cessation of benefits. These exceptions apply only rarely. For further information, see the sources at the end of this chapter.

The frequency with which SSA will review an individual's disability status depends on the permanence of the impairment that was the basis for the finding of disability. If SSA expected the impairment to improve to the extent that it would no longer be disabling, the reviews will generally be held at intervals from 6 to 18 months after the decision was made that the person was disabled or still disabled. If improvement is possible but cannot be predicted, the case will be reviewed every 3 years. If improvement is not expected, the case will be reviewed every 5 to 7 years. SSA may also reclassify a beneficiary's status when it reviews the claim, and there are some exceptions to the general rules for when reviews are conducted.

Individuals who are found to be no longer disabled based on a continuing disability review may appeal. The appeal steps are the same as for initial applications. However, at the reconsideration level, the beneficiary has a right to request a face-to-face "disability hearing" with a special employee called a disability hearing officer at the DDS. This hearing does not take the place of an ALJ hearing; if the individual is dissatisfied with the outcome of the reconsideration, he or she still has the right to request a hearing before an ALJ.

Beneficiaries who believe that their disabilities have not ended may also elect to continue to receive benefits during their appeals at the reconsideration level and at the ALJ hearing level until the ALJ issues his or her decision. If the appeal is not successful, the individual may have to repay these benefits. The beneficiary must request continuation of benefit payments during appeal within 10 days of the notice telling him or her that disability has ended and must do so at each separate level of appeal in order to keep receiving benefits. However, as with the provisions for filing appeals within 60 days of the notice, there are provisions for good cause for later filing.

RETURN TO WORK

Many people with disabilities want to work, and the Act provides a number of incentives for SSDI and SSI beneficiaries to try working. There are many different kinds of work incentives under both programs, including a number of amendments to the law made by the Ticket to Work and Work Incentives Improvement Act of 1999 (Public Law 106–170). There are protections for disabled individuals against losing entitlement or eligibility on the basis of work. There are various rules for disregarding income so that some individuals can work or go to school and continue to receive benefits. There are also incentives that provide continuing Medicare entitlement or Medicaid eligibility to individuals with disabilities whose earnings are too high to receive cash benefits. For some individuals, there are provisions that allow reentitlement without having to reapply and that provide the protection of the medical improvement review standard used in continuing disability reviews.

It is important for disability beneficiaries to understand that they can still receive cash or medical benefits, or both, while they test their ability to work. SSA asks people who represent or deal with SSDI or SSI beneficiaries who are working or who are interested in working to contact them about work incentives and how they can affect their benefits.

Summary

The information provided thus far has been somewhat technical and offers a broad view of the Social Security disability programs. How this process comes into play when a patient (claimant) submits an application for benefits can be approached from two perspectives—the patient's and the physician's.

The Patient's Point of View

When a patient files for disability, he or she completes a number of forms, detailing medical history, medical sources, and work history. What happens next?

1. The DDS sends a request for existing medical evidence to the named medical sources.
2. When the DDS receives medical evidence, the evaluation process described earlier in the chapter begins.
3. When the evidence received is sufficient and any inconsistencies or conflicts therein have been resolved, a decision is made.
4. This process can take several months to complete. The patient and SSA appreciate anything the physician can do to speed up the process, such as sending in the requested information promptly.

The Physician's Point of View

The physician may have suggested that a patient file for disability or may first learn of the application on receipt of a request for medical records from the DDS. In any event, the physician receives the request and perhaps several forms to complete. What should the physician do?

1. Complete any forms received to the best of his or her ability, giving full details wherever known.
2. Submit the completed forms and the requested medical records, including all pertinent test results (labs, imaging, etc.), as soon as possible.
3. Remember that any medical opinion he or she gives, either on a form or in a narrative report to the DDS, will be considered based on how well it is supported by the total evidence.
4. Remember that the decision on whether any individual is disabled under the Social Security law is reserved to the Commissioner and his or her agents, including the DDS or an ALJ. Thus any opinion the physician offers on whether the individual is disabled will be considered but does not direct the final decision.

5. Sometimes, the physician may be recontacted for clarification of some point. This may be by telephone, letter, or fax. Such requests should be responded to promptly. These requests are not a reflection on the physician. Sometimes there are conflicts in the evidence from two sources or there is a seeming inconsistency in the records.
6. Most of all, remember that this is not being done for SSA or the DDS, but for the patient.

CONCLUSION

Despite the length of this chapter, the authors have given only a small taste of the complex and interesting features of these important programs that help individuals and families, and of the various roles that medical professionals play in the disability evaluation process. They have attempted to provide a better understanding of the scope of the legal definition of disability, how the determination whether a person is disabled is made, and what needs to be done to make correct and timely decisions.

The most important lesson provided in this chapter is the importance to SSA of good, detailed medical information and opinions from a claimant's own treatment sources. Medical sources are often asked why their patients or clients were denied benefits or why SSA simply did not accept their statements that their patients were disabled. The program has both medical and legal requirements and it is SSA's responsibility to make the determination of disability, but SSA considers medical providers to be primary sources of information for its determinations. It is important for medical providers to explain their findings and opinions as well as possible. This is critical when the disability is not evident from the objective medical data alone, such as when pain, fatigue, or other symptoms are the essential cause of disability.

The authors have attempted to provide a sense of the massive job the thousands of men and women who work for SSA and the state DDSs have undertaken and how the physician can help in that process. The task of gathering evidence and processing millions of claims quickly and correctly is, to say the least, a daunting one. Mistakes are made, but improvement is ongoing. For example, many listings and other disability rules are currently being reviewed to bring them as up-to-date as possible and to make them easier to understand and use.

As we mentioned earlier in this chapter, SSA intends to implement a process in which some cases will not be decided by teams in the DDSs. We believe that this process would make more effective and efficient use of disability examiner and medical and psychological consultant resources. SSA is also considering ways to refine the initial claim and appellate processes to reduce the time that it takes for all claimants to receive final agency decisions on their claims.

Perhaps when the next edition of this book is issued there will be different story to tell. In the meantime, answers to questions about any aspect of SSA's disability programs can be provided by the following sources.

FOR FURTHER INFORMATION

1. General information—Information about SSA's disability programs is available from any local Social Security field office or from SSA's toll-free numbers (1–800–772–1213 and TTY 1–800–325–0778). These sources have many free pamphlets and fact sheets as well as representatives who can answer questions.

   The single best source of information on SSA's programs is SSA's Internet site, SSA Online (http://www.ssa.gov). The site provides a wealth of nontechnical and technical information and data for every aspect of SSA's disability programs. It also includes most of the documents listed in the following. There are links to all of SSA's pamphlets and fact sheets for the disability programs at this site, as well as a number of other publications, including the Social Security Handbook, the Social Security Act, all of SSA's regulations and rulings, and some of the forms used in the disability application process. There is also information about how to contact SSA field offices and various departments within SSA, as well as state DDS contact information. Follow the links to "Disability," "Employment support for people with disabilities," "Medicare information," "Policy, research, and statistics," and the links under "Laws, regulations, rulings." To find out about employment at a DDS and agency professional relations activities, including when SSA representatives will be available at professional conferences, click on "Disability," then "Professional relations."
2. Regulations and Social Security Rulings—SSA's disability regulations are set out in the Code of Federal Regulations, Title 20, Parts 400–499. The basic disability regulations for SSDI are in Subpart P of Part 404 (the regulations that begin with the number 404.1500); for SSI, the basic regulations are in Subpart I of Part 416 (the regulations that begin with the number 416.900). This reference is available at libraries and for purchase from the U.S. Government Printing Office (202–512–1800). It can also be accessed at no charge at SSA's Web site. Follow the link to "Current rules and regulations." This link also contains more recently pub-

lished regulations (including listings) that have not yet been published in book form and proposed regulations on which SSA has asked for public comments.

3. The Listing of Impairments (the listings)—The only official publication of the listings is in SSA's regulations. The listings are included in Appendix 1 of Subpart P of Part 404 of the regulations. (Although the listings apply to SSI cases too, they are not reprinted in Part 416. Instead, to save space, the regulations in Part 416 cross-refer to the listings printed in the SSDI regulations.)

   SSA also publishes the listings in a handbook entitled Disability Evaluation Under Social Security, which can be read and downloaded on the Internet at www.ssa.gov/disability/professionals/bluebook. This handbook, often called the Blue Book, is widely distributed to physicians and mental health professionals; several chapters in this book make reference to it. It also includes brief information about other aspects of the disability evaluation process. The Web site is updated whenever we revise the listings, so it is important to check back from time to time to see if we have made changes.

4. The Social Security Handbook, 13th edition (SSA Pub. No. 65–008, ICN 958392, August 1997)—This book provides more detailed information about SSA's disability programs than is provided by pamphlets and other public information SSA publishes, but in less technical form than in the Act and regulations. The book is available for purchase from the Government Printing Office and may be read at SSA's Web site. Go to http://www.ssa. gov/disability, where there are links to this book and many other disability publications.

5. Work incentives—SSA publishes many pamphlets addressing the various incentives available to people with disabilities who would like to try to work. A summary of the incentives is published in a booklet called The Red Book. This short "book" may be read or downloaded on the Internet. Go to www.ssa.gov/work and click on "Resources Toolkit."

References

1. There are two Social Security trust funds: the Old-Age and Survivors Insurance (OASI) trust fund, which pays benefits to retirees and their families, and the Disability Insurance (DI) trust fund, which pays disability benefits. In addition, a portion of FICA taxes goes to a trust fund for Medicare.
2. The Act also provides another benefit that is not a cash benefit, called a period of disability. A period of disability protects a disabled person's insured status and may affect the amount of benefits a person may receive in the future. All people who receive disability insurance benefits also have a period of disability, but the converse is not necessarily true: it is sometimes possible to have a period of disability without disability insurance benefits. This is a very technical provision and is not addressed in this chapter.
3. The normal retirement age for Social Security began to increase beginning in January 2000. Although 62 remains the earliest age at which individuals can retire and collect reduced benefits, the age for collecting full Social Security benefits will gradually increase from age 65 to 67 over a 22-year period. For those born in 1940 (age 62 in 2002) the new retirement age is 65 and 6 months. The increase in the retirement age was included in the Social Security Amendments of 1983.
4. Widows, widowers, and surviving divorced spouses may receive benefits at age 60 regardless of whether they are disabled. Therefore, applicants for this disability benefit are usually between age 50 and 60.
5. Under current law, some individuals, known as qualified aged aliens, may have to show that they are disabled when they are 65 or older. Occasionally, other individuals who are at least 65 years old must establish that they are disabled to satisfy certain complex SSI rules or to receive higher benefits from their states.
6. When photocopies of a chart are submitted they must be legible. This means not only in terms of the quality of the photocopy but in terms of handwriting. Whereas physician penmanship has been the butt of many jokes, illegible handwriting is a real and serious problem in a system that adjudicates so many claims each year and in claims that may eventually have to be read by judges and lawyers without assistance from medical professionals.
7. Sections 223(d) and 1614(a). See also section 216(i).
8. The regulations are in Title 20 of the Code of Federal Regulations (20 CFR) at 20 CFR §§ 404. 1520 and 416.920.
9. For SSDI programs, the current substantial gainful activity threshold for individuals who are statutorily blind is $1300 per month in 2002. This threshold increases annually based on the cost of living. See 20 CFR § 404.1584(d). (Under SSI, statutorily blind individuals do not have to show that they are unable to work to qualify, so there is no substantial gainful activity threshold for them.) Under SSDI and SSI, the substantial gainful activity threshold for the nonblind was $500 per month for many years. On July 1, 1999, SSA increased the level to $700. See 64 FR 18566 (4/15/99), corrected at 64 FR 22903 (4/28/99); 20 CFR §§ 404.1574 and 416.974.
10. Under SSA's regulations, laboratory findings include the results of psychological tests.
11. 20 CFR, Appendix 1 of Subpart P of Part 404.
12. In technical, legal language, the rules take administrative notice of the existence of numerous unskilled occupations that exist in the national economy at various levels of exertion. See 20 CFR §§ 404.1568, 404.1569, 416.968, 416.969, and Appendix 2 of Subpart P of the Regulations Part 404.
13. 493 U.S. 521 (1990).
14. See 56 FR 5534 (2/11/91) and 58 FR 47532 (9/9/93). SSA's Web site also contains several links in nontechnical language explaining the prior rules and the provisions of current law and regulations.
15. Public Law No. 104–193, August 22, 1996.
16. Act, section 1614(a)(3)(C)(i).
17. Balanced Budget Act of 1997 (August 5, 1997), Public Law 105–33, section 4913. Section 1902(a)(10)(A)(i)(II) of the Act.
18. The major regulations for evaluating SSI childhood disability are set out at 20 CFR §§ 416.924 through 416.924b and

416.926a. The last of these regulations provides the detailed rules for evaluating functional equivalence. See 65 FR 54747 (9/11/2000).

19. 20 CFR § 416.9269. 65 FR 54782 (9/11/2000); 65 FR 80308 (12/21/2000).
20. SSA field offices also confirm periodically that beneficiaries continue to meet the nondisability requirements for entitlement or eligibility. Beneficiaries are instructed to report a number of changes and events that may affect their status, such as going back to work or moving. SSI beneficiaries must report their income and resources at regularly scheduled redeterminations. However, these reviews are separate from the continuing disability reviews conducted by the DDSs.
21. For adults, see 20 CFR §§ 404.1594 and 416.994. For SSI child beneficiaries, the process is different, but there must still be a showing of medical improvement and a finding about whether a child who has medically improved is currently disabled. See 20 CFR § 416.994a.

CHAPTER

7

The Medical–Legal Interface

LAWRENCE P. POSTOL, JD

The interface between physicians and the legal world is not always an easy one. Confusion between the professions requires that care must be taken any time the law and medicine interface. Both are complex fields, with many important decisions being made, and neither field is an exact science. However, if the physician has a minimum level of understanding of the legal system, and the lawyer has an adequate understanding of medical facts and the limits of medical science, the medical–legal interface can be a successful one.

The Role of the Physician in the Legal World

Some physicians are too fearful of interacting with the legal world, and some are not cautious enough. Those physicians who see a potential lawsuit at every corner, and thus refuse to give a written opinion or hesitate to identify a malingerer, are too cautious. Those who assume they can do whatever they want, relying either on bluffing or on their malpractice insurance, are also mistaken. Both the lack of caution and over-cautiousness come from a lack of knowledge of the legal world.

Although, in theory, anyone who can pay the filing fee can sue another, lawsuits are rarely filed unless there is some minimal basis for the claim. Most such lawsuits are taken on a contingent fee basis—the lawyer only gets paid if he or she wins. Thus a lawyer will not take such a case unless he or she believes he or she has a chance to win. Although the physician can never guarantee that he or she will never be sued, he or she can take some steps to greatly reduce the risk of becoming a defendant in litigation. That is, if certain precautions are taken, a lawsuit against the physician will look less attractive to lawyers, thus reducing the risk of a lawsuit.

Conversely, if a physician is so cautious that he or she never gives a definitive opinion, he or she is useless to the legal system. The key for the physician, in addition to focusing on the medical questions, is to understand the legal issues, how the physician's opinion interfaces with them, and what the physician's role is in answering the legal issues.

Testifying in Court

It is important to recognize that when a physician testifies in court, he or she is usually offering a medical opinion as an expert witness. The courts have grappled with minimum standards for an expert witness's opinions, so that "junk science" can be excluded from the courtroom. Thus, a physician must have a minimum scientific basis for an opinion before he or she will be allowed to testify in court (see also Chapter 8).

The United States Supreme Court recently addressed when an expert, and in particular, when a medical expert, can offer an opinion into evidence. In Daubert v Merrell Dow Pharmaceuticals Inc., 509 U.S. 579, 113 S. Ct. 2786, 125L. Ed. 2nd 508 (1993), the Supreme Court was faced with the admissibility of medical experts' opinions that the prenatal ingestion of bendectin can cause birth defects. The Court held that a medical expert's opinion is admissible only if it is based on "scientific validity;" that is, if it is based on scientific methods that have tested its validity. Put another way, the person offering expert opinion must have "a reliable basis in the knowledge and experience of his discipline." The Supreme Court noted that trial judges, in order to test scientific validity, must initially determine whether the theory or technique in question "can be (and has been) tested," whether it has been "subjected to peer review and publication," its "known or potential error rate," the "existence and maintenance of standards controlling its operation," and finally, whether it has attracted "widespread acceptance" within a relevant scientific community. The Court emphasized that the heart of scientific methodology is "testing [theories] to see if they can be falsified." The Court also noted that "a known technique that has been able to attract only minimal support . . . may properly be viewed with skepticism." Of course, the expert's theory must be properly applied to the facts of the claim in dispute; that is, the theory must be relevant to the claim.

Although there was some dispute whether Daubert applied to all experts, in Kumho Tire Co. v Carmichael, U.S., 119 S. Ct. 1167 (1999), the Supreme Court ruled that the Daubert standard for determining whether an expert's opinion was reliable applied to all kinds of experts.

In most cases, the medical opinion will not be questioned as to its admissibility, as in a diagnosis of cancer. However, when a physicians testifies in a controversial area, especially on causation, he or she can expect that his or her opinion will be challenged as to whether it is even admissible; that is, whether it can be presented to the jury, to be weighed against other experts' opinions.

Definitions

Lawyers use legal terminology that is often foreign to physicians. It is curious that a lawyer often requests that a physician acting as an expert witness spend hours explaining the details of the doctor's professional opinion to the lawyer, yet the lawyer rarely takes the time to explain certain simple, but critical, legal terminology to the physician who is acting as an expert witness. The following are some of the legal terms that a physician might encounter in dealing with lawyers.

The Law

"The Law" is a term lawyers often use to refer to the controlling rules of the litigation. The law is made up of statutes, regulations, and common law. Statutes and regulations are written documents that explicitly define certain rules and duties, although they are often subject to differing interpretations. The common law is simply prior judicial (court) decisions (precedents) that impose obligations and liability on certain persons. For example, if a shop owner is negligent in not shoveling the sidewalk and a person slips on it and falls, the shop owner is liable for the damages to that person. Although certain legal principles are fairly uniform, the law does vary from state to state, and from state courts to federal courts.

An Expert

An expert is defined in most jurisdictions as any person who by "knowledge, skill, experience, training, or education" has "scientific, technical, or other specialized knowledge" that will aid the judge or jury in determining the facts at issue in a lawsuit (Federal Rule of Evidence 702). The knowledge must be of a type not normally possessed by the general public, or for which the expert has some specialized expertise such that his or her opinion will aid the judge or jury. An expert may be retained simply to assist an attorney in preparing a case, or may provide testimony at the hearing.

Discovery

A party is entitled to "discover" the relevant facts of a case and the evidence the other party has before the trial. Cases are not to be tried by surprise. The primary mechanisms for obtaining discovery are interrogatories (written questions), requests for production of documents, depositions (a lawyer questioning a witness in the presence of a court reporter and the opposing lawyer), and subpoenas. If an expert is hired but his or her opinion is not going to be used at trial (for example, where the opinion does not support the party's position), his or her opinion is usually not discoverable.

Interrogatories

A party may pose written questions to the other party in litigation; these questions are called interrogatories. The interrogatories may relate to the facts of the case as well as potential evidence at the trial. For expert witnesses, a party usually will send an interrogatory requesting the subject matter on which the expert is expected to testify and the substance of the facts and opinions to which the expert is expected to testify as well as a summary of the grounds for each opinion. For cases in federal court, a party using an expert witness must produce a report by the expert that discloses his or her opinions and the basis for those opinions. The expert must also disclose his or her qualifications, including a list of his or her publications in the past 10 years, his or her compensation for his opinion, and any cases he or she has testified in (at trial or by deposition) in the prior 4 years (Federal Rule of Civil Procedure 26[a][2][B]).

Deposition

A deposition is an oral examination of a person taken outside the courtroom and before the trial. A party may take the deposition of any witness, including an expert witness, to discover what he or she will say at trial. If a witness is unavailable at trial, his or her deposition testimony may be offered into evidence. In addition, if a witness testifies at trial, the deposition can be used to impeach him or her if he or she makes statements that are inconsistent with prior deposition testimony.

A deposition may be taken at any location, but it is usually held at an attorney's office or the witness's place of business. The attorneys for both sides, as well as a court reporter, will be present, and the court reporter will transcribe the attorney's questions and witness's answers. If an attorney objects to a question, he or she states the objection so that the judge can rule on the objection at a later date when the judge reads the deposition testimony. The witness must still answer the question, unless the attorney who represents him or her instructs him or her not to answer the question, as when a privileged attorney–client matter is involved.

Request for Production of Documents and Subpoena

A party may ask the other side to produce certain documents. Similarly, a subpoena can be sent to nonparties to compel them to produce documents, appear at a deposition or trial, and give testimony.

Evidence

Evidence is the testimony that has been heard at trial and the documents admitted at trial. The judge or jury must base their decision only on the evidence admitted. In selecting a physician's writings for admission into evidence, counsel and the physician should be certain that these writings properly explain their client's position.

Hearsay

Hearsay is a statement that is offered into evidence by someone other than the person who made the statement; it is normally not admissible. Thus, a paper written by John Doe cannot be offered into evidence by Dick Smith. There are certain exceptions to the hearsay exclusion rule. Of critical importance, business records that are made in the ordinary course of business are admissible into evidence. Moreover, an expert can base an opinion on facts that are not in evidence, if the facts are "of a type reasonably relied upon by experts in the particular field in forming opinions or inferences upon the subject" (Federal Rule of Evidence 703). However, whatever facts an expert relies upon must be disclosed to the other side if a proper discovery request is made.

The Physician As An Expert Witness

A physician may be questioned by a lawyer as to the treatment given in the ordinary practice of medicine. In such a case, he or she is a witness, similar to a bystander witnessing a car accident. For example, a physician may treat a patient for carpal tunnel syndrome, and only learn after the fact that the patient has a workers' compensation claim. Nevertheless, the physician can be called as a witness to describe the care and treatment of the injury. More often than not, however, the medical provider will know ahead of the treatment that there is a legal issue, and that he or she will be called as an expert witness. The minimum skills required of an expert are the knowledge, skill, experience, training, or education needed to qualify to give an expert opinion on the issue in the case. Any expert witness, including a physician, is judged by credentials, independence, and ability to convince a judge or jury that his or her opinion is correct.

When a physician is called as an expert witness by one party, the physician can expect that the other side will have its own expert witness who will disagree with the opinion of the first expert. Judges and juries usually resolve the battle of the experts by selecting the expert who has the most impressive credentials, who appears to be least biased, and whose opinion seems most logical and rational. It is with this background in mind that attorneys select a physician as an expert witness.

The lawyer will try to select someone who is a true expert—an individual who practices full-time in the medical field in question and who is recognized by his or her peers as a true authority. Preferably, the physician will have written extensively on the relevant subject and will have performed research in the field in question. Appointments by associations or organizations of fellow professionals to positions of prestige are important. Certification by recognized boards is a minimum qualification. Awards and honors are helpful. Affiliations with universities and teaching positions are impressive to judges and juries, who assume the universities attract the best and that such teachers keep up with current scientific knowledge. In short, whatever demonstrates a thorough knowledge of the field, and recognition of such knowledge by others, is helpful.

The issue of bias is always raised with respect to experts because they are being paid for their time, and the misperception is that their opinion has been bought. In order to combat this problem, lawyers look for experts who appear to have some independence. Thus, most lawyers try to avoid hiring professional witnesses—individuals who spend a great deal of time testifying in litigation as experts. The lawyer would rather try to find an individual who does not testify frequently. In addition, when a physician has previously testified on a medical issue, it helps if he or she has testified on both sides of the fence—for both plaintiffs and defendants—thus showing independence. Of course, the attorney must be careful to make sure that the expert does not have any prior damaging testimony that conflicts with his or her opinion in the case at hand.

Attorneys favor a physician who is recognized by peers as a true expert; such a position helps explain to the judge or jury why the lawyer has called him or her as a witness and thus helps refute the charge that he or she is a hired gun. Similarly, the attorney wants a physician whose charges are reasonable. If an expert's fees are high, the impression is created that his or her opinion is in fact for hire.

Finally, a physician is worthless as an expert witness unless he or she can communicate knowledge to a judge and jury. The judge and jury will follow an expert's opinion only if they understand it and are persuaded by it. Thus, a physician must be able to explain technical knowledge to nonmedical persons in a fashion that they can understand. Moreover, the presentation must appear to be based on adequate knowledge, be given in an unbiased manner, and withstand a nonmedical person's test of reasonableness—does it sound right and make sense? If an opinion is given in a manner in which it does not sound right or make sense, the judge or jury will simply reject it. The physician must have the ability to teach the judge or jury about his or her field of medicine in a convincing manner.

Attorney-Expert Relations

When an attorney requests a physician to testify as an expert witness in a case or provide assistance to the attorney in litigation, the attorney should communicate the nature of the physician's duties and the attorney's expectations. The attorney must give directions in a neutral manner so that the physician's independence will not be compromised. The physician must assure that he or she has all available relevant information, including all past medical records and reports, depositions, and claim-related documents and correspondence, and that his or her research is thorough and his or her opinion is unimpeachable.

Physicians often receive calls from attorneys at a very late stage of litigation, and the parameters of an attorney–expert relationship are not well defined. Certain ground rules should be spelled out at the beginning of the relationship. The amount of the fee to be paid by the attorney, and when it will be paid, should be established. Most physicians charge an hourly rate and send a bill after they have testified, although for prolonged cases, interim billing is appropriate and avoids surprises. Moreover, the physician may want to give an estimate of how much time he or she will need to prepare the opinion, so that the attorney will not be shocked by the bill.

The physician must remember that whatever information he or she obtains or relies upon in forming an opinion will be subject to discovery by the other side. Thus, the physician does not want any explicit directions from the attorney as to the final outcome of the expert's opinion, for fear it will appear that he or she is being led around by the attorney. Similarly, the physician does not want to review any document that will "prejudice" his or her opinion, such as the attorney's client's position paper. Rather, the physician should expect only to receive all information relevant to his or her inquiry, and that the outer limits of the investigation should be set forth by the attorney. Of course, this should include all of the medical records of the case.

A physician must be thorough in investigation and analysis. The physician must make sure he or she has obtained all relevant documents, performed all appropriate tests, and fully researched available medical literature. A good attorney will help a physician obtain all appropriate information and assure that the investigation has been thorough. In preparing for trial, the attorney will often play devil's advocate in a mock questioning session and test the physician's opinion.

A question often arises as to whether the opposing attorney can talk to the patient's physician. If the physician is hired by the patient's attorney and is initially retained as an expert witness, the answer is no, except via a formal deposition with the patient's attorney being present. If the physician's treatment occurred before the litigation was filed and was in the ordinary course of business (a treating physician), then most jurisdictions hold that the opposing attorney can engage in an *ex parte* interview with the doctor, if the doctor is so inclined, in the same manner that any witness in a litigation can be interviewed. In this circumstance, as a treating physician, he or she is not an expert witness for either the patient or for the party the patient is suing. Thus, similar to a witness to a car crash, either side's attorney can try to interview the doctor and get a witness statement or report from the doctor. Some courts, however, have taken a contrary view, ruling that the physician—patient relationship is special; those courts do not allow *ex parte* contacts, but rather limit the patient's adversary to a formal deposition in order to determine the doctor's opinion.

The Physician's Report

The physician acting as an expert witness presents his or her opinion in two forms: the report and the direct examination testimony at the trial when he or she is questioned by the hiring attorney. Because this presentation is the key to the physician's assistance to the lawyer, the presentation must be well prepared and flawless.

The physician must be extremely careful in preparing the written report, because once he or she has put something in writing, he or she will be discredited if he or she later varies from the report. Moreover, the physician usually only has one opportunity to prepare a report, as a good opposing attorney will discover if any drafts of the report were prepared. For these reasons, many attorneys prefer to receive oral reports and request that the physician either not prepare a written report or do so only after conferring with the attorney. On the other hand, if there is extensive contact with the attorney, the inference is that the attorney unduly influenced the physician's opinion. Each attorney will have a unique approach for dealing with this situation. Usually, however, a skilled and experienced attorney will trust the expert to prepare a report without interference. If, however, the report is harmful to the attorney's case, he or she will not use it and will simply hire another physician as the expert witness. The report of an expert witness who was retained for but not used in litigation is normally not discoverable by the other side.

Direct Examination of the Physician

Whether a report is prepared or not, the physician may testify at trial. The attorney will ask the physician questions, and the expert will answer them. One cannot lead one's own witness; the questions cannot suggest the answer. Thus the attorney and expert must rehearse the physician's testimony so that there will be no surprises and to ensure that the testimony is clear and convincing.

Where there is an expert on the other side, the physician will have to not only convince the judge or jury of the appropriateness of his or her opinion but also that the opinion is more credible than the views of the opposing expert. This can be achieved by explaining the thoroughness of the investigation, detailing the literature that supports the analysis, pressing the logical nature of the opinion, and attacking (in a low key manner) the opponent's expert's opinion by highlighting the flaws in his or her investigation and analysis.

Cross-Examination

Every expert witness will be cross-examined by the other side's attorney, who will attempt to discredit the expert witness. The opponent's attorney will attack the physician's credentials, independence, thoroughness, and analysis. The attorney in his or her cross-examination may become hostile and even angry with the physician. It is at this point that the good expert witnesses are separated from the bad ones. The good expert will keep composure and not only repel the attack calmly but also use the opportunity to reinforce in the mind of the judge or jury the propriety of his or her opinion.

The opposing attorney will do his or her best, through questioning, to demonstrate that the physician is stupid, is ill-informed, did not have all relevant facts necessary to evaluate the situation, was improperly paid off by the hiring attorney, and provided an analysis that is illogical and contrary to established scientific principles. To achieve this result, the opposing attorney will use any prior writings or testimony of the physician as well as any available scientific literature.

During the cross-examination, the physician must not lose sight of the key factors that are used to evaluate him or her: credentials, independence, and expertise. Thus, the physician should be prepared for all questions and respond with informed answers. The physician does not want to appear to be trying to avoid a question, to be hiding anything, or to be ignorant. He or she must not argue with the attorney, but rather must directly answer the attorney's questions without appearing to be an advocate. A dispassionate and direct answer is called for by the physician. However, the witness is allowed to answer any question fully. Thus, if an answer gives a false or misleading impression, the physician can and should fully answer the question by not only providing the information requested but by adding his or her explanation of why the information is incomplete or gives a false impression. In this manner, the expert witness can not only stand up to the questioning but also can use the cross-examination to continue to press for the acceptance of his or her opinion.

Finally, the physician should realize that no matter how prepared he or she is, he or she may still encounter a surprise question. At this point, the physician must remember to answer the question in a direct, straightforward manner, and that it is the lawyer's job to win the case. Thus, no matter what the question and its apparent adverse inference, the expert witness must always follow the cardinal rule for every witness: be truthful and candid. No witness has ever failed when following this simple rule. Juries can see when a witness tries to avoid a question or gives an incredible answer. Such a response taints the expert's entire testimony.

The Physician's Status in Answering Medical–Legal Questions

The first thing a physician must do is clarify his or her status. If the physician is a treating physician, then there is a physician–patient relationship, which means that the physician owes a duty of care to the patient and that communications between the physician and patient are confidential, although, as noted in the following, the confidentiality can be waived. If the patient goes directly to the physician, there is no question as to the existence of the physician–patient relationship. An examinee may present via a referral from an employer or insurer, and there may still be a physician–patient relationship. For example, in approximately half the states, under workers' compensation laws, the employer selects the treating physician. Nevertheless, the selected physician owes the same duty of care to the injured worker as to any other patient. If the physician has any question as to whether he or she is a treating physician or provider, the source of the referral should be consulted as well as the patient. It is important that all three (the physician, referral source, and patient) have the same understanding.

Often, the physician is not hired by the patient, but rather is conducting an examination for another party. This occurs in pre-employment physicals and in the so-called independent medical examination (IME). When a physician performs an IME, he or she is an expert witness for the person or entity who retained him or her. If a person puts his or her medical condition into issue (e.g., a car accident lawsuit or a workers' compensation claim), then the defendant/employer is entitled to have a physician of his or her choice perform an examination. In such situations, the physician owes his or her duty to the hiring entity, and not the examinee. The physician must, however, clarify his or her status with the individual. Thus the physician should inform the individual that there is no physician–patient relationship and that he or she will not report his or her findings to the individual (any privilege extends only to the referring party).

If the physician is clearly not treating the examinee and the physician has no duty toward the worker (e.g., pre-employment physicals or an IME), it is of critical importance that the examinee be informed of this information up front and that he or she sign a document recognizing and agreeing to this arrangement. For example, the examinee might sign a statement as follows: "I recognize that Dr. XXX is performing a pre-employment physical examination on me at the request of YYY Inc. I understand that Dr. XXX is not my physician, I am not his patient, and he owes no duty to me to look for, or disclose, any medical condition I may have. I further understand and release Dr. XXX to disclose any findings to YYY Inc. and I agree that these findings will not be disclosed to me since the examination conducted by Dr. XXX was at the request and expense of YYY Inc."

What if the physician, performing an IME, discovers a correctable life-threatening condition? Can he or she inform the examinee of it? Obviously, most defendants and employers would never restrict the IME physician from giving the examinee this information. However, if the IME physician has any concern, he or she should make it clear to the defendant or employer, when he or she is retained, that he or she will be permitted to disclose such information to the examinee.

Potential Malpractice Liability

Physicians dealing with disability, like any other physicians, commit malpractice if their treatment or actions do not follow a reasonable standard of care. Of particular concern are the failure to notify a worker of an adverse condition or of risk of future problems and the premature return to the job or return without adequate work restrictions.

Workers' compensation is the exclusive remedy only between the employee (the first party) and the employer and its agents or other employees (the second party). If any third party negligently contributes to a worker's injury, the employee may sue that third party in civil court, outside the workers' compensation system. For example, if a crane collapses at work and injures a worker, the worker can recover workers' compensation from the employer and sue the manufacturer of the crane for building a defective crane. The most famous lawsuits of this type are by insulators who handled asbestos in their jobs. Millions of dollars have been recovered from the manufacturers of asbestos. In the same manner, a physician who negligently injures a worker when treating a work injury can be sued for malpractice. The malpractice action for that physician will be no different from a malpractice action against a physician who improperly cared for a non-work-related illness. Moreover, if the employee does not sue, the employer or insurance carrier, who paid the increased workers' compensation benefits caused by the doctor's malpractice, may be entitled to sue the physician for the increased workers' compensation benefits paid as a result of the physician's malpractice.

Failure to Notify the Worker of an Adverse Condition or of an Increased Risk

If there is a physician–patient relationship, then the physician owes a duty to the patient to disclose any adverse condition and to notify the patient of any risks of future health problems related to the condition. For the physician involved in a disability evaluation, this area of liability is often overlooked (see Chapter 1 for the definitions of impairment and disability).

When an injury causing an impairment is known to the physician, he or she may use too narrow a focus when examining the patient. For example, if a chest roentgenogram is being read to determine whether the injured worker suffered a broken rib, there may still be a duty on the part of the physician to look for any nodule that might represent a tumor. Certainly, the physician does not want to be in the position where the lesion is discovered a year later, and the lesion can be seen clearly on the chest roentgenogram taken for the work injury a year earlier. To a trial jury, that failure is clearly malpractice.

Conversely, if the physician is treating the worker for a sprained small toe, there is no obligation to take a chest roentgenogram and look for other abnormalities. Physicians must, of course, use common sense. They must recognize that workers can suffer illnesses and injuries outside the workplace. The patient must be looked at not only as a worker but also as a patient. In addition, the physician should carefully document the patient's complaints and what the physician did and did not investigate. Indeed, unless it is absolutely clear, the physician should inform the patient that the examination and treatment are limited to the work injury, or the disability at issue, and that the physician did not perform a complete physical examination.

Similarly, the physician should be careful to advise the patient of any risk that the current condition involves. For example, if a worker is recovering from disc surgery, and the worker is being returned to manual labor, the risk of a recurrent disc problem should be carefully explained to the patient. As with all patients, the doctor should assume nothing. Rather, care should be taken to explain the condition fully to the patient and explain in detail (and preferably in writing) what the patient can and cannot do and the risks involved. Of course, the physician should also advise the patient of what problem signs to look for that may indicate the need for further medical evaluation.

Premature Return to Work or Inadequate Work Restrictions

The physician should be especially concerned with the possibility that a worker will allege that the physician returned the employee to work prematurely or with inadequate work restrictions. In the context of a workplace injury, employers are motivated to return the injured worker to work as soon as possible, with the minimum level of work restrictions possible. Conversely, some employees want to stay out of work as long as possible and, when they return to work, they want their duties to be as light as possible. The effort some employees put into not working can surprise even the most hardened soul in this field.

Suffice it to say that the prudent physician should avoid being caught between these two tensions. The physician should carefully document any actions taken and explain them to the employee as well as to the employer. If the employee objects to the physician's actions or shows signs of being a malingerer, the physician may want to refer the patient for a second opinion so that the return to work cannot reasonably be challenged.

A second opinion has the advantage of covering the initial physician's opinion. With a second opinion in hand, the physician is no longer alone in his or her assessment. Moreover, if the physician is an in-house doctor, for workers' compensation litigation the employer will often want a second opinion from an independent outside physician. Although a second opinion is not needed in every case, the experienced physician can usually spot the problem cases: excessive subjective complaints, extreme reluctance to return to work, desire for overly severe work restrictions, an unusually frequent history of minor injuries, or engagement in physician-shopping. In such cases, wise employers realize that a second opinion is appropriate preparation for litigation over the disability claim.

Liability for Unauthorized Release of Information (Libel and Slander and Contractual Interference)

A physician evaluating a disability has a general duty to keep information concerning patients confidential. Of course, when a worker files a workers' compensation claim or a law-suit to recover for an injury, this usually waives any privilege of confidentiality and allows the employer/defendant to be informed of the patient's treatment. Indeed, in most jurisdictions, in the case of work injuries, the treating physician must file medical reports with the industrial commission and the employer. Similarly, in many jurisdictions, state statutes require that gunshot wounds or contagious diseases must be reported.

In the absence of a waiver or statutory duty to disclose information, the physician has a duty to protect the patient's confidences and the confidentiality of any treatment given. The physician's breach of this trust can result in liability for invasion of privacy or breach of the patient—physician relationship.

Although the physician may have a defense for disclosure based on a duty imposed by law to file a report, or a duty to the public interest, the physician should be sure of his or her position before making the disclosure. It is generally safer to obtain a consent form, after disclosing to the patient all relevant facts, including to whom the disclosure is being made and what records will be disclosed. A second option is to have the employer or defendant obtain a subpoena for the records.

The hardest cases are ones where there are conflicting duties toward the patient and the public and there are no clear statutory or regulatory directives as to which duty should prevail. Unfortunately, when the physician must act, only later will the court tell the physician if he or she made the right choice. As a general rule, common sense is the best guide.

In emergency situations, the physician should make the minimum disclosure necessary to protect others. Thus, if emergency personnel are about to treat a cut on a patient with AIDS, the physician should advise the personnel that the Occupational Safety and Health Administration requires medical workers to use gloves and that they should follow similar universal precautions. However, if it can be avoided, the physician should not disclose that the reason for the precautions is AIDS.

Physicians should also be aware of federal and state regulations that protect certain medical records, even limiting the release of alcohol and drug abuse records. Physicians must remember that they with consent can be sued for libel and slander. Although opinions are not actionable and testimony in court is privileged, physicians should always be cautious about how they make negative statements and to whom.

Truth is always a defense to an action for libel (written defamation) or slander (oral defamation), but it can often be an expensive process to litigate the truth of a statement. Thus physicians must be careful of what they say and to whom. Generally, libel and slander laws only protect one's reputation. For example, if a physician makes a false statement (e.g., that worker is a liar) and it injures the worker's reputation, then the defamatory statement is actionable. Diagnostic opinions generally would not affect one's reputation and thus would not be actionable under the law of libel and slander.

In the psychiatric arena, the fields of medicine and libel law overlap. Courts have held that psychiatric reports that state that a worker is mentally unfit to work are actionable because mental illness reflects on one's reputation and ability to work. Whether this principle would be extended to calling a worker a malingerer or simply physically unfit to work is unclear.

The physician's statement, even if defamatory and untrue, may still be protected if privileged. There is an absolute privilege for any testimony in a court of law. Moreover, there is generally a qualified privilege if a statement is made in a reasonable manner and for a proper purpose. Generally, a physician's statement to an employer as to the fitness of a worker to perform his or her job enjoys a qualified privilege. This privilege is qualified because it is lost if the physician acts with malice—knowing the statement is false or with reckless disregard for its truth.

Thus, generally, physicians cannot be sued for their opinions concerning a worker's ability to work unless the statement made was false and was made with recklessness. This is a hard standard for a worker to meet. Nevertheless, physicians should make sure they have taken steps such that their conduct is far from reckless, and thus they will not have to prove the truth of their statements via expensive litigation.

Physicians can also be sued for negligent interference with a contractual relationship, which is a relatively new but developing doctrine. Thus, even if there is no physician—patient relationship, the physician may still owe a duty to the worker not to interfere negligently with the worker's relationship with the employer. For example, if a physician performing an examination of a worker for a job application is negligent and incorrectly states that the worker is in poor health, the physician could arguably be held liable to the worker for negligent interference with the worker's contractual relationship–getting a job with the employer.

Insurance Coverage

Many physicians do not worry about their potential liability because they have malpractice insurance. There are two problems with this attitude. First, a claim may cause an increase in the doctor's insurance premium or even cancellation of the policy. Secondly, not all claims are covered by all policies. An insurance policy is a contract. The insurance company says it will defend against and pay certain types of claims when certain conditions are met. Thus a physician must carefully examine the policy to see what is and is not covered and what the limits are. This is much like a homeowner's policy, which may not cover damage from floods, or an automobile insurance policy that does not cover the driver if he or she is legally drunk or that only pays a maximum of $300,000 in all cases.

If a physician has a malpractice policy, it may not cover libel or slander. It may not cover the physician in acting as an independent medical examiner, or when a report is written based on a review of records without seeing the patient. This may not be considered the practice of medicine so as to trigger coverage. Rather, an errors or emissions policy may be needed. The physician should read the policy carefully and have any questions answered in writing by the insurance company. It is critically important that the physician know what coverage has and has not been purchased.

Returning a Worker to Work

One of the critical and most demanding tasks of a medical provider is deciding when a worker can return to work. A premature return to the job can result in an aggravation of the original injury and longer impairment. An unnecessarily delayed return results in increased workers' compensation costs and an unhappy employer. A balance is achieved when the physician understands the patient and communicates effectively with the employer.

In the rush to have a high-volume practice, some physicians sometimes forget that not all patients are alike. Some employees like their work and want to be with their friends on the job; they are eager to return to work. Some patients believe it shows strength to work while hurt, much like a football player who plays while hurt. Some workers just want to get out of the house and away from their spouse.

Other workers are overly concerned with their health and have unfounded, but real, fears about becoming reinjured. They wrongly equate minimal pain with permanent injury. Some are unrealistically unwilling to accept the slightest amount of pain, despite the fact that their work is no more physically stressful than getting dressed in the morning and engaging in the normal activities of life.

Finally, there are those workers who believe that they deserve a free ride because they were injured and those who simply want to cheat the system. It is almost beyond belief the efforts some people make not to work. If their energies could be channeled into their job, they would be highly productive workers. Some workers will stay out of work without pay for over a year without any adverse condition, just so they can obtain a workers' compensation settlement. They believe that their cheating and lying is justified because they were hurt and deserve money.

A physician loses credibility and effectiveness if he or she does not understand that these different types of persons exist. The physician's care and opinions must take into account the individuality of the patient. For the "tough" worker, the physician must take care not to recommend injurious activities. The physician must carefully explain to the employee why he or she must remain out of work and why, when he or she returns, he or she will need light duty restrictions for a short time. The key is to emphasize that if he or she tries too much too early, reinjury may occur and permanently disability may result.

For the hypochondriac (and most people have a degree of hypochondria at one time or another), the physician must explain to the worker why it is safe to return to work and how the activity of work is a form of therapy that will help the recovery. The physician should explain how the light-duty restrictions will protect the worker and that minimal pain should be tolerated.

For the malingerer, the physician should inform the employer and release the employee to return to work. Of course, the physician should be sure of this opinion, but it is often easy enough to verify by observing the patient and questioning persons in contact with the patient. The physician should not avoid the issue by simply referring the patient to another doctor or a pain clinic.

In working with employers, the most critical step is for the physician to recognize the nature of the employee and explain this to the employer. Most employers do not want to treat their employees unfairly; they want to do the right thing. However, many physicians believe whatever their patients say and do whatever the patient wants, which has caused many employers to lose faith in the credibility of physicians.

A physician should not simply hand out disability slips whenever a worker asks that his or her time be covered and still expect the respect of the employer. Yet some physicians cover time out despite a lack of objective findings and without seeing the patient during the covered time period. Similarly, a physician should not excuse a worker from a job without knowing the actual physical demands of the job. Likewise, advice on work restrictions should be clear and realistic. A doctor should not say a worker cannot bend; one must bend in order to go to the bathroom. Rather, the doctor should say excessive bending would be unwise, or better yet, should quantify exposure to bending, such as suggesting no more than five spine flexions per hour.

Employers understand rational and clear medical analysis. Yet most doctors are afraid to communicate with the employer, or they simply refuse to take the time to do so. This not only results in an unhappy employer, but it can reduce the effectiveness of the physician's care. In returning a worker to the job, the doctor must know what the job is, as well as what light-duty alternatives and work restrictions are practical. Communication with the employer is the key. Often the worker is a poor historian and communicator. A 2-minute call to the employer can give the physician invaluable information and result in a satisfied employer.

If a physician engages in prudent medical care, and explains the reasons for his or her decisions to the patient and employer, all except the malingerers will be happy. However, if a physician simply believes all subjective complaints of a patient, in the absence of any objective findings, then the employer will be unhappy and in the long run the physician will have done a disservice to the patient.

In returning a worker to work, the physician must also consider the Americans with Disabilities Act (ADA) requirements on the employer (see Chapter 47). In order to reduce workers' compensation costs and prevent injured workers from getting used to being at home but on the payroll (so-called "workers' compensation syndrome"), many employers have reserved light-duty work for employees injured on the job. Other employers, ignoring the economic effect of workers' compensation liability have refused to take injured employees back if they had any work restrictions. Many employers would not accommodate work restrictions if a personal injury or illness is not covered by workers' compensation. The ADA has changed all of this.

The return to work of an injured worker used to be simple. The worker returned to the employer with a light-duty slip or work restrictions from his or her physician. The employer could have refused to take back a worker with such restrictions or could have claimed that there was no work within the work restrictions. There were no means for the employee to challenge the employer's decision. The ADA now requires much more. First, the employee can challenge—in court—the employer's decision and the physician's work restrictions. Second, the employer must make reasonable accommodations that will allow the employee to return to work despite work restrictions. Although the employer need not create light-duty jobs per se, the reasonable accommodations of part-time or modified work schedules, job restructuring, and reassignment to vacant positions come close to being equivalent to such a light-duty mandate.

To assure compliance with the ADA, the following procedure is recommended. Physicians must provide substantial detail and quantification in their work restrictions. Full-page forms are available that quantify by-the-hour activities such as standing, walking, and sitting. When a worker brings in his or her work restrictions, the employer should send the worker to his or her manager or supervisor. The manager or supervisor should then compare the restrictions to the worker's written job description and circle those aspects of the job that the worker is prohibited from performing. The manager or supervisor should then send the circled job description to the physician and ask him or her to confirm that the interpretation of the work restrictions is correct and that the doctor agrees the worker cannot safely perform the circled duties and that the work restrictions are based on the ADA safety standard—designed only to preclude probable injuries, not merely possible injuries.

The physician should confirm that the correct standard was used, and the employer should confirm that any of the circled precluded tasks are essential functions of the job. The manager or supervisor (or the personnel, safety, or medical department) must then consider reasonable accommodations that would allow the worker to perform the essential functions of the job (for a discussion of the concept of "essential functions," see Chapter 47). Only when the employer determines how many tasks the worker cannot perform can that evaluation be made.

For example, a common work restriction is "no bending." If a supervisor applied the restriction literally, he or she would disqualify a worker who had to bend once a day to pick up a pencil. Subsequently, if the case went to trial, and the physician took the witness stand, he or she would in all likelihood testify that he or she really meant no excessive bending; or no bending with the back, but that bending with the knees is fine; or no bending and lifting heavy objects. It is best to clarify this before the employer spends tens of thousands of dollars in legal fees preparing for trial.

The next step, which most companies have never considered, is reasonable accommodations. Someone must evaluate them, even though that task does not fall neatly into the framework of the traditional management departments—personnel, safety, medical, or production. Continuing with the example of the "no bending" restriction, possible reasonable accommodations might include purchasing a crane to lift objects, having an assistant put an object on the workbench, or reassigning the lifting to another worker (if it is a nonessential function). All these options must be considered and discussed with the worker. It is wise, of course, to document all such efforts to consider and make reasonable accommodations.

Occupational Physicians' and Nurses' Status: Co-Employee Immunity and the Physician–Patient Relationship

Many medical providers are in-house nurses or doctors; they are employees of the injured worker's employer. Thus, the injured worker and the physician are co-employees. Under normal circumstances, an injured worker's exclusive remedy against the employer and its agents and employees (i.e., coworkers) is the workers' compensation remedy. Neither the employer nor co-workers can be sued for negligence; thus being an employee may reduce the medical provider's risk of a lawsuit by coworker employees.

This general rule has normally been applied to company doctors and nurses who are true employees of the employer of the injured worker. Thus even if the company physician–employee errs in treating the injured worker, the worker cannot sue the physician for malpractice. Rather, the sole remedy is workers' compensation benefits. Company physicians should not, however, blindly assume that this general rule applies to them. At least four states currently recognize exceptions to this rule, and instituting these exceptions appears to be a trend.

Both California and Georgia courts recognize the dual capacity doctrine. Under this doctrine, the company physician–employee is said to have two separate capacities: as a company employee (i.e., coworker of the injured worker) and as the injured worker's physician. In this second capacity, the injured worker may sue the company physician if he or she commits malpractice.

At least two other jurisdictions have used a combination of the dual capacity doctrine and semantics to hold company physician–employee liable for malpractice. Both Indiana and Louisiana have held that a physician, in terms of malpractice liability, is always an independent contractor (as opposed to an employee) because a corporation cannot practice medicine and thus direct the work of the physician. As an independent contractor, the physician cannot benefit from workers' compensation exclusivity.

The dual-capacity independent contractor doctrines highlight one of the potential pitfalls that exist in all jurisdictions: even in those jurisdictions that apply the coworker immunity to company physician employees, the company physician must be a true employee of the corporation. For example, the fact that the patient was referred to the physician, or that the company requested an opinion from the physician, does not make the physician a company employee. Rather, the physician would be an independent contractor, and thus liable for any malpractice. To be an employee, withholding taxes, Social Security taxes, and similar employee status actions would have to have been applied to the physician. Conversely, at least one court has held that the fact that the company physician is a part-time employee does not mean the coworker immunity is inapplicable.

Similarly, the company physician may be able to argue that, although not an employee of the employer, he or she was its agent, and, as such, the workers' compensation exclusivity bar applies. The question then becomes whether the physician was an agent of the employer or whether the actions were taken independently of the employer and in the status as a physician.

There is one exception to the workers' compensation exclusivity bar that applies to everyone. Workers' compensation is a replacement system for negligence lawsuits. It is not designed to replace liability for intentional torts. Thus the exclusivity bar does not prevent an action for an intentional tort. The classic example is an employee who, dissatisfied with a recent raise, strikes the foreman. The employee's assault is an intentional tort, and thus the foreman can sue the employee. Moreover, for intentional torts, the victim can recover punitive damages as well as compensatory damages. Of concern to physicians, libel and slander are intentional torts.

In addition, willful and wanton disregard for safety concerns is also considered, in some jurisdictions, to be an intentional tort. Thus employers have been held liable, outside the workers' compensation system, for ignoring unsafe levels of airborne lead particles and fraudulently concealing the hazards of asbestos, as well as for intentionally concealing the fact that a worker had asbestosis and that further exposure would be harmful. Although in most cases the employer is the target of the lawsuit, a company physician who has aided in defrauding the workers can be and has been named as a defendant.

Even if the physician does not benefit from the coworker workers' compensation exclusivity bar, it is possible to escape liability if there is no physician–patient relationship. For example, some courts have held that when a physician performs a pre-employment physical for an employer and gives no report or advice to the worker, there is no physician–patient relationship with the worker, and thus the worker cannot sue the physician for malpractice. That is, if there is no physician–patient relationship, the physician owes no duty to the worker, and the worker has no reasonable expectations of the physician. Of course, the physician's actions may create other causes of action, such as for libel and slander or negligent interference with a contract (between the employer and the worker).

Occupational physicians thus need to be aware of the applicable legal doctrines in their state, and must define clearly their relationship with the patient and the employer: Is the physician an employee of the employer or an independent contractor? Is the physician the employer's agent or the patient's treating physician? What, if any, other duties does the physician owe the employee?

Conclusion

If a physician understands the legal issues at stake, and his or her role in resolving them, he or she will be much more effective in providing an opinion, and significantly reduce his or her exposure to potential liability.

CHAPTER

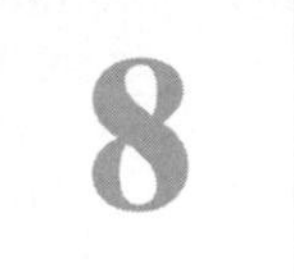

The Physician as a Witness

LYNN C. SLABY, JD

Cross-examination is an art, not a science. *Black's Law Dictionary* defines cross-examination as "the examination of a witness upon a trial or hearing, or upon taking a deposition, by the party opposed to the one who produced him, upon his evidence given in chief, to test its truths, to further development, or for other purposes."[1] The specific purpose for cross-examining a witness is to test the truthfulness of that witness's testmony. The cross-examining attorney is attempting to challenge the truthfulness of the witness and the opinion.

Witness testimony is evidence that will be heard and evaluated by a trier of fact. That trier of fact can be a judge or a jury. The Rules of Civil Procedure and the Rules of Evidence control what witnesses can testify to.

> The purpose of these rules is to provide procedures for the adjudication of causes to the end that the truth may be ascertained and proceedings justly determined. The principles of the common law shall supplement the provisions of these rules, and the rules shall be construed to state the principles of the common law unless the rule clearly indicates that a change is intended. These rules shall not supersede substantive statutory provisions.[2(p399)]

By standardizing the rules of evidence, the State has created a level playing field for all litigants.

Although the rules establish standard procedures for witnesses, there are exceptions. Expert testimony is one such exception. The exception for expert testimony is specifically carved out within the rules themselves and the expert witness is thus governed by the rules specifically set forth in these provisions.[3]

Certifying an Expert and Guiding the Testimony

Certification as an Expert

Before an expert witness is permitted to testify, he or she must first be qualified as an expert. The judge will make this determination. The judge will also determine if the information to be relayed by the expert witness is relevant, and if relevant, if the information is privileged. The Supreme Court of the United States has set out criteria to be used by federal judges to determine both the qualifications and the reliability of an expert. This case is known as the Daubert decision.[4] Although not followed in all states, the Daubert decision sets up criteria for defense counsel to follow when attacking the reliability of an expert opinion. Judges in the federal court system will be the evaluators of whether an expert may testify. There are four factors federal courts will consider[5]:

1. Testing
2. Peer review
3. Error rates in the methodology employed by the witness
4. The general scientific acceptability of the opinions elicited

Experts testifying in state courts may not be challenged under the Daubert decision. However, that does not mean that an attorney will not cross-examine the expert on each of the four criteria. There have also been several articles written about what the judges will look for when arriving at a decision to exclude an expert's testimony. The federal courts and the states that follow Daubert do so to prequalify an expert.[6] That is, the judge will make a determination before the expert has the opportunity to testify before a jury. The use of Daubert may save valuable jury time.

Professor Daniel Capra, in "The Daubert Puzzle,"[7] set out five red flags that indicate a serious admissibility question under Daubert:

1. Improper extrapolation—drawing an unsupported conclusion from an accepted premise
2. Reliance on anecdotal evidence—basing an opinion solely on personal experience with patients or on a few case studies
3. Reliance on temporal proximity—basing a conclusion about causation on the short time span between exposure to a substance and the subsequent injury
4. Failure to consider other causes
5. Subjectivity—not being able to explain a methodology in objective terms

Knowing that judges will be looking for these red flags, attorneys will cross-examine the expert on these specific items.

Experts can still be challenged in the state courts that do not follow Daubert. The attorneys will cross-examine the expert on all the issues in Daubert. The attorneys will point out the weaknesses of the expert to the judge in an effort to get the expert disqualified. If that does not work, the attorney will use apparent weaknesses in argument to get the jury to disbelieve the expert's opinion.

Typically, witnesses are prohibited from testifying to any fact or matter of which they do not have personal knowledge. The general rule is that the witness must be testifying to something that his or her own senses perceived.[8] Additionally, under the rules, a lay witness cannot give his or her opinion. This is because conclusions based on the evidence are left to the province of the trier of fact. However, it is not unusual for attorneys to seek medical opinions by experts who have no firsthand knowledge of the facts in the litigation. Rendering opinion evidence is what distinguishes the expert witness from the lay witness.

Of course, there are exceptions to each rule. A lay witness may testify to an opinion under two circumstances. These exceptions are limited to the following[9]:

Opinions rationally based on the perception of the witness

Opinions helpful to a clear understanding of the testimony or the determination of a fact in issue

Outside of these limited exceptions, in order to render an opinion a witness must be certified as an expert. A witness may testify as an expert if all of the following apply[10]:

Either the witness's testimony relates to matters beyond the knowledge or experience possessed by laypersons, or it dispels a misconception common among laypersons.

The witness is qualified as an expert by specialized knowledge, skill, experience, training, or education regarding the subject matter of the testimony.

The witness's testimony is based on reliable scientific, technical, or other specialized information. To the extent that the testimony reports the result of a procedure, test, or experiment, the testimony is reliable only if all of the following apply:

The theory upon which the procedure, test, or experiment is based is objectively verifiable or is validly derived from widely accepted knowledge, facts, or principles.

The design of the procedure, test, or experiment reliably implements the theory.

The particular procedure, test, or experiment was conducted in a way that will yield an accurate result.

On consideration of these criteria and the potential expert's credentials, the court will determine whether to certify the witness as an expert.

An expert witness must be competent to testify. *Black's Law Dictionary* defines competency as "the presence of those characteristics, or the absence of those disabilities, which render a witness legally fit and qualified to give testimony in a court of justice."[11(p257)] Competency differs from credibility. Competency to testify must be considered before the witness can give the opinion. Credibility concerns the degree of credit to be given to the testimony. Competency denotes the personal qualifications of the witness. Credibility deals with the witness's veracity. A witness may be competent and give incredible testimony. The witness could be incompetent to testify and yet the evidence, if received, could be perfectly credible. There are different rules in different states regarding competency.[12]

In some states, a psychiatrist would be competent to testify as to a mental deficiency, but a psychologist may not be.[13] In Ohio, a person is presumed to be competent to testify. The exceptions are young individuals or specific situations such as testimony in medical malpractice cases. In Ohio, for example, the rule on competency limits expert testimony in a civil action against a physician, podiatrist, or hospital arising out of the physician's, podiatrist's, or hospital's diagnosis, care, or treatment of any person. In order to be competent to testify in these matters, the expert must devote at least one-half of his or her professional time to active clinical practice in his or her field of licensure or to its instruction in an accredited school.[14]

The importance of the relevancy of the evidence testified to by an expert witness cannot be overstated. Evidence is relevant when it has "any tendency to make the existence of any fact that is of consequence to the determination of the action more probable or less probable than it would be without the evidence."[15] For example, if a cardiologist testifies to an opinion about a patient's a broken leg, such testimony would not normally be relevant. The further the expert strays from his or her field of expertise, the less relevant the evidence becomes.

Content of the Expert Opinion

An expert can give an opinion on facts or data of which he or she has personal knowledge. The expert can also testify as to facts that have been admitted into evidence but have not personally been observed by the expert. The expert may testify in terms of opinion or inference based on the facts presented to the expert. The opinion may be in response to a hypothetical question. The facts in the hypothetical question must either be personally known by the expert or have been introduced into evidence before they are used as the basis for the expert's opinion. Judges, however, often allow attorneys to present facts to the expert if the attorney states that the facts will be offered in later testimony. The expert should be careful in responding to a hypothetical question. If the attorney presents facts that are not personally known to the expert, the expert should point out that the opinion is based on something of which he or she is not aware.[16] An example of some questions follows:

> Question: Doctor, you testified that, in your opinion, based on A, B, C, D, E, and F, you have come to your professional conclusion. Now, doctor, if we add S, T, U, and V, would that change your opinion?
>
> Answer: It may; however, I was not aware of S, T, U, or V when making my diagnosis.
>
> Question: Well, Doctor, if you based your opinion on A, B, C, D, E, and F, what if you didn't have C and D—would that change your opinion?
>
> Answer: It may; however, I had to consider all of the factors that I had before me at the time of my diagnosis.

The expert will testify to facts of which he or she has personal knowledge. Then, based on that knowledge, the expert will give an opinion on what conclusions he or she has developed. The expert's background, training, experience, and education allow an expert to perceive facts and draw conclusions from those facts. The expert will testify that to a reasonable degree of medical certainty the conclusion is more likely than not to be what the opinion says. The nonexpert can only testify to the facts themselves.

Legal Standards

Expert opinion testimony is either given to help a party meet the burden of proof in the case or used by an opponent to disprove the theory propounded. Whether an expert is testifying for the plaintiff or for the defense, it is important to understand the role of the burden of proof.

The burden of proof in a case is generally upon the plaintiff. The plaintiff is the party who is attempting to be made whole, usually with money damages. The plaintiff has the responsibility to establish who, what, where, how, and when he or she was injured. These are negligence tort claims. The burden in negligence cases is "beyond a preponderance of the evidence."[17] That is, the plaintiff must show that there is more evidence on his or her side of the case than there is on the defendant's side. The plaintiff must prove that there was an injury, that the defendant did or did not do something and that act or omission was the direct cause of the injury, and that there was a monetary loss.

The plaintiff in a tort case has the burden of establishing the following[18]:

1. There was a duty owed by the defendant to the plaintiff.
2. That duty was breached.
3. Because of that breach the plaintiff was injured.
4. There was a direct relation between the breach of the duty and the injury (this is known as proximate result of the breach).
5. There was actual injury with a value that can be measured by a monetary loss.

Preponderance of the evidence is the greater weight of the evidence; that is, evidence that is believable because it outweighs or overbalances the evidence opposed to it. A preponderance means evidence that is more probable, more persuasive, or of greater probative value. Consider scales of justice. If the scales are tipped to one side, that side is the side that has the preponderance of the evidence. The scales tipped to one side have the greater weight. It is the quality of the evidence that must be weighed. Quality may or may not be identical to quantity.[19] Beyond a preponderance of the evidence is more than 50%; it is greater than or equal to 51%. The key phrase to remember when testifying in these cases is that the conclusion is "more likely than not." "A very strong chance" is not sufficient to get over the 50% mark; however, an expert does not have to establish beyond all doubt that a certain injury resulted from a particular event. It is the quality of the expert's opinion that will make the difference in any given case.

An expert can determine if his or her opinion is going to satisfy the 51% rule by asking him- or herself true or false questions. For example, he or she can ask him- or herself: Is it possible? Almost all things are possible. Therefore, the answer is true. Then, he or she can ask: Is it 100% certain? All things are subject to some doubt. Therefore, the answer would be false. Then, he or she can ask: Is it likely? If the answer is more likely true, that will get the expert beyond the 51% rule.

Consider the following continuum:

Less than likely→50%→More than likely

The further to the right of the 50% mark, the more likely the 51% rule is to be met.

An expert may be certain in his or her mind beyond all doubt that the opinion he or she is about to give could be no other. This may be true in a minority of cases. However, attorneys will push the expert to the point of saying that it is an absolute certainty. Once the expert is locked into this position, it is easy for the attorney to present a hypothetical question that will take the opinion out of the absolute certainty classification. Once this is done, the expert opinion will be subject to question. Experts sometimes fear that if their opinion is not an absolute certainty that another expert will undermine their opinion. There is practically nothing in this world that is an absolute certainty. Experts need to keep in mind that their opinion is based on facts that they were presented with. Different facts, as in a hypothetical situation, will have different consequences.

There are two other burdens of proof placed upon plaintiffs in different types of cases: clear and convincing evidence and proof beyond a reasonable doubt. The burdens of proof can be demonstrated by the following continuum:

Less likely→50%→More likely→Clear and convincing→Beyond reasonable doubt

There are some cases that require clear and convincing evidence. To be clear and convincing, the evidence must have more than simply a greater weight than the evidence opposed to it and must produce a firm belief or conviction about the truth of the matter.[20] This is the burden of proof in cases where the courts have determined that an erroneous verdict in favor of the plaintiff would be most egregious. Generally, medical experts would not be testifying in this type of case. However, the criteria given previously are still applicable. It is the quality of the evidence that will convince the trier of fact to have a firm belief or conviction about the truth of the matter.

The highest burden of proof is only required in criminal cases. The burden in a criminal case is proof beyond a reasonable doubt. Reasonable doubt is present when the jurors, after they have carefully considered and compared all the evidence, cannot say they are firmly convinced of the truth of the charge. It is a doubt based on reason and common sense. Reasonable doubt is not mere possible doubt, because everything relating to human affairs or depending on moral evidence is open to some possible or imaginary doubt. Proof beyond a reasonable doubt is proof of such character that an ordinary person would be willing to rely and act upon it in the most important of his or her own affairs.[21]

A doctor does not have to be a pathologist to find him- or herself testifying in a criminal case. A general practitioner may be called upon to give an opinion on the state of health of a patient just prior to death. A cardiologist may be called upon to give expert testimony as to the health of a patient's heart just prior to death. These cases can arise when a person dies as a result of a criminal act other than by violence against the deceased. Expert testimony is also needed in cases concerning automobile accidents that appear to have been caused by driving under the influence but may have been naturally caused. Psychologists may be called to testify as to the suicidal tendencies of a deceased person.

Whatever the burden of proof for the particular case, the expert opinion must be relevant, reliable, factual, honest, and, most importantly, credible. Although the expert opinion is important in a given case, the expert cannot make the whole case or carry the entire burden of proof. Experts should not try to overstate their opinion. After all, neither "beyond the preponderance of the evidence" nor "beyond a reasonable doubt" means beyond all doubt. The opinion of the expert will be admitted and accepted by the trier of fact if it is honest and credible.

How does an expert present an opinion that is not an absolute certainty? There are some key words or phrases that an expert should keep in mind when testifying. In order to have an opinion that will be admissible, the opinion must be based on a reasonable degree of medical certainty. This standard will be applicable in administrative hearings as well as trials. Remember that only more than a 51% possibility must be shown. The key phrase is "it is more likely than not" that a certain fact produced a certain result. When an expert testifies about a result, the expert must make it clear that the opinion is based on more than a 50% probability. Many cases are lost because the expert has rendered an opinion without being clear that there is a greater than 50% probability that the result was caused by the facts alleged. An example of where a problem can arise is contained in the following question:

Question: Doctor, in your opinion, did the negligent act cause the resulting injury to this patient?

Answer: In my opinion, it is probable.

This is the wrong answer. The correct answer would be: "It is more likely than not that the act caused the resulting injury."

An expert may be concerned that anything but an absolute will harm his or her opinion. Once an expert acknowledges that the results of the opinion are not 100% absolute, the attorney will press for a definite percentage. This may cause some concern for the expert. However, the key is not the exact percentage, but that the final opinion is going to put the resulting probability at or above the 51% bar.

Legal Arenas Where an Expert Opinion May Be Rendered

Expert testimony can be given in several legal arenas. Specifically, expert testimony is often offered through depositions, in administrative hearings, and at trials.

Depositions

Although depositions are the least structured and most informal of the proceedings mentioned above, in this process the opposing attorney will begin to explore all "fluffing." The attorney will want to know everything about the expert's education, experience, honors, and publications. Additionally, the opposing attorney will generally question how often the expert has testified and for whom. A word of caution is necessary at this juncture. Although it is easy for an expert attempting to stress his or her expertise to stretch the truth, this can be a critically dangerous venture. Once an expert stretches the truth or facts to make a point, credibility becomes an issue and all testimony can be called into question.

The evidence given in a deposition is very important. Once an expert has been deposed, his or her testimony is essentially cast in stone. This testimony will be transcribed verbatim. The opposing attorney will go over the testimony with a fine-tooth comb. The attorney may use any publications mentioned at the deposition to educate him- or herself on the subject. The attorney will also use sources cited in the articles to find those experts in a particular field who disagree with the opinion rendered. The attorney will often use the publications referred to in the deposition for cross-examination. The next time the expert will see anything that was said at the deposition will be either at an administrative hearing or at trial.

Administrative Hearings

An administrative hearing is a semi-informal proceeding through which a fact-finder accepts evidence in a matter. A magistrate generally conducts administrative hearings. The magistrate has all the powers of a judge during the hearing. The magistrate usually hears the same types of cases over and over. This means that the magistrate may already be familiar with the various opinions of experts in the field. The magistrate is the finder of fact in these hearings. It is his or her responsibility to make a determination as to what the facts are. This clearly means the magistrate decides to either accept or reject an expert opinion. The fact that the magistrate may be aware of experts and their opinions can be helpful to the expert who is truthful and stays within his or her field of expertise. Although all rules of evidence should be followed in administrative hearings, most magistrates will allow some leeway to these rules. If the magistrate believes that the expert is going beyond his or her field, the magistrate may allow the cross-examination to go beyond the rules. If the magistrate does not believe the expert is credible, he or she may allow the cross-examination to clearly establish this in the record. This extensive cross-examination will make a clear record of the evidence to be preserved if the case is appealed.

An expert should not let the informality of the deposition or administrative hearing distract his or her attention from the goal of expressing the opinion and having that opinion admitted into evidence. The relaxed atmosphere should not relax the expert. The opposing counsel will attempt to attack the credibility of the expert during these proceedings. Therefore, it is important for the expert to stay within his or her field of expertise. Once the expert strays beyond his or her field of expertise, the door is opened to attacks on the credibility of the expert.

Workers' compensation hearings are typical of the type of administrative hearings in which expert testimony is rendered. These hearings are fraught with the potential for an expert to go beyond his or her field. This is especially true in cases requiring the establishment of causation, because although the expert may be well qualified in an area, the scientific area connecting the injury to its cause may require a different type of expertise. In cases where the injury is clear, the key is to convince the hearing officer that it is more likely than not that the injury came from work-related activity. For example, in a case where an individual is trying to establish a workers' compensation case for carpal tunnel syndrome, an expert may be an excellent orthopedic hand and wrist surgeon, but if the expert has not had additional education, training, and experience on the causal relationship of the injury, the expert may not be qualified to render that opinion.

One of the advantages for an expert at an administrative hearing, such as a workers' compensation hearing, is that the magistrate usually has had enough experience to quickly qualify an expert and will accept the legal standard of proof. Juries, on the other hand, may not be so readily receptive to the expert's opinion. Additionally, juries may have difficulty accepting the more than 50% standard. However, the judge and not the expert is the one to control the jury. It is the judge who is responsible for properly instructing the jury on the applicable standards.

Following cross-examination at an administrative hearing, the expert will generally not have to undergo cross-examination again at any subsequent point in the administrative appeal process. Although a losing party may appeal the findings of the magistrate, the appeal will only be on legal issues. It will not be a rehearing on the facts. An expert may, however, find that there will be an administrative hearing as well as a trial of the same issues. This can happen when an employee alleges a work-related injury. Soon after the alleged injury, the employee may be discharged for absenteeism. The employee will have the right to a hearing on the workers' compensation claim and the employee may have a claim for wrongful discharge. Both will have their basis in the same incident. The expert may find it necessary to be deposed, testify in an administrative hearing, and then testify at trial.

Trials

Trials in the common pleas court are the most formal of legal proceedings. These are cases that could not be resolved in an administrative hearing. These cases usually will have a number of experts on both sides. These are cases such as malpractice and negligence cases that resulted in severe damages. All the rules of evidence will be followed. The expert must be aware that at trial anything that he or she testified to in the deposition can be used to attack the credibility of the expert's opinion. The expert can also be cross-examined on any testimony given at an administrative hearing.

Most experts are concerned about making a good impression before juries. They want to be the most "expert" in their field. The key, however, is not being the most expert, but the most credible expert. The foundation for being the most credible began back at the time of deposition. If the expert tried to pad his or her curriculum vitae, he or she can be attacked on that basis. If the foundation for the expert being qualified to render an opinion is assailed, the opinion likewise falters.

It is important for an expert to prepare adequately to testify at trial. The best defense is a good offense. The expert should thoroughly review his or her deposition prior to testifying at trial. Additionally, it is important to know what other experts are saying in the particular field. The expert should know the following:

1. The most published experts in the field
2. The most recently published experts
3. The effect, if any, the most recent publications would have on the opinion the expert is about to give

All parties to the litigation, in order to either support or discredit the opinion rendered by the expert, will frequently question the expert. The questions may come from either attorney.

Question: Doctor, are you familiar with other authorities in this area?

Answer: Yes.

Question: Who are they?

Answer: [List of the authorities with whom the Doctor is familiar.]

Question: Doctor, are there others in this field who have published articles on this subject?

Answer: There may be but I am not familiar with them.

Question: Doctor, are you familiar with Doctor X?

Answer: Yes.

Question: Doctor X has written an article that would differ from your conclusions, hasn't he, Doctor?

Answer: Yes.

A cross-examining attorney may stop there. This would leave the jury with the impression that there is clearly an opposite opinion on the subject or diagnosis.

If the expert is not familiar with Doctor X in the previous scenario, a line of questioning like the following may occur:

Question: Doctor, are you familiar with Doctor X?

Answer: No.

Question: Well, Doctor, I have an article written on this subject by Doctor X. Doctor X would disagree with your opinion. Have you read this article, Doctor?

Answer: No.

Question: Do you avoid reading articles by those who do not agree with you, Doctor?

(or)

Question: Doctor, this article was written last month—do you not keep up to date on new research in your field?

Two-way communication between the expert and the attorney is extremely important when an expert has been hired to give an opinion. If the opinion sought is even slightly outside a particular field of expertise, the attorney should know that fact. If there are publications or articles that have been published that differ from the expert's opinion, the attorney should know this. These publications may not have any effect on the opinion itself, but they may give the appearance of attacking the credibility of the expert. If these publications or other authorities appear to differ from the testimony of the expert, the attorney should know this. If the attorney is aware of the differences and why the differences exist, the attorney can prevent attacks on the expert opinion by bringing these differences out on direct examination rather then having them brought out on cross-examination. The hiring attorney can then avoid being placed on the defensive and can instead stay one step ahead of the opposition. Additionally, this avoids the appearance that the expert is trying to hide unsupportive authority because it differs from the expert's opinion.[22]

This two-way communication is as much a responsibility of the physician as it is of the attorney. The physician has the responsibility of advising the attorney of the strengths as well as the weaknesses of the physician's analysis. Most attorneys would rather reach a settlement of a case rather than go to trial on a case. Whenever a case goes to trial, the attorney loses control. Juries are an unknown quantity. Therefore, the physician must educate the attorney on the alternative possibilities of the physician's analysis.

The physician must also educate the attorney on the specific disease or injury. The more the attorney knows the better the attorney can protect his or her client and the physician. Attorneys are not physicians. They must be educated on both the specific medical problems and the general field of medicine in a particular case. The attorney must know the experts and publications in the field. The expert must also educate the attorney about the experts who may be disclosed to the attorney from the other side. If medical history could make a difference, the physician should inform the attorney.

Experts will sometimes attempt to outguess the attorney during cross-examination. This can be very dangerous. The general trend of opposing attorneys is to begin to attack the credibility of the expert from the point of his or her credentials. The attorney will go over the curriculum vitae point by point. It is an attorney's dream to have an expert who publishes and teaches because there is always another expert who publishes or teaches on the subject. Therefore, it is almost always possible to find an expert who will differ in some aspects in the field of expertise. The more the expert has written, lectured, and spoken on a particular subject, the more an attorney can cross-examine. The attorney will then present other experts' publications on the same subject.

Medical experts, especially, may believe that their opinion will win the day. Attorneys will attempt to get doctors to be argumentative on cross-examination. The more argumentative the doctor becomes, the less credible the opinion becomes. It is the responsibility of the attorney who offers the doctor as an expert to prevent this from happening. The attorney is responsible for pointing out that the cross-examining attorney is the one who is arguing with the expert. Arguing makes the expert appear stubborn and unwilling to change his or her opinion under any circumstances. It is better to avoid getting into an argument when testifying.

The expert who holds him- or herself to be the world's leading expert in a particular field may be the most susceptible to cross-examination. There are always going to be other experts who will have different opinions. The opposing attorney will attempt to make the so-called world's leading expert appear to be an egotist whose own self-image would prohibit him or her from being objective about flaws in his or her opinion. As pointed out previously, everything is subject to some doubt. A question concerning who is the world's leading authority on the subject at hand can be expected.

> Question: Doctor, who would you consider to be the world's leading expert in this field?
> Answer: I am.

This is the wrong answer. It gives the expert the appearance of not being willing to listen to other authorities in the field. A better answer would be as follows:

> Answer: I am not certain. I would like to think of myself as one of them, but I know there are others.

An expert can expect to be asked about texts, articles, or studies done by others recognized in the field. The authors of these other articles may not have the credentials of the expert testifying. However, the cross-examining attorney will attempt to make it appear to the judge or jury that these are authoritative studies that disagree with the opinion of the expert witness. This is merely another attempt to discredit the expert's opinion.

The cross-examining attorney will also look for biases. If an expert consistently testifies only for plaintiffs or a particular insurance company, that expert may have a bias. It is not unusual for an expert to be asked to testify on the same subject repeatedly once that expert has successfully testified. This does not necessarily show a bias. However, the attorney will indicate to the jury or judge that this expert clearly has a bias toward one side or the other.

Whereas repetitive testimony is often used to show bias, the opposite is also true. This repetitive testimony solidifies the expertise of the expert. The expert should not simply rely on past successes, however. The opposing attorney will have other experts reviewing the analysis closely. Scientific techniques change, tests change, and the testifying expert must keep up with these changes in order to address them in cross-examination.

Experts who testify frequently have an advantage. This can also work against them. The attorney will have reviewed the cases where the expert has testified. The attorney will also review all the articles published as well as the teaching cases presented by the expert. If the expert has testified consistently for one side or the other, the attorney will point out a bias. If the expert has testified on both sides of an issue, the attorney will use prior testimony to attempt to impeach the expert in a case. The expert should be aware that testifying on both sides of an issue could show that the expert is fair and unbiased. That is as long as the fees charged for the testimony and opinions are the same for both positions. It may be difficult for an expert to remember the exact facts of the previous case. The expert should be quick to point out that the facts differ in each case and that the facts in the previous case were not the same as in the current case. Different facts call for different conclusions.

There are experts who solicit business. Experts who find themselves testifying more often for the plaintiff or defendant should be extremely careful when being cross-examined. This type of expert runs the risk of being more familiar with the strengths of one side and the weaknesses of the other side, giving the appearance of being myopic or having a stubborn streak that would not allow the expert to appreciate any other view. These experts are usually referred to on cross-examination as "hired guns." Related questions will generally be in conjunction with questions on compensation.

> Question: Doctor, have you testified more often for insurance companies than for victims of serious accidents?
>
> Answer: Yes.
>
> Question: In fact, Doctor, you have advertised in professional journals that you are an expert in this field, haven't you?
>
> Answer: Yes.
>
> Question: Doctor, how much are you getting paid for your opinion today?
>
> Answer: I am not getting paid for my opinion; I am getting paid for my time.
>
> Question: Doctor, how much did you get paid the first time you testified on this subject?
>
> Answer: (It will be a lot less than the current fee.)
>
> Question: Doctor, have you become a hired gun?

An expert can expect an attorney to attempt to impeach him or her by using articles or publications that have been released very recently. The expert may or may not have read all the articles that have been published within the last couple of weeks. If the expert has not, the attorney may argue that the expert is not keeping up on the most recent developments in the field of study.

When an attorney asks about an article in a journal published last week, the expert can reply that he or she has not seen the article published in any of the journals he or she reads regularly. This can raise doubt concerning the acceptability of the article, author, or publication. If the attorney uses it for a hypothetical, the expert can again point out that the theory has not been generally recognized or accepted.

Questions about recent articles may be answered in a couple of different ways. The following is an example:

> Question: Doctor, have you read the recent article in the ABC professional journal?
>
> Answer: That is not a publication I read regularly.
>
> Question: Is that because you do not keep current on all the medical journals?
>
> Answer: I subscribe to and read the journals with the most recognized authorities.
>
> Question: But, Doctor, in this article Doctor X points out that even the most recognized authorities may be wrong. Would you like to read it?
>
> Answer: That may be true; however, the author is not a recognized authority on this subject, and the theory is not yet accepted as being within a certain degree of medical certainty. My opinion is based on a degree of medical certainty founded on recognized and acceptable theory.

An expert can expect to be cross-examined on whether he or she is being paid and who is paying for the expert testimony. Attorneys will explore who is paying the bill and how much is being paid. They will also want to know what percentage of the expert's income is derived from testifying. If the expert does not know, the attorney will ask who would have this information. Certainly, someone, such as an accountant or clerk, should know. The attorney may even want to see the books to verify a percentage when it is given. Judges generally will not let the attorney go that far; however, not knowing or not willingly turning over financial records could imply a bias. This is especially true if a large portion of the expert's income comes from testifying for one party. Questions on the percentage of income derived from testifying should be anticipated.

> Question: Doctor, what percentage of your annual income is derived from testifying?
>
> Answer: I am not sure.
>
> Question: Well, Doctor, can you give us a guess?
>
> Answer: Without my records before me to give an accurate answer, I would not want to guess.
>
> Question: Well, Doctor, who can we call to get those records?
>
> Answer: My office manager.
>
> At this point there should be an objection. However, if there is not, the name of the person should be given.
>
> Question: Doctor, we really do not need a precise answer. Can you give just an approximation?
>
> Answer: [The percentage.] But that is a pure guess—unlike my opinion, which is based on documented facts.
>
> Question: Doctor, is all your extra income derived from insurance companies? (This could also be asked if the expert is testifying most often for plaintiffs.)
>
> Answer: Because of my education, experience, and training, insurance companies (or plaintiffs' attorneys) have come to recognize my opinions as being thorough and objective.

Besides attacking the expert witness him- or herself, attorneys will attack the fact basis upon which the expert reached his or her determination. Attorneys will ask the expert about every piece of paper that was generated during an investigation of a particular case. It is not unusual for the expert not to have seen everything generated when reviewing a case for an opinion. Hopefully, the expert will have seen everything that is relevant to the matter. However, it is not uncommon for the attorney to ask the expert if he or she has seen item "A"—an item previously overlooked or an item excluded from the materials presented to the expert. When the expert says no, the attorney will ask if that item would have made a difference in his or her opinion. Without having seen the item, the expert cannot be sure. The attorney will then ask the expert if he or she wants to see the item. The expert has to say yes because the document may reinforce the opinion or help to eliminate other possible opinions. The attorney will then give the expert the item. The expert must try to review the document and put the information into perspective with his or her opinion. The expert must exercise caution when reviewing this new information and be certain to give it a thorough review before answering any questions concerning the material or the impact it may have on the opinion. However, once the expert has had a chance to look at the documentation, he or she can say that the documentation is beyond the scope of the opinion to be rendered. Even if the item has no relevance, the attorney may continue to ask questions to make it appear that the only reason the evidence does not have relevance to the expert is that the expert does not want it to because it might undermine the expert's opinion.

Physicians should always respond by letter to attorneys regarding exactly what was reviewed and how the information provided was reviewed, describing all that was reviewed and the exact significance of each item. If there is other information that is normally reviewed, the expert should also ask in writing for this information. The attorney may not know that a history from the patient's primary physician is necessary to know if there was a prior debilitating injury or history. The physician should educate the attorney on the importance of this information.

The cross-examining attorney will also try to get the expert to come close to his or her position. The other tactic will be to try to get the expert to go beyond his or her particular field of expertise. The attorney will attempt to get the expert to agree that there are other experts in the field with the same or better credentials, although the existence of others in the field does not mean that an expert's opinion is not valid on certain facts and in certain circumstances.

Sometimes, if the attorney knows of more than one opinion that differs from that of the expert testifying, the attorney will attack the opinion head on. The attorney will ask the expert why there are more opinions on the other side of the issue. The answer is that the other experts may not be as detailed in their analysis. There may also be differences in exactly what was asked of the experts. The attorney will again ask if the expert really believes in his or her opinion. Once the expert says "absolutely," the attorney will have the expert in an untenable position. A better answer is: "To a reasonable degree of medical certainty."

Doctors can put themselves in a precarious position by being absolutely certain of their position without other support. Questions may go like this:

> Question: Doctor, I know that you have testified that asbestos exposure can increase the risk of getting lung cancer. However, most authorities in this field believe that only those individuals who have asbestosis as a reflection of their asbestos inhalation will have an increased risk of getting lung cancer. Why is it that you are testifying that anybody with asbestos inhalation is at risk?
>
> Answer: Because this reflects the material that I have read, the education I have received, and continuing medical education courses that I have attended.
>
> Question: I understand that, Doctor. However, I am still asking you the question: Why is it that there are no published reports that would support your side of the argument?
>
> Answer: Oh, I am sure that I have read a few of these.
>
> Question: Doctor, you had the chance to provide these articles following your deposition. However, they were not forthcoming. Do you still believe that your position is true?
>
> Answer: Absolutely.

The doctor has now placed him- or herself in the situation of not having any other authority to support his or her position and has failed to support the position with anything other then a self-serving statement. The doctor expects the jury to believe that his or her opinion is the only opinion that could be given; the jury could believe anything other than that opinion by the time the cross-examination is over.

The expert must try to avoid testifying in such a manner that the information relayed is lost on the general citizen owing to its complexity. Most attorneys will have just enough knowledge of the subject matter to be dangerous. They will sound like they are experts to the jury. Juries are made up of ordinary citizens. Attorneys are taught to present a case as if they were addressing individuals with a sixth-grade education. Experts are there to help the juries understand concepts that are not within their common knowledge. If an attorney cannot get the expert to waffle on his or her opinion and cannot get the expert to go outside of the field of expertise, the attorney may try to get the expert to get so detailed that the jury will feel lost. The attorney will then make the expert appear to be on an ego trip so that the jury will lose faith in the credibility of the expert's opinion.

The expert is responsible for educating the attorney, judge, and jury. This is not an easy task. The expert must explain his or her opinion and position clearly enough for a 12-year-old to understand. One way for an expert to test his or her testimony is to practice on a spouse or children. If children do not understand it, juries will discount it.

Hypotheticals are used to confuse the expert and the jury. Usually they are very long and complicated. The general rule is that the parties may not cross-examine on evidence that has not been or will not be presented. However, the hypothetical can be so long and involved that the judge may allow such cross-examination simply because it might have relevance. These are very dangerous questions. The opposing attorney will begin to subtly change some of the facts of the hypothetical. If the hiring attorney does not object, the expert may find him- or herself admitting that certain facts could change his or her opinion. The expert should not be afraid to acknowledge that based on certain facts his or her opinion would be different. However, the expert should quickly point out that these were not the facts in the current case.

There are different approaches that can be used to prevent confusion for both the expert and the jury. An expert can restate the hypothetical as he or she understands it. The expert can write down the hypothetical as it is being given. Then the expert can point out to the attorney how the hypothetical differs from the facts of the current case. This can give the jury the impression that the expert really knows the facts, and then the jury will look to the cross-examining attorney's expert to understand the differences as well. The expert can ask the attorney to repeat the hypothetical and specifically ask the attorney to clarify what the attorney perceives to be different from the previous hypothetical.

Long, complicated hypothetical questions become dangerous because they are difficult for a witness to remember. The attorney will have the luxury of being able to read the hypothetical; however, the expert does not have this benefit. The expert must try to keep the original hypothetical in mind and spot any changes made by the opposing attorney when the hypothetical posed differs from the actual facts that were presented. Frequently, the cross-examining attorney will merely give the facts and then a conclusion. The attorney will then ask for a yes or no answer as to the conclusion. These types of questions often do not allow for an explanation as to the differences between the facts presented and the facts of the case. The expert must rely on the attorney to permit the expert to explain on redirect examination.

Attorneys may ask a hypothetical, and then ask, "What if only a part is changed?"—without repeating the entire hypothetical. The expert can ask the attorney to repeat the whole hypothetical with the change so the expert completely understands the question. If the expert has written down the first hypothetical, he or she should repeat the entire hypothetical so the jury understands there is a difference. The jury will also be more aware of the thoroughness of the expert. Different facts will lead to different conclusions.

The expert must be cautious and listen carefully to hypothetical questions. The attorney may start out with a fact pattern very similar to the case at hand and then subtly change small details. The attorney who begins with a fact pattern close to the facts of the case will often lead the expert down a path to a point where the opinion will change. If the expert's opinion does not change, the attorney may use the hypothetical to lead the expert beyond his or her field and then attack that portion of the opinion that is outside the field of expertise. This does not mean that the original opinion would not still be valid. However, once any part of the opinion or hypothetical is called into question, the whole opinion may seem suspect.

The opposing attorney may, however, start out with facts that clearly would result in a different opinion. The attorney who begins with such a hypothetical will then begin to narrow the facts. The attorney will be looking for a point where the expert will come back to the same conclusion and opinion as based on the facts of the case. The attorney will then begin to work back to a point where the expert has to find a different result. The purpose of this type of cross-examination is to get the expert to flip-flop on the opinion rendered. The jury then becomes confused; the result is that the expert is unable to help the jury understand that which is outside their general knowledge.

Attorneys may simply get the expert to admit that there are other reasons for a resulting injury and then stop the cross-examination. This puts the expert in a position of having to rely on the hiring attorney to go further into the basis of the opinion and has the effect of putting the hiring attorney on the defensive. Once this is done, it can open doors for re–cross-examination. The purpose is that the attorney in closing arguments can honestly say that the expert him- or herself admitted that there are other reasons for the resulting injury. This would not be a misstatement of the evidence. This tactic would also enhance the attorney's position that the opinion may be in question.

Experts should consider alternate reasons for resulting injuries. The expert may not be able to eliminate all possible reasons for resulting injuries, but the fact that the expert considered them lends credibility to the expert's opinion. The expert should point out that the alternatives, although possible, would be less likely than not; therefore, the 51% criterion would not be met. Questions asked about alternative theories may be approached in the following manner:

> Question: Doctor, did you consider the possibility that the injury may have been the result of another intervening cause?
>
> Answer: Yes. However, it is less likely than not to be the cause.
>
> Question: But, Doctor, it is possible, isn't it?

Answer: I have considered various possibilities, but they are all less likely than not to be the cause. The only one that is more likely than not is the opinion I just gave.

The primary reason for the expert to stay within his or her field is so that any hypothetical or any other documentation that is presented will have a minimum impact. If something is presented that will have an effect on the opinion, the hiring attorney will have alerted the expert in the beginning, provided there was good two-way communication.

Trick Questions and Trial Tactics

There are a variety of techniques that an attorney may use when cross-examining an expert. These can be broken down into the following four broad categories:

1. Credentials
2. Biases
3. Analysis and preparation techniques
4. Conclusions

The attorney may begin by asking a series of questions about education. These may include questions about the recognition of the schools attended by the expert as well as the expert's class rank. The attorney may cross-examine the expert on the schools' competitiveness and accreditation. The expert will want to know if the hospital with which the expert is associated is a teaching hospital and will inquire into its accreditation. The expert can expect questions on everything from residency to specialized training. The attorney will try to show that the expert did not go to the top ranked school, did not graduate first in the class, has not written the most articles, has not been published the most, and has not taught as much as some other experts. If the expert is young, the attorney may ask questions concerning lack of experience. If the expert is older, the attorney may inquire into the most recent teaching techniques.

Attorneys will want to know the names of the national experts in the field. They will ask questions such as the following:

Have you heard of Doctor X?
Is Doctor Y of UCLA recognized as an expert in this area?
What are the primary textbooks in this area?
Have you published anything on this type of case?
How many articles have you written on this issue?
How many books have you published on this issue?
Have you ever instructed physicians or students on this issue?
Are you aware of the most recent articles written on this subject?

Attorneys will also ask questions about an expert's practice:

Do you see patients on a daily basis?
What are your hospital affiliations?
Have you ever been denied hospital rights, or had your rights taken away?
Do you maintain an office with other doctors? If so, what are their practices? Do they see more patients than you do? How often do they testify on this issue? If they testify more, why aren't they here? If they testify less, why do you spend so much time testifying?

The answers to these types of questions should be straightforward and truthful. These types of questions will not disqualify the expert from giving the ultimate opinion. The medical expert should provide straightforward answers to these questions.

These questions will generally be asked after the expert has been qualified to testify. The questions are designed to attempt to get the expert to become defensive. An expert should not be defensive about his or her education, training, or experience.

The second area on which attorneys will focus is bias. Attorneys will ask questions that may lead a jury to believe that the opinion is based on a bias. The questions may begin with a question such as the following: "Why are you here today, Doctor?" The answer is as follows: "I was asked to give my opinion on the issue." "Do you always testify for the defendant (or plaintiff)?" If the answer is no, then the attorney will follow up with a question concerning how many times the expert has testified for the defendant or plaintiff. If the expert does not know, the attorney will ask how many times the expert has testified in total. Then the attorney will follow up with questions concerning what percentage of the time the expert testifies for one side or the other. This is an attempt to show that the expert testifies more often for one side. If the expert does not know the number or the percentage of times, the attorney will ask for a guess. This seems like something an expert can do. However, later a question will arise regarding the expert's opinion, concerning whether the opinion is a guess, like the one made about the number of times testifying. The expert should not guess. The answer to "best guess" questions is as follows: "Because I do not have my records or specific information in front of me as I did in forming my opinion, it would only be a guess and have little or no significance."

An expert may be asked if he or she has ever refused to testify for or against an insurance company.

An expert's bias will also emerge during questioning about compensation. The expert can expect a question such as the following: "How much are you getting paid for your opinion?" The answer is: "I am not getting paid for my opinion. I am getting paid for my time." "Who is paying you? How much are you getting paid? Doctor, the people in the jury box only make a small fraction of that kind of money. How do you justify that expense?" The answer is that the fee is based on more than just the time in court. All costs must be factored in—office, overhead, insurance, conference time, educational updates, and lost billable time in the office. The charges are based on what it cost the expert—his or her knowledge, skills, and ability in the field. "Doctor, how much did you earn last year testifying?" If the expert does not know, he or she will be asked who does know and whether he or she can bring the records to refresh the expert's memory. The expert may be asked to guess and should avoid guessing for any answer. It is better to answer "I don't know" than to guess. Guessing can only bring trouble later.

The third area the attorney will attack is the fact basis or the method of the expert's analysis. Attorneys will ask if the expert had all the medical records and will ask the expert to list the records he or she had to review. If a record is missed, the expert will be asked if he or she saw record X. If the expert did not see a record, he or she will be asked if he or she would have liked to see the missing record. If the answer is no, the jury will believe no facts would change the expert's mind. If the answer is yes, the attorney will hand over the record for the expert to review while sitting on the stand. The expert should answer that he or she based his or her opinion on the records that were provided or that could be obtained independently. This is why communication between the attorney and the expert is so important in the early stages of a case. Everything that would affect the expert's opinion must be provided.

The expert who testifies on cause and effect must be especially careful. Questions to the expert may go like this:

> Question: Doctor, you have testified to a degree of medical certainty that Ms. Jones has carpel tunnel syndrome.
>
> Answer: Yes.
>
> Question: Doctor, you have also testified that she has acute and chronic pain with this; isn't that true?
>
> Answer: Yes.
>
> Question: Doctor, the extent of pain is within an individual's state of mind, isn't it?
>
> Answer: Yes.
>
> Question: Doctor, I didn't see in your vitae that you were certified in psychology or psychiatry, did I?
>
> Answer: No.

The expert will be asked if he or she discussed the case with the attorney. "Did you meet with counsel to prepare your testimony? Do you normally prepare with a lawyer to tell the truth?" The answer is: "I met and prepared with the attorney so that my opinion will be clearly understood by non-physicians. It is a complex issue that I want to help make clear." If the expert is not the treating physician, he or she will be asked if he or she consulted with the treating physician. If not, the attorney may ask: "Did you receive summaries of the medical records in this case? If they were just summaries, how do you know that there was not something else? If there was something omitted, could that affect your opinion? Did you ever see the plaintiff personally? If you didn't have a personal consultation, you couldn't ask if there were other factors that might have influenced your opinion, could you?"

If the physician is not the primary care physician or did not have personal contact with the plaintiff, a series of questions on the notes provided can be expected. The expert who is the primary care physician or who has seen the plaintiff personally may also get questions on notes. The questions may be as follows: "Doctor, did you see the plaintiff personally? Did you talk with other doctors about the plaintiff? Did you make notes about the plaintiff's condition? Did you make any notes when talking with the attorney about this case? If you talked with the plaintiff personally, did you make any notes about what the plaintiff told you? If you didn't, how could you fully evaluate the plaintiff's condition? If you did, do you have your notes with you today, Doctor? If yes, can I see them? If no, why not, or what did you do with them? If they are in the file back at the office, can someone get them for you and bring them here? If you don't have the notes, why don't you? If you destroyed them, aren't you destroying evidence, or at least hiding evidence?" The expert could answer that he or she did not need them anymore. However, this would give the appearance that the expert only wanted the jury to know part of what was involved in the evaluation. Notes can be discoverable and should not be destroyed. The expert may be required to bring them to court. Therefore, the notes should reflect what was done and how conclusions were reached.

The expert will be asked to summarize the history of this case. "When did you obtain this history? When did you form your opinion in this case? Was it before or after talking with the attorney? What medical research, if any, did you review in conjunction with this case? How many hours did you spend reviewing this case? Did you personally talk with the other physicians? Did you get a complete history of the plaintiff from the primary physician? Have you ever told an attorney that your opinion would not support the client's claim?" The answer to these questions is that the expert spent a number of hours reviewing the case, applied knowledge and skill, and rendered a truthful opinion to the attorney.

The fourth broad area of attack is the opinion itself. The expert will hear hypothetical questions. These questions will either attack the opinion head on or begin to make changes that would alter the opinion. If the facts are different from those in the current case, the opinion may be different based on the different facts. The expert should reply that the hypothetical facts were not before him or her while he or she was forming an opinion. The expert will be asked: "Is the opinion a guess, like the number of cases you testified in?"

The expert should be cautious when rendering opinions on the proximate result of an act or the failure to act. The cause of a resulting injury will involve an additional discipline other than the specific medical field. Injury owing to a car accident may involve accident reconstruction. The expert may know something about accident reconstruction but not qualify as an expert in the field. The attorney will try to get the doctor to go outside his or her field of expertise by testifying about the accident and its cause. This may be guessing or speculating on the cause. Once the expert guesses or speculates on something outside the field of expertise, the opinion also begins to look like speculation.

If the plaintiff has chronic pain, the expert may be asked to describe what that means. If the physician begins to talk about the mental state or stress of the patient, the attorney may state that he or she does not see a psychology or psychiatry degree in the expert's biography. The answer may be that the expert has the training in the specific area of illness and pain to make such a diagnosis. However, he or she must be prepared to address the basis of the expertise of rendering the opinion of proximate result. There must be a connection and that connection is not just a diagnosis of the specific injury. If there is another expert who will testify to the relationship between the act and the injury, the expert should not guess, speculate, or hypothesize on that relationship.

If the expert's opinion differs from another expert's opinion, he or she must be prepared to answer how that can be. The answer is that the experts may have had different materials to review. The experts may not have the same knowledge and experience. The other expert may not have taken as much time to review the facts. The expert only knows that based on his or her knowledge, skill, and experience that to a reasonable degree of medical certainty his or her opinion is correct.

Conclusion

Experts are rendering opinions to help, not confuse. It is important to stay within one's own field and be completely honest and direct. The expert cannot be afraid to say "That is not within my field," "That is not what I was hired to do," "What you presented me was not within the scope or purpose of my review," "These are not the facts of this case study," or "There are others within the field who may not agree with me; however, they may not have had what I had to review." The bottom line is being honest and accepting that juries may not follow or agree with an expert's opinion. The expert will want to be called upon to give another opinion another day; it is not unusual for a defense attorney to hire the expert he or she has put through a grueling cross-examination if he or she believes the expert is honest and credible.

References

1. Black HC: Blacks Law Dictionary, 5th Edition. St Paul, MN, West Publishing Co, 1979, p 339.
2. Ohio Rules of Court: Coordinated Research in Ohio from West Group. Eagen, MN, West Publising Co, 2000, p 185.
3. American Jurisprudence, (ed 2): Federal Rules of Evidence, Rochester, NY. The Lawyers Co-operative Publishing Company, 1982, Volume 32B, p 791.
4. Capra DJ: The Daubert Puzzle, 32 Ga Law Rev 699, 1998.
5. Daubert v Merrill Dow Pharm, Inc 509 U.S. 579, 113 S Ct 2786, 125 L. Ed. 2nd 508, 1993.
6. The Kansas Journal of Law and Public Policy, Lawrence, Kansas, University of Kansas School of Law, Volume IX, Number 1, Fall 1999.
7. Capra DJ: The Daubert Puzzle, 32 Georgia Law Review 699, 1998.
8. American Jurisprudence, (ed 2): Federal Rules of Evidence, Rochester, NY. The Lawyers Co-operative Publishing Company, 1982, Volume 32B, p 705.
9. American Jurisprudence, (ed 2): Federal Rules of Evidence, Rochester, NY. The Lawyers Co-operative Publishing Company, 1982, Volume 32B, p 706.
10. Ibid.
11. Black HC: Blacks Law Dictionary, 5th Edition. St Paul, MN, West Publishing Co, 1979, p 257.
12. Federal Rules of Court: Coordinated Research in Ohio from West Group. Eagen, MN, West Publishing Co, 2000, Rule 601, p 136.
13. American Jurisprudence, (ed 2): Federal Rules of Evidence, Rochester, NY. The Lawyers Co-operative Publishing Company, 1982, Volume 32B, p 791.
14. Ohio Rules for Court: Coordinated Research in Ohio from West Group. Eagen, MN, West Publishing Co, 2000, Rule 601, p 190.
15. Black HC: Blacks Law Dictionary, 5th Edition. St Paul, MN, West Publishing Co, 1979, p 1160.
16. American Jurisprudence, (ed 2): Federal Rules of Evidence, Rochester, NY. The Lawyers Co-operative Publishing Company, 1982, Volume 32B, p 797.
17. Ohio Jury Instrutions: Ohio Jury Instructions Committee of the Ohio Judicial Conference 2000. Cincinnati, OH, Anderson Publishing Co, Volume One, Ch 3.5, p 112.
18. Black HC: Blacks Law Dictionary, 5th Edition. St Paul, MN, West Publishing Co, 1979, p 1335.
19. Ohio Jury Instruction: Ohio Jury Instructions Commitee of the Ohio Judicial Conference 2000. Cincinnati, Ohio, Anderson Publishing Co, Volume One, Ch 3.5, p 112.
20. Ibid, p 113.
21. Page's Ohio Revised Code Annoted. Cincinnati, Ohio, Anderson Publishing Co, 1999, ORC 2901 05(D).
22. Ohio Association of Civil Attorneys, Quarterly Review: Direct Examination of the Defendant Doctor in a Medical Malpractice Case. Forrest Norman III, Esq Winter 2000, Issue No 1, p 39.

CHAPTER

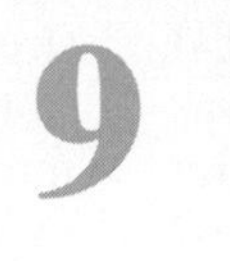

Evidence-Based Medical Dispute Resolution

TEE L. GUIDOTTI, MD, MPH

A disability evaluation does not occur in a vacuum and is not driven by the patient's diagnosis. It is driven by claims of injury, qualification for benefits, and the need to assess a person's remaining capabilities. These issues are inevitably subject to dispute. One of the biggest disputes of all centers on causation. These disputes place the physician or other health professional in the role of expert witness in litigation and medical advisor in adjudication.

Medical testimony used for dispute resolutions is an old and venerable function of health professionals. The law, in general, respects their opinion. However, junk science and the spectacle of dueling experts have provoked a backlash. In past years, the informed judgment of health professionals carried a greater weight than it does today. Recent legal trends in the United States, led by the landmark Daubert decision, have put a greater emphasis on defensible arguments based on empirical data and less emphasis on expert judgment. The ability to base testimony on evidence is more important in today's courtroom. How does the expert witness or medical advisor meet these elevated expectations?

Today, the time is right for an evidence-based approach to legal evidence, whether provided as testimony in a courtroom or input into the adjudication of a claim. About 20 years ago, the movement known variously as critical appraisal and clinical epidemiology, gave rise to evidence-based medicine, which revolutionized medical practice. Something similar could happen in the realm of the court and the expert witness. Adjudication mechanisms that are supported by expert consultants, such as workers' compensation tribunals, have already adopted in practice such an evidence-based approach, in theory. The application of medical knowledge in law may be called evidence-based medical dispute resolution.[6]

The term "evidence-based medical dispute resolution" (EBMDR) is not ideal. First, the qualifier "evidence-based" is intended to evoke parallels with evidence-based medicine and public health, a concept that is meaningful to health care practitioners and epidemiologists, but not necessarily to lawyers. Second, "medical" is used here broadly to refer to issues of health and health care, and is not intended to exclude public health or the application of medical knowledge to public policy. Unfortunately, there is no simple and commonly understood inclusive adjective in the English language for the applied health sciences. Third, "dispute resolution" is a term meaningful to lawyers but not necessarily to health practitioners. Putting these words together, the result is a clunky name for a fairly simple but elusive concept—the evaluation of evidence from the biomedical and population health sciences in the application to law and the resolution of social issues.[6]

Dispute Resolution

There are three alternatives for deciding a case under the law. The first is criminal prosecution, which is only applicable when a law has been violated. The second is litigation and applies when there is a dispute among parties. The third is adjudication, when the responsibility for deciding a case is delegated to a presumably impartial adjudication mechanism. Adjudication is the usual way to resolve issues involving workers' compensation claims, claim appeals, labor–management conflicts, citations for occupational health and safety violations, disability under Social Security, and pension benefits. It may also be required by contract to be used in the first instance to deal with real estate disputes—for example, in California—and may be used by some professional organizations, such as medical licensing bodies, to settle complaints to avoid formal proceedings.

Informal and voluntary adjudication is a growing field as parties seek to avoid the expense of litigation. Adjudication is both a means of reducing the burden and cost of such decisions by diverting them away from the civil litigation system and a mechanism to ensure some degree of consistency in the decisions. Voluntary adjudication systems are usually entered into by contract. Administrative adjudication is a delegation of authority to an administrative officer or tribunal to decide disputes within a circumscribed area of authority, such as workers' compensation claims or insurance benefits. Administrative adjudication systems such as workers' compensation appeals are, in effect, based on tort principles adapted to the circumstances. For example, in workers' compensation the benefit of the doubt is given to the claimant but in tort litigation the benefit of the doubt is on the side of the defendant.

Criminal cases require a certainty beyond reasonable doubt, not unlike scientific certainty. The criteria for adjudications are generally consistent with those of civil law. In civil law, a balance of probabilities is sufficient to decide the case. Applied in adjudication, the usual criterion is a balance of probabilities, or more than 50% certainty, that the putative cause is responsible for the outcome. The usual criterion applied in the workers' compensation arena for accepting an association as causal is that the disease in question is more likely than not associated with the occupational exposure; in cases of doubt, the benefit of the doubt will be given to the claimant.

Causation

Causation is important in disability cases for many reasons, including the following:

- To establish responsibility on the part of whomever allowed it to happen, such as the employer or manufacturer
- To counsel the worker to avoid future exposure
- To prevent the exposure of others, where possible, now or in the future
- To establish the work relationship of a condition for purposes of compensation
- To establish eligibility for workers' compensation, disability insurance, or employment insurance, which are insured services that provide income replacement, each under certain employment-related conditions
- To establish eligibility for social security or welfare, or other entitlement programs that provide income support when the cause of the impairment is judged not to be work-related
- To determine the degree of work injury–related impairment and therefore, indirectly in combination with information on employability, the degree of disability
- To determine whether such impairment is temporary or permanent
- To determine whether exposure standards and regulations governing working conditions have been violated
- To determine whether trends for this disorder in general are improving or worsening as an indication of general working conditions in the industry

Assessment of causation is as critical to a complete evaluation as is diagnosis, prognosis, and disability evaluation. Whenever possible, it is necessary to establish the following:

- The relationship between the disorder and workplace exposure
- The relationship between workplace exposure and specific employment
- The extent to which the worker is impaired owing to the disorder
- The portion of the total impairment narrowly attributable to the work-related component of the disorder
- How likely it is that the degree of impairment is either stable or changing
- Whether others in the same workplace are likely to be exposed to the same hazard to a degree likely to result in the same condition

In most adjudication proceedings, the standard for assessing causation is that it must be more likely than not that a given exposure or action resulted in the adverse outcome, such as an occupational disease or work-related impairment. This is not quite the same as the idea that the prior risk (a priori) was at least somewhat in excess of the risk conferred by any other factor and by all other risk factors in combination, including the risk factors extant in the general population. A priori risk is meaningful only before the event has occurred. After the event has occurred and its causes must be sorted out, the risks must be put into the context of an individual risk profile. The test is whether the likelihood that the outcome was the result of the action in question is at least equal to the likelihood that the outcome might have occurred from all other possible causes. This is not the same as being the most likely possible cause; if there are a number of possible causes, the most likely is not necessarily most probable.

These statements of certainty can be interpreted as descriptions of whether a particular factor was the cause of a particular disorder. This is true only when the assumption is made that there is only one sole and sufficient cause of the outcome. There may be several possible causes, but the argument proceeds on the basis of which cause is more likely to be responsible. This is a common situation, as in cases disputing whether exposure to a carcinogen was sufficient to cause cancer, whether or not there were other causes. In this situation, it is sufficient to determine that the evidence suggests that the cause in question is sufficient and more likely than any and all of the other possibilities.

A related issue arises when exposure to a cause is necessary but not sufficient. For example, consider the situation where a particular exposure raises the risk of a heart attack, but only in persons with high blood pressure. The claimant, who has hypertension, experienced the exposure and sustained a heart attack. To accept the claim, it should be demonstrated that the available evidence shows it to be more likely than not that but for the exposure the person would not have had a heart attack, regardless of the cause of his or her underlying hypertension. It is enough to show that the necessary exposure is present at a level, more likely than not to provoke the effect, once the sufficient grounds are shown to be present.

These statements of certainty can also be applied to incomplete causes. They describe how sure one is with respect to whether some factor was a cause at any level. Some adjudication systems admit liability in circumstances where causation is incomplete. For example, if an occupational exposure contributed to the development of a disease, the fact of that contribution alone is sufficient to define eligibility for compensation under the policies of many workers' compensation boards. However, one must still decide whether it is more likely than not that the factor in question contributed anything to the causation of the outcome.

Causation analysis is, in part, a technical problem. The assessment of causation informs social mechanisms that must operate with equity and fairness. In order to ensure consistency, there must necessarily be a certain amount of standardization and regularity to the evaluation. The consensus approach used for impairment assessments, which has resulted in the AMA Guides, has had no counterpart in causation analysis. Recent legal trends are now forcing this consensus.

Levels of Certainty

A tort is an injury sustained by one person at the hands of another, for which the injured party sues for compensation. The party who sues is the plaintiff and the party sued is the defendant. In principle, the claimant or the plaintiff is challenging the status quo and must provide information necessary to establish his or her claim and to upset the status quo. The burden of proof rests on the plaintiff and the standard employed is proof on the balance of probabilities, which roughly translates to a greater than 50% likelihood.[1] This standard is also adopted in adjudication systems that are based on the model of torts or that substitute for civil litigation, such as workers' compensation, except for the usual provision that the benefit of the doubt is given to the claimant, applicant, or worker.

These ideas work on two levels: the development of a theory or hypothesis concerning an individual claim and the application of a scientific theory to resolving a disputed claim.

There are three levels of certainty that must be satisfied in a medical, or any other, legal dispute[4]:

Burden of proof
Preponderance of evidence
Standard of persuasion or belief

The burden of proof is the responsibility to establish those facts that must be proven if the case is to be resolved. In theory, the burden of proof falls to the claimant in an adjudication. However, in practice, the workers' compensation system requires the claimant only to put forward a proportion of the facts of the case. The defense then rebuts that proportion in the adjudication process as if it bore the burden of proof. Ultimately, no matter who shoulders the burden of proof, it comes down to the fact of causation: Did the exposure cause the damage or not? This is a dichotomy, a true or false proposition. The burden of proof is a statement of fact, not supposition.

The preponderance of evidence in favor of one interpretation or another reflects the weight of evidence used to establish the burden of proof. In other words, in order to establish the facts, evidence must be presented if available. This evidence may be strong, weak, absent, or false and will be rebutted and examined by the other side. At the end of the proceedings, there will be evidence on both sides, each piece of which will carry some weight. In cases of a new association or a poorly documented problem, there may be very little evidence and the evidence may be soft on both sides. In the case of an extensively documented problem, such as asbestos exposure or tobacco smoking, the evidence may be very strong and carry exceptionally high weight. Whichever the situation, what ultimately matters is the preponderance of evidence when the evidence of both sides is reviewed. The preponderance of evidence is described by statements of certainty, such as probable, more likely than not, and possible, the latter term implying less than 50% and therefore being likely to lose the case.

The standard of persuasion or belief is the degree of confidence imparted to the adjudicator and internalized by him or her in making the decision. It is a psychological factor for the adjudicator. The standard of persuasion reflects the uncertainty that the adjudicator may have over the decision and whether the apparent evidence is actually concordant with what really happened. It is a statement about the security of supposition in the face of the unknowable. Terms that may be used to describe what is essentially a state of mind may include beyond reasonable doubt, convincing, more likely than not, most likely among the possibilities, and possible, the latter term implying conceivability but not persuasiveness and usually losing the case.

Gold has pointed out that the statements of probability about burden of proof, evidence, and persuasion are often conflated into a general statement of likelihood.[4] He notes that this confusion distorts the proper analysis of the case in several ways. It devalues the preponderance of evidence because it confuses the notions of weight of evidence and the most convincing, or most likely to make an impression. It makes it difficult to sort through complicated chains of logic, each step of which is associated with a conditional probability, in which the more likely than not standard must either apply to each sequential step in the logic (relaxing the expected rigor of the testimony) or to an overall summation of the argument (increasing the standard for accepting the testimony). Collapsing also tends to favor certain types of evidence, such as epidemiologic studies, that yield clear statements of probabilities and estimates, whereas the standard for resolving medical disputes is making a conclusion about an individual case for which there may be particular circumstances. It also tends to promote fixation on a particular estimate or probability when a range or set of values may be more appropriate to the case. Finally, Gold points out that decisions are made on the basis of persuasion, not by the other levels of certainty. These are of course critical in arriving at the final level of persuasion, but it is ultimately the confidence in the mind of the adjudicator that decides the case.

Implications of Daubert

In the United States, a court decision has clarified the standard for applying scientific information to dispute resolution. The decision in Daubert v Merrell Dow Pharmaceuticals, Inc., 509 U.S. 579, 113 S. Ct. 2786, 125 L. Ed. 2nd 508 (1993), [AU1]attempts to set a new and higher standard for federal courts in reviewing scientific evidence. The effect of this decision was that judges presiding over technically complicated cases have assumed a new gatekeeping function, monitoring scientific evidence that they cannot be expected to have mastered.

In keeping with an earlier trend in some state high courts and general trends in adjudication bodies, Daubert requires federal courts to examine the quality and logic of scientific testimony in arriving at their decisions and to apply the standards of science to scientific testimony. Its influence has been felt throughout the legal system, resulting in higher expectations for rigor and persuasiveness in the opinions offered by expert witnesses.[7]

This new development in tort litigation brings this area of civil litigation in line with the procedures more commonly used in administrative adjudication, where specific technical arguments within a well-circumscribed body of knowledge are the norm. The difference is that the scope of civil litigation is much broader. Civil courts were intended to be the arena for impartial trial of a case based on the information that arises from testimony during the trial. Civil courts were not designed to acquire specialized knowledge to deal with highly technical cases before they come to trial. Now, however, the court must have some prior understanding of the intricacies of the evidence if it is to fulfill its mandate to determine what is admissible.

Prior to 1993, the precedent that determined the standard for admissibility of scientific testimony in most American courts was Frye v. United States, 293 Fed. 1013 (App. D.C. 1923). This case involved the testimony of an expert witness regarding the results of a primitive form of lie detector test. The court refused to admit the testimony on the grounds that the test had not gained "general acceptance in the particular field in which it belongs." The so-called Frye test, as it was then construed, required that the opinions of expert witnesses reflect predominant scientific opinion. Theoretically, idiosyncratic and individualistic opinions were not admissible.[7] The actual text of the Frye decision, referring in ambiguous syntax to "the thing from which [a] deduction is made," might just as well have been construed to refer to the general acceptability of the logic of an opinion, but historically it has not been.[2] Instead, it was assumed to hold the expert witness to testimony that reflected the state of the then-current art, not the cutting edge or the most recent theory or method. The advantage of this system was that the mechanisms of science decided what was acceptable in court and admissible as evidence.

After 30 years, a legal backlash began, supported by arguments that the test was too conservative, was unresponsive to the rapid development of science, and was overly deferential to scientific orthodoxy. The Federal Rules of Evidence, enacted in 1975, undermined the test by omitting it from mention and in effect supplanting it in federal court. The new rule was that if scientific testimony was useful in assisting in finding the facts, it was admissible. This meant that it was up to the jury to decide whether an opinion was sound once the credentials of an expert witness had been established. Even so, many state courts retained the Frye test and were not bound by federal rules of evidence. In cases such as Ferebee v Chevron Chemical Co., 736 F.2d 1529 (1984), juries were entitled to accept or reject the opinions of expert witnesses on faith, having satisfied themselves that one set of witnesses was better qualified or more believable than the other.

In the two decades that followed, the mounting wave of increasingly technical tort litigation made this rule increasingly difficult to sustain. There was a strong perception by the public and among scientists that expert witnesses were free to express any opinion, supported or otherwise, and that "junk science" was allowed in the courtroom.[1,3] The issue came to the forefront in litigation over the risk of birth defects associated with the antepartum antinausea drug Bendectin. In this case, the opinions of many medical experts offered the subjective opinion that the drug was likely to cause birth defects, as opposed to a considerable body of scientific evidence that the drug was not associated with an increased risk. The merits of the case itself are another matter; the legacy of lasting importance was the decision in Daubert v Merrill Dow regarding the admissibility of scientific evidence.

In Daubert, the Supreme Court declared that courts had a responsibility to make a preliminary assessment of the reasoning, premises, and methodology of scientific testimony in order to determine whether the reasons behind the opinion are scientifically valid and useful as applied to the facts of the case. This decision may be made in many ways, including determining whether the theory or method is falsifiable or testable, has been described in peer-reviewed journals, has a demonstrably acceptable error rate, and has received general acceptance among scientists. The basic thrust is to require the court to judge the opinions of expert witnesses by the standards that are applied within the discipline in which the expert witness works.

The Daubert decision imposed a great burden on courts. Few judges and clerks are prepared to assess scientific data independently and few have staffs equipped to do this knowledgeably. Most lawyers will agree that law school was never designed to prepare them for technical issues in science. Some will even go so far as to say that they went into law to avoid science. In the rare instance in which a judge has had access to a consultant capable of rendering an independent assessment, there have been concerns that the in-house expert could unduly affect the decision by manipulating the assessment and by inadvertently supplanting the role of the judge.[6]

The Role of the Medical Advisor

The need to demonstrate a balance of probabilities on the basis of evidence creates two primary responsibilities for the medical advisor in adjudication or the expert witness in court: to provide a clear rationale behind the opinion and to articulate it in a manner that is useful to the adjudicating body. The expert witness in a tort case or the medical advisor in an adjudication hearing has always been expected to express a sound opinion in a comprehensible fashion. However, they are now also expected to provide solid grounds and a coherent chain of logic for the opinion expressed, and to place the opinion in a context that assists the adjudicator in arriving at an informed decision. This discussion approaches evidence-based medical dispute resolution from a general, more theoretical level and looks at how fundamental principles apply to workers' compensation adjudication and appeals.[6]

The medical advisor is expected to reflect either a professional consensus or a well-accepted minority opinion with considerable backing in the scientific community. A personal or idiosyncratic interpretation of the facts contributes little and may undermine one's credibility.

There is nothing unethical about holding one opinion with respect to the legal interpretation of a set of findings and another with respect to the scientific interpretation. Sometimes, the scientific evidence for an association is strong but not conclusive. In such cases, it is entirely reasonable and responsible for an expert witness to maintain on the witness stand that there is or is not an association on the basis of an interpretation of "the weight of evidence," but maintain in a scientific forum that the association is not proven because it has not been proven beyond a reasonable doubt. What counts in the end is the weight of what evidence exists, not how strong the body of evidence is in its entirety.[8]

Independent Medical Examination

Causation assessment and disability evaluation are often conducted by physicians who are hired as independent medical examiners (IME)—neutral and disinterested parties whose role is to determine the facts and to come to a conclusion. The role of the IME is to apply a systematic approach to the evaluation of suspected occupational and environmental disorders. This means taking a fresh and detailed history, reviewing medical records in detail, conducting a new and directed physical examination, understanding but questioning the basis for an existing diagnosis, and addressing the causation issues in the case. IMEs are most often used to assess causation and to determine impairment.

IMEs are growing in importance as lawyers, workers' compensation carriers, and insurance companies see the advantages in objective opinions rendered by a physician who does not have an ongoing relationship with the patient and is not involved in his or her treatment or care. Different health care professionals see the injured worker, for example, in different ways. The person may be a patient with whom the physician has a long-term relationship, a case to be interpreted by experience, a diagnostic dilemma, or an example of frustrated management. Not infrequently, the relationship between the injured worker and the treating health care professional complicates the process, leads to conflicts in interpretation, and interferes with prompt resolution of the claim submitted to the workers' compensation carrier. Part of the current trend toward referring such cases to designated IMEs reflects recognition that a more comprehensive and unified approach expedites care and adjudication and usually results in more consistent management of similar claims. The IME is not cast in a physician–patient relationship with the injured worker and has no role in treatment or management.

In California, the workers' compensation system uses an "agreed medical examiner"(AME). The health care provider serving as the AME is agreed upon in advance by both sides. Similar provisions are found in other states. By contrast, the traditional IME may act as the agent of one side or another.

Epidemiology

Epidemiology is fundamentally a science of generalizations. The basic approach of epidemiology in estimating risk is to measure the experience of a population of individuals with the expectation that, all other things being equal, the overall risk for the group will be a valid estimate for most members of the group. As it is treated in conventional inferential statistics, the risk reflected by the group experience is an estimate for a hypothetical set of similar groups under similar circumstances, not an accurate prediction for an individual member of the group. This estimate may be misleading if there is considerable variation or heterogeneity in the population.[6] (See also Appendix A.)

Population Risk versus Individual Risk

Multiple risk estimates will tend to cluster around a value that represents what some epidemiologists might consider the "true" frequency. However, this is misleading. The toxicologist and occupational physician know how heterogeneous the workers who constitute the population are and how variable the distribution of risk factors may be. They may quite fairly consider the estimate to be rather arbitrary, reflecting the distribution of exposure opportunity among group members as much as it does an exposure–response relationship.

Epidemiology gives the most likely estimates and a statement of uncertainty for larger populations or for certain subgroups, whereas legal proceedings and adjudication are obliged to resolve individual cases. Epidemiology is a population science, but what is most needed in the courts and in claims adjudication is an individualized decision.

Epidemiology is an invaluable aid to interpreting individual cases and claims, but it is only a guide. Estimates of risk derived from epidemiology are limited in their usefulness in individual cases by the methodology of epidemiology.

Concepts of Population Risk

Population risk is only an estimate for the individual within the population and the precision of this estimate depends on epidemiologic methods and the stability of the risk in the population under study. Risks from the experience of a past population may not apply to future risk if determinants of risk have changed.

Individual risk may be very different from its estimate by population studies if the individual differs in characteristics from the profile of the population on average. It is a mistake to take a risk from epidemiologic literature and apply it uncritically to all members of the group.

Measures of Risk Consistent With "More Likely Than Not"

Epidemiology is a science. As such, it adopts the scientific standard of proof, which can be generally characterized as ≥95% sure. However, civil litigation and adjudication hold to a different standard. How does one apply epidemiology when the standard is "50 + 1%"?

There are two separate questions to be considered in evaluating the association between a claim for a possibly work-related condition and occupational exposure when population risk data are to be extrapolated to individual cases: 1) How strong is the evidence for an association? and 2) How strong is the association itself? For population risk data to be useful when applied to the individual, some indication must be given that the individual risk, inferred from the strength of the association in the population, is as least as great as that from other causes not associated with the occupation cause. This is a necessary criterion that must be met before it can be concluded that an occupational cause is likely to be causal in an individual case.

For a cause to meet the criterion of more likely than not, the risk associated with the cause (attributable risk) must exceed the risk that would occur without the operation of the cause. In epidemiology, this corresponds to a relative risk or odds ratio greater than 2.0 or an attributable risk fraction greater than 100%. If there is to be a balance of probabilities that is tipped in favor of the claimant, the risk associated with the occupation or cause in the equation must equal the baseline risk of others in the population. In epidemiologic terms, the attributable risk must be 1.0, or 100% of the expected risk, or greater. A standardized mortality ratio (SMR) of 200 is equal to an attributable risk of 100% of expected. Likewise, the odds ratio—a different way of expressing the same idea—must be 2.0 or more. This corresponds to an overall probability of 50% or greater that the condition was due to the exposure in the population under study and is applied as an estimate of risk due to exposure in the individual.

Limitations of Epidemiology

Epidemiology is subject to numerous sources of bias and error. The key studies on which a case rests must be examined critically with attention to these issues. For a rare cause of death, especially for young workers, the power of any cohort study to detect a true excess risk in the population corresponding to a SMR of 200 is usually much less than 0.80, far less even than the power of most studies to detect lung cancer, and is often less than 15%. That means that even a well-designed study may not detect the true risk.

Statistical Treatment is a priori, not post hoc

Conventional statistics for risk derived from epidemiologic research and applied to an individual assume that the individual's experience is in the future and will be similar to the group experience previously described. There are many logical fallacies in this construct. Clinical medicine has adopted another statistical approach, called the Bayesian approach, which looks at the probability of an event after it has occurred. This approach fits the needs of causation analysis better than the conventional approach. Although the Bayesian approach is not difficult, it is unfamiliar and the logic less accessible to laypersons.

Evaluation of the Literature

The evidence accumulated that bears on the question of causation may be evaluated by various criteria, of which the most accepted among epidemiologists are those developed in 1965 by Sir Austin Bradford Hill. The traditional Hill criteria are used by epidemiologists to assess whether an association may be causal, but not whether the risk factor being evaluated is the strongest, the most frequent, or the most necessary for a disease to occur. The Hill criteria address causation in general but not causation in a given situation. Following are the criteria proposed by Hill for accepting an epidemiologically demonstrated association as causal:

- Strength of the association
- Consistency among studies, especially by different techniques
- Specificity of outcome
- Exposure preceding disease outcome
- Dose–response relationship (epidemiologic)
- Plausibility of a biological mechanism
- Coherence of chain of evidence
- Experimental association, especially dose–response (toxicologic)
- Analogy to similar effect produced by a similar agent

The criteria are important in establishing an epidemiologic association but cannot meaningfully be applied to the individual case.

Apportionment

Workers' compensation boards in all jurisdictions are faced with an expanding challenge in the management of claims related to occupational disease. Questions of causation, the presence of multiple risk factors, and modifications of the characteristic presentation of occupational diseases greatly complicate adjudication.[6]

The process of adjudicating workers' compensation claims involves a differentiation between occupational and nonoccupational causes of disease and injury. Although in practice this can be exceedingly difficult and in some cases impossible, the imperative of establishing causation is an integral part of the philosophy of workers' compensation. That is because workers' compensation systems are mandated to resolve individual claims on the best evidence, not to generalize to groups.

Faced with a large number of difficult occupational disease cases, workers' compensation agencies have considered apportionment by cause. Apportionment by cause is the estimation in an individual case of the relative contribution to an outcome, such as a multifactorial disease, of several risk factors or potential causal exposures that are present in the case and that are known to be associated with the outcome. Apportionment by cause is a way of apportioning responsibility and contribution to the final outcome. In the tort system, the equivalent concept is apportionment of harm (meaning responsibility for causing harm) but because workers' compensation is a no-fault insurance system, the assignment of blame or responsibility is not as useful.

Apportionment by cause must be performed on the individual case, which may vary from the population as a whole. Often, apportionment cannot be determined with certainty and epidemiologic data may then be used to derive an estimate of the relative contribution of a risk factor in an individual claim. However, this must be understood to be a derived estimate, not to be confused with the apportionment of impairment or its social derivative, disability, which can be done by specific measurement in the individual case.

The benefits of fair and accurate apportionment, when it can be done, are obvious: adjudication may be simpler, adjudication may be fairer to employers and some injured workers, and financial resources would be conserved for workers with greater impairment. Workers might be encouraged to take responsibility for their own health, fiscal exposure would be more fairly shared among health care funding agencies, and the relative contribution to disability benefits for permanent impairment could be divided among payers, such as provincial health care plans, Social Security or Canada Pension, and workers' compensation.

Although apportionment is an attractive option for adjudication in compensation, it has many drawbacks and uncertainties. The single greatest obstacle to apportionment is the availability of data and limitations on the methodology of assessment of relative contribution to the disease outcome. A new generation of biomarkers of exposure and effect may provide an approach to the apportionment of causation resulting from recent exposures. Clinical medicine and, soon, genomics and the study of gene–toxicant interactions may provide insights that can be used to derive reasonable estimates of apportionment in the individual case. Barring a major technical breakthrough in biomarkers, these will always be rough estimates. However, even at the current crude state of the art, they may be used as the basis for a consensus on apportionment, not unlike the AMA Guides which represents a consensus on impairment.

In most jurisdictions, workers' compensation carriers are required to accept claims in their totality if a substantial component of the disease is work related. However, defining what constitutes a substantial, significant, or even minimal component is often difficult.

A special case of apportionment is presumption. This is the assumption that because the majority of cases of a disease or outcome in a given occupation or population can be attributed to the cause or risk factor in question, any such case for which a claim is filed will be routinely accepted unless there is a direct challenge, or rebuttal, that presents facts to the contrary. Many presumptions are written into law, often without good evidence, such as the presumption in California for heart disease among firefighters and police officers. Others are "scheduled," or designated on lists. Presumption logically requires both strong evidence of an association and a risk that is at least doubled, as described previously. A simple association can be accepted at a more than 50% level of certainty for the occupational group overall at whatever degree of association, but a simple association is not the same as presumption. A presumption involves the same degree of certainty but an actual proportion of the disease (attributable fraction) compatible with at least 50% in the occupation or population overall. At such a high frequency, it is statistically likely that for any one individual drawn from that population (and submitting a claim) who presents with the disease or outcome in question, the occupational cause would be the risk factor. For example, firefighters have a much higher risk of kidney cancer than the general population but their risk of lung cancer is only elevated by about 50%. One can justify a presumption for kidney cancer, but not for lung cancer. Any firefighter with kidney cancer probably would not have been at risk if he or she were not in that occupation.

Among the most common forms of apportionment in lung disease is assessing the contribution to causation from cigarette smoking compared to occupational exposures. The usual practice has been to compare the magnitude of risk imposed by exposures, or demonstrated in studies of groups, compared to the undeniably high risk of disease associated with cigarette smoking. However, in workers' compensation, there is a principle that one "takes the worker as they come." This principle means that once a worker is hired, the employer is responsible for injuries or illness arising from work regardless of the worker's personal health history or lifestyle. If a worker who smokes is hired, because there is no policy against hiring smokers, the employer is responsible for disorders arising out of work regardless of whether smoking played a role. This means that the relevant comparison is not the degree of risk imposed by cigarette smoking compared to the usually lesser degree of risk imposed by the occupational exposures. Logically, it means that the employer is responsible if the worker's risk due to exposure is substantially increased compared to other smokers who are not occupationally exposed. In practice, however, the simpler comparison between smokers and nonsmokers is usually the only one considered. This is one example of how principles in workers' compensation are often applied inconsistently.

Asbestos-related diseases are particularly problematic in this regard and illustrate these problems well. The example of asbestos-related disease illustrates the fundamental issues associated with the adjudication of multifactorial diseases. Among these fundamental issues is the relative contribution of different causes, such as cigarette smoking or asbestos exposure, to the risk of a disease such as lung cancer or to overall impairment from an outcome such as chronic obstructive airway disease. It is generally easier to distinguish occupational from nonoccupational disease when characteristic outcomes are specific to the exposure, as occurs with pneumoconioses such as asbestosis, or when the association is so great that a presumption is reasonable, as in mesothelioma. However, when the outcomes are not specific, and especially when they may also be caused by other common environmental exposures such as cigarette smoking, defining causation can be problematic. The first step is to determine that a relationship to asbestos exposure exists. The second would be to assess the relative contribution of the asbestos exposure.

Cigarette smokers may be at greater risk for lung cancer from their cigarette smoking habit, in isolation, than their asbestos exposure, in isolation, but such exposures usually do not occur in isolation. The more relevant fact is that in combination, exposure to asbestos raises the risk of lung cancer among smokers in comparison to other, nonexposed smokers to such a degree that by the standards of civil litigation it should be considered more likely than not that the asbestos exposure was responsible. Because employers almost never required that workers be nonsmokers at the time of hire, the system must logically "take the workers as they come" and assess their risk as smokers, not compared to nonsmokers.

Conclusion

Health and medical knowledge are essential to the resolution of disputes in legal and administrative applications (such as workers' compensation) and provide essential input into public policy decisions. There are no socially agreed-upon rules for the application of this knowledge except in the law. On a practical level, the legal system lacks the capacity to evaluate the validity of knowledge as evidence and therefore relies heavily on expert opinion. A similar problem once existed for the clinical practice of medicine. Over the last 20 years, an approach called critical appraisal has established norms for the acceptance of evidence in clinical practice that are now almost universally accepted. Critical appraisal is a systematic approach to evaluating the evidence based on clinical epidemiology; evidence-based medicine is the practice of medicine justified by valid studies correctly interpreted. A project to develop a framework for applying the knowledge of health and medicine similar to the concept of critical appraisal but conducted within the dominant framework of dispute resolution in society—the law—is being developed.[6] One critical issue is how to apply scientific evidence when the standard is "more likely than not," rather than scientific certainty. Another is how the generalizations drawn from epidemiology and population-based sciences are interpreted and individualized, as they must be, for the case at hand. Two related issues are how risk is interpreted for an individual after the fact, when conventional probability treats risk before the fact and that conventional biostatistics apply primarily to populations. This emerging approach is being called evidence-based medical dispute resolution.[6]

References

1. Boden LI, Miyares Jr, Ozonoff D: Science and persuasion: Environmental disease in U.S. courts. Soc Sci Med 27:1019–1029, 1988.
2. Black B: Evolving legal standards for the admissability of scientific evidence. Science 239:1508–1512, 1988.
3. Burger EJ Jr: Scientific information in judicial and administrative systems. Soc Sci Med 27:1031–1041, 1988.
4. Gold S: Causation in toxic torts: Burdens of proof, standards of persuasion, and statistical evidence. Yale Law J 96:376–402, 1986.
5. Guidotti TL: Considering apportionment by cause: Its methods and limitations. Journal of Workers' Compensation 7:55–73, 1988.
6. Guidotti TL, Rose SG (eds): Science on the Witness Stand: Scientific Evidence in Law, Adjudication, and Policy. Beverly Farms, Mass, OEM Health Information, 2001.
7. Levy DM: Scientific evidence after Daubert. Litigation 22:48–52, 1995.
8. Rose S: Landmark legal cases in epidemiology. In Bernier RH, Mason V (eds): Episource: A Guide to Resources in Epidemiology. Roswell, GA, The Epidemiology Monitor, 1991, pp 786–826.

CHAPTER

10

Causality

ELIZABETH GENOVESE, MD, MBA

The independent medical examiner is expected to address causality unless it has already been accepted by the insurer, is presumptive (i.e., automatically accepted based on case law or legislation), or has been established through litigation. Causality always must be addressed when the referral source has significant doubts regarding the legitimacy of a claimant's complaints as related to the initial injury (or alleged injury). Even in the presence of a clear causal relationship between an accident and subsequent physical pathology, one may need to state whether an exacerbation, recurrence, or aggravation of a prior condition occurred and apportion liability accordingly.

When examining a claimant who seems credible and insists that one or several medical problems were caused by a given event or exposure, many physicians accept this as fact, even though a careful analysis of the situation would clearly indicate otherwise. The independent examiner is hired to evaluate the claimant objectively, and is expected to base determinations of causality upon commonly accepted physiologic, epidemiologic, and statistical principles, rather than make decisions empirically or based solely on the claimant's history and the apparent believability thereof. Multiple definitions of causation and their application are discussed in the AMA Guides fifth,[9] and in greater detail in the Guides companion, Master the Guides Fifth.[10]

Fundamentals

Medical causality is imputed when the association between a medical condition and a given exposure (physical, biologic, or chemical) is such as to lead one to believe that the condition would not have occurred in the absence of the exposure (Table 10–1). The temporal relationship between the exposure or injury and the medical condition (or symptoms suggestive of the condition) is the first factor that must be assessed. The illness or disease should occur after the exposure (referred to as "temporal ordering") and within a time period that is reasonable given the nature of the exposure (temporal

TABLE 10–1

Criteria for Asserting the Existence of a Causal Relationship

Temporal Relationship	Cause should come before effect. The interval between the two should be consistent with waht is found in reports or studies of similar exposures/injuries.
Mechanism	Must be anatomically and physiologically plausible.
Contiguity (Dose-Response/Duration)	Should be a clear relationship between cause and effect, with an increase in exposure (dose or duration) leading to an increaes in effect.
Consistency	Exposure should consistently cause the disease or injury under investigation.
Specificity	Should be a relative absence of other factors or conditions which "explain" the disease.
Coherence	Presumption of work-relatedness in an individual case should be consistent with the medical literature.

contiguity). In certain situations (such as asbestos, lead, and benzene exposure) there is a long latency between the time of exposure and the appearance of disease. Hence, regardless of whether a temporal relationship appears to be present, determining causality also requires one to assess whether a causal relationship is biologically plausible.

A causal relationship is biologically plausible when:

1. The relationship between the medical condition and the exposure or injury can be explained anatomically or physiologically.
2. The duration, intensity, or mechanism of exposure or injury was sufficient to cause the illness or injury in question.
3. There is evidence suggesting that the exposure is consistently or reliably associated with the process under investigation in the population under investigation or in peer-reviewed literature.
4. Cause and effect are contiguous—i.e., there is a readily understandable relationship between the two, in which an increase in the magnitude of the exposure reliably leads to an increase in the severity of its alleged effect upon the injured or exposed person, and vice versa.
5. There is literature providing biologic or statistical evidence indicating that the symptoms or disorder could develop as a result of the exposure (coherence).[1]
6. There is specificity of the association for the injury (i.e., the absence of other factors, especially preexisting disease, that could have caused or contributed to the problem).

The independent examiner is obligated to evaluate the validity and strength of all postulated causal mechanisms. Mechanisms that appear weak, or are clearly flawed, must be identified as such and accepted as likely only when at least two other criteria for biologic plausibility have been met. Optimally one would wish to satisfy all criteria. There are, however, circumstances when contiguity cannot be demonstrated, as some exposures lead to disease in a noncontiguous fashion. Specificity of association is also difficult to illustrate definitively given the multifactorial nature of many disease processes. Literature supportive of causality is generally available, but must be closely scrutinized before relying upon it as it is often of poor quality.

Literature Review

The criteria of temporal relationship and mechanism of exposure or injury must be met in any reference purporting to establish a causal exposure between the outcome under investigation and a given event. Furthermore, when using citations from the literature as the basis for imputing causality, one must be careful to differentiate between experimental studies demonstrating cause and effect and epidemiologic studies demonstrating association, because the existence of an association between two events does not necessarily mean that they are causally related.

The assessment of study design is the most critical task one must perform in evaluating whether statements regarding causality in the literature are sound. Studies can be experimental or observational. Experimental, randomized controlled studies are the best method for assessing if an exposure leads to a given outcome, because one can randomize the choice of subjects and control for those variables that might be etiologic for the disease. One can also control the intensity and duration of exposure and the interpretation (single blind, double blind) of data. The studies utilized in the assessment of causality in humans are usually observational and epidemiologic rather than experimental (Table 10–2).

Epidemiology is defined as "The science concerned with the study of factors determining and influencing the frequency and distribution of disease, injury, and other health-related events in a defined human population."[2] It is primarily descriptive and identifies the presence or absence of associations between disease and exposure in the population or populations studied. Epidemiologic studies, however, are only as good as their design and analysis. It is consequently mandatory for those involved in the assessment of causality to be able to evaluate these

TABLE 10–2

Experimental vs. Observational Studies

Study Characteristics	Experimental	Observational
Single – Blind (Subject unaware of exposure)	Generally	Rarely
Double – Blind (Subject/investigator unaware)	Sometimes	Never
Investigator controls "dose"	Yes	No
Subjects randomly selected	Yes	No
Possible selection bias	No	Yes
Possible recall bias	No	Yes
Possible confounders (non-causal)	Sometimes	Often
Suggests "cause and effect" if positive	Yes	Rarely
Only suggests "association" if positive	No	Yes

studies critically before automatically accepting their conclusions as valid. Furthermore, "as confident as one might be that the conclusions of an epidemiological study are scientifically sound, there is always a possibility that new discoveries or even new analyses of old data will alter those conclusions."[3]

In observational studies, researchers do not control exposure and do not randomly select subjects. They instead must work with existing data, which makes these studies subject to bias (a systematic or measurement error in the design or analysis of a study that leads to an erroneous conclusion or judgment regarding the strength and significance of a given association). Selection bias (a bias in which groups differ in ways other than just their exposure to a given factor) is a common problem affecting observational studies. Recall bias (a bias that occurs when members in one group [generally the one with the disease] are more likely to recall certain events or exposures than are those in the control group) is also common. Other common biases are information bias (which occurs when information is collected differently from the exposed and unexposed groups), nonresponse bias (which occurs when there are differences between those who do or do not follow-up with a survey or treatment), and detection bias (which occurs when a problem is detected at an earlier stage in the group that is screened than it would have been otherwise).

Observational studies can be descriptive or analytic. Case reports and case series are examples of descriptive studies. In these studies, the author simply describes a study of a given process among a group of individuals, attempting to ascertain what factor the individuals had in common that could explain the disease. This type of study does not include individuals without the condition. Consequently, although one can look at the affected population and generate hypotheses regarding similar exposures that might be reflective of causality, they are not suitable to evaluate whether a given exposure truly led to the disease in question (Table 10–3).

Analytic studies are designed to evaluate hypotheses. There are three types of studies that do so: prevalence, case–control, and cohort studies. Data can be collected either at a single point in time, as in prevalence and case–control studies, or longitudinally, as in cohort studies and case–control studies that use incident cases (i.e., that wait for cases to occur). In these studies, direct testing of causal hypotheses is possible because the exposure of the group with the disease is compared to that of the unaffected group.

In prevalence (or cross-sectional) studies, the prevalence of a condition in a population at a point in time is analyzed. The presence of suspected risk factors is assumed to be present in those with and without the condition of interest. Because the cases studies are prevalent and not incident, the relationship of cause and effect due to the exposure cannot be readily determined. In particular, it is common for individuals with clusters of risk factors, rather than a single risk factor, to end up in the same group. When the data are analyzed, one cannot definitively state that the association between the condition under investigation is reflective of a particular risk factor or if the association is artifactual. Prevalence studies are most effectively used as a means of assessing the distribution of disease in a population; distribution patterns may then suggest etiological hypotheses that can be tested first by case-control and then by prospective studies.[4]

TABLE 10–3

Comparison of Observational Studies

Study Characteristics	Cross Sectional	Case Control	Historical Cohort	Nested Case Control	Prospective Cohort
Data collected at single point in time	Yes	Yes	Yes	Y/N: cases are incident	No
Data collected longitudinally	No	Y/N incident	Yes	Yes	Yes
Work "backward" to identify exposures	Yes	Yes	Yes	No	No
Used to calculate disease incidence	Yes	No	Yes	Yes	Yes
Prone to recall bias	Yes	Yes	No(?)	No	No
Prone to artifactual associations	Yes	Yes	No	No	No
Suitable for rare disease processes	Yes	Yes	Yes	Yes	No
Appropriate for diseases with long latency	Yes	Yes	Yes	Yes	No
Expense	Low	Low	Low	Medium	High
Strength of evidence regarding etiology	Low	Low	Medium	Medium	Good

In case–control studies, individuals with signs and symptoms of a disease are matched to controls according to various characteristics, after which the two groups are comparatively analyzed. There are usually predetermined and equal numbers of cases and controls. In order for the study to be valid, cases and controls must be matched for all factors and characteristics except the one under evaluation. To the extent that this does not occur, the analysis of the data may be flawed.

The ideal epidemiologic study is a longitudinal prospective study of a group (or cohort) of healthy people in a well-defined source population, followed over a period of time. Baseline information about the persons under evaluation and their risk factors is collected before the disease occurs. One then observes the cohort over time to see if, and in whom, the disease occurs. Cohort studies offer the best evidence regarding etiology because they most closely approximate a randomized controlled trial. However, before performing this type of study, it is best to have data (from prior descriptive or cross-sectional studies) that lead one to suspect that a particular exposure causes the disease of interest, because they can be too expensive to do otherwise.

The terms "relative risk" and "odds ratio" are used to characterize the degree to which a given disease is associated with potentially causative factors. Statistically significant risk estimates that are greater than or equal to 2.0 are considered indicative of a strong association.[5] Likewise, a relative risk ratio less than one would suggest that an exposure is protective. Statistical significance is present if the occurrence of a given exposure leads to a prevalence (or incidence) of the medical condition under evaluation that is greater than 2 to 3 (depending on the P value one is using). Standard deviations in the control group outside the mean are outside the realm of what was expected (see Appendix A). A confidence interval can also be calculated from the data and the probability can be determined of the mean value falling inside this interval. If the mean does not fall into the predetermined confidence interval, then one hypothesizes that the external event or situation was a causal factor in shifting the confidence interval away from the "true" mean. In this situation, the results are reflective of an association rather than an absolute proof of causality.

As implied in the discussion of bias, the existence of an association between two events does not automatically imply that they are causally related. Associations can be causal but they can also be noncausal, artifactual, or reflective of multiple causations. Artifactual associations occur when the studies or analyses on which the assumption of causality is based fail to appropriately consider sources of bias or are flawed in their statistical analysis of the data. Noncausal relationships can be mistakenly imputed as indicative of causality when there is a third, or "confounding," factor or variable. A confounding factor is a variable that is independently related to the outcome of interest and is more likely to be present in one group of subjects than another; and potentially confuses or "confounds" the results,[6] or is associated with both the exposure and the disease. A classic example was the initial description of an association between coffee drinking and heart disease—ultimately determined to reflect the indepedent association of cigarette smoking with both. In summary, although experimental studies are the best way to establish cause and effect, the studies on which physicians tend to base their opinions are generally observational or epidemiologic in nature. Case reports and cross-sectional or prevalence studies are fraught with potential sources of error. Cohort studies, especially if prospective, minimize errors but are difficult to perform and may lead, via selection bias, to noncausal or artifactual associations, or be reflective of multiple causation.

Multiple causation is common in medicine and occurs when a given disease is, or can be, due to one or more processes. Specificity of association cannot be claimed if multiple causations are operative. One is then obliged to estimate the degree to which each of the multiple potential causal factors led to the disease in question. It is in this situation where the various aspects of apportionment—precipitation, acceleration, aggravation, and exacerbation—become relevant.

Specificity of Association and Apportionment

Most medical conditions are multifactorial in etiology; i.e., they are reflective of more than one physiologic or environmental process. Evaluation of the results of epidemiologic studies via regression analysis (which weighs the contribution of various factors both individually and in combination on a given event or events) provides data that can be applied when reaching conclusions regarding the degree to which one would expect a given factor to contribute to the medical condition under evaluation but never can provide definitive answers regarding apportionment.

It is impossible to accurately evaluate to what extent a given factor or exposure was the contributing cause in a multifactorial disease process. Likewise, in certain situations (such as heart disease), the genetic predisposition of the affected individual is a considerable, if not primary, determinant of causality. Assessing the specificity of association is consequently often the most difficult aspect of causality analysis.

There is a great deal of legal terminology focused on establishing, and labeling, the degree to which an event or injury has led to a particular outcome. The legal determination of causality uses, but does not necessarily rely upon, the medical evidence that supports or refutes a causal relationship between a given event and outcome. Furthermore, it is often societal decision, and not scientific method, that determines the degree of certainty required to reach conclusions about the presence or absence of a causal relationship.[7] Using the legal definitions of causality, a relationship between an event and a given outcome is classified as "probable" or "possible." It is probable if the chance of them being related is greater than 50%. It is possible if the chance of a relationship is deemed to be less than 50%. The skill of the attorneys arguing the case, the credibility of the claimant and his or her physician, the ability of the medical expert to present the medical information regarding causality, and the existence of case law (which may have established the de facto existence of a causal relationship unless definitively proven otherwise) all influence the ultimate determination. Statements are often made regarding the probability or possibility of a causal relationship between an event and an outcome in the absence of any objective epidemiologic or biologic rationale for the determination. While the Supreme Court, in the Daubert case, held that testimony must be grounded in the methods and procedures of science and based on more than simply subjective belief or unsupported speculation to be held as relevant and reliable,[8] this standard is not routinely used in many jurisdicitons. Thus the use of the legal terminology alone can imply a degree of certainty that may be completely unfounded.

The concept of apportionment reflects the understanding that legal definitions of causality are often not medically supportable, as medical decisions regarding causality generally require certainty in excess of 95% in order to be valid. Apportionment is necessary when multiple causal factors lead to a given level of symptoms, disease, impairment, or disability and involves determining to what extent the current condition is related to a particular event or events, injury, preexisting conditions, or unrelated disease processes. Under these circumstances, apportionment requires the examiner not only to understand the temporal factors, biologic plausibility, and literature in support of the alleged association between the exposure or injury and the disease, but also to know the claimant's medical history, the usual natural history of the medical condition under investigation, the legal background or constraints under which the claim is being investigated, and, if two injuries have occurred, the contribution that each may have made to the claimant's current condition.

The concept of apportionment also requires an understanding of the terms precipitation, acceleration, aggravation, exacerbation, and recurrence (Table 10–4). Precipitation implies that the injury or exposure caused a disease process for which the claimant was at risk, but that had not yet (and possibly never would have) become manifest. In acceleration, the exposure hastens, or is claimed to hasten, the course of the disease; i.e., the disease would have eventually become symptomatic but did so more rapidly as a result of the injury or exposure. When a given event accelerates the manifestation of a given disease process, it is not necessarily any worse than it would have been in the absence of the injury or exposure—it just occurs earlier. This is different from aggravation, which is the permanent worsening of a prior condition by a particular event or exposure. This can include those situations where a process was without symptoms, or allegedly without symptoms, until the event under investigation occurred. Exacerbation is the transient worsening of a prior condition by an injury or illness, with the expectation that the situation will eventually return to baseline. The issue, of course, is when one might expect this to occur. A recurrence is similar to an exacerbation, but generally involves the reappearance of signs or symptoms attributable to a prior injury with minimal or no provocation—i.e., in the absence of definable injury. A detailed description of the context in which symptoms appeared is mandatory when recurrence is suspected, as are medical records from the claimant's primary physician.

Causality Assessment

Before making any impairment or disability determination, the physician is obligated to understand how an organ system (or body part under study) normally functions in the absence of disease. This is then coupled with a thorough understanding of the mechanism of the disease process under investigation. Causality is possible—i.e., biologically plausible—if the nature of the adverse effects produced by a given physical, chemical, biologic, or psychological stressor is sufficient to alter the anatomy or physiology of the system or body part involved in a fashion that results in the disease under investigation. There also must be an appropriate temporal relationship between the alleged causal event and the disease manifestations. Furthermore, in situations where there is trauma, the mechanical forces involved must be sufficient to cause the alleged physiologic or anatomic stress.

TABLE 10–4

Terminology Utilized in Apportionment

Precipitation	Injury or exposure causes a "latent" or potential disease process to become manifest
Acceleration	Injury or exposure hastens clinical appearance of an underlying disease process
Aggravation	Permanent worsening of a prior condition by a particular event or exposure
Exacerbation	Temporary worsening of a prior condition by a exposure/injury
Recurrence	Signs of symptoms attributable to a prior illness or injury occur in the absence of a new provacative event

One should then look for studies supporting the causal relationship between the type of exposure or injury the claimant sustained and the disease process or injury under investigation in the medical literature. If they exist, the next step is to assess whether the epidemiologic and statistical principles used in these studies suggest that the casual association is real, or whether these studies are merely anecdotal or otherwise without scientific basis or validity. If the association between an exposure or injury and the postulated "effect" meets epidemiologic, physiologic, and mechanistic criteria for imputing causality, or the injury is a clear sequela of direct trauma, it is then reasonable to assume that a causal relationship between an alleged exposure or injury and the disease process actually exists.

These types of determinations must not be made solely on the basis of the claimant's history. The medical records provide a more accurate and defensible history and must support the occurrence of the injury and the appearance of symptoms or signs of pathology within a time frame that is consistent with the disease process under investigation. Those records from immediately after the injury are best for this purpose, as they are generally the most accurate source of information regarding the claimant's status both before and after a trauma, and often provide the most accurate description of what actually occurred. Emergency room records, police and accident reports, and the employer's report of occupational injury or disease (for workers' compensation claims) are examples of documents that are particularly useful in this regard. If these records are not available or are ambiguous, it is best to describe the assessment of causality as provisional rather than definitive, even if the mechanism of injury, the physical examination, and the literature review indicate that a causal relationship may indeed be present.

Combinations of direct trauma and a preexisting disease process are more difficult to assess for causality and apportionment. One must determine, again, if the requirements of temporal relationship, biologic plausibility, literature support, and sufficient injury have been met. This includes an assessment of whether the trauma would have caused the disease in the absence of the preexisting process or whether the injuries caused by the trauma or exposure would ordinarily decrease over time, because these answers provide grounds for apportionment. It is equally important to assess whether the preexisting process would have progressed on its own accord to a point where the claimant would have had the same clinical presentation; if so, one can argue that the accident only caused an acceleration of an inevitable process.

When dealing with preexisting conditions, it is mandatory to examine all the records carefully, paying particular attention to the records of those providers who treated the claimant immediately after the accident. These are often the most accurate rendition of the incident and treatment that can be found. Records prior to the accident are even more critical, as they may be the only source of information regarding preexisting conditions. When there are no medical records from before and immediately after an accident, one cannot definitively establish that a causal relationship between current complaints and the accident exists—only that the claimant's history supports the causal relationship. If the examiner believes that additional information, records, or tests are needed to support conclusions regarding relatedness, then it is necessary to state this and to describe exactly what information or testing is required.

In conclusion, the examiner can only provide an accurate determination of causality if he or she applies commonly accepted principles of causality assessment, within an objective framework, in which the claimant's statements have validity only to the extent that they are supported by the medical records. In those instances where the medical record is inadequate, the examiner can make preliminary conclusions regarding causality, especially if the elements of temporal relationship and biologic plausibility have been met, but should reserve final judgment until the entire relevant medical record is available for review.

References

1. Harris J (ed). Occupational Medicine Treatment Guidelines. American College of Occupational and Environmental Medicine. Beverly, Mass, OEM Press, 1997.
2. Dorland's Medical Dictionary 28th Edition. Philadelphia, WB Saunders, 1994.
3. Macklin R: Ethics, epidemiology and law: the case of silicone breast implants. Am J Public Health 89:487–489, 1999.
4. Morton RF, Hebel JR, McCarter RJ: A Study Guide to Epidemiology and Biostatistics. Aspen Publishers, Gaithersburg, Maryland, 1990.
5. Bombardier C, Kerr MS, Shannon HS, Frank JW: A guide to interpreting epidemiologic studies on the etiology of back pain. Spine 19:2047S–2056S, 1994.
6. Dawson-Saunders B, Trapp RG: Basic and Clinical Biostatistics, 2nd edition. Appleton and Lange, Norwalk, Connecticut, 1994.
7. Harber P, Shusterman D: Medical causation analysis heuristics. J Occ Env Med 38:577–586, 1996.
8. Annas GJ: Burden of proof: judging science and protecting public health in (and out of) the courtroom. Am J Public Health 89:490–493, 1999.
9. Cocchiarella L, Andersson GBJ (eds): Guides to the Evaluation of Permanent Impairment, 5th ed. Chicago, American Medical Association, 2001.
10. Cocchiarella L, Lord SJ Master the AMA Guides Fifth: A Medical and Legal Transition to the Guides to the Evaluation of Permanent Impairment, Fifth Edition. First Edition. Chicago, American Medical Association, 2001.

CHAPTER

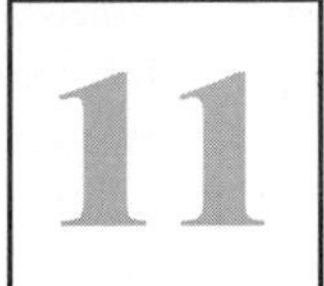

Contrasting the Standard, Impairment, and Disability Examination

STEPHEN L. DEMETER, MD, MPH

As discussed in Chapter 1, there are fundamental differences between a disability examination (DE) and an impairment evaluation (IE). The goal for a DE is to determine an individual's ability to perform a certain task or tasks. These tasks are generally (but not always) in the work setting and may include issues concerning the individual's ability to travel to and from work, participate in the work environment, and interact with coworkers. The goal of an IE is to determine deviations in health status and to quantify those deviations.

Just as there are fundamental differences between a DE and an IE, there are fundamental differences between these two types of examinations and a standard medical examination (ME). Most physicians approach IEs and DEs by extrapolating from the knowledge and experience gained in their own specialty. IEs and DEs are emerging, if not as specialties in their own right, then as fields requiring specialized knowledge and skills. This chapter explores the fundamental differences between the standard ME that a practitioner performs in his or her own specialty area and the IE and DE required in that field.

TABLE 11–1

Similarities Between a Disability or Impairment Evaluation and a Standard Medical Examination/Practice

1. Gather the patient's history
2. Perform a physical examination
3. Order appropriate laboratory tests
4. Apply the information obtained in steps 1 to 3
5. Report the information from steps 1 to 3
6. Act ethically
7. Establish a practice

TABLE 11–2

Goal of an Impairment Examination

1. Identify issue(s) requiring clarification by the referring source
2. Obtain, be familiar with, and use appropriate rating systems
3. Determine if the claimant has reached maximum medical improvement (MMI)
4. Rate the impairment(s) requested by the referring source
5. Apportion the various causes of the impairment, if requested

Impairment Evaluations

Similarities Between the IE, DE, and ME

See Table 11–1 for similarities between an IE and a standard ME or practice. Table 11–2 shows goals of the IE.

History

The history is the single most important facet of every patient encounter. It has been stated that 90% of all diagnoses are based on the history alone. For the ME, physical examinations and laboratory tests rarely change the initial impressions and are used primarily to confirm and quantitate diagnostic abnormalities. This is also true for IE, although to a lesser degree because the diagnosis of a problem is not really the goal in an IE as it is in the standard ME. A physician often assumes the role of a detective in the standard ME. In the IE the physician works to obtain an impairment rating wherein the diagnosis is often known, and proceeds to evaluate the functional impact of the impairments. Thus the history takes on the role of documenting an injury or quantitating the effects on a person's lifestyle or capabilities.

Depending on the type of examination performed and the expected treatment recommendation, some MEs also focus on documentation and quantitation (for example, to determine whether surgery is needed for a patient with spinal stenosis) and some IEs are oriented toward arriving at a proper diagnosis (for example, determining whether a person exposed to potentially toxic fumes has a resultant asthma if hyperventilation syndrome is the cause for the shortness of breath). In general, the history either assists in diagnosis or provides documentation and quantitation.

Physical Examination

A sound and skillful physical examination is a necessary component of the standard ME and the IE. As with the history, the evidence obtained with a physical examination supports or refutes a diagnosis, documents abnormalities, and quantitates pathologic changes. In the IE, however, the next step, that of evaluating the impact of an impairment, is the focus. In addition, for an IE, certain examinations may be limited to conform to a particular rating system (see later discussion and Chapter 12).

Laboratory Testing

As with the history and physical examination, laboratory tests assist in making a diagnosis, documenting a problem, or quantitating an abnormality. During an IE, the types of tests ordered and performed may differ from those used in a standard ME, depending on the rating system used.

Applying Information

Regardless of the emphasis, knowledge is obtained about the individual's abnormalities and limitations and the expected future of that individual vis-a-vis those abnormalities and limitations. The critical difference between the IE and the standard ME lies in the application of that knowledge versus its acquisition.

Reporting Information

Once knowledge is derived, a report is prepared to summarize the knowledge and finalize the conclusion. In the standard ME these conclusions may be verbal or written down in a listing of diagnostic conclusions or therapeutic recommendations; alternately, a written report may be prepared. The IE and DE use the written report exclusively.

Ethical Considerations

The earliest and best-known standard of medical ethics is found in the Hippocratic Oath. Physicians are expected to act compassionately and always in the best interest of their patients, to be honest and sincere, to be knowledgeable about their particular field and its limitations, and be willing to refer patients to other physicians when their limitations are exceeded. Just as a physician is morally bankrupt if he or she intentionally falsifies diagnoses or makes recommendations for inappropriate treatment, so too is the physician who provides a biased report that overestimates or underestimates an impairment rating in his or her role as a plaintiff's or defense physician when performing an IE. The end result of an IE is usually a monetary award for the examinee rather than an operative or therapeutic intervention, but the requirement to be honest applies as much in an IE as in a standard ME. An inequitable monetary outcome from a purposely biased IE may affect a person as profoundly as any false diagnosis made in a standard ME and should be equally condemned.

Establishment of a Practice

Physicians accept compensation for applying their knowledge and skills in patient care. Toward this end, practices are established. Many physicians supplement their medical practice by performing IEs, and some physicians specialize in this area. Semiretired physicians, especially those formerly involved in fields where the cost of malpractice insurance is high, are particularly drawn to this area.

Differences

In addition to the subtle changes in the emphasis in an otherwise similar situation, true differences between standard MEs and IEs exist and are detailed here. See Table 11–3.

Goals

As noted earlier, although the IE and the standard ME start with a history, physical examination, and laboratory testing to arrive at a diagnosis or assessment, the standard ME has the goal of formulating a therapeutic recommendation, whereas the IE moves toward an impairment rating and an evaluation of the functional impact that results. Occasionally the physician performing an IE will be asked to comment on the effects of treatment, provide an assessment of permanency, or make recommendations regarding future treatment (medical or surgical) or the effects of rehabilitation. However, none of these elements are the same as the recommendations regarding therapeutic approaches or treatments formulated by the treating physician in a standard ME. The treating physician takes an active role with regard to the recommended treatment and actively reassesses the results of treatment and then further rec-

TABLE 11–3
Differences Between a Disability or Impairment Evaluation and a Standard Medical Examination/Practice

1. Goals
2. Opportunities for examination
3. Treatment recommendations
4. Work history
5. Rating system requirements
6. End results
7. Peripheral issues
8. Reliance on nonmedical personnel
9. Specific issues addressed
10. Extrapolation regarding causation
11. Legal responsibilities and malpractice coverage
12. Source of referrals

ommends either continuation or alteration in the treatment plan. The physician doing an IE merely extrapolates from the knowledge acquired through the examination to predict future outcomes, in a passive fashion. Thus, once information is acquired, there is a wide divergence regarding its application, with the physician assuming an active role in the standard ME and a passive one in the IE.

Opportunity for Examination

A standard ME is rarely limited to a single patient encounter, whereas this is normal for the IE and, at times, in the DE. This important difference creates a situation where the impairment examiner must, by necessity, be more through than a medical examiner, who will generally have further opportunities to ask the patient questions that were missed, overlooked, or underemphasized while taking the initial history, to perform additional elements of the physical examination or to obtain additional laboratory tests. The impairment evaluator must rely on the expectations of the requesting party to adequately address the completeness or comprehensiveness of the examination. For example, in performing entry-level evaluations for the Bureau of Workers' Compensation, the examination might be completed within 15 to 20 minutes and address only a single issue. In contrast, examinations providing the basis for testimony in cases expected to go to trial can take as long as 3 or 4 hours for the history and physical examination alone. Clearly, performing an in-depth examination is appropriate for the latter situation but would be inappropriate for the former. A good rule to remember when performing IEs is to do what is expected, which requires a preknowledge of the depth necessary for completing a competent examination as determined by the requesting party. This should be clarified with the requesting party before the examination is performed.

Treatment Recommendations

As already discussed, the major difference between the standard ME and the IE is that the physician adopts an active role or a passive role in relation to the examinee's medical problems—a crucial legal difference. Any recommendations given by the physician to the examinee regarding the findings derived from the IE can be considered as "treatment" and should be avoided. No prescriptions are given. These issues are more completely developed in Chapter 7.

Work History

Work histories are important in a standard ME, particularly in attempting to establish a causation for a particular problem or illness. However, they assume a more important and vital role in the IE. Except for very brief IEs, examinees should list all jobs that they have ever held (starting with babysitting or delivering papers as a teenager). The examinee can prepare this part of the history before the examination or after checking in with the receptionist. This list is reviewed with the examinee to clarify dates, job titles or descriptions, and exposures or injuries. This information is crucial in correlating an impairment rating with the future employment evaluation, which constitutes the IE.

Rating System Requirements

In addition to establishing the expectations of the referring source, it is vital that the physician be aware of which rating system will be used for an IE. The various systems have varying rules about specific elements in the history or physical examination. Of greater importance, however, are the restrictions placed on the laboratory tests that are accepted, acceptable, and paid for. Additionally, mandatory prerequisites are often set before some tests are performed.

Illustrations of Ratings Systems

An individual presents for a pulmonary impairment rating and an IE. If the individual is being tested for the Social Security System, the name of the manufacturer of the spirometer and the model number must be included in the report (see Chapter 22). The paper speed, height of the graphs, and conditions of the test are all clearly stated in the Social Security Handbook (SSA Listings).[5] The following points are noted:

1. A volume-time curve is recommended even though this is an outdated test. When a flow-volume loop is used to measure the forced vital capacity and the forced expiratory volume (FEV_1), volume calibrations at 30, 60, and 180 L/min must be performed and included in the report. (These

regulations represent an improvement in the testing protocol because flow-volume loops were considered invalid tests as recently as the previous [1992] edition of the listings.[4])

2. If the examinee is wheezing or if the airflow rates are low, a spirometric test is acceptable only after a bronchodilator has been given. To use preboncho-dilator data is unacceptable when using the SSA Listings.

The AMA Guides allow the use of only those machines approved by the American Thoracic Society, but flow-volume loops are acceptable. Postbronchodilator results are also used under circumstances similar to those found in the Social Security System.[2] However, the third edition (revised) of the AMA Guides states that "an individual should be evaluated after he or she has received optimum therapy or is in optimum health,"[1(p13)] whereas the fourth edition states, "a patient may decline treatment with a surgical procedure, a pharmacological agent, or other therapeutic approach. The view of the Guides fifth is that if a patient declines therapy for a permanent impairment, that decision should neither decrease nor increase the estimated percentage of the patient's impairment."[6] This issue was not addressed in the 1992 Social Security System Listings, but the 1994 edition states that the spirometric values to be used exist "during the individual's most stable state of health."[5] Thus a person who just finished smoking a pack of cigarettes or who refuses to take prescribed bronchodilators could be evaluated under the fourth or fifth edition of the AMA Guides and the 1992 Social Security Listings, but not under third edition of the AMA Guides and only under the 1994 Social Security Listings if this represents that person's stable state of health (as long as the spirometric rules were followed regarding bronchodilator administration).

Arterial blood gas levels can be valuable measures of pulmonary impairment. They represent a crucial component of an examination performed under the Black Lung Law, are deemed usually unnecessary under the AMA Guides, and are performed only "in a clinically stable condition on at least two occasions, three or more weeks apart within a 6 month period"[5] under the Social Security System. Furthermore, the Pao_2 is stratified according to the $Paco_2$, altitude of the testing facility, and the presence or absence of obesity under the Social Security Listings;[5] by the $Paco_2$ only in the Black Lung Regulations;[3] and by none of these measures in the AMA Guides.[2]

In assessing impairment resulting from coronary artery disease, the Social Security System will only pay for the electrocardiogram (ECG) or a thallium stress test, although it will accept the results of a coronary angiogram if independently obtained. Very specific requirements are found with regard to treadmill speed, the ECG strips, and interpretations. The AMA Guides are less strict on technical details.

Thus the physician must be aware of the proscriptions, limitations, and requirements of the various components of the history, physical examination, and laboratory tests based on the rating system used for each IE. Lack of awareness can create improper and insupportable results.

End Results

The end result of an IE is a rating that expresses the impact of the patient's impairment on his or her life. In a standard ME, the diagnosis serves as the springboard to therapeutic recommendations. It must again be emphasized that the rating derived from an IE directly reflects the rating system used as determined by the requesting source. The types of examinations used in deriving this rating are system-specific, as are the final results of the rating itself.

Peripheral Issues

There are circumstances where the requesting source will appreciate, request, or expect peripheral information. Examples include a detailed job description (especially the present job) and personal and demographic information concerning the examinee (place in family; information on parents or siblings, including medical problems, education, jobs, and home life; present family; prior families/marriages; economic information; prior occupation-related injuries or litigation; education and training; hobbies; travel; or physical status of the home). Knowledge of the expectations of the referring source as well as the nature of the IE helps in deciding how deeply to delve into these aspects.

Reliance on Nonmedical Personnel

Disability is directed toward the concept of the ability to sustain remunerative employment. Impairment is a limitation caused by a medical problem. Therefore a truly comprehensive impairment or disability report may include evaluations performed by nonmedical personnel, such as industrial hygienists, occupational safety experts, environmental engineers, social workers, occupational rehabilitationists, physical rehabilitationists, vocational rehabilitationists, and accountants (see Chapters 12, and 43 to 52). Rarely will a physician need to include these contributions in a standard ME, although these circumstances arise occasionally and the physician should be aware of these professionals' contributions.

Specific Issues Addressed

It must be remembered that the physician is requested to examine and report on one or more specific issues in an IE or DE. These should be explored and documented to the depth appropriate to the request. Other issues, medical or otherwise, may be inappropriate for the final report.

Extrapolation Regarding Causation

What does one do when examining an individual with a low back problem when that problem (injury) represents only one of many similar problems? How does one determine an impairment rating for the second of four low back injuries? How much of this impairment was caused by the situation in question? For example, how much of an individual's pulmonary problems are attributable to working in a coal mine and how much to a two-pack-a-day cigarette smoking habit? These questions, obviously separate an IE from a standard ME, where no such issues ever arise. There are no simple solutions to the dilemmas of causation involving multiple injuries or factors. Occasionally old records or laboratory tests help, but guesses can be the only answer-educated guesses based on all the knowledge, skill, and experience that physicians, specializing in certain areas, as well as in the area of disability examination, can offer. The resolutions to these requests involve honest, ethical, and educated estimates.

Legal Responsibilities and Malpractice Coverage

As mentioned earlier, the impairment evaluator must never cross the line and become a treating physician. Such an action places the physician into the legal and malpractice liability role shared by treating physicians. Therefore a medical malpractice insurance policy may not be of value in a disability evaluating practice; a general policy or specific liability coverage may be more appropriate. These legal issues are beyond the scope of this chapter, and the physician should consult Chapter 7, a lawyer, or his or her malpractice carrier.

Source of Referrals

A medical practice relies on patient, physician, or third-party referrals in order to maintain an adequate patient base. A disability examination practice has similar needs but the referral sources are generally different, including governmental agencies (Social Security Department, state Workers' Compensation boards, the Veterans Administration, or the Federal Aviation Agency, for example), insurance companies, attorneys, and employers. As in a medical practice, referral sources are maintained by providing satisfactory work. However, the results of examinations must not be biased to satisfy the referring source. Vigilance and honesty are the only safeguards against such a bias.

Disability Examination

As previously mentioned, there are fundamental differences among the standard ME, DE, and IE. The DE occupies a place somewhere in the middle of the standard ME and the IE. Some DEs are more impairment oriented and some are more standard medically oriented. The goal of the examiner is to determine the location along that spectrum of information requested by the referring source and to provide the information required. Table 11–4 illustrates some goals of the DE. As noted previously, the IE utilizes a physician's knowledge and skills based on his or her specialty but requires specialized training and knowledge to produce an impairment rating. The IE, for that reason, is rarely performed well by a physician without that specialized training. The DE, by contrast, is often performed by the attending physician (AP). It also calls for specialized training and skills but this is only infrequently recognized by the AP. Often, work release forms are sent to the AP, who fills them out based on his or her knowledge of the patient and his or her specialty. The frustration that most APs experience when filling out these forms is based on a subliminal acknowledgement that he or she does not possess the skills or training to fill out these forms adequately. This section explores the difference between the standard ME and the DE in order to create that awareness.

Because the DE falls somewhere on the line separating the standard ME and the IE, it follows that many of the comments made regarding IEs hold true for DEs and are not reiterated here. The fundamental goals of the DE are addressed. These are the elements that separate the DE from both the IE and the standard ME. Many of these issues are also addressed in Chapters 12 and 42.

TABLE 11–4

Goals of a Disability Examination

1. Establish diagnosis or diagnoses
2. Quantify impairment
3. Determine if examinee is capable of performing specified tasks
4. Determine if examinee can attend work
5. Determine if examinee can work in the occupational environment
6. Determine if worker poses a threat to others in the workplace
7. Make recommendations regarding job modifications
8. Extrapolate into the future
   a. Recommend treatment
   b. Derive a time course
   c. Specify how treatment/time will change points 1 through 7

Establish Diagnosis

The first issue addressed in a DE is what is wrong with the examinee. The goal of a DE is to determine if the examinee is capable of performing certain tasks—usually within the workplace. Usually, the physician is asked to address this issue concerning a specified injury or illness. It is usually presumed that because the examinee participated in the work setting before the illness or injury, absent that medical problem (or on resolution of the illness or injury), that the examinee can return to work and perform in a similar fashion after recovery from an illness or injury. That is usually the case for a young, healthy worker who suffers an acute medical condition, but it may be more problematic for the older or less healthy worker who has other medical conditions other than the acute injury or illness. In order to address the issue of return to work (RTW) competently, the certifying physician should be aware of the examinee's diagnoses, medications, and general medical condition. For this reason, the AP is usually the person asked to perform this job.

If the examiner is not the AP, then that person should become as familiar as the AP regarding the examinee's total medical condition. Thus the DE moves toward the standard ME end of the scale. If the examiner is the AP, specialized skills are needed to address the issues of RTW, thus moving the DE more toward the IE end of the scale. In the end, both elements must be addressed competently by the disability evaluator—complete knowledge of the examinee's medical condition and how to assess that condition vis-a-vis the demands of the workplace.

Quantify Impairment

The first step in making the RTW recommendation is, as discussed, determining what and how much is wrong with the examinee. For example: Does the examinee have asthma? If so, how bad is it? Is it controlled with only an as-needed inhaler or is the examinee still symptomatic despite 4 or 5 medications? What are the side effects of the medications that he or she is taking? Are there other diagnoses (such as heart or liver disease) that impact upon the primary problem, which will then affect the examinee's ability to return to work? The assessment of the degree of impairment will address these concerns. It should be noted that an impairment rating is not needed at this point. Rather, the information (medical conditions or diagnoses and determination of the level of severity for each condition) is.

Determine if the Examinee Is Capable of Performing Specified Tasks

A disability evaluation is designed to provide information regarding the examinee's capabilities to perform certain tasks based on the limitations of his or her medical impairments to the referring source. This topic is covered in the chapter on functional capacity assessment (see Chapters 51, 52, 54, and 55). However, for the examiner to provide this type of information, it is necessary for the examiner to have a description, from the referring source, of the tasks that the examinee is expected to perform. The greater the detail of these tasks, the more precise the examiner can be when submitting the final report. In many circumstances, this information is not provided. Obtaining the duties of the examinee's job from the examinee him- or herself is a poor substitute for asking the referring source for the information. Since the passage of the Americans with Disabilities Act (see Chapter 47), this information is usually known and can be obtained from the human resources department of the employer on request.

Determine if the Examinee Can Attend Work

Physical or mental impairments may preclude an otherwise capable person from being at the workplace. The worker who has a private cubicle and does a desk job but who has two fractured femurs or severe agoraphobia may not be able to be physically present in the workplace despite having no limitations in performing the specific tasks of the job. Likewise, the examinee who requires hemodialysis or physical therapy for an injury may require significant amounts of time away from the worksite.

Determine if the Examinee Can Work in the Occupational Environment

These topics are covered more fully in Section III. Briefly, to address this issue, the examiner must be aware of what the occupational environment is like. For the examinee with a visual impairment, what is the lighting like? For the examinee with asthma, are the levels of dust, fumes, smoke, or extremes of temperature high enough to provoke an asthmatic reaction? For the examinee with a psychiatric impairment, are there high stress levels?

Determine if the Worker Poses a Threat to Others in the Workplace

Does the worker with a bad back pose a threat to his or her coworkers who are required to lift heavy objects with the examinee? Does the examinee with a psychiatric impairment pose either a direct or an indirect threat to the productivity or well-being of fellow workers?

Make Recommendations Regarding Job Modifications

In some circumstances, an examinee with a medical impairment will be able to compensate, to some degree, for that impairment by using special devices. When these devices are used exclusively and frequently by the examinee, then the examinee is said to have a handicap. Examples include hearing aids, glasses, wheelchairs, and canes. A job can also be modified so that the examinee can perform a certain task more safely (e.g., using a hoist so that bending and lifting becomes less necessary for the examinee with a bad back). However, that person is not normally considered handicapped, despite the use of an assistive device. The recommendations in this part of the report will not be familiar to the examiner except for the occupational physician. There are resources that the physician may draw upon, such as the human resources department, occupational safety specialists, vocational rehabilitationists, and others (see Chapters 44 and 45). If "reasonable" (see Chapter 47), the company is obligated to make these job modifications to accommodate the worker with a medical impairment.

Extrapolate Into the Future

Physicians perform this function as a matter of course in their medical practices. A surgeon can and should delineate such issues as the expected benefit from the operation, the expected time to recovery, the risks, the complication rate, and alternatives. Those statistics are, of course, derived from population studies and may not be applicable to a given patient. That patient may have a complication requiring a more prolonged hospitalization with less than the expected results. So, too, in this section, should the examiner look into the future and provide information, when available, regarding treatment outcomes, time necessary to reach maximum medical improvement (MMI), and the expected changes in the degree of impairment found on the present examination. References are often useful and take the report out of the realm of one person's opinion, placing it in the realm of established medical care.

References

1. American Medical Association: Guides to the Evaluation of Permanent Impairment, 3rd ed rev. Chicago, American Medical Association, 1990.
2. American Medical Association: Guides to the Evaluation of Permanent Impairment, 4th ed. Chicago, American Medical Association, 1993.
3. Department of Labor, Employment Standards Administration: Standards for determining coal miners total disability or death due to pneumoconiosis. Federal Register 45:13678–13712, 1980.
4. Social Security Administration: Disability evaluation under Social Security, 1992. Washington, DC, U.S. Department of Health and Human Services, 1992.
5. Social Security Administration: Disability evaluation under Social Security, 1994. Washington, DC, U.S. Department of Health and Human Services, 1994.
6. Cocchiarella L, Andersson GBJ (eds): Guides to the Evaluation of Permanent Impairment, 5th ed. Chicago, American Medical Association, 2001.

PART II

Impairment

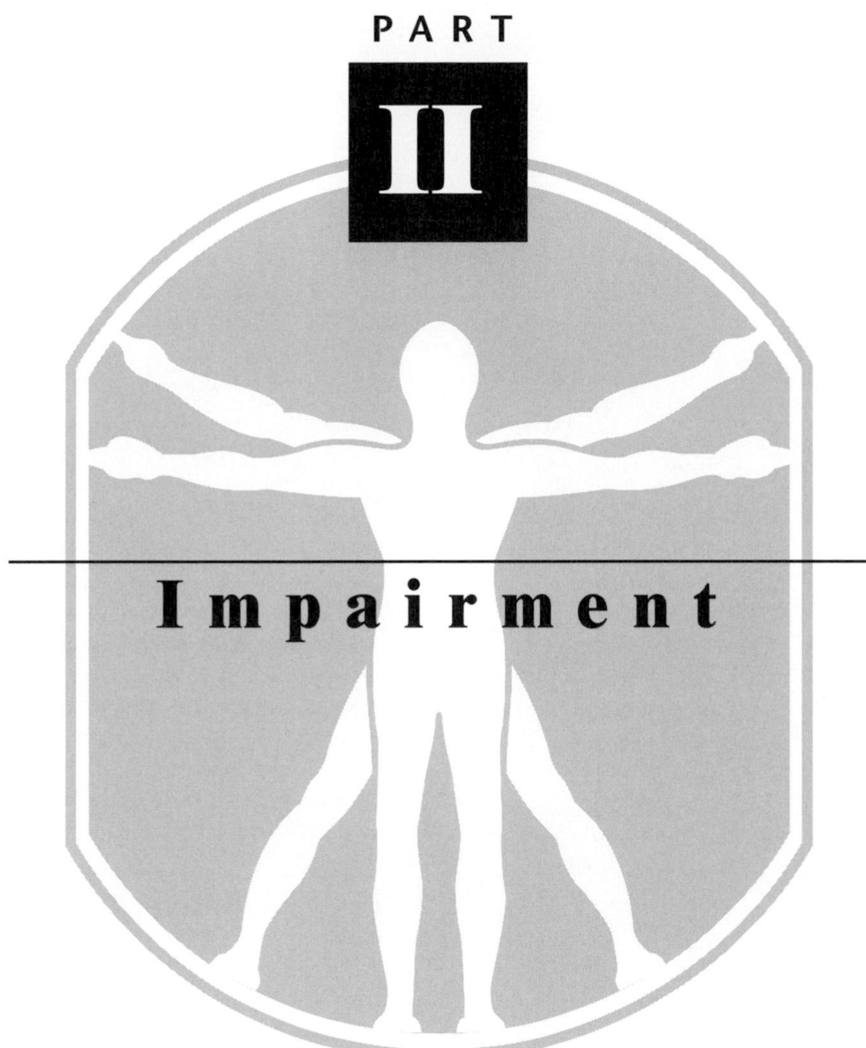

CHAPTER

12

The Impairment-Oriented Evaluation and Report

STEPHEN L. DEMETER, MD, MPH ■ RONALD J. WASHINGTON, MD, FAADEP

Just as there are major orientation differences between the standard medical examination and the impairment evaluation, the reports generated by each procedure differ in orientation.

The purpose of an impairment evaluation is to measure, define, and determine the status of the claimant's health at a particular point in time. Any deviation from population norms or from the claimant's prior health status is then translated into an impairment rating. The purpose of this rating is usually to determine a financial remuneration to the claimant by a third party. That third party may be an entity that created the deviation in the health status of the claimant (e.g., personal injury) or an employer (e.g., work-related injury or illness). The third party may also be an insurance company that previously "guaranteed" a certain level of health based on issuing a disability/dismemberment/injury policy.

An impairment report differs from a disability report (see Chapters 1 and 43). The purpose of a disability report is to assess an individual's ability to perform certain tasks in the workplace within the limitations created by an individual's health status. Thus, although these two reports examine and report on many of the same aspects, there is a major orientation difference between them. The impairment evaluation, like-wise, deviates from a standard medical report (see Chapter 11) wherein the goal of the medical report is to diagnose and assess an individual's health status and make recommendations regarding factors that would change (usually positively) that person's health. In an impairment evaluation, the diagnosis is usually known. In some circumstances, the future health status and factors influencing it are irrelevant to the impairment evaluation. The major orientation of the impairment evaluation is, again, the assessment and measurement of the deviation of an individual's health status from population norms or from the individual's prior health status. The guidelines offered in this chapter are comprehensive and may be used as a general background reference or as a checklist depending on the preferences and needs of the physician and the referral source.

Parts of this chapter have been adapted from the previous chapter in the first edition, which was also coauthored by George M. Smith. The boxes found in this chapter are very comprehensive. It is not anticipated that a physician will need to use every element for his or her evaluation or report. The item used will reflect the expressed needs and concerns of the requesting source.

COMMUNICATION

The first principle in preparing an impairment report focuses on communication with the referral source regarding the purpose of the evaluation, the expectations concerning the issues to be addressed, the completeness of the documents provided, the rating system to be used, and the expectations regarding testing and disclosure (Box 12–1). Some referring sources are specific and some are vague. Deviations from the stated expectations are seldom appreciated.

If the introductory letter to the physician states that the evaluation is an impairment evaluation of an individual who was injured in a motor vehicle accident, the referring source should be asked if the purpose of the examination is to assess an individual's health status globally or to focus on the effects of the injury. Either report may be the desired one but, as can be expected, there will be major differences regarding the scope of the history, physical, and testing necessary for each examination. The referring source may not be willing to pay for the global assessment nor need that amount of information.

BOX 12–1 Steps in Preparation for an Impairment Examination by the Examiner

I. Verify the purpose(s) of the evaluation with the requesting source(s)
  A. Impairment evaluation
  B. Disability determination (see Chapter 43)
II. Determine evaluating system used (refers to United States only)
  A. Workers' compensation
    1. AMA Guides
      a. Which edition?
    2. State-specific system
    3. Hybrid system
  B. Social Security system
    1. Disability evaluation under Social Security
  C. Federal employee
    1. Federal Employee's Compensation Act (FECA)
    2. AMA Guides
  D. Coal workers' pneumoconiosis
    1. Federal Coal Mine Health and Safety Act
  E. Longshoremen, shipbuilding workers
    1. Longshore and Harbor Workers' Compensation Act (LSA)
    2. AMA Guides
  F. Military/veterans
    1. Veterans Administration: Physician guide; Title 38, Part 4 of the Code of Federal Regulations
  G. Railroad workers
    1. Federal Employer's Liability Act, 45 US code annotated §§51–60 (FELA)
  H. Seamen
    1. Jones Act (extends FELA [see G] to seamen)
  I. Medical malpractice (tort system)
  J. Injury-related (tort system)
  K. Disability insurance
III. Clarify issue regarding maximum medical improvement
  A. Temporary partial examination
  B. Temporary total examination
  C. Permanent partial examination
  D. Permanent total examination
IV. Obtain the forms desired by the requesting party
  A. Review prior to the evaluation
    1. This may dictate specific choices in the examination methods, testing, etc.
  B. If unclear, communicate with the referring source prior to the evaluation
V. Obtain and review nonmedical records
  A. Workers' compensation records of present injury
    1. Accident/incident report
    2. Employee's and employer's first report of injury
    3. Employee's and employer's supplemental statements
    4. Employee's and employer's job description
    5. Employee's and employer's claim form
  B. Other workers' compensation records
  C. Other injury, disability, impairment records
    1. Off-work and return to work forms by attending physician(s)
    2. Restrictions placed on injured worker for above issues from attending physician(s)
    3. Records from insurance company
    4. Other independent medical evaluations

Box continued on opposite page

BOX 12–1 Steps in Preparation for an Impairment Examination by the Examiner *Continued*

- D. Legal records
  1. Depositions
  2. Workers' compensation decisions
  3. Court decisions
- E. Personnel records from human resources department
  1. Employment application
  2. Past and present job descriptions from employer(s)
  3. Performance appraisals
  4. Attendance records
  5. Employee relations records
     - a. Counseling memos
     - b. Written notices and warnings
     - c. Termination notice

VI. Obtain and review medical records
- A. Medical office records
- B. Hospital records
- C. Emergency room and urgent care center records
- D. Reports by consulting physicians
- E. Reports by other independent medical examinations
- F. Results of testing
  1. Laboratory
  2. Radiology
  3. Psychological
  4. Functional capacity assessments
  5. Others

EXAMPLE

One of the authors was once asked to perform an impairment evaluation of a police officer for low back strain. Thus a specific body part was to be assessed; a global evaluation was not desired. The officer had been injured in a motor vehicle accident while on duty. No documents were provided. When queried, the officer stated that he was in his cruiser, stopped at a light, and was rear-ended by another car. When asked how he injured his low back, he stated that he did not; rather, he had a whiplash injury. The referring source was called and the circumstances were discussed. What they wanted and what was performed was an examination of the low back (it was normal) and the report was submitted accordingly. The referring source was adamant that the examination was not to be for the cervical spine. That report, which from a medical perspective was more appropriate, was neither desired nor expected. The officer, then, had a 0% impairment of the whole person based on the stated allowed injury; namely, low back strain.

In this example, several points were made that need to be stressed in the impairment evaluation examination and report:

1. The referring source dictates to the physician (and not the physician to the referring source) exactly what is to be done. The physician and the report are part of a process. As noted in Chapter 1, this is a major orientation shift that takes place, and unless the physician is aware of his or her role in the process, he or she can become frustrated with these types of examinations.
2. The "correct" report, addressing the whiplash injury, was neither desired nor expected. Had it been submitted, the referring source might have been disinclined to pay, would have needed to have the claimant examined again, and would hesitate to hire the same physician as an examiner in the future.
3. Communication is the key element in preparing an acceptable report. If the claimant states that certain tests were performed documenting results supporting a claim and those documents were not provided, communication with the referring source is necessary to obtain those documents. If the goals of the assessment are vague, communica-

BOX 12–2 Steps in Preparation for an Impairment Evaluation by the Referring Source

I. Be specific about what you are asking for
   A. Is this an impairment or a disability-oriented report (or both)?
   B. Specify the rating system/method to be used
   C. Do you want to know if the claimant is at maximum medical improvement (MMI)?
      1. If not, do you want to know what is necessary to attain MMI?
         a. Do you want a projected timeline?
         b. Do you want to know the costs?
         c. Do you want an estimate of impairment when the claimant reaches MMI?
   D. Is this for a permanent/temporary impairment or is it for a complete/partial impairment?
   E. Do you want specific forms filled out?
   F. Do you want references to the medical literature?

II. Provide sufficient records for the examiner to review
   A. Many records will be unnecessary
      1. Do not touch on present case (e.g., a different medical condition)
      2. Are superfluous (e.g., full hospital records for a claimant being assessed for the effects in a particular injury; these may be critical, however, in a malpractice review)
   B. Provide those that will assist the examiner (see the lists under V and VI, Box 12–1)
   C. Communicate with examiner if some materials exist but are not being provided to determine if the examiner desires these documents
   D. Remember that the examiner can prepare an opinion only on the material that is furnished

III. Provide information on how to contact you
   A. Phone and fax numbers
   B. E-mail (if desired)
   C. Hours

IV. Clarify if you want a verbal report prior to anything committed to paper

V. Tell the examiner what to do with the provided material when the case is finished
   A. Return
   B. Keep
      1. For how long?
   C. Dispose
      1. Shred?

VI. Be specific regarding the fee
   A. The agreed price
      1. Hourly
      2. Per case
   B. How and when to bill
   C. How soon to expect payment after receiving the invoice
   D. Your anticipated figure (if necessary)
   E. If research is necessary, do you prefer to do some or all for the examiner?
      1. If not, are you prepared to pay for this service?

VII. If travel is necessary, indicate whether you will pay the cost
   A. Type of transportation
   B. Class of transportation
   C. Hotel/meal reimbursements
   D. Who makes the travel arrangements, hotel reservations, etc.?

tion with the referring source will define the exact goals of the examination. If the prior health status is irrelevant to the current examination, that should be known before the report is prepared.

4. As discussed in Chapter 1, the physician's role in an impairment evaluation is no longer at the top of the decision making pyramid. There are several layers above him or her. One of those individuals is the claimant's attorney. This is the person responsible for correcting the mistake in this claimant's forms—not the physician. Just as it is inappropriate for the physician to fill the role of the pathologist/nurse/radiology technician in a hospital setting, so too is it inappropriate for the physician in an impairment evaluation to usurp the role of another person who occupies a higher position in the decision-making pyramid.

Just as it is important for the examiner to understand what the referring source wants and expects from the evaluation, it is also important for the referring source to adequately equip the examiner with the necessary materials to provide that evaluation (Box 12–2). As discussed in Chapter 1, communication in a language that both parties can understand is the key to mutual satisfaction. Also, as discussed in Chapter 1, role awareness on the part of the examiner is crucial for the successful completion of an impairment evaluation. Box 12–3 can assist the examiner in that role awareness and provides additional data points in the communication link between the examiner and the referring source.

The second major principle in communication is to request and review all appropriate medical and nonmedical documents (Box 12–4). The evaluating physician's primary task is to define the examinee's current health status thoroughly and accurately. First, the evaluating physician analyzes the medical information contained in the clinical records, which reflect past evaluations and treatments. The object is to determine whether there is a medical foundation on which to base the diagnosis and management of the examinee. To review, analyze, and comment appropriately on past and present medical history, the examining physician must have access to all existing medical records, reports, and results of tests and diagnostic procedures dating from at least the onset of the medical condition for which the evaluation is being performed. Omission of these records renders the impairment report incomplete and potentially places the acceptability of the conclusions in jeopardy. The impairment report must be complete with records supplied by the treating physicians. Differences in clinical findings, especially any recent findings, must be addressed and properly accounted for.

If the information contained in the records is insufficient to justify a diagnosis or a medical management plan and additional clinical information must be acquired, the desired approach is to record all positive and pertinent negative findings derived from the medical history, the physical examination, and the tests and diagnostic procedures. Box 12–4 provides a checklist of the elements essential to a complete medical evaluation.

Once the history is established, the examining physician must ensure that the clinical examination addresses all the relevant clinical issues. This section of this book details the clinical evaluation of each body system. Careful attention to the information contained in the clinical chapters will maximize the evaluating physician's ability to achieve the objective of thoroughness in the medical aspects of the evaluation. Although the evaluating physician may be a medical specialist performing an evaluation that focuses on a particular body part, system, or function, the individual should always be considered as a whole.

THE REPORT

A properly constructed impairment evaluation report addresses the needs and requests of the referring source and is as comprehensive as the referee desires. The report analyzes the supporting information and reconciles it with the current examination, points out discrepancies between the written record and the claimant's historical interview and determines if these points are viable issues, and reviews prior diagnoses and treatments and comments on accuracy, completeness, and appropriateness.

In some circumstances, the impairment evaluation seeks to address two further issues. First, is the claimant at maximum medical improvement? Second, does the claimant have the capacity to perform certain tasks? This second issue is the basis of the disability report and is covered in Chapter 43. Although there are differences in orientation of the examination and report of impairment and disability, both examinations can be performed simultaneously. Either two separate reports can be prepared or, in the assessment and conclusion of the report, each issue can be addressed separately. It is confusing and inappropriate to mix these two concepts together. Bold-facing, highlighting, separating paragraphs, or separating sections are ways of distinguishing these two elements.

To address the issue of MMI, the physician is extrapolating into the future. This calls on the physician's best judgment and demands the clinical skills and experience that the physician has garnered during training and years of practice. Supporting documentation or medical references are often desirable. This serves the purpose of taking what could be merely an opinion and buttressing it with medical fact. Any change in the

BOX 12–3 Understanding and Responding to the Needs of the Referral Source in an Impairment Evaluation*

I. What functions does the medical advisor/consultant/evaluating physician perform for the referral source?
   A. Professional/technical function—Assess and explain the probative value of medical information
   B. Clinical function—Perform an impairment or disability-oriented medical evaluation
   C. Communications function—Analyze and explain, both orally and in writing, enough about medical issues and their relationship to nonmedical issues so that the referral source feels comfortable with the information and confident in making necessary decisions

II. What critical questions must the medical advisor/consultant/evaluating physician ask of the referral source?
   A. What are the issues of this case?
   B. What is the purpose of the evaluation?
   C. What are you asking me to do?
   D. What questions do you want me to answer?
   E. Will you ask me to help you prepare for and assist in depositions of the claimant's physicians?
   F. Is it likely that I will be deposed?
   G. Will there be a trial if the case is not resolved?
   H. If so, will there be a jury?
   I. Will you ask me to serve as a witness if there is a trial?
   J. If so, will I be a fact witness or an expert witness?

III. What critical question must the medical advisor/consultant/evaluating physician answer personally?
   A. Beyond the information requested, what information does the referral source need?

IV. What information does the evaluating physician need?
   A. Dates
      1. Date of birth
      2. Date of hire
      3. Date of the incident
      4. Date of onset of the medical condition
      5. Date of onset of (alleged) disability
      6. Date of the first medical examination
      7. Critical employment-related dates
   B. Definitions
      1. Impairment—deviation in anatomic structure, physiologic function, intellectual capability, or emotional status from what the individual possessed prior to an alteration in those structures or functions or from what is expected from population norms
      2. Disability—medical impairment that prevents an individual from performing specified intellectual, creative, adaptive, social, or physical functions; inability to complete a specific task that the individual was previously capable of completing or that most members of society are capable of completing owing to a medical or psychological deviation from an individual's prior health status or from the status expected of most members of a society
      3. Workers' compensation/insurance
         a. Medical condition
         b. Temporary/permanent
         c. Partial/complete
      4. Accommodation—Americans with Disabilities Act: modification of a job or work situation that enables an individual to meet the same job demands and conditions of employment as any other individual in a similar job
      5. Occupational disability—medical condition precluding travel to and from work, being at work, or performing appropriate tasks and duties while at work, with or without accommodation

Box continued on opposite page

BOX 12–3 Understanding and Responding to the Needs of the Referral Source in an Impairment Evaluation* *Continued*

C. Clear statement of the burden of proof the claimant must meet
   1. Law
   2. Regulations
   3. Insurance policy contract
   4. Employer's policy
   5. Labor management agreement

D. Relevant medical information from primary clinical source documents—Documents containing information obtained or communicated for the purpose of documenting the medical history and clinical findings and for managing a patient's clinical care
   1. Emergency room records or other first encounter records
   2. Medical office records
   3. Hospital inpatient records
   4. Consultation reports
   5. Physical therapy/occupational therapy records
   6. Reports of the results of laboratory tests
   7. Reports of the results of diagnostic tests and procedures
   8. Any other documents related to medical management of the claimant

Note 1—Letters to addresses not involved in the clinical management of the claimant (e.g., claims examiners, lawyers, disability evaluating physician) are not medical source documents. They have the quality of testimonial statements only.

Note 2—Reports of independent medical evaluation(s) or disability evaluation(s) by a physician who is not a treating physician are not primary clinical source documents.

Note 3—Unless you are a treating physician, your report is not a primary medical source document.

E. Relevant information from nonmedical primary source documents
   1. Injury report
   2. Employer's first report
   3. Physician's first report
   4. Personnel records
      a. Employment application/employment history
      b. Performance appraisals
      c. Counseling memos/disciplinary actions
      d. Awards and commendations
      e. Dates of changes in employment situation
         (1) Promotion/demotion
         (2) Transfer
         (3) New supervisor
         (4) New work assignment
   5. Legal documents
      a. Complaints
      b. Briefs
      c. Interrogatories
      d. Depositions
      e. Affidavits
   6. Case-related correspondence

Note—If you perform an evaluation:
   1. Verify the examinee's understanding of the purpose of the evaluation
   2. Ensure that it is clinically complete with respect to the medical condition regardless of what is requested

*Parts of this box were taken from Chapters 1 and 11 of the first edition, co-authored by George M. Smith, MD, MPH.

BOX 12–4 Components of the Impairment Examination

I. Identify the needs/requests of the requesting source
II. Determine the evaluating system to be used
   A. Often will dictate specific physical examination tests to be used/not used
   B. Often will dictate specific laboratory tests that are approved/not approved
III. Review the reports provided
   A. May assist the focus of the examination
   B. May identify missing parts that need to be explored in greater detail
   C. May identify contentious issues that need particular care
IV. Perform a careful history
   A. Pay specific attention to injury/illness of concern
   B. Full review of systems
   C. Family history
   D. Work history
      1. To include all jobs
      2. Identify duties in those jobs
      3. Duration of each job
      4. Potential hazards of each job
      5. Other work-related injuries including medical leaves/workers' compensation claims
   E. Social history
      1. Include habits such as alcohol use, smoking, recreational drug use
      2. Include home environment (heating, humidity, air filtration devices, air conditioning, smokers, animals, stairs/levels of home and site of residence, presence of elevators where applicable)
      3. Travel history (when needed)
      4. Recreational/hobby history
      5. Social circumstances (when needed, such as education, home life, spouse/children status, income levels, and others)
   F. Present medications
   G. Allergies
   H. Medical history
      1. Surgeries
      2. Hospital admissions
      3. Significant outpatient care such as physical therapy, psychological counseling
      4. Other illnesses/injuries
      5. Complete list of current/past diagnoses
V. Perform a careful physical examination
   A. Mental status examination (if appropriate and needed; otherwise, a comment on memory and cooperativeness is all that is necessary)
   B. Physical examination
      1. Full/limited based on request from referring source
      2. Specific examinations dictated by impairment system
VI. Recommend/perform appropriate laboratory tests
   A. Based on communication with referring source
   B. Based on impairment system
VII. Recommend further medical evaluation as medically warranted and approved by referring source
VIII. Prepare report

BOX 12–5 Structure of the Impairment Report

I. Identifying remarks
   A. Purpose of examination
   B. Referring source
   C. Time and place of examination
   D. Attendees (other than the claimant and examining physician)
   E. Time spent with claimant (better—time at the start of the interview and time at the end of the examination)
   F. Whether the process was recorded for sound/video plus sound
II. Records available for review
   A. Separate line for each record
   B. Specify the particulars of each record
      1. Prepared by whom
      2. Prepared for whom
      3. Date
      4. Site of report generation
      5. Purpose of the record
   C. (Possibly) list records not available for review
III. Rating method
IV. History
   A. Obtained by examiner
V. Physical examination
   A. Obtained by examiner
VI. Results of laboratory testing
   A. Obtained by examiner
   B. Comment on reliability (accuracy of test by examinee)
VII. Analysis of record review
   A. History
   B. Physical examination(s)
   C. Laboratory tests
      1. Include comment on reliability and accuracy of tests
   D. May lump or split
      1. Results of A, B, C for each examination performed in the past in a separate paragraph for each
      2. Results of all histories in one paragraph, all physical examinations in next paragraph, and all laboratory tests in the next paragraph
   E. Reconcile the results of the history, physical examination, and test results obtained by record review with the current history, physical examination, and test results
      1. State congruencies
      2. State discrepancies
         a. Cite appropriate parts of statements in the history
            (1) Use quotations and references
         b. Describe reliability, accuracy, and validating tests used in the various physical examinations
         c. Give reasons for divergence of laboratory tests
            (1) Comment on reliability/accuracy of each discrepant test
            (2) Provide statistical review of tests (i.e., sensitivity, specificity, positive predictive value, etc.; see Appendix A on biostatistics and epidemiology)

Box continued on following page

impairment rating, based on anticipated change in future function, can then be commented upon.

An important point is that the examiner should use the guidelines offered by the rating system. It is inappropriate to use the AMA Guides when conducting a Social Security report. This seems an obvious point but it can be overlooked. More importantly, the examiner must be aware of the technical specifications of the

BOX 12–5 Structure of the Impairment Report *Continued*

VIII. Assessment
- A. Should be one paragraph long for each issue noted in Part VII
- B. Should summarize all congruencies and discrepancies found in Part VII
- C. Reference to medical literature provided in this part

IX. Summary and conclusions
- A. Summarize in a short paragraph
- B. Provide impairment rating

X. Recommendations
- A. Further tests needed to enhance reliability/accuracy of present report
- B. Possible changes in present report based on:
  1. Reviewing records not provided
  2. Obtaining new tests
- C. Repeat examination when claimant reaches maximum medical improvement
  1. Owing to change in lifestyle
  2. Owing to change in medications, surgery, or rehabilitation (vocational, occupational, physical, cardiac, pulmonary)
  3. Owing to change in job or work environment
- D. Describe process of addendum report (if needed)
  1. If report can be generated solely by reviewing new records—either from a review of old records or new tests
  2. If claimant needs to be examined again
  3. Time frame
  4. Additional fees for addendum report

BOX 12–6 Content of the Impairment Report

I. Introduction
- A. Identifying information
- B. Referral source
- C. Purpose of the evaluation
- D. For each disability system:
  1. Cite applicable law or regulations
  2. Cite the criteria for disability or impairment employability
- E. Date of the initial evaluation and dates of all follow-up visits
- F. Complete list of all information used as the basis of the report (excluding the present examination), including:
  1. All records, reports, x-rays, results of special tests and diagnostic procedures, and laboratory test results, with source and date for each
  2. All verbal communication with employer/attorneys/others working with or part of the referring source including dates, times, names, and other appropriate identifying information, including who gave permission for the communication (if necessary)
- G. Presence of attendees at the examination (excluding the physician and the claimant), including:
  1. Family members
  2. Legal representatives
  3. Medical witnesses (e.g., female office staff member during an examination between a male physician and a female examinee)
  4. Others

Box continued on opposite page

BOX 12–6 Content of the Impairment Report *Continued*

- II. Results of the clinical evaluation
  - A. History of the medial condition(s)
    1. Method by which the history was obtained
    2. Identity of the history taker(s)
    3. Narrative description of the history, including reference to all positive and pertinent negative results:
       - a. As extracted from the records and reports
       - b. As obtained from the examinee
    4. Comments regarding agreement and discrepancies within and between the sources
  - B. Findings from physical examination and mental status examination
    1. Positive and pertinent negative clinical findings
    2. Validation signs (as appropriate)
    3. Ability to dress and undress, get on and off the examining table
    4. For each body part, system, and function, report observations that are required under the criteria of the disability system of record
  - C. Findings from laboratory tests and diagnostic procedures
  - D. Results of medical specialty evaluations
- III. Clinical impressions
- IV. Assessment of current health status
  - A. Explain the basis for a conclusion that the clinical information is or is not sufficient to assess the individual's current health status
  - B. Explain whether each medical condition has become static or well-stabilized with reference to past records and current findings to support each conclusion
  - C. If improvement or deterioration of any medical condition is expected, explain the basis for the conclusion, the expected course of the condition, and the time frame within which the improvement or deterioration is likely to take place
  - D. Explain any impact on life activities
    1. Personal activities
       - a. Self-care (personal hygiene, dressing, food preparation and eating)
       - b. Personal business (maintaining a bank account, paying bills, entering into contracts such as leases, loans, or insurance)
    2. Social activities
    3. Leisure and recreational activities
- V. Medical management plan (if appropriate)
  - A. Recommendations for further diagnostic testing
  - B. Referral for medical specialty evaluation
  - C. Periodic reevaluation of active treatment
  - D. Rehabilitation/reconditioning
  - E. Follow-up impairment evaluation
  - F. Anticipated costs and timeline (if requested)
- VI. Synthesis of information
  - A. Review and analyze documentation
    1. Note consistency of information from various healthcare providers
    2. Evaluate sufficiency of the information on which diagnoses and medical management plans are based
    3. If the examinee was off work, include:
       - a. Why examinee stopped working
       - b. Duration
       - c. If still absent from work, why examinee has not returned
  - B. Analyze the accumulated medical information
    1. Medical history
       - a. Historical interview, clinical findings, treatment, and response to treatment
       - b. Any conspicuous omissions of information

Box continued on following page

BOX 12–6 Content of the Impairment Report *Continued*

2. Conclusions
   a. The examinee's medical condition has or has not become static or well-stabilized
   b. The examinee is or is not likely to suffer subtle or sudden incapacitation
   c. The examinee is or is not likely to suffer injury, harm, or aggravation of the medical condition by engaging in specific work-related and nonwork-related activities
   d. Risk avoidance or therapeutic value associated with restricting the examinee from particular activities, both on and off the job
3. Life situation factors

C. Assess the medical and nonmedical information in relation to the following factors:
1. Likelihood that the circumstances could have caused or contributed to the onset or aggravation of the medical condition
2. Consistency or inconsistency in records, reports, history, and previous clinical findings
3. Validity of the diagnosis with respect to established medical diagnostic criteria
4. Appropriateness of the treatment and medical management with respect to generally accepted medical principles and practices
5. Assessment of the degree to which the medical condition has or has not adversely affected the examinee's nonwork-related life activities (driving, use of public transportation, shopping, self-care, leisure activities)
6. Likelihood that the examinee will suffer sudden or subtle incapacitation, noting:
   a. How soon
   b. How suddenly
   c. How severely
   d. The probable consequences in terms of injury or harm to the individual or others and aggravation of the medical condition
   e. The degree to which the medical condition has or has not become static or well-stabilized
7. The need for further treatment and the nature of such treatment
8. Likelihood that the medical condition will change
9. Potential restrictions or job modifications to:
   a. Enable the examinee to carry out essential job functions
   b. Reduce to an acceptable level the risk of sudden or subtle incapacitation; injury, harm or aggravation of the condition; or injury or harm to others (see discussion of "direct threat" in Chapters 7 and 47)
10. Degree to which the individual meets the criteria of the disability system under which the evaluation is conducted

VII. Conclusions and impairment rating

A. Based on the disability system used
1. The burden of proof is met based on the rating system
   a. Identify the specific items that conform to the elements required for proof
2. The burden of proof is not met based on the rating system
   a. Identify the specific items necessary to establish proof
      (1) Missing documents
      (2) Further testing
   b. Explain sequence of events necessary to establish proof
      (1) Addendum report after review of missing documents, completion of tests, etc.
      (2) Need for second examination of the claimant

B. Apportionment if appropriate

C. Factors that could change the impairment rating
1. Types of factors
2. Likelihood of change
3. Degree to which the impairment rating will change
4. Time course

BOX 12–7 Recommendations for Producing a Well-written Disability Report

1. Use short paragraphs.
2. Provide space (two or three lines between headings).
3. Avoid surplus words such as compound prepositions and word-wasting idioms when simple, concise words suffice.
4. Employ active verbs. Passive verbs require a supporting verb (was) followed by a preposition (by).
5. Generally, use short sentences, especially when comparing items. Vary sentence length somewhat for variety, which improves readability.
6. Guide your reader. Begin sentences with names and dates. Place new information or important facts at the beginning of a sentence or paragraph.
7. Arrange your words with care, following the normal English word order of placing the subject first followed by the verb and then the object. Avoid wide gaps among the subject, the verb, and the object.
8. Present material in tables when appropriate. Tables present complicated bits of information clearly and concisely.
9. Use commonly understood English phrases and clearly defined terms. For example, instead of using terms like inspection, palpation, percussion, and auscultation, chose verbs (inspect, palpate, percuss, auscultate). Lay language is preferable: I observe, I see, I feel.
10. Avoid language quirks, habits, current catch phrases, and jargon. Maintain neutrality and objectivity. Make no attempt at humor.
11. Document all sources of information, both medical and nonmedical. Present these materials chronologically, identifying the date, source, recipient, and subject matter.
12. Carefully proofread and edit your report. Typographic errors and other easily corrected mistakes diminish the impact of the report. Rephrase passages that seem unclear on the second reading. Make sure that your report has successfully translated medical language into good English.
13. Use headings, underlining, and boldface print for emphasis and organization. Strive for a professional format that presents information clearly.
14. Be precise.
15. Be terse in the assessment/conclusion parts of your report.
16. Use phrases such as "within a reasonable degree of medical certainty," "more likely then not," and others where and when appropriate.
17. Provide a list of references as needed. If appropriate, enclose a copy of one or two articles with appropriate passages highlighted. This adds power and credibility to your report.

rating system. As discussed in Chapter 11, not all systems use, accept, or pay for the same test. Certain systems are, a priori, global assessment systems (Social Security, for example); others can be injury or disease specific (AMA Guides, for example). If the rules, regulations, specifications, and technical requirements of the rating system are unknown, these can be requested from the referring source prior to the examination. (Chapter 4 provides the rating system and addresses of many of the federal programs and may be used as a reference.)

Finally, to meet the needs of nonmedical users, the report must use nontechnical terms to explain the medical opinions while being responsive to the administrative or legal issues involved. The user must understand the rationale underlying the conclusions and be able to adopt that rationale in formulating a plan of action. Recommendations regarding the specific writing of the report are given in Boxes 12–5, 12–6, and 12–7. Each evaluation should reflect the four "R"s of any successful report (Box 12–8).

BOX 12–8 THE FOUR "Rs" OF ANY SUCCESSFUL REPORT

1. A *responsive* report fulfills the request of the referring source. The report begins with an introductory statement assuring the requestor that his or her interests will be addressed.
2. *Readable* means that the visual appearance and structure (introduction/body/summary) make the report easy to follow.
3. A *relevant* report provides information that supports or disproves an issue and explains contradictions.
4. The summary ends a well-*reasoned* report and draws impartial conclusions that fit and follow from the reasons offered in the body of the report. These *reasons* flow from established medical science to support or refute specific issues. The results of this analysis are unique to, and specific for, the questions posed by the requesting party.

SECTION

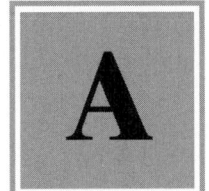

Musculoskeletal Impairment Assessment

CHAPTER

13

Range of Motion Evaluation

TOM G. MAYER, MD

Testing range of motion (ROM) as a clinical measurement of impairment remains an accepted method of musculoskeletal assessment in the AMA Guides to the Evaluation of Permanent Impairment.[4] Challenges to use of this methodology have emerged, centered on debate concerning the relationship among mobility deficits, functional loss, and impairment; consideration of age-related changes; challenges in establishing normative data; questions concerning ability to evaluate patient effort; and inexact accuracy of measurements in specific joints or spinal regions. These questions have led to exploration in other directions, based on the fundamental AMA Guides' principle that impairment evaluation should be based on gauging functional loss. However, concerns about a "diagnosis-only" assessment system has encouraged continued use of ROM as a component of musculoskeletal impairment assessment in the spine and extremities.

In some cases, human performance testing involving greater complexity, incurring greater cost, and requiring greater patient cooperation has been advocated for assessing impairment (e.g., pulmonary function, strength, endurance, lifting capacity, or other activities of daily life simulations). On the other hand, use of the "diagnostic category" has gained greater popularity for a number of reasons.[46] Using the diagnosis as a substitute for performance testing makes the assessment easier, allowing a larger number of treating or evaluating physicians to perform these assessments. The convenience and ease of diagnostic model application has opened the field of impairment assessment to other providers, including nurses, therapists, and chiropractors. Determination of impairment usually entails a nonmedical outcome (for distributing financial benefits) utilizing a medical "gatekeeper process." Operational simplicity represents a compelling objective, particularly to external payors and jurisdictions.

However, involvement of a medical gatekeeper introduces equally justifiable concern. An administrative process that is scientifically valid must adhere to sound medical principles, in fact as well as appearance. This is especially important if the vital interests of the patient being evaluated are to be best served. There is obvious validity in the link between impairment and the loss of specific functions such as mobility and strength, even when correlation with a medical diagnosis may be limited. A single diagnosis may be associated with wide variations of functional impairment, handicap, and disability. This is particularly true in controversial, but common, musculoskeletal disorders, such as those involving the spine and upper extremities. However, the problems inherent in human performance measurement may be accentuated in controversial cases, particularly when claimants know that fiscal rewards will be greater for lesser performance. ROM evaluation represents a microcosm of the controversy created by the differing goals of the various parties represented in a disability claim, including the employer, the injured worker, his or her legal representative, the insurance company, the regulatory agency, and the physician.

A rudimentary understanding of the terms impairment, disability, handicap, and employability is required for full assimilation of these issues (see also Chapter 1). Disability is an administrative term that refers to an individual's inability to perform certain activities of daily life, such as gainful employment or recreation, which are customarily accessible to the average, healthy individual. Impairment is a medical term that represents an alteration of the patient's usual health status that is evaluated by medical means. Handicap occurs as a consequence of an impairment, representing a barrier to performance of an activity of daily living, but one that may be overcome by reasonable accommodation or adaptation.

Accommodation refers to modification of the environment to suit the needs of the handicap and decrease the degree of disability. Adaptation by the individual achieves the same goal by enhancing residual capabilities to replace those that may have been lost. Employability represents another administrative process affected by disability and handicap. Any decrease in employability as a consequence of an injury may result in economic loss to the patient, leading to a compensatory monetary award whose numerical value must be determined statutorily. One factor in this award is the evaluation of perceived damage to the patient's health status (or impairment), for which the physician is generally deemed responsible. If a numerical value is to be placed on impairment, an administrative methodology must respond to a number of sometimes contradictory objectives (Table 13–1).

TABLE 13–1

Considerations in Selecting an Impairment Methodology

Principle	Considerations
Objectivity	Validity, intratester reliability, accuracy. Relevance preferred.
Consistency	Intertester reliability. Small range of normal human variability preferred.
Fairness	Relationship between numerical impairment rating and true alteration of health status and physical function.
Accuracy	Precision, signal-to-noise ratio, specificity, sensitivity; potential to discriminate, intraindividual and interindividual alterations in health status.
Relevance	Correlation between assessment technique and alteration of health status from normal. Requires comparison to normal functioning.
Convenience	Test must be easy to perform, preferably with techniques known to all potential evaluators. Limited educational requirements. Limited time required for assessment.
Cost	Minimum desirable by parties requesting assessment but not at the price of significantly increased variability. Shortest possible time commitment of expert evaluators. Minimize variability to minimize disputes generally considered worth paying for.

ROM testing in impairment evaluation is essentially a quantitative component of the physical examination. The most abbreviated musculoskeletal physical examination almost always includes a qualitative assessment of mobility during the initial, interim, and terminal visits to assess progress. Regardless of the extremity or spinal area involved, or the specific pathology, the mobility of joints adjacent to the injury site is always a relevant outcome measure for return of function or functional loss in musculoskeletal medical care. When a patient reaches a plateau, it is often assumed that all temporary impairment in the ROM has resolved. If there is loss of mobility, it is generally believed that it should be correlated in some way with a component of the permanent impairment. In the absence of optimum rehabilitation and effort, this assumption may be untrue. When a quantitative assessment is required, in order to provide a numerical component of the administrative process of disability evaluation, a deeper understanding of the principles and methodology of mobility assessment is needed.

Evaluation of impairment, as noted, presumes a temporal factor; that is, there will be a temporary component of mobility loss during a period of healing, intervention, and rehabilitation, followed in some cases by a permanent component. With acute injury or illness, joint or para-articular swelling affecting soft tissues is frequently accompanied by some temporary loss of motion. Loss of mobility may be one of the only clinical signs leading to a correct diagnosis, particularly in situations in which visualization of superficial structures (to detect in-tissue consistency, color, or temperature changes) may be absent. In most cases, resolution of an acute infection or inflammatory process, if properly treated, results not only in complete symptomatic recovery, but also in full restoration of mobility in adjacent joints.

In situations involving episodic or repetitive trauma, continuous use (or cumulative stress), or systemic arthritis or severe joint derangement, internal and external joint scarring and contracture may occur, and lead to residual stiffness. Whereas the accompanying loss of motion may infrequently be painless, there is usually a correlation between persistent pain and loss of motion, with episodes of increasing pain-associated symptoms that correlate with the waxing and waning mobility deficits. These correlations of temporary functional loss with synovitis in acute exacerbations are most easily recognized in hemophilic arthropathy or systemic arthritis.[1,35,77] However, they accompany many other inflammatory conditions, as well as most musculoskeletal chronic pain syndromes.

In the same way, alteration of ROM at the time of maximum medical improvement (or the point at which the condition becomes permanent and stationary) may bear some relationship to the degree of permanent impairment sustained by that individual as a treatment outcome. The measurement of mobility may then assist the clinician in evaluating one of the critical functional outcomes of natural healing, medical intervention, and physical rehabilitation.[50]

The complex relationship between pain and loss of motion is worth exploring in more detail. Pain is a crucial symptom that represents the major reason formerly healthy individuals seek medical assistance. In the musculoskeletal system, this relationship is even more common. Yet because pain is perceived exclusively by the subject with the painful condition, pain is the least verifiable symptom a patient can experience. In cases of acute infection or trauma, signs of swelling, heat, or induration may provide objective evidence for subjective pain complaints. In most disability evaluations, however, coming at the termination of medical treatment, a report of pain is usually viewed as subjective, particularly because it is prone to exaggeration. Financial secondary gain is often cited as the reason for untruthful statements by a claimant regarding his or her pain. Great effort may be expended on identifying signs of psychological distress, called nonorganic signs, which may be used (or misused) subsequently to discredit complaints of the claimant.

Loss of motion, on the other hand, has the advantage of being observable and quantitatively measurable. It lacks objectivity only insofar as it is prone to voluntary restriction through suboptimal effort, as in any human performance test. Involuntary mobility loss owing to joint pain has been experienced by every human adult. By itself, loss of motion may create functional loss (e.g., joint contractures). However, when joint motion is both restricted and painful, the impairment is compounded. The relationship is further complicated because pain itself may lead to restriction of joint motion, whether voluntarily, involuntarily, or both. Perhaps the greatest paradox and challenge to be dealt with in impairment evaluation is that this varied relationship between pain and loss of mobility presents both the greatest correlational advantage and worst confounder of the process. At this time, mobility that is simply inhibited by pain is considered to have a lesser degree of permanence than motion deficits created by contracture. The future usefulness of motion measurement, as with any quantitative human performance test, will depend on measurement procedures that can stratify, insofar as is possible, the interrelated impairments to pain from those to rigidity or ankylosis. Both may exist concurrently, and both may be important in functional loss.

PRINCIPLES OF MOBILITY TESTING

Neutral Zero Method and Terminology

Two parallel goals in musculoskeletal impairment evaluation are to achieve objectivity and consistency. One crucial factor in meeting these goals is standardized terminology and measurement protocols to enhance both intratester and intertester reliability. The neutral zero concept is the most generally accepted of these concepts.[13,29] The principle begins with a zero starting position, equivalent to an individual standing erect with hands by the side in a military-attention posture. All movement is then recorded from this starting position in the three planes intersecting at 90° angles: sagittal, coronal, and axial. Figure 13–1 demonstrates the three planes,[4] differing from the neutral zero position only in that the forearms are held in the anatomic supine position.[29]

The most common sagittal plane terms, flexion and extension, will be addressed first. This terminology may be confusing if one fails to recognize that there is a difference between the neutral zero position (from which the numerical starting point is derived) and the supine anatomic position (from which the named direction of motion is derived). The difference is only relevant in the upper extremity distal to the elbow (Fig. 13–1). Beginning in the supine anatomic position, all sagittal motion is termed flexion/extension. One must view the femur as the dividing line, above which flexion increases as the volar angle decreases; distal to the femurs, volar angle increase is termed extension. All axial motion is termed pronation/supination or rotation

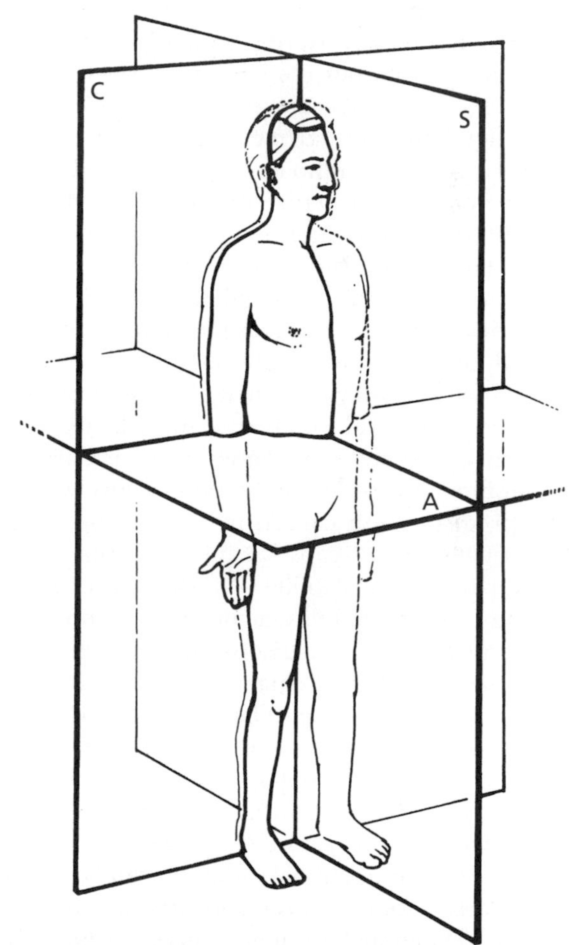

Figure 13–1. Body planes for measuring motion. S, Sagittal plane: a vertical plane that divides the body into right and left parts. A, Axial plane: a crosswise plane that divides the body into upper and lower parts and is perpendicular to the sagittal and frontal planes. C, Coronal plane: a vertical plane that divides the body into anterior and posterior parts. (Modified from Cocchiarella L, Andersson GBJ (eds): Guides to the Evaluation of Permanent Impairment, 5th ed. Chicago, American Medical Association, 2001, and Gerhardt JJ, Cocchiarella L, Lea RD: The Practical Guide to Range of Motion Assessment, First Edition. Chicago, American Medical Association, 2002.)

(either left/right or internal/external). Coronal motion is described by a large number of terms, including abduction/adduction, eversion/inversion, deviation (e.g., ulnar/radial), or lateral bend (e.g., left/right spinal).

Regardless of direction of measurement, the neutral zero position always represents the zero degree position, whether at end-range or some intermediate point for the joints or regions under consideration. Numerical values of ROM are generally expressed in the angle through which a joint passes from the neutral zero position to its terminal position. In some joints, such as the elbow, knee, and fingers, the neutral zero position is essentially in full extension, and all the recorded motion is in flexion. Loss of extension mobility is termed flexion contracture. In other joints, the neutral zero position is at some midpoint of the planar range. Ankylosis refers to complete joint immobility and is expressed as a specific angle in the terminology of the planes involved (e.g., ankle ankylosed at 10° [plantar-] flexion). More commonly, some residual joint motion persists, but the joint is limited in reaching the usual extreme of the range. Because it is generally acknowledged that impairment is greater when the neutral zero position can no longer be achieved, the presence of a flexion contracture in a joint like the elbow, knee, or fingers is of greater significance than loss of terminal planar motion when the neutral zero position is preserved (for example, retained cervical spine motion from 30° flexion to 30° extension). Contractures in joints with a midpoint neutral zero position may also be administratively termed ankylosed when there is remaining motion, but the neutral zero point cannot be reached.[3]

The term hyperextension connotes a potentially pathologic condition of hypermobility that may involve either a genetic predisposition caused by or from ligamentous laxity or ligament and capsular injury creating residual post-traumatic joint instability.[15,88] When an extremity is affected in terms of mobility, a contralateral normal side is often available for comparison. This is not true in the spine, so that a normative database must be developed if deviations from normal are to be identified. When quantitative, rather than qualitative, expressions of these deviations are needed introducing the requirement to account for normal human variation in performance measurements, including such factors as age, gender, weight, or joint laxity. Even occupational variations can be identified in some joints, although it remains unclear whether the presumed occupational influence causes the mobility difference or there is an accompanying genetic predisposition selecting for the occupation, or both.[67]

ROM can be measured either actively (AROM) or passively (PROM). AROM, generally acknowledged as a safer method of measurement, requires the patient's voluntary cooperation using active muscle contraction. This method may have the unintended side effect of limiting terminal motion, as when a cocontraction is stimulated. PROM requires the intervention of the examiner moving a joint to a terminal position, which is generally considered more objective because the movement is free of control by the examinee. Distal extremity joints lend themselves more readily to this type of measurement. Even under conditions of maximum effort, AROM may be different from PROM, as is the case when pain inhibits active (increased loading) motion or when muscle weakness prevents full active motion against gravity. Whenever possible, the examiner should evaluate both AROM and PROM.

Measurement Techniques

Quantitative measurement in most joints, particularly in the extremities, is facilitated by use of the simple two-armed goniometer.[31] As the goniometer is essentially a hinge, it is particularly useful whenever a typical hinge or ball-and-socket joint is being measured in a single plane (Fig. 13–2, A and B). Measurement is also facilitated by the presence of a contralateral side, easy palpation of bony landmarks, and experience of the test administra-

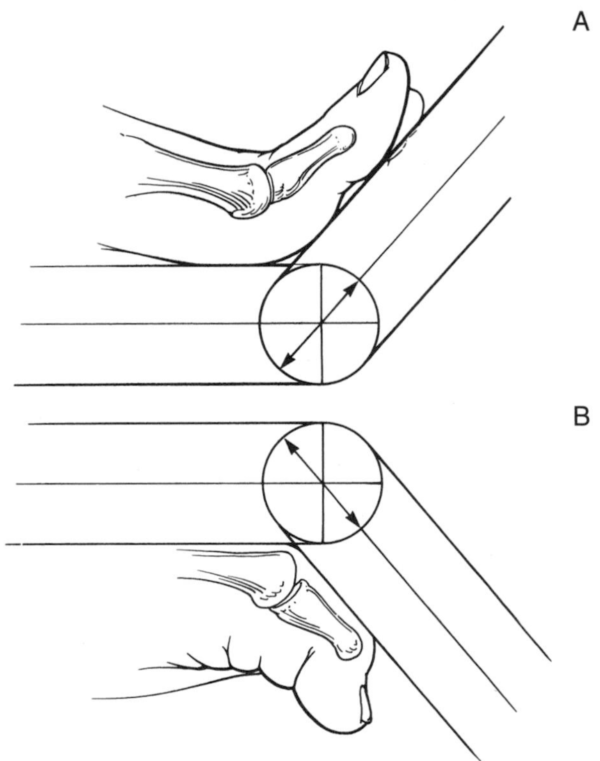

Figure 13–2. Evaluating the range of motion of the metatarsophalangeal (MTP) joint of the great toe. A, Extension. The goniometer is under the MTP joint, and its angle is read as a baseline. The patient extends (dorsiflexes) the toe maximally, and the angle subtending the maximum arc of motion is read; the baseline angle is subtracted. B, Flexion. The goniometer is placed over the MTP joint. The baseline angle is read. The patient plantar flexes the MTP joint maximally. The angle subtending the maximum arc of motion is read, and the baseline angle is subtracted. (From Cocchiarella L, Andersson GBJ (eds): Guides to the Evaluation of Permanent Impairment, 5th ed. Chicago, American Medical Association, 2001.)

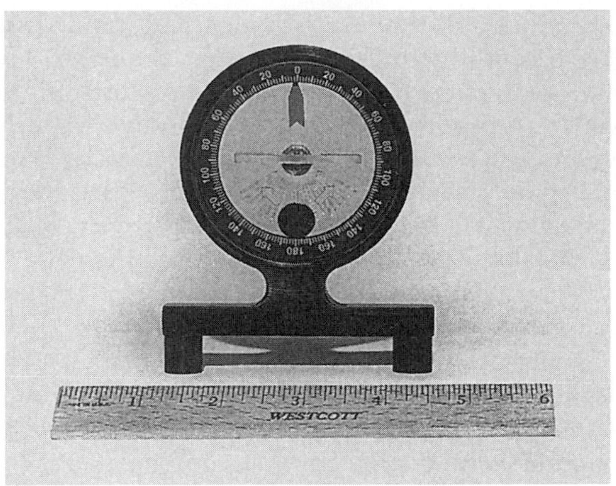

Figure 13–3. A mechanical inclinometer. (From Cocchiarella L, Andersson GBJ (eds): Guides to the Evaluation of Permanent Impairment, 5th ed. Chicago, American Medical Association, 2001.)

tor. In contrast, however, overlying soft tissue, obesity, and lack of contralaterality or regional movements (e.g., in the spine) make use of the goniometer less preferable owing to decreasing accuracy, relevance, or objectivity. For special situations, smaller flat-surface goniometers have been developed (e.g., finger measurements).[32]

Inclinometers are versatile tools that have evolved from the simple carpenter's level. Small, inexpensive versions of these devices, with reasonable accuracy, can be obtained at any hardware store (Fig. 13–3). Because two-arm goniometry is ineffective in spine measurement, inclinometers are preferred for use in these regions.[29,40,42,52,83] A dual inclinometer technique has been developed for measuring each of the specific spinal regions. Subtraction of the motion of the lower inclinometer from that of the upper inclinometer leads to a true spinal motion measurement (Fig. 13–4).[36,45,52] It is customary to measure true cervical motion from the occiput to T1, thoracic from T1 to T12, and lumbar from T12 to the sacrum. Accurate measurements may be obtained with these simple devices if attention is paid to proper training of test administrators, to good human/device contact, and to the location of bony landmarks.[24,39,44,49]

Beyond the simple tools, a multitude of other motion measurement devices have been devised. A magnetic compass may be utilized to measure inclination out of the gravitational plane.[17,42,55] Flexicurves and kyphometers have been used for specialized spinal regional measurements and are designed to overcome some of the limitations of other measurement tools in these areas.[11,33] Various electrogoniometers or electronic inclinometers have been developed as tools for more accurately assessing spinal motion in a gravitational plane. Unfortunately, excellent device accuracy may be offset in routine spinal evaluation by inexperience, lack of training, and other determinants.[29,45,61,90] Finally, a variety of computerized goniometers have been utilized, primarily

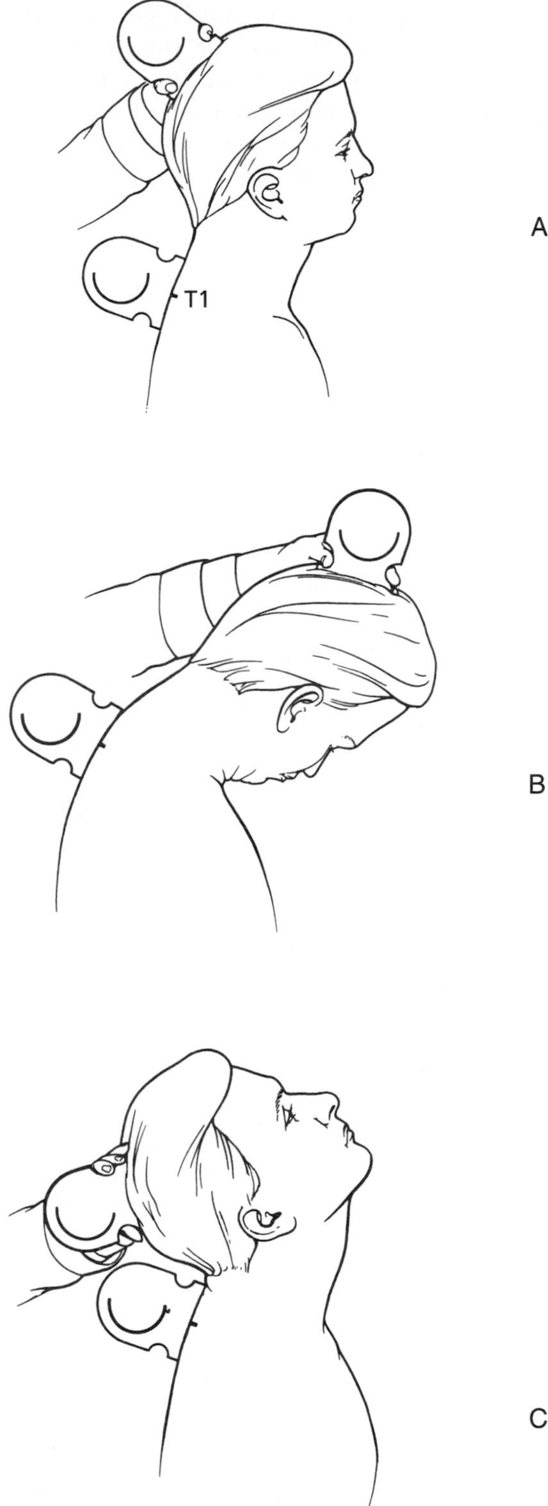

Figure 13–4. Two-inclinometer measurement technique for cervical flexion and extension. A, The subject is sitting with the head in the neutral position, and the inclinometers are held over the occiput and T1. B, With the subject flexing the neck fully, determine the lower inclinometer angle. Then subtract the lower angle from the upper angle. C, With the patient extending the neck, read the two angles and subtract the T1 angle to determine the extension angle. (From Cocchiarella L, Andersson GBJ (eds): Guides to the Evaluation of Permanent Impairment, 5th ed. Chicago, American Medical Association, 2001.)

for research purposes, to obtain very precise motion measurements. These include such devices as three-dimensional digitizers, computerized inclinometers, optical scanners, video combined with light emitting diodes, and various multiposition x-ray techniques. The expense of these approaches precludes their general medical use (see also Chapter 18).[9,18,60,62,63,75,78,79,86]

Accuracy, Reliability, and Validity

The term accuracy refers to how close a measured value approaches the "real" or "actual" value. It is limited by the precision of the measurement, which is determined by the smallest increment of measurement indicated by the scale on the device (5° on most simple goniometers or 1° on most electronic inclinometers). The reliability or reproducibility refers to the ability of a clinical measurement to equal a previous or prior series of measurements. Reliability is a complex concept that depends on a multitude of factors (Table 13–2). Reliability testing is the most common method for assessing the utility of a measurement system, because it is easy to evaluate statistically. Its disadvantage is that it originates from a somewhat imprecise social sciences conceptual framework, rather than from physics-based measurement principles commonly used in engineering science. Reliability measures the reproducibility of repeated measures, but it cannot quantitatively identify the factors or sources of error that compromise test repeatability. Validity is another social sciences concept that refers to the usefulness of a measurement system (as opposed to a device) in evaluating a clinical paradigm. It may consist of many types of validity (such as face validity, content validity, construct validity, and consensual validity).

TABLE 13–2

Factors Important in Testing Reliability and Clinical Utility Involving Devices for Human Performance Measurement

Principle	Considerations
Device accuracy/precision	The ability of the device to repeatably produce the same value.
Human/device interface	The reliability component based on applying the device appropriately to the individual being measured, depending commonly on factors such as bony landmarks, overlying soft tissues, parallax, skin adhesion, and relationship between skin movement and underlying bony movement.
Test administrator training	The skill and training of the test administrator recognizing the multiple potential sources of error, usually evaluated by comparing intratester and intertester reliabilities.
Normal human variability	Variability associated with factors such as age, gender, weight, occupation, training, and culture, which can be anticipated even with perfect device and measurement validity.
Errors unique to subjects undergoing impairment evaluation	Limited effort and cooperation; secondary gain for poor performance; effect of pain; threat of litigation and adversarial environment.

Considering all the potential sources of error, ±5° is the commonly acknowledged variability that may be encountered before any "real" change in motion can be accepted as valid.[2,3,8] Additionally, it is axiomatic that inclinometers or goniometers should be checked periodically against a reference standard such as a wall or floor. Whereas the device accuracy of a simple two-armed goniometer is usually limited only by its precision, its reliability in a measurement system is generally conceded to be good, although intertester reliability is usually less than intratester reliability. This appears to be more a function of test administrator training than an issue related to the device itself.[8,23,32,49,70,73] Reliability testing for inclinometers provides a confusing mixture of impressions for the reader, as most investigators have failed to recognize that assessment of inclinometric measurements in a measurement system like the spine raises all the possible sources of error noted in Table 13–2.

The device error for inclinometers is usually found to be very low, with the device accuracy generally determined by its precision. This is usually about ±5° for inexpensive fluid-filled inclinometers, decreasing to 0.5° for electronic inclinometers with optical–electronic scanners. Limitations in reliability testing noted in multiple clinical studies are usually on the basis of sources of error other than the device. Common pitfalls are improper identification of bony landmarks, inadequate warm-up of subjects, improper use of the device with the subject, and lack of recognition of the motion endpoint.[7,12,16,20,28,30,36,45,49,56,65,68,69,76,87,89] In general, examiners interested in maximizing reproducibility of their spinal measurement skills should concentrate on expertise with the device chosen, ability to find bony landmarks, and firm application of the device to the subject's body. The AMA Guides Practical Guide to Range of Motion Assessment teaches the examiner a standardized approach to range of motion assessment through a pictoral, self instructional style.[29]

Normal Human Variability and Databases

Age is definitely a factor in ROM. Due to intrauterine compression, significant alterations in ROM of neonates can be demonstrated, particularly in the shoulders, elbows, ankles, knees, and hips.[27,34] Generally speaking, mobility is higher in children than in adults and progressively declines with age, due to a number of factors including genetics, training, trauma, occupation, and gender.[6,15,72,81,88] Age-related changes tend to occur symmetrically in the extremities if they are not accompanied by factors that act unilaterally, such as injury. As such, the importance of age-related change is greater in the spine, where lack of contralaterality implies that quantitative impairment evaluation using ROM must rely on a normative database. There have been several studies looking at age-related change over the past few years, and decrease of mobility over age 60 is found uniformly. However, in a working population between 20 and 60 years of age, findings are highly variable.[19,21,38,45,59,80,89] Normal values depend on a multitude of factors, many of which have been assessed and demonstrated.[36,45,47,48] Other studies have tested chronically impaired patients before and after rehabilitation to document the physical progress in overcoming temporary impairment to reach their final status of residual permanent impairment.[14,37,41,51] Other changes related to age have been well-documented in the literature.[19,20,57,80,84] Gender plays a small role in mobility except in cases of ligamentous laxity and normal human variability seen with training effects in women engaged in activities involving stretching. Only cervical extension mobility and hamstrings extensibility (effecting hip flexion in the straight leg raising test) appear to be consistently greater in magnitude for women.[25,45,53,54,66,80,89] Cultural differences related to childhood positioning or customary postures (e.g., "hunkering" in many Asian cultures) may be the reason for significant variability of motion in lower-extremity joints such as the hip and ankle.[19,36,80]

The concept of normal values is especially noteworthy in relation to spine measurements. Normal spine measurements can be very useful for impairment ratings, because the patient's less-than-optimum effort can be anticipated when greater financial reward is associated with poorer performance. Many studies have looked at normal ROM with a variety of techniques and are available for the preparation of mobility-based impairment systems.[14,22,26,43,58,64,67,71,74,81,82] Although some consider the concept of normal values biased, with or without use of normalizing factors, there are no studies that demonstrate significant variation from normal in any cohort of asymptomatic subjects.

Relationship of Motion to Impairment

Impairment evaluation is performed by a physician using medical means, and is most commonly used in determining awards related to permanent injury. This need for medical determination occurs most commonly in the industrial setting (e.g., workers' compensation cases). An increasing number of workers' compensation venues have chosen to use impairment-based administrative systems rather than those based on wage loss or demonstration of inability to work (disability-based systems). Because spinal disorders represent a majority of the workers' compensation permanency awards, and musculoskeletal claims account for nearly 80% of these awards, much of the controversy has focused on human performance measurements in this organ system. These contentious and multifactorial indemnity contests bring a social rather than a scientific/medical bias to the debate over the "scientific evidence" documenting the relationship between impairment and ROM. Such debate really hinges on the relationship between any form of musculoskeletal impairment, regardless of the rating method, and the perceived disability caused by the injury for which society will reward the claimant. The complexity of the situation is compounded in a variety of different ways, including attempts to relate spine flexibility in uninjured workers to the possibility of future back pain complaints, and is further illustrated by the variable relationship between pain and motion.[5]

Under ideal circumstances, there would be perfect correlation between physical impairment as measured by some functional human performance test and the complaints of pain and work impairment, or other type of impairment. This impairment number then might be converted to a numerical rating of disability by using a few well-selected social factors such as age, education, and skills. Unfortunately, such a construct has been, and no doubt will continue to be, elusive. In a classic study, looking at a multitude of important factors, Waddell et al found a number of variables to coincide with an independent measure of impairment. The majority of the relevant measures were related to active or passive ROM measurements.[85] However, others have continued to focus attention on the limitations of standardized techniques of ROM measurement in assessing spinal impairment, particularly as related to age changes.[22,41] Further complicating the situation is that increasing age may produce musculoskeletal soft tissue diseases and injuries on a microtrauma level, which may lead to painful alterations of function without any objective change in AROM or PROM. Declines in mobility with age are usually accompanied by changes in the mechanical properties of ligaments and increasing stiffness associated with these changes. However, normative testing in older-age populations has generally ignored this potentially correctable stiffness due to inactivity, which is to be differentiated from uncorrectable age-related change.[10]

Even more disconcerting is the episodic nature of "permanent" mobility loss, which increases with inflammation and often is accompanied by greater levels of pain. Disability may also be increased by environmental factors, such as the need to bend, climb, run, or reach overhead, creating episodic increases in impairment or disability. This may occur in an individual who had previously achieved a stable balance in functioning through reasonable accommodation combined with physical adaptation. The social imperatives of protecting impaired workers yet providing incentives to maintain productivity can only be achieved by recognizing the advantages and limitations of the most sophisticated functionally based methodologies for assessing impairment.

Limited Effort and Cooperation

This chapter has reviewed some of the issues involved in clinical measurement of ROM for impairment evaluation purposes. Current literature demonstrates that accurate, precise ROM measurements can be obtained if the examiner is familiar with pitfalls in measurement. These pertain to proper use of the device, identification of anatomic landmarks for correct device application, and experience and skill in the use of the measurement system. The examiner must also be aware of normal human variation, as influenced by age, gender, occupation, and culture. In the situation in which ROM measurement is being used for impairment evaluation, another set of factors apply, with which the sophisticated examiner should be familiar (Table 13–2). Because the financial award is intimately tied to the quantitative functional performance measurement, the claimant's motivational disincentives often will prevail over the need for maximum effort. Several methods may be used to neutralize this potential behavior. In the extremities, and even in the cervical spine, gentle PROM can be used to validate AROM. The medical records must be carefully surveyed to be certain that the evaluee has cooperated adequately with his or her rehabilitation. Otherwise, the evaluator cannot be certain that the decreased mobility noted at the time of the examination exists and is an actual reflection of permanency, rather than being a sign of temporary impairment or the result of voluntarily limiting ROM.

It is a paradox that noncompliant and unmotivated evaluees often receive greater financial rewards, regardless of the impairment evaluation methodology used (diagnosis, surgical procedures, mobility testing). If the examinee demonstrates suboptimal effort, impairment higher than that expected for the degree of pathology, or limited evidence for rehabilitation compliance, then he or she may not be at the state of maximum medical improvement. In some cases, the claimant may be rehabilitated before being remeasured. If this is not possible, or if the claimant has refused or abandoned appropriate rehabilitation, the examining physician must estimate what the ROM would have been had he or she received and cooperated with treatment that resolved the temporary impairment component. Alternatively, the claimant may simply be denied a rating for the components of the examination that require prior rehabilitation or test effort (motion, strength, neurological deficit).

Finally, another useful discriminating validity factor for the physician is to determine whether there is a correlation between the pathologic state (as measured by other factors) and the ROM. For example, an individual showing only 20% of normal lumbar spine motion and no history of systemic disease, spinal surgery, or previous injury, and who has supposedly been fully rehabilitated, is demonstrating functional changes inconsistent with that degree of pathology. Small deficit variations from normative values may be anticipated in nonoperated cases after completion of treatment. Even in operated cases, when only one or two spinal levels are involved, full mobility of the remaining joints should create only mild deficits of total regional mobility. In the case of spinal fusion, where complete immobility of one or more spinal joints has occurred, more significant loss of mobility may be anticipated. Because these changes also create higher biomechanical loading on adjacent joints, and because these changes have been shown to hasten the degenerative process at the adjacent joints, higher impairment ratings for loss of motion, as well as for the anatomic changes produced, are justifiable.

SUMMARY

Ultimately, we must question the wisdom and propriety of utilizing any functional measure for assessing a nonmedical, indemnity-based construct like impairment or disability. It is not surprising that administrators, attorneys, and legislators are attempting to abandon many of the older methods of disability evaluation to escape the morass of social disincentives to productive social behaviors created by rewarding disability. In the past half-century, economic philosophies in the industrialized world have favored relatively high unemployment, which has made disability a convenient method for providing minimum incomes for displaced workers, irrespective of the cost. Musculoskeletal injury, particularly involving the spine, is a favored route of entry into this system. The administration of financial awards by subjective determination of wage loss or inability to work provided a convenient politically influenced mechanism for abetting the post-Depression economic model. The drastic economic changes in the United States over the past decade, culminating in the lowest unemployment since World War II, and the corresponding upsurge of employment in the entire industrialized world, has altered the paradigm. The shift into using medically determined impairment for social purposes, and turning the physician-evaluator into the gatekeeper for this system, is a parallel development. However, use of medical impairment evaluation produces a misleading impression of scientific validation for what is essentially an economic issue. Therefore, the place of ROM measurement for permanent impairment rating will continue to remain controversial. The value of ROM, however, as a scientific measure of real musculoskeletal physical impairment and performance remains high. It is useful for making an initial diagnosis, measuring progress of treatment, and recognizing limitations associated with maximum improvement. Motion assessment has far greater ability to discriminate between musculoskeletal life functions in individual cases than a diagnostic category. It remains unclear whether these medical activities quantifying ROM can be reconciled with nonmedical socioeconomic forces that seek to place aspects of social policy under a mantle of scientific respectability.

References

1. Altman R: Criteria for the classification of osteoarthritis of the knee and hip. Scand J Rheumatol 65 (Suppl. 0): 31–39, 1987.
2. American Medical Association: Guides to the Evaluation of Permanent Impairment, 3rd ed. Chicago, American Medical Association, 1988.
3. American Medical Association: Guides to the Evaluation of Permanent Impairment, 3rd ed, rev. Chicago, American Medical Association, 1990.
4. Cocchiarella L, Andersson GBJ (eds): Guides to the Evaluation of Permanent Impairment, 5th ed. Chicago, American Medical Association, 2001.
5. Battie M, Bigos S, Fisher L, et al: The role of spinal flexibility in back pain complaints within industry: A prospective study. Spine 15:768–773, 1990.
6. Baxter M: Assessment of normal pediatric knee ligament laxity using the genucom. J Pediatr Orthop 9:546–550, 1988.
7. Boline P, Keating J, Haas M, Anderson A: Interexaminer reliability and discriminant validity of inclinometric measurement of lumbar rotation in chronic low-back pain patients subjects without low-back pain. Spine 17:335–338, 1992.
8. Boone D, Azen S, Lin C-M, et al: Reliability of goniometric measurements. Phys Ther 58:1355–1390, 1978.
9. Brown R, Burstein A, Nash C, Schock C: Spinal analysis using a three-dimensional radiographic technique. J Biomech 9:355–365, 1976.
10. Buckwalter A, Goldberg V, Woo S: Musculoskeletal Soft-tissue Aging: Impact on Mobility. Chicago, American Academy of Orthopaedic Surgeons Symposium, 1993.
11. Burton A: Regional lumbar sagittal mobility: Measurement by flexicurves. Clin Biomech 1:20–26, 1986.
12. Capuano-Pucci D, Rheault W, Aukai J, et al: Intratester and intertester reliability of the cervical range of motion device. Arch Phys Med Rehab 72:338–340, 1991.
13. Cave E, Robert S: A method for measuring and recording joint function. J Bone Joint Surg 18:455–465, 1936.
14. Chen J, Solinger A, Poncet J, Lantz C: Meta-analysis of normative cervical motion. Spine 24: 1571–1578, 1999.
15. Cheng J, Chan P, Hui P: Joint laxity in children. J Pediatr Orthop 11:752–756, 1991.
16. Clapper M, Wolf S: Comparison of the reliability of the Orthoranger and the standard goniometer for assessing active lower-extremity range of motion. Phys Ther 68:214–218, 1988.
17. Dillard J, Trafimow M, Andersson G, Cronin K: Motion of the lumbar spine: Reliability of two measurement techniques. Spine 16:321–324, 1991.
18. Dopf C, Mandel S, Geiger D, Mayer P: Analysis of spine motion variability using a computerized goniometer compared to physical examination: A prospective clinical study. Spine 19:586–595, 1994.
19. Dvorak J, Antinnes J, Panjabi M, et al: Age and gender related normal motion of the cervical spine. Spine 17(Suppl.):393–398, 1992.
20. Dvorak J, Panjabi M, Novotny J, Antinnes J: In vivo flexion/extension of normal cervical spine. J Orthop Res 9:828–834, 1991.
21. Dvorak J, Vajda G, Grob D, Panjabi M: Normal motion of the lumbar spine as related to age and gender. Eur Spine J 4:18–23, 1995.
22. Einkauf D, Gohdes M, Jensen G, Jewell M: Changes in spinal mobility with increasing age in women. Phys Ther 67:370–375, 1987.
23. Elveru R, Rothstein J, Lamb R: Goniometric reliability in a clinical setting: Subtalar and ankle joint measurements. Phys Ther 68:672–677, 1988.
24. Ensink F, Saur P, Frese K, et al: Lumbar range of motion: Influence of time of day and individual factors on measurements. Spine 21:1339–1343, 1996.
25. Esola M, McClure P, Fitzgerald G, Siegler S: Analysis of lumbar spine and hip motion during forward bending in subjects with and without a history of low back pain. Spine 21:71–78, 1996.
26. Fitzgerald G, Wynveen K, Rheault W, et al: Objective assessment with establishment of normal values for lumbar spinal range of motion. Phys Ther 63:1776–1781, 1983.
27. Forero N, Okamura L, Larson M: Normal ranges of hip motion in neonates. J Pediatr Orthop 9:391–395, 1989.
28. Gajdosik R, Bohannon R: Clinical measurement of range of motion: Review of goniometry emphasizing reliability and validity. Phys Ther 67:1867–1872, 1987.
29. Gerhardt JJ, Cocchiarella L, Lea RD: The Practical Guide to Range of Motion Assessment, First Edition. Chicago, American Medical Association, 2002.
30. Gill K, Krag M, Johnson G, et al: Repeatability of four clinical methods for assessment of lumbar spinal motion. Spine 13:50–53, 1988.
31. Greene W, Heckman J: The Clinical Measurement of Joint Motion. Chicago, American Academy of Orthopaedic Surgeons, 1994.
32. Hamilton G, Lachenbruch P: Reliability of goniometers in assessing finger joint angle. Phys Ther 49:465–469, 1986.
33. Hart D, Rose S: Reliability of a noninvasive method for measuring the lumbar curve. J Orthop Sports Phys Ther 8:180–184, 1986.
34. Hoffer M: Joint motion limitation in newborns. Clin Orthop 148:94–96, 1980.
35. Johnson R, Babbitt D: Five states of joint disintegration compared with range of motion in hemophilia. Clin Orthop 201:36–42, 1985.
36. Keeley J, Mayer T, Cox R, et al: Quantification of lumbar function 5: Reliability of range-of-motion measures in sagittal plane and in vivo torso rotation measurement techniques. Spine 11:31–35, 1986.
37. Kohles S, Barnes D, Gatchel R, Mayer T: Improved physical performance outcomes following functional restoration treatment in patients with chronic low-back pain: Early versus recent training results. Spine 15:1321–1324, 1990.
38. Kuhlman K: Cervical range of motion in the elderly. Arch Phys Med Rehabil 74:1071–1079, 1993.
39. Lea R, Gerhardt J: Current concepts review: Range of motion measurements. J Bone Joint Soc 77:784–798, 1995.
40. Loebl W: Measurements of spinal posture and range in spinal movements. Ann Phys Med 9:103, 1967.
41. Lowery W, Horn T, Boden S, Wiesel S: Impairment evaluation based on spinal range of motion in normal subjects. J Spinal Disability Assessment 5:398–402, 1992.
42. MacRae I, Wright V: Measurement of back movement. Ann Rheum Disability Assessment 28:584–589, 1969.

43. Mallon W, Brown H, Nunley J: Digital ranges of motion: Normal values in young adults. J Hand Surg 73A:882–887, 1991.
44. Mayer R, Chen I, Lavender S, et al: Variance in the measurement of sagittal lumbar spine range of motion among examiners, subjects, and instruments. Spine 20:1489– 1493, 1995.
45. Mayer T, Brady S, Bovasso E, et al: Noninvasive measurement of cervical triplanar motion in normal subjects. Spine 18:2191–2195, 1993.
46. Mayer T, Dowdle J: Impairment/disability evaluation. An Assoc Orthop Surg Bull 40:12–13, 1992.
47. Mayer T, Gatchel R, Keeley J, et al: A male incumbent worker industrial database. Part I—Lumbar spinal physical capacity. Spine 19:755–761, 1994.
48. Mayer T, Gatchel R, Keeley J, et al: A male incumbent worker industrial database. Part II—Cervical spinal physical capacity. Spine 19:762–764, 1994.
49. Mayer T, Kondraske G, Beals S, Gatchel R: Spinal range of motion: Accuracy and sources of error with inclinometric measurement. Spine 22:1976–1984, 1997.
50. Mayer T, Mooney V, Gatchel R: Contemporary Conservative Care for Painful Spinal Disorders: Concepts, Diagnosis and Treatment. Philadelphia, Waverly Press, 1991.
51. Mayer T, Pope P, Tabor J, et al: Physical progress and residual impairment quantification after functional restoration. Part I—Lumbar mobility. Spine 18:389–394, 1994.
52. Mayer T, Tencer A, Kristoferson S, Mooney V: Use of noninvasive techniques for quantification of spinal range-of-motion in normal subjects and chronic low-back dysfunction patients. Spine 9:588–595, 1984.
53. McClure P, Esola M, Schreier R, Siegler S: Kinematic analysis of lumbar and hip motion while rising from a forward flexed position in patients with and without a history of low back pain. Spine 22:552–558, 1997.
54. McGregor A, McCarthy I, Hughes S: Motion characteristics of the lumbar spine in the normal population. Spine 20:2421–2428, 1995.
55. Mellin G: Method and instrument for noninvasive measurements of thoracolumbar rotation. Spine 12:28–31, 1987.
56. Miller S, Mayer T, Cox R, Gatchel R: Reliability problems associated with the modified Schober technique for true lumbar flexion measurement. Spine 17:345–348, 1992.
57. Moll J, Wright V: Normal range of spinal mobility. Ann Rheum Disability Assessment 30:381–386, 1971.
58. Morrey B, Askew L, Chao E: A biomechanical study of normal functional elbow motion. J Bone Joint Surg 63A:872–877, 1988.
59. Netzer O, Payne V: Effects of age and gender on functional rotation and lateral movements of the neck and back. Gerontology 39:320–326, 1993.
60. Ordway N, Seymour R, Donelson R, et al: Cervical sagittal range of motion analysis using three methods—cervical range of motion device, 3 space, and radiography. Spine 22:501–508, 1997.
61. Paquet N, Malouin F, Richards C, et al: Validity and reliability of a new electrogoniometer for the measurement of sagittal dorsolumbar movements. Spine 16:516–519, 1991.
62. Pearcy M: Measurement of back and spinal mobility. Clin Biomech 1:44–51, 1986.
63. Pearcy M, Portek I, Sheperd J: The effect of low-back pain on lumbar spine movements measured by three dimensional x-ray analysis. Spine 10:150–153, 1985.
64. Petherick M, Rheault W, Kimble S, et al: Concurrent validity and intertester reliability of universal and fluid-based goniometers for active elbow range of motion. Phys Ther 68:966–969, 1988.
65. Portek I, Pearcy M, Reader G, et al: Correlation between radiologic and clinical measurement of lumbar spine movement. Br J Rheumatol 22:197–205, 1983.
66. Porter J, Wilkinson A: Lumbar–hip flexion motion: A comparative study between asymptomatic and chronic low back pain in 18- to 36-year-old men. Spine 22:1508–1514, 1997.
67. Reid D, Burnham R, Saboe L, et al: Lower extremity flexibility patterns in classical ballet dancers and their correlation to lateral hip and knee injuries. Am J Sports Med 15:347–352, 1987.
68. Reynolds P: A measurement of spinal mobility: A comparison of three methods. Rheumatol Rehab 14:180–185, 1975.
69. Rheault W, Miller M, Nothnagel P, et al: Intertester reliability and concurrent validity of fluid-based and universal goniometers for active knee flexion. Phys Ther 78:1676–1678, 1988.
70. Riddle D, Rothstein J, Lamb R: Goniometric reliability in a clinical setting: Shoulder measurements. Phys Ther 67:688–693, 1987.
71. Roaas A, Andersson G: Normal range of motion of the hip, knee and ankle joints in male subjects, 30–40 years of age. Acta Orthop Scand 53:205–208, 1982.
72. Roach K, Miles T: Normal hip and knee active range of motion: The relationship to age. Phys Ther 71:656–665, 1991.
73. Rothstein J, Miller P, Roettger R: Goniometric reliability in a clinical setting: Elbow and knee measurements. Phys Ther 63:1611–1615, 1983.
74. Ryu J, Cooney W, Askew L, et al: Functional range of motion of the wrist joint. J Hand Surg 16A:409–419, 1991.
75. Salisbury P, Porter R: Measurement of lumbar sagittal mobility: A comparison of methods. Spine 12:190–193, 1987.
76. Shirley F, O'Connor P, Robinson M, MacMillan M: Comparison of lumbar range of motion using three measurement devices in patients with chronic low back pain. Spine 19:779–783, 1994.
77. Spiegel T, Spiegel J, Paulus H: The joint alignment and motion scale: A simple measure of joint deformity in patients with rheumatoid arthritis. J Rheumatol 14:887–892, 1987.
78. Steffen T, Rubin R, Baramki H, et al: A new technique for measuring lumbar segmental motion *in vivo*: Method, accuracy, and preliminary results. Spine 22:156–166, 1997.
79. Stokes I, Wilder D, Frymoyer J, Pope M: Assessment of patients with low-back pain by biplanar radiographic measurements of intervertebral motion. Spine 6:233–240, 1980.
80. Sullivan M, Dickinson C, Troup J: The influence of age and gender on lumbar spine sagittal plane range of motion: A study of 1126 healthy subjects. Spine 19:682–686, 1994.
81. Svenningsen S, Terjesen T, Auflem M, et al: Hip motion related to age and sex. Acta Orthop Scand 60:97–100, 1980.
82. Swanson A, Goran-Hagert C, de-Groot-Swanson G: Evaluation of impairment in the upper extremity. J Hand Surg 12A:896–926, 1987.
83. Troup J, Hood C, Chapman A: Measurements of sagittal mobility of the lumbar spine and hips. Ann Phys Med 9:308–313, 1968.
84. Twomey L, Taylor J: Age changes in the lumbar articular triad. Aust J Physiother 31:106–112, 1985.
85. Waddell G, Somerville D, Henderson I, et al: Objective clinical evaluation of physical impairment in chronic low-back pain. Spine 17:617–628, 1992.
86. Whittle M: Calibration and performance of a three-dimensional television system for kinematic analysis. J Biomech 15:185–196, 1982.
87. Williams R, Binkley J, Bloch R, et al: Reliability of the modified-modified Schober and double inclinometer methods for measuring lumbar flexion and extension. Phys Ther 73:26–36, 1993.
88. Wynne-Davies R: Familial joint laxity. Proc R Soc Med 64:689–690, 1971.
89. Youdas J, Carey J, Garrett T: Reliability of measurements of cervical spine range of motion—comparison of three methods. Phys Ther 71:98–106, 1991.
90. Zaki A, Goldberg M, Khalil T, et al: Comparison between the one and two inclinometer techniques for measuring body ranges of motion using the Orthoranger II. In: Das B (ed): Advances in Industrial Ergonomics and Safety II. New York, Taylor & Francis, 1990, pp 135–142.

CHAPTER

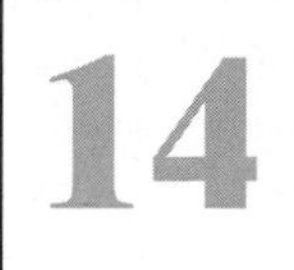

The Role of Radiologic Imaging in the Orthopedic Impairment Evaluation

RICHARD J. HERZOG, MD ■ J. BRUCE KNEELAND, MD

During the course of the evaluation of patients who have acute, subacute, or chronic injuries that limit their occupational capacity or activities of daily living (ADL), a clinician will frequently order diagnostic tests to determine if there is objective evidence of tissue dysfunction. Because injuries to the musculoskeletal system are a frequent cause of impairment, it is important for the clinician working with these patients to understand the efficacy of the diagnostic tests that are available to assess these clinical problems. Radiologic imaging studies have been heavily utilized to document objective pathologic changes in the musculoskeletal system, but to use these tests effectively it is necessary to understand their strengths and limitations. The efficacy of these tests is not only affected by the quality of the study but by the expertise of the individual who interprets the examination. The additional data provided by these tests only become useful clinical information when integrated with the patient's history, physical examination, and other diagnostic tests.

The radiologic studies that are frequently ordered in the evaluation of the musculoskeletal disability include standard plain films, magnetic resonance imaging (MRI), radionuclide studies, ultrasound (US), and computed tomography (CT). This chapter will focus on the application of plain films, MRI, US, and CT in impairment evaluation. Both plain films and CT have played a major role in the detection of osseous abnormalities in the body, whereas MRI has been particularly useful in the assessment of soft tissue injury (e.g., cartilage, muscles, tendons, and ligaments). In addition, MRI is particularly sensitive to detect abnormalities of cancellous bone. The application of US is limited to the assessment of superficial soft tissue structures. A basic understanding of the physics and the technical factors involved in these different modalities is needed in order to facilitate the selection of the appropriate imaging modality for different diagnostic problems.

PHYSICS AND TECHNICAL FACTORS OF RADIOLOGIC STUDIES

The musculoskeletal system has long been studied with plain film radiographs. In fact, the first anatomic images ever taken by Roentgen were of the human hand. Radiographs are projection images in which the contrast arises from the differential attenuation (i.e., scattering and absorption of x-rays by different structures). This type of image demonstrates the anatomy of the cortical and cancellous bone at high resolution, as well as the abnormalities that affect them. The visualization of bony detail results from the strong attenuation of the x-ray beam by calcified structures. Metallic appliances and clips used for surgical procedures on the musculoskeletal system attenuate x-rays even more effectively than calcium and are also well seen. The capacity of this technique to demonstrate abnormalities in the soft tissues of the musculoskeletal system is exceedingly limited owing to small differences in attenuation by different soft tissues. Soft tissue abnormalities may be detected as a vague increase in density due to replacement of fat by water-density structures, distortion of the surface contour, and the presence of calcifications or gas. Plain films are inexpensive and readily available. They do, however, carry the small but finite risks associated with the use of any ionizing radiation; in particular, the induction of neoplasms.[50,228,261]

CT utilizes x-rays to generate cross-sectional images in which the intensity is proportional to the degree of attenuation of the x-ray beam. As with plain films, the strong scattering of x-rays by the calcium permits a relatively detailed visualization of bony detail in cross-section. In contradistinction to plain films, the extremely pronounced attenuation of the x-ray beam by metallic appliances gives rise to streak artifacts that can obscure large parts of the image. CT gives more detailed information regarding the soft tissues than do plain films, although it is still limited by the relatively small differences in x-ray scattering present among different soft tissues. Differences in soft tissue attenuation can, in many cases, be increased by the intravenous administration of iodine-containing contrast agents. Iodine strongly attenuates x-rays, and differences in delivery of the contrast agent to a given region (e.g., due to differences in perfusion of the tissues or permeability of the vessels) can result in differences in attenuation of the x-rays that are detectable by CT. The planes of section that can be imaged with CT are limited by both the physical geometry of the gantry and the constraints of patient positioning within the gantry, although there is clearly more flexibility in positioning the extremities than the chest or abdomen. CT also poses the previously noted small but finite risks associated with ionizing radiation.[96]

US forms images by transmitting pulses of high frequency sound and detecting the reflected pulses. The images so formed are dependent on both the strength of the reflected wave as well as the distance traveled by the reflected wave. Sound waves do not penetrate the bones and cannot be used to evaluate these structures. They can, however, demonstrate the morphology of the more superficial soft tissues of the musculoskeletal system. US is widely available, relatively inexpensive, and believed to be completely safe. US of the musculoskeletal system, however, although reported to be successful in the hands of some investigators, is technically demanding and has not gained widespread acceptance.[201]

Radionuclide bone scanning, which is usually performed with Tc-99 m MDP, provides low resolution projection images, or with the use of single photon emission computed tomography (SPECT), crosssectional images of the skeletal system. The degree of uptake at a given location is proportional to the blood flow and to the amount of new bone formation. The bone scan is exquisitely sensitive to the presence of any process that increases the amount of new bone formation such as neoplasm, trauma, or osteoarthritic hyperostosis. Its sensitivity to all of these diseases, however, renders it nonspecific as to the nature of the disease present in any given case.[43,180]

MRI is a method of forming cross-sectional images of the body that uses the magnetic properties of the hydrogen nuclei of "mobile" water molecules. Mobile water molecules are those molecules that are not tightly bound to macromolecules. In order to create MR images the subject must first be placed in a strong static magnetic field. This induces a difference in the energy levels of the hydrogen nuclei whose magnetic moments are pointed in the direction of the static field and those that are pointed in the opposed direction. Transitions between these levels are then induced by irradiating the nuclei with an additional magnetic field that is oscillating at the "resonant" frequency of the hydrogen nucleus. As the excited nuclei return to their original state they emit a brief pulse of energy. This emitted pulse can be detected and constitutes the MR signal. Spatial localization of the MR signal is achieved by superimposing on the strong static magnetic field a relatively weak magnetic field with a known spatial variation called a gradient field. The characteristic "banging" noise associated with MRI results from turning these gradient fields off and on. The signal intensity in MRI arises from the number of mobile water nuclei present per unit of tissue volume and, more importantly, from properties of the nuclei called the T1 and T2 relaxation times. These latter two quantities characterize the rate of recovery of the nuclei from the excited to the unexcited states (T1) and the decay of the MR signal (T2). It is the relaxation times that are altered from their normal values by the presence of disease. The precise method used to excite the nuclei determines whether the signal intensity and hence the image contrast are more dependent on differences in T1 (T1-weighted) or on differences in T2 (T2-weighted) among the different tissues. The soft tissue contrast afforded by differences in relaxation times is far greater than the differences seen in the attenuation of x-rays that determines contrast in CT, and for this reason the contrast between normal and abnormal tissue seen with MRI is generally much greater. Intravenous contrast agents are used in MRI to further enhance contrast. MR contrast agents produce their result by shortening the T1 relaxation times and, as with the CT contrast agents, alter the contrast to different regions based on differences in vascular perfusion or permeability. Another strength of MRI resides in its direct multiplanar capabilities. CT is limited to obtaining scans only in the plane of the gantry. Any additional multiplanar CT images are constructed by a computer algorithm that results in some loss of image detail.[34]

MRI is generally safe for subjects, although certain patients are at risk and must not be imaged. These include patients with cardiac pacemakers, neurostimulatory devices, certain types of intracranial aneurysm clips, radiographically visible metallic fragments within the orbits or spinal canal, and certain types of prostheses. Although MRI probably provides the greatest amount of information compared to other radiologic imaging techniques, it is also the most expensive and probably the most complex method of imaging available.[219]

SPINAL DYSFUNCTION

Lumbosacral Spine

Because back pain is the second leading cause of work absenteeism and the number one cause of Workers' Compensation claims, it is important to understand the appropriate role of radiologic imaging in the assessment of spinal dysfunction. The goal of any imaging study is to define accurately the pathomorphologic changes in a specific tissue, organ, or part of the body. Objective categorization of pathologic changes facilitates the interpretation and communication of abnormalities detected on a test, and these same criteria can be used on follow-up evaluation to assess the effects of different forms of therapy (e.g., surgical intervention or nonoperative rehabilitation). The reproducibility and the reliability of all objective diagnostic criteria must be rigorously evaluated in prospective blinded studies prior to their implementation.[36,215,221,265]

Patients with neck or low-back pain (LBP) are a challenge to the physician who desires a precise pathoanatomic diagnosis prior to the initiation of therapy. Back pain and neural dysfunction are a frequent symptom complex for many processes afflicting the lumbar spine and paraspinal tissues. For this reason, a clinician assessing a patient after a work-related injury must consider and exclude a large number of potential causes to explain a patient's symptoms. Fortunately, most episodes of back pain are self-limited, and no diagnostic tests are needed. However, if pain persists or becomes worse, it is usually necessary to order a diagnostic test to provide the additional clinical information needed to choose rationally the appropriate therapeutic modality. Prior to ordering any diagnostic test, a clinician must determine how the information provided by the test will affect patient management and mentally compare projected test costs and expected benefits. The more precise the information provided by a diagnostic test, the greater will be its impact on directing patient care. The value of different tests depends on their sensitivity, specificity, accuracy, risk, cost, and availability.

Prior to 1970, plain film radiography was the primary radiologic study available to evaluate patients with neck or back pain. Plain films provide direct information only on the morphology of the osseous components of the spinal motion segments (i.e., the vertebral bodies and the facet joints at each disc level). Any pathologic process that precipitates osseous destruction, degeneration, or remodeling can be detected on plain films if a sufficient amount of bone is affected by the pathologic process. When a worker has symptoms of acute or chronic LBP or sciatica, disc disease or spinal stenosis must be excluded as a potential cause of the worker's symptomatology. Plain film findings that are indicative of disc degeneration include decreased disc height, a disc vacuum phenomenon, end-plate ridges and sclerosis, and a degenerative olisthesis (Fig. 14–1). Unfortunately, these changes occur relatively late in the natural history of disc degeneration and most of them represent adaptive changes of the bone to the abnormal biomechanics of a degenerating disc. The only plain film findings indicative of an acute disc herniation would include an acute Schmorl node, displacement of calcified disc material, or a limbus vertebra (i.e., a fractured vertebral body rim secondary to displaced disc material). To determine that these represent an acute finding, a prior set of normal spine radiographs would be needed.

In order to determine the value of plain radiographs in the work-up of back or radicular pain, it is necessary to know the spectrum of findings detected on plain films of asymptomatic patients. Frymoyer et al[75] evaluated the plain films of 292 subjects, including 96 with no history of back pain, 134 with a history of previous or current moderate back pain, and 62 with a history of prior or current severe back pain. In the three groups, the frequency of transitional vertebrae, Schmorl nodes, disc vacuum phenomenon, "claw" spurs, and disc space narrowing at the L3–4 and L5–S1 disc levels were similar. Traction spurs or disc space narrowing at the L4–5 level had a positive correlation to severe LBP. Only end-plate spurs increased in incidence with aging. Spurs and disc narrowing had no correlation with occupation. Dabbs et al[51] evaluated disc height on the plain films obtained on 51 asymptomatic and 86 symptomatic subjects. Both groups of patients had evidence of decreased disc height and there was no significant difference between the two groups. Witt et al[264] also compared the plain film findings in patients with and without back pain. There was no difference in the prevalence of disc degeneration or spondylosis comparing the 238 patients with LBP and sciatica to 68 asymptomatic patients. The incidence of both disc degeneration and spondylosis increased with age in both groups.

In contrast to the studies that have demonstrated limited value of plain films in the assessment of patients with LBP, Torgerson et al[238] evaluated 217 asymptomatic patients between the ages of 40 and 70 and 387 symptomatic patients in the same age range. Fifty-six percent of the symptomatic patients had plain film evidence of disc degeneration, compared to 22% of the asymptomatic patients. Even though this difference may be significant, the findings of disc degeneration lack specificity to explain symptomatology considering their common occurrence in both the symptomatic and the asymptomatic groups. Torgerson et al also found a higher incidence of spondylolysis and spondylolisthesis in the symptomatic patients. In addition, they reported that osteophyte formation had no direct correlation to back pain.

Considering the increasing age of the workforce, it is important to determine the value of plain films in

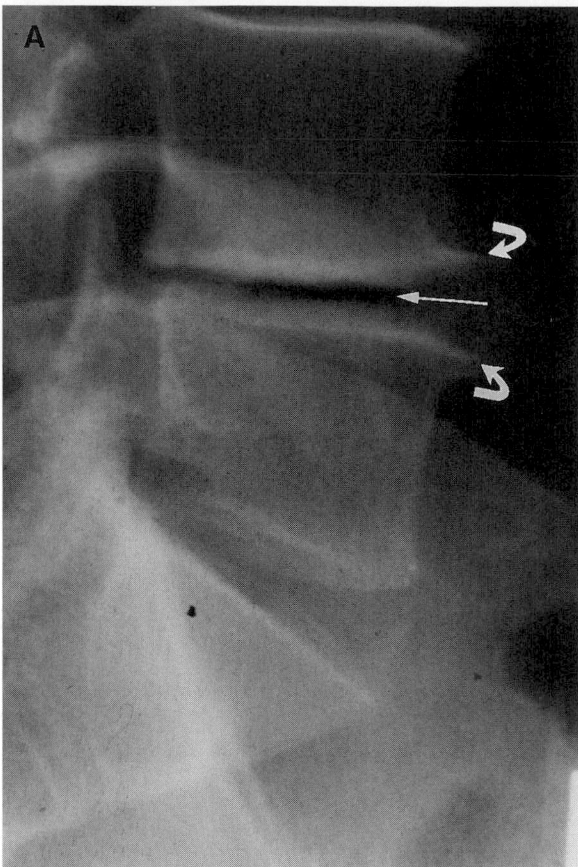

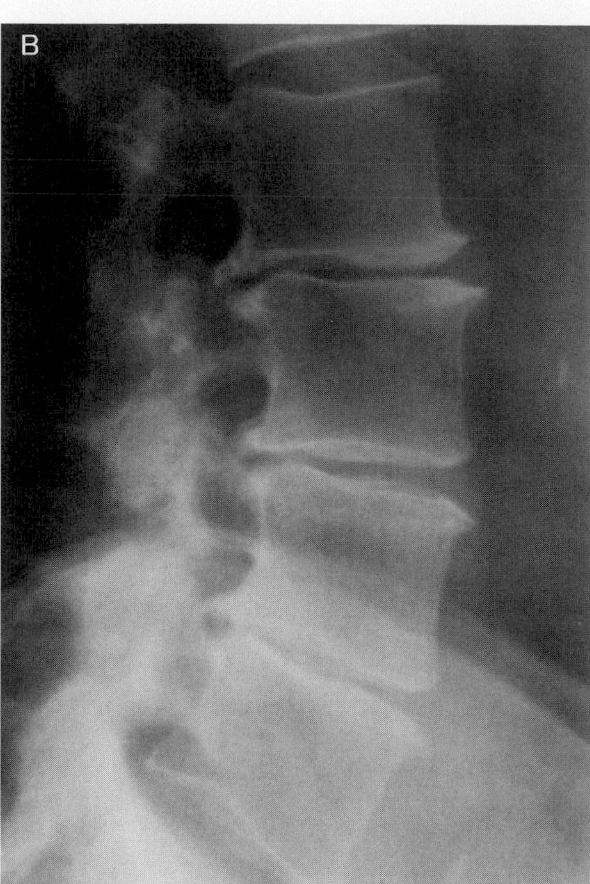

Figure 14–1. On that spot lateral radiograph of the lumbosacral junction (*A*) at the L4–5 disc level there is decreased disc height, a disc vacuum phenomenon (*straight arrow*), anterior end-plate ridges (*curved arrows*), and end-plate sclerosis. On the full lateral radiograph of another patient (*B*) there is evidence of multilevel disc degeneration with decreased disc height, both anterior and posterior end-plate ridges, end-plate sclerosis, and a minimal retrolisthesis at the L2–3 disc level.

the older patient population. Biering-Sorensen et al[19] reported on the plain films findings of 666 60-year-old men and women taking part in a general population survey. Evidence of disc degeneration was significantly more common in individuals reporting LBP compared to those without pain. L4–5 disc degeneration was the only radiologic abnormality correlated to work absence due to LBP. The authors calculated the predictive value of a positive or negative finding of L4–5 disc degeneration in relation to LBP within the last 10 years. The predictive value of a positive finding was 64% and the predictive value of no disc degeneration was 49%, clearly indicating the limited value of the radiologic findings.

When comparing the data from studies reporting on patients with back or neck pain, the precise characteristics of the cohort group must be specified (e.g., physical condition, social and work history, and psychological status if relevant). The value of plain film studies also depends on the reliability of the interpretation of the spine radiographs. Coste et al[47] have reported on the variability of the interpretations by rheumatologists who were assessing plain spinal films obtained on patients with benign LBP. A significant variability of interpretation was observed for findings considered by the author to be important in the assessment of patients with LBP. There were low levels of agreement in the diagnosis of Schmorl nodes, apophyseal joint abnormalities, spondylolysis, and structural deviations. The highest levels of interobserver agreement were for the detection of disc abnormalities. The authors concluded that better standardized criteria are needed to improve the reliability of plain film interpretation of the spine. Andersson et al[7] reported on the influence of spinal motion segment orientation and reader variability in the measurement of disc height. Three orthopaedic surgeons and three radiologists, using the same measurement criteria, assessed disc height on lateral spinal radiographs. Differences of up to 50% of the nominal disc height were observed between different readers. Spinal orientation also affected the accuracy of the measurements, and the authors concluded that accurate measurements cannot readily be made on routine spine radiographs.

Considering the limitations of spinal radiographs in the assessment of patients with LBP, in what clinical situations are they indicated? Liang et al[143] performed a cost-effective analysis of plain films in the assessment of primary-care patients with back pain. The cohort group included patients aged from 18 to 60 with acute LBP but no symptoms or signs suggesting serious disease (e.g., cancer or infection). The authors concluded that the risks and costs of obtaining lumbar x-rays at the initial patient visit compared to performing x-rays 8 weeks later for patients with persistent symptoms did not seem to justify the relatively small associated benefit of an earlier x-ray examination. This was based on the assumption that the probability of diseases requiring specific therapy was 0.2% in this patient population. The probability of disease may be different in referral practices. Deyo et al[57] also assessed the value of lumbar spine films in a primary-care facility. They developed a selective group of indications for ordering early radiographs that included age greater than 50, significant trauma, neuromotor deficits, unexplained weight loss, suspicion of ankylosing spondylitis, drug or alcohol abuse, history of cancer, use of corticosteroids, temperature greater than 100°F, recent visit for same problem that had not improved, and patients seeking compensation for back pain. Using these criteria, 40% of 227 patients presenting with one of these indications had x-ray findings that could explain their symptoms, compared to 12% of the patients who lacked these indications. The indication with the highest diagnostic yield was age greater than 50. Whereas their data support the safety and value of applying selective x-ray ordering criteria, it is apparent that their indications are limited to patients presenting to a primary-care facility and not for an impairment evaluation.

When a patient presenting with back or leg pain requires further diagnostic evaluation, the question arises as to what constitutes a complete radiologic study, where should it be performed, and who should provide the diagnostic interpretation of the study. Even with its limited sensitivity and specificity, plain film radiography should be the initial screening examination when radiologic evaluation is indicated. Scavone et al[210] attempted to determine what constitutes an adequate lumbar spine examination. They evaluated 993 radiographic studies performed on 782 patients presenting with a variety of problems. Anteroposterior (AP), lateral, oblique, and spot lateral radiographs constituted the standard study for all patients. The authors initially interpreted only the AP and lateral radiographs on each patient. This was followed by an evaluation utilizing all five radiographs. In 97.9%, the diagnoses could be made using only the AP and lateral radiographs. In 2.4% of the patients, the diagnoses were missed. The 19 missed diagnoses included unilateral spondyloyses (68%), bilateral spondylolyses (26%), and congenital anomalies (5%). The value of oblique radiographs focuses on the evaluation of the pars interarticularis and the facet joints. The authors found that although the oblique views provided the best evaluation of the facet joints, the degenerative changes of the facets could also be seen on the AP and lateral radiographs. The additional information obtained on the oblique views concerning facet degenerative changes did not change the patient diagnosis or therapy. The authors concluded that the oblique views should be obtained if there is a questionable abnormality on the AP and lateral views, and possibly in the evaluation of patients with major trauma. The limited x-ray study (i.e., the AP and lateral radiographs) was also appropriate for the evaluation of patients with chronic symptoms.

In addition to the utilization of spinal radiographs for the evaluation of patients with acute and chronic back or leg pain, radiographs have also been used as part of pre-employment evaluations to screen job applicants. Bigos et al[20] reported on the value of pre-employment x-rays for predicting acute and chronic back injury claims. The prevalence of spina bifida occulta, spondylolysis, spondylolisthesis, transitional vertebrae, Scheuermann disease, facet tropism, straightening of the lumbar spine, or evidence of degenerative disc disease was determined. The radiographic study included full AP and lateral views of the spine, along with a spot lateral view of the lumbosacral junction. The data indicated that the radiographs were not helpful in predicting who is more likely to make a back claim injury nor in detecting the worker who becomes disabled for more than 6 months. The authors concluded that the radiation exposure is not justified due to the limited predictive value of pre-employment screening radiographs.

The diagnostic value of any imaging study is highly dependent on the quality of the examination. Rueter et al[205] reported on the quality of radiographs of the lumbar spine performed in hospitals and other facilities. A critical factor affecting the quality of a radiograph is film processing. If film is underprocessed, then additional x-ray exposure to the patient would be needed to achieve the same density on a film that has been processed normally. Underprocessing also degrades image quality. The authors found that 33% of hospitals, 25% of radiology facilities, and 48% of chiropractic facilities underprocessed lumbosacral spine radiographs. It is evident from this report that there is currently a need to improve the quality of radiographic studies at all facilities performing routine spinal x-rays. This is important considering that the quality of spinal radiographs directly affects the accuracy of x-ray interpretation. Shaffer et al[218] conducted a series of experiments to assess the consistency and the accuracy of sagittal translation measurements from x-rays of varying quality. The authors found that high-quality radiographs were more accurately evaluated than the lower-quality examinations. They also demonstrated a high false-positive and false-negative rate using different methods of measurement in the experimental setting, along with inconsistencies in the interpretations of the clinical flexion-extension studies.

With the cross-sectional imaging capabilities of both CT with multiplanar reconstruction (CT/MPR) and MRI it is possible to evaluate the paraspinal musculature in patients presenting with back pain. Alaranta et al[4] recently evaluated the fat content of lumbar extensor muscles in patients with disabling LBP. They found a positive correlation between the fat content of the lower lumbar paraspinal muscles and the severity of self-reported disability in men. It is not possible from their study to determine if the muscle atrophy was the cause or the result of back pain. The possibility of paraspinal muscle compartment syndromes as a potential etiology of back pain has also been reported and both CT[41] and MRI[59] were used to document edematous changes with the muscles.

Cervical Spine

Although neck pain is not as frequent as back or leg pain as a cause for disability claims, it is frequently the symptom of patients experiencing spinal pain after a vehicular injury or a fall. Workers performing overhead activities or who carry loads that may strain the neck muscles may also have debilitating neck or arm pain. There is little question on the value of radiographs as the initial screening examination to detect fractures or malalignment in patients who have experienced major neck trauma (Fig. 14–2). Their value in the assessment of patients with minor trauma or with chronic neck symptoms is less clear. To assess the efficacy of cervical x-rays it is first necessary to determine their accuracy and then to compare the findings on plain films obtained on asymptomatic and symptomatic patients.

Friedenberg et al[72] correlated the findings observed on radiographs of a cadaveric cervical spines to anatomic findings. Anteroposterior, lateral, and oblique views of the cervical spine were performed prior to dissection. They found a 67% correlation between the radiographic and the anatomic manifestations of disc degeneration. Disc space narrowing was the most common x-ray finding and even minor narrowing of the disc space on the x-ray correlated with anatomical disc degeneration. Posterior osteophytes were most easily seen on the oblique projections and they were always associated with disc space narrowing. Only 57% of large posterior osteophytes detected on dissection were identified on the spinal radiographs. Evaluation of the apophyseal joints was difficult on the radiographs and only 32% of the anatomical abnormalities were identified on the radiographs. It is evident that cervical spine radiographs, like lumbar radiographs, lack sensitivity in the detection of early degenerative changes, but they are very specific for degenerative disease once they become positive.

The radiographic findings of the cervical spine in asymptomatic patients were reported by Gore et al.[82] They evaluated the incidence and severity of degenerative changes of the cervical spine on lateral radiographs obtained on 200 asymptomatic men and women. Age correlated significantly with the severity of disc space narrowing, end-plate sclerosis, anterior and posterior osteophytes, and the degree of lordosis. The severity of each type of degenerative change correlated with the severity of the other types of degeneration at the same disc level. By the age of 40, 35% of the individuals had evidence of degenerative changes and this increased to 83% by the age of 60. In the older age groups, evidence of disc degeneration was more prevalent in men compared to women.

Friedenberg et al[73] compared the findings of radiographs performed on 92 asymptomatic and symptomatic patients. Degenerative changes were most common at the C5–6 and the C6–7 disc levels in both groups. Sixty-two percent of the symptomatic patients had changes at the C5–6 level, compared to 35% of the asymptomatic individuals. This difference was statistically significant. Similar to the findings by Gore et al[82] degenerative changes in the cervical spine increased with age in asymptomatic individuals. Comparing the two groups with respect to foraminal stenosis and facet arthrosis, there were no significant difference in the severity of the degenerative changes. The authors concluded that the value of cervical spine radiographs in determining the clinical significance of degenerative disease of the spine was limited and, at best, radiographs could provide information on the severity of the degenerative process.

Gore et al[83] evaluated the predictive value of cervical radiographs to detect patients who may develop chronic neck pain after the onset of cervical symptoms. Two hundred five patients with neck pain were followed clinically for a minimum of 10 years after the onset of symptoms. Thirty-two percent of the patients had moderate or severe neck pain on follow-up evaluation. The only clinical feature that was of value to predict outcome was a history of an injury associated with the severe neck pain. The presence or severity of the pain was not correlated with the degree of degenerative changes, the sagittal spinal canal diameter, the degree of cervical lordosis, or to any change in these measurements detected on spine radiographs during the follow-up period. At the time of the initial evaluation, 57% of the patients with injuries and 42% of the patients without injuries had normal cervical x-rays. The authors also compared the radiographic findings between these symptomatic patients and a group of age-matched asymptomatic patients. They found that anterior osteophyte formation was the only degenerative change that was present more frequently in the symptomatic patients who were over the age of 35 and had a history of neck injuries. The authors concluded that the treating physician must be

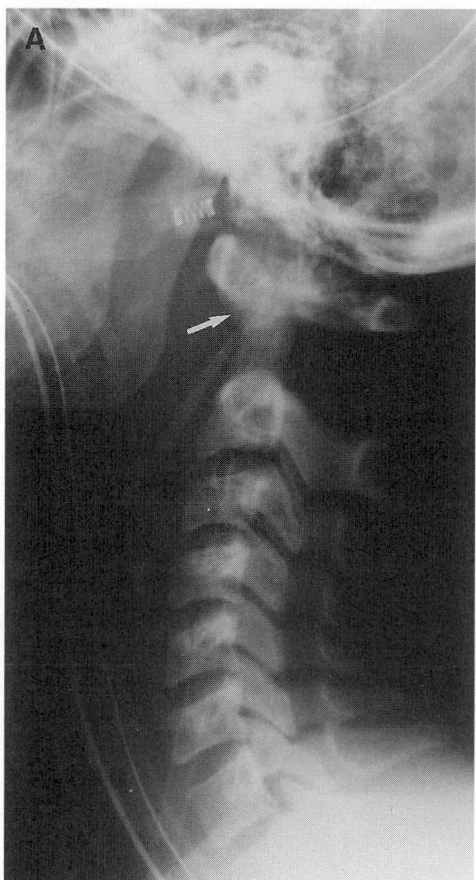

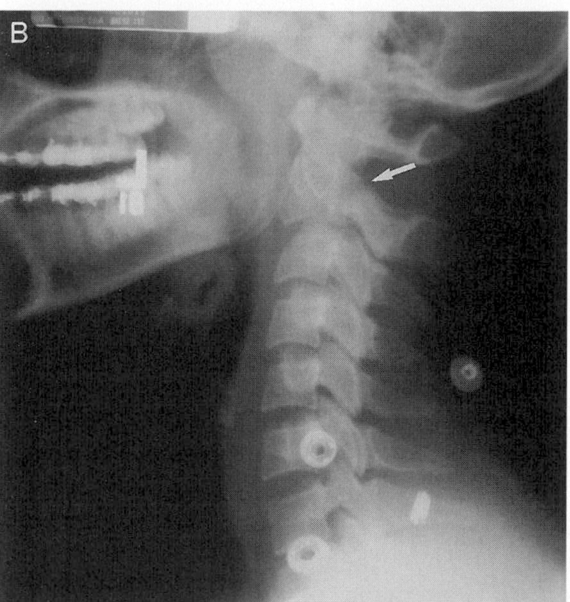

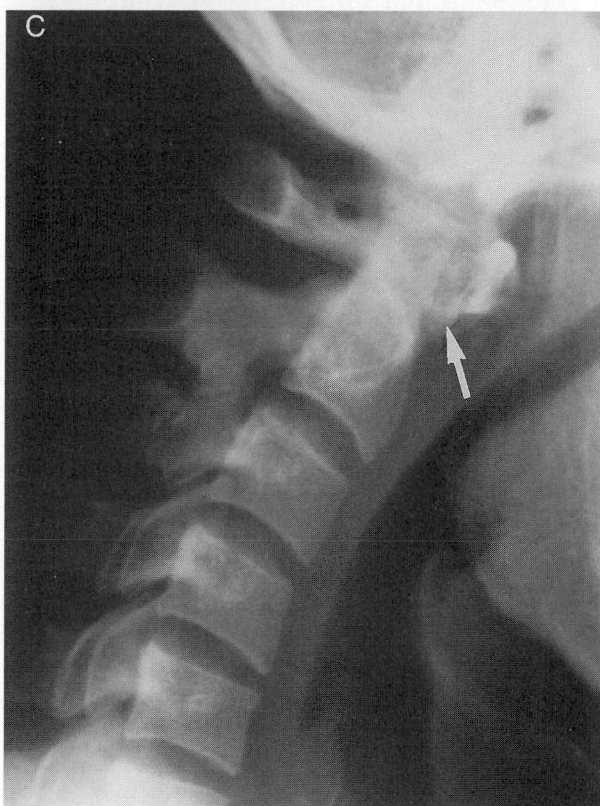

Figure 14–2. On the lateral radiograph of a patient, who was involved in a motor vehicle accident (*A*) there is marked distraction and anterior subluxation at the C1–2 motion segment (*arrow*). In another patient (*B*), who experienced an extension injury, there is a fracture of the posterior arch of C2 (*arrow*). The flexion lateral radiograph of a third patient (*C*), who was injured in a football game, demonstrates instability at the C1–2 motion segment with increased space between the anterior arch of C1 and the odontoid process (*arrow*).

cautious in making a prediction of the final outcome based on the findings on cervical radiographs.

Radiographic Imaging of Disc Disease and Spinal Studies

Plain films provide a global assessment of the severity of degenerative spinal disease, but they are extremely limited in determining the precise location of a pathologic process to explain a patient's symptoms. With the development and implementation of cross-sectional imaging studies (e.g., MRI and CT/MPR) it became possible to evaluate directly the soft tissue and osseous components of each spinal motion segment. Degenerative disc disease, which includes the osseous adaptive changes induced by the biomechanically abnormal disc, is probably the most common etiology of back or leg pain when a precise etiology can be defined. Kirkaldy-Willis[127] was one of the first investigators who stressed the importance of the progressive nature of disc degeneration and herniation.

Degenerative spinal disease is a continuous subclinical process that frequently does not cause symptoms. Abnormalities detected on CT or MRI studies in asymptomatic individuals[25,27] do not represent false positive findings but actual structural or pathologic changes of spinal structures that are not evoking symptoms and, therefore, are not clinically important. In other words, the significance of these morphologic changes can only be determined by correlating the test results to the patient's symptoms. Both CT/MPR and MRI provide excellent delineation of morphologic changes of disc degeneration. The major difference between the imaging modalities resides in the ability of MRI to delineate pathoanatomic and physiochemical changes in a degenerating disc prior to alterations of the disc contour. Both the nucleus pulposus and annulus fibrosus consist of water, collagen, and proteoglycans, with the major differences between the two being the relative amount of these components, level of hydration, and the particular type of collagen that predominates.[78] With MRI, it is possible to delineate different parts of disc architecture. On T2-weighted images, the high signal intensity in the central position of the disc originates from both the nucleus pulposus and the inner annular fibers.[269] The outer annular fibers demonstrate very low signal intensity, as do the adjacent anterior and posterior longitudinal ligaments[183] (Fig. 14–3). The signal intensity in the disc is related to its state of hydration and the physicochemical state of the disc's tissue.[79,99] With aging, there is gradual breakdown of proteoglycans in the nucleus, gradual desiccation of the mucoid nuclear material, and loss of anatomic delineation between the nucleus and inner annular fibers.[154] Over the age of 30, an intranuclear cleft, which represents ingrowth of fibrous tissue,[2] can be identified in normal discs on T2-weighted MR images.

Both experimentally and clinically, the occurrence of a radial annular tear may be a step in the development of disc degeneration and herniation.[144,270] It is now possible with MRI to delineate small tears in the outer annulus with T2-weighted[9,270] or gadolinium-DTPA (Gd-DTPA) enhanced T1-weighted images[202,229] (Fig. 14–4). Annular tears may be present in the periphery of a disc and not communicate with the nucleus pulposus. These tears have been referred to as rim tears and occur at the insertion site of the outer annular fibers into the vertebral body end-plates.[179] Osti et al[178] reported on the possible significance of these peripheral tears as a source of

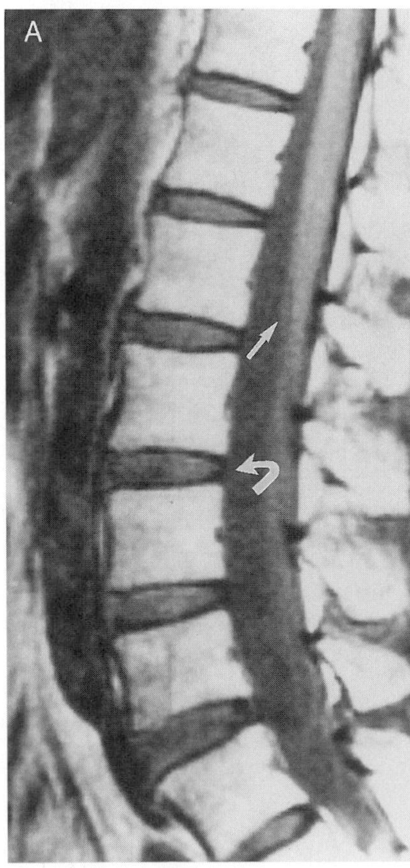

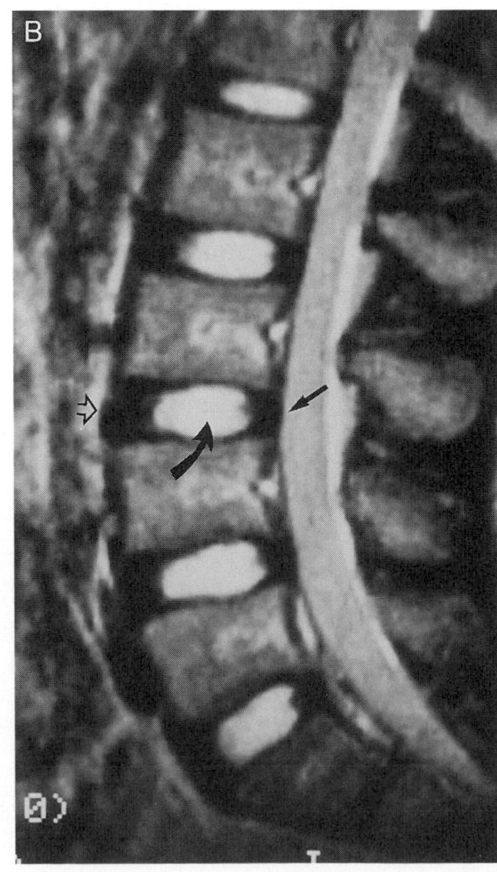

Figure 14–3. On the sagittal T1-weighted image of the lumbar spine (*A*) there is excellent delineation of the conus medullaris (*straight arrow*). The intervertebral disc space is well delineated, but the posterior margin of the disc is not well defined due to the similar signal intensity of the posterior outer annular fibers and the adjacent cerebrospinal fluid (*curved arrow*). On the sagittal T2-weighted image (*B*) there is increased signal intensity in the cerebrospinal fluid and excellent delineation of the posterior margin of the disc (*straight arrow*). There is increased signal intensity within the central portion of the disc (*curved arrow*) that represents a combination of the nucleus pulposus and the inner annular fibers. The anterior annular fibers (*open arrowhead*) are also delineated. (From Physical Medicine and Rehabilitation: State-of-the-art Reviews, vol 4, no 2. Hanley & Belfus, Inc., 1990.)

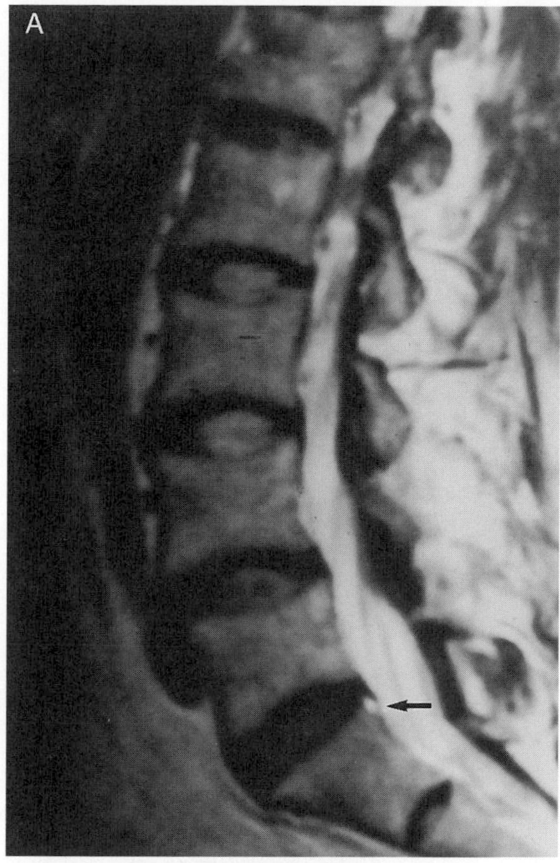

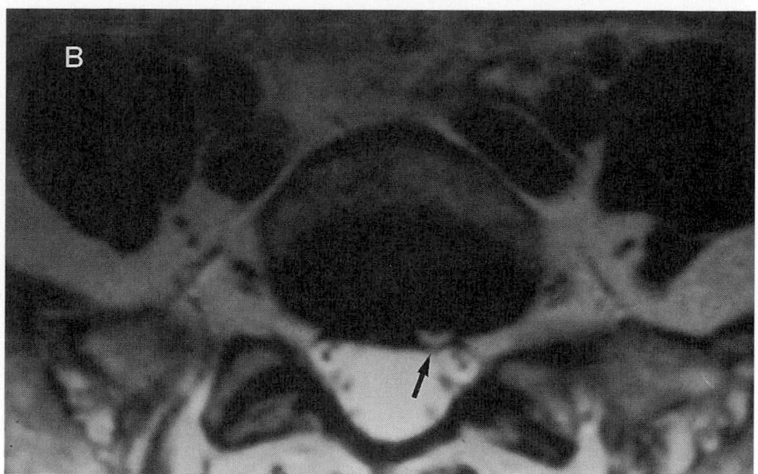

Figure 14–4. On the spin-echo T2-weighted sagittal (*A*) and axial (*B*) images there is a small focus of high signal intensity in the outer annular fibers (*arrow*) representing a small annular tear.

acute back pain. As a disc ages, there may be coalescence of these peripheral tears and delamination of the annular fibers. This may precipitate a generalized bulge of the disc contour due to the loss of the tensile strength of the outer segment of the disc.

If a radial tear develops and communicates with the nucleus pulposus, the disc will begin to degenerate and demonstrate decreased signal intensity on T2-weighted images. Disc herniations result from the displacement of nuclear, annular, or end-plate material through these communicating radial tears. Displacement of the disc material into the region of the outer annular-posterior longitudinal ligament complex will cause altered morphology of the periphery of the disc, resulting in a focal protrusion of the disc beyond the margin of the vertebral body endplates. A contained disc herniation represents displaced discal material that is still bound by the outer annular fibers and/or the posterior longitudinal ligament. Both CT/MPR and MRI provide excellent delineation of these contour changes[118,262] (Fig. 14–5).

In some patients, the development of annular fissures may lead to internal disc disruption[23] or intervertebral disc resorption[112] without the displacement of discal material. MRI is helpful in the evaluation of these patients because it demonstrates altered signal intensity in the abnormal disc. Unfortunately, it is relatively common to detect discs with decreased signal intensity in patients who are asymptomatic.[25] For this reason, some patients with persistent back pain who have had an MRI study delineating decreased signal intensity at one or more disc levels are sometimes further evaluated with discography and CT discography. These studies are performed at some centers for the preoperative evaluation of a patient with multilevel disc degeneration to localize which disc level generates the patient's pain, or for a patient with refractory mechanical back pain who has had a normal MRI study. In addition to the information these tests provide on the abnormal morphology of the disc, the discogram is a provocative test to demonstrate the patient's pain response when the disc is injected. When performing lumbar discography, it is routine to inject the suspected abnormal disc level and the contiguous disc levels, even when these discs appear normal on the MRI evaluation. There have been several reports documenting discs with normal signal intensity on MRI that were abnormal morphologically on discography.[18,273] Discography cannot detect peripheral annular tears that do not communicate with the nucleus pulposus.[268] Although some studies have reported on the advantages of discography, its value in the workup of patients with back or radicular pain is still controversial.[1,8,255]

With the superb soft tissue resolution of MR imaging, it may be possible to determine whether a disc herniation is contained by the outer annular-posterior longitu-

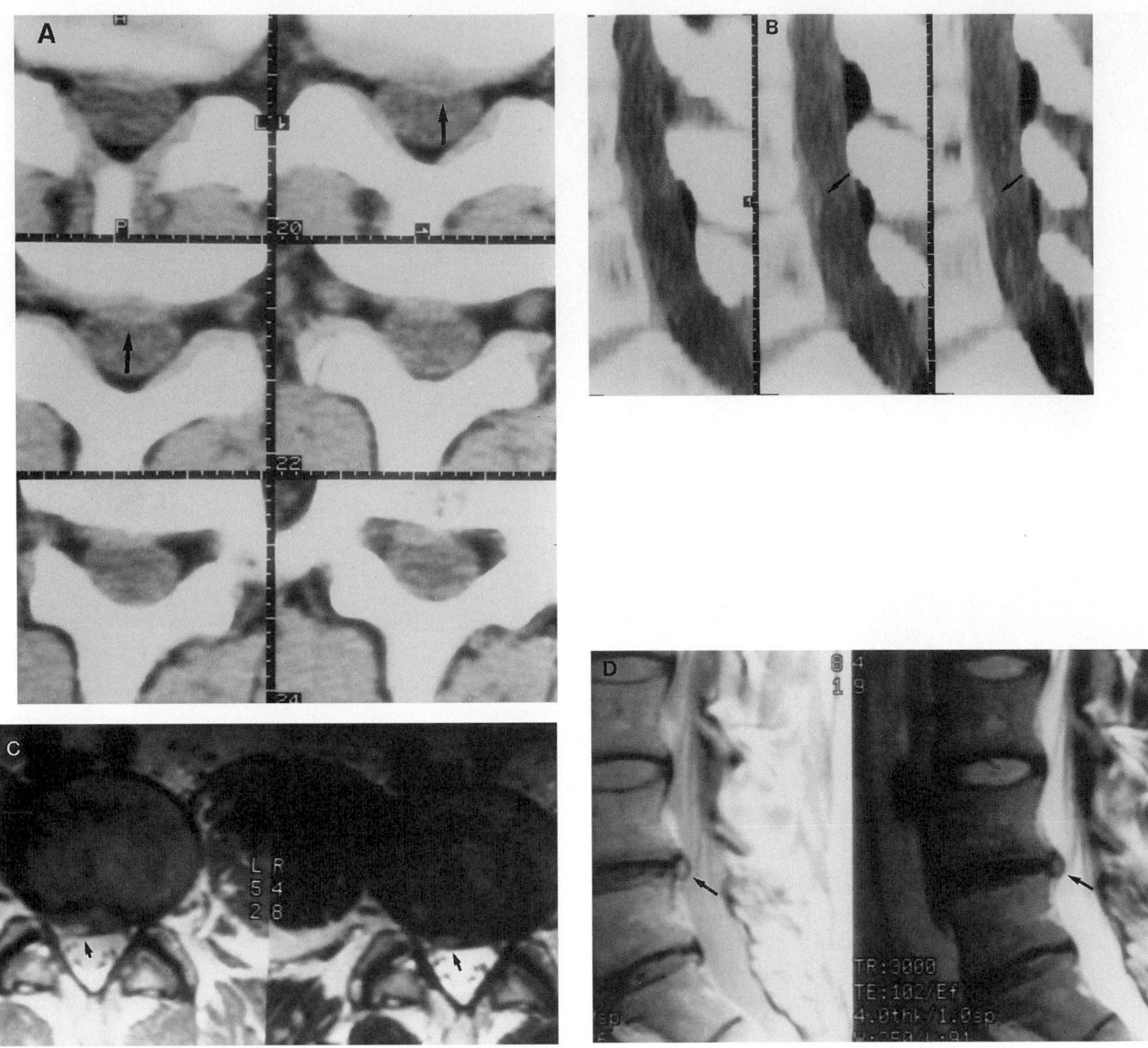

Figure 14–5. A small contained disc herniation (*arrow*) is delinated on the axial (*A*) and sagittal (*B*) images of a CT/MPR study. On another patient, on the axial (*C*) and sagittal (*D*) images of an MRI study, there is a small contained disc herniation (*arrow*).

dinal ligament complex or has extruded through this complex, becoming an extruded, noncontained herniation[87] (Fig. 14–6). This information is needed for the successful application of percutaneous discectomy[155] and chemonucleolysis. It is also important as an indicator of surgical outcome for lumbar disc herniation.[109] The diagnosis of disc extrusion from CT studies is dependent on the configuration of the herniated disc.[74,81] Axial images are always needed on either an MRI or CT/MPR study to evaluate neural displacement or impingement and to detect posterolateral or lateral disc herniations.

Herniated disc material may separate from the disc of origin and become a sequestered fragment. MRI is useful in differentiating between a disc extrusion and a sequestration. Sequestered disc fragments usually generate increased signal intensity on T2-weighted images compared to the degenerated disc of origin. In one prospective study, the accuracy of MRI in differentiating sequestered disc fragments from other forms of lumbar disc herniation was 85% compared to a 65% accuracy for CT myelography.[149] The differential diagnosis of a sequestered disc fragment includes epidural abscess,[187] extradural tumor,[232] conjoined nerve root,[184] nerve root sheath tumor or cyst,[84] synovial cysts,[271] and epidural hematoma.[142]

Following herniation, the disc will continue to degenerate, and on an MRI study, the degenerated disc will demonstrate decreased signal intensity on the T2-weighted sequence. To date, there has been no prospec-

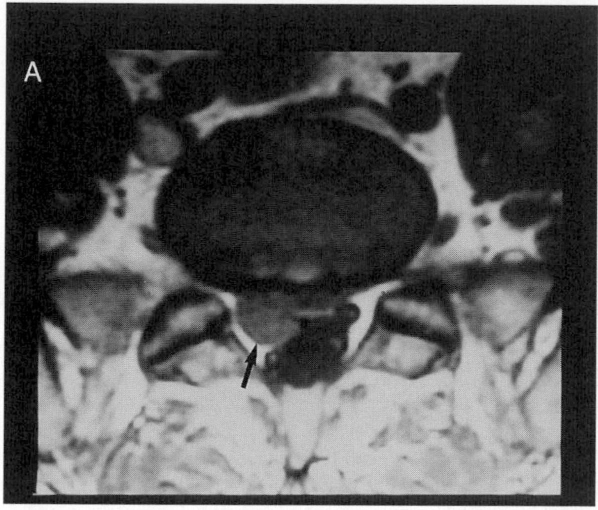

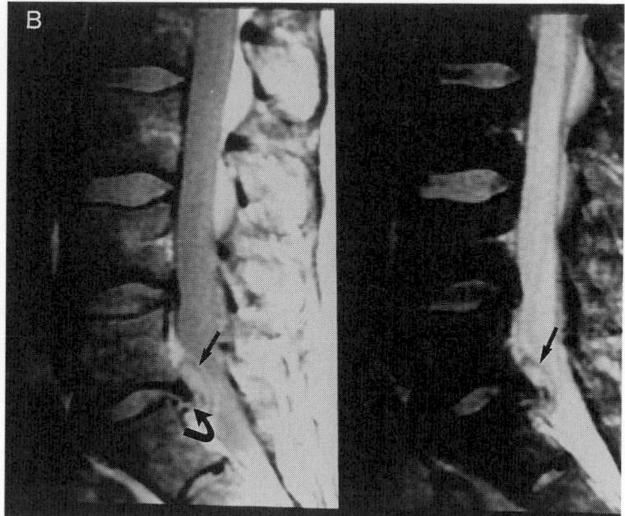

Figure 14–6. At the L5–S1 disc level, a disc extrusion (*straight arrow*) is identified on the MRI axial (*A*) and sagittal (*B*) images. There is interruption of the posterior outer annular/posterior longitudinal ligament complex (*curved arrow*).

tive study in humans to determine the length of time necessary for a normally hydrated disc to become desiccated after it herniates. Therefore, it is not possible to date the exact occurrence of a disc herniation if a prior imaging study is not available for comparison. Even when secondary degenerative changes are identified (e.g., end-plate osteophytes), a disc herniation still may represent an acute process superimposed on a chronic degenerative state. In cases of longstanding disc degeneration, fluid containing fissures may be present in the degenerative disc along with the ingrowth of granulation tissue.[49] These pathologic changes may result in increased signal intensity in the disc on T2-weighted images, and this should not be confused with an inflammatory process[166] (Fig. 14–7). Calcification or gas in the disc may be difficult to detect on T2-weighted images due to the decreased signal intensity in the severely degenerated disc and the absence of an MR signal from the calcium or gas. T1-weighted or gradient echo images have been found to be more useful in delineating a vacuum phenomenon or disc calcification.[163]

With the excellent characterization of normal and abnormal discs by MRI and CT/MPR, it is now possible to study noninvasively the natural history of disc degeneration and herniation. Several studies have reported on the high accuracy of these studies in diagnosing disc disease.[60,66,70,74,94] In addition, MRI and CT have been utilized to document the resorption of disc herniations in patients treated nonoperatively.[3,32,38] Bozzao et al[32] demonstrated that 63% of the patients with disc herniations showed at least a 30% reduction in the size of their herniations, with the greatest size reduction occurring in the larger herniations. Bush et al[38] documented that 76% of disc herniations of nonoperatively treated patients showed partial or complete resolution.

Forristall et al[70] compared MRI and CT myelography in the evaluation of 25 patients with a suspected disc herniation who underwent surgery. Compared to the surgical findings, the accuracy of MRI was 90.3% and CT myelography 77.4%. Recently, Bischoff et al[21] compared CT myelography, MRI, and standard myelography in the evaluation of 57 patients for a disc herniation or spinal stenosis. Compared to the surgical findings, CT myelography was the most accurate test (76.4%), and plain myelography the most specific test (89.2%) in diagnosing a disc herniation. For the diagnosis of spinal stenosis, CT myelography and MRI were the most accurate (85.3%) and the most sensitive (87.2%), and plain myelography was the most specific (88.9%) However, this study had some methodologic limitations and only with a prospective study, where all three modalities are performed routinely, will it be possible to compare the relative accuracy of the different tests.

It is important to remember when evaluating the clinical aspects of different imaging tests of the spine that evidence of herniated discs and spinal stenosis is present in many healthy individuals (Chapter 21). Myelograms, CT imaging, and MRI studies show that disc herniations are anatomically present in 25% or more of asymptomatic individuals. The percentage of abnormal findings increases when the population is older. In a recent MRI study of 98 asymptomatic subjects by Jensen et al,[114] 52% had bulging discs, 27% a disc protrusion (herniation), and 1 subject an extrusion. Stenosis was present in 14%. Only 38% were found to have normal MRI findings. Studies of the cervical spine have shown similar results.[27,235] Clearly this means that imaging must be cor-

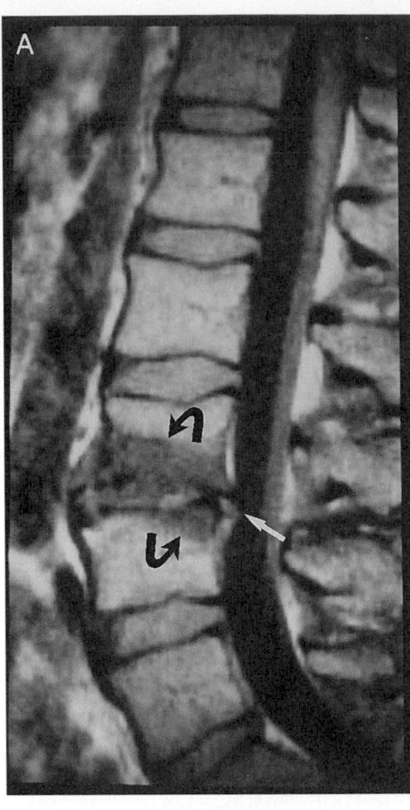

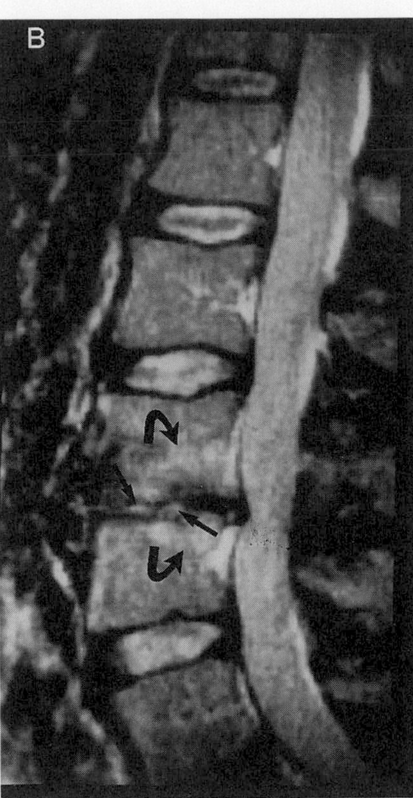

Figure 14–7. At the L3–4 disc level, on the MRI sagittal T1 (*A*) and T2 (*B*) weighted images, there are changes of chronic disc degeneration. On the T1-weighted sagittal image, there is decreased disc height, posterior protrusion of the disc, and spondylotic ridges (*straight arrow*). There is decreased signal intensity in the cancellous bone adjacent to the end-plates (*curved arrows*) due to the presence of fibrovascular tissue. On the T2-weighted sagittal image there is increased signal intensity in the cancellous bone adjacent to the end-plates (*curved arrows*) and in the disc (*straight arrows*) due to the presence of granulation tissue. The vertebral body end-plates on the T2-weighted image are well defined, which helps to differentiate chronic degenerative changes from infection. With infection, the abnormal signal intensity in the vertebral body cancellous bone is usually more extensive than what is identified with chronic degenerative changes.

related to clinical symptoms and signs for a meaningful interpretation.[6,16,31]

It is not infrequent that patients who have undergone disc surgery will experience recurrent back pain when they return to work. If conservative management does not relieve the patient's symptoms, an MRI study is the optimal imaging examination to evaluate the operative site. When performing an MRI study to evaluate a postoperative patient, the length of time between surgery and the MRI examination is an important factor in determining the significance of MRI findings. In two studies, there was no correlation between the immediate postoperative appearance on an MRI examination and symptoms.[14,203] In the first few postoperative months, the changes detected on an MRI study reflect the reparative response to the operative procedure. An MRI study in the immediate postoperative period may not help to diagnose the etiology of a patient's persistent pain. Even 1 year after successful disc surgery, an MRI examination may show persistent posterior contour abnormalities of the disc causing a mass effect on the thecal sac or nerve roots.[53] Tullberg et al[241] evaluated 36 patients 1 year after lumbar disc resection and found no consistent correlation between postoperative back or radicular pain and the MRI findings. The value of an MRI study in assessing patients with recurrent back pain or failed back surgery syndrome centers on the differentiation of epidural scar versus disc after at least 2 to 3 months have transpired since disc surgery. Epidural fibrosis is frequently present at an operative site. Recurrent disc herniations are typically contiguous with the disc space, are well-marginated, and, compared to the disc of origin, display isointensity or hypointensity on T1-weighted images and isointensity or hyperintensity on T2-weighted images. The intravenous administration of Gd-DTPA is particularly helpful in differentiating disc material from fibrosis[42,108] (Fig. 14–8).

As a result of disc degeneration and herniation, there will be altered biomechanics of the motion segment. End-plate degenerative changes are frequently associated with degenerative disc disease. MRI is extremely sensitive to detecting degenerative changes in the adjacent vertebral body end-plates, and Modic et al[164] have described the pathologic alterations in the vertebral body marrow adjacent to discs undergoing degeneration. With Type I end-plate degeneration, there is decreased signal intensity in the subchondral cancellous bone on a T1-weighted image and increased signal intensity on a T2-weighted image compared to normal bone marrow. The region of altered signal intensity pathologically represents prominent fibrovascular tissue in the marrow adjacent to the vertebral body end-plate. Type II end-plate degenerative changes, which pathologically represent increased fat in the subchondral bone marrow, display signal hyperintensity on T1-weighted images and slight hyperintensity or isointensity

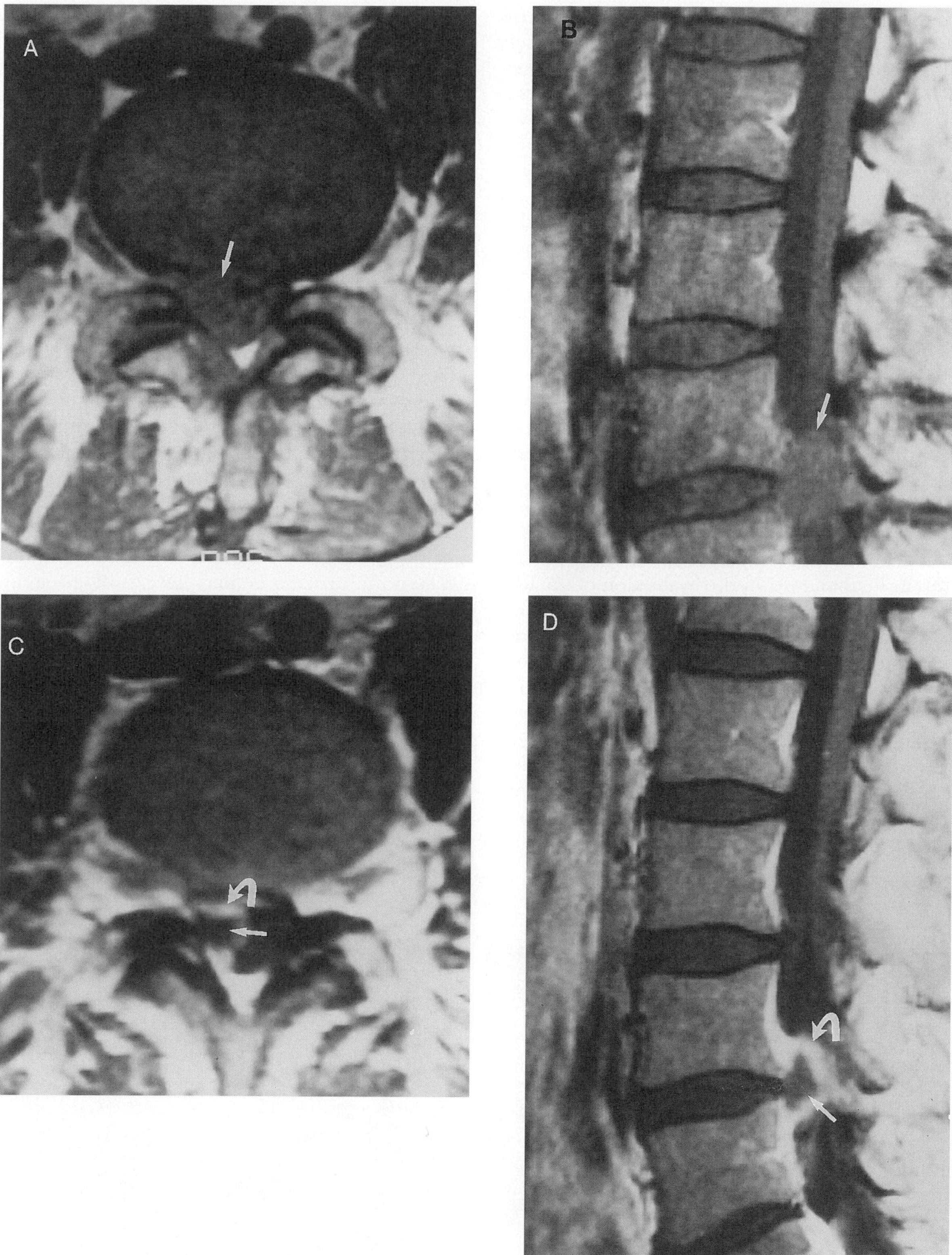

Figure 14–8. On the MRI study in a postoperative patient presenting with recurrent right leg symptoms, on the T1-weighted axial (A) and sagittal (B) images, there is a poorly defined soft tissue mass (*arrow*) positioned in the right side of the spinal canal. On the sagittal image the mass is contiguous with the disc space. After the intravenous injection of Gd-DPTA, on the repeat T1-weighted axial (C) and sagittal (*D*) images, there is enhancement of the vascularized fibrous tissue (*curved arrow*) surrounding the herniated disc material (*straight arrow*).

on T2-weighted images compared to normal marrow. Type III end-plate degenerative changes represent coarsening and thickening of the subchondral trabeculae, which is depicted on T1- and T2-weighted images as decreased signal intensity. Gradient echo sequences are frequently part of the routine MRI evaluation of the lumbar spine. These sequences are not as sensitive to the signal intensity changes within the disc or in the adjacent vertebral body marrow associated with disc degeneration[162] as are standard spin echo T1- and T2-weighted sequences. On CT/MPR evaluation, only end-plate sclerosis can be delineated, and this is not necessarily correlated to Type III changes identified by MRI. On the T1-weighted image, the MRI signal intensity of the vertebral body is predominantly determined by the amount of fat present in the marrow. It is therefore possible to maintain normal signal intensity in a vertebra with thickened trabeculae if there is still a critical amount of residual fat present in the marrow.

End-plate osteophytosis is frequently associated with disc degeneration. With CT's excellent delineation of osseous structures and its superior spatial resolution, it is more accurate than MRI in the evaluation of the location and size of end-plate osteophytes. CT permits accurate delineation of the position of end-plate proliferative changes in relation to neural structures and differentiation of ridges from disc material. With MRI, it may be difficult to separate an osseous ridge from herniated disc material due to the hypointensity of both structures on T1- and T2-weighted sequences. This is not uncommon in the neural foramina where posterolateral disc herniations are frequently associated with osteophytes projecting off the vertebral body end-plates.

Hypertrophy and hyperplasia of connective tissue of the spinal motion segment are frequently precipitated by disc degeneration. The degenerative tissue may encroach into the central spinal canal and compress the neural structures. Spinal stenosis is defined as a local, segmental, or generalized narrowing of the central or intervertebral canals by bony or soft tissue elements that may lead to encroachment on the neural structures. The narrowing may involve the bony canal alone, or the dural sac, or both.[10] The degenerative changes most often associated with central stenosis include osteophytes projecting off the vertebral body end-plates, hypertrophy and bony proliferation of the facet joints, and hypertrophy of the ligamenta flava and anterior facet capsules.[193,213] The purpose of MRI and CT/MPR in the evaluation of a patient presenting with back pain, radiculopathy, or intermittent claudication is not just to demonstrate the presence of stenosis, but to define the relative contributions of each component in the stenotic process (Fig. 14–9).

In the lumbar spine, it has become clear that patients of any age may have disc degeneration superimposed on a stenotic process or may have isolated stenosis as a cause of leg or back pain.[37,93] In order to obtain the true diameter of the central spinal canal, axial images orthogonal to the long axis of the spinal canal or midline sagittal images must be performed. With its excellent spatial resolution of osseous structures, CT/MPR provides the optimal technique to ascertain precise osseous spinal measurements. The classification of spinal stenosis as congenital, developmental, or acquired is extremely helpful when evaluating a small spinal canal.[250,252] Congenital stenosis is due to dis-

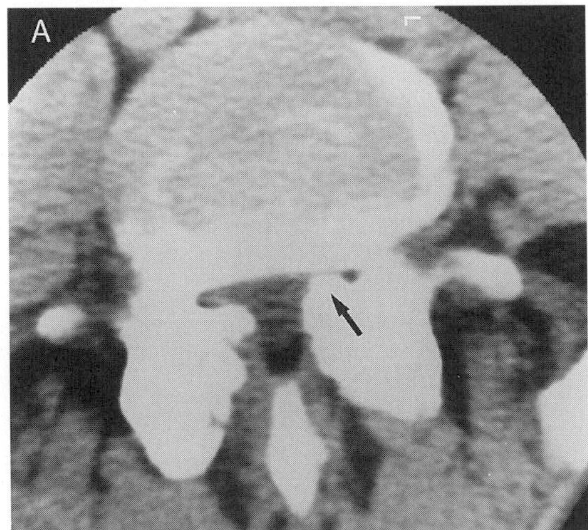

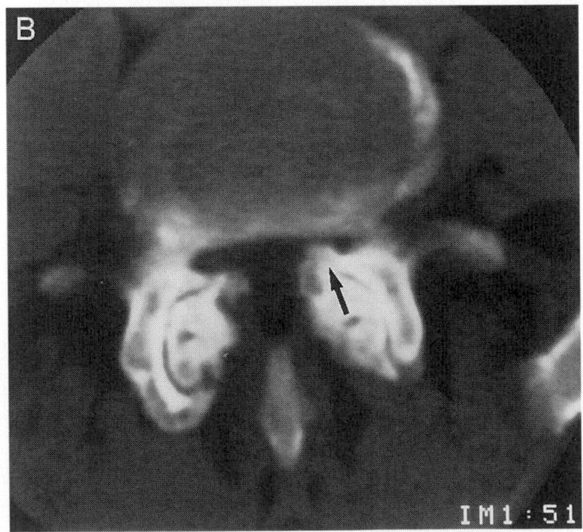

Figure 14–9. At the L4–L5 disc level, on the axial CT images (*A* and *B*), there are severe degenerative changes of the facet joints with prominent osteophytes causing stenosis of the subarticular and lateral recesses of the central spinal canal. The proliferative changes of the left facet joint (*arrow*) are causing severe stenosis of the left subarticular lateral recess. (From Physical Medicine and Rehabilitation: State-of-the-art Reviews, vol 4, no 2. Hanley & Belfus, 1990.)

turbed fetal development and may occur as one element of a congenital malformation of the lumbar spine. Developmental stenosis is a growth disturbance of the posterior elements, involving the pedicles, lamina, or articular processes, resulting in decreased volume of the spinal canal.[199] A true midline osseous sagittal diameter measuring less than 12 mm is considered as relative stenosis and a diameter of less than 10 mm is considered as absolute stenosis.[251] This diameter is measured from the middle of the posterior surface of the vertebral body to the point of junction of its spinous process and laminae. With relative stenosis, the reserve capacity of the spinal canal is reduced, thus predisposing the neural elements to impingement or compression by a small disc herniation or mild degenerative changes. Porter et al[185] reported that patients with a small spinal canal, detected with ultrasonography, do not have a greater prevalence of back pain, but if they do experience back pain, it will be of greater severity compared to patients with a normal-sized canal. Acquired stenosis is the narrowing of the central or intervertebral canals by degenerative changes of the discovertebral joints, facet joints, and ligamenta flava.[211,213,250]

In a prospective study, 60 patients with suspected lumbar disc herniations and/or spinal central stenosis were studied with first generation MRI, standard CT, and/or myelography, and the results were compared to the findings at surgery. The surgical diagnosis of stenosis agreed with MRI in 77% of the cases, CT in 79%, and myelography in 54%.[165] This study did not differentiate between central or intervertebral canal stenosis and the CT study did not include multiplanar reformations, which are extremely helpful in the evaluation of stenosis.[138,150] Schnebel et al[211] compared MRI with CT myelography in the diagnosis of spinal stenosis and demonstrated a 96.6% agreement between the two tests.

The importance of intervertebral foraminal stenosis as a cause of radicular symptoms[186] and its significance in failed back surgery has been well-documented.[37] Considering that all neural foramina in the spinal column have a vertical and horizontal dimension, as well as a length (up to 12 mm at the L5-S1 disc level), the foramen is truly a three-dimensional structure (i.e., a canal). Pathologic changes of any component of the foramen may impinge or compress the exiting nerve root. The foramen at the L5-S1 disc level is unique in its morphometry and due to its length, it may be stenotic at its entrance, mid, or exit zone. The most common etiology of stenosis at this level is an osteophytic ridge projecting off the inferior end-plate of L5 and, less commonly, the superior endplate of S1.[30,193] Degenerative changes of the facet joint or the anterior facet capsule may lead to decreased volume of the posterior and superior compartment of the foramen, potentially causing neural compression. Extraforaminal (far-out) stenosis[263] may also occur at the L5-S1 disc level in young patients with spondylolisthesis or elderly patients with disc degeneration and scoliosis.[90] The stenosis is secondary to the apposition of the base of the junction of the transverse process and pedicle of L5 to the adjacent sacral ala. In addition, osseous ridges may project off the lateral margin of the vertebral body endplates of L5 and S1 and may impinge the L5 nerve root in the paravertebral gutter (far-far out stenosis). The pathoanatomy of the intervertebral foramen can be assessed by both CT/MPR and MRI (Fig. 14–10).

Degenerative spondylolisthesis is an important cause of central canal stenosis and most frequently involves the L4–5 disc level.[148] Disc degeneration along with degenerative changes of sagittally oriented facet joints[209] predispose the motion segment to an anterolisthesis that rarely progresses beyond a Grade I slip due to the intact neural arch. The combination of hyperostotic ridges projecting off the anteromedial margin of the facet joints, hypertrophy of the ligamenta flava, annular redundancy, and an anterolisthesis can result in severe central canal and subarticular lateral recess stenosis. There is usually at least mild narrowing of the neural foramina in the cephalocaudal direction secondary to the decreased disc height and the anterolisthesis.

Both disc degeneration and spinal stenosis are frequently detected in patients with isthmic spondylolisthesis. The occurrence of disc herniation has been reported both at the spondylolytic level[233] and at the superjacent motion segment.[86,204] Foraminal stenosis at the L5-S1 disc level is also relatively common due to the decreased cephalocaudal dimension of the canal secondary to the anterolisthesis. This predisposes the L5 nerve root to dynamic impingement and entrapment by osseous ridges encroaching on the foramen.

Conclusions

Both CT/MPR and MRI are excellent noninvasive imaging studies to delineate pathomorphologic changes of the spinal motion segment. The transformation of the data from these examinations into useful clinical information necessitates precise correlation of the examination's results to the patient's clinical condition and any additional diagnostic tests (e.g., electromyographs) that have been performed. Proliferative osseous degenerative changes occur concurrently with disc degeneration and herniation. Therefore, it is necessary that all components of the spinal motion segment be completely evaluated in each patient presenting with back or leg pain in order to determine the pathoetiology of his or her symptomatology. A precise anatomic diagnosis is needed to provide a rational basis for therapeutic decisions. An important question that has not been resolved is which study, CT or MRI, should be ordered when additional information is needed in

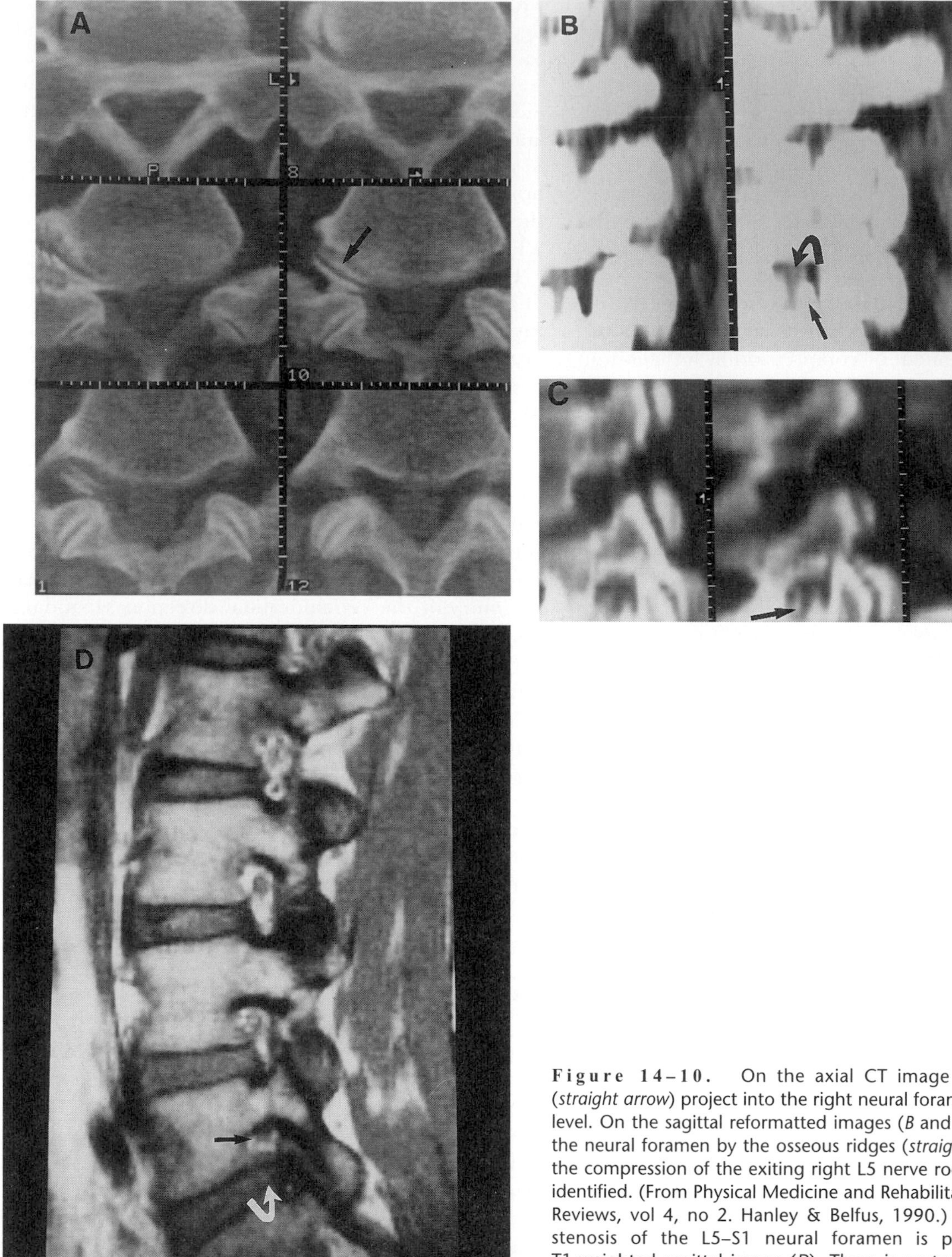

Figure 14–10. On the axial CT image (*A*), osseous ridges (*straight arrow*) project into the right neural foramen at the L5–S1 disc level. On the sagittal reformatted images (*B* and *C*), the narrowing of the neural foramen by the osseous ridges (*straight arrow*), along with the compression of the exiting right L5 nerve root (*curved arrow*), are identified. (From Physical Medicine and Rehabilitation: State-of-the-art Reviews, vol 4, no 2. Hanley & Belfus, 1990.) On another patient, stenosis of the L5–S1 neural foramen is present on the MRI T1-weighted sagittal image (*D*). There is protrusion of the disc and osteophytes into the neural foramen (*curved arrow*). A small amount of fat is present around the L5 nerve root (*straight arrow*).

the evaluation of a patient with spinal symptoms. Thornbury et al[237] reported on the relative efficacy of MRI, CT myelography, and plain CT to evaluate patients with acute LBP that clinically was suspected to be related to neural compression by a herniated disc. Ninety-five patients with acute low back and radicular pain underwent MRI and either CT (34%) or CT myelogram (66%). Patients were followed for at least 6 to 12 months. Fifty-six patients underwent surgery and 39 received conservative treatment. The results of the study demonstrated no statistically significant difference in the diagnostic accuracy of the three modalities to detect a herniated disc that was causing neural compression. The authors concluded that factors such as cost, radiation dose, and invasiveness should influence the selection of modality. They suggest that MRI should replace CT myelography, but that it should not replace plain CT because of the extra cost of the MRI study. In this study, the cost of a plain CT was $534, for a CT myelogram $1104, and for an MRI $1135. The recent marked decline in the cost of MRI studies would have a significant impact on the study's cost-benefit analysis. Although the design of the study was rigorous and well controlled, its results only apply to a narrow spectrum of patients presenting with a very specific clinical problem. Considering the high rate of surgery for the patients in the study (almost 60%), it is evident that they do not represent the spectrum of patients typically presenting with back or radicular pain (74% of the patients in this study were referred from a neurosurgical clinic). There is still a need to compare the three imaging modalities for the evaluation of back pain, tumor, trauma, arthritis, and infection prior to recommending which test is optimal in different clinical situations. The age range and symptoms of patients presenting for impairment evaluation are quite broad; therefore, the optimal imaging study must be able to detect a broad spectrum of pathologic conditions. Whichever technique is used, clinical correlation is essential to interpret correctly the significance of any findings.

SOFT TISSUE INJURIES

Injuries to the soft tissues of the body are probably the most frequent cause of musculoskeletal dysfunction. With the recent development and implementation of MRI, it is now possible to evaluate noninvasively all the soft tissue structures in the body (e.g., muscles, tendons, ligaments, and cartilage) that may be responsible for a patient's symptoms. Ultrasonography is also used to assess soft tissue disorders of the musculoskeletal system.[91,121] The major advantage of US is its availability, safety, and lower cost compared with MRI. It is limited to the evaluation of tissues that transmit sound waves; thus osseous structures or soft tissues shielded by osseous tissue cannot be evaluated. Compared with the other imaging modalities the efficacy of US is heavily dependent on the operator of the equipment, but this should not preclude its use in appropriate clinical situations. Considering its cost and availability, the role of US may grow as staff in more centers become proficient in its application. This is already true in many European countries where US is heavily used in the evaluation of musculoskeletal disorders.[12,176] The following sections present the role of radiologic imaging in the assessment of patients with musculoskeletal injuries.

MUSCLE INJURIES

Muscle Contusions and Tears

Muscle injuries may result from a direct or indirect application of force to the muscle. A direct blow to a muscle may cause a muscle contusion with disruption of muscle fibers. Acute disruption of muscle fibers and capillaries may precipitate soft tissue hemorrhage and a hematoma along with a secondary inflammatory response. With the acute pain associated with muscle injury, it may be difficult on a physical examination to determine the precise location, extent, and severity of an injury. Prior to the implementation of MRI, radiologic imaging studies were of little value in the evaluation of acute muscle injuries. On plain films there may be obscuration of the fat planes surrounding an injured muscle secondary to the perimuscular edema. With CT there may be an alteration of the size or contour of a muscle but detection of intramuscular hemorrhage, edema, or a hematoma is difficult. With the excellent soft tissue contrast resolution provided by MRI, it is now possible to obtain the following important clinical information related to a muscle injury: (1) the extent of muscle edema and/or hemorrhage; (2) if a focal hematoma is present, including its size and location; (3) the degree and extent of muscle fiber disruption; (4) if there is complete disruption of the muscle, whether there is associated muscle retraction; (5) whether there is interruption of the overlying fascia and if there is a muscle herniation; (6) the degree of muscle swelling and the detection of a possible concomitant compartment syndrome; and (7) whether single or multiple muscles are injured. Muscle contusions occur most frequently in the lower extremities, particularly involving the quadriceps mechanism.[207]

On an MRI examination, a muscle contusion is detected by abnormal signal intensity and morphology of the muscle. On spin-echo sequences, normal muscle demonstrates intermediate signal intensity on T1-weighted sequences and intermediate to low signal intensity on T2-weighted or short tau inversion recovery (STIR) sequences. In a contused muscle, the interstitial edema or hemorrhage will be detected as high signal intensity on T2-weighted sequences. Because hemorrhage infiltrates through the muscle, and mixes with the interstitial edema, it is not possible to separate it from the edematous muscle tissue. With a grade 1 contusion (i.e., microstructural fiber failure) there may be a slight increase in the size of the muscle and the margins of the muscle may have a feathery appearance due to the extension of interstitial edema into the perimuscular tissue.[54,156] Edematous changes in the adjacent subcutaneous fat are also frequently detected. With a grade 2 muscle contusion (i.e., partial tear) there will be a focus of disrupted muscle fibers in addition to the altered

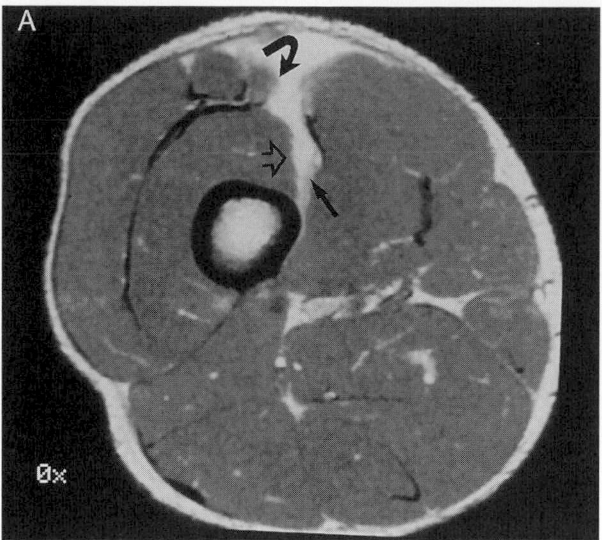

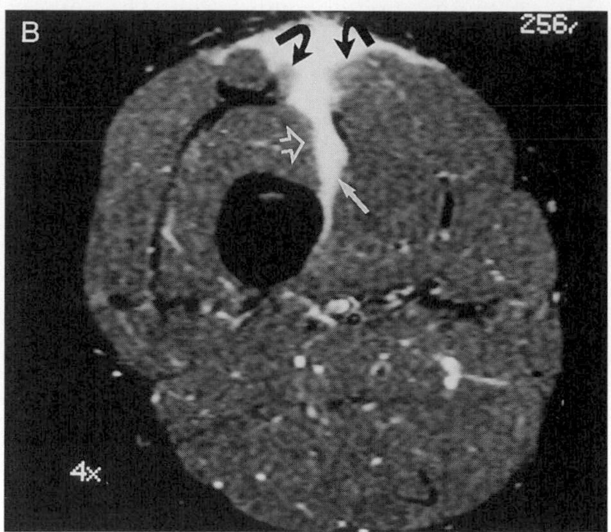

Figure 14–11. After a direct blow to the thigh, on the proton density weighted (*A*) and STIR (*B*) axial images, there is a tear of the quadriceps muscle involving both the vastus medialis (*curved arrows*) and the vastus intermedius (*open arrowheads*) muscles. Hemorrhage/edema (*straight arrow*) extends to the femur.

signal intensity from the interstitial edema and hemorrhage (Fig. 14–11). A grade 3 muscle contusion will appear similar to a grade 2 contusion, except there will be complete disruption of the muscle fibers. With a muscle hematoma, there will be a focal accumulation of blood within a muscle. A hematoma demonstrates intermediate or high signal intensity on a T1-weighted sequence, depending on the chemical composition of the hematoma, and high signal intensity on a T2-weighted sequence. The sequelae of a muscle contusion may include muscle atrophy, fibrosis, calcification, or ossification.

The role of plain films and CT in the evaluation of these potential complications has focused mainly on the detection of muscle calcification or ossification. Myositis ossificans is a benign ossifying soft tissue mass typically located within skeletal muscle. A history of prior trauma is present in approximately 50% of cases; frequently the episode of trauma is of a minor degree. Plain radiographs show faint calcification within the muscle from 2 to 6 weeks after the onset of symptoms and a well-circumscribed osseous mass in approximately 6 to 8 weeks. The lesion will then mature over the next 6 months and become smaller. In the early stages of the lesion, prior to bony maturation, the margins of the ossified mass may be poorly defined on plain films. If there is a history of only a minor injury or no trauma, the possibility of a soft tissue malignancy (e.g., osteosarcoma) is sometimes entertained after obtaining the plain films. If a CT scan is obtained at 4 to 6 weeks, it will demonstrate a rim of mineralization surrounding a central area of decreased attenuation. On an MRI examination, the characteristics of myositis ossificans are highly dependent on the age of lesion. On a T2-weighted sequence, an early lesion usually has well-defined margins and inhomogeneous intermediate to high signal intensity within the lesion. Perilesional edema is also identified with an acute lesion. As the lesion matures, it will develop a rim of mature bone.[133] Mature lesions are well defined with inhomogeneous signal intensity similar to fat. The most important finding on all of these imaging modalities is that the areas of ossification are most mature at the periphery of the lesion and the central core contains the immature cellular components. This is in contrast to a soft tissue osteosarcoma that is most mature centrally and immature peripherally. A few months of watchful waiting will demonstrate the normal maturation of myositis ossificans.

Muscle Strains

Muscle strains are probably the most common type of injury to the myotendinous unit (MTU). A muscle strain is an acute stretch-induced injury secondary to excessive indirect force generated by eccentric muscular contraction. Muscle strains may occur anywhere in the body, but the most frequent muscles involved are the quadriceps femoris, biceps femoris, semimembranosus, semitendinosus, and gastrocnemius-soleus complex. Muscles that cross two joints and have a high proportion of fast twitch fibers are more prone to muscle strains. Muscle strains may also involve the muscles stabilizing the hip, shoulder, and elbow joints. The pain elicited from an acute muscle strain is typically experienced during an athletic activity or immediately at its termination.[171] The pathologic changes in an acutely strained muscle include disruption of the muscle fibers near the myotendinous junction along with edema and hemorrhage. The grade of a muscle strain depends on the degree of fiber disruption and the clinical findings.

The appearance of a grade 1 muscle strain on MRI is similar to the findings of a grade 1 muscle contusion. There may be enlargement of the muscle due to interstitial edema and hemorrhage and, on a spin-echo T2-weighted or STIR sequence, there will be increased signal intensity within the muscle (Fig. 14–12). Muscle strains are frequently located near the muscle's myotendinous junction. The tendon of a multipennate muscle extends into the muscle belly; therefore, the symptoms elicited by a strain may be located anywhere within a muscle and not merely at its ends. MRI has provided excellent documentation of the extent and position of these injuries. Fleckenstein et al[69] reported on the MRI appearance of the natural history of acute muscle strains. Acutely, the abnormal signal intensity was identified throughout the muscle, but on follow-up studies the abnormal signal intensity was most prominent in the periphery of the muscle. In one patient there was persistent abnormal signal intensity within the muscle after complete resolution of symptoms.

A grade 2 muscle strain manifests clinically as muscle pain associated with a loss of strength. Pathologically there is a macroscopic partial tear of the MTU. On an MRI study, there will be a partial tear of the muscle fibers associated with edema and/or hemorrhage. With a grade 3 strain there is a complete disruption of the MTU. Plain films provide little useful information in the evaluation of most muscle strains. Only if there is a grade 3 strain that results in gross instability or malalignment (e.g., a quadriceps rupture) will plain films be helpful. CT has also been used to evaluate muscular strain injuries, but it provides less useful clinical information compared to an MRI examination.[224]

In addition to the evaluation of acute or delayed muscle injuries, MRI is an ideal imaging modality to follow the evolution of the inflammatory and reparative processes within a muscle. With MRI it is possible to detect any sequelae from a MTU injury (e.g., muscle atrophy or fibrosis).[85] Clinically it can be extremely difficult to determine when a muscle has completely healed, and if an athlete or worker returns to his or her athletic activity or job too soon after injury, he or she may be predisposed to repeat injury. MRI has detected acute MTU injuries that were superimposed on subacute or chronic injuries that may have predisposed the muscle to reinjury.

Compartment Syndromes

Another recent application of MRI in the assessment of muscle injury is in the evaluation of patients for the possibility of acute or chronic compartment syndromes. An acute compartment syndrome developing after a fracture may be secondary to an accumulation of blood or interstitial edema in a closed fascial compartment. Acute compartment syndromes most frequently involve the lower extremity, but MRI may be of benefit in demonstrating pathologic changes in any muscle. In a patient with an acute paraspinal lumbar compartment syn-

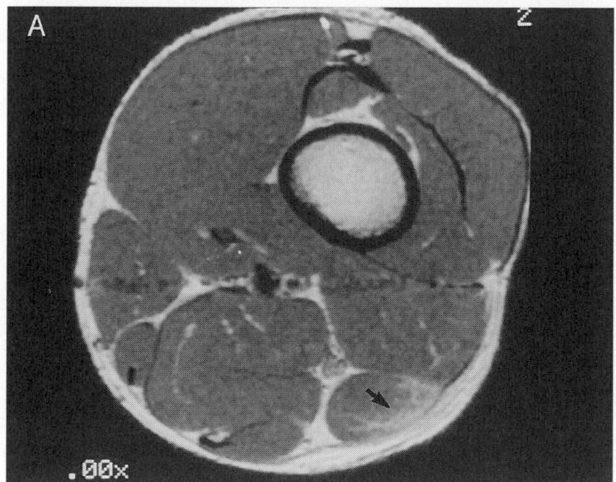

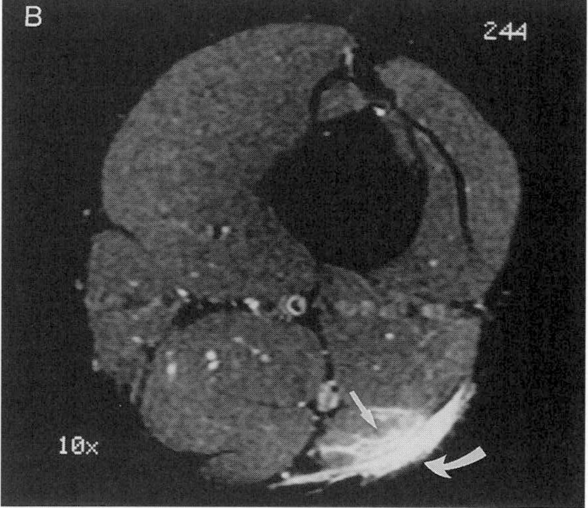

Figure 14–12. While exercising, a patient experienced the acute onset of pain in the region of the hamstring muscles. On the MRI study obtained after injury, on the T1-weighted axial image (*A*), there is a subtle increased signal intensity within the periphery of the biceps femoris muscle (*straight arrow*), which is much easier to detect on the axial STIR image (*B*). On the STIR image the edematous changes in the muscle (*straight arrow*) and in the subcutaneous tissue (*curved arrow*) are delineated.

drome, an MRI study demonstrated increased signal intensity in the symptomatic paraspinal muscles that also had abnormal intracompartmental pressures.[59] Resolution of the abnormal signal intensity paralleled the improvement of the patient's symptoms. MRI has also been used in the evaluation of patients with chronic compartment syndromes. Amendola et al[5] demonstrated that in five patients with a positive clinical history for chronic compartment syndromes and who also had elevated postexercise pressures, four demonstrated abnormal MRI signal intensity within the muscle. Patients who were initially thought to have a chronic compartment syndrome, but whose pressure measurements were normal, also had a normal MRI examination.

Conclusions

Although MRI is extremely sensitive in detecting pathologic changes within a muscle due to accumulation of fluid, it lacks specificity. Any pathologic process that incites an inflammatory response or increases muscle hydration will present with abnormal signal intensity. Other muscular conditions that may appear similar to muscle injury on MRI include metabolic myopathies,[113] dermatomyositis,[98,182] diabetic muscular infarction,[172] vasculitis, viral myositis,[97] sarcoid myopathy,[135] and acute rhabdomyolysis.[220] Fibromyalgia, however, presents with a normal MRI.[134] Even a benign procedure such as an intramuscular injection can be detected on an MRI examination as a focus of abnormal signal intensity in the muscle and perifascial tissue.[196] It is quite apparent that the clinical significance of any abnormal finding on an MRI examination can only be determined by close correlation with the patient's history and physical examination. The value of a negative MRI may also be important in reaching an accurate diagnosis or directing treatment.

TENDON INJURIES

The function of a tendon is to transmit the force from its muscle of origin to the bone where it inserts. Tendons are stressed by muscle contractions and the highest stress on a tendon is generated with eccentric muscle contractions. Excessive acute or chronic stress on a tendon may precipitate fiber disruption and induce pain. Disruption of a tendon may occur anywhere along its length. Avulsion of a tendon from its bony insertion may or may not be associated with a bony avulsion.

There have been a variety of terms used to describe tendon injuries. To classify tendon injuries it is necessary to know whether an injury is related to an acute traumatic event or to chronic overload. The duration of a patient's symptoms must also be considered. An acute injury to a tendon may precipitate fiber failure (i.e., a strain) that is classified as grades 1 to 3 depending on the degree of fiber disruption. Although the term tendinitis is frequently used when a patient has pain related to a tendon or to the peritendinous tissue, only an injury that acutely precipitates failure of tendon fibers along with disruption of vascularized peritendinous connective tissue can produce an acute inflammatory response in a tendon (i.e., tendinitis).[139] Tendinitis may be acute, subacute, or chronic depending on the duration of a patient's symptoms. If an acute injury incites an inflammatory response only in the soft tissue surrounding a tendon (e.g., the peritendon or the paratenon) without disruption of the tendon fibers, then the terms peritendinitis or paratenonitis are the more appropriate to describe a patient's symptomatology.[139,188]

Chronic microtrauma to a tendon, frequently secondary to chronic eccentric overload, may precipitate intrasubstance fiber failure. There is typically no history of an acute injury and the symptoms have an insidious onset. The chronic pathologic changes identified within the substance of a chronically overloaded tendon include fibrillar degeneration, angiofibroblastic proliferation, fiber necrosis with myxoid and hyaline degeneration, fibrosis, and occasionally chronic inflammation.[194] The term tendinosis has been employed to describe these chronic pathologic changes.[144] Tendinosis may represent an abortive healing response of a tendon from chronic overload. It is possible to have changes of tendinitis or peritendinitis superimposed on changes of tendinosis.

A normal tendon is composed predominantly of collagen fibers and it appears as a structure with minimal or no signal intensity on MRI spin-echo or STIR sequences. It is necessary to understand the spectrum of the appearance of normal tendons with MRI prior to attempting to diagnose pathologic changes.[120,272] Certain tendons (e.g., the posterior tibial tendon[62,214] and the rotator cuff[160]) will demonstrate increased signal intensity within normal segments of the tendon. This may be related to the orientation of a tendon with respect to the direction of the magnetic field used for MR imaging.

With peritendinitis, pathologically there will be increased fluid in the peritendinous tissue secondary to an inflammatory process. This will be detected on an MRI spin-echo T2-weighted or STIR sequence as a focus of high signal intensity surrounding a normal tendon. With tendinosis, a focus of myxoid degeneration or angioblastic proliferation within the substance of a tendon will generate increased signal intensity within the tendon on a spin-echo T1-weighted or STIR sequence. On a T2-weighted sequence, the abnormal signal intensity may persist, but usually not as brightly as it was on the T1-weighted sequence. The signal intensity within a degenerated tendon frequently appears normal on a T2-weighted sequence. Persistent high-signal intensity on a T2-weighted or STIR sequence may be seen if there is inflammatory or degenerative tissue within a tendon. A high-grade partial tear of a tendon provides a mechanism whereby fluid or inflammatory tissue can extend into the substance of a tendon. STIR or other fat suppression sequences have been particularly useful to evaluate tendon disruptions.

In addition to the abnormal signal intensity identified within inflamed or degenerated tendons, altered morphology is also frequently identified (e.g., hypertrophy or attenuation of a tendon). A grading system of disorders of the posterior tibialis tendon has been reported.[214] A hypertrophied tendon containing abnormal signal intensity has been classified as grade 1 degeneration or partial tear, an attenuated tendon containing abnormal signal intensity as grade 2 degeneration or partial tear, and a complete tear of the tendon is classified as grade 3.

With the direct multiplanar capabilities of MRI, it is possible to evaluate the condition of any tendon in the body. MRI provides a very sensitive test to detect tendon disorders, but unfortunately it lacks specificity. It is not possible on an MRI study to determine whether a focus of abnormal high signal intensity within a tendon is secondary to acute inflammation or chronic degeneration. If abnormal tendon morphology is also detected (e.g., with an acute partial tendon tear), then it may be inferred that some of the abnormal signal intensity is secondary to an acute inflammatory process. But these acute changes may be superimposed on chronic degenerative changes of a tendon. For this reason, the term tendinopathy (i.e., a pathologic condition of a tendon) is probably more appropriate in describing an abnormal tendon detected on an MRI study that demonstrates abnormal signal intensity and is not partially or completely torn. In the assessment of the abnormal signal intensity surrounding a tendon, it is also not possible to determine whether the altered tissue hydration is associated with an inflammatory infiltrate. Therefore, these edematous changes should be described, but not considered as proof for the presence of an inflammatory response.

MRI has had a major impact in the advancement of our understanding of the natural history of tendon failure. With MRI it is possible to detect subclinical injuries (e.g., pathologic changes in a tendon resulting from chronic microtrauma or aging). These injuries by definition do not incite symptoms, but they may predispose a tendon to future dysfunction or failure. When the tendons of patients with acute complete tendon rupture are studied histologically, changes of chronic tendon degeneration are usually demonstrated adjacent to the area of an acute rupture. Even a great percentage of nonruptured tendons in healthy individuals demonstrate pathologic changes of chronic degeneration.[119] These abnormalities can be detected with MRI by the demonstration of abnormal signal intensity or altered morphology of a tendon. These abnormal foci detected on an MRI study are not false-positive findings because they represent true pathologic changes in the tendon that do not evoke symptoms. The detection of subclinical tendon injury or degeneration may provide important information with respect to changing training or rehabilitative techniques or to job-related activities that may be overloading a tendon.

The location of tendon degeneration and/or tear depends on the etiology of fiber failure. An acute tendon rupture may occur at the myotendinous junction, within the main segment of the tendon, or at the tendon insertion site (Fig. 14–13). The nature of the force, the position of the joint at the time of injury, and with any predisposing factors that may have weakened the tendon, will all affect the site of rupture. If failure is secondary to extrinsic impingement (e.g., by a degenerative osseous ridge), the location of the tendon failure will occur where the tendon impinges against this

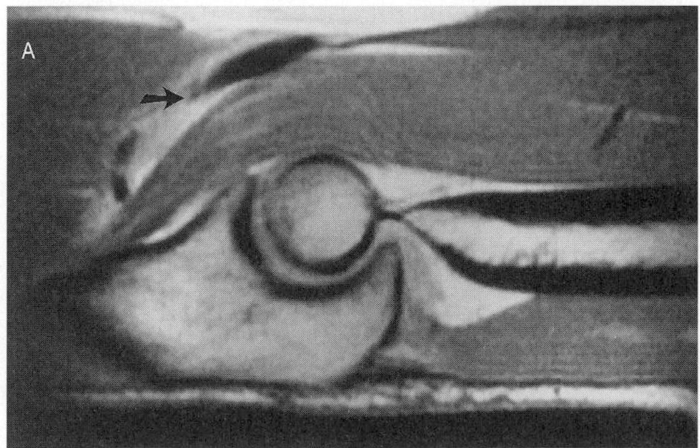

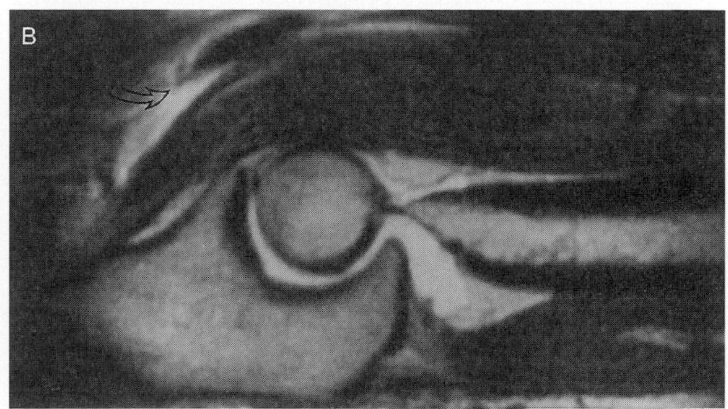

Figure 14–13. On the MRI evaluation of a patient who fell on an outstretched arm, there is a complete tear of the biceps tendon (*arrow*) on the proton density (*A*) and T2-weighted (*B*) images. (From Magn Reson Q 9, 1993.)

extrinsic structure. Chronic overload injuries to a tendon, frequently secondary to eccentric muscle contraction, may cause microstructural damage within the substance of a tendon at its insertion site (e.g., the quadriceps, patellar, or posterior tibial tendons). Extrinsic impingement or intrinsic overload of a tendon may be amplified if there is also instability of a joint that precipitates external friction or increased tension of a tendon when the MTU is active. With MRI it is possible to determine the exact location and extent of an injury to a tendon. Equally important, an MRI examination provides a comprehensive evaluation of all the peritendinous structures that may impinge a tendon and precipitate failure. US has been extensively used in the evaluation of tendon degeneration or tears,[117,153] but provides little or no information about the status of a tendon where it is located beneath an osseous structure. It also has limited use in defining abnormal osseous structures that may cause extrinsic impingement of a tendon. US is most valuable in the assessment of a superficially located tendon (e.g., the Achilles[115,116] or patellar tendon).

Chronic intrinsic overload of a tendon is probably the most frequent cause of fiber failure and tendon degeneration in a young or middle-aged individual with tendon dysfunction. Lateral epicondylitis and medial tendinosis are discussed in Chapter 17.

Achilles Tendon

Dysfunction of the Achilles tendon is a frequent cause of debilitating ankle pain. There is no tenosynovial sheath surrounding the Achilles tendon; therefore, if acute pain is associated with inflammation in the peritendinous soft tissues, it involves the paratenon or peritendon. MRI has proven to be very useful in the evaluation of patients with refractory Achilles pain or an acute rupture. Intrasubstance partial tears or degeneration of a tendon are detected as foci of increased signal intensity on spin-echo and STIR sequences due to the increased hydration of the pathologic tissue. Thickening of the tendon is also usually detected. With a partial tear that interrupts the peripheral fibers of the tendon, or with a complete tear, focal fiber disruption is identified (Fig. 14–14). The MRI examination can be performed with the patient's foot in both dorsiflexion and plantar flexion to assess the size of the gap between the ends of a torn tendon. Weinstabl et al[258] reported on 28 patients with suspected tendon injury. Of the 13 patients who required operative treatment, all partial and complete tears detected at surgery were correctly diagnosed on an MRI study. Ultrasonography was also performed on 10 of the 28 patients; 1 patient with a partial rupture at surgery had a false-negative US. Kalebo et al[116] recently reported on the diagnostic value of ultrasonography in the assessment of patients with partial ruptures of the Achilles tendon. The overall sensitivity for US was 0.94, the specificity was 1.00, and the accuracy was 0.95 in this highly selected group of patients. The authors concluded that the advantages of US are its availability, low cost, and real-time imaging capabilities compared to MRI studies.

Patellar Tendon

Like the Achilles tendon, the patellar tendon is prone to chronic overload injuries.[65] Both US and MRI have been used to evaluate the pathologic changes within the tendon in symptomatic patients. Even though pain and dysfunction of the patellar tendon is usually referred to as patellar tendinitis, pathologic changes detected within the tendon frequently demonstrate changes of fiber disruption, chronic myxoid degeneration, and focal fibrinoid necrosis.[28] If a patient does not respond to conservative care, an imaging study is frequently ordered to corroborate the presumptive clinical diagnosis and to assist in preoperative planning. With MRI it is possible to determine the exact location and extent of the pathologic changes within the patellar tendon (Fig. 14–15).[216] It is difficult to determine the true accuracy or efficacy of US, MRI, or CT, particularly in the detection of small lesions of the patellar tendon. If only large lesions are refractory to conservative therapy, then the detection of small lesions may not be important, but this will have to be proven with a long-term prospective study.

Rotator Cuff

The rotator cuff is one of the largest tendinous structures in the body and, because of its functional demands, it is prone to degeneration and failure. The two primary mechanisms of injury to the cuff are extrinsic primary impingement and intrinsic chronic overload. The impingement syndrome presents as painful dysfunction of the shoulder, particularly with overhead activities. The pain is precipitated by entrapment or abrasion of the rotator cuff mechanism (i.e., the rotator cuff and the peritendinous soft tissue) under a degenerated acromioclavicular (AC) joint or under the coracoacromial arch (i.e., the arch formed by the coracoid process, the coracoacromial [CA] ligament, and the acromion). In the supraspinatus outlet, the rotator cuff mechanism may impinge against a thickened CA ligament, an enthesophyte projecting off the anteroinferior margin of the acromion at the insertion of the CA ligament, or against a curved or hooked acromion. Repetitive abrasion of the rotator cuff mechanism can precipitate bursal inflammation, peritendinous inflammation, or tendon degeneration.[217] Fiber disruption secondary to cuff abrasion will be associated with edema and/or hemorrhage in the cuff and the peritendinous tissues. With MRI it is possible to define precisely the anatomy of the AC joint and the supraspinatus outlet and to detect any evidence of a degenerative process affecting these structures (Fig. 14–16). It is possible to define the location where the cuff may be impinging against areas of bony proliferation or ligamentous hypertrophy. It is also possible to detect evidence of bursal inflammation. Impingement (i.e., to push against) is a physical phenomenon and can be detected by an MRI examination; but the diagnosis of an impingement syndrome, which is a painful symptom complex secondary to the repetitive abrasion and inflammation of the cuff and/or the peritendinous tissue resulting from impingement, can only be made clinically. With continued injury to a cuff, a focal partial tear or full thickness cuff tear may develop. In young patients, degenerative changes of the AC joint or the acromion are rarely present. Cuff failure is more likely to be secondary to intrinsic overload of the cuff and fatigue failure of the tendon fibers. With the decreased tensile strength of the cuff, further stress may precipitate a partial or full-thickness tear. If biomechanical imbalance results from a torn rotator cuff, or is present secondary to primary shoulder instability, secondary impingement of the cuff may also be present and elicit symptoms.

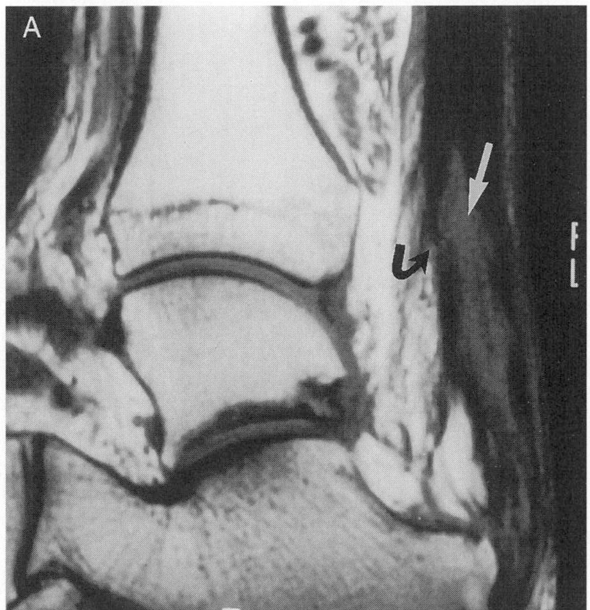

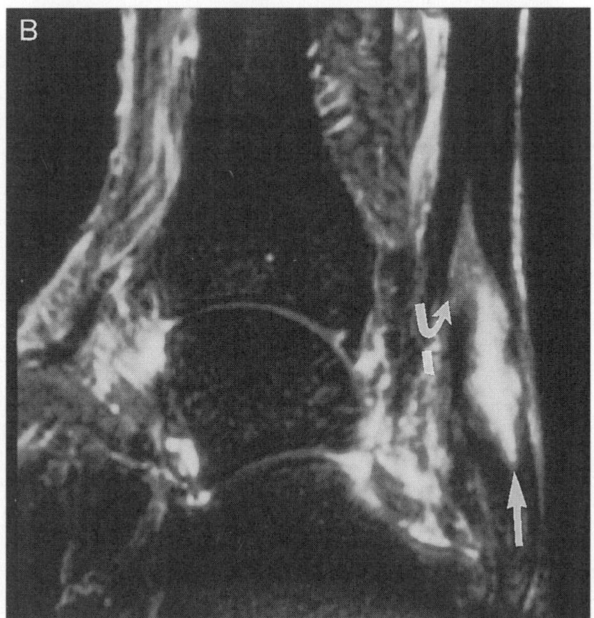

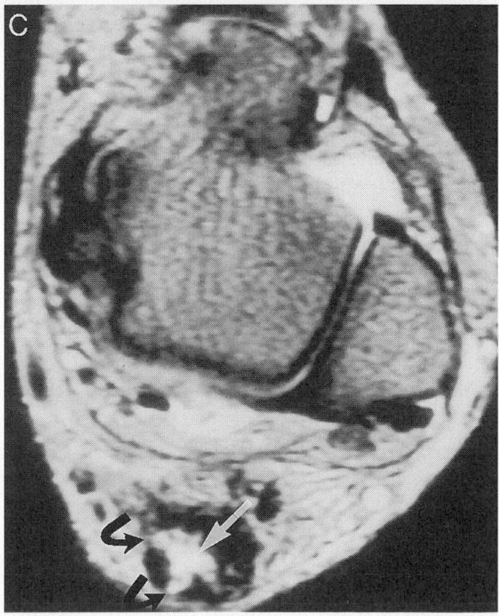

Figure 14–14. During exercising, a runner developed acute pain over the Achilles tendon in an area where he had previously experienced mild chronic pain. On the T1-weighted (*A*) and STIR (*B*) sagittal images and on the T1-weighted (*C*) axial image, there is diffuse thickening of the tendon along with a long tubular focus of intratendinous high signal intensity (*straight arrow*). A partial tear of the peripheral margins of the tendon is also identified (*curved arrows*).

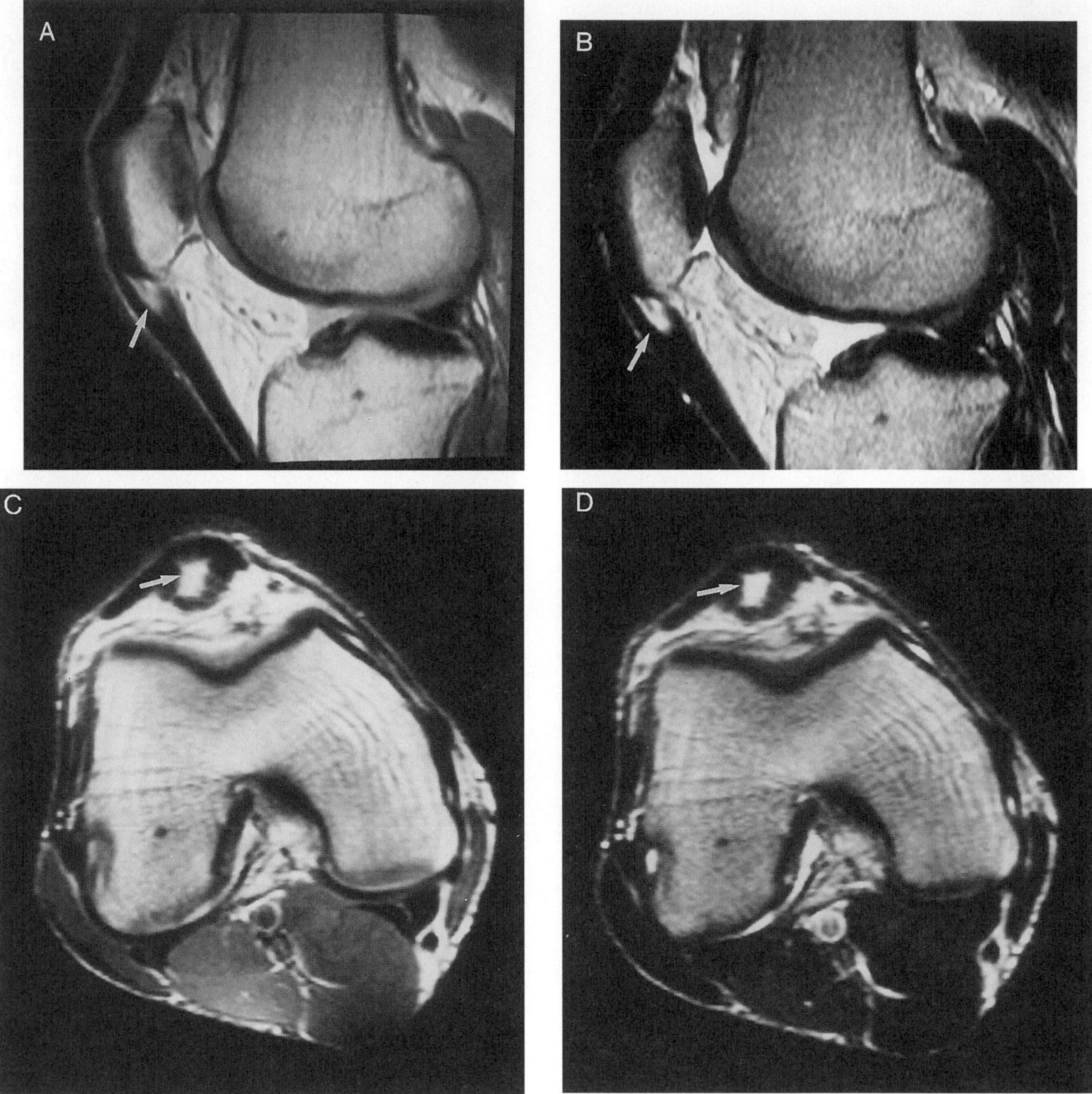

Figure 14–15. A patient was experiencing chronic pain over the patellar tendon. On the MRI evaluation, on the proton density (*A*) and T2-weighted (*B*) sagittal images, and on the proton density (*C*) and T2-weighted (*D*) axial images, there is hypertrophy along with a focal area of high signal intensity in the center of the proximal segment of the tendon at its insertion site (*arrow*). At the time of tendon repair, tissue histology revealed chronic degenerative changes within the tendon at this location.

Imaging studies of the rotator cuff are frequently obtained after an unsuccessful trial of conservative therapy for a rotator cuff impingement or tear. Prior to the development of US and MRI, plain films were the primary diagnostic imaging tool to evaluate the shoulder for rotator cuff dysfunction. Although plain films are helpful in the evaluation of osseous anatomy and pathology, they provide no direct and only limited indirect evidence of rotator cuff pathology. The best indicator for a torn rotator cuff on plain films is when the distance between the humeral head and the acromion is less than 6 mm on an AP view of the shoulder with the arm in neutral rotation.[257] Unfortunately this is a very late finding in the natural history of cuff degeneration and when it is present, there is usually a very large or massive tear of the cuff. The supraspinatus outlet view has recently been implemented to assess the shape of the acromion. Because a plain film is a two-dimensional projection of a three-dimensional structure, it is frequently difficult to determine the true shape of the acromion. Interobserver variability is also a problem with the interpretation of this projection. Special views

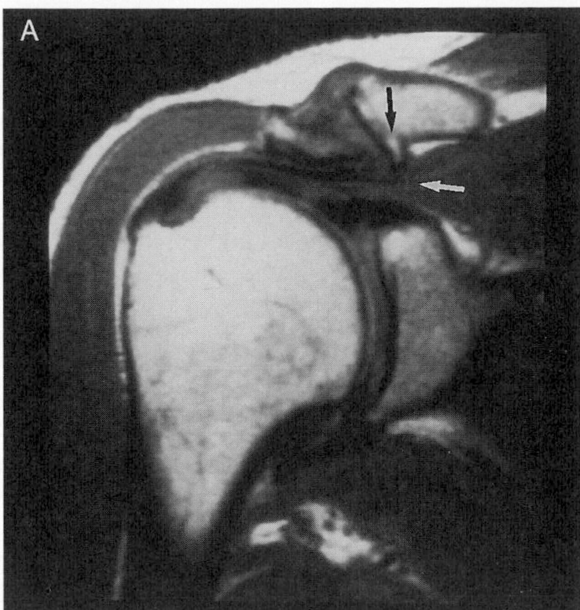

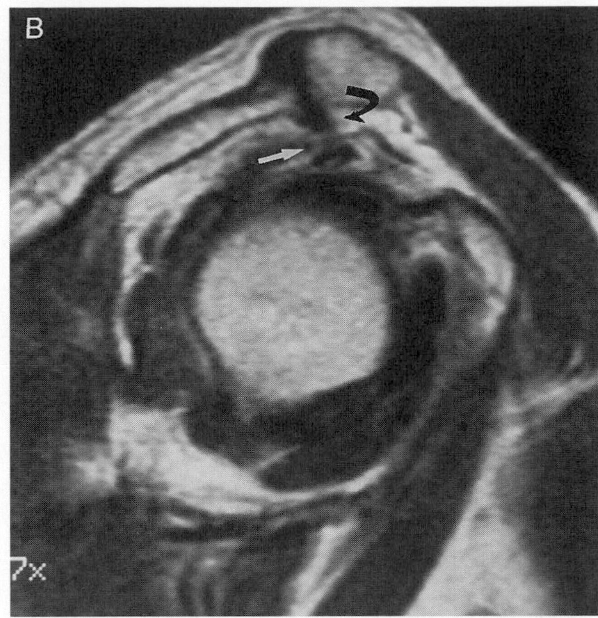

Figure 14–16. On the MRI examination of a patient experiencing shoulder pain with overhead activity, on the proton density weighted oblique coronal (*A*) and oblique sagittal (*B*) images, degenerative changes of the AC joint are identified with an osseous ridge projection off the inferior margin of the head of the clavicle (*straight black arrow*) and the inferior surface of the acromion (*curved black arrow*). The supraspinatus myotendinous junction is impinged by the osteophytes (*white arrow*).

have also been developed to detect osseous ridges projecting off the anteroinferior margin of the acromion.[177]

The integrity of the rotator cuff can be assessed by arthrography, which is an invasive procedure. After the instillation of contrast into the shoulder joint, one may detect full-thickness cuff tears by the leakage of contrast. The sensitivity of arthrography to detect full-thickness tears measuring over 1 cm is probably over 90%, but the study is less sensitive in detecting small full-thickness tears or partial tears of the articular surface of the cuff. It is insensitive in the detection of partial tears on the bursal side of the cuff that may result from extrinsic impingement. Arthrography provides little information on the status of the cuff fibers (e.g., evidence of degeneration or attrition) and provides no information on the assessment of the CA arch and the supraspinatus outlet. The detection of a full-thickness cuff tear may occur in asymptomatic elderly patients and in asymptomatic individuals who have undergone a surgical repair of the cuff. Calvert et al[39] performed arthrography on 20 patients after rotator cuff repair and demonstrated leakage of contrast indicating a full-thickness cuff tear in 18 of the patients. Seventeen of the 18 patients were asymptomatic at the time of arthrography.

US and MRI are noninvasive tests performed to evaluate the rotator cuff and the surrounding soft tissue structures. One advantage of US is the capacity to study the cuff with the arm in different positions. This may be particularly useful in the evaluation of patients with shoulder impingement syndrome.[63] There have been several reports on the value of US to detect tears of the rotator cuff.[33,147,260] Weiner et al[260] reported on a group of 225 patients who had preoperative sonography and compared the results of US to the surgical findings. The abnormalities detected on the US included partial and full-thickness cuff tears. US findings were surgically confirmed in 92% of the cases. Misamore et al[161] recently reported a prospective study of 32 patients who had degeneration of the rotator cuff and who required surgery. Preoperatively US and arthrography were both performed. Of the 20 patients who had a full-thickness tear, arthrography detected 100% and US detected 35%. Of the 7 patients with a partial-thickness tear, arthrography was accurate in 3, and US in 2 of the cases. Arthrography was accurate in all 5 patients who did not have a tear and US was accurate in 3 of the cases. Both studies had methodologic problems, which introduced potential sources of bias. It appears from the reports in the literature that in some centers US provides useful information for a certain subset of patients. The efficacy of US cannot be deduced from these studies as to its application as a screening examination for rotator cuff disorders.

MRI is the optimal imaging modality to provide a comprehensive evaluation of the shoulder in a patient with shoulder dysfunction. The strengths of MRI are its direct multiplanar capabilities, excellent soft tissue contrast resolution, and ability to evaluate completely both the normal and abnormal osseous architecture of the shoulder girdle. Whereas US has received criticism for its operator dependence, the efficacy of MRI in the assessment of the shoulder is highly dependent on the imaging protocols employed and the expertise of the radiologist interpreting the study. Like all structures in the body, there is a spectrum in the appearance of normal anatomy that must be appreciated.[160,170] The pathoetiology of abnormalities detected on an MRI study can only be determined by precisely comparing the findings on an MRI study to those detected at arthroscopy, arthrotomy, or to tissue histology obtained from cadavers.

The appearance of a normal rotator cuff is similar to that of other tendons in the body. With its high collagen content, it demonstrates minimal signal intensity on spin-echo or STIR sequences. Abnormalities of the rotator cuff are detected by altered cuff morphology along with abnormal signal intensity. Complete assessment of the soft tissues and osseous structures surrounding the cuff is mandatory in order to achieve a comprehensive evaluation of a shoulder. Imaging of the shoulder in three orthogonal planes should be performed on all patients. The axis of the different scan planes is determined by the orientation of the supraspinatus tendon and the scapula. The coronal sequence is oriented parallel to the long axis of the body of the scapula and the supraspinatus tendon. The sagittal sequence is oriented perpendicular to the coronal sequence. Both the coronal and sagittal sequences are oriented obliquely to the coronal and sagittal planes of the body due to the normal rotation of the scapula on the chest wall. Therefore, these sequences are referred to as oblique coronal or oblique sagittal sequences. The axial sequence is oriented perpendicular to the face of the glenoid, and depending on the degree of scapular rotation, it may be necessary to perform an oblique axial sequence with respect to the horizontal plane of the body. Spin-echo T1- and T2-weighted sequences are standard for the evaluation of the shoulder, and additional sequences (e.g., gradient-echo or STIR) may be performed to provide supplemental information.

With a partial tear of the rotator cuff on an MRI study, there will be a focal area of fiber disruption on the bursal or articular surface of the cuff or within the substance of the cuff. With a full-thickness cuff tear, there will be complete discontinuity of the cuff fibers (Fig. 14–17). Spin-echo T2-weighted sequences are optimal to diagnose partial- or full-thickness tears by the detection of fluid in the cuff defect. Optimally, to diagnose a full-thickness cuff tear, fluid should be detected extending from the articular to the bursal surface of the cuff along with the presence of fluid in the adjacent subdeltoid bursa. Unfortunately, this is not always detected with a full-thickness tear, particularly when a tear is chronic and has generated a fibrous reaction in the peritendinous tissue. In these cases, assessment of cuff morphology or the detection of cuff retraction may provide the necessary information to reach an accurate diagnosis. With a complete evaluation of a cuff tear in at least two imaging planes, it is possible to accurately measure the size and location of a tear. In some reported series the size of a cuff tear appears to have prognostic significance as to which patients will be improved by operative intervention. Full-thickness cuff tears usually first involve the supraspinatus segment of the cuff posterior to the rotator interval. Isolated full-thickness tears of the subscapularis segment of a cuff may be difficult to detect clinically, but MRI provides an excellent means to detect these tears.[77] With MRI it is also possible to determine the degree of cuff retraction and whether there is associated atrophy of the rotator cuff musculature. The status of the rotator cuff musculature may be important in the type of postoperative rehabilitation selected for a patient. The size of recurrent cuff tears also appears to be related to the degree of a patient's dysfunction.[92] The same MRI evaluation performed preoperatively can be employed in the postoperative evaluation of the cuff.

Iannotti et al[110] reported on the efficacy of MRI of the shoulder in the evaluation of 91 patients who required an operative procedure for shoulder dysfunction and for 15 asymptomatic volunteers. In the detection of a complete cuff tear, MRI was 100% sensitive and 95% specific. Tendinitis was defined arthroscopically as an area of hyperemia on the undersurface of the cuff or as a thickening of the subacromial bursa. Degeneration or partial tear of the cuff was defined arthroscopically as fraying or fibrillation of the cuff. For the differentiation between cuff tendinitis and degeneration, the sensitivity of MRI was 82% and the specificity was 85%. In differentiating a normal tendon from one showing signs of impingement, the sensitivity of MRI was 93% and specificity 87%. The authors concluded that high-resolution MRI is an excellent noninvasive tool in the diagnosis of disorders of the rotator cuff mechanism. Both the administration and interpretation of the MRI examinations in the study were performed by musculoskeletal radiologists with extensive experience with MRI. In addition to this study, there have been several other reports on the high accuracy of MRI to detect fill-thickness cuff tears.[64,103,190,240]

The sensitivity of MRI to detect partial cuff tears is considerably lower than its detection rate for full-thickness tears. In two studies that compared MRI to the findings at arthroscopy, Traughber et al[240] reported that 4 of 9 partial tears were not detected on an MRI study, and Hodler et al[103] reported that only 1 of 13 partial tears was detected on an MRI study. Holder et al[103] also performed MR arthrography on these patients and 6 of the partial tears were detected. Both Palmer et al[181] and Karzel et al[123] have recently reported on the improved detection rate of MR arthrography compared to standard MRI to detect partial- and full-thickness rotator cuff tears. Because MR arthrography is a more invasive, costly, and time-consuming examination compared to a standard MRI study, its efficacy will have to be proven in well-designed prospective studies before it can be recommended.

LIGAMENT INJURIES

The most common ligament sprain involves the lateral ligamentous complex of the ankle (i.e., the anterior and posterior talofibular ligaments and the calcaneofibular

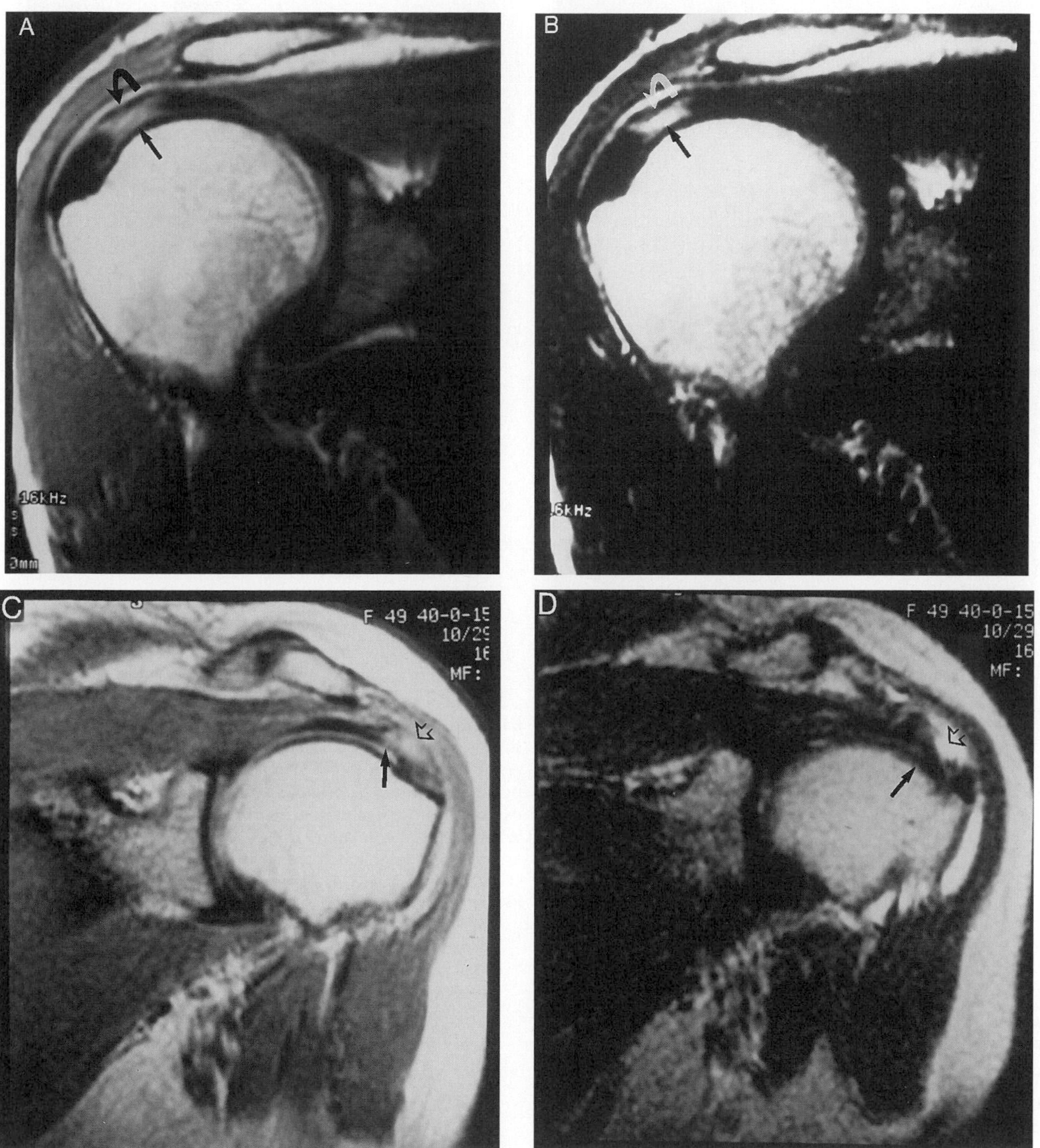

Figure 14–17. A partial tear of the rotator cuff is identified on the MRI proton density (*A*) and T2-weighted (*B*) oblique coronal images. There is discontinuity of the articular surface of the cuff (*straight arrow*) but not the bursal side of the cuff (*curved arrow*). On the MRI study performed on another patient with chronic shoulder pain there is a partial tear of the bursal surface of the cuff (*open arrowhead*) on the proton density (*C*) and T2-weighted (*D*) oblique coronal images. The articular surface of the cuff is intact (*straight arrow*). *Figure continues on following page*

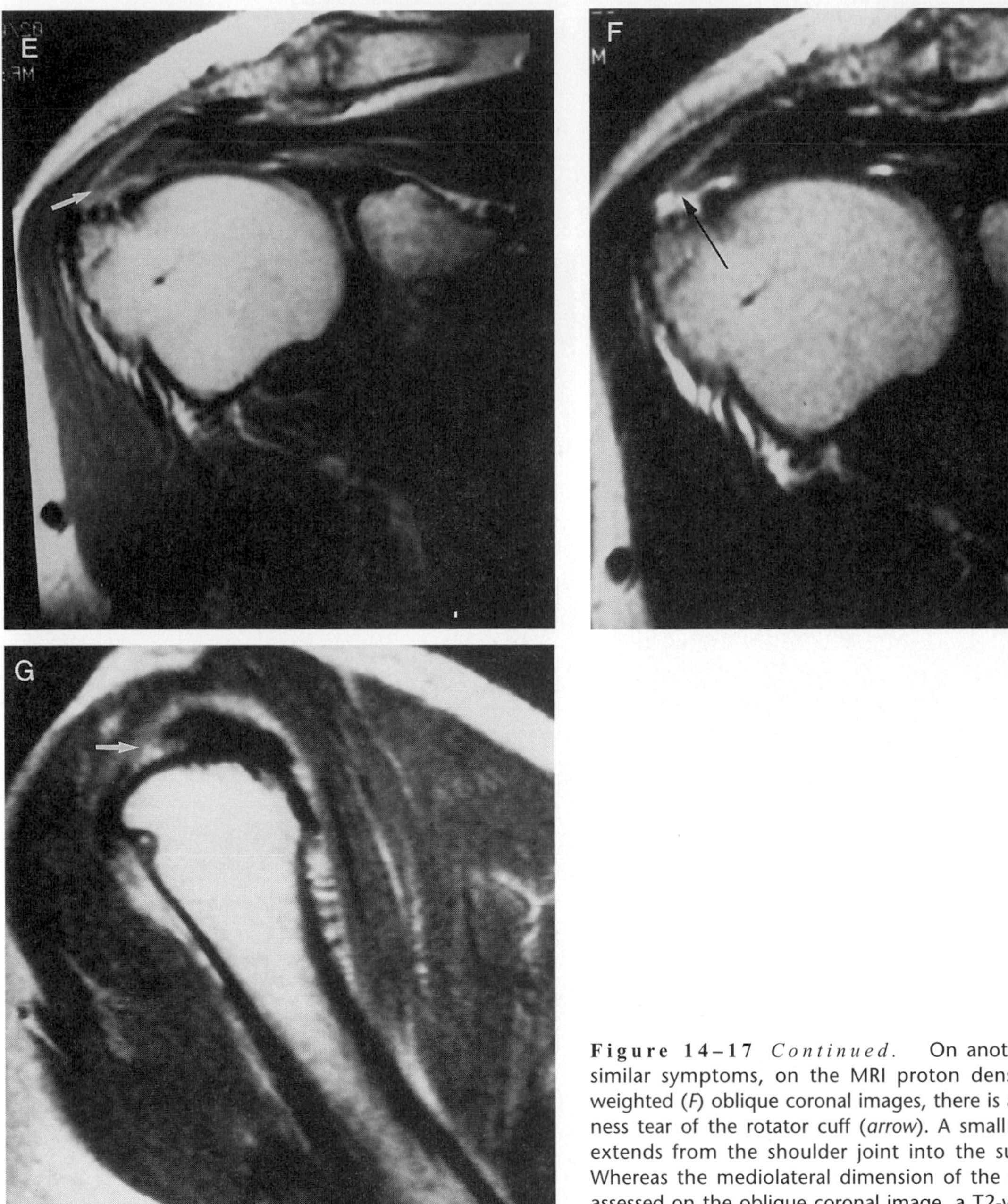

Figure 14–17 *Continued.* On another patient with similar symptoms, on the MRI proton density (*E*) and T2-weighted (*F*) oblique coronal images, there is a small full-thickness tear of the rotator cuff (*arrow*). A small amount of fluid extends from the shoulder joint into the subdeltoid bursa. Whereas the mediolateral dimension of the cuff tear can be assessed on the oblique coronal image, a T2-weighted oblique sagittal image (*G*) is needed to evaluate the anteroposterior extent of the tear (*arrow*).

ligament). Plain films are frequently obtained after an acute ankle sprain to evaluate the integrity of the ankle mortise and to detect the presence of a possible avulsion fracture. Stress radiography can also be performed to assess the integrity of the ligaments if the physical examination is inconclusive[189] and if this information is needed to guide therapy.[13] The accuracy of MRI in the detection of ankle ligamentous tears has been reported in several studies.[40,197,212,253] The use of thin sections and three-dimensional imaging techniques seems to improve the accuracy of an MRI examination. Prior to obtaining an MRI study to assess the ankle ligaments, it is important to determine how the results of an MRI examination will affect clinical care. The information provided by an MRI study may be useful for preoperative planning, but it provides no indication of the degree of joint instability because it is not a functional examination. To date, there have been no prospective studies to determine the impact of MRI on the outcome of patients with ankle ligamentous dysfunction.

Plain film evaluation is also used to detect evidence for injury of the anterior cruciate ligament (ACL). Positive findings include the detection of bony avulsions or osseous impactions. Overall, plain films are extremely insensitive in detecting ACL injuries. Plain film findings that have a high specificity for ACL tears (e.g., a Segond fracture or gross malalignment of the knee joint) are rarely present with most ACL injuries. Stress radiography[71] may have a role in the assessment of ACL ligamentous dysfunction, but it provides no information on the presence of concomitant knee injuries that may be associated with an ACL tear.

The initial application of MRI in the assessment of ligamentous dysfunction focused on the evaluation of the ACL. In the last few years, there have been many reports documenting the high accuracy of MRI in detecting complete tears of the ACL.[80,111,141,159,195,244] With MRI, it is possible to determine the precise location of an ACL tear (e.g., proximal, midsubstance, or distal) (Fig. 14–18). Although several studies have reported on the value of secondary signs detected in knees with a torn ACL,[45,152,230,245] the diagnosis of an ACL tear should be primarily based on the appearance of the ACL on the MRI study.[242] Improvement in the detection of ACL tears is accomplished by imaging the knee in three orthogonal planes.[68] In addition to detecting a torn ACL, it is equally important to determine whether there are concomitant injuries to the meniscus, cartilage, bone, or other ligaments of the knee, which may cause similar symptoms and affect knee stability.[136] This information is needed when trying to prognosticate the long-term outcome of patients with an ACL injury.[174,223]

Oberlander et al[173] have reported a prospective study that assessed the accuracy of the clinical examination of the knee. The diagnostic accuracy of the clinical examination for intra-articular knee injuries was determined by comparison to arthroscopic findings. An overall correct diagnosis for the clinical examination was present in 56% of the cases, an incomplete diagnosis in 31%, and an incorrect diagnosis in 13%. When a single lesion was present, diagnostic accuracy was 72%, but when more than two abnormalities were present, the accuracy of the clinical examination fell to 30%. Lesions most difficult to diagnose were cartilage fractures, tears of the ACL, and loose bodies. The strength of an MRI examination in the evaluation of an acutely or chronically symptomatic knee is its ability not only to assess the integrity of a single structure in the knee (e.g., the ACL) but to provide a comprehensive evaluation of the entire knee. This is particularly important in the clinical situation where pain or locking limits the diagnostic capacity of a physical examination. Complete evaluation of the other ligaments of the knee (e.g., the posterior cruciate ligament,[67,88,89] the medial collateral ligament,[54,157] and the lateral collateral ligament[157,256]) can be achieved with

Figure 14–18. After a patient's ski injury, there is a complete tear of the mid-segment of the anterior cruciate ligament (*arrow*) on the MRI proton density (*A*) and T2-weighted (*B*) sagittal images.

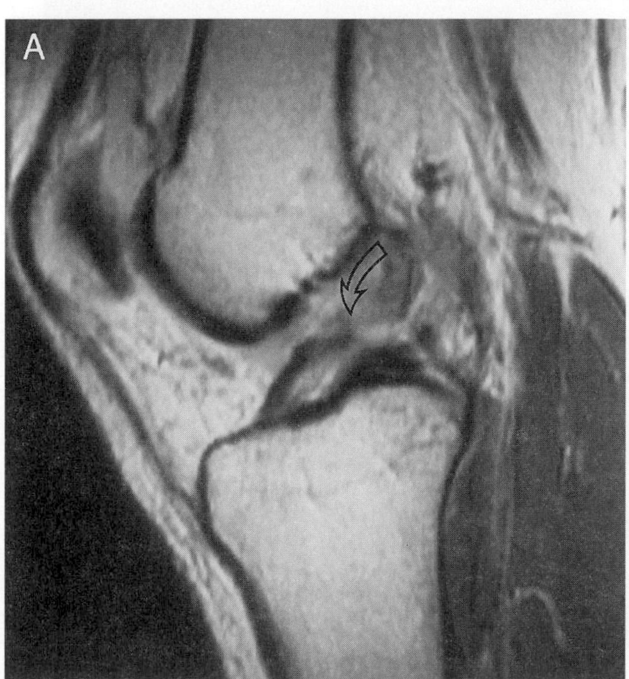

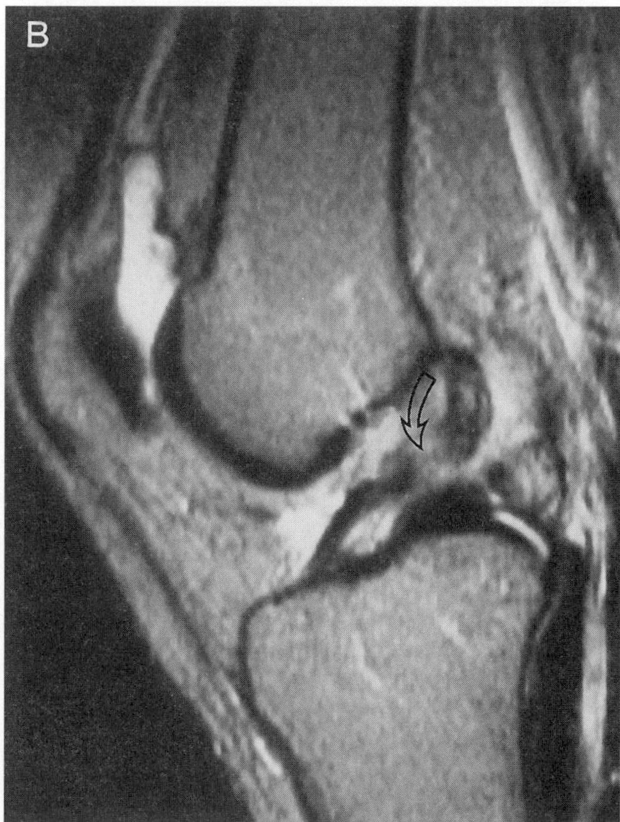

an MRI examination. The same diagnostic criteria applied to ACL tears are applied in the assessment of these ligaments.

In addition to detecting acute ligamentous injuries, it is possible with MRI to assess the degree of ligamentous healing with follow-up studies. We have followed the course of healing of acute grade 3 MCL injuries in several athletes. On the initial study, diffuse maceration of the ligament was detected, not a focal avulsion of the ligament at its bony insertion site. On the MRI study the ligament demonstrated diffuse increased signal intensity on the spin-echo and STIR sequences. There was no evidence of normal ligamentous fibers spanning from the femur to the tibia. In addition, prominent thickening of the ligament secondary to the fiber disruption and concomitant edema and hemorrhage was present. On the follow-up MRI studies the ligament became well-defined, thickened, and demonstrated decreased signal intensity compatible with collagenous repair (Fig. 14–19). The MRI examination provides direct information documenting the structural restoration of a ligament but cannot determine its functional integrity. In the process of healing, a medial collateral ligament is composed of a greater percentage of Type III collagen and is weaker than a normal ligament composed of Type I collagen. Currently, it is not known whether the MR signal characteristics of Type I collagen are different from Type III collagen.

MRI has also been applied in the evaluation of ACL reconstructive surgery. The MRI appearance of a neoligament composed of gracilis and semitendinous tendons[44,107] and the patellar tendon[191,266] has been reported. The neoligaments typically demonstrate increased signal intensity in the first few months after surgery, reflecting the increased hydration and vascularity of the structure. On follow-up MRI studies, there may be a varied appearance of the morphology and the signal intensity of the ligament. Yamato et al[266] reported on the assessment of 15 patients with a clinically stable patellar bone-tendon-bone autograft from 3 months to 3 years and 3 months after reconstructive surgery. Only in two patients did the entire ligament appear as a band of low signal intensity. Rak et al[191] reported on the MRI evaluation of 37 patients with an ACL reconstruction using patellar bone-tendon-bone autografts. On 43 of 47 MR examinations they identified a well-defined ligament with low signal intensity. The correlation between the clinical examination and MRI was 92% and between the MRI and a second-look arthroscopy was 100%. Coupens et al[48] reported on the follow-up MRI evaluation of the native patellar tendon after it had been used to supply the autograft for ACL reconstruction. They evaluated 20 patients up to 18 months after harvesting the patellar bone-tendon-bone autograft. By 18 months the signal intensity in the residual patellar tendon appeared normal, but there was a significant increase in the thickness of the tendon on all follow-up studies.

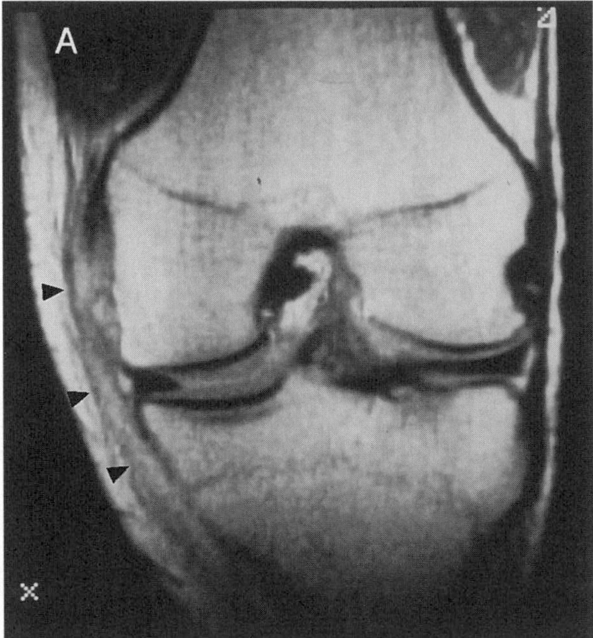

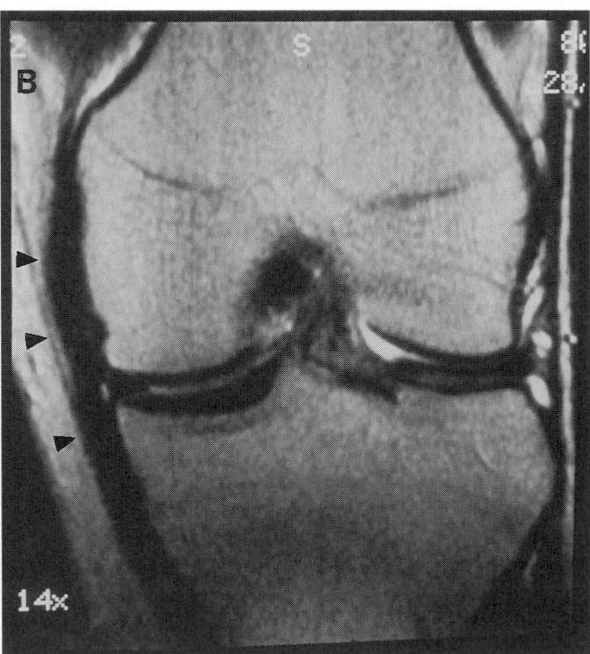

Figure 14–19. On the MRI evaluation of a patient who experienced an acute valgus injury to the knee, on the proton density weighted coronal image (*A*), there is diffuse maceration of the medial collateral ligament (MCL) (*arrowheads*). On the follow-up MRI (*B*) obtained approximately 8 months after injury, on the T2-weighted coronal image there is a completely healed, hypertrophied MCL (*arrowheads*).

CARTILAGE INJURIES

Damage to articular cartilage due to an acute traumatic injury or to chronic microtrauma may be an important component in the pathoetiology of joint dysfunction. Prior to the development of MRI, the radiologic detection of cartilage abnormalities on plain films was based on indirect evidence of cartilage damage (e.g., joint space narrowing or secondary osseous degenerative changes). Cartilaginous injury or degeneration can be directly evaluated with arthrography or CT arthrography. The sensitivity of arthrography is limited, owing to the difficulty in evaluating the curved articular surfaces that are present in most joints. The tomographic capability of CT arthrography improves the detection of cartilaginous lesions[101] but, like standard arthrography, it has limited applications and is a relatively invasive procedure.

With the excellent soft tissue resolution provided by MRI, it was initially hoped that it would be the ideal study for the assessment of cartilage disorders. In addition to excellent contrast resolution, a high degree of spatial resolution is needed to detect cartilage abnormalities considering that most articular cartilage ranges in thickness from 2 to 3 mm. Because the thickness of the patellar articular cartilage is approximately 5 mm, the initial effort to optimize MRI sequences for the evaluation of articular cartilage has focused on the assessment of normal and abnormal patellar cartilage.

Disorders of the patellar articular cartilage are considered a potential source of pain in many patients presenting with knee dysfunction (e.g., young athletes with parapatellar pain syndrome or workers whose jobs require repetitive or long periods of kneeling). Therefore, an accurate noninvasive test to detect these abnormalities would have a significant impact on patient care. The clinical efficacy of MRI in the detection of chondromalacia of the patella was reported by Conway et al.[46] The authors concluded that MRI was relatively sensitive and had a high predictive value in the detection of grades 3 and 4 chondromalacic lesions, even though no statistical analysis of the data was reported. There was also no discussion concerning the preoperative evaluation of these patients or the criteria employed to determine the indications for arthroscopy. McCauley et al[151] evaluated the appearance of the articular cartilage of the patella in 52 patients who underwent knee arthroscopy after an MRI examination. Twenty-nine of these patients had findings of chondromalacia at arthroscopy and the remaining 23 patients had normal patellar articular cartilage. The MRI studies were reviewed retrospectively by two radiologists without knowledge of the arthroscopic findings. An MR diagnosis based on focal signal or contour abnormalities detected on an axial spin-echo proton-density or T2-weighted sequence had a sensitivity of 86%, a specificity of 74%, and an accuracy of 81%. The sensitivity, specificity, and accuracy to detect chondromalacia was higher in the patients without joint fluid compared to patients with effusions. This finding is at odds with other clinical studies,[225] but the imaging techniques used in the different studies are dissimilar. The authors concluded that thinner sections may improve the accuracy to detect chondromalacia, but this will have to be proven with a prospective blinded study.

In addition to the evaluation of hyaline cartilage, one of the initial applications of MRI was in the evaluation of fibrocartilage (e.g., the knee meniscus and the intervertebral disc). The normal knee meniscus is a triangular fibrocartilaginous structure that generates no signal on an MRI study. Abnormal signal intensity within a meniscus is graded 1, 2, or 3, depending on the shape of the abnormal signal and whether it extends to the articular surface of a meniscus. Grade 1 is a globular focus of increased signal intensity that does not extend to the meniscal articular surface. Grade 2 is a linear focus of increased signal intensity that does not extend to the meniscal articular surface, but may extend to the meniscocapsular junction. Grade 3 is any focus of increased abnormal signal intensity that extends to the meniscal articular surface. Several studies have demonstrated the high accuracy of MRI to detect meniscal tears.[29,67,80,111,132] With aging, horizontal meniscal tears are frequently detected in asymptomatic patients,[132] therefore making it more difficult to determine their significance in a symptomatic patient. The standard criteria used to diagnose a meniscal tear on an MRI study are not as accurate in the assessment of the meniscus in older individuals.[102]

The diagnosis of a meniscal tear is more difficult in the postoperative knee because of the altered morphology and signal intensity of the meniscus.[55] An MRI is most valuable if only a small portion of the meniscus has been resected. It is possible to perform an MR arthrogram with Gd-DPTA to improve the detection rate of postoperative tears, but the MRI study then becomes a relatively invasive and more expensive procedure. In the future, other possible applications of MRI with respect to the meniscus may include kinematic MRI studies to assess meniscal stability and three-dimensional examinations to create templates for meniscal implant surgery.

One question that frequently arises when discussing the optimal MRI examination of the knee is whether a high-field strength MR system (i.e., > 1.0 T) is needed for accurate diagnosis. Barnett[15] has reported on the effect of field strength on the efficacy of MRI diagnosis. The MRI findings in 118 consecutive patients who underwent an MRI examination with a 0.5 T system were compared to the arthroscopic findings. The accuracy for the detection of medial meniscus tears was 92%, lateral meniscal tears 93%, and complete tears of the anterior cruciate ligament 97%. These results are not significantly different compared to the use of high-field strength systems. The examination times were longer on the 0.5 T system than on a high-field strength system. Potential sources of bias in this study were that the arthroscopists probably knew the results of the MRI examination prior to the arthroscopic procedure, and the fact that all these patients required arthroscopy indicates that a greater severity of knee dysfunction was present, which may inflate the accuracy of the MRI examination. As noted by the author, it is difficult to eliminate the second potential source of bias if arthroscopy is used as the gold standard.

In a prospective study from England, Spiers et al[226] reported on 58 patients with suspected internal derangement of the knee who had an MRI examination followed by arthroscopy. They found that their preoperative clinical assessment had a sensitivity of 77% and specificity of 43%, and the MRI had a sensitivity of 100% and a specificity of 63%, when compared to the arthroscopic findings. The authors concluded that acceptance of the MRI findings could have resulted in a 29% reduction in the arthroscopic procedures without missing any significant meniscal lesion. Similar results were found by Boden et al[26] and Ruwe et al.[206]

OSSEOUS INJURIES

In the evaluation of acute skeletal trauma, plain films should be the initial radiologic study obtained to detect the presence of an osseous infraction and to determine the nature and extent of bony disruption. With acute fractures of the skeletal system that involve cortical bone, standard x-rays are usually adequate to determine whether there is an acute cortical injury. Plain films are optimal to assess angulation, rotation, and distraction of the fracture fragments and to evaluate the integrity of the adjacent joints. At least two orthogonal x-ray views (i.e., 90° perpendicular to each other) are required to accurately assess the extent and alignment of a fracture. To optimize the detection of traumatic changes with plain films, it is important that the relevant clinical history is available at the time of plain film interpretation. Berbaum et al[17] reported on how the knowledge of the location of a patient's symptoms and signs affected the detection rate of fractures. Analysis of receiver-operator characteristic parameters indicated that the clinical information improved the detection rate of fractures. The improvement was based on an improved true-positive rate, without an increased false-positive rate.

With complex fractures, plain films are frequently not adequate to determine the nature and extent of an osseous injury. In these cases, CT is the ideal study to perform after the initial plain film evaluation. With CT, it is possible to determine the precise number and relationship of the different fracture fragments. It also is excellent in determining whether a fracture extends into contiguous joints, information that is critically needed in presurgical planning. Several studies have reported on the value of CT in the assessment of shoulder,[126] pelvis, tibial,[58] and calcaneal fractures.

Plain films are also the standard examination to follow fracture healing, by detecting the presence and extent of callus formation.[200] Early detection of a delayed union or nonunion is delineated with plain films. If there is a clinical concern about the degree of healing, conventional or computed tomography can be performed to determine the extent of fracture healing. Smith et al[222] reported on the prediction of fracture healing of the tibia by quantitative radionuclide imaging. The test had a sensitivity of 70% and a specificity of 90%. In cases where internal fixation had been applied, the assessment of fracture healing was more difficult.

Chronic osseous microtrauma may result in fractures of the cortical or cancellous bone, if the cumulative load exceeds the cell-matrix adaptive capacities. This may occur at the insertion site of tendons into bone (e.g., apophyseal traction injuries[145]) or at sites of mechanical overload related to increased physical activity[61] (e.g., march fractures). Chronic stress fractures are referred to as fatigue fractures if they result from excessive load applied to normal bone or as insufficiency fractures if they result from the application of physiologic stress to weakened bone.[52,124] Bone normally responds to new functional demands by remodeling, but if the rate of tissue disruption exceeds tissue repair, failure may result. Because the pathologic process involves both bone resorption and healing, the stress fractures that develop will initially have indistinct margins and are difficult to detect with plain films. If a stress fracture involves the cortical bone, periosteal new bone formation may be detected at the fracture site. If the fracture involves the cancellous bone, subtle areas of linear sclerosis may be detected in regions of trabecular compaction or callus formation. It usually takes 5 to 6 weeks for an x-ray to become positive after the onset of symptoms, and even then, the findings on plain films may be extremely subtle. If the findings on plain films are indeterminate, additional studies (e.g., CT or bone scintigraphy) may be needed to evaluate the bony changes.[208] CT has proven useful in the assessment of stress fractures of the tarsal navicular[130] and of the pars interarticularis of the spine. CT has also been employed to differentiate between stress fractures and bone tumors (e.g., osteoid osteomas).

As a result of the active bone remodeling at the site of a stress fracture, a bone scan will usually be positive soon after the onset of symptoms, particularly in a young patient. A positive bone scan will occur with any process that increases bone metabolism and therefore its specificity is limited. In addition, there is limited spatial resolution with a bone scan and it may be difficult to localize precisely the position of an abnormality and to determine if adjacent soft tissues or joints are involved by a pathologic process. There also have been case reports of negative bone scans in patients with stress fractures.[125,231]

MRI is also extremely sensitive in detecting stress fractures or any pathologic process that replaces the normal medullary fat in the cancellous bone by edematous tissue or a cellular infiltrate.[106] In both the inflammatory and reparative phases of a fracture, there will be increased fluid and cellular infiltration at the fracture site. These changes will be detected on a spin-echo T1-weighted sequence as a focus of intermediate signal intensity compared to the high signal of the normal fat, and on a T2-weighted or STIR sequence as a focus of high signal intensity. The strength of MRI compared to a bone scan is its excellent spatial resolution, direct multiplanar capabilities, high soft tissue contrast resolution, and the fact that it requires no exposure to ionizing radiation. With an MRI, it is usually possible to localize precisely the position of an abnormality. In cases where other diagnoses are being considered in addition to a stress fracture (e.g., infection or tumor), Gd-DTPA can be used to enhance the value of an MRI study. The results of an MRI study are also immediately available after the completion of an examination which facilitates optimal patient care.

The major drawbacks of MRI compared to bone scans are its higher cost, lower accessibility, and that it is contraindicated for certain patients. One way to curtail MRI costs is to perform a limited MRI study only, and this has proven to be extremely valuable in the detection of subtle femoral neck fractures in elderly patients.[198] Deutsch et al[56] employed a coronal spin-echo T1-weighted sequence in the evaluation of 23 patients in whom there was a high clinical suspicion of fracture and who had normal plain films. A fracture was demonstrated by MRI in 9 of 9 patients who, on follow-up x-rays, had fractures and the MRI excluded a fracture in 14 of 14 patients without fractures. In the same study, radionuclide scans were positive in 4 of 4 patients with a fracture and equivocal in one patient who did not have a fracture. The authors concluded that MRI can provide rapid, cost-effective, and anatomically precise diagnoses of hip fractures in patients with normal or equivocal plain films. Bone scans are also used to detect insufficiency fractures of the femoral neck in older patients,[239] but it may take several days before the scan becomes positive. It also may be difficult with a bone scan to differentiate between a fracture and severe arthritis.

After a direct injury to an extremity, it is fairly common for an individual to experience pain involving an osseous structure. Prior to the application of MRI, the precise etiology of this pain was unclear considering that plain films were usually negative. With the exquisite sensitivity of MRI to detect bone marrow edema, it quickly became apparent that many patients with acute trauma had areas of edematous cancellous bone at the site of an osseous injury.[140,146,158,267] The focal areas of bone marrow edema are most likely secondary to trabecular microtrauma (i.e., bone contusions or bruises) in the cancellous bone. They may occur secondary to an extrinsic impaction injury or may be secondary to bones impacting against one another as a result of acute instability or malalignment.

One of the first injuries where bone contusions were frequently detected was in patients with acute tears of the ACL.[122,167,227] The osseous contusions are typically located in the cancellous bone of the lateral femoral condyle superjacent to the condylar-trochlear sulcus and in the cancellous bone of the posterosuperior segment of the lateral tibial condyle (Fig. 14–20). There are several potential reasons why the detection of these bone contusions is important. Clinically a patient may

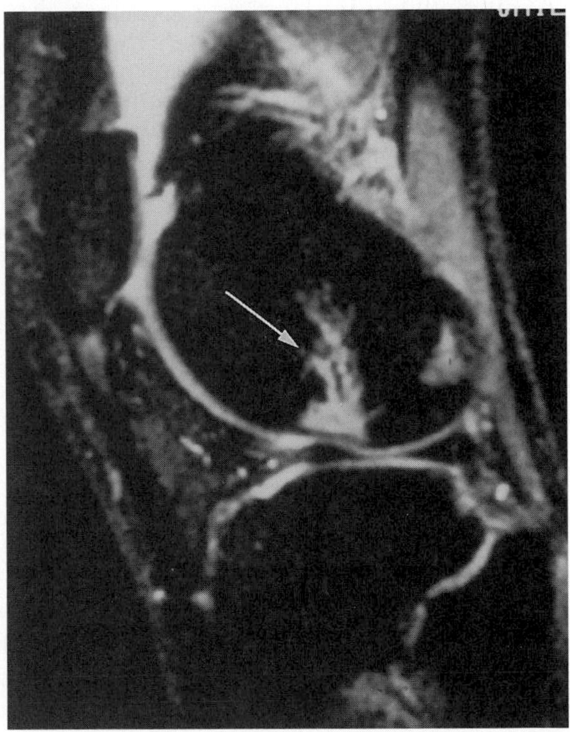

Figure 14–20. An MRI study was performed on a patient who incurred an acute ACL tear while skiing. The patient presented with lateral joint-line pain and the clinician suspected a tear of the lateral meniscus. On the STIR sequence there is high signal intensity in the cancellous bone of the lateral femoral condyle (*arrow*). There was no tear of the lateral meniscus on the routine MRI spin-echo sequences or at arthroscopy.

have lateral joint line pain and the possibility of a torn lateral meniscus must be considered as a potential source of this pain. With an MRI examination, it is not only possible to assess the appearance of the meniscus, but MRI also clarifies the etiology of the pain by demonstrating the presence of a bone contusion. The fact that the contusion exists also means that the overlying articular cartilage and/or meniscus also sustained a focal impaction force at the time of the injury. Cartilage tears are difficult to detect on an MRI, but the presence of a contusion should alert the radiologist to evaluate critically the articular cartilage overlying the region of the contused bone. Vellet et al[249] reported on a group of 21 patients with acute hemorrhagic knee effusions who underwent an MRI study and arthroscopy. Bone contusions adjacent to the subchondral plate were detected on the MRI in these patients, but at arthroscopy the overlying articular cartilage was normal. When these individuals were reevaluated at 6 to 12 months after the injury with a repeat MRI examination, 67% had developed osteochondral abnormalities. It is possible that when bone contusions are detected at the time of the initial injury, rehabilitation should be directed to prevent further overload to the articular cartilage, perhaps by an extended period of nonweight bearing. This should be investigated by appropriate long-term prospective studies.

By the detection of the position of bony contusions, it is possible to determine the exact location of the bone subjected to an extrinsic force. This information may help clarify the manners and mechanisms of different injuries and help to diagnose the precise etiology of knee pain when the history and physical examination are indeterminate. The diagnosis of patellar dislocation may be difficult if the patella relocates immediately. A patient may present with parapatellar pain and swelling and with a history of the knee giving out. MRI can be particularly helpful in these cases by detecting bone bruises on the anterolateral nonarticular margin of the lateral femoral condyle and in the medial facet of the patella.[129,137,254] The bony contusions are secondary to impaction of the medial facet of the patella against the lateral femoral condyle when the patella translates medially in the process of relocation. It is also possible to detect injuries of the lateral patellar facet and the lateral facet of the femoral trochlea if they impact against each other as the patella translates laterally. Kirsch et al[129] reported on the findings of transient lateral patellar dislocation in 26 patients. Partial or complete disruption of the medial patellar retinaculum was detected in 96%, a contusion of the lateral femoral condyle in 81%, osteochondral injuries in 58%, lateral patellar tilt or subluxation in 92%, and a joint effusion in 100%. Patellar dislocation had not been suspected prior to the MRI study in 73% of the patients. Axial images revealed the constellation of abnormalities present with transient lateral patellar dislocation. As many of these patients are being imaged for knee dysfunction without the clinical suspicion of transient lateral dislocation, it is mandatory that an axial sequence be part of a standard MRI evaluation for all patients with acute knee dysfunction. From these reports, it appears that the spin-echo[129] and STIR[137] sequences are optimal to detect these abnormalities.

Another important application of MRI in the evaluation of pathologic changes in bone is in the detection of osteonecrosis (ON). STIR and fat suppressed spin-echo T2-weighted sequences are probably optimal to detect marrow edema. The pathoetiology (e.g., atraumatic or traumatic) and the stage of evolution of ON will determine its appearance on an MRI study. Atraumatic ON is an evolving process, whether associated with medications such as steroids or as part of a clinical disorder causing ischemia to the femoral head, such as sickle cell or marrow storage diseases. Intermittent ischemia will precipitate microinfarcts with secondary inflammation and repair. The inflammatory and reparative processes are associated with increased fluid in the marrow that may elevate the marrow pressure due to the constraints of the surrounding bone.[116] It appears that the earliest change of ON depicted on a routine MRI is the detection of marrow edema, which explains why the study would be negative in detecting ON secondary to acute vascular disruption.[11] It is possible that both dynamic radionuclide and dynamic MRI studies with Gd-DPTA,[168] which can assess the perfusion status of the femoral head, may be able to detect perfusion abnormalities of the femoral head after a femoral neck fracture. The presence of decreased perfusion to the femoral head does not necessarily mean that ON will develop.

The detection of bone marrow edema on an MRI study is not a specific finding for ON but can be found with other disorders causing increased marrow hydration (e.g., ischemia,[248] fracture, transient bone marrow edema syndrome,[95,247] infection, or malignancy). Once there is osseous repair and/or replacement of the necrotic trabeculae with new bone, a characteristic "double line" can be detected at the interface between the necrotic and viable bone. On an MRI spin-echo T2-weighted sequence there will be a zone of high signal intensity secondary to the reparative tissue, surrounded by a zone of low signal intensity representing the repaired thickened trabecular bone. Any area of fibrosis or mineralized tissue will appear on the T2-weighted sequence as a focus of low signal intensity. Contrast-enhanced MRI studies may help differentiate between viable and nonviable marrow at this stage of ON.[246] With progression of ON, fracture and/or collapse of the femoral head can be detected with MRI, but CT is helpful to delineate small areas of cortical disruption or subchondral fractures. The location and extent of the osteonecrotic bone may be of prognostic value in predicting whether the femoral head will collapse[175,234]; therefore, both sagittal and coronal sequences are needed to calculate the extent of ON. Because MRI is noninvasive, it is possible to follow patients who are at high risk for developing ON[76,236] or patients who have undergone core decompression[104,169] to determine the status of their femoral heads. Plain films are insensitive in detecting early ON,[243] and by the time a subchondral fracture or collapse of the femoral head is detected on a plain film, the value of a core decompression may be limited.

In addition to the detection of ON of the hip, MRI is useful in detecting ON of the knee,[22] shoulder, wrist, or ankle. With the exquisite sensitivity of MRI to detect abnormalities of bone marrow, it was hoped that it could also be applied in assessing patients with reflex sympathetic dystrophy (RSD). Three-phase radionuclide bone scans have a reported 100% sensitivity, 80% specificity, 54% positive predictive value, and 100% negative predictive value for the detection of RSD of the foot.[105] Koch et al[131] reported on the MRI findings of 17 patients with RSD. Ten of 17 were normal on MRI, 6 of 17 had nonspecific soft-tissue changes or bone marrow sclerosis, and 1 of 17 showed changes of abnormal signal intensity. The fact that an MRI is negative with RSD may help elucidate the pathophysiology of RSD. It seems likely that the increased marrow perfusion detected on radionuclide studies may not be associated with concomitant marrow edema.

CONCLUSION

Musculoskeletal dysfunction occurs when the capacity of the cell-matrix complex to adapt to biomechanical force is exceeded. Whether this is an acute or chronic process will determine the nature of an injury and the secondary tissue response, including inflammation or degeneration. By understanding the initial mechanism of injury and the spectrum of tissue reaction to structural failure, it is possible to predict the manifestations of myriad musculoskeletal disorders on any type of imaging study. Each radiologic imaging examination, such as plain films, CT, MRI, and ultrasonography, encodes a different physical property of tissue; therefore each study should be used in specific clinical situations. Redundant studies must be eliminated if the costs of health care are to be controlled. Prospective controlled studies must be performed comparing the various imaging modalities to determine their cost-effectiveness. It is also possible that certain imaging studies may decrease medical costs by eliminating more expensive diagnostic procedures such as arthroscopy.[35,192,206,226]

References

1. Abdelwahab F, Gould ES: The role of diskography after negative postmyelography CT scans: Retrospective review. Am J Neuroradiol 9:187–190, 1988.
2. Aguila LA, et al: The intranuclear cleft of the intervertebral disk: Magnetic resonance imaging. Radiology 155:155–158, 1985.
3. Ahn S-H, Ahn M-W, Byun W-M: Effect of the transligamentous extension of lumbar disc herniations on their regression and the clinical outcome of sciatica. Spine 25:475–480, 2000.
4. Alaranta H, Tallroth K, Soukka A, Heliovaara M: Fat content of lumbar extensor muscles and low back disability: A radiographic and clinical comparison. J Spinal Disord 6:137–140, 1993.
5. Amendola A, Rorabeck CH, Vellett FD, et al: The use of magnetic resonance imaging in exertional compartment syndromes. Am J Sports Med 18:29–34, 1990.
6. Amundsen T, Weber H, Lilleas F, et al: Lumbar spinal stenosis: Clinical and radiologic features. Spine 20:1178–1186, 1995.
7. Andersson GBJ, Schultz A, Nathan A, Irstam L: Roentgenographic measurement of lumbar intervertebral disc height. Spine 6:154–158, 1981.
8. Anti-Poika I, Soini J, Tallroth K, et al: Clinical relevance of discography combined with CT scanning. J Bone Joint Surg 72(B):480–485, 1990.
9. Aprill C, Bogduk N: High-intensity zone: A diagnostic sign of painful lumbar disc on magnetic resonance imaging. Br J Radiol 65:361–369, 1992.
10. Arnoldi CC, et al: Lumbar spinal stenosis and nerve root entrapment syndromes: Definition and classification. Clin Orthop 115:4–5, 1976.
11. Asnis SE, Gould ES, Bansal M, et al: Magnetic resonance imaging of the hip after displaced femoral neck fractures. Clin Orthop 298:191–198, 1994.
12. Aspelin P, Ekberg O, Thorsson O, et al: Ultrasound examination of soft tissue injury of the lower limb in athletes. Am J Sports Med 20:601–603, 1992.
13. Auletta AG, Conway WF, Hayes CW, et al: Indications for radiography in patients with acute ankle injuries: role of the physical examination. Am J Roentgenol 157:789–791, 1991.
14. Balagura S, Neumann J: Magnetic resonance imaging of the postoperative intervebral disc: The first eight months—clinical and legal implications. J Spinal Disord 3:212–217, 1993.
15. Barnett MJ: MR diagnosis of internal derangements of the knee: Effect of field strength on efficacy. Am J Roentgenol 161:115–118, 1993.
16. Beattie PF, Meyers SP, Stratford P, et al: Associations between patient report of symptoms and anatomic impairment visible on lumbar magnetic resonance imaging. Spine 25:819–828, 2000.
17. Berbaum KS, El-Khoury GY, Franken EA, et al: Impact of clinical history on fracture detection with radiography. Radiology 168:507–511, 1988.
18. Bernard TN Jr: Lumbar discography followed by computed tomography: Refining the diagnosis of low-back pain. Spine 15:690–707, 1990.
19. Biering-Sorensen F, Hensen FR, Schroll M, Runeborg O: The relation of spinal X-ray to low-back pain and physical activity among 60-year-old men and women. Spine 10:445–451, 1985.
20. Bigos SJ, Hansson T, Castillo RN, et al: The value of preemployment roentgenographs for predicting acute back injury claims and chronic back pain disability. Clin Orthop 283:124–129, 1992.
21. Bischoff RJ, Rodriguez RP, Gupta K, et al: A comparison of computed tomography-myelography, magnetic resonance imaging, and myelography in the diagnosis of herniated nucleus pulposus, and spinal stenosis. J Spinal Disord 6:289–295, 1993.
22. Bjokengren AG, Airowaih A, Lindstrand A, et al: Spontaneous osteonecrosis of the knee: Value of MR imaging in determining prognosis. Am J Roentgenol 154:331–336, 1990.
23. Blumenthal SL, et al: The role of anterior lumbar fusion for internal disc disruption. Spine 13:566–569, 1988.

24. Boden S, Davis DO, Dina TS, et al: The incidence of abnormal lumbar spine MRI scans in asymptomatic patients: A prospective investigation. J Bone Joint Surg 72A:1178–1184, 1989.
25. Boden SD, David DO, Dina TS, et al: Abnormal magnetic resonance scans of the lumbar spine in asymptomatic subjects. J Bone Joint Surg 72A:403–408, 1990.
26. Boden SD, Labropoulos PA, Vailas JC: MR scanning of the acutely injured knee: Sensitive, but is it cost effective? J Arthro Surg 6:306–310, 1990.
27. Boden SD, McCowin PR, Davis DO, et al: Abnormal magnetic resonance scans of the cervical spine in asymptomatic subjects. J Bone Joint Surg 72A:1178–1183, 1990.
28. Bodne D, Quinn SF, Murray WT, et al: Magnetic resonance images of chronic patellar tendinitis. Skeletal Radiol 17:24–28, 1988.
29. Boeree NR, Watkinson AF, Ackroyd CE, et al: Magnetic resonance imaging of meniscal and cruciate injuries of the knee. J Bone Joint Surg 73B:452–457, 1991.
30. Bohatirchuk F: The aging vertebral column (macro- and histo-radiographical study). Br J Radiol 28:389–404, 1955.
31. Boos N, Rieder R, Schade V, et al: The diagnostic accuracy of magnetic resonance imaging, work perception, and psychosocial factors in identifying symptomatic disc herniations. Spine 24:2613–2625, 1993.
32. Bozzao A, Gallucci M, Masciocchi C, et al: Lumbar disk herniation: MR imaging assessment of natural history in patients treated without surgery. Radiology 185:135–141, 1992.
33. Brenneke SL, Morgan CJ: Evaluation of ultrasonography as a diagnostic technique in the assessment of rotator cuff tendon tears. Am J Sports Med 20:287–288, 1989.
34. Bronskill MJ, Sprawls P: The Physics of MRI: 1992 AAPM Summer School Proceedings. American Institute of Physics, Woodbury, NY, 1993.
35. Bui-Mansfield L, Youngberg RA, Warme W, et al: Potential cost saving of MR imaging obtained before arthroscopy of the knee: Evaluation of 50 consecutive patients. Am J Roentgenol 168:913–916, 1997.
36. Burstein AH: Editorial: Fracture classification systems: Do they work and are they useful? J Bone Joint Surg Am 75A:1743–1744, 1993.
37. Burton CV, et al: Causes of failure of surgery on the lumbar spine. Clin Orthop 157:191–199, 1981.
38. Bush K, Cowan N, Katz DE, Gishen P: The natural history of sciatica associated with disc pathology: A prospective study with clinical and independent radiologic follow-up. Spine 17:1205–1212, 1992.
39. Calvert PT, Packer NP, Stoker DJ, et al: Arthrography of the shoulder after operative repair of the torn rotator cuff. J Bone Joint Surg Br 68B:147–150, 1986.
40. Cardone BW, Erickson SJ, Den Hartog, Carrera GF: MRI of injury to the lateral collateral ligamentous complex of the ankle. J Comput Assist Tomogr 17:102–107, 1993.
41. Carr D, Gilbertson L, Frymoyer J, et al: Lumbar paraspinal compartment syndrome: A case report with physiologic and anatomic studies. Spine 10:816–820, 1985.
42. Cavanagh S, Stevens J, Johnson J: High-resolution MRI in the investigation of recurrent pain after lumbar discectomy. J Bone Joint Surg 75B:524–528, 1993.
43. Chandra R: Introductory Physics of Nuclear Medicine. Philadelphia, Lea and Febiger, 1976.
44. Cheung Y, Magee TH, Rosenberg ZS, Rose DJ: MRI of anterior cruciate ligament reconstruction. J Comput Assist Tomogr 16:134–137, 1992.
45. Cobby MJ, Schweitzer ME, Resnick D: The deep lateral femoral notch: An indirect sign of a torn anterior cruciate ligament. Radiology 184:855–858, 1992.
46. Conway WF, Hayes CW, Loughran T, et al: Cross-sectional imaging of the patellofemoral joint and surrounding structures. RadioGraphics 11:195–217, 1991.
47. Coste J, Paolaggi JB, Spira A: Reliability of interpretation of plain lumbar spine radiographs in benign, mechanical low-back pain. Spine 16:426–428, 1991.
48. Coupens SD, Yates CK, Sheldon C, Ward C: Magnetic resonance imaging evaluation of the patellar tendon after use of its central one-third for anterior cruciate ligament reconstruction. Am J Sports Med 20:332–335, 1992.
49. Coventry MB, Ghormley RK, Kernohan JW: The intervertebral disc: Its microscopic anatomy and pathology: Part II—changes in the intervertebral disc concomitant with age. J Bone Joint Surg 27:233–247, 1945.
50. Curry TS III, Dowdey JE, Murry RC Jr: Christensen's Physics of Diagnostic Radiology. Philadelphia, Lea and Febiger 1990.
51. Dabbs VM, Dabbs LG: Correlation between disc height narrowing and low-back pain. Spine 15:1366–1369, 1990.
52. Daffner RH, Pavlov H: Stress fractures: Current concepts. Am J Roentgenol 159:245–252, 1993.
53. Deutsch AL, et al: Lumbar spine following successful surgical discectomy. Spine 18:1054–1060, 1993.
54. Deutsch AL, Mink JH: Articular disorders of the knee. Magn Reson Imaging 1:43–56, 1989.
55. Deutsch AL, Mink JH: The postoperative knee. In: Mink JH, Reicher MA, Crues JV, et al (eds): Magnetic Resonance Imaging of the Knee, 2nd ed. New York, Raven Press, 1993, p 237.
56. Deutsch AL, Mink JH, Waxman AD: Occult fractures of the proximal femur: MR imaging. Radiology 170:113–116, 1989.
57. Deyo RA, Diehl AK: Lumbar spine films in primary care: Current use and effects of selective ordering criteria. J Intern Med 1:20–25, 1986.
58. Dias JJ, Stirling AJ, Finlay DBL, Gregg PJ: Computerised axial tomography for tibial plateau fractures. J Bone Joint Surg Br 69B:84–88, 1987.
59. DiFazio FA, Barth RA, Frymoyer JW: Acute lumbar paraspinal compartment syndrome. J Bone Joint Surg Am 73A:1101–1103, 1991.
60. Edelman RR, et al: High-resolution of surfacecoil imaging of lumbar disk disease. Am J Roentgenol 144:1123–1129, 1985.
61. Eisele SA, Sammarco GJ: Fatigue fractures of the foot and ankle in the athlete. J Bone Joint Surg Am 75A:290–298, 1993.
62. Erickson SJ, Cox JH, Hyde JS, et al: Effect of tendon orientation on MR Imaging signal intensity: A manifestation of the "magic angle" phenomenon. Radiology 181:389–392, 1991.
63. Farin PU, Jaroma H, Harju A, Soimakallio S: Shoulder impingement syndrome: Sonographic evaluation. Radiology 176:845–849, 1990.
64. Farley TE, Neumann CH, Steinbach LS, et al: Full-thickness tears of the rotator cuff of the shoulder: Diagnosis with MR imaging. Am J Roentgenol 158:347–351, 1992.
65. Ferretti A, Ippolito E, Mariai P, Puddu G: Jumper's knee. Am J Sports Med 11:58–62, 1983.
66. Firooznia H, et al: CT of lumbar spine disk herniation: Correlation with surgical findings. Am J Roentgenol 5:91–96, 1984.
67. Fischer SP, Fox JM, De Pizzo W, et al: Accuracy of diagnoses from magnetic resonance imaging of the knee. J Bone Joint Surg 73A:2–10, 1991.
68. Fitzgerald SW, Remer EM, Friedman H, Rogers LF: MR evaluation of the anterior cruciate ligament: Value of supplementing sagittal images with coronal and axial images. Am J Roentgenol 160:1233–1237, 1993.
69. Fleckenstein JL, Weatherall PT, Parkey RW, et al: Sports-related muscle injuries: Evaluation with MR imaging. Radiology 172:793–798, 1989.
70. Forristall RM, Marsh HO, Pay NT: Magnetic resonance imaging and contrast CT of the lumbar spine: Comparison of diagnostic

methods and correlation with surgical findings. Spine 13:1049–1054, 1988.

71. Franklin JL, Rosenberg TD, Paulos LE, et al: Radiographic assessment of instability of the knee due to rupture of the anterior cruciate ligament: A quadriceps-contraction technique. J Bone Joint Surg Am 73A:365–372, 1991.
72. Friedenberg ZB, Edeiken J, Spencer HN, Tolentino SC: Degenerative changes in the cervical spine. J Bone Joint Surg 41A:61–70, 1959.
73. Friedenberg ZB, Miller WT: Degenerative disc disease of the cervical spine. J Bone Joint Surg 45A:1171–1178, 1963.
74. Fries JW, et al: Computed tomography of herniated and extruded nucleus pulposus. J Comput Assist Tomogr 6:874–887, 1982.
75. Frymoyer JW, Newberg A, Pope MA, et al: Spine radiographs in patients with low-back pain: An epidemiological study in men. J Bone Joint Surg 667:1048–1105, 1984.
76. Gennuso R, Zappulla RA, Strenger SW: A localized lumbar spinal root arteriovenous malformation presenting with radicular signs and symptoms. Spine 14:543–546, 1989.
77. Gerber C, Krushell RJ: Isolated rupture of the tendon of the subscapularis muscle: Clinical features in 16 cases. J Bone Joint Surg Br 73B:389–394, 1991.
78. Ghosh P (ed): The Biology of the Intervertebral Disc, vol. I. Boca Raton, Fla, CRC Press, 1988, p 245.
79. Ghosh P (ed): The Biology of the Intervertebral Disc, vol. II. Boca Raton, Fla, CRC Press, 1988, p 207.
80. Glashow JL, Katz R, Schneider M, Scott WN: Double-blind assessment of the value of magnetic resonance imaging in the diagnosis of anterior cruciate and meniscal lesions. J Bone Joint Surg 71A:113–119, 1989.
81. Glenn WV Jr, et al: Multiplanar display computerized body tomography applications in the lumbar spine. Spine 4:282–294, 1979.
82. Gore DR, Sepic SB, Gardner GM: Roentgenographic findings of the cervical spine in asymptomatic people. Spine 11:521–524, 1986.
83. Gore DR, Sepic SB, Gardner GM, Murray P: Neck pain: A long-term follow-up of 205 patients. Spine 12:1–5, 1987.
84. Goyal RN, et al: Intraspinal cysts: A classification and literature review. Spine 12:209–213, 1987.
85. Greco A, McNamara MT, Escher MG, et al: Spin-echo and STIR MR imaging of sports-related muscle injuries at 1.5 T. J Comput Assist Tomogr 15:994–999, 1991.
86. Grenier N, et al: Isthmic spondylolysis of the lumbar spine: MR imaging at 1.5 T. Radiology 170:489–493, 1989.
87. Grenier N, et al: Normal and disrupted lumbar longitudinal ligaments: Correlative MR and anatomic study. Radiology 171:197–205, 1989.
88. Gross ML, Grover JS, Bassett LW, et al: Magnetic resonance imaging of the posterior cruciate ligament. Am J Sports Med 20:732–737, 1992.
89. Grover JS, Bassett LW, Gross ML, et al: Posterior cruciate ligament: MR imaging. Radiology 174:527–530, 1990.
90. Grubb SA, Lipscomb HJ, Coonrad RW: Degenerative adult onset scoliosis. Spine 13:241–245, 1988.
91. Harcke HT, Grissom LE, Finkelstein MS: Evaluation of the musculoskeletal system with sonography. Am J Roentgenol 150:1253–1261, 1988.
92. Harryman DT, Mack LA, Wang KY, et al: Repairs of the rotator cuff: Correlation of functional results with integrity of the cuff. J Bone Joint Surg 73A:982–989, 1991.
93. Hasso AN, et al: Computed tomography of children and adolescents with suspected spinal stenosis. J Comput Assist Tomogr 11:609–611, 1987.
94. Haughton VM, et al: A prospective comparison of computed tomography and myelography in the diagnosis of herniated lumbar disks. Radiology 142:103–110, 1982.
95. Hayes CW, Conway WF, Daniel W: MR imaging of bone marrow edema pattern: Transient osteoporosis, transient bone marrow edema syndrome, or osteonecrosis. RadioGraphics 13:1001–1011, 1993.
96. Hendee WR: The Physical Principles of Computed Tomography. Boston, Little, Brown, 1983.
97. Hernandez RJ, Keim DR, Chenevert TL, et al: Fat-suppressed MR imaging of myositis. Radiology 182:217–219, 1992.
98. Hernandez RJ, Sullivan DB, Chenevert TL, Keim DR: MR imaging in children with dermatomyositis: Musculoskeletal findings and correlation with clinical and laboratory findings. Am J Roentgenol 161:359–366, 1993.
99. Hickey DS, et al: Analysis of magnetic resonance images from normal and degenerate lumbar intervertebral discs. Spine 11:702–708, 1986.
100. Hitselberger WE, Witten RM: Abnormal myelograms in asymptomatic patients. J Neurosurg 28:204–206, 1968.
101. Hodge JC, Ghelman B, O'Brien SJ, Wickiewicz TL: Synovial plicae and chondromalacia patellae: Correlation of results of CT arthrography with results of arthroscopy. Radiology 186:827–831, 1993.
102. Hodler J, Haghighi P, Pathria MN, et al: Meniscal changes in the elderly: Correlation of MR imaging and histologic findings. Radiology 184:221–225, 1992.
103. Hodler J, Kursunoglu-Brahme S, Snyder SJ, et al: Rotator cuff disease: Assessment with MR arthrography versus standard MR imaging in 36 patients with arthroscopic confirmation. Radiology 182:431–436, 1992.
104. Hofmann S, Engel A, Neuhold A, et al: Bonemarrow oedema syndrome and transient osteoporosis of the hip: an MRI-controlled study of treatment by core decompression. J Bone Joint Surg Br 75B:210–216, 1993.
105. Holder LE, Cole LA, Myerson MS: Reflex sympathetic dystrophy in the foot: Clinical and scintigraphic criteria. Radiology 184:531–535, 1992.
106. Hosten N, Schorner W, Neumann K, et al: MR imaging of bone marrow: Review of the literature and possible indications for contrast-enhanced studies. Adv MRI Contr 1:84–98, 1993.
107. Howell SM, Clark JA, Blasier RD: Serial magnetic resonance imaging of hamstring anterior cruciate ligament autografts during the first year of implantation: a preliminary study. Am J Sports Med 19:42–47, 1991.
108. Hueftle M, et al: Lumbar spine: Postoperative MR imaging with Gd-DTPA. Radiology 167:817–824, 1988.
109. Hurme M, Alaranta H: Factors predicting the result of surgery for lumbar intervertebral disc herniation. Spine 12:933–938, 1987.
110. Iannotti JP, Zlatkin MB, Esterhai JL, et al: Magnetic resonance imaging of the shoulder. Magn Reson Imaging 73A:17–29, 1991.
111. Jackson DW, Jennings LD, Maywood RM, Beger PE: Magnetic resonance imaging of the knee. Am J Sports Med 16:29–38, 1988.
112. Jaffray D, O'Brien JP: Isolated intervertebral disc resorption: A source of mechanical and inflammatory back pain? Spine 11:397–401, 1986.
113. Jehenson P, Leroy-Willig A, de Kerviler E, et al: MR imaging as a potential diagnostic test for metabolic myopathies: Importance of variations in the T2 of muscle with exercise. Am J Roentgenol 161:347–351, 1993.
114. Jensen MC, Brant-Zawdzi MN, Obuchowski N, et al: Magnetic resonance imaging of the lumbar spine in people without back pain. N Engl J Med 331:69–73, 1994.
115. Kainberger FM, Engel A, Barton P, et al: Injury of the achilles tendon: Diagnosis with sonography. Am J Roentgenol 155:1031–1036, 1990.
116. Kalebo P, Allenmark C, Peterson L, Sward L: Diagnostic value of ultrasonography in partial ruptures of the Achilles tendon. Am J Sports Med 20:378–381, 1992.

117. Kalebo P, Karlsson J, Sward L, Peterson L: Ultrasonography of chronic tendon injuries in the groin. Am J Sports Med 20:634–639, 1992.
118. Kambin P, et al: Annular protrusion: Pathophysiology and roentgenographic appearance. Spine 13:671–675, 1988.
119. Kannus P, Jozsa L: Histopathological changes preceding spontaneous rupture of a tendon: A controlled study of 891 patients. J Bone Joint Surg Am 73A:1507–1525, 1991.
120. Kaplan PA, Bryans KC, Davick JP, et al: MR imaging of the normal shoulder: Variants and pitfalls. Radiology 184:519–524, 1992.
121. Kaplan PA, Matamoros A, Anderson JC: Sonography of the musculoskeletal system. Am J Roentgenol 155:237–245, 1990.
122. Kaplan PA, Walker CW, Kilcoyne RF, et al: Occult fracture patterns of the knee associated with anterior cruciate ligament tears: Assessment with MR imaging. Radiology 183:835–838, 1992.
123. Karzel RP, Snyder SJ: Magnetic resonance arthrography of the shoulder. Clin Sports Med 12:123–136, 1993.
124. Kathol MH, El-Khoury GY, Moore TE, Marsh JL: Calcaneal insufficiency avulsion fractures in patients with diabetes mellitus. Radiology 180:725–772, 1991.
125. Keene JS, Lash EG: Negative bone scan in a femoral neck stress fracture: a case report. Am J Sports Med 20:234–236, 1992.
126. Kilcoyne RF, Shuman WP, Matsen FA, et al: The Neer classification of displaced proximal humeral fractures: Spectrum of findings on plain radiographs and CT scans. Am J Roentgenol 154:1029–1033, 1990.
127. Kirkaldy-Willis WH: The pathology and pathogenesis of low back pain. In: Managing Low-back Pain. New York, 1988, Churchill Livingstone, pp 49–75.
128. Kirkaldy-Willis H, et al: Pathology and pathogenesis of lumbar spondylosis and stenosis. Spine 3:319–328, 1978.
129. Kirsch MD, Fitzgerald SW, Friedman H, Rogers LF: Transient lateral patellar dislocation: diagnosis with MR imaging. Am J Roentgenol 161:109–113, 1993.
130. Kiss ZS, Khan KM, Fuller PJ: Stress fractures of the tarsal navicular bone: CT findings in 55 cases. Am J Roentgenol 160:111–115, 1993.
131. Koch E, Hofer HO, Sialer G, et al: Failure of MR imaging to detect reflex sympathetic dystrophy of the extremities. Am J Roentgenol 156:113–115, 1991.
132. Kornick J, Trefelner E, McCarthy S, et al: Meniscal abnormalities in the asymptomatic population at MR imaging. Radiology 177:463–465, 1990.
133. Kransdorf MJ, Meis JM, Jelinek JS: Myositis ossificans: MR appearance with radiologic-pathologic correlation. Am J Roentgenol 157:1243–1248, 1991.
134. Kravis MMM, Munk PL, McCain GA, et al: MR imaging of muscle and tender points in fibromyalgia. J Magn Reson Imaging 3:669–670, 1993.
135. Kurashima K, Shimizu H, Ogawa H: MR and CT in the evaluation of sarcoid myopathy. J Comput Assist Tomogr 15:1004–1007, 1991.
136. Lahm A, Erggelet C, Steinwachs, Reichelt A: Articular and osseous lesions in recent ligament tears: Arthroscopic changes compared with magnetic resonance imaging findings. Arthroscopy, 14:597–604, 1998.
137. Lance E, Deutsch AL, Mink JH: Prior lateral patellar dislocation MR imaging findings. Radiology 189:905–907, 1993.
138. Lancourt, JE, Glenn WV Jr, Wiltse LL: Multiplanar computerized tomography in the normal spine and in the diagnosis of spinal stenosis: A gross anatomic-computerized tomographic correlation. Spine 4:379–390, 1979.
139. Leadbetter WB: Cell-matrix response in tendon injury. In Renstrom AFH, Leadbetter WB (eds): Clinics in Sports Medicine: Tendinitis–Basic Concepts. Philadelphia, WB Saunders 1992 p 533.
140. Lee JK, Yao L: Occult intraosseous fracture: magnetic resonance appearance versus age of injury. Am J Sports Med 17:620–623, 1989.
141. Lee JK, Yao L, Phelps CT, et al: Anterior cruciate ligament tears: MR imaging compared with arthroscopy and clinical tests. Radiology 166:861–864, 1988.
142. Levitan LH, Wiens CW: Chronic lumbar extradural hematoma: CT findings Radiology 148:707–708, 1983.
143. Liang M, Komaroff AL: Roentgenograms in primary care patients with acute low back pain. Arch Intern Med 142:1108–1112, 1982.
144. Lipson SJ, Muir H: Proteoglycans in experimental intervertebral disc degeneration. Spine 6:194–210, 1981.
145. Lombardo SJ, Retting AC, Kerlan RK: Radiographic abnormalities of the iliac apophysis in adolescent athletes. J Bone Joint Surg Am 65A: 444–446, 1983.
146. Lynch TCP, Crues JV, Morgan FW, et al: Bone abnormalities of the knee: Prevalence and significance at MR imaging. Radiology 171:761–766, 1989.
147. Mack LA, Gannon MK, Kilcoyne RF, Matsen FA: Sonographic evaluation of the rotator cuff: Accuracy in patients without prior surgery. Clin Orthop 234:21–27, 1988.
148. NacNab I: Spondylolisthesis with an intact neural arch, the so-called pseudo-spondylolistheses. J Bone Joint Surg 32B:325–333, 1950.
149. Masaryk TJ, et al: High-resolution MR imaging of sequestered lumbar intervertebral disks. Am J Roentgenol 150:1155–1162, 1988.
150. McAfee PC, et al: Computed tomography in degenerative spinal stenosis. Clin Orthop 161:221–234, 1981.
151. McCauley TR, Kier R, Lynch KJ, Jokl P: Chondromalacia patellae: Diagnosis with MR imaging. Am J Roentgenol 158:101–105, 1992.
152. McCauley TR, Moses M, Kier R, et al: MR diagnosis of tears of anterior cruciate ligament of the knee: importance of ancillary findings Am J Roentgenol 162:115–119, 1994.
153. Middleton WD, Reinus WR, Totty WG, et al: Ultrasonographic evaluation of the rotator cuff and biceps tendon. J Bone Joint Surg 68A:440–450, 1986.
154. Miller JAA, Schmatz C, Schultz AB: Lumbar disc degeneration: Correlation with age, sex and spine level in 600 autopsy specimens. Spine 13:173–178, 1988.
155. Mink JH: Imaging evaluation of the candidate for percutaneous lumbar discectomy. Clin Orthop 238:83–103, 1989.
156. Mink JH: Muscle injuries. In Mink JH, Reicher MA, Crues JH, et al: Magnetic Resonance Imaging of the Knee, 2nd ed. New York, Raven Press, 1993, p 401.
157. Mink JH: The cruciate and collateral ligaments. In Mink JH, Reicher MA, Crues JV, et al: Magnetic Resonance Imaging of the Knee, 2nd ed. New York, Raven Press, 1993, p 141.
158. Mink JH, Deutsch AL: Occult cartilage and bone injuries of the knee: Detection, classification, and assessment with MR imaging. Radiology 170:823–829, 1989.
159. Mink JH, Levy T, Crues JV: Tears of the anterior cruciate ligament and menisci of the knee: MR imaging evaluation. Radiology 167:769–774, 1988.
160. Mirowitz SA: Normal rotator cuff: MR imaging with conventional and fat-suppression techniques. Radiology 180:735–740, 1991.
161. Misamore GW, Woodward C: Evaluation of degenerative lesions of the rotator cuff: A comparison of arthrography and ultrasonography. J Bone Joint Surg 73A:704–706, 1991.
162. Modic MT, Masaryk TJ, Ross JS: Magnetic Imaging of the Spine. Chicago, Year Book Medical Publishers, 1989.
163. Modic MT, Masaryk TJ, Ross JS, Carter JR: Imaging of degenerative disc disease. Radiology 168:177–186, 1988.
164. Modic MT, et al: Degenerative disc disease: Assessment of changes in vertebral body marrow with MR imaging. Radiology 166:193–199, 1988.

165. Modic MT, et al: Lumbar herniated disc disease and canal stenosis: Prospective evaluation by surface coil MR, CT, and myelography. Am J Roentgenol 147:757–765, 1986.
166. Modic MT, et al: Vertebral osteomyelitis: Assessment using MR. Radiology 157:157–166, 1985.
167. Murphy BJ, Smith RL, Uribe JW, et al: Bone signal abnormalities in the posterolateral tibia and lateral femoral condyle in complete tears of the anterior cruciate ligament: A specific sign? Radiology 182:221–224, 1992.
168. Nadel SN, Debatin JF, Richardson WJ: Detection of acute avascular necrosis of the femoral head in dogs: Dynamic contract-enhanced MR imaging vs. spin-echo and STIR sequences. Am J Roentgenol 159:1255–1261, 1992.
169. Neuhold A, Hofmann S, Engel A, et al: Bone marrow edema of the hip: MR findings after core decompression. J Comput Assist Tomogr 16:951–955, 1992.
170. Neumann CH, Holt RG, Steinbach LS, et al: MR imaging of the shoulder: Appearance of the supraspinatus tendon in asymptomatic volunteers. Am J Roentgenol 158:1281–1287, 1992.
171. Noonan TJ, Garrett WF: Injuries at the myotendinous junction. Clin Sports Med 11:783–806, 1992.
172. Nunez-Hoyo M, Gradner CL, Motta AO, Ashmead JW: Case report—skeletal muscle infarction in diabetes: MR findings. J Comput Assist Tomogr 17:986–988, 1993.
173. Oberlander MA, Shalvoy RM, Hughston JC: The accuracy of the clinical knee examination documented by arthroscopy: A prospective study. Am J Sports Med 21:773–778, 1993.
174. O'Brien WR: Degenerative arthritis of the knee following anterior cruciate ligament injury: Role of the meniscus. Sports Med Arthroscopy Rev 1:114–118, 1994.
175. Ohzono K, Saito M, Takaoka K, et al: Natural history of non-traumatic avascular necrosis of the femoral head. J Bone Joint Surg Br 73B: 68–72, 1991.
176. O'Keeffe D, Mamtora H: Ultrasound in clinical orthopaedics. J Bone Joint Surg Br 74B:488–494, 1992.
177. Ono K, Yamamuro T, Rockwood CA: Use of a thirty-degree caudal tilt radiograph in the shoulder impingement syndrome. J Shoulder Elbow Surg 1:246–252, 1992.
178. Osti OL, Fraser RD: MRI and discography of annular tears and intervertebral disc degeneration: A prospective clinical comparison. J Bone Joint Surg Br 74B:431–435, 1992.
179. Osti OL, Veron-Roberts B, Moore R, Fraser RD: Annular tears and disc degeneration in the lumbar spine: A post-mortem study of 135 discs. J Bone Joint Surg Br 74B:678–682, 1992.
180. Palmer EL, Scott JA, Straukse HW: Practical Nuclear Medicine. Philadelphia, WB Saunders, 1992.
181. Palmer WE, Brown JH, Rosenthal DI: Rotator cuff: Evaluation with fat-suppressed MR arthrography. Radiology 188:683–687, 1993.
182. Park JH, Vansant JP, Kumar NG, et al: Dermatomyositis: Correlative MR imaging and P-31 MR spectroscopy for quantitative characterization of inflammatory disease. Radiology 177:473–479, 1990.
183. Pech P, Haughton ML: Lumbar intervertebral disk: correlative MR and anatomic study. Radiology 156:699–701, 1985.
184. Peyster RG, Teplick JG, Haskin M: Computed tomography of lumbosacral conjoined nerve root anomalies: Potential cause of false-positive reading for herniated nucleus-pulposus. Spine 10:331–337, 1985.
185. Porter RW, Bewley B: A ten-year prospective study of vertebral canal size as a predictor of back pain. Spine 19:173–175, 1994.
186. Porter RW, Hibbert C, Evans C: The natural history of root entrapment syndrome. Spine 9:418–421, 1984.
187. Post MJD, et al: Spinal infection: Evaluation with MR imaging and intraoperative US. Radiology 169:765–771, 1988.
188. Puddu G, Ippolito E, Postacchini F: A classification of Achilles tendon disease. Am J Sports Med 4:145–150, 1976.
189. Raatikainen T, Putkonen M, Puranen J: Arthrography, clinical examination, and stress radiograph in the diagnosis of acute injury to the lateral ligaments of the ankle. Am J Sports Med 20:2–12, 1992.
190. Rafii M, Firooznia H, Sherman O, et al: Rotator cuff lesions: Signal patterns at MR imaging. Radiology 177:817–823, 1990.
191. Rak KM, Gillogly SD, Schaefer RA, et al: Anterior cruciate ligament reconstruction: Evaluation with MR imaging. Radiology 178:553–556, 1991.
192. Rangger C, Klestil T, Kathrein A, et al: Influence on magnetic resonance imaging on indications for arthroscopy of the knee. Clin Orth 330:133–142, 1996.
193. Rauschning W: Normal and pathologic anatomy of the lumbar root canals. Spine 12:1008–1019, 1987.
194. Regan W, Wold LE, Conrad R, Morrey BF: Microscopic histopathology of chronic refractory lateral epicondylitis. Am J Sports Med 20:746–749, 1992.
195. Remer EM, Fitzgerald SW, Friedman H, et al: Anterior cruciate ligament injury: MR imaging diagnosis and patterns of injury. RadioGraphics 12:901–915, 1991.
196. Resendes M, Helms CA, Fritz RC, et al: MR appearance of intramuscular injections. Am J Roentgenol 158:1293–1294, 1992.
197. Rijke AM, Goitz HT, McCue FC, Dee PM: Magnetic resonance imaging of injury to the lateral ankle ligaments. Am J Sports Med 21:528–534, 1993.
198. Rizzo PF, Gould ES, Lyden JP, Asnis SE: Diagnosis of occult fractures about the hip: Magnetic resonance imaging compared with bone-scanning. J Bone Joint Surg 75A:395–401, 1993.
199. Roberson GH, Llewellyn HJ, Taveras JM: The narrow lumbar spinal canal syndrome. Radiology 107:89–97, 1973.
200. Rogers LF, Hendrix RW: Radiography of fracture healing. Current Imaging 2:194–200, 1990.
201. Rose JL, Goldberg B: Basic Physics in Diagnostic Ultrasound. New York, Wiley, 1979.
202. Ross JS, Modic MT, Masaryk JJ: Tears of the anulus fibrosus: Assessment with Gd-DTPA-enhanced MR Imaging. Am J Roentgenol 154:159–162, 1990.
203. Ross J, et al: Lumbar spine: Postoperative assessment with surface-coil MR imaging. Radiology 164:851–860, 1987.
204. Rothman SLG, Glenn WV Jr: CT multiplanar reconstruction in 253 cases of lumbar spondylolysis. Am J Neuroradiol 5:81–90, 1984.
205. Rueter FG, Conway BJ, McCrohan JL, et al: Radiography of the lumbosacral spine: Characteristics of examinations performed in hospitals and facilities. Radiology 185:43–46, 1992.
206. Ruwe PA, Wright J, Randall RL, et al: Can MR imaging effectively replace diagnostic arthroscopy? Radiology 183:335–339, 1992.
207. Ryan JB, Wheeler JH, Hopkinson WJ, et al: Quadriceps contusions. Am J Sports Med 19:299–304, 1991.
208. Satku K, Kumar VP, Chacha PB: Stress fractures around the knee in elderly patients: A cause of acute pain in the knee. J Bone Joint Surg 72A: 918–922, 1990.
209. Sato K, et al: The configuration of the laminas and facet joints in degenerative spondylolisthesis and clinicocardiologic study. Spine 14:1265–1271, 1989.
210. Scavone JG, Latshaw RF, Weidner WA: Anteroposterior and lateral radiographs: An adequate lumbar spine examination. Am J Roentgenol 136:715–717, 1981.
211. Schnebel B, Kingston S, Watkins R, Dillin W: Comparison of MRI to contrast CT in the diagnosis of spinal stenosis. Spine 14:332–337, 1989.
212. Schneck DC, Mesgarzadeh M, Bonakdarpour A: MR imaging of the most commonly injured ankle ligaments: Part II—ligament injuries. Radiology 184:507–512, 1992.
213. Schneck DC: The anatomy of lumbar spondylosis. Clin Orthop 193:20–37, 1985.

214. Schweitzer ME, Caccese R, Karasick D, et al: Posterior tibial tendon tears: Utility of secondary signs for MR imaging diagnosis. Radiology 188:655–659, 1993.
215. Scott WW, Lethbridge-Cejku M, Reichle R, et al: Reliability of grading scales for individual radiographic features of osteoarthritis of the knee: The Baltimore longitudinal study of aging atlas of knee osteoarthritis. Invest Radiol 28:497–501, 1993.
216. Scranton PE, Farrar EL: Mucoid degeneration of the patellar ligament in athletes. J Bone Joint Surg 74A:435–437, 1992.
217. Seeger LL, Gold RH, Bassett LW, Ellman H: Shoulder impingement syndrome: MR findings in 53 shoulders. Am J Roentgenol 150:343–347, 1988.
218. Shaffer WO, Spratt KF, Weinstein J, et al: The consistency and accuracy of roentgenograms for measuring sagittal translation in the lumbar vertebral motion segment: An experimental model. Spine 15:741–750, 1990.
219. Shellock FG: Safety. In Stark DD, Bradley WG: Magnetic Resonance Imaging. St. Louis, Mosby-Year Book, 1992, pp 522–544.
220. Shintani S, Shiigai T: Repeat MRI in acute rhabdomyolysis: Correlation with clinicopathological findings. J Comput Assist Tomogr 17:786–791, 1993.
221. Sidor ML, Zuckerman JD, Lyon T, et al: The Neer classification system for proximal humeral fractures: An assessment of interobserver reliability and intraobserver reproducibility. J Bone Joint Surg 75A:1745–1750, 1993.
222. Smith MA, Jones EA, Strachan RK, et al: Prediction of fracture healing in the tibia by quantitative radionuclide imaging. J Bone Joint Surg Br 69B:441–447, 1987.
223. Sommerlath K, Lysholm J, Gillquist J: The long-term course after treatment of acute anterior cruciate ligament ruptures: A 9 to 16 year follow-up. Am J Sports Med 19:156–162, 1991.
224. Speer KP, Lohnes J, Garrett WE: Radiographic imaging of muscle strain injury. Am J Sports Med 21:89–96, 1993.
225. Speer KP, Spritzer CE, Goldner JL, Garrett WE: Magnetic resonance imaging of traumatic knee articular cartilage injuries. Am J Sports Med 19:396–402, 1991.
226. Spiers ASD, Meagher T, Ostlere SJ, et al: Can MRI of the knee affect arthroscopic practice? J Bone Joint Surg Br 75B:49–52, 1993.
227. Spindler KP, Schils JP, Bergfeld JA, et al: Prospective study of osseous, articular, and meniscal lesions in recent anterior cruciate ligament tears by magnetic resonance imaging and arthroscopy. Am J Sports Med 21:551–557, 1993.
228. Sprawls P Jr: Physical Principles of Medical Imaging. Gaithersburg, MD, Aspen Publishers, 1987.
229. Stadnik TW, Lee RR, Coen HL, et al: Annular tears and disk herniation: Prevalence and contrast enhancement on MR images in the absence of low back pain and sciatica. Radiology 206:49–55, 1998.
230. Stallenberg B, Gevenois PA, Sintzoff SA, et al: Fracture of the posterior aspect of the lateral tibial plateau: Radiographic sign of anterior cruciate ligament tear. Radiology 187:821–825, 1993.
231. Sterling JC, Webb RF, Meyers MC, Calvo RD: False-negative bone scan in a female runner. Med Sci Sports Exerc 25:179–185, 1993.
232. Sze G, et al: Malignant extradural spinal tumors: MR imaging with gadolinium-DTPA. Radiology 167:217–223, 1988.
233. Szypryt EP, et al: The prevalence of disc degeneration associated with neural arch defects of the lumbar spine assessed by magnetic resonance imaging. Spine 14:977–981, 1989.
234. Takatori Y, Kokubo T, Ninomiya S, et al: Avascular necrosis of the femoral head: Natural history and magnetic resonance imaging. J Bone Joint Surg Br 75B:217–221, 1993.
235. Teresi LM, Lufkin RB, Reicher MA, et al: Asymptomatic degenerative disc disease and spondylosis of the cervical spine: MR Imaging. Radiology 164:83–88, 1987.
236. Tervonen O, Mueller DM, Matteson EL, et al: Clinically occult avascular necrosis of the hip: Prevalence in an asymptomatic population at risk. Radiology 182:845–847, 1992.
237. Thornbury JR, Fryback DG, Turski PA, et al: Disc-caused nerve compression in patients with acute low-back pain: Diagnosis with MR, CT myelography, and plain CT. Radiology 186:731–738, 1993.
238. Torgerson WR, Dotter WE: Comparative roentgenographic study of the asymptomatic and symptomatic lumbar spine. J Bone Joint Surg 58A:850–853, 1976.
239. Tountas AA: Insufficiency stress fractures of the femoral neck in elderly women. Clin Orthop 292:202–209, 1993.
240. Traughber PD, Goodwin TE: Shoulder MRI: Arthroscopic correlation with emphasis on partial tears. J Comput Assist Tomogr 16:129–133, 1992.
241. Tullberg T, Grane P, Isacson J: Gadolinium-enhanced magnetic resonance imaging of 36 patients one year after lumbar disc resection. Spine 19:176–182, 1994.
242. Tung GA, Davis LM, Wiggins ME, Fadale PD: Tears of the anterior cruciate ligament: Primary and secondary signs at MR imaging. Radiology 188:661–667, 1993.
243. Turner DA, Templeton AC, Selzer PM, et al: Femoral capital osteonecrosis: MR findings of diffuse marrow abnormalities without focal lesions. Radiology 171:135–140, 1989.
244. Vahey TN, Broome DR, Kayes KJ, Shelbourne KD: Acute and chronic tears of the anterior cruciate ligament: Differential features at MRI imaging. Radiology 181:251–253, 1991.
245. Vahey TN, Hunt JE, Shelbourne KD: Anterior translocation of the tibia at MR imaging: A secondary sign of anterior cruciate ligament tear. Radiology 187:817–819, 1993.
246. Vande Berg B, Malghem J, Labaisse MA, et al: Avascular necrosis of the hip: Comparison of contrast-enhanced and nonenhanced MR imaging with histologic correlation (work in progress). Radiology 182:445–450, 1992.
247. Vande Berg BE, Malghem JJ, Labaisse MA, et al: MR imaging of avascular necrosis and transient marrow edema of the femoral head. Radio-Graphics 13:501–520, 1993.
248. Vande Berg B, Malghem J, Labaisse MA, et al: Apparent focal bone marrow ischemia in patients with marrow disorders: MR studies. J Comput Assist Tomogr 17:792–797, 1993.
249. Vallet AD, Marks PH, Fowler PJ, Munro TG: Occult post-traumatic osteochondral lesions of the knee: Prevalence, classification, and short-term sequelae evaluated with MR imaging. Radiology 178:271–276, 1991.
250. Verbiest H: Fallacies of the present definition, nomenclature, and classification of the stenosis of the lumbar vertebral canal. Spine 1:217–225, 1976.
251. Verbiest H: Results of surgical treatment of idiopathic development stenosis of the lumbar vertebral canal. J Bone Joint Surg 59B:181–188, 1977.
252. Verbiest H: Words images knowledge, and reality: Some reflections from the neurosurgical perspective. Acta Neurochirurgica 69:163–193, 1983.
253. Verhaven EFC, Shahabpour M, Handelberg FWJ, et al: The accuracy of three-dimensional magnetic resonance imaging in the diagnosis of ruptures of the lateral ligaments of the ankle. Am J Sports Med 19:583–587, 1991.
254. Virolainen H, Visuri T, Juusela T: Acute dislocation of the patella: MR findings. Radiology 189:243–246, 1993.
255. Walsh TR, Weinstein JN, Spratt KF, et al: Lumbar discography in normal subjects. J Bone Joint Surg 72A:1081–1088, 1990.
256. Weber WN, Newmann CH, Barakos JA, et al: Lateral tibial rim (segond) fractures: MR imaging characteristics. Radiology 180:731–734, 1991.
257. Weiner DS, Macnab I: Superior migration of the humeral head: A radiological aid in the diagnosis of tears of the rotator cuff. J Bone Joint Surg 52B:524–527, 1970.

258. Weinstabl R, Stiskal M, Neuhold A, et al: Classifying calcaneal tendon injury according to MRI findings. J Bone Joint Surg Br 73B:683–685, 1991.
259. Wiesel SE, Tsourmas N, Feffer H, et al: A study of computer-assisted tomography: The incidence of positive CAT scans in an asymptomatic group of patients. Spine 9:549–551, 1984.
260. Wiener SN, Seitz WH: Sonography of the shoulder in patients with tears of the rotator cuff: accuracy and value for selecting surgical options: Am J Roentgenol 160:103–107, 1993.
261. Whalen JP, Balter S: Radiation Risks in Medical Imaging. Chicago, Year Book Medical Publishers, 1984.
262. Williams AL, et al: Computed tomographic appearance of the bulging annulus. Radiology 142:403–408, 1982.
263. Wiltse L: Far-out syndrome. In Rothman LG, Glenn WV (eds): Multiplanar CT of the Spine. Baltimore, University Park Press, 1985, pp 384–393.
264. Witt I, Vestergaard A, Rosenklint A: A comparative analysis of x-ray findings of the lumbar spine in patients with and without lumbar pain. Spine 9:299–300, 1984.
265. Wright JG, Feinstein AR: Improving the reliability of orthopedic measurements. J Bone Joint Surg 74B:287–291, 1992.
266. Yamato M, Yamagishi T: MRI of patellar tendon anterior cruciate ligament autografts. J Comput Assist Tomogr 16:604–607, 1992.
267. Yao L, Sinha S, Seeger LL: MR imaging of joints: Analytic optimization of GRE techniques at 1.5 T. Am J Roentgenol 158:339–345, 1992.
268. Yasuma T, Ohno R, Yamauchi Y: False-negative lumbar discograms: Correlation of discographic and histological findings in postmortem and surgical specimens. J Bone Joint Surg 70A:1279–1290, 1988.
269. Yu S, et al: Progressive and regressive changes in the nucleus pulposus: Part II—the adult. Radiology 169:93–97, 1988.
270. Yu S, et al: Criteria for classifying normal and degenerated lumbar intervertebral discs. Radiology 170:523–526, 1989.
271. Yuy WTC, Drew JM, Weinstein JN, et al: Intraspinal synovial cysts: Magnetic resonance evaluation. Spine 16:740–745, 1991.
272. Zeiss J, Saddemi SR, Ebraheim NA: MR imaging of the quadriceps tendon: Normal layered configuration and its importance in cases of tendon rupture. Am J Roentgenol 159:1031–1034, 1992.
273. Zucherman J, et al: Normal magnetic resonance imaging with abnormal discography. Spine 13:1355–1359, 1988.

CHAPTER

Cumulative Trauma

THOMAS J. ARMSTRONG, PhD

This chapter is concerned with cumulative trauma disorders of the upper limb. Cumulative trauma disorders are defined as disorders that are caused, precipitated, or aggravated by repeated exertions or movements of the body. This definition reflects the philosophy of most workers' compensation laws in the United States (see Chapters 4 and 5) and most Western countries. Whether work is a primary cause or an aggravating cause of these disorders is not always clear; however, the way the laws are written, the employer will generally be held responsible unless there is clear and convincing evidence to the contrary. From a disability or an occupational health perspective, the question is not "what causes" but "what might cause" cumulative trauma disorders.

CHARACTERISTICS

The term cumulative trauma disorder is a general name used for disorders with similar characteristics.[7] The most commonly affected tissues of the body include muscles, tendons, and nerves. Frequent diagnoses are myalgia, tendinitis, and carpal tunnel syndrome. A detailed description of the signs and symptoms of these disorders is beyond the scope of this chapter; however, they are often poorly localized, nonspecific, and episodic. Symptoms tend to develop over periods of weeks, months, or even years and recovery similarly requires long periods. These traits often make it difficult to determine the exact time of onset or specific causes of the disorders. Cumulative trauma disorders may go unreported. Workers may not associate their symptoms with specific job-related activities. They may be afraid to report them to management. Workers can be very resourceful in finding ways of coping so that cases go unreported.

The causes of upper limb cumulative trauma disorders are not fully understood, but they are believed to involve multiple factors. The World Health Organization (WHO)[109] has recognized upper limb disorders as being both "personal" and "work related." Personal factors refer to characteristics of the individual (e.g., sex, age, body size and composition, acute and chronic diseases). Work factors refer to characteristics of the job (e.g., work rates, duration, forces, locations, environments). Work-related factors appear to involve common mechanical and physiologic mechanisms.[7,83,84,108]

Upper limb cumulative trauma disorders are a major cause of worker impairment and disability. Some people refer to cumulative trauma disorders as the epidemic of the 1990s; however, Ramazzini described these disorders in 1713[92]:

> Various and manifold is the harvest of diseases reaped by certain workers from the crafts and trades that they pursue. All the profit that they get is fatal injury to their health, mostly from two causes. The first and most potent is the harmful character of the materials they handle ... The second, I ascribe to certain violent and irregular motions and unnatural postures of the body, by reason of which, the natural structure of the vital machine is so impaired that serious diseases gradually develop therefrom.

Ramazzini went on to describe and trace the causes of these problems among various kinds of workers of his time, such as scribes, bakers, and weavers[92]:

> The maladies that afflict the clerks aforesaid arise from three causes: First, constant sitting, secondly the incessant movement of the hand and always the same direction, thirdly the strain on the mind from the effort not to disfigure the books by errors or cause loss to their

employers when they add, subtract, or do other sums in arithmetic.

The modern-day scribe would most likely use a computer, but still would be exposed to "constant sitting," "incessant movement of the hand," and "strain on the mind." Likewise, most bakers no longer hand-mix bread, but they are exposed to similar physical stresses in the handling of ingredients and packaging of products. Also, workers in the upholstery, plastic, and rubber industries are exposed to similar stresses. In addition to "unnatural postures," these stresses include forceful exertions, repeated or sustained exertions, and mechanical contact stresses.

Ramazzini characterized most musculoskeletal disorders as swelling and fatigue, which was disabling in some cases[92]:

> An acquaintance of mine, a notary by profession, still living, used to spend his whole life continually engaged in writing, and he made a good deal of money by it; first he began to complain of intense fatigue in the whole arm but no remedy could relieve this, and finally the whole right arm become completely paralyzed. In order to offset this infirmity he began to train himself to write with the left hand, but it was not very long before it too was attacked by the same malady.

There may be a tendency to question the validity of worker complaints of pain or other subjective symptoms. There may be suspicion that the worker is motivated by secondary gain. One wonders what secondary gain could have motivated the eighteenth-century workers described by Ramazzini.

Fatigue is an accepted side effect of work in most situations and is not considered compensable; however, chronic muscle, tendon, and nerve disorders should not be accepted and may be compensable. Nearly all human activities involve some pain. The question is how much is too much and when are work or medical interventions warranted. It can be shown that the incidence and severity of pain increases with certain physical activities, but there is not yet a standard for how much pain is excessive.[24,26,95] Only the individual experiencing the pain can say how much is too much for him- or herself. Identification and control of musculoskeletal disorders can be very frustrating if there is no trust among workers, employers, and health care providers. Cailliet[20] describes chronic pain as the "most serious disabling condition of humans" and suggests that pain should be considered a disease, not merely a symptom. He also suggests that trauma and inflammation of soft tissue figure heavily into the cause of musculoskeletal pain[20]: "All musculoskeletal pain may be considered a sequela of soft tissue injury, irritation, or inflammation. Trauma in the broadest concept of the term is the greatest cause of soft tissue pain and functional impairment."

Pain may be accompanied by objective physiologic signs that can be evaluated using objective tests, including range of motion tests, provocative tests, and nerve conduction testing (see also Chapters 33 and 39). Standardized protocols have helped to improve the objectivity of diagnostic criteria for specific muscle, tendon, and nerve disorders.[32,35,52,58,105] These tests are often used for epidemiologic studies.

There have been some attempts to evaluate these tests quantitatively by comparing them with so-called "objective" tests.[34,51] Katz[51] compared diagnostic results based on the criteria used by the National Institute for Occupational Safety and Health (NIOSH) for carpal tunnel syndrome with those based on nerve conduction studies. Nerve conduction studies are generally regarded as the gold standard for diagnosing carpal tunnel syndrome. Katz found that 67% of all persons meeting the NIOSH criteria[51,72] had carpal tunnel syndrome using objective nerve conduction tests, 58% of those with negative findings had negative nerve conduction tests, and the test could predict only 50% of the population with positive or negative nerve conduction findings. Studies by Homan et al[47] also found a poor correlation among electrodiagnostic abnormalities, physical findings, and symptoms. These studies raise questions about what is carpal tunnel syndrome. Franklin et al[33] proposed that carpal tunnel syndrome identified from workers' compensation reports was less severe than that reported in clinical case series. Rempel et al[94] proposed consensus criteria for the classification of carpal tunnel syndrome in epidemiologic studies. Normal objective test findings may be a small consolation to a worker in pain. Similarly, a patient with no symptoms and positive nerve conduction tests may be a dilemma to the healthcare provider or employer. Pain and other fatigue-like symptoms are likely to continue as a major issue in the diagnosis and treatment of upper limb musculoskeletal disorders.

MORBIDITY PATTERNS

The earliest estimates of the incidence and prevalence of cumulative trauma disorders came from insurance records or clinical case series reports. Zollinger[111] reported some 1927 cases of crepitant tenosynovitis from Swiss insurance records. Obolenskaja and Goljanitzki[85] suggested that high rates of work, 7600 to 12,000 exertions per shift, were a major factor in 189 cases of tenosynovitis of the upper extremities among a group of 700 packers in a tea factory.[59] Conn[25] reported that tenosynovitis accounted for approximately 1% of lost days in the Ohio rubber industry in 1930.

Clinics specializing in services to employers and inplant medical departments are another source of information about musculoskeletal morbidity patterns. Reed and Harcourt[93] reported that 70 persons with tenosynovitis accounted for 0.54% of all visits to the Indianapolis Industrial Clinic and resulted in 1222 lost days in a 12-month period. Thompson et al[102] reported that 466 of 544 patients with peritendinitis crepitans and simple tenosynovitis, seen between 1941 to 1950 at a British hospital and outpatient service, were manual workers and agricultural workers. They also reported 40 cases annually with an average absence of 21 days at the Vauxhall Motors Company, which employed 12,000 persons. Hymovich and Lindholm[48] described 66 cases of repetitive trauma disorders reported during a 6-year period in 160 persons employed in the manufacturing of electrical-mechanical products. This corresponds to an incidence rate of 6.6 cases per 100 workers per year or per 200,000 work hours. Fine et al[31] showed that the incidence rates of cumulative trauma disorders at two similar and nearby automobile assembly plants, based on required Occupational Safety and Health Association (OSHA) records, were significantly lower than those based on workers' compensation reports (0.03 to 0.15 versus 0.29 to 0.45 cases per 200,000 work hours) and rates based on personal medical absences (0.3 to 0.4 versus 3.0 to 1.8 cases per 200,000 work hours). They found that incidence rates of plant medical visits varied significantly between the two plants (2.0 and 14.0 cases per 100 workers per year) and that at one plant the incidence rate was less than the rate based on personal medical absences. Failure to report all likely cases on the OSHA records has been a cause of OSHA litigation.[27]

Threat of OSHA action and clarification of OSHA recordkeeping requirements along with increased awareness of possible work relatedness has no doubt contributed to increased reports of musculoskeletal disorders as a work-related problem. According to the Bureau of Labor Statistics,[18] the incidence of "repeated motion" disorders was 3 per 10,000 workers per year from 1978 to 1984. Since then it has increased steadily to nearly 30 cases per 10,000 workers per year. Franklin et al[33] reported an incidence rate of 17.4 cases of carpal tunnel syndrome per 10,000 full-time equivalent (FTE) workers in the state of Washington from 1984 to 1986. They reported that the highest rates were among workers in food processing (100 to 250 cases per 10,000 FTE workers) and those in carpentry, wood products, and logging (60 to 110 cases per 10,000 FTE workers). Other studies have attempted to identify specific causes of cumulative trauma disorders by examining the association among morbidity patterns, work patterns, and worker attributes.

By systematically selecting workers based on work exposure and personal attributes, morbidity patterns can be used to identify common risk factors or to test hypothesized associations between disorders and risk factors. Duncan and Ferguson[29] compared the work behavior of 90 male telegraphers with diagnosed myalgia to a group without this disorder to test the hypothesis that there is an association between certain work postures and myalgia. Subjects were matched by sex, age, duration of service, and status. The authors concluded that differences in keyboard design and work height resulting in different operating postures were factors in the myalgia. To test the hypothesis that repetitive work is a factor in tenosynovitis, Luopajarvi et al[69] compared a group of 163 female assembly line packers who performed machine-paced work with up to 25,000 cycles per day to 143 female retail shop assistants who performed nonrepetitive cashier work. The prevalence of hand and wrist tenosynovitis was 56% among the group performing high-repetitive work versus only 14% among the group performing low-repetitive work. By comparing keyboard operators with repetitive strain disorders and job-matched operators without injuries, Oxenburgh[88] concluded that repetitive strain injuries were associated with use of keyboards for more than 5 hours per shift. Using a longitudinal study design, Waersted et al[103] later reported that short work shifts appeared to delay but not prevent musculoskeletal disorders.

Silverstein et al[96] and Armstrong et al[8] found repetition and force were both associated with the prevalence of carpal tunnel syndrome and hand and wrist tendinitis. Their cross-sectional study design entailed identification of four job categories at each of seven worksites. They then randomly selected at least 20 workers from each job category while maintaining overall sex and age balance across the study groups. They studied a total of 652 workers (89.7% participation rate). The prevalence of carpal tunnel syndrome and hand-wrist tendinitis was determined from interviews and physical examinations of all workers. Avocation activities were investigated, but none was found to be significant.

Nathan et al[78] compared the prevalence of carpal tunnel syndrome using electrodiagnosis among five job classes of "repetition" and "resistance." The prevalence of persons with impaired median sensory conduction increased significantly from the lowest to the highest job-stress class; the prevalence of persons with bilateral slowing increased from the lowest to the second highest job-stress class but decreased for the highest-stress class job. This led them to conclude that carpal tunnel syndrome is not related to work. The low prevalence in the highest job-stress class suggests a "healthy worker" effect in which workers who are adversely affected by physical work stresses associated with a given job leave that job by going onto disability, transferring into another less-stressful job, or quitting—in each case only the survivors are available for study. The results also could be affected by sampling biases, age, and sex, which were not discussed.

Barnhart et al[12] also utilized a cross-sectional study design to evaluate the relationship between repetition and carpal tunnel syndrome among workers at a ski manufacturing plant. They reported a significantly higher prevalence of electrodiagnostic and physical signs among persons performing repetitive work than among those performing nonrepetitive work (15.4% versus 3.1%).

Latko et al[60] found a strong relationship between repetitive work and carpal tunnel syndrome based on symptoms, symptoms plus electrodiagnostic findings, tendonitis symptoms, and nonspecific musculoskeletal pain. Repetition was assessed using a 0 to 10 rating scale much like engineers use to develop time standards.[61] The prevalence of symptoms was found to increase in proportion to increases in repetition and did not suggest a threshold below which the risk was zero.

Stevens et al[98] examined medical records from the Mayo Clinic from 1961 through 1980. Because the Mayo Clinic was the only provider of medical services in the Rochester, Minnesota area, it was assumed that these cases represented all of the cases in the community. An age-adjusted incidence rate of 52 and 149 cases per 100,000 person-years was reported for males and females, respectively. It was found that the incidence increased with age, but peaked for women between the ages of 45 and 54. A similar study was performed at the Marshfield Clinic in Wisconsin by Nordstrom et al,[82] who reported an incidence rate for newly diagnosed or probable carpal tunnel syndrome of 346 cases per 100,000 person-years. Further analysis identified associations between both personal and work-related factors and carpal tunnel syndrome. The most significant personal factors pertained to body weight. Work factors included the use of power tools and worker control over the job. The study specifically did not include keyboard work. DeKrom et al[28] reported a prevalence of 5.6% in male and female respondents in a community-based study in Maastricht, The Netherlands. When comparing persons with symptoms to those without symptoms, they found carpal tunnel syndrome to be associated with working with a flexed or extended wrist, hysterectomy with oophorectomy, menopause, and obesity. Tanaka et al[100] are among the few investigators to study an upper limb musculoskeletal disorder other than carpal tunnel syndrome. Using the Occupational Health Supplement Data of the 1988 National Health Interview Survey, they found that 0.46% of the 127 million people who had worked during the proceeding 12 months reported that they experienced "prolonged" hand discomfort, which was called tendinitis, synovitis, tenosynovitis, de Quervain disease, epicondylitis, ganglion cyst, or trigger finger by medical personnel. The actual prevalence may have been higher as many persons with hand injuries do not seek medical attention. Twenty-eight percent of these cases were thought to be work-related by the medical assessor. Bending or twisting of the hands or wrists at work and female sex were associated with these disorders.

These studies show that the incidence rate of musculoskeletal disorders and particularly carpal tunnel syndrome in community populations is high. The rate variation from study to study is likely due to differences in reporting, diagnostic criteria and awareness, and attitudes of patients and health care providers.

Available morbidity studies show that the prevalence of cumulative trauma disorders increases with increasing exposures to work-related physical stresses; however, it is important to recognize that there appears to be background prevalence even for the lowest levels of repetitive work. These data can be characterized as an exposure-response relationship between repetitions (Fig. 15–1).[60,96] This relationship is critically important for development of work design specifications. Further studies are required to reach agreement on definitions of risk factors and diagnostic criteria and to then determine the point where risk is significantly elevated. Such studies will need to consider not only the effects of repetition, but also interactions with force, posture, vibration, and other physical work stresses.

Personal factors (e.g., systemic diseases, nutrition, fitness, weight, age, sex, pregnancy) are also important in the cause of these disorders.[1,22,28,33,79,80,106] Theoretically, it should be possible to evaluate workers and work for these factors and control them through selection, training, or job redesign. There are several barriers to control through selection. Present U.S. regulations place a high burden on the employer to demonstrate that the worker has a condition that has a high likelihood of resulting in illness or injury and that it is not possible to accommodate that worker through job modifications.[3] None of the factors are perfect predictors of risk (i.e., their sensitivities and specificities are all below 100%).[44,51] Even if a given factor has a high sensitivity and specificity, it will discriminate against some qualified workers. For example, consider a potential population of 100 people. Assume that 10% of the

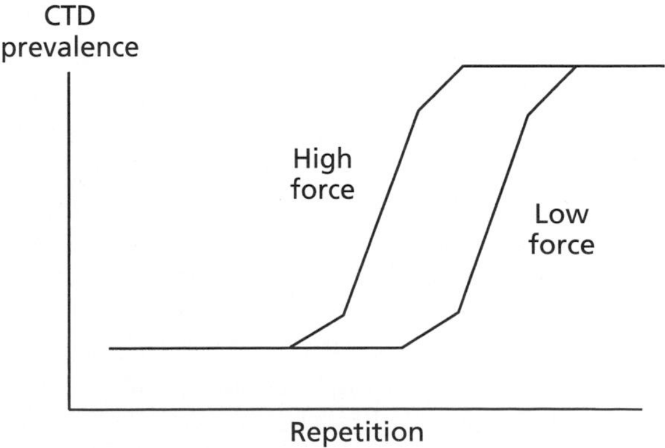

Figure 15–1. Generic exposure–response relationship for repetition, force, and cumulative trauma disorders (CTD).

population has a condition that is predictive of a future disorder. If the factor has a sensitivity and specificity both equal to 90%, then it will correctly identify 9 of the 10 people at risk who would develop disorders, but it would also falsely identify 9 out of 90 people who would not develop disorders. If a factor has a sensitivity of 90% but a specificity of only 50%, it would still identify 9 of the 10 people at risk, but it would also falsely identify 45 people out of 90 as at risk. Most studies of personal risk factors are based on clinical populations. These cases would represent the extreme cases included in the low exposure end of the curve shown in Figure 15–1. It is doubtful that reliable and legal studies that can identify persons who will develop cumulative trauma disorders, as a result of work before they are hired, will be available in the foreseeable future.

MECHANISMS

The mechanisms underlying the development of upper-limb disorders are not fully understood. Armstrong et al[7] proposed a multistage model in which exposure to work activities produces a series of mechanical and physiologic events. Mechanical mechanisms involve the transmission of forces through the body to counteract gravity, inertial and drag forces on work objects, and the body itself. The tissues of the body, like any material, deform when subjected to a force. The direction and magnitude of the deformation depend on the direction and magnitude of the force and the tissue characteristics.

Figure 15–2 shows a simplified longitudinal view of the wrist. Contraction of the forearm flexor muscles pulls on the finger flexor tendons; this pull force is transmitted through the tendons to the second and third phalanges.[17] Newton's second law states that exertion of a force on an object will cause that object to accelerate in the direction of the force and in proportion to its mass. This means that the tendon will move and the phalanges will rotate toward the contracting muscle. Contraction of the finger flexor muscles causes the joints to rotate in a direction that closes the fist. Contraction of the extensor muscles causes the joint to rotate in a direction that opens the fist. The position of the hand is controlled by a very delicate mechanical equilibrium between those forces that open the fist and those that close the fist.[17] If the moments closing the fist exceed those opening the fist, the interphalangeal joints will rotate in a direction that closes the fist. This rotation will occur until the fingers come into contact with an external object or with another part of the body. As the fingers press against another surface, moments will be produced that oppose those produced by the contracting muscle. This can be seen by tightly closing the fist around a handle or against itself. If the fingers do not encounter another object the joints will rotate until the limits of joint motion are reached. As the joint reaches the limits of its range of motion, it becomes very stiff and resists further rotation. This can be seen by opening the fist to its full extent.

In addition to the forces produced by muscles, acceleration, and passive joint rotation, there are also friction forces on tendon and joint tissues. Friction forces are proportional to velocity. The moving parts of the body, such as tendons, are generally well-lubricated; however, certain disorders result in increased friction. In extreme cases, adhesions may form between tendons and adjacent structures that further impair function.

Forces are classified according to the direction of their action and tissue deformation.[62,89] Pull forces that act perpendicular to the surface and cause tissue elongation are classified as tensors. Push forces that act perpendicular to the surface and cause tissue shortening are classified as compressors. Forces that act parallel to the surface, such as those produced by friction, are classified as shear forces which cause angular deformation of tissue. The effect of a force is related to the area over which it is distributed; therefore, forces are normally expressed as a stress or force per unit area. Similarly, deformations are generally related to the size of the object over which the stress is acting; therefore, deformations are normally expressed as a strain, or the deformation divided by the size of the object. Strains due to compressive and tensile stresses are often expressed as percent shortening or lengthening. Strains due to shear stress are expressed in angular units. The amount of strain produced for a given amount of stress is related to the stiffness of the material. The stiffness of biological tissues increases as they are stretched. Some tissues, such as skin, may stretch several percent before their stiffness increases significantly.[5] This characteristic of skin tends to equalize stress concentrations over the external surface of the body. The stiffness of other tissues, such as tendons, increases very rapidly with the application of a stress.[40] This characteristic facilitates the

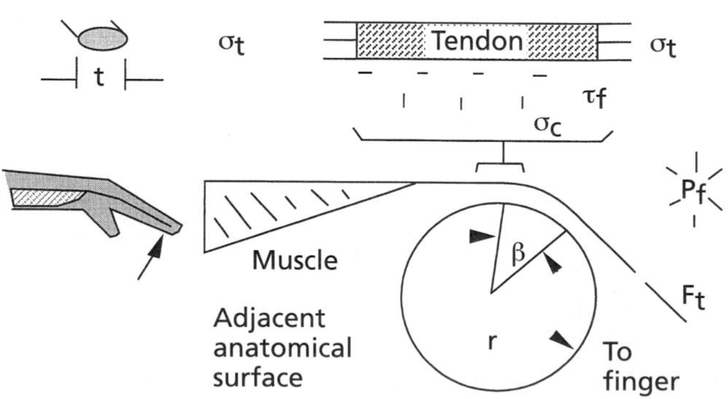

Figure 15–2. The tendons in the wrist can be characterized as a belt stretched around a pulley and subjected to fluid pressure (P_f) and tensile (σ_t), compressive (σ_c), and shear stresses (τ_f).

transmission of force from muscles to the skeletal system.

In addition to the tension forces produced by muscles on the tendon, the tendons are also exposed to compressive forces. The finger flexor tendons in the carpal tunnel are of particular interest because of their possible involvement in carpal tunnel syndrome. These tendons and their adjacent anatomic structures inside the carpal tunnel (Fig. 15–2) have been characterized as anatomic belts and pulleys.[10,62] It can be shown that pressures sufficient to interfere with nourishment of tendon, synovial, and nerve tissues are produced by maximum exertions of the hand. Most workers do not maintain maximum exertions for prolonged periods; however, prolonged exertions at even a few percent of maximum strength are sufficient to affect these tissues adversely. Because these forces are exerted only between the tendon and supporting structure, the nerve is affected by this mechanism only in flexion. Exertion with the flexed wrist forms the basis of the well-known Phalen or wrist flexion test.[90,97]

Compressive stresses also result from increased fluid pressure. Muscles and tendons are arranged in compartments that can be characterized as fluid-filled sponges encased in a distensible membrane. Fluid pressure is uniformly distributed on the surfaces of the compartment and its contents. Fluid pressure may also be increased by an enlarged fluid volume associated with past trauma.[6] Although the mechanics of these complex structures have not been well described, the magnitude of fluid pressure change is related to the change in compartment shape and volume.[16]

There now have been a number of studies of intracarpal canal pressures using catheters inserted into the carpal canal. These studies demonstrate that the pressure can be increased by certain postures and repetitive exertions. Pressures as high as 4.0 kilopascals (30 mm Hg) have been reported in extension of the wrist.[54,107] Wrist extension appears to reduce the cross-sectional area of the carpal canal and draw the ends of the flexor muscles into the carpal canal. Although fluid pressure changes inside the carpal tunnel are not as high as the stress produced by contact between the tendons and the walls of the carpal tunnel, they affect the nerve regardless of posture. Also, increased fluid pressure may occur without exertion of force while a worker is seemingly at rest.

Fluid pressure inside the carpal tunnel can be increased by external contact or pressure. This occurs when the wrist is exerted against an external object such as a hand tool or work surface. These stresses are related to the contact force divided by the area of contact. Lundborg et al[67,68] demonstrated that pressures of 8 and 12 kPa (60 and 90 mm) produced by pressure on the base of the wrist were sufficient to impair nerve viability and function.

Rempel et al showed that mouse use is associated with increased intercarpal canal pressure that may play a role in increased risk of carpal tunnel syndrome for jobs that require mouse use.[94]

Friction or shear stresses are produced in dynamic exertions at locations where the tendons slide against adjacent anatomic surfaces.[62] Because shear forces act parallel to the surface of the tissue, they are not directly comparable to fluid or compressive stresses. The movement of tendons past adjacent surfaces is lubricated by synovial fluid produced by the synovial sheaths. Synovial fluid also nourishes the tendons and plays a role in repair of tendon damage.

Tensile, compressive, and shear stresses all cause some degree of elastic or viscous deformation in biological tissues. Elastic deformation occurs immediately as a stress is applied or removed. Viscous deformation occurs after the load is applied or removed.[40,77,101] If the recovery time between successive exertions is not long enough for a given force and duration, the recovery will not be complete and the tendon will be stretched further with each successive exertion. Critical recovery times for given work-rest profiles have not yet been determined.

It has been shown that excessive stress will result in mechanical failure or yielding of tendons. In addition to acute mechanical effects resulting from high, prolonged, or repeated exertions, there may be delayed effects involving physiologic mechanisms. For example, Z-line disruption can be seen immediately after eccentric muscle loading, but elevation of serum creatine kinase and muscle pain may be delayed.[36,41–43,81] Wound healing following microrupture of muscle connective tissue or tendons is characterized by three stages[104]: 1) the inflammatory stage, which includes infiltration of polymorphonuclear cells, capillary budding, and exudation; 2) the reparative stage, which includes accumulation of fibroblasts that produce randomly oriented and attached collagen fibers and begins in about 1 week; and 3) the remolding stage which includes realignment of collagen fibers with normal alignment and begins in about a month and possibly continues for several months. This healing process is characterized as extrinsic because it involves infiltration of cells from other tissues. Gelberman and others have put forth an intrinsic healing model for tendons that does not involve external tissues but does involve a series of cellular changes that proceed over a similar time frame.[37]

Mechanical forces interfere with normal physiologic processes well before mechanical damage occurs. Exertions above 15% of maximum strength are sufficient to impair muscle circulation and accelerate fatigue.[11,63] Intramuscular pressure and distortion of the vascular bed appear to increase with increasing muscle tension. Studies of skin show that cutaneous circulation will be restricted by much lower tensions than are required for mechanical tissue failure. Kenedi et al[55] suggested that physiologic limits are more meaningful than mechanical limits. Increased intramuscular pressure may also impair perfusion of adjacent tendons and contribute to ischemic tendon damage.[45,46] The mechanisms of nerve entrapments also appear to involve an ischemic mechanism due to external pressure.[67] Pressure may be due to the acute effects of repeated exertions or certain postures, or to a secondary effect due to thickening of the adjacent tissues.[65,90,97,99] Thickening of the flexor synovium in the carpal tunnel is a common finding in patients with carpal tunnel syndrome.[6,90,110]

In addition to muscles and tendons, ligaments are important load-bearing tissue in certain work activities. Basmajian[13] showed that in certain arm positions the muscles of the shoulder relax and transfer the weight of the upper limb to ligaments. Later studies showed that force-induced pain in these ligaments is a limiting factor of work performance.[14,30] The mechanism of pain was not proposed, but it most likely entailed mechanical strain. Gamekeeper's thumb is perhaps the most extreme example of mechanical failure of a ligament caused by repetitive force.[21]

Muscle contraction triggers a series of physiologic processes. These processes entail the consumption of substrate (e.g., creatine phosphates, oxygen, glycogen, fatty acids) and the accumulation of by-products (e.g., lactates and heat)—all of which contribute to fatigue.[14,19,23] Increased intramuscular circulation is required to restore substrates and remove by-products. Sufficient circulation is not possible at high levels of contraction due to disruption of the vascular bed. In addition, muscle contraction entails the release of calcium and potassium into the interstitial spaces; there is evidence that elevated calcium ion concentrations attack cell membranes and increase their susceptibility to damage by free radicals produced during reoxygenation of hypoxic tissue.[49,66] Further studies are necessary to determine the short- and long-term physiologic limits for tendon and nerve loading in order to plan safe work schedules.

RECOMMENDATIONS

Sufficient data have not been accumulated to develop work-design guidelines based on a given level of risk for a given disorder. In the absence of such data and in the presence of regulations regarding worker safety and health, workers' compensation, and nondiscrimination, employers must be vigilant in recognizing work factors that might cause cumulative trauma disorders and workers who might be experiencing cumulative trauma disorders. Suspect jobs and workers can then be evaluated. The available data provide insight into the development of interventions, but it is essential that all work and medical interventions be evaluated to ascertain their effectiveness.

There are currently no national ergonomics standards. The U.S. Department of Labor/OSHA has a recordkeeping requirement, but there is a moratorium on reporting musculoskeletal and hearing injuries. The General Duty Clause Section 5(a)(1) of the Occupational Safety and Health Act of 1970[87] specifies that each employer " ... shall furnish to each of his employees employment and a place of employment which are free from recognized hazards that are causing or are likely to cause death or serious physical harm to his employees ... " In addition, Section 8(c)(2), Record Keeping, specifies that each employer[87] " ... shall make, keep and preserve, and make available to the Secretary ... such records regarding his activities relating to this Act." The General Duty Clause has been used in the past to encourage employers to develop ergonomic programs for preventing musculoskeletal disorders. Records of these citations and the latest OSHA guidelines can be found on their Web site www.osha.gov.

Many employers have developed their own programs for control of upper-limb cumulative trauma disorders.[36,76] Programs are generally designed to fit the needs of each organization.[2] A generic organization chart that can be adapted to most employers is shown in Figure 15–3. A program plan should state the objectives and lay out the necessary tasks, steps, and schedules for achieving them. The organizational aspects of an

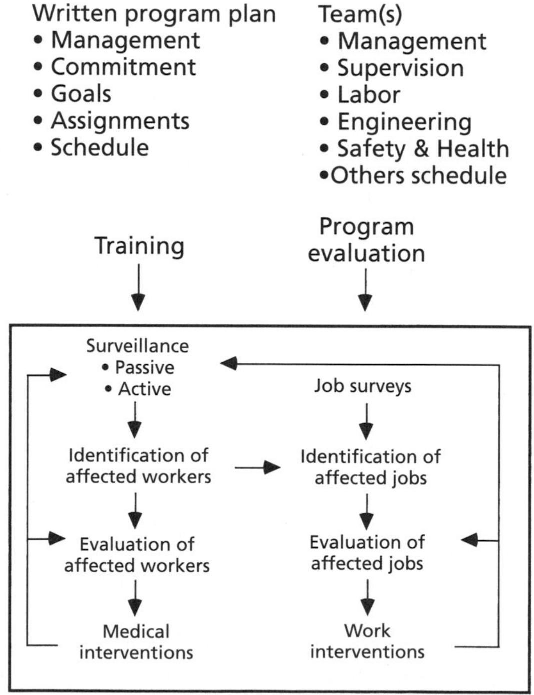

Figure 15–3. Components of a generic ergonomics program that should be tailored to meet the needs of each organization.

ergonomic program will vary from one work setting to another depending on the size of the work force, the type of work processes involved, the administrative structure of the organization, and the professional services (e.g., health care and engineering) available on site or in the community. Each program should include objectives that are as specific as possible as well as achievable. Elimination of all upper-limb disorders may be desirable, but it probably is not achievable. Achieving a rate of upper-limb disorders at the level of those not performing repetitive or stressful handwork is more realistic. Other objectives might specify implementation of a surveillance program, implementation of a training program, a review of jobs for the presence of risk factors for upper limb disorders, and the development of new technologies to reduce work stresses. The plan should also take into consideration the organizational structure and the available resources for the work setting where it is to be implemented. The plan should be reviewed periodically to determine if all the goals are being achieved. If they are not achieved, it should be determined if the goals are appropriate or if other methods are necessary for achieving them. If the goals are appropriate, the cause for failing to meet the goals should be determined and remedied.

Active and passive surveillance methods are utilized to identify cumulative trauma disorders. Active surveillance entails the use of questionnaires, surveys, and physical examinations. Several questionnaires and physical examinations have been proposed that may be adapted to a given setting.[32,35,51,52,58,72,91] Active surveillance is not just a matter of passing out questionnaires for workers to answer at their convenience. Workers must be given a time, place, and sufficient instructions for meaningful participation. Care should be exercised to avoid biasing the results through the inclusion or exclusion of possible participants. It is also important to avoid leading or suggestive questions.[75] Some investigators eschew questionnaires and interviews in favor of objective tests based on nerve conduction or quantitative sensory testing; however, these so-called "objective" tests only detect disorders of nerves—not those of muscles or tendons. Nerve conduction testing is considered the most definitive test for carpal tunnel syndrome and is used to determine sensitivities and specificities of other tests (see Chapters 16 and 33). At present, other tests compare poorly with nerve conduction testing[34,47,51]; however, just because a worker does not fit an established diagnostic criterion for carpal tunnel syndrome does not mean that there is nothing wrong with the worker's hands and wrists.

Passive surveillance entails analysis of available data sources (including OSHA records, workers' compensation reports, personal medical claims, and company medical visits). There are several components of an effective passive surveillance monitoring system. There must be a mechanism for workers to report problems. Resources vary from plant to plant. Some plants do not have on-site medical resources. In those cases it is necessary to work with the referral health care provider or with local clinics to identify possible causes. Employers need to understand that worker health records are confidential and that the health care provider may be able to give them only general feedback in which individuals cannot be identified. Reporting will be affected based on either a hostile or a supportive attitude by management toward injured workers. Reporting can also be affected by the attitude of the local medical community. In some communities, health care providers work closely with local industry by visiting the workplace to observe jobs and discussing possible work restrictions; in others, there may be no such interaction.

Workers need to understand that if persistent discomfort interferes with activities of work or daily living, then they should see a health care provider for an evaluation. They also should understand that some discomfort may be normal. Workers may need guidance about where to go to report their problems and to get help, but they must not feel threatened that reporting will affect their job security or earnings. This can be a problem in plants where wages are based on an incentive system.

OSHA has attempted to facilitate passive surveillance by specifying standardized reporting criteria[86]:

1. At least one physical finding (e.g., positive Tinel, Phalen, or Finkelstein test); or swelling, redness, or deformity; or loss of motion; or
2. At least one subjective symptom (e.g., pain, numbness, tingling, aching, stiffness, or burning), and at least one of the following:
   a. medical treatment (including self-administered treatment when made available to employees by their employer),
   b. lost work days (includes restricted work activity), or
   c. transfer or rotation to another job.

These reporting guidelines are sensitive because they identify persons with any kind of upper limb problem that causes them to seek help. They are not very specific because they do not discriminate between various disorders, and they can identify unaffected workers as having cumulative trauma disorders.

It is necessary to have a plan for managing workers identified through passive or active surveillance. All possible cases need to be evaluated. In some cases it may be found that the worker has fatigue and requires rest and reassurance. Reassurance may come in the form of an explanation and monitoring of the problem. Other workers may need medical interventions, such as physical therapy, medications, or even surgery. The work should always be evaluated for possible risk factors in

TABLE 15–1
Work Improvements

Alteration	Improvement
Adjust production standards	R, S, D
Incentives	R, S, D
Rotations	R, S, D
Work enlargement	R, S, D
Mechanical aids	
Tools	R, S, D, F, P, C, V, T
Supports	S, F, P
Hoists and articulating arms	S, F, P
Motion economy	R, S, D
Weight of job work objects/materials	F
Friction	F
Gloves	F, V, T
Balance	F
Handles	F, C
Tool torque	F
Tool shape	F, P
Bits	F
Blades	F
Adjustable work surfaces	P
Isolation devices	V
Air temperature	T
Air leaks	T
Air line attachments	F, T

R = repetition; S = static exertions; D = work duration; F = force; P = posture; C = contact stress; V = vibration; T = temperature.

order to accommodate the affected worker and prevent future cases.

Specification and interpretation of work restrictions is a common source of frustration for both the health care provider and the employer. In some cases restrictions are vague, and workers may be laid off or unwittingly given alternative work that is worse that the original. A restriction that says "avoid forceful exertions" may leave an employer wondering what is too forceful. A restriction that says "do not lift more than 20 pounds" does not consider the fact that 20 pounds close to the body is not as bad as 20 pounds at arm's length from the body. A work restriction should be based on knowledge of the operations at the place of the affected worker's employment. By observing or discussing jobs with management, it may be possible to locate jobs or tasks that entail elements that appear to contribute to a given disorder.

A thorough job analysis should be performed for all affected workers. The analysis should include a description of work standards, methods, materials, equipment, and environment. It should delineate the frequency and severity of generic risk factors (e.g., repeated and sustained static exertions, forces, postures, contact stresses, and exposures to vibration and low temperatures). It is desirable that the analysis also indicates the cause of major stresses (job-specific factors) (e.g., flexing wrist six times per minute is caused by driving screws in a horizontal surface 1 m above the floor). Table 15–1 includes a list of job-specific factors associated with generic cumulative trauma disorder factors. This information will help plant personnel develop work interventions to accommodate the restricted worker (see also Chapter 48 and Appendix B).

In some cases it is not possible to visit the worksite or even get a good analysis of the jobs. In those cases, the treating physician may obtain the information from a worker or someone at the plant. Table 15–2 lists some of the information that will be helpful for planning restrictions.

By focusing the restriction on a specific aspect of the job, it may be possible for the employer to develop a workplace modification that would facilitate returning the worker to the same job and preventing future occurrences in other workers. For example, if the restriction focuses on torque associated with use of a hand tool, it may be possible for the employer to find an alternative tool with a lower torque reaction force to use as an articulating arm to eliminate the torque from the worker. A general list of factors associated with risk factors is summarized in Table 15–2. It is essential that all interventions be evaluated to ascertain their effectiveness.

Several schemes have been proposed for analyzing jobs. These include checklists,[56,73] open-ended observational-based systems,[4,57] instrumental systems using goniometers and surface electromyography,[9,50,64,70,71] and a number of traditional interview and observational methods.[75] In 2001, the American Conference of Governmental Industrial Hygienists published a threshold limit value for preventing work-related musculoskeletal disorders in mono-task hand work.[2] The proposed standard includes recommendations for assessing repetition and force. Descriptions of job analysis methods are beyond the scope of this discussion.

Control of cumulative trauma disorders entails participation and training of persons from many parts of the organization. A commitment is required from all levels of management to provide leadership and support for others in the organization. Commitment entails stating goals, assigning responsibilities, and maintaining accountabilities. It also entails allocating necessary time and monetary resources. Managers need training to understand the characteristics and causes of cumulative trauma disorders, their responsibility for providing workers with a safe and healthful workplace, the components of a control program, and the necessary resources.

Workers' participation is required to report possible health and job problems and to cooperate in implementing control measures. Workers need training on the characteristics and causes of cumulative trauma disorders, when and where they should report health and work problems, and how they can prevent cumulative trauma disorders via work methods and workplace adjustments.

TABLE 15-2

Job Information Needed for Developing Work Restrictions

Documentation
- Job title (including all jobs through which a worker may rotate)
- Information on what the worker does
- Information on work standard
- Information on pay and incentive system

Lists and descriptions
- List of steps necessary to perform the job along with the work objects and locations
- List of the work objects along with their size, weight, or other force information (e.g., torque, insertion force)
- Description of the range of environments in which the job is performed (e.g., inside at room temperature, outside at ambient temperature)
- List of personal protective equipment (e.g., gloves)

Assessment of physical stresses
- Does the worker have difficulty making production or keeping up with the line?
  ——Always ——Sometimes ——Never ——Why?
- Does the worker work overtime?
  ——Always ——Sometimes ——Never ——Why?
- Does the worker maintain the same position or hold a work object for prolonged periods?
  ——Always ——Sometimes ——Never ——Why?
- Does the worker assume unnatural or awkward postures to perform the job?
  ——Always ——Sometimes ——Never ——Why?
- Does the worker have difficulty exerting the force required to perform the job?
  ——Always ——Sometimes ——Never ——Why?
- Do any work objects rub or create stress concentrations on the surface of the body?
  ——Always ——Sometimes ——Never ——Why?
- Does the worker hold or touch anything that shakes or vibrates?
  ——Always ——Sometimes ——Never ——Why?
- Does the worker hold or touch anything cold (less than 70°F)—tools, parts, air?
  ——Always ——Sometimes ——Never ——Why?

Answering the question "why" will help determine the feasibility of interventions.

Supervisors often are the first to hear of a worker's problem or to see a problem with equipment or materials. They must be vigilant in recognizing these problems and cooperate with the implementation of interventions. Supervisors need training on the characteristics and causes of cumulative trauma disorders, what they should do when workers report problems, and the need for work equipment to be set up and adjusted properly.

Engineering participation includes fixing equipment, identifying material and method problems as they are identified, and developing new designs that minimize physical work stresses. Engineers need training on the characteristics and causes of cumulative trauma disorders—especially with respect to the design of work equipment and methods. They need to be able to identify physical work stresses. They need to appreciate the range of physical and behavior differences in the working population and where to find work design information. Engineers need to appreciate the need to perform user trials on equipment before designs are finalized.[74]

The role of health care providers in surveillance and medical management has already been described. Providers may need additional training to appreciate the unique properties of cumulative trauma disorders and the use and limitations of surveillance methods, as well as to interpret job analysis information and develop recommendations.

Other health and safety personnel (such as the occupational safety expert) often participate through training and the analysis of data for injury and illness trends. Also, they may work with purchasing agents to be sure that new equipment and material acquisitions are reviewed for the risk of avoidable stresses to workers. They need training on the characteristics and causes of cumulative trauma disorders, the organizational aspects of ergonomics programs, regulatory issues, and work analysis and design. The depth of their training will vary according to the role they play in the plant program. Often, safety and health personnel set up, run, and evaluate preventive programs for workplaces. Other members of the organization may participate as necessary, and they should receive sufficient training regarding their role in the program.

Training should be tailored to each industry and setting. The training requirements of a large office facility will be different from those of a small manufacturing plant. Training should be an ongoing process. This can often be done in conjunction with a review of various program aspects or when technical assistance is needed for specific problems.

Because a control program for cumulative trauma disorders draws on a number of different skills, the assistance of one or more teams may facilitate preventive efforts. The team should be provided with training on the characteristics and causes of upper limb disorders. They also should be given training on how to analyze jobs. The team should meet at regular intervals to review new and existing cases. At that time the team may review the progress toward goals and recommend necessary program enhancements. Written records should be kept to document team activities so that its progress can be evaluated. These records will also provide institutional memory of problems and solutions and will be useful in the future. Employers should be aware that some team activities may be a violation of the National Labor Relations Act of 1935.[15] They should consult with their personnel managers before setting up teams.

SUMMARY

Cumulative trauma disorder refers to a group of muscle, tendon, and nerve disorders that can be caused, precipitated, or aggravated by repeated exertions or movements of the hand. Reports of these disorders dating back nearly 300 years demonstrate that they are a major cause of worker impairment and disability in some occupations. Causes of cumulative trauma disorders include personal and work-related factors. Contemporary regulations regarding worker safety and health, workers' compensation, and nondiscrimination obligate employers to identify and remedy hazardous work situations before disorders occur and to identify affected workers before they develop long-term consequences. This is best achieved by implementation of an ongoing program that includes a written plan tailored to the needs of each organization, surveillance, analysis and design of jobs, management of affected workers, a team approach, and training for the team members.

References

1. Amadio PC: Carpal tunnel syndrome, pyridoxine, and the workplace. J Hand Surg 12A5(Part 2):875–881, 1987.
2. American Conference of Governmental Industrial Hygienists: Hand Activity Level. 2001 Threshold Limit Values for Chemical Substances and Physical Agents and Biological Exposure Limits. Cincinnati, American Conference of Governmental Industrial Hygienists, 2001, pp 110–111.
3. The Americans With Disabilities Act of 1990 (Public Law: 110th Congress HR). Washington, DC, 1990.
4. Armstrong TJ: Ergonomics and cumulative trauma disorders. In Kasdan M (ed): Hand Clinics. Philadelphia, WB Saunders, 1986.
5. Armstrong TJ: Mechanical considerations of skin in work. Am J Ind Med 8:463–472, 1985.
6. Armstrong TJ: Some histological changes in carpal tunnel contents and their biomechanical implications. J Occup Med 26:197–201, 1984.
7. Armstrong TJ, Buckle P, Fine L, et al: A conceptual model for work-related neck and upper-limb musculoskeletal disorders. Scand J Work Environ Health 19:73–84, 1993.
8. Armstrong TJ, Fine L, Goldstein S, et al: Ergonomic considerations in hand and wrist tendinitis. J Hand Surg 12A5(Part 2):830–837, 1987.
9. Armstrong TJ, Foulke J, Joseph B, Goldstein S: Investigation of cumulative trauma disorders in a poultry processing plant. Am Ind Hyg Assoc J 43:103–116, 1982.
10. Armstrong TJ, Chaffin DB: Some biological aspects of the carpal tunnel. J Biomech 12:567–570, 1979.
11. Barcroft H, Greenwood B, Whelan R: Blood flow and venous oxygen saturation during sustained contraction of the forearm. J Physiol 168:848–856, 1963.
12. Barnhart S, Demers PA, Miller M, et al: Carpal tunnel syndrome among ski manufacturing workers. Scand J Work Environ Health 17:46–52, 1991.
13. Basmajian JV: Weight-bearing by ligaments and muscles. Can J Surg 4:166–170, 1961.
14. Basmajian JV, DeLuca CJ: Muscles Alive, Their Functions Revealed by Electromyography, 5th ed. Baltimore, Williams & Wilkins, 1985.
15. Bernstein A: Making teamwork work—and appeasing Uncle Sam. Bus Week 101, 1993.
16. Brain WR, Wright AD, Wilkinson M: Spontaneous compression of both median nerves in the carpal tunnel. Lancet 8:277–282, 1947.
17. Brand PW: Clinical Mechanics of the Hand. St. Louis, CV Mosby, 1985.
18. Bureau of Labor Statistics, US DOL: Occupational Injuries and Illnesses in the United States by Industry. Washington, DC, U.S. Government Printing Office, 1994.
19. Bystrom S, Sjogaard G: Potassium homeostasis during and following exhaustive submaximal static handgrip contractions. Acta Physiol Scand 142:59–66, 1991.
20. Cailliet R: Soft Tissue Pain and Disability. Philadelphia, FA Davis, 1977.
21. Campbell CS: Gamekeeper's thumb. J Bone Joint Surg 37B:148–149, 1955.
22. Cannon LJ, Bernacki EJ, Walter SD: Personal and occupational factors associated with carpal tunnel syndrome. J Occup Med 23:255–258, 1981.
23. Caplan A, Carlson B, Faulkner J, et al: Skeletal muscle. In Woo SL, Buckwalter JE (eds): Injury and Repair of the Musculoskeletal Soft Tissues. Park Ridge, IL, American Academy of Orthopaedic Surgeons, 1988.
24. Chaffin DB: Localized muscle fatigue—definition and measurement. J Occup Med 15:346–354, 1973.
25. Conn HR: Tenosynovitis. Ohio State Med J 27:713–716, 1931.
26. Corlett EN, Bishop RP: A technique for assessing postural discomfort. Ergonomics 19:175–182, 1976.
27. Courtney TK, Smith GD, Armstrong TJ: Ergonomics and OSHA: A chronological overview of enforcement and regulation development. In Kumar S (ed): Advances in Industrial Ergonomics and Safety—IV. London, Taylor & Francis, 1992, pp 1313–1320.
28. DeKrom MC, Kester AD, Knipschild PG, Spaans F: Risk factors for carpal tunnel syndrome. Am J Epidemiol 132:1102–1110, 1990.
29. Duncan J, Ferguson D: Keyboard operating posture and symptoms in operating. Ergonomics 17:651–662, 1974.
30. Elkus R, Basmajian JV: Endurance in hanging by the hands. Am J Phys Med 52:124–127, 1973.
31. Fine LJ, Silverstein B, Armstrong T, Anderson C: The detection of cumulative trauma disorders of the upper extremities in the workplace. J Occup Med 28:674–678, 1986.
32. Fine LJ, Silverstein BA: Work–related disorders of the neck and upper extremity. In Levy B, Wegman D (eds): Occupational Health: Recognizing and Preventing Work-related Disease, 3rd ed. Boston, Little, Brown, 1995.
33. Franklin GM, Haug K, Heyer N, et al: Occupational carpal tunnel syndrome in Washington state—1984–88. Am J Public Health 81:741–746, 1991.
34. Franzblau A, Werner W, Valle J, Johnston E: Workplace surveillance for carpal tunnel syndrome: A comparison of methods. J Occup Rehab 3:1–14, 1994.
35. Franzblau A, Werner RA, Albers JW, et al: Workplace surveillance for carpal tunnel syndrome using hand diagrams. J Occup Rehab 4:185–198, 1994.
36. Friden J, Sjostrom M, Ekblom B: A morphological study on delayed muscle soreness. Experientia 37:506–507, 1981.
37. Gelberman RH, Goldberg V, An K-N, et al: Tendon. In Woo SL, Buckwalter JE (eds): Injury and Repair of the Musculoskeletal Soft Tissues. Park Ridge, IL, American Academy of Orthopaedic Surgeons, 1988.
38. Gelberman RH, Hergenroeder PT, Hargens AR, et al: The carpal tunnel syndrome: A study of carpal tunnel pressures. J Bone Joint Surg 63A:380–383, 1981.
39. Gelberman RH, Szabo RM, Williamson RV, Dimick MP: Sensibility testing in peripheral-nerve compression syndromes. J Bone Joint Surg 65A:632–638, 1983.
40. Goldstein SA, Armstrong TJ, Chaffin DB, Matthews LS: Analysis of cumulative strain in tendons and tendon sheaths. J Biomechanics 20:1–6, 1987.
41. Hagberg M: Local shoulder muscular strain—symptoms and disorders. J Hum Ergol 11:99–108, 1982.

42. Hagberg M: Occupational musculoskeletal stress and disorders of the neck and shoulder: A review of possible pathophysiology. Int Arch Occup Environ Health 53:269–278, 1984.
43. Hagberg M: Work load and fatigue in repetitive arm elevations. Ergonomics 24:543–555, 1981.
44. Hennekens CH, Buring JE: Epidemiology in Medicine. Boston, Little, Brown, 1987.
45. Herberts P, Kadefors R, Andersson G, Peterson I: Shoulder pain in industry: An epidemiological study on welders. Acta Orthop Scand 52:299–306, 1981.
46. Herberts P, Kadefors R, Hogfors C, Sigholm G: Shoulder pain and heavy manual labor. Clin Orthop 191:166–178, 1984.
47. Homan MMA, Franzblau A, Werner RA, et al: Agreement between symptom surveys, physical examination procedures and electrodiagnostic findings for the carpal tunnel syndrome. Scand J Work Environ Health 25:115–124, 1999.
48. Hymovich L, Lindholm M: Hand, wrist and forearm injuries: The result of repetitive motions. J Occup Med 8:573–577, 1966.
49. Jackson MJ, Jones DA, Edwards RHT: Experimental skeletal muscle damage: The nature of the calcium-activated degenerative processes. Eur J Clin Invest 14:369–374, 1984.
50. Jonsson B: The static load component in muscle work. Eur J Appl Physiol 57:305–310, 1988.
51. Katz JN: Validation of a surveillance case definition of carpal tunnel syndrome. Am J Public Health 81:189–193, 1991.
52. Katz JN, Larson MG, Sabra A, et al: The carpal tunnel syndrome: Diagnostic utility of the history and physical examination findings. Ann Intern Med 112:321–327, 1990.
53. Keir PJ, Bach JM, Rempel DH: Effects of computer mouse design and task on carpal tunnel pressure. Ergonomics 42:1350–1360, 1999.
54. Keir PJ, Bach JM, Rempel DH, et al: Effects of finger posture on carpal tunnel pressure during wrist motion. J Hand Surg [Am] 23:1004–1009, 1998.
55. Kenedi RM, Gibson T, Daly CH: Bioengineering studies of the human skin. In Kenedi RM (ed): Symposium on Biomechanics and Related Bio-engineering Topics, Proceedings. Glasgow, Pergamon Press, 1964, pp II-147–II-158.
56. Keyserling WM, Stetson DS, Silverstein BA, Brouwer ML: A checklist for evaluating ergonomic risk factors associated with upper extremity cumulative trauma disorders. Ergonomics 36:807–831, 1993.
57. Keyserling WM, Armstrong TJ, Punnett L: Ergonomic job analysis: A structural approach for identifying risk factors associated with overexertion injuries and disorders. Appl Occup Env Hyg 6:353–363, 1991.
58. Kuorinka I, Jonsson B, Kilbom A, et al: Standardised Nordic health questionnaires for the analysis of musculoskeletal symptoms. Appl Ergonomics 18:233–237, 1987.
59. Kurppa K, Waris P, Rokkanen P: Peritendinitis and tenosynovitis: A review. Scand J Work Environ Health 5(Suppl. 3):19–24, 1979.
60. Latko WA, Armstrong TJ, Franzblau A, et al: Cross-sectional study of the relationship between repetitive work and the prevalence of upper limb musculoskeletal disorders. Am J Ind Med 36:248–259, 1999.
61. Latko WA, Armstrong TJ, Foulke J, et al: Development and evaluation of an observational method for assessing repetition in hand tasks. Am Ind Hyg Assoc J 58:278–285, 1997.
62. LeVeau B: Williams and Lissner Biomechanics of Human Motion, 3rd ed. Philadelphia, WB Saunders, 1992.
63. Lind AR, McNicol GW, Donald KW: Circulatory adjustments to sustained (static) muscular activity. Proc Symp Phys Activity Health Dis 38–63, 1966.
64. Linderhed H: A new dimension to amplitude analysis of EMG. Int J Ind Ergonomics 11:243–247, 1993.
65. Louis DS: The carpal tunnel syndrome. In Millender LH, Louis DS, Simmons BP (eds): Occupational Disorders of the Upper Extremity. New York, Churchill Livingstone, 1992.
66. Lovlin R, Cottle W, Pyke I, et al: Are indices of free radical damage related to exercise intensity? Eur J Appl Physiol Occup Physiol 56:313–316, 1987.
67. Lundborg G: Nerve Injury and Repair. New York, Churchill Livingstone, 1988.
68. Lundborg G, Rank F: Experimental intrinsic healing of flexor tendons based upon synovial fluid nutrition. J Hand Surg 3:21–31, 1978.
69. Luopajarvi R, Kourinka I, Virolainen M, et al: Prevalence of tenosynovitis and other injuries of the upper extremities in repetitive work. Scand J Work Environ Health 5(Suppl. 3):48–55, 1979.
70. Marras WS, Schoenmarklin RW: Wrist motions in industry. Ergonomics 36:341–351, 1993.
71. Mathiassen SE, Winkel J: Quantifying variation in physical load using exposure-vs-time data. Ergonomics 34:1455–1468, 1991.
72. Matte TD, Baker EL, Honchar PA: The selection and definition of targeted work-related conditions for surveillance under SENSOR. Am J Public Health 79:21–25, 1989.
73. McAtamney L, Corlett EN: RULA: A survey method for the investigation of work-related upper limb disorders. Appl Ergonomics 24:91–99, 1993.
74. McClelland I: Product assessment and user trials. In Wilson JR, Corlett EN (eds): Evaluation of Human Work: A Practical Ergonomics Methodology. New York, Taylor & Francis, 1990.
75. McCormick E: Job and task analysis. In Salvendy G (ed): Handbook of Industrial Engineering. New York, John Wiley & Sons, 1982.
76. McKenzie F, Storment J, Van Hook P, Armstrong T: A program for control of repetitive trauma disorders associated with hand tool operations in a telecommunications manufacturing facility. Ind Hyg Assoc J 46:674–678, 1985.
77. Moore JS: Function, structure, and responses of components of the muscle–tendon unit. Occup Med 7:713–740, 1992.
78. Nathan PA, Meadows KD, Doyle LS: Occupation as a risk factor for impaired sensory conduction of the median nerve at the carpal tunnel. J Hand Surg 13B:167–170, 1988.
79. Nathan PA, Keniston RC, Myers LD, Meadows KD: Obesity as a risk factor of sensory conduction of the median nerve in industry. J Occup Med 34:379–383, 1992.
80. Nathan PA, Meadows KD, Doyle LS: Relationship of age and sex to sensory conduction of the median nerve at the carpal tunnel and association of slowed conduction with symptoms. Muscle Nerve 11:1149–1153, 1988.
81. Newham DJ, Jones DA, Edwards RHT: Plasma creatine kinase changes after eccentric and concentric contractions. Muscle Nerve 9:59–63, 1986.
82. Nordstrom DL, Vierkant RA, Layde KA, Smith MJ: Comparison of self-reported and expert-observed physical activities at work in a general population. Am J Ind Med 34:29–35, 1998.
83. National Research Council: Work-related Musculoskeletal Disorders: A Review of the Evidence. Washington, DC, National Academy Press, 1998.
84. National Research Council and Institute of Medicine: Musculoskeletal Disorders and the Workplace: Low Back and Upper Extremities. Washington, DC, National Academy Press, 2001.
85. Obolenskaja AJ, Goljanitzki IA: Die serose tendovaginitis in der klinik und im experiment. Deutsch Z Chir 201:388–399, 1927.
86. Occupational Safety and Health Administration: Ergonomics Program Management Guidelines for Meatpacking Plants (OSHA-3121). Washington, DC, Bureau of National Affairs, 1990.

87. Occupational Safety and Health Administration: Occupational Safety and Health Act of 1970, Public Law 91–596. Washington, DC, U.S. Department of Labor, 1970.
88. Oxenburgh M: Musculoskeletal injuries occurring in word processor operators. In Adams A, Stevenson M (eds): Proceedings of the 21st Annual Conference of the Ergonomics Society of Australia and New Zealand. Sydney, 1984, pp 137–143.
89. Ozkay A, Nordin M: Fundamentals of Biomechanics, Equilibrium, Motion and Deformation. New York, Van Nostrand Reinhold, 1991.
90. Phalen GS: The carpal-tunnel syndrome: Seventeen years' experience in diagnosis and treatment of six hundred fifty-four hands. J Bone Joint Surg 48A:211–228, 1966.
91. Putz-Anderson V: Cumulative Trauma Disorders—A Manual for Musculoskeletal Diseases of the Upper Limbs. New York, Taylor & Francis, 1988.
92. Ramazzini B: Diseases of Workers (de morbis artificum). Chicago, University of Chicago Press, 1713.
93. Reed JV, Harcourt AK: Tenosynovitis: An industrial disability. Am J Surg 62:392–396, 1943.
94. Rempel D, Evanoff B, Amadio PC, et al: Consensus criteria for the classification of carpal tunnel syndrome in epidemiologic studies. Am J Public Health 88:1447–1451, 1998.
95. Saldana N, Herrin G, Armstrong T: A computerized method for assessment of musculoskeletal discomfort in the workforce: A tool for surveillance. Ergonomics 37:1097–1112, 1994.
96. Silverstein BA, Fine LJ, Armstrong TJ: Occupational factors and carpal tunnel syndrome. Am J Ind Med 11:343–358, 1987.
97. Smith EM, Sonstegard DA, Anderson WH: Carpal tunnel syndrome: Contribution of flexor tendons. Arch Phys Med Rehabil 58:379–385, 1977.
98. Stevens JC, Sun S, Beard CM, et al: Carpal tunnel syndrome in Rochester, Minnesota, 1961 to 1980. Neurology 38:134–138, 1988.
99. Szabo RM, Chidgey LK: Stress carpal tunnel pressures in patients with carpal tunnel syndrome and normal patients. J Hand Surg 14A:624–627, 1989.
100. Tanaka S, Petersen M, Cameron L: Prevalence and risk factors of tendinitis and related disorders of the distal upper extremity among U.S. workers: Comparison to carpal tunnel syndrome. Am J Ind Med 39:328–335, 2001.
101. Taylor DC: Viscoelastic properties of muscle–tendon units: The biomechanical effects of stretching. Am J Sports Med 18:300–309, 1990.
102. Thompson AR, Plewes LW, Shaw EG: Peritendinitis crepitans and simple tenosynovitis: A clinical study of 544 cases in industry. Br J Ind Med 8:150–160, 1951.
103. Waersted M, Bjorklund RA, Westgard RH: Shoulder muscle tension induced by two VDU–based tasks of different complexity. Ergonomics 34:137–150, 1991.
104. Wahl S, Renstrom P: Fibrosis in soft-tissue injuries. In Leadbetter WB, Buckwalter JA, Gordon SL (eds): Sports Induced Inflammation: Clinical and Basic Science Concepts. Park Ridge, IL, American Academy of Orthopaedic Surgeons, 1990.
105. Waris P, Kuorinka I, Kurppa K, et al: Epidemiologic screening of occupational neck and upper limb disorders: Methods and criteria. Scand J Work Environ Health 5(Suppl. 3):25–38, 1979.
106. Werner RA, Albers JW, Franzblau A, Armstrong J: The relationship between body mass index and the diagnosis of carpal tunnel syndrome. Muscle Nerve 17:632–636, 1994.
107. Werner R, Armstorng TJ, Bir C, Aylard M: Intracarpal canal pressure: The role of finger, hand, wrist, and forearm position. Clin Biomech 12:44–51, 1997.
108. Winkel J, Mathiassen SE: Assessment of physical work load in epidemiologic studies: Concepts, issues, and operation considerations. Ergonomics 37:979–988, 1994.
109. WHO: Identification and control of work related diseases, Report of a WHO Expert Committee, WHO Technical Report 714, p 9, Geneva: WHO, 1985.
110. Yamaguchi DM: Carpal tunnel syndrome. Minn Med 22–33, 1965.
111. Zollinger F: A few remarks on the question of tubercular tendovaginitis and bursitis after an accident. Arch Orthopadische Unfall-Chirurgioe 24:456–467, 1927.

CHAPTER

16

Joint Systems

Hand and Wrist

MARK S. COHEN, MD ■ DAVID M. KALAINOV, MD

ENTRAPMENT NEUROPATHIES

Carpal Tunnel Syndrome

Anatomy/Pathophysiology

The median nerve passes across the wrist through an unyielding fibroosseous canal called the carpal tunnel. Compression of the median nerve within this canal is termed carpal tunnel syndrome. The condition occurs owing to a mismatch between the volume of the canal and the canal contents; namely, the median nerve and the nine digital flexor tendons (Fig. 16–1). The typical histologic appearance involves edema and fibrous hypertrophy of the synovial lining of the flexor tendons (tenosynovium) with minimal inflammation.[23]

Carpal tunnel syndrome is associated with several medical conditions, including diabetes, hypothyroidism, rheumatoid arthritis, and renal failure. Other contributory risk factors include wrist fractures, obesity, and pregnancy.[4,76] In the workplace, carpal tunnel syndrome has been associated with repetitive use of the wrist and digits, repeated impact on the palm, and the operation of vibratory tools.[11,21,50,52,53] Mechanically disadvantaged wrist positions such as extremes of flexion and extension have been shown experimentally to increase pressures within the carpal canal.[25] However, the mechanisms by which task-related factors contribute to carpal tunnel syndrome are poorly understood.[35,76,79]

Diagnosis

The diagnosis of carpal tunnel syndrome relies initially on the patient history. Symptoms may include numbness (on the palmar surface of the radial three and one-half digits), tingling, burning, and decreased dexterity of the hand. The symptoms correspond to the sensory and motor distributions of the median nerve. Prolonged wrist extension while driving or flexion during sleep will often aggravate the condition and nocturnal paresthesias with awakening are a frequent complaint. Symptoms of advanced median nerve compression include diminished sensation (in the radial three and one-half digits) and atrophy of the thenar eminence muscles (abductor pollicis brevis, flexor pollicis brevis, opponens pollicis).

The physical examination is very important in establishing the diagnosis of carpal tunnel syndrome. Thenar muscle bulk and strength are evaluated and sensibility testing is performed. Two-point discrimination refers to the ability to distinguish two points on the pulp of the

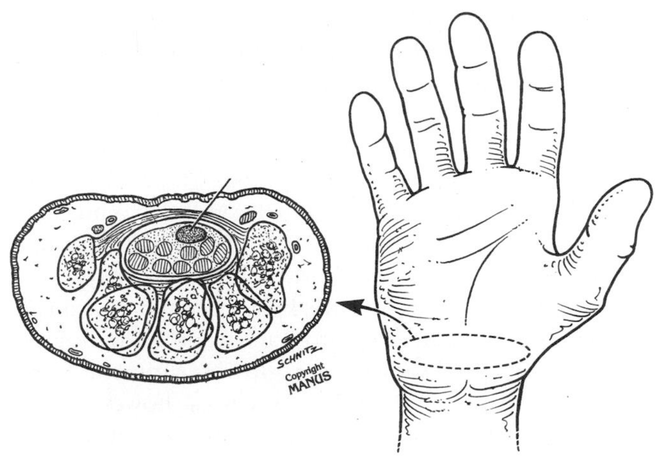

Figure 16–1. Cross-section of the carpal tunnel at the level of the wrist (carpal bones). The median nerve lies beneath the transverse carpal ligament with the flexor tendons of the digits. Compression of the median nerve within this canal leads to carpal tunnel syndrome. (Courtesy of the Indiana Hand Center, Indianapolis, Indiana.)

digit at decreasing distances.[54] Monofilaments are used as a quantitative sensory threshold test to assess light touch in the median nerve distribution.[27] Dryness or unusual texture of the radial digits signifies disruption of the sympathetic fibers carried by the median nerve.

A variety of provocative tests are used to reproduce or accentuate the symptoms of carpal tunnel syndrome. These tests have varying sensitivities and specificities (Table 16–1). Phalen test refers to placing the wrist in a fully flexed posture.[63] Tinel test refers to percussion of the median nerve over the wrist.[74] The median nerve compression test involves direct pressure on the median nerve over the carpal canal and is the most sensitive and specific.[18] One or more of these tests should reproduce the symptoms in patients with carpal tunnel syndrome.

An electrodiagnostic study is often used to confirm the diagnosis of carpal tunnel syndrome and is helpful in quantifying the degree of median nerve involvement. The test is also beneficial in assessing for a coexisting polyneuropathy or other site of upper extremity nerve compression.[66] However, there is a documented 8% to 12% false-negative rate for the diagnosis of carpal tunnel syndrome with electrodiagnostic testing.[33,49] Furthermore, approximately 15% of the normal asymptomatic population will test positive for carpal tunnel syndrome by electrical criteria.[4] The results therefore need to be carefully correlated with the patient's clinical symptoms and physical examination.

TABLE 16–1

Sensitivity and Specificity of Tests Used in Diagnosing Carpal Tunnel Syndrome

Test	Sensitivity	Specificity
Two-point discrimination	33%	100%
Phalen test	71%	80%
Tinel percussion	44%	94%
Semmes-Weinstein monofilaments	91%	80%
Monofilaments with Phalen	82%	86%
Median nerve compression test	87%	90%

Sensitivity expresses the fraction of patients with carpal tunnel syndrome who are correctly identified by the test. Specificity expresses the fraction of normal patients (without carpal tunnel syndrome) who are correctly identified as normal. Whereas expanded two-point discrimination in the median nerve distribution (≥6 mm) and the Tinel percussion test are the most specific findings in carpal tunnel syndrome, they are the least sensitive tests. The monofilament and median nerve compression tests appear to have the best combined sensitivity and specificity.[18,28,43]

Treatment

Initial treatment for carpal tunnel syndrome, in the absence of diminished sensation, muscle atrophy, or denervation potentials on an electrodiagnostic study, involves splinting the wrist in neutral alignment. This position relaxes the median nerve and maintains a low pressure in the carpal canal. Associated systemic diseases such as diabetes and hypothyroidism should be appropriately managed. Cortisone injection into the carpal canal is a useful adjunctive modality. The injection can be very helpful in confirming the diagnosis and may be curative in patients with mild symptoms. It also has prognostic significance as patients who experience temporary relief following an injection are more apt to obtain similar relief from carpal tunnel release surgery.[32] Ergonomic changes in the workplace should be considered for general patient comfort and satisfaction, including appropriate upper extremity positioning and posture. Other recommended measures, however, such as specially designed desk chairs and computer keyboards, have not been scientifically proven to prevent or ameliorate symptoms of carpal tunnel syndrome.

If patients experience partial or only temporary relief with conservative treatment measures and continue to have significant symptoms, carpal tunnel decompression may be considered. Surgery is also indicated in the presence of thenar muscle atrophy, electrical denervation, and diminished sensation. The procedure is typically performed under local or regional anesthesia on an outpatient basis. Motion of the fingers is encouraged in the immediate postoperative period to diminish tendon adhesions and digital stiffness. Newer approaches such as limited incision carpal tunnel releases[6,9,46,55] and releases performed endoscopically have been developed to decrease palm discomfort and quicken the return to activities and employment. The endoscopic technique has been found to shorten the recovery period when compared to a standard open decompression. However, it has been associated with a higher incidence of complications (including nerve injury) and the results of both surgical techniques are essentially equivalent at 3 months.[1,10,13]

Results

Splinting and injection will provide short-term relief of symptoms in over 75% of patients with carpal tunnel syndrome when evaluated at 6 weeks.[24] These measures may result in continued symptomatic relief in 13% to 40% of patients followed for 1 year who had early diagnosis and milder disease. Conservative care may also diminish symptoms, obviating the need for carpal tunnel surgery in a much greater percentage. Good prognostic indicators for success include the presence of symptoms for less than 12 months, intermittent numbness, age over 40, male sex, absence of advanced sensory changes, and normal thenar muscle bulk.[24,37,40,83]

Operative release will reliably diminish pain and paresthesias. Improvements in numbness and weakness are less predictable. In patients with severe, chronic nerve compression, it is not unusual to have permanent low-grade symptoms following a successful carpal tunnel release.[26] Individuals involved in strenuous labor may also experience residual symptomatology.[87] Palm sensitivity around the scar, referred to as pillar pain, is quite common following median nerve decompression. Scar desensitization performed by an occupational therapist can be helpful in this regard when symptoms warrant. Scar tenderness characteristically resolves by 3 to 6 months but may take longer in some individuals. The use of an antivibration glove is often helpful in this situation. Activity restrictions are typically recommended for a period of 6 to 8 weeks following surgery in manual laborers. Grip strength measurements predictably improve over the first 6 months but can continue to improve for up to 1 year.[17,29,45] Most patients are eventually able to return to their previous employment activities with maximum medical improvement anticipated between 3 and 6 months postoperatively.

TENOSYNOVITIS/TENDINITIS

Tenosynovium functions as a low friction envelope around tendons, enhancing gliding through tendon sheaths and around bony prominences. Tenosynovitis refers to inflammation and proliferative changes in this lining, typically associated with an inflammatory disease process. Etiologies include rheumatoid arthritis, infection (septic tenosynovitis), gout, and amyloidosis.[84] A more frequently encountered condition, termed stenosing tenosynovitis or tendovaginitis, involves reactive thickening of the tendon and overlying retinacular sheath with less inflammatory changes.[14,84] Continuous motion of a tendon through the fibroosseous sheath is thought to lead to thickening and nodular formation. The tendon sheath may hypertrophy in response. Increased frictional forces leads to impaired tendon gliding, which manifests clinically as limited mobility, soft tissue swelling, and discomfort with active motion. Tendinitis is a more general term often used interchangeably with tenosynovitis in describing a variety of painful tendon conditions.[3]

De Quervain Disease

Anatomy/Pathophysiology

The dorsal wrist is comprised of six synovial-lined compartments that encompass the extensor tendons of the wrist and hand. The first compartment contains the abductor pollicis longus (APL) and the extensor pollicis brevis (EPB) tendons and is located directly over the styloid process of the distal radius (Fig. 16–2). This compartment is an unyielding fibroosseous tunnel approximately 1 to 2 cm in length with proximal and distal synovial extensions. Painful restricted motion of the thumb tendons through this compartment is referred to as de Quervain disease, or stenosing tenosynovits of the first extensor compartment.

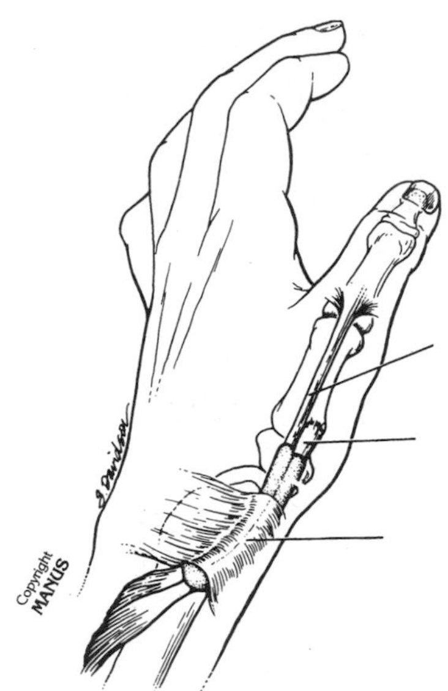

Figure 16–2. The first dorsal compartment of the wrist contains the abductor pollicis longus tendon and the extensor pollicis brevis tendon. These tendons pass through a fibro-osseous tunnel that lies over the styloid process of the radius. Edema and thickening of tissues within this compartment leads to de Quervain disease. (Courtesy of the Indiana Hand Center, Indianapolis, Indiana.)

De Quervain disease is often associated with activities involving forceful grasping or pinching motions with the wrist flexed or ulnarly deviated. Women are more frequently affected than men by a ratio of 6:1. The condition can be associated with direct trauma, as well as rheumatoid arthritis, gout, and diabetes mellitus.[84] A subdivision of the compartment by a septum separating the APL and EPB tendons is thought to predispose some individuals to the development of this condition.[48]

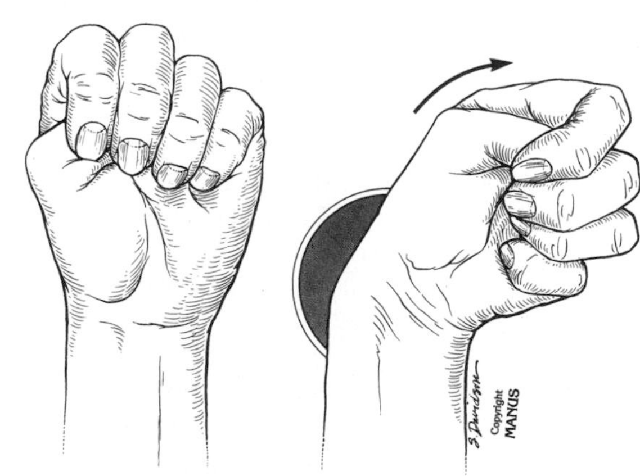

Figure 16–3. The Finkelstein test for de Quervain disease involves ulnar deviation of the wrist with the thumb flexed into the palm. This increases the excursion of the first dorsal compartment tendons and leads to pain in individuals with this condition. (Courtesy of the Indiana Hand Center, Indianapolis, Indiana.)

Diagnosis

Patients with de Quervain disease present with symptoms of pain and tenderness over the radial styloid and base of the thumb. Motions of the wrist and thumb are often limited by swelling and narrowing of the first extensor compartment. Crepitation with thumb flexion and extension is occasionally palpable, as are small cysts (ganglia) arising from the diseased compartment.

The Finkelstein test is the best objective tool in making the diagnosis of de Quervain disease.[20] The patient is instructed to make a fist over a flexed thumb followed by ulnar deviation of the wrist (Fig. 16–3). This maneuver maximizes excursion of the tendons through the stenotic first dorsal compartment, producing significant discomfort if the condition is present. The differential diagnosis of de Quervain disease includes thumb basilar joint arthritis, trigger thumb, intersection syndrome, and flexor carpi radialis tendinitis.

Treatment

Cortisone injections into the first dorsal compartment constitute the mainstay of conservative treatment for de Quervain tenosynovitis. Often several injections are required over several weeks to months. A short arm thumb spica splint may be considered for comfort, but splinting has not been shown to provide additional benefit when combined with a cortisone injection.[82] Nonsteroidal anti-inflammatory medication and ice may also be of benefit.[44] Temporary job modifications are often recommended during the initial course of treatment. The success rate for conservative treatment ranges between 50% and 80%.[84]

When conservative measures fail to relieve symptoms adequately, surgical release of the first extensor compartment may be considered. Surgery involves incision of the fibrotic tendon sheath under local or regional anesthesia. Care must be taken to protect the dorsal sensory branches of the radial nerve and to cut through all visualized septa within the compartment separating the tendon slips.[48] Shortly after surgery, range of motion exercises of the thumb and wrist are encouraged. Interval splinting is used if required for comfort and support initially.

Results

Release of the first dorsal compartment is curative in the majority of cases. The primary concern of most patients after surgery relates to scar tenderness. Branches of the dorsal radial sensory nerve typically course directly over the first extensor compartment. Simple retraction of these nerves intraoperatively may cause peri-incisional pain or numbness. A therapist can often help to desensitize the area and assist the patient in regaining motion and strength. Patients are generally able to return to unrestricted employment within a period of 4 to 8 weeks after surgery.

Trigger Finger

Anatomy/Pathophysiology

Stenosing tenosynovitis of the digital flexor tendons is referred to as trigger finger and trigger thumb. The digital flexor tendons enter an intricate set of pulleys that begin at the palmar metacarpophalangeal joint level (distal palmar flexion crease). The pulleys prevent bowstringing of the flexor tendons, thereby increasing the tendons' mechanical advantage during flexion. The first annular pulley acts as a fulcrum about which the flexor tendons bend. Thickening of the flexor tendon and its sheath at this level leads to a mechanical obstruction to normal tendon gliding, with "catching or locking" of the digit (Fig. 16–4).[67] Once symptoms of triggering have developed, repeated attempts to pull the thickened tendon through the stenotic pulley aggravate the condition.

Primary or idiopathic stenosing tenosynovitis is the most common type of trigger digit and is accompanied by a paucity of inflammation. In the workplace, the condition may be associated with repetitive gripping and microtrauma to the palm. Secondary trigger digits are accompanied by both tenosynovial proliferation and inflammation and occur in patients with rheumatoid arthritis, gout, diabetes, and renal failure.[84]

Diagnosis

Primary trigger digits develop more frequently in women than men and typically present in late middle age. The most commonly affected digit is the ring finger followed in order by the thumb, middle, index, and small fingers.[67] Premonitory symptoms may be experienced prior to triggering and include pain in the region of the first annular pulley and discomfort with digital flexion and extension. Examination reveals tenderness over the distal palm and a palpable nodularity that moves with excursion of the digit. The inability to completely extend the finger represents a "locked" or incarcerated trigger finger.

Treatment

Conservative care of trigger digits involves activity modification and corticosteroid injection into the digital flexor tendon sheath. With primary trigger digits, a cortisone injection has a high probability for success. Single digit involvement, a discreet palpable nodule, and a short duration of symptoms are favorable prognostic indicators.[56] Digital splinting of the metacarpophalangeal joint in extension for a brief period may be

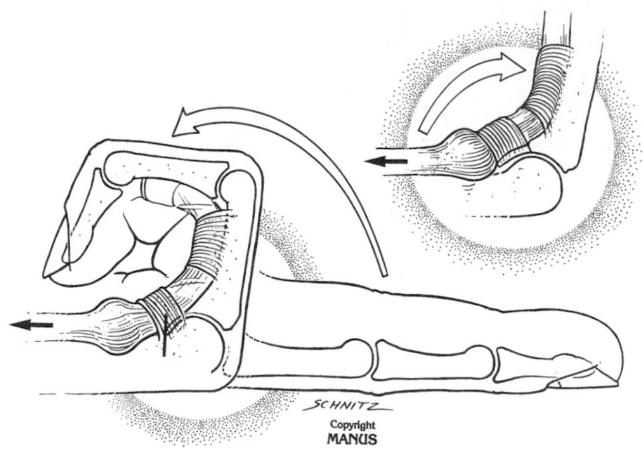

Figure 16–4. Stenosing tenosynovitis (trigger finger) involves the formation of a nodule on the flexor tendon that becomes restricted through a stenotic first annular pulley. Mechanical obstruction of the tendon ensues with "catching or locking" during digital motion. (Courtesy of the Indiana Hand Center, Indianapolis, Indiana.)

added to the treatment regimen. In individuals whose symptoms are aggravated by the use of small narrow-handled tools, modification of these instruments to distribute forces over a greater area and require less digital flexion may be beneficial.

If conservative management fails (including one cortisone injection) and symptoms warrant, surgical treatment is appropriate.[7] Surgery is also indicated for an irreducibly locked digit. The operation consists of releasing the stenotic first annular pulley through a small palmar incision under local anesthesia. The procedure may alternatively be performed percutaneously in the office setting with great care taken to avoid injury to the digital neurovascular bundles.[34,60] Patients are asked to actively flex and extend their fingers immediately after the release to ensure adequate pulley incision. The postoperative dressing allows for digital range of motion, which is encouraged.

Results

Following corticosteroid injection, the majority of patients note a gradual decrease in triggering over the first 1 to 2 weeks. Reported cure rates following an injection range from 60% to 84%.[22,58,78] Persistent or recurrent triggering, however, is not uncommon, particularly when the symptoms have been present for several months. Surgical release carries a 98% cure rate. Palmar incisional tenderness is a frequent complaint and usually improves with an occupational therapy scar program. A therapist can also assist the patient in regaining finger motion and with improving grip strength. The majority of patients will return to unrestricted work activities between 4 and 8 weeks postoperatively. Maximum medical improvement is anticipated by 3 months. Patients with secondary trigger digits often require a more extensive procedure (e.g., tenosynovectomy for rheumatoid arthritis[19]) with an expected delay in recovery and a potentially worse prognosis.

Other Tendonopathies of the Wrist/Hand

Pain and inflammation can involve several other tendons in the wrist and hand. Intersection syndrome refers to tenosynovitis of the second dorsal compartment tendons.[84] Symptoms are localized to an area three to four fingerbreadths proximal to the wrist, where the first dorsal compartment tendons (APL and EPB) cross the second dorsal compartment tendons (extensor carpi radialis longus and extensor carpi radialis brevis) (Fig. 16–5). This syndrome is occasionally seen in association with activities involving frequent and repetitive wrist movements. Patients exhibit inflammation and tenderness well proximal and ulnar to the radial styloid process where it is seen in de Quervain disease. Palpable crepitation with wrist flexion and extension is not uncommon.

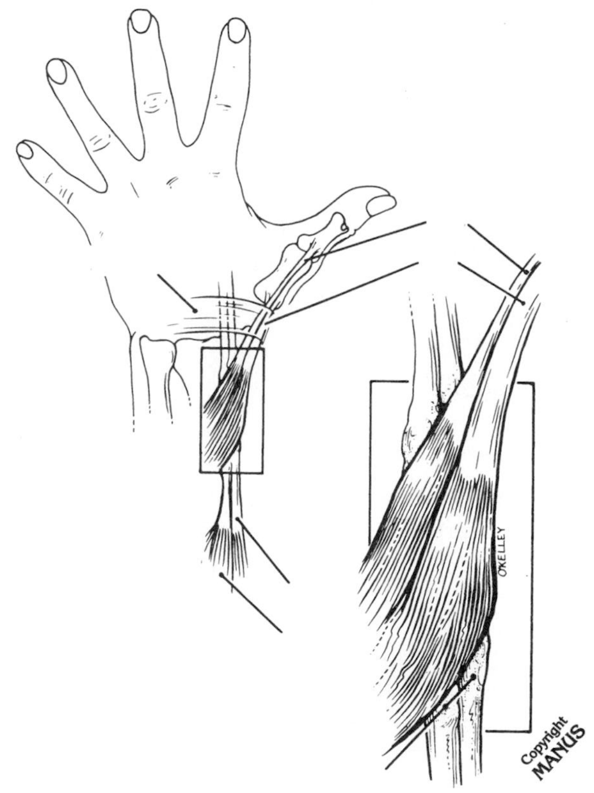

Figure 16–5. Intersection syndrome involves inflammation at the intersection of the first and second dorsal wrist compartment tendons. Swelling and discomfort localize to an area several centimeters proximal to the radiocarpal joint. Crepitation is frequently palpable with wrist flexion and extension. (Courtesy of the Indiana Hand Center, Indianapolis, Indiana.)

Other wrist and digital tendons occasionally involved in inflammation and stenosis include the flexor carpi ulnaris (over the volar-ulnar wrist flexion crease), the flexor carpi radialis (over the volar-radial wrist), the extensor carpi ulnaris (dorsal to the ulnar head), and the extensor pollicis longus (adjacent to Lister tubercle on the dorsal distal radius). Each of these conditions may present in a fashion similar to de Quervain disease with pain and limited range of motion. Treatment measures are comparable with splinting, ice, anti-inflammatory medication, activity modification, and steroid injection. Nonoperative treatment is usually effective in these less common conditions. However, early surgery may be considered for tendonitis of the extensor pollicis longus tendon when associated with a distal radius fracture due to increased risk for rupture.[84]

GANGLIA

Ganglia are fluid-filled structures that arise from a joint, tendon, or tendon sheath. They contain lubricating fluid called mucin, which is similar in content but more viscous than the fluid found in joints and tendon sheaths. Ganglia can emanate from almost any anatomic region, but they are most common at the wrist, the distal interphalangeal joints, and the proximal margins of flexor tendon sheaths. The cysts communicate with these structures through one or more ducts that account for their intermittent fluctuation in size.[69] The etiology of ganglia remain speculative. Histologically, they represent myxoid and mucinous degeneration of the normal capsular tissues or tendon sheath.[2]

Carpal Ganglia

Anatomy/Pathophysiology

Ganglia of the wrist occur most frequently over the dorsal radiocarpal joint near the midline of the wrist. They present less commonly at the palmar radial border of the carpus, adjacent to the flexor carpi radialis tendon (Fig. 16–6). Dorsal ganglia typically arise from the scapholunate interosseous ligament, whereas palmar ganglia most often originate at the scaphotrapezial or radiocarpal joints. The cysts may be multiloculated and much larger than clinically apparent, extending far from their point of origin.[77]

Diagnosis

Patients with carpal ganglia may report activity-related aching or vague wrist discomfort exacerbated by activity. Limitation of active wrist motion secondary to discomfort is infrequent. Occasionally an "occult" dorsal carpal ganglion will be too small to palpate.[71] More commonly, a ganglion can be palpated as a firm mass or fullness in the affected region. Palmar flexion of the wrist will help accentuate the dorsally located cyst. If the diagnosis is in question, a needle aspiration will confirm the diagnosis of a cyst with the expression of clear or blood-tinged viscous material from the mass.

Treatment

Although wrist ganglia can cause symptoms, they are frequently asymptomatic. Patients often request evaluation of a wrist lump noted only incidentally. These ganglia may be tender to direct palpation, but they do not cause exertional discomfort or limit activities. No intervention is necessary for either asymptomatic or minimally symptomatic carpal cysts.

For a symptomatic dorsal wrist ganglion, aspiration of the cyst and injection of cortisone is successful in less than 50% of cases.[2,64] Aspirations/injections are relatively contraindicated for palmar wrist ganglia owing to the close proximity of the radial artery. Temporary splinting of the wrist and the use of a nonsteroidal anti-inflammatory medication may lead to symptomatic improvement. Surgical excision of wrist ganglia is indicated only if symptoms warrant. The necessary dissection can be fairly extensive and involves removal of the cyst along with a small amount of normal tissue surrounding its origin. Volar wrist ganglia typically displace and envelop the radial artery and occasionally the palmar cutaneous branch of the median nerve and are especially tedious to excise.

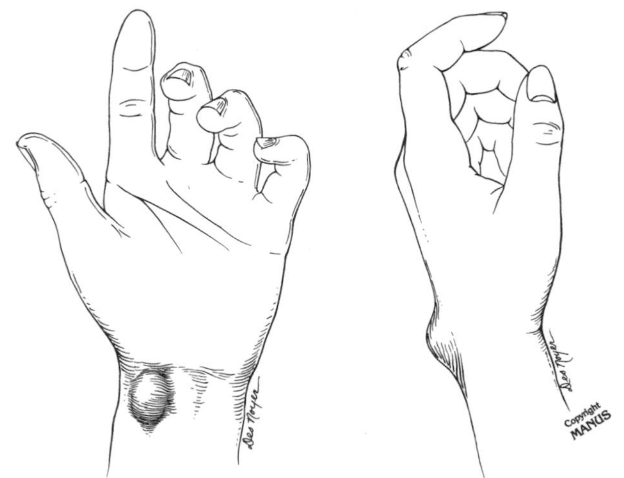

Figure 16–6. Carpal ganglia commonly arise over the dorsum of the wrist at the radiocarpal joint and at the palmar aspect of the wrist adjacent to the flexor carpi radialis tendon. Ganglia can be multiloculated and more extensive than apparent on clinical examination. (Courtesy of the Indiana Hand Center, Indianapolis, Indiana.)

Results

Surgical excision will result in cure of the cyst in over 95% of cases. The procedure is usually performed open but an arthroscopic technique for excising dorsal ganglia has been described.[8,57] Failure to excise the deep soft tissue attachments is associated with a 30% to 50% recurrence rate, with the majority of recurrences noted within the first 3 months.[2] Volar wrist ganglia are especially prone to recurrence.[86] Wrist range of motion and strength return slowly and usually require a supervised occupational therapy program. This is especially the case for dorsal cysts that require excision of part of the dorsal wrist capsule. Early rehabilitation is recommended for these patients and a minor loss of terminal wrist flexion is not uncommon. Many patients report continued low-grade aching pain for weeks to months following ganglion excision. Maximum medical improvement is anticipated 8 to 12 weeks postoperatively.

Retinacular Cysts

Ganglia arising from the digital flexor tendon sheath are termed volar retinacular ganglia or retinacular cysts. These appear as a small lump at the base of a digit adjacent to the palmar digital flexion crease. The ganglia are attached to the tendon sheath and do not move with the tendon as would trigger finger nodules.

Retinacular cysts are problematic owing to their location on the palmar side of the digit. They commonly cause discomfort during activities that require gripping or holding objects in the palm. These ganglia need no treatment if they are asymptomatic. When they cause pain with use of the hand, they can be treated with needle aspiration and injection, with a higher rate of success than carpal cysts.[2,64] Alternatively, surgical excision is performed under local anesthesia and is usually curative.

Mucous Cysts

Cysts that arise from the distal interphalangeal joint are termed mucous cysts. These are invariably associated with osteoarthritis of the distal finger joint. Histologically, mucous cysts resemble ganglia and are believed to result from herniation and degeneration of joint synovium and capsular tissues.[39,41] Because of their location, mucous cysts can disrupt the germinal matrix of the nail bed and lead to longitudinal nail plate grooves and ridges (Fig. 16–7). Mucous cysts can also become quite tender when enlarged.

Aspiration and instillation of a corticosteroid may be attempted with mucous cysts, but this treatment is rarely curative. Aspiration may also increase the likelihood of septic arthritis as the joint is immediately beneath the skin surface. Simple cyst excision carries a recurrence rate of 25% or greater.[39] The cyst is related to joint degeneration and osteophytes, which must be removed to limit recurrence. Excision of the joint marginal osteophytes with the cyst is successful in over 95% of cases.[39,41] Recovery following mucous cyst excision is relatively rapid and unrestricted use of the hand should be possible within 3 to 6 weeks.

Other Ganglia

Ganglion cysts occasionally arise from other tendons and joints in the wrist and hand. They may be seen overlying an extensor tendon on the dorsum of the hand, along the dorsal margin of a proximal interphalangeal joint, or adherent to a carpometacarpal joint.[2] Treatment principles are similar to those discussed for carpal, retinacular, and mucous cysts.

OSTEOARTHRITIS

Osteoarthritis is a slowly progressive joint disease of multifactorial etiology.[31,51] Cartilage degeneration and osteophyte formation are often seen in association with advancing age and characteristically affect the hands in a symmetrical pattern. The distal interphalangeal joint of the finger is the most commonly involved hand joint followed by the thumb basilar joint. In contradistinction to autoimmune arthritic conditions such as rheumatoid arthritis, the metacarpophalangeal joints are typically spared. Hand involvement is more prevalent in women and there appears to be a hereditary component.

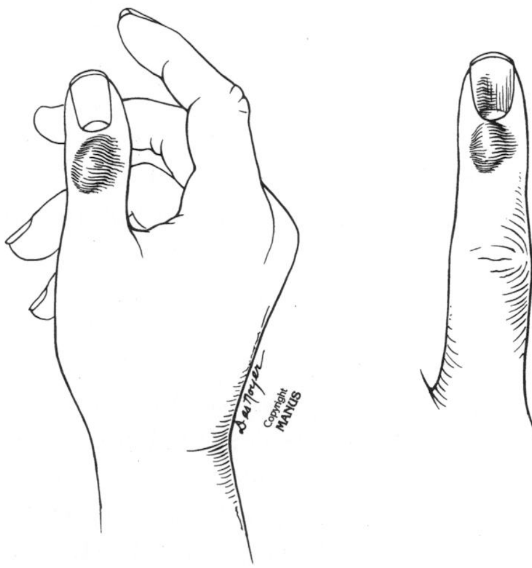

Figure 16–7. Mucous cysts are ganglia that arise from the distal interphalangeal joint. These cysts can compress the germinal nail matrix and lead to ridges or grooves in the nail plate. (Courtesy of the Indiana Hand Center, Indianapolis, Indiana.)

Several studies discuss "overuse" as having an influence on the development of osteoarthritis in the wrist and hand.[59,62] However, the relationship of osteoarthritis to work activities remains uncertain.

Wrist

Anatomy/Pathophysiology

Unlike the finger interphalangeal and thumb basilar joints, osteoarthritis of the wrist typically occurs secondary to a traumatic event. Intra-articular fractures of the distal radius, malunited scaphoid fractures, scaphoid nonunions, and intercarpal ligamentous injuries all predispose the wrist to degeneration. Calcium pyrophosphate deposition disease has also been implicated in the development of wrist degenerative arthritis.[12,36] In many cases, however, a cause is not readily identifiable.

An orderly sequence of joint deterioration has been described following ligamentous injury, scaphoid nonunion, and pyrophosphate deposition disease. This has been termed the SLAC (scapholunate advanced collapse) pattern of arthritis and is reportedly seen in over 70% of cases of osteoarthritis of the wrist.[81] Degeneration initially occurs at the distal radioscaphoid articulation, progressing to the proximal radioscaphoid joint and eventually to the capitolunate joint. The radiolunate joint is characteristically preserved. A second degenerative pattern is occasionally seen at the scaphoid, trapezium, and trapezoid articulations.

Diagnosis

Patients with wrist osteoarthritis report pain, loss of mobility, and weakness. Crepitation during motion or loading activities and swelling over the dorsal carpus are common in advanced disease. Examination reveals tenderness that is initially localized to the tip of the radial styloid process at the radioscaphoid joint. Tenderness later becomes more diffuse. Limitation of wrist motion is common as is diminished grip strength. The diagnosis is confirmed on roentgenograms. Degeneration of the distal radioulnar joint is less common and manifests primarily as pain with occasional restriction of forearm rotation.

Treatment

For early degenerative disease of the wrist, conservative measures are frequently successful. These include nonsteroidal anti-inflammatory medication, wrist immobilization, activity modification, and steroid injection into the carpus. Once significant degenerative arthritic changes have developed, there is typically some degree of permanent impairment and often activity and job modifications are required. Intermittent use of a wrist splint may be helpful during more strenuous activities. Surgery is only indicated if conservative treatment measures fail and symptoms warrant. Various procedures have been described and include proximal row carpectomy (excision of the three most proximal carpal bones), partial intercarpal fusions, and total wrist arthrodesis. Surgical decision-making involves an assessment of the location and degree of degenerative arthritis as well as the needs and expectations of the individual patient. The period of postoperative immobilization varies depending on the surgical procedure performed, typically averaging 6 to 10 weeks for a fusion procedure.

Results

Similar to other joints affected by degenerative arthritis, conservative therapy is more successful in less advanced cases. Results of surgical treatment for wrist arthritis are favorable in terms of pain relief. Motion retaining procedures such as partial wrist fusions and proximal row carpectomy require a considerable amount of therapy following cast removal.[15] Grip strength and range of motion generally plateau by 6 months but may continue to improve for up to 1 year. Total wrist fusion may be the most reliable in terms of relieving pain, but at the expense of all wrist motion.

Work restrictions following wrist surgery must be determined on an individual basis, taking into account the degree of residual impairment and the specific job requirements. Maximum medical improvement is anticipated 4 to 6 months postoperatively.

Thumb Basilar Joint

Anatomy/Pathophysiology

The basilar joint of the thumb consists of the thumb metacarpal and trapezium. The unique saddle-shaped configuration of the articulation affords the thumb exceptional mobility. The joint not only permits freedom of motion in several planes but also provides a significant load-bearing function during pinch and grasp activities.[5] Arthritis of the basilar thumb joint is the second most common site for degenerative joint disease in the hand (preceded only by the distal interphalangeal joint). The condition is more frequent in women (10:1) and has been attributed to laxity of the important stabilizing ligaments of the thumb base.

Diagnosis

Patients with basilar thumb joint arthritis have pain at the base of the thenar muscles with occasional proximal and distal radiation. The pain is exacerbated by pinching and gripping activities. It is characteristic for patients to have problems opening jars and turning doorknobs. As the condition advances, pinch and grip strength are diminished and thumb range of motion becomes limited.

Examination reveals a tender, prominent basilar joint. In advanced cases, a stiff adduction deformity of the thumb metacarpal may occur with compensatory hyperextension of the thumb metacarpophalangeal joint. Pain is reproduced when the joint is palpated on its radial and dorsal aspects. Stress applied to the joint through axial grinding and shearing of the metacarpal base exacerbates the pain (Fig. 16–8). This may also elicit instability and crepitation. The Finkelstein test is usually negative, which helps to distinguish basilar joint arthritis pain from de Quervain disease. The diagnosis is confirmed by roentgenograms. These images should include both a lateral projection and a pronated anteroposterior Robert view of the trapeziometacarpal joint (Fig. 16–9).[72]

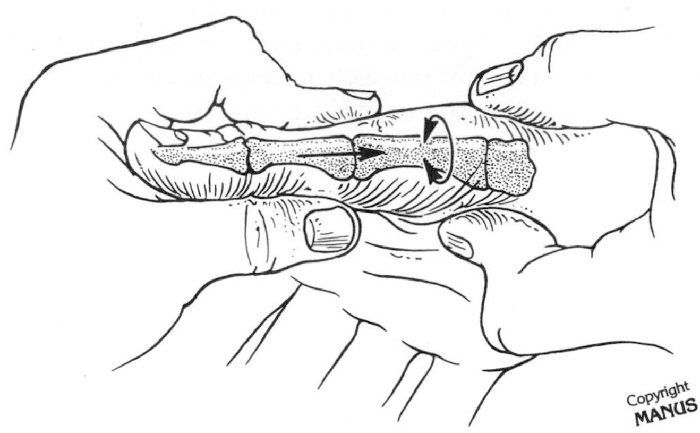

Figure 16–8. A thumb carpometacarpal joint "grind test" involves axial compression of the thumb metacarpal with rotation of the basilar joint. This maneuver exacerbates the discomfort associated with basilar joint arthritis. (Courtesy of the Indiana Hand Center, Indianapolis, Indiana.)

Treatment

Initial treatment of basilar joint osteoarthritis includes activity modification, splint immobilization (leaving the interphalangeal joint free for writing and light activities), nonsteroidal anti-inflammatory medication, thenar muscle strengthening exercises, and steroid injection. Splint wear is advocated full time for a period of 2 to 3 weeks.[5]

When patients' symptoms are not satisfactorily relieved by conservative means, surgical intervention may be considered. The basilar thumb joint is the most common joint in the hand requiring surgery for osteoarthritis. Most surgical procedures involve partial or total excision of the diseased trapezium with stabilization of the thumb metacarpal base using local tendon graft or transfer.[5,65] Significant hyperextension of the thumb metacarpophalangeal joint may necessitate concomitant fusion of this joint in some cases. The postoperative course involves a 4- to 6-week period of immobilization followed by a supervised therapy program.

Results

Pain relief with surgery is common, but symptoms may persist for several months even in successful cases. Thumb motion, grip, and pinch strength may continue to improve for up to 1 year postoperatively.[65] Activity modifications in the workplace may be indicated for an extended period of time following basilar thumb reconstructive surgery. Maximum medical improvement is anticipated at approximately 6 to 8 months.

Fusion of the thumb basilar joint is most commonly reserved for younger individuals involved in manual labor. Arthrodesis provides excellent pain relief and improved strength at the expense of thumb mobility.[42] Fusion will result in a small degree of permanent impairment secondary to the loss of motion at the basal joint. However, individuals with a successful joint fusion are often capable of returning to heavy manual labor. Arthrodesis is contraindicated in the presence of concomitant scaphotrapezial degenerative arthritis.

Proximal Interphalangeal Joints

Anatomy/Pathophysiology

Osteoarthritis of the proximal interphalangeal joint is relatively rare in comparison to the distal joint. When arthritic changes develop in this joint, they typically

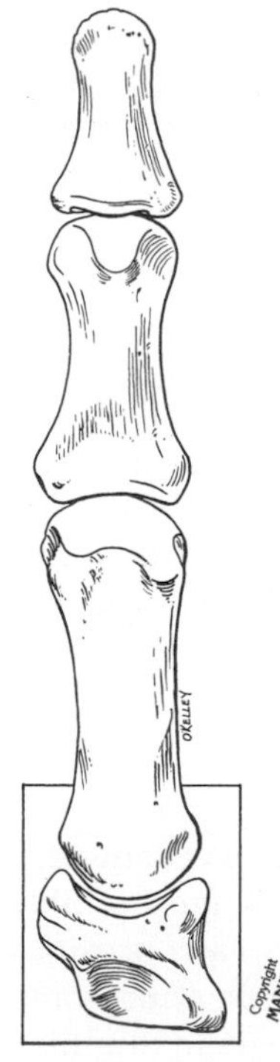

Figure 16–9. The Robert view of the trapeziometacarpal joint (basilar joint) is taken with the arm fully pronated, the shoulder internally rotated, and the thumb abducted. This position provides a true anteroposterior view of the joint. (Courtesy of the Indiana Hand Center, Indianapolis, Indiana.)

occur in conjunction with distal interphalangeal joint degeneration.[73] Isolated degeneration of a proximal interphalangeal joint is usually post-traumatic in nature, following a dislocation or intra-articular fracture.

Diagnosis

Swelling and morning stiffness are the first signs of early degenerative arthritis. Limited proximal interphalangeal joint motion follows with the development of marginal osteophytes (Bouchard nodes.) Late joint degeneration leads to angular deformity and joint instability (Fig. 16–10). A progressive loss of motion usually occurs although many severely involved joints will continue to function well with little associated discomfort. Roentgenograms confirm the diagnosis and document the degree of joint destruction (Fig. 16–11).

Treatment

Conservative treatment measures include nonsteroidal anti-inflammatory medication, activity modification, and short-term splinting. Steroid injections can be helpful in ameliorating pain early in the degenerative process. They are more effective, however, in inflammatory arthritic conditions (e.g., rheumatoid arthritis). If these measures fail and considerable symptoms persist, surgical intervention may be considered. Surgical alternatives include arthrodesis and silastic replacement arthroplasty.[73,75]

Arthrodesis is the most reliable method of eliminating pain and is superior in restoring pinch strength to the index finger. Fusion of the ulnar digits at the proximal interphalangeal joint level impairs grip strength and dexterity to a greater degree than the radial digits. Silicone arthroplasty preserves mobility but provides little stability to laterally directed forces. Both procedures can be performed under a local or regional anesthetic block. Fusions are performed with pins, wires, or screws. Patients are protected postoperatively from heavy loading for approximately 6 to 10 weeks, or until fusion is confirmed on roentgenograms. Arthroplasties of the proximal interphalangeal joint should never be subjected to high stress or lateral shear forces given the potential for implant breakage. Silicone replacement is therefore typically reserved for older individuals and those who will place low demand on the implant.

Results

Fusion rates vary from 84% to 100% with excellent pain relief.[47] Joint deformity is corrected and finger stability is improved. Silicone replacement arthroplasty provides pain relief with the added benefit of preserving some joint motion.[73,75] However, mobility appears to diminish with time. Furthermore, arthroplasty carries attendant risks of joint instability and implant breakage, which may necessitate future surgery.[61]

Maximum medical improvement is expected 3 to 6 months postoperatively following either procedure. Impairment following fusion primarily involves loss of

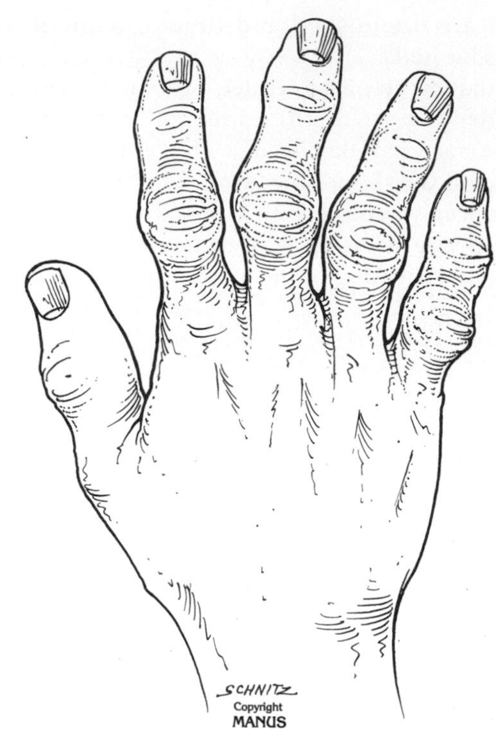

Figure 16–10. Late appearance of degenerative joint disease of the proximal interphalangeal joints. Osteophyte formation (Bouchard nodes) leads to joint enlargement. Asymmetrical destruction leads to instability and angular deformity of the digits. (Courtesy of the Indiana Hand Center, Indianapolis, Indiana.)

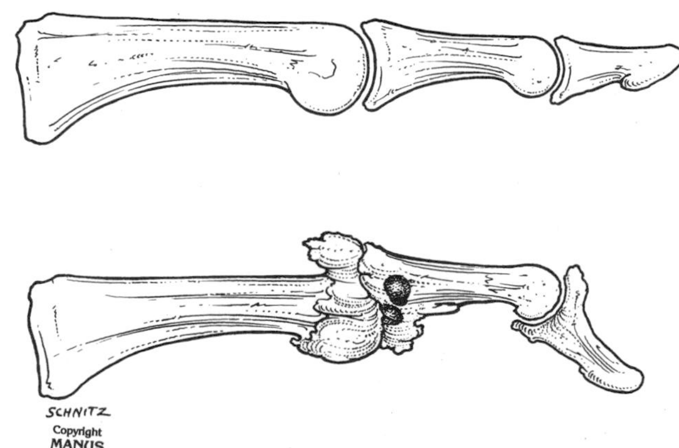

Figure 16–11. Proximal interphalangeal joint arthritis manifests as joint space narrowing and marginal osteophyte formation. Degenerative cysts and subchondral sclerosis are also prominent features of the degenerative process. (Courtesy of the Indiana Hand Center, Indianapolis, Indiana.)

joint motion. Grip strength may also be diminished, especially if the fusion involves the ulnar digits, which greatly contribute to grip strength.

Distal Interphalangeal Joints

Anatomy/Pathophysiology

The distal interphalangeal joints of the fingers are the most frequently affected joints in the body in patients with osteoarthritis. Degeneration commonly involves multiple digits in a symmetrical distribution. In most cases, symptoms are mild and functional impairment is minimal. Isolated distal interphalangeal joint degeneration is usually the sequela of previous trauma to the joint (e.g., mallet fracture).

Diagnosis

Swelling and stiffness are common in early joint degeneration. These symptoms typically occur in the morning or after prolonged use of the involved fingers. As the disease progresses, distal interphalangeal joint enlargement is seen secondary to osteophyte formation (Heberden nodes), and painful limited motion results. Late in the disease joint deformity occurs with angular and rotational deformities at the fingertip. Roentgenograms again confirm the diagnosis and document the severity of joint destruction. Advanced disease is compatible with adequate function and minimal symptoms in most cases.

Treatment

Conservative care is successful in the majority of individuals. Treatment measures include nonsteroidal anti-inflammatory medication, activity modification, and occasional short-term splinting. Cortisone injections can also be of benefit. Surgery is reserved for late degenerative disease that does not respond to conservative measures and is causing significant pain, deformity, or instability. Distal interphalangeal joint arthrodesis is the procedure of choice, although silastic arthroplasty may be considered in special cases.[16,68] Both procedures can be effectively performed with digital block anesthesia. Fusions are accomplished using screws or Kirschner wires. Postoperative protection from heavy loading is required for approximately 6 to 10 weeks, or until fusion is confirmed radiographically.

Results

Fusion reliably relieves pain, restores stability and strength, and improves the appearance of the digit. Successful distal interphalangeal joint fusion rates vary from 80% to 100%, with arthrodesis providing predictable long-lasting results.[38] Incisions placed at the pulp tip for screw insertion are frequently sensitive, requiring scar desensitization. Arthroplasty maintains some distal interphalangeal motion while providing pain relief. Similar to the proximal interphalangeal joint, instability and breakage of the implants are potential complications. Maximum medical improvement is expected 3 to 6 months postoperatively. Impairment following successful distal joint fusion or arthroplasty is minimal.

REFLEX SYMPATHETIC DYSTROPHY

Anatomy/Pathophysiology

Reflex sympathetic dystrophy is a neurogenic disorder characterized by pain out of proportion to the level anticipated, swelling, vasomotor changes (autonomic dysfunction), and joint stiffness.[30,70] In the past, a variety of terms have been used to describe this condition, including causalgia, Sudeck atrophy, and shoulder-hand syndrome. Recently, the condition has been renamed type I chronic regional pain syndrome (CRPS) and incorporated into a broader classification scheme of chronic pain syndromes.[85] CRPS can occur following any traumatic event to the upper extremity. Alternatively, the condition can develop following a relatively simple surgical procedure.

The pathogenesis of CRPS remains poorly understood. Autonomic hyperactivity and nerve injuries are implicated in the development of CRPS, and psychological factors seem to play a role in many cases. Some clinicians believe in a diathesis or constitutional predisposition with dystrophy patients being more anxious, insecure, hysterical, passive-aggressive, and over-reactive to pain. Whether patient personality characteristics predispose to the condition or are secondary is debatable. In either event, psychological factors clearly aggravate the symptom complex when present.

In many cases, full-blown reflex dystrophy progresses through a series of loosely defined stages. Initially pain, swelling, restricted motion, and vasomotor changes (hyperhidrosis, erythema, excessive warmth) predominate the symptom complex. Later, after several months, pain remains the dominant feature and swelling changes from a soft to a hard brawny edema. The hand eventually becomes dry, stiff, and atrophied. After many months to years, the skin assumes a shiny, glossy appearance and stiffness becomes marked with fixed contractures. However, not all cases of CRPS fit this temporal scheme. The condition represents a continuum with a variable presence and intensity of symptoms.

Diagnosis

The diagnosis of reflex sympathetic dystrophy is made primarily on clinical examination but may be confirmed by a variety of objective tests. Diffuse pain out of proportion to the initial injury, diminished hand function secondary to stiffness or pain, and sympathetic dysfunction (edema, hyperhidrosis or anhidrosis, atrophy of skin, hair or nail changes, warmth or coolness, discoloration of skin) are present in varying degrees. The pain is frequently described as burning and intense and may be exacerbated with a light touch of the skin. Roentgenograms frequently reveal diffuse osteopenia secondary to demineralization within 3 to 5 weeks after the onset of symptoms. Three-phase bone scans show characteristic diffuse uptake in the involved areas. Sympathetic blockade of stellate ganglia remains the most definitive means of establishing the diagnosis; immediate symptom improvement confirms the presence of CRPS.

Treatment

The key to successful treatment of reflex sympathetic dystrophy is prompt diagnosis and intervention to break the pain cycle. Treatment should be initiated as soon as the diagnosis is suspected to prevent the full-blown syndrome. The appearance and persistence of inordinate postoperative pain may be the first sign of early CRPS. Care should be taken to eliminate any potential painful stimuli (wound hematoma, cast compression).

Supervised active range of motion exercises, edema control, and interval splinting are initiated by an experienced therapist. A stress-loading program consisting of active traction and compression exercises has been shown to be helpful.[80] Transcutaneous electrical nerve stimulation is occasionally useful in controlling pain in the early stages of CRPS. Pharmacologic intervention involves the use of oral corticosteroids, alpha-adrenergic blocking agents, calcium channel blockers, and antidepressants. Sympathetic blocks (e.g., stellate ganglion blocks and intravenous regional blocks) provide immediate pain relief and are an integral component of treatment. They often must be repeated to break the cycle of CRPS pain. Occasionally, a continuous stellate ganglion block is utilized.

Surgical intervention in CRPS must be considered cautiously. Only if an identifiable pathologic condition is present and thought to be contributing to the condition is this considered. Examples include a painful neuroma or compressive neuropathy that may have precipitated the condition. Surgery should not be performed if motion and function are improving. Perioperative sympathetic blockade is useful to thwart a possible flare-up of symptoms. Surgical sympathectomy is sometimes required in refractory cases.

Results

The earlier intervention is instituted, the better the chance for a successful result. However, a significant percentage of patients may still complain of pain, cold intolerance, nail and hair growth changes, sensory disturbances, swelling, hand weakness, and stiffness years later.[88] Once the chronic stages of reflex sympathetic dystrophy have occurred, results are even less favorable, with varying degrees of permanent upper extremity impairment.

References

1. Agee JM, McCarroll HR, Tortosa RD, et al: Endoscopic release of the carpal tunnel: A randomized prospective multicenter study. J Hand Surg 17A:987–995, 1992.
2. Angelides AC: Ganglions of the wrist and hand. In Green DP, Hotchkiss RN, Pederson WC (eds): Green's Operative Hand Surgery, 4th ed. Philadelphia, Churchill Livingstone, 1999, pp 2171–2183.
3. Armstrong TJ, Fine LJ, Goldstein SA, et al: Ergonomic considerations in hand and wrist tendonitis. J Hand Surg 12A:830–837, 1987.
4. Atroshi I, Gummesson C, Johnson R, et al: Prevalence of carpal tunnel syndrome in the general population. JAMA 282:153–158, 1999.
5. Barron OA, Glickel SZ, Eaton RG: Basal joint arthritis of the thumb. J Am Acad Orthop Surg 8:314–323, 2000.
6. Bensimon RH, Murphy RX Jr: Midpalmar approach to the carpal tunnel: An alternative to endoscopic release. Ann Plast Surg 36:462–465, 1996.
7. Benson LS, Ptaszek AJ: Injection versus surgery in the treatment of trigger finger. J Hand Surg 22A:138–144, 1997.
8. Bienz T, Raphael JS: Arthroscopic resection of the dorsal ganglia of the wrist. Hand Clin 15:429–434, 1999.
9. Bromley GS: Minimal-incision open carpal tunnel decompression. J Hand Surg 19A:119–120, 1994.
10. Brown RA, Gelberman RH, Seiler JG, et al: Carpal tunnel release: A prospective randomized assessment of open and endoscopic methods. J Bone Joint Surg 75A:1265–1275, 1993.
11. Bystrom S, Hall C, Welander T, et al: Clinical disorders and pressure–pain threshold of the forearm and hand among automobile assembly line workers. J Hand Surg 20B:782–790, 1995.
12. Chen C, Chandnani VP, Kang HS, et al: Scapholunate advanced collapse: A common wrist abnormality in calcium pyrophosphate dihydrate crystal deposition disease. Radiology 177:459–461, 1990.
13. Chow JC: Endoscopic release of the carpal ligament for carpal tunnel syndrome: A 22-month clinical result. Arthroscopy 6:288–296, 1990.
14. Clark MT, Lyall HA, Grant JW, et al: The histopathology of de Quervain's disease. J Hand Surg 23B:732–734, 1998.
15. Cohen MS, Kozinn SH: Degenerative arthritis of the wrist: proximal row carpectomy versus scaphoid excision and four-corner arthrodesis. J Hand Surg 26A:94–104, 2001.
16. Culver JE, Fleeger ES: Osteoarthritis of the distal interphalangeal joint. Hand Clin 3:385–402, 1987.
17. DeStefano F, Nordstrom DL, Vierkant RA: Long-term symptom outcomes of carpal tunnel syndrome and its treatment. J Hand Surg 22A:200–210, 1997.
18. Durkam JA: A new diagnostic test for carpal tunnel syndrome. J Bone Joint Surg 73A:535–538, 1991.
19. Ferlic DC: Rheumatoid flexor tenosynovitis and rupture. Hand Clin 12:561–572, 1996.
20. Finkelstein H: Stenosing tenosynovitis of the radial styloid process. J Bone Joint Surg 30A:509, 1930.
21. Franklin GM, Haug J, Heyer N, et al: Occupational carpal tunnel syndrome in Washington State, 1984–1988. Am J Public Health 81:74, 1991.

22. Freiberg A, Mulholland RS, Levine R: Nonoperative treatment of trigger fingers and thumbs. J Hand Surg 14A:553–558, 1989.
23. Fuchs PC, Nathan PA, Myers LD: Synovial histology in carpal tunnel syndrome. J Hand Surg 16A:753–758, 1991.
24. Gelberman RH, Aronson D, Weisman MH: Carpal tunnel syndrome: Results of a prospective trial of steroid injection and splinting. J Bone Joint Surg 62A:1181–1184, 1980.
25. Gelberman RH, Hergenroeder PT, Hargens AR, et al: The carpal tunnel syndrome: A study of carpal tunnel pressures. J Bone Joint Surg 63A:380, 1981.
26. Gelberman RH, Rydevik BL, Pess GM, et al: Carpal tunnel syndrome: A scientific basis for clinical care. Orthop Clin North Am 19:115–124, 1988.
27. Gelberman RH, Szabo RM, Williamson RV, et al: Sensitivity testing in peripheral-nerve compression syndromes. J Bone Joint Surg 65A:632–638, 1983.
28. Gellman H, Gelberman RH, Tan AM, et al: Carpal tunnel syndrome: An evaluation of the provocative diagnostic tests. J Bone Joint Surg 68A:735–737, 1986.
29. Gellman H, Kan D, Gee V, et al: Analysis of pinch and grip strength after carpal tunnel release. J Hand Surg 14A:863–864, 1989.
30. Gellman H, Nichols D: Reflex sympathetic dystrophy in the upper extremity. J Am Acad Orthop Surg 5:313–322, 1997.
31. Goldring MB: The role of the chondrocyte in osteoarthritis. Arthritis Rheum 43:1916–1926, 2000.
32. Green DP: Diagnostic and therapeutic value of carpal tunnel injection. J Hand Surg 9A:850–854, 1984.
33. Grundberg AB: Carpal tunnel decompression in spite of normal electromyography. J Hand Surg 8:348–349, 1983.
34. Ha KI, Park MJ, Ha CW: Percutaneous release of trigger digits. J Bone Joint Surg 83B:75–77, 2001.
35. Hadler NM: Repetitive upper-extremity motions in the workplace are not hazardous. J Hand Surg 22A:19–29, 1997.
36. Harrington RH, Lichtman DM, Brockmole DM: Common pathways of degenerative arthritis of the wrist. Hand Clin 3:507–525, 1987.
37. Irwin LR, Beckett R, Suman RK: Steroid injection for carpal tunnel syndrome. J Hand Surg 21B:355–357, 1996.
38. Jones BF, Stern PJ: Interphalangeal joint arthrodesis. Hand Clin 10:267–275, 1994.
39. Kasdan ML, Stallings SP, Leis VM, et al: Outcome of surgically treated mucous cysts of the hand. J Hand Surg 19A:504–507, 1994.
40. Katz JN, Losina E, Amick BC III, et al: Predictors of outcomes of carpal tunnel release. Arthritis Rheum 44:1184–1193, 2001.
41. Kleinert HE, Kutz JE, Fishman JH, et al: Etiology and treatment of the so-called mucous cyst of the finger. J Bone Joint Surg 54A:1455–1458, 1972.
42. Klimo GF, Verma RB, Baratz ME: The treatment of trapeziometacarpal arthritis with arthrodesis. Hand Clin 17:261–270, 2001.
43. Koris M, Gelberman RH, Duncan K, et al: Carpal tunnel syndrome: Evaluation of a quantitative provocational diagnostic test. Clin Orthop Rel Res 251:157–161, 1990.
44. Lane LB, Boretz RS, Stuchin SA: Treatments of de Quervain's disease: Role of conservative management. H Hand Surg 26B:258–260, 2001.
45. Leach WJ, Esler C, Scott TD: Grip strength following carpal tunnel decompression. J Hand Surg 18B:750–752, 1993.
46. Lee WPA, Plancher KD, Strickland JW: Carpal tunnel release with a small palmar incision. Hand Clin 12:271–284, 1996.
47. Leibovic SJ, Strickland JW: Arthrodesis of the proximal interphalangeal joint of the finger: Comparison of the use of Herbert screw with other fixation methods. J Hand Surg 19A:181–188, 1994.
48. Leslie BM, Ericson WB Jr, Morehead JR: Incidence of a septum within the first dorsal compartment of the wrist. J Hand Surg 15A:88–91, 1990.
49. Louis DS, Hankin FM: Symptomatic relief following carpal tunnel decompression with normal electromyographic studies. Orthopedics 10:434–436, 1987.
50. Mackinnon, SE, Novak CB: Repetitive strain in the workplace. J Hand Surg 22A:2–18, 1997.
51. Martel-Pelletier J: Pathophysiology of osteoarthritis. Osteoarthritis and Cartilage 6:374–376, 1998.
52. Masear VR, Hayes JM, Hyde AG: An industrial cause of carpal tunnel syndrome. J Hand Surg 11A:222–227, 1986.
53. Miller RF, Lohman WH, Maldonado G, et al: An epidemiologic study of carpal tunnel syndrome and hand-arm vibration syndrome in relation to vibration exposure. J Hand Surg 19A:99–105, 1994.
54. Moberg E: Objective methods of determining functional value of sensibility in the hand. J Bone Joint Surg 44:454, 1958.
55. Nathan PA, Meadows KD, Keniston RC: Rehabilitation of carpal tunnel syndrome patients using a short surgical incision and an early program of physical therapy. J Hand Surg 18A:1044–1050, 1993.
56. Newport ML, Lane LB, Stuchin SA: Trigger finger treated by steroid injection. J Hand Surg 15A:748–750, 1990.
57. Osterman AL, Raphael J: Arthroscopic resection of dorsal ganglion of the wrist. Hand Clin 11:7–12, 1995.
58. Otto N, Wehbe MA: Steroid injections for tenosynovitis in the hand. Orthop Rev 15:290–293, 1986.
59. Palmieri TJ, Grand FM, Hay EL, et al: Treatment of osteoarthritis in the hand and wrist. Hand Clin 3:371–381, 1987.
60. Patel MR, Moradia VJ: Percutaneous release of trigger digit with and without cortisone injection. J Hand Surg 22A:150–155, 1997.
61. Pelligrini VD, Burton RI: Osteoarthritis of the proximal interphalangeal joint of the hand: Arthroplasty or fusion? J Hand Surg 15A:184–209, 1990.
62. Peyron JG: The epidemiology of osteoarthritis. In Moskowitz R, Howell D, Goldberg V, et al (eds): Osteoarthritis: Diagnosis and Management. Philadelphia, WB Saunders, 1984, pp 9–27.
63. Phalen GS: The carpal tunnel syndrome: Seventeen years experience in diagnosis and treatment of 654 hands. J Bone Joint Surg 48A:211–228, 1966.
64. Richman JA, Gelberman RH, Engber WD, et al: Ganglions of the wrist and digits: Results of treatment by aspiration and cyst wall puncture. J Hand Surg 12A:1041–1043, 1987.
65. Robinson D, Aghasi M, Halperin N: Abductor pollicis longus tendon arthroplasty of the trapezial-metacarpal joint: Surgical technique and results. J Hand Surg 16A:504–509, 1991.
66. Robinson LR: Role of neurophysiologic evaluation in diagnosis. J Am Acad Orthop Surg 8:190–199, 2000.
67. Saldana MJ: Trigger digits: Diagnosis and treatment. J Am Acad Orthop Surg 9:246–252, 2001.
68. Snow JW, Boyes JG, Greider JL: Implant arthroplasty of the proximal interphalangeal joint of the finger for osteoarthritis. Plast Reconstr Surg 60:558–560, 1977.
69. Soren A: Pathogenesis and treatment of ganglions. Clin Orthop 48:173, 1966.
70. Soucacos PN, Diznitsas LA, Beris AE, et al: Reflex sympathetic dystrophy of the upper extremity: Clinical features and response to multimodal management. Hand Clin 13:339–354, 1997.
71. Steinberg BD, Kleinman WB: Occult scapholunate ganglion: A cause of dorsal radial wrist pain. J Hand Surg 24A:225–231, 1999.
72. Steinberg DR: Management of the arthritic hand. In Chapman MW (ed): Operative Orthopaedics, 2nd ed. Philadelphia, JB Lippincott, 1993, pp 1571–1578.
73. Stern PJ, Ho S: Osteoarthritis of the proximal interphalangeal joint. Hand Clin 3:405–412, 1987.
74. Stewart JD, Eisen A: Tinel's sign and the carpal tunnel syndrome. Br Med J 2:1125–1126, 1978.
75. Swanson AB, Maupin BK, Gajjar NV, et al: Flexible implant arthroplasty in the proximal interphalangeal joint of the hand. J Hand Surg 10A:796–805, 1985.

76. Szabo RM: Entrapment and compression neuropathies. In Green DP, Hotchkiss RN, Pederson WC (eds): Green's Operative Hand Surgery, 4th ed. Philadelphia, Churchill Livingstone, 1999, pp 1404–1447.
77. Thornburg LE: Ganglions of the hand and wrist. J Am Acad Orthop Surg 7:231–238, 1999.
78. Turowski GA, Zdankiewics PD, Thomson JG: The results of surgical treatment of trigger finger. 22A:145–149, 1997.
79. Vender MI, Kasdan ML, Truppa KL: Upper extremity disorders: A literature review to determine work-relatedness. J Hand Surg 20A:534–541, 1995.
80. Watson HK, Carlson L: Treatment of reflex sympathetic dystrophy of the hand with an active "stress loading" program. J Hand Surg 12A:779–785, 1987.
81. Watson HK, Vender MI: Wrist and intercarpal arthrodesis. In Chapman MW (ed): Operative Orthopaedics, 2nd ed. Philadelphia, JB Lippincott, 1993, pp 1363–1377.
82. Weiss APC, Akelman E, Tabatabai M: Treatment of de Quervain's disease. J Hand Surg 19A:595–598, 1984.
83. Weiss AP, Sachar K, Gendreau M: Conservative management of carpal tunnel syndrome: A re-examination of steroid injection and splinting. J Hand Surg 19A:410–415, 1994.
84. Wolfe SW: Tenosynovitis. In Green DP, Hotchkiss RN, Pederson WC (eds): Green's Operative Hand Surgery. Philadelphia, Churchill Livingstone, 1999, pp 2022–2044.
85. Wong GY, Wilson PR: Classification of complex regional pain syndromes: New concepts. Hand Clin 13:319–325, 1997.
86. Wright TW, Cooney WP, Ilstrup DM: Anterior wrist ganglion. J Hand Surg 19A:954–958, 1994.
87. Yu GZ, Firrell JC, Tsai TM: Preoperative factors and treatment outcome following carpal tunnel release. J Hand Surg 17B:646–650, 1992.
88. Zyluk A: The sequelae of reflex sympathetic dystrophy. J Hand Surg 26B:151–154, 2001.

CHAPTER

17

Joint Systems

Shoulder and Elbow

ANTHONY A. ROMEO, MD ■ BRIAN S. COHEN, MD

Occupational disorders of the shoulder and elbow affect a substantial segment of the workforce in the United States, with employment-related upper extremity and shoulder impairment occurring in more than 500,000 workers per year.[97] After back and knee conditions, the shoulder is the most common site of long-term impairment. Injuries to the shoulder area are usually related to overexertion, direct trauma, or a fall.[142]

When evaluating occupational-related disorders, and their potential for impairment, the common goal is to develop scenarios where prevention is the focus. "Identifying the extent to which a disorder may have a sudden or gradual onset (or both) has important implications for improving prevention."[130] Reductions in duration, frequency, and intensity have a greater impact in preventing gradual onset type or overuse injuries, whereas sudden onset or traumatic type disorders are better prevented with safety adjustments; for example, machine guarding or nonslippery surfaces.

The evaluation of workers' compensation claimants is often difficult because of the unspoken issues of secondary gains. There is a concern "that the prognosis for compensation patients would be consistently poor" based on their "underlying" motives.[134] However, there are many studies that indicate no difference between pain intensity and pain descriptors reported by compensation patients as compared to a noncompensation patient population.[75,85,86,139] It is important for the health care provider to approach these individuals in an unbiased fashion.

Conditions of the shoulder and elbow resulting in impairment can be divided into two main categories: mechanical and nonmechanical. Nonmechanical problems are characteristically not related to specific activities or positions. They are difficult to localize and are frequently accompanied by sensations of hot or cold, numbness, and intermittent swelling. Nonmechanical conditions are difficult to categorize into specific diagnostic groups and therefore make the evaluation and treatment more complex.

Mechanical conditions characteristically become symptomatic during certain activities and positions. They are reproducible, well localized, and described by the patient in terms such as weakness, stiffness, slipping, or catching. For example, a muscle tear will be associated with weakness, whereas arthritis is generally associated with stiffness. Mechanical conditions often have typical signs and symptoms, leading to well-recognized diagnostic categories for which evaluation and management strategies have been developed.

SHOULDER DISORDERS

The shoulder is inherently an unstable joint. Normal shoulder function is dependent on a reciprocating relationship between glenohumeral mobility and stability. A large humeral head articulating with a small glenoid socket permits unrestricted motion at the shoulder, but compromises the integrity of the joint. Glenohumeral stability has been extensively researched, and is the responsibility of the static and dynamic stabilizers.[12,62] Static stability is derived from many different components of the shoulder. The conformity of the articulating surfaces between the humeral head and the glenoid socket provides the baseline from which glenohumeral stability is founded. This is accomplished by providing a platform for a very secure concavity-compression environment.[41] This is enhanced by the fibrous labrum, which increases the depth and surface area of the articulation.[62] The glenohumeral ligaments (Fig. 17–1) impart

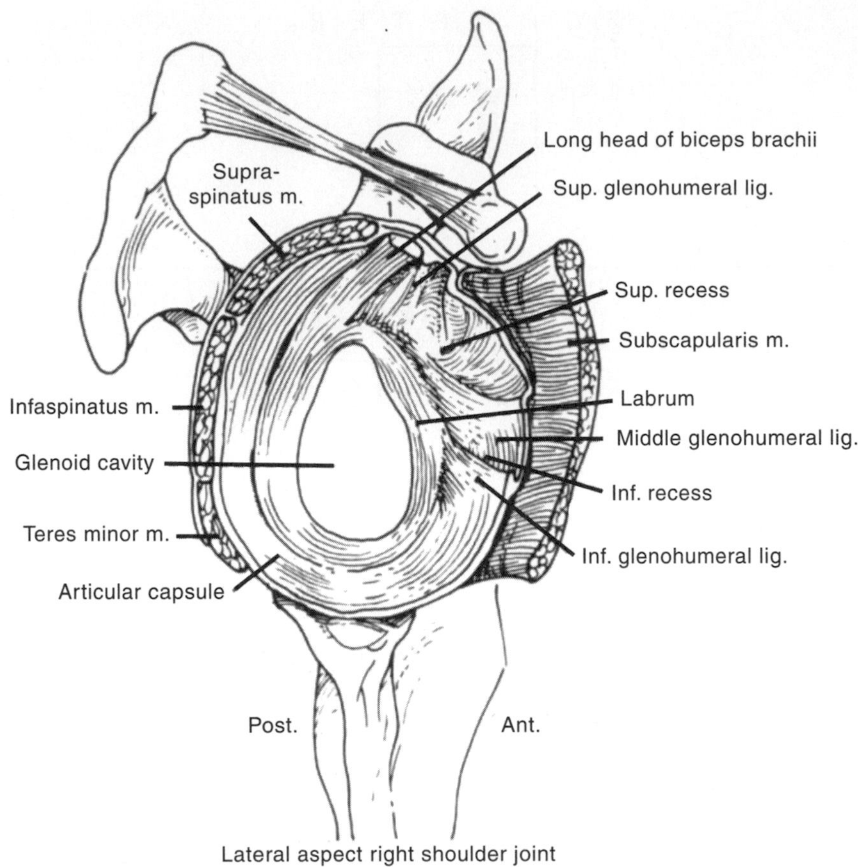

Figure 17–1. Glenohumeral ligaments and the rotator cuff stabilizers of the glenohumeral joint. (From Morrey BF, Itoi E, An K: Biomechanics of the shoulder. In Rockwood CAJ, Matsen FA III [eds]: The Shoulder. Philadelphia, WB Saunders, 1998, pp 233–276.)

static stability during the end ranges of shoulder rotation. They function as check-reins, reciprocally tightening and loosening in a load-sharing fashion, controlling humeral head rotation and translation.[147]

The dynamic stabilizers include the muscles of the rotator cuff, the long head of the biceps brachii, and the scapular stabilizing muscles. Through active muscle contraction of the rotator cuff and to a much lesser extent the long head of the biceps, stability of the glenohumeral joint is enhanced by ligament dynamization and by increasing the joint compression forces during the midranges of motion.[23] Proper positioning of the scapula—i.e., the glenoid—is also important for shoulder stability and is accomplished by the coordinated activity of the scapula stabilizing musculature.

A simple explanation for shoulder instability is failure of the humeral head to remain centered in the glenoid socket. This can be the result of trauma, the most extreme situation being a shoulder dislocation, or the result of muscle malfunction, as seen with rotator cuff tendonitis where the muscle is too inflamed to function normally, or, in the more traumatic situation, a rotator cuff tear. After inflammation is controlled, nonoperative and if necessary operative management focuses on restoring the central position of the humeral head within the glenoid socket. Only when this is successfully accomplished can the patient expect to achieve pain-free shoulder stability and function.

Normal shoulder function requires the coordinated movements of the sternoclavicular, acromioclavicular, and glenohumeral joints, as well as the scapulothoracic articulation and the motion interface between the rotator cuff and overlying coracoacromial arch. Successful elevation of the arm requires a minimum of 30 to 40 degrees of clavicular elevation and at least 45 to 60 degrees of scapula rotation. Motion across these articulations is accomplished by "the delicate interaction of approximately 30 muscles."[93] Pathologic changes in any portion of the complex may disrupt the normal biomechanics of the shoulder. Therefore, pain and/or weakness in one area can adversely affect the muscle-tendon units in another area of the complex. For example, pathology in the area of the subacromial space can cause significant discomfort in the area along the medial scapula (scapular stabilizing musculature) and/or pain going up into the neck (trapezius muscle). The importance of this is to understand that when treatment is instituted evaluation and management of the entire shoulder complex is required.

Injuries around the shoulder can be broken down into acute or sudden onset type or gradual or overuse related injuries. In general, basic treatment concepts should initially be implemented for both injury types, but in the end, adjustments in shoulder mechanics or work responsibilities (duration, frequency, and intensity) may be needed to avoid a recurrence of an overuse type injury.

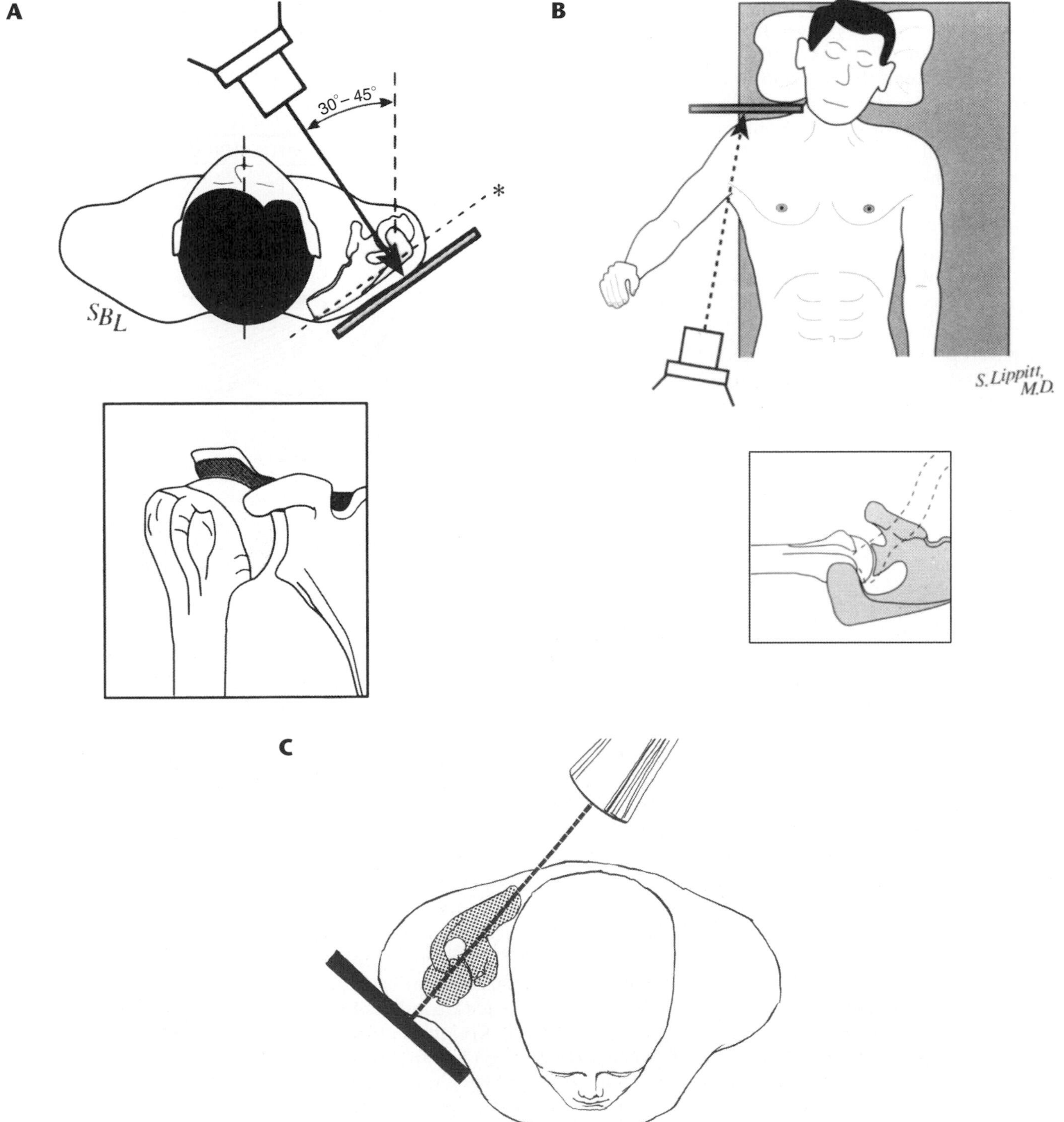

Figure 17–2. Trauma series: (a) anteroposterior view in the plane of the scapula, (b) an axillary lateral view, and (c) a scapulolateral view.

Acute injuries to the shoulder include contusions, ligamentous sprains, muscular strains or tendon tears, dislocations, and fractures. Treatment should be initiated within an hour of the initial injury and should include rest, ice, compression, and elevation (RICE) as well as nonsteroidal anti-inflammatory medication (NSAIDs). This regimen provides relief of pain by decreasing inflammation and swelling. The physician evaluation should include a careful history and physical examination. The patient history should focus on the mechanism of injury, including the damaging forces involved and the position of the arm at the time of injury. It is also important to document any previous past history of problems related to the involved shoulder. As with athletic injuries, an early, thorough physical examination is crucial.[145] The ability to evaluate the patient prior to the onset of significant inflammation and swelling is critical for developing an early, accurate diagnosis. A complete shoulder evaluation should also include a comprehensive radiographic assessment of the shoulder. This is best accomplished with a shoulder trauma series (an anteroposterior view in the plane of the scapula, an axillary lateral view, and a scapulolateral view) (Fig. 17–2).[119]

If the radiologic evaluation of the shoulder is negative for a separation, dislocation, or fracture, and the patient's primary complaints are pain and soreness, the physician should initiate the RICE treatment protocol along with a short course of NSAIDs. Newer COX-2 anti-inflammatory medications have the added benefit of reduced gastrointestinal side effects and no platelet inhibition, which makes the medications more tolerable to the patient and more beneficial in a traumatic related injury.[7] In addition, physical therapy can be instituted early to help control pain and swelling. This is accomplished by utilizing modalities such as cold and heat therapy, ultrasound, electrical stimulation, and iontophoresis. The therapist should also focus on maintaining shoulder motion and restoring strength in an effort to return the patient back to the preinjury condition safely and expeditiously.[129] Most of these conditions improve within 4 to 6 weeks. If symptoms persist, particularly mechanical symptoms, then consideration of specific shoulder conditions should ensue.

Impingement Syndrome

The most complex issue in the diagnosis of shoulder disorders relates to the diagnosis of the impingement syndrome.[98–100] Patients will complain of pain in the upper arm, pain with overhead activity, and pain at night. The pain in the upper arm is the result of referred pain from irritation of the rotator cuff; the pain with overhead activities is caused by the pinching of tissue between the greater tuberosity of the humerus and the undersurface of the acromion; the pain at night is also related to this phenomenon because the weight of the arm and gravity are neutralized.

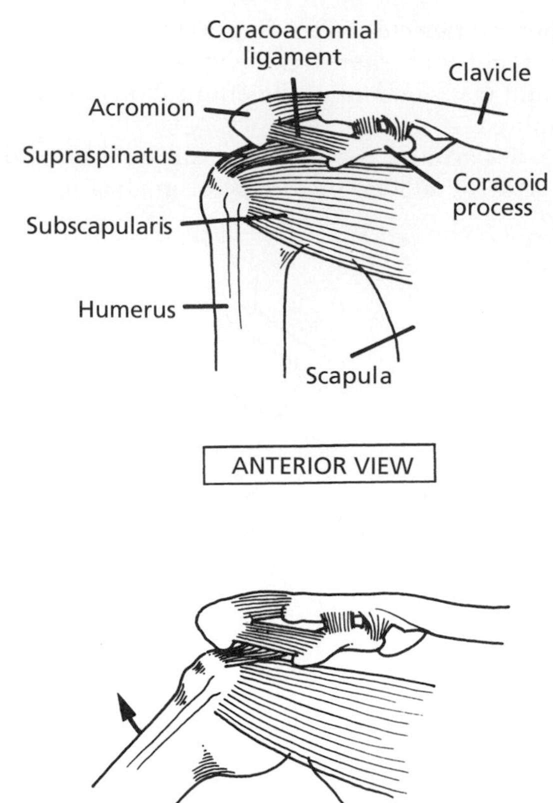

Figure 17–3. Anatomy of the rotator cuff and acromion as it pertains to the impingement syndrome. Notice the potential abutment of the acromion on the rotator cuff when the arm is maximally elevated.

The proposed pathophysiology is abutment of the proximal humerus and rotator cuff against the anterior acromion when the arm is in forward elevation (Fig. 17–3). Encroachment of the subacromial space either by anterior, superior migration of the humeral head or by undersurface spur formation on the acromion makes impingement more likely (Fig. 17–4). The impingement syndrome is generally divided into three stages based on characteristic pathology and age. Stage I consists of reversible edema and hemorrhage in the rotator cuff tendon and subacromial bursa, usually seen in patients under the age of 25. Stage II consists of fibrosis and tendonitis of the rotator cuff (primarily the supraspinatus), typically in patients between 25 and 40 years of age. The pathology may not be reversible, and recurrence of pain with activity is common. Stage III includes acromion spur formation with associated

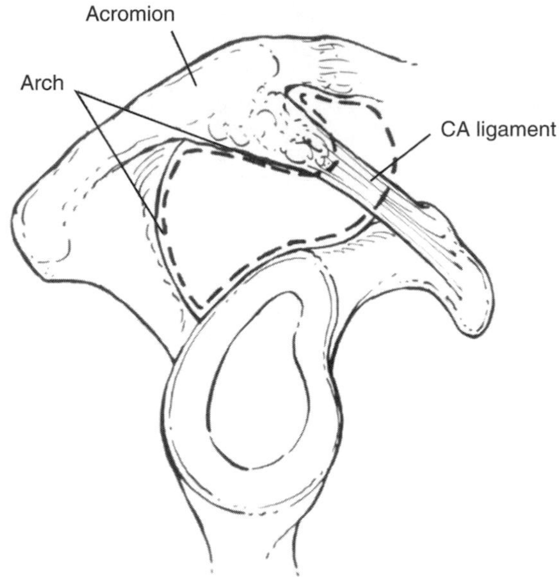

Figure 17–4. Schematic representation of spur formation on the undersurface of the acromion compromising the patency of the subacromial space.

rotator cuff tendon ruptures, usually in patients over the age of 40. Hawkins et al[57] and Ellman[35] modified the Neer stages of impingement to include subgroups of Stage II impingement characterized by partial supraspinatus tendon tears, which may actually represent the subset of this group that has recurrence of pain with activity.

A component of impingement syndrome is often tightness of the posterior capsule that results in the humeral head being displaced anteriorly and superiorly, further compromising the patency of the subacromial space and increasing the risk of rotator cuff and/or bursal impingement. Secondary impingement is easily identified in patients who have a loss of internal rotation and cross-body adduction representing tightness of the posterior shoulder capsule. Recognition is essential for treating the problem, and failed treatment is usually the result of failure to identify and treat posterior capsule tightness.

Unfortunately, the physical examination of patients with impingement syndrome in and of itself may not be diagnostic, but it can be highly suggestive of the source of the problem. Inspection is the key to determining obvious reasons for shoulder pain. Utilizing the normal shoulder as a template, side-to-side comparisons can help highlight obvious problems. In the case of impingement syndrome, evaluation of the supraspinatus and infraspinatus fossas may help to delineate evidence of a chronic rotator cuff injury defined by atrophy of either or both muscles. Observation of the patient's active motion should include forward elevation in the plane of the scapula, external rotation with the arm at the side and in abduction, cross-body adduction, and internal rotation with the arm in abduction and internal rotation up the back. Once again comparison to the normal shoulder is important to understand the patient's baseline level. Both shoulders should be brought through the same motions passively. Differences in active and passive ranges of motion may be related to a rotator cuff tear or rotator cuff weakness secondary to inflammation. Asymmetric scapular motion can also contribute to the impingement phenomenon. Documentation of side-to-side strength differences throughout the different motions is also important. Loss of strength associated with pain may be the result of a painful rotator cuff tear or can be attributed to a significantly inflamed muscle tendon unit. Loss of cross-body adduction and internal rotation are indicative of tightness of the posterior shoulder capsule and need to be noted and treated because of the displacing effect on the humeral head. Pain with resisted forward elevation, external rotation, or internal rotation is not diagnostic but is indicative of rotator cuff tendonitis and is referred to as a positive tendon sign.

Special tests that are performed to help in the diagnosis of impingement syndrome include Neer's impingement sign and Hawkins impingement examination. Neer's impingement sign is performed when the examiner stabilizes the patient's scapula with one hand and then elevates the patient's humerus in slight internal rotation (Fig. 17–5).[101] This allows the greater tuberosity to progress directly under the anterior acromion and "supposedly causes the critical area of the supraspinatus tendon to be impinged against the anterior inferior acromion."[56] The sign is positive when the maneuver produces pain, and often elicits a grimacing facial expression. Hawkin's impingement maneuver is performed with the humerus forward flexed to 90 degrees followed by forcible internal rotation of the shoulder (Fig. 17–6).[56] This will also result in impingement of the supraspinatus tendon on the anterior acromion and is positive if pain is elicited.

Neer's impingement test may be both diagnostic and in some instances therapeutic.[101] As described, it is performed when 10 mL of 1% Xylocaine is injected into the subacromial space. We perform this from a posterior approach under sterile conditions (Fig. 17–7). Resolution of a positive impingement sign following the injection constitutes a positive impingement test. Additional information can be gained from patients who have a recovery of rotator cuff strength. Patients who were previously found to be painfully weak with certain resisted motions and now have no discernible side-to-side strength differences may have their weakness attributed to an inflamed tendon rather than a torn rotator cuff. Patients who have pain-free weakness following the injection have a high likelihood of having an associated rotator cuff tear as the cause of their weakness. The impingement test can become therapeutic if a

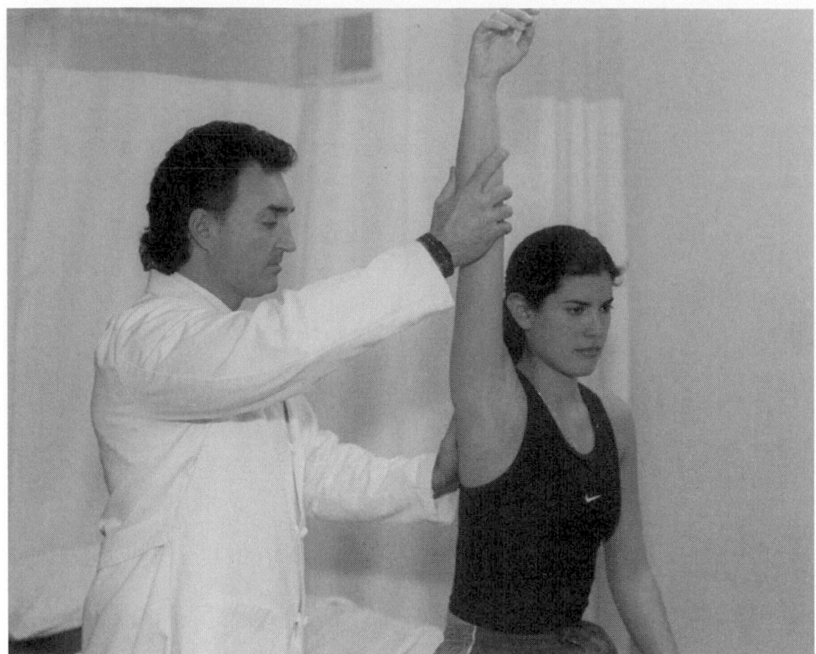

Figure 17–5. Neer's impingement sign: The examiner stabilizes the patient's scapula with one hand, and then elevates the patient's humerus in slight internal rotation.

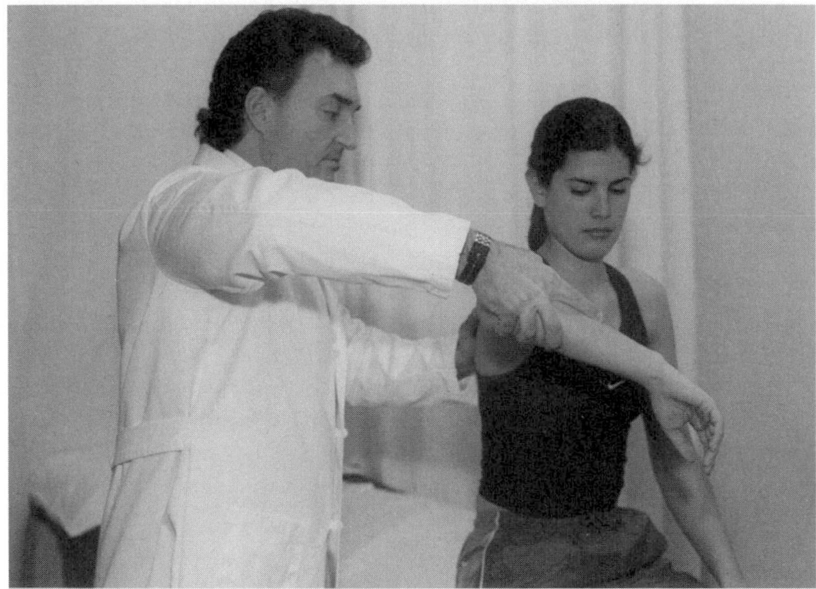

Figure 17–6. Hawkin's impingement maneuver: Hawkin's impingement maneuver is performed with the humerus forward flexed to 90 degrees followed by forcible internal rotation of the shoulder.

corticosteroid is added to the injection. The medication should only be added in patients where there is a low suspicion of a rotator cuff tear, because of the negative effect that the steroid has on healing tissue. We do not perform more than three injections, and never within 6 weeks of each other. The injection delivers a high dose of anti-inflammatory medication to the source of the problem, and is very beneficial for patients who are experiencing significant discomfort from the inflammation. In addition, patients who are intolerant of NSAIDs can benefit significantly and safely from the corticosteroid injection. It is important to educate patients on the fact that it often takes about 2 days for the medication to become effective; this will help avoid confusion when there is little pain relief in the first 48 hours.

Treatment

Initial treatment for impingement syndrome should always begin with nonoperative management. In addition to the anti-inflammatory effect provided by the subacromial injection, a short course of NSAIDs can also help decrease inflammation in the shoulder, helping with pain relief. A well-focused physical therapy program is the key to a successful outcome. Treatment should first focus on pain relief by decreasing inflammation. Appropriate utilization of the different modalities such as cold and heat therapy, ultrasound, electrical stimulation, and iontophoresis is important and should be tailored to each patient appropriately. Recovery of motion is essential, especially in patients with loss of internal rotation. Focused stretching of the posterior capsule with internal rotation and cross-body adduction exercises will help loosen the shoulder capsule. Avoidance of provocative maneuvers such as forward elevation and abduction during the first 7 to 10 days of therapy will help with resolution of inflammation by avoiding the effects of repetitive trauma. Strengthening of the rotator cuff with the arm at the patient's side will help to re-educate the rotator cuff to accomplish its centering effect on the humeral head within the glenoid socket. This is accomplished with isotonic internal and external rotation strengthening exercises with TheraBands and subsequent advancement to lightweight strengthening. Strengthening of the scapular stabilizing musculature is also important to achieve coordinated movement of the scapulothoracic joint with the glenohumeral joint as asymmetric motion can also result in secondary impingement.[127] There is a paucity of literature on the natural history of the impingement syndrome or the outcome of nonoperative management such as physical therapy, but most physicians believe that the majority of patients with this diagnosis improve without surgical management.[55,94]

Plain radiographic studies are obtained to rule out any contributing causes to impingement-like symptoms, such as calcific tendonitis or a type III acromion (Fig. 17–8). Standard radiographic evaluation of the shoulder should always include a true anteroposterior view of the glenohumeral joint, a scapulolateral view, and an axillary lateral view.[119] These three views will provide sufficient information for a thorough radiographic evaluation of the shoulder in the majority of patients. Supplementary views for the impingement syndrome are directed toward better visualization to the acromion and include the supraspinatus outlet view as well as the 30° caudal tilt view.[119] Radiographic studies are often noncontributory, especially in patients under the age of 40. Associated, nonspecific findings may include greater tuberosity sclerosis and cyst formation, acromial spurring, and degenerative changes of the acromioclavicular joint.

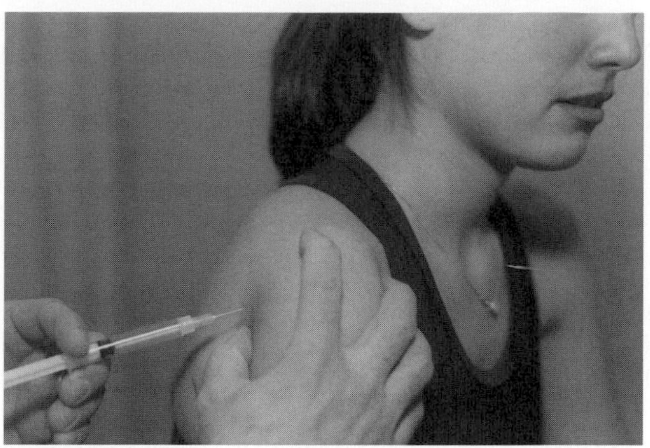

Figure 17–7. Author's method of choice for a subacromial injection.

If a well-motivated patient does not respond to physical therapy after 6 to 8 weeks of rehabilitation, a study to image the rotator cuff is indicated. Double-contrast arthrography of the glenohumeral joint is the historical gold standard for imaging the rotator cuff. The escape of dye from the glenohumeral joint into the subacromial or subdeltoid bursa is indicative of a rotator cuff tear with an accuracy greater than 95%.[49,89,119]

Ultrasonography is being utilized more often as an effective method to image the rotator cuff. It has the advantage of being "safe, rapid, noninvasive and inexpensive and has the benefit of the ability to evaluate and compare both shoulders."[119] It can reliably demonstrate full thickness rotator cuff tears in the range of 92

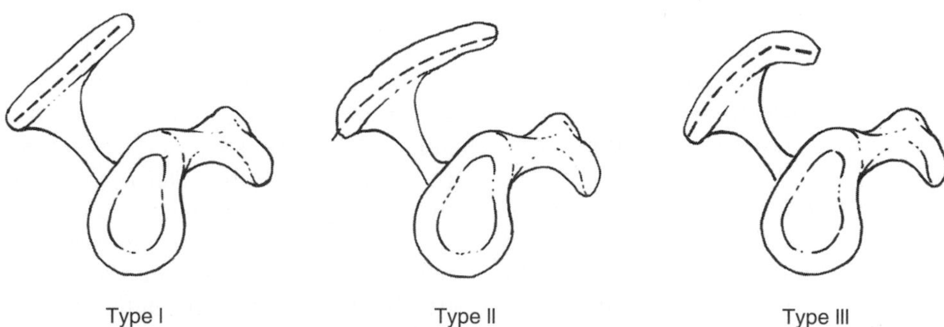

Figure 17–8. The three types of acromion morphology defined by Bigliani and Morrison. (From Bigliani LU, Morrison DS, April EW: The morphology of the acromion in its relationship to rotator cuff tears. Orthopaedic Transactions 10:228, 1986.)

to 95%.[60,81] In one study, ultrasound had a sensitivity of 100% and an overall accuracy of 96% in diagnosing full-thickness rotator cuff tears.[141] Magnetic resonance imaging (MRI) has become the most frequently used imaging study of the shoulder after plain radiographs. MRI has replaced shoulder arthrograms in most centers after initial reports demonstrated sensitivity of 100% and specificity of 95% in the diagnosis of full-thickness rotator cuff tears.[6,61,63] However, MRI may not be able to discriminate among rotator cuff tendonitis, partial thickness tears of the rotator cuff, and small full-thickness tears of the rotator cuff. The studies are often over-read, leading to a significant rate of false-positive results (i.e., full-thickness rotator cuff tear), especially in younger patients.[88] These false-positive reports encourage surgical intervention in a patient population that would be expected to have a high success rate with conservative management. MRI appears to have its greatest value at the two ends of the rotator cuff disease spectrum: no abnormalities or complete tears of the rotator cuff. For patients who present with MRI findings of a partial thickness rotator cuff tear and have no history of trauma, we recommend that, prior to proceeding to surgical management, a full course of conservative management including anti-inflammatory medication and a well-organized/supervised physical therapy program be completed to avoid operating on patients with false-positive studies.

The timing of surgical management for impingement syndrome is not well defined. Surgical intervention is indicated in patients with persistent impairment who fail appropriate conservative management, which also includes a well-motivated effort to eliminate stiffness.[2,36,44,52,59,78,82,98,99,113,120] Patients under the age of 40 must be carefully selected before proceeding with operative management, because rotator cuff pathology is less common in this population than in an older one.[59,82]

Positive prognostic indicators of surgical success include well-motivated patients over the age of 40, the absence of posterior shoulder stiffness, the presence of reproducible subacromial crepitance, and pain relieved by the subacromial injection of lidocaine.[82,121] Poor prognostic factors include age under 40, stiffness, lack of relief by subacromial injection, attribution of the problem to occupation, concomitant evidence of glenohumeral instability, and neurogenic rotator cuff muscle weakness.

The surgical technique of subacromial decompression has been well described, whether performed through an open shoulder incision or arthroscopically (Fig. 17–9 *A–D*).[36,44,52,55,59,82,99,113] We utilize an arthroscopic approach and recommend the cutting-block technique as described by Caspari and Thal.[18] A comparison of patients who have undergone an open versus an arthroscopic acromioplasty reveal patients in the arthroscopic group to have a greater benefit during the first 3 months with regards to better motion, less discomfort, and a quicker return to work and activities of daily living (ADLs), but at 1 year of follow-up, both groups had a similar successful rate of recovery.[2,44,126] An earlier return to work in patients following an arthroscopic subacromial decompression has the potential to ease the negative economic impact that results from people being out of work for significant periods of time.

Postoperative rehabilitation begins with an early range of motion program. During the first month, patients who have undergone an open procedure are started on a passive range of motion program, while patients who have undergone an arthroscopic procedure are advanced quickly to an active-assisted range of motion program. After 1 month, the two groups are rehabilitated at a similar pace. By 8 weeks, a full range of motion should be achieved. The expected return to work is within 3 months, with maximum medical improvement achieved by 3 to 6 months in well-motivated patients. If favorable preoperative prognostic factors are present, the procedure is predictably effective; however, workers' compensation patients generally demonstrate results that are inferior to nonworkers' compensation patients.[55,59,113] In fact, approximately 25% of workers' compensation patients who are treated with an acromioplasty will demonstrate permanent impairment prohibiting return to their previous occupation. Furthermore, if a workers' compensation patient continues to have unresolving shoulder pain for 9 months or more following an acromioplasty, the likelihood of return to the previous occupation is less than 15%, even if a revision acromioplasty is performed.[58] Diagnoses that are often associated with or mislabeled as an impingement syndrome include partial-thickness rotator cuff injury, full-thickness rotator cuff injury, and early adhesive capsulitis or frozen shoulder.

Partial Rotator Cuff Injury

The rotator cuff is defined by the coalescence of tendons from the subscapularis, supraspinatus, infraspinatus, and teres minor as they insert on the proximal humerus adjacent to the articular surface (Fig. 17–10). Its function is paramount to normal shoulder function, although other muscles may compensate remarkably in the absence of the rotator cuff. The rotator cuff is highly resistant to injury in people under the age of 40; however, increasing age and disuse are associated with its failure. Symptomatic partial tears of the rotator cuff usually occur in younger patients between the ages of 30 and 50.[84] They are almost always associated with tearing of the supraspinatus tendon, most commonly on the undersurface of the tendon.[22] Patients commonly report an injury where an unexpected or overwhelming eccen-

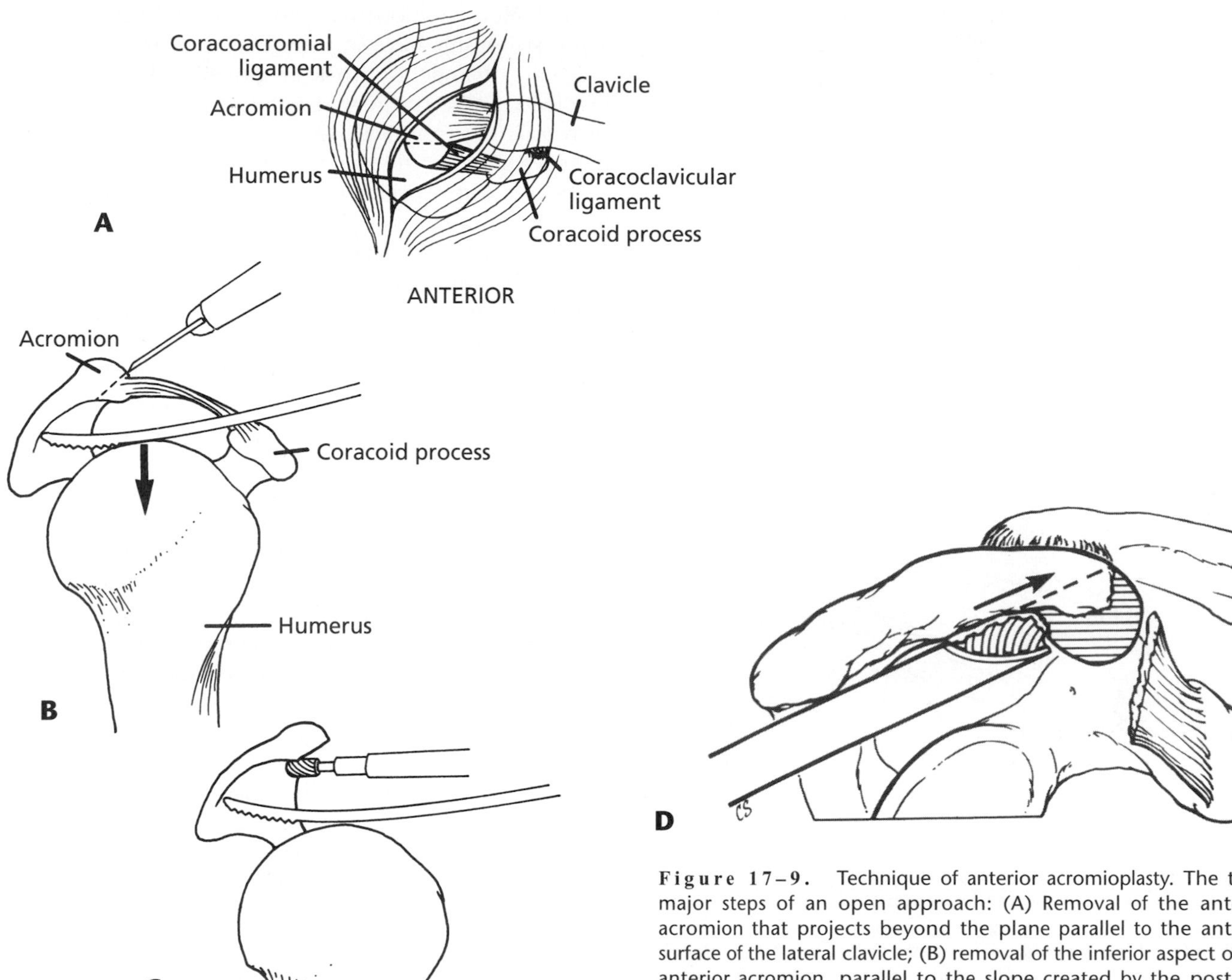

Figure 17–9. Technique of anterior acromioplasty. The three major steps of an open approach: (A) Removal of the anterior acromion that projects beyond the plane parallel to the anterior surface of the lateral clavicle; (B) removal of the inferior aspect of the anterior acromion, parallel to the slope created by the posterior acromion; and (C) final smoothing of the undersurface of the acromion with a burr or rasp. (D) View from the lateral portal of a completed arthroscopic acromioplasty.

tric load was applied to the arm, resulting in shoulder pain. Mechanical symptoms include difficulty in active elevation, especially against resistance.

The physical examination must be effective in eliminating other diagnoses while focusing on the rotator cuff. The most sensitive provocative test is the impingement sign, which is frequently positive in various shoulder conditions.[99,102] The most specific sign of rotator cuff pathology is weakness of the rotator cuff.[14,83,100] The strength of the cuff muscles can be tested by resisted elevation of the arm at 90° and resisted external rotation with the elbow at the patient's side. External rotation weakness may be directly related to cuff deficiency.[14] Patients are generally able to move the shoulder through a substantial arc of motion, but resisted external rotation and abduction results in increased pain and is consistent with rotator cuff pathology (positive cuff signs).[84] Associated findings with partial rotator cuff tears include mild atrophy of the supraspinatus muscle belly (located in the supraspinatus fossa of the scapula) and crepitation emanating from the subacromial space when the arm is internally and externally rotated in abduction. Also, stiffness of the posterior shoulder is frequently demonstrated. The patient will have limited internal rotation and cross-body adduction, signifying posterior shoulder stiffness.

Although the diagnosis of partial-thickness rotator cuff tears may be strongly suspected from the history and physical examination, it must be differentiated from small full-thickness tears. This distinction is important as the management of the two conditions differs. Plain radiographs are of little benefit in differentiating partial-thickness tears from small full-thickness tears. Double-contrast arthrography of the glenohumeral joint has the ability to distinguish partial thickness from full thickness tears, and was considered the gold standard

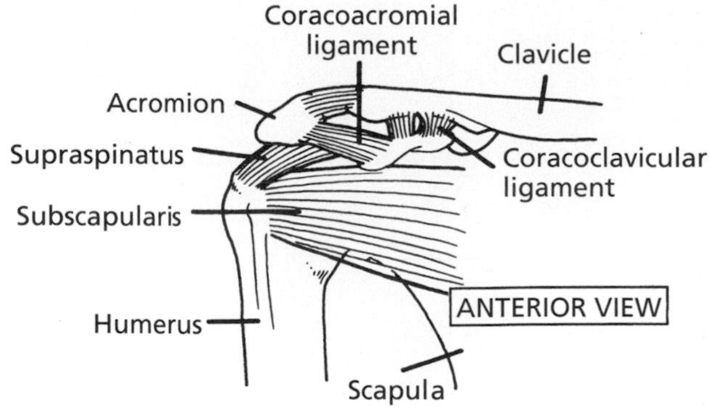

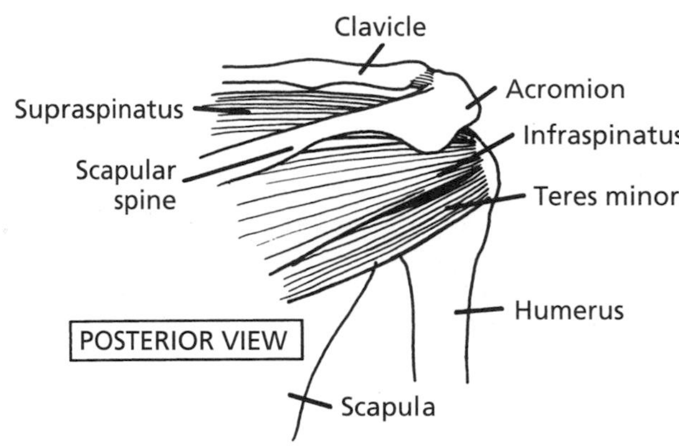

Figure 17–10. Rotator cuff anatomy. The rotator cuff is formed by the coalescence of the tendons from the supraspinatus, infraspinatus, teres minor, and subscapularis as they insert on the tuberosities of the humerus. The supraspinatus is most commonly involved in pathologic process es that affect the rotator cuff. Note its position in relationship to the anterior acromion.

for imaging the rotator cuff.[89] The value of MRI in the determination of partial-thickness tears appears to be similar to double-contrast arthrography at this time. The integrity of the rotator cuff should be evaluated with an advanced imaging study if there is a poor response to treatment after 6 weeks. Additionally, if 80% of preinjury level of function has not been achieved by 3 months, an imaging study is recommended.

The management of partial-thickness rotator cuff tears begins with the RICE protocol. Nonsteroidal anti-inflammatory mediation is useful for decreasing symptoms of pain and inflammation. Physical therapy is essential due to the associated stiffness that frequently accompanies this condition. The therapist needs to specifically instruct the patient to work on flexibility of the posterior aspect of the shoulder. Internal rotation and cross-body adduction, as well as the traditional motions of forward elevation and external rotation, must be stressed.[83,84] Most patients experience a substantial reduction in their shoulder symptoms within 6 weeks.[94] Return to one-handed work can begin after the acute symptoms have improved (1 to 2 weeks), with a gradual advance of work responsibilities using the involved limb. If the patient is well motivated and responds to physical therapy, maximum medical improvement should be achieved by 3 months.

Despite appropriate management and a motivated patient, symptoms may persist well beyond the 3 months. One reason that a patient may fail to improve is that a partial thickness rotator cuff tear has progressed to a larger tear or a full-thickness tear. This has been seen in over two-thirds of partial rotator cuff tears evaluated by arthrography in one study.[152] Only 7% of the partial thickness rotator cuff tears evaluated showed evidence of healing.[152] These symptomatic, partial-thickness rotator cuff tears pose a dilemma for the patient, the physician, and the workers' compensation system. There is good evidence that these conditions continue to improve beyond 3 months, and that very few patients need surgery if appropriate management continues for up to 1 year.[55,59,82,94,98,99,113] However, employers and insurance companies are generally not willing to accept limitations for up to 1 year. Six months of nonoperative management is generally accepted. If a patient has a partial-thickness cuff tear, or if the patient does not improve by 6 months, surgery can be considered. If a full-thickness tear is demonstrated on the imaging studies, surgical repair is indicated.

Surgical treatment of partial-thickness rotator cuff tears includes acromioplasty, with or without a repair of the torn section of the rotator cuff. The gold standard was an acromioplasty performed through an open incision as previously discussed. Recent reports have indicated that arthroscopic acromioplasties may return the patient's function sooner than open acromioplasties.[2,44] However, the arthroscopic procedure remains technically demanding, and 6-month comparisons of patient results, even in the hands of experienced arthroscopists, have not demonstrated a clear advantage. For many orthopaedic surgeons, an open acromioplasty may provide better results.[55,94,78,113] One potential advantage of arthroscopic surgery is the ability to carefully visualize the rotator cuff from both the articular side and the bursal side. Repair of partial-thickness tears of the rotator cuff remains controversial, but when more than 50% of the rotator cuff tendon thickness is involved, completion of the tear and surgical repair is recommended.[150] When the tear involves less than 50% of the rotator cuff thickness, debridement of the partial-thickness tears combined with an acromioplasty yields a satisfactory result in the majority of patients (Fig. 17–11).[2,44]

Range of motion exercises are started immediately following surgery. Some patients benefit from continuous passive motion devices following surgery, but the final outcome may not be improved over patients who exercise consistently.[26,42,66,104] Patients treated with completion and repair of the partial thickness rotator cuff tear are restricted from active motion exercises (usually forward elevation because the supraspinatus is the cuff tendon that is most often affected) for the first 6 weeks. This allows for the tendon to heal securely to its insertion on the greater tuberosity. Patients treated with cuff debridement progress from passive to active range of motion exercises over the first 1 to 2 weeks. Strengthening of the deltoid and rotator cuff is started between 4 and 6 weeks for patients following debridement, and at about 10 to 12 weeks for patients following rotator cuff repair. Light manual labor work can begin between 8 and 12 weeks for patients following debridement and 14 and 16 weeks for those following repair, with a gradual advancement of their work status after 3 and 4 months, respectively. Maximum medical improvement is usually achieved by 6 months, although patients may continue to improve in strength for more than a year.

Full-thickness Cuff Tear

Full-thickness tears of the rotator cuff are potentially labor-ending injuries, even when appropriate management is provided. Although full-thickness cuff tears are often treated as the end-stage of the impingement syndrome, acute work-related injuries are responsible for a substantial number of full-thickness tears. The incidence

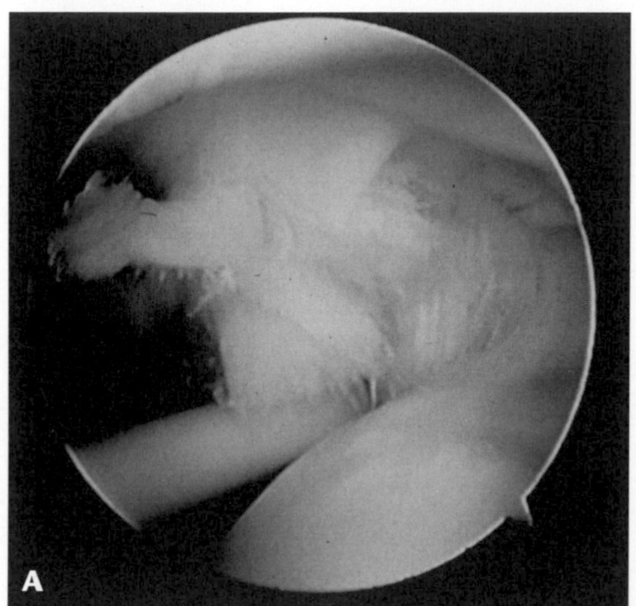

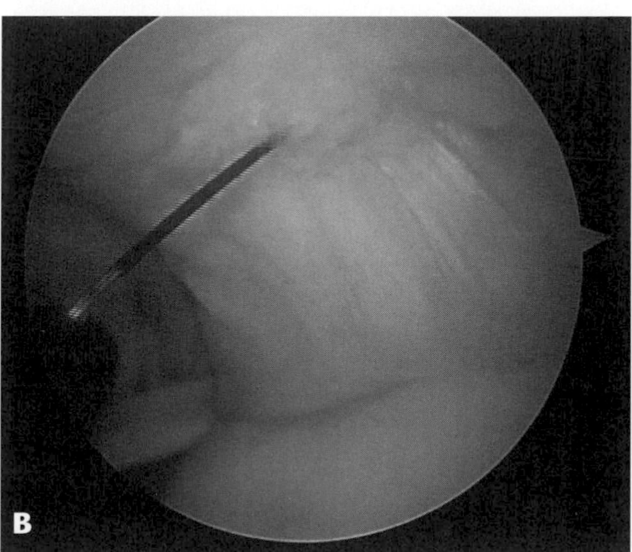

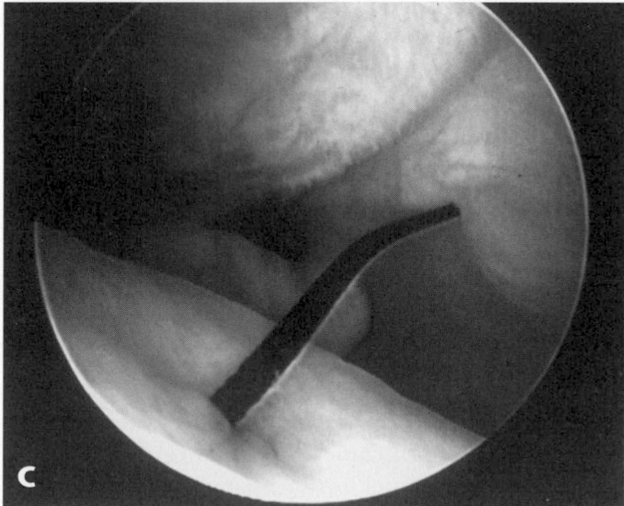

Figure 17–11. Arthroscopic evaluation and treatment of a partial thickness rotator cuff tear of the supraspinatus tendon. (A) Evaluation of the partial thickness tear of the supraspinatus tendon from the articular side; (B) debridement and suture localization of the torn cuff tissue; (C) evaluation of the area of concern from the bursal side.

of rotator cuff disease increases with age, with the "prevalence of partial or full-thickness tears increasing markedly after 50 years of age."[87] The diagnosis should be obtained within the first 6 weeks following the injury as the outcome of chronic tears (greater than 3 months) is less successful than that of acute tears.[5]

In the general population, the typical age of patients with full-thickness rotator cuff tears is between 48 and 75 years.[84] Patients under the age of 60 are more likely to suffer a full-thickness rotator cuff tear after a major eccentric load occurs to the arm, such as in a fall or with a sudden forceful above-shoulder movement or lift. Work-related full-thickness rotator cuff tears are commonly associated with these injury mechanisms. Patients older than 60 often have the insidious onset of shoulder pain with a gradual decrease in shoulder function, particularly in overhead activities. In these older patients, the tear of the rotator cuff tendon may be relatively atraumatic, occurring secondarily to the attrition of cuff tissue, either by disuse or from progression of the impingement disease.

Physical examination findings may include atrophy of the rotator cuff musculature within the supraspinatus or infraspinatus fossas, and are usually seen in patients with chronic cuff tears. Patients may also have palpable tenderness at the greater tuberosity, the most common site being the supraspinatus tendon insertion.[22] This can be palpated on examination by locating the proximal aspect of the bicipital groove, then advancing 1 cm laterally. More specific findings on examination include deficit in active motion when compared to passive motion, weakness of elevation of the arm, weakness of external rotation, weakness of internal rotation, and frequently, painful crepitation in the subacromial region with internal and external rotation in abduction. Weakness of external rotation with the elbow by the patient's side appears to be the most sensitive indicator of the extent of rotator cuff disease.[14] As indicated previously, weakness associated with pain can be the result of significant rotator cuff tendon inflammation, and can be differentiated from an actual cuff tear if, following a subacromial injection with 1% Xylocaine, there is a resolution of pain and restoration of strength.

Specialized imaging studies are recommended if the history, physical examination, and radiographs are consistent with a substantial injury to the rotator cuff, or when patients do not respond to 6 to 8 weeks of rehabilitation exercises. The historical gold standard for specialized evaluation of the rotator cuff integrity is the double-contrast arthrogram. However, most physicians have replaced shoulder arthrograms with MRI. MRI is very accurate in determining whether a full-thickness rotator cuff tear is present. However, partial-thickness tears challenge the interpretative skills of radiologists, as the images of tendonitis, partial-thickness rotator cuff tears, and small full-thickness rotator cuff tears can be similar. MRI findings other than complete full-thickness rotator cuff tear should be interpreted with caution. Surgical management should be strongly supported by the history and physical examination, or by an arthrogram.

Patients seen with chronic symptoms of rotator cuff disease are initially treated in the same way as patients with partial-thickness cuff tears: RICE, anti-inflammatory medications, occasionally a subacromial injection of a corticosteroid, and physical therapy focused on improving shoulder motion. Special attention is directed toward the posterior shoulder stiffness that frequently accompanies rotator cuff conditions. Chronic, symptomatic tears that do not respond to therapy should be treated with the primary goal of pain relief. Improvement in strength is less predictable.

Acute full-thickness tears of the rotator cuff are repaired soon after the diagnosis is confirmed. Repair within 6 weeks of the initial injury is recommended.[5] Preoperative factors suggestive of a good postoperative prognosis include the acute onset of symptoms, specific injury to the shoulder, younger age, good maintenance of external rotation strength (Grade 3 or 4), and normal radiographs.[5,37,83] Poor postoperative function is associated with a longer duration of pain, older patients, severe weakness (<Grade 3) of abduction and external rotation, decreased acromiohumeral interval on plain radiographs, and revision rotator cuff repairs.[29,37,52]

It is well recognized that surgical repair of symptomatic rotator cuff tears results in predictable improvement in pain relief primarily with restoration in function secondarily.[9,46,79,106,110,125,140] It has also been shown that arthroscopic acromioplasty and cuff debridement alone for full-thickness rotator cuff tears is predictably unsuccessful in active patients.[38,153] Therefore, a secure cuff repair is the key for a successful outcome, and it is the integrity of this repair over time that has been shown to correlate with better motion and better function.[47,54]

There are three surgical approaches available to effectively repair the rotator cuff: classic-open, mini-deltoid split, and arthroscopic.[83] The surgeon should utilize the technique that is most consistently reproducible in his or her hands. Arthroscopic cuff repair is the latest surgical treatment for the management of rotator cuff tears and has grown as a successful technique as arthroscopic technology has advanced (Fig. 17–12).[123] We have reviewed our arthroscopic population in a similar manner as Harryman et al[54] and found similar results in relation to preoperative tear size and postoperative cuff integrity as well as better motion and function in those patients with an intact repair.[124] This supports the fact that it is still the effectiveness and durability of the cuff repair itself and not the surgical approach that translates into a successful patient outcome. It is the responsibility of the surgeon to select the repair technique with which he or she is most comfortable and that affords the opportunity to consistently repair the rotator cuff tendon securely.

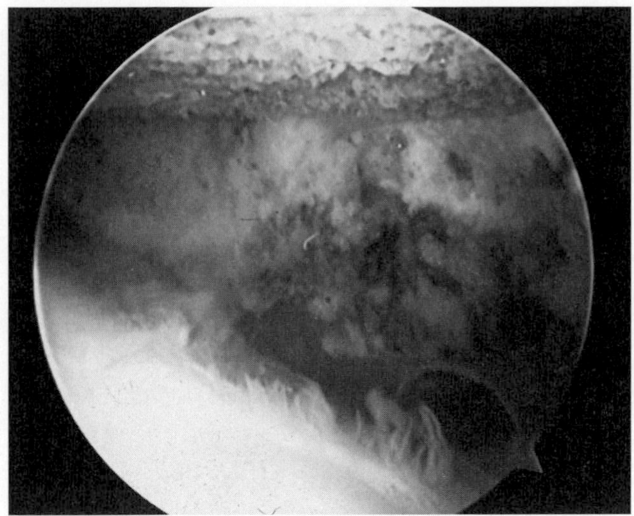

Figure 17–12. Arthroscopic rotator cuff repair.

Regardless of which surgical technique is utilized to repair a torn rotator cuff, the biology of healing tissue is not changed. Protection of the repair for at least 6 to 10 weeks is required to allow appropriate healing of the tendon to its insertion. Following rotator cuff repair, the shoulder is protected with a sling during the first 4 to 6 weeks. The rehabilitation program begins either on the day of surgery or the following morning. Although patients will experience substantial discomfort that requires appropriate pain management, the benefit of early mobilization has been documented.[8,83,84,64] For the first 6 to 8 weeks, the primary goal of therapy is to re-establish motion of the shoulder. This is accomplished through passive range of motion exercises. The size of the tear and the comfort of the repair dictate how aggressive the surgeon will allow the rehabilitation program to be following surgery. In general a great deal of information can be obtained in the operating room following the tendon repair. Shoulder motion on the table will give the surgeon an idea of the safe ranges of motion through which the repair is minimally stressed. Based on the fact that tears come in different shapes and sizes means that the quality of the repair will be variable; therefore there is not one answer with regards to a rehabilitation protocol following all rotator cuff repairs. Motions to avoid early on include extension, direct abduction (with either internal or external rotation), and cross-body adduction.

Active assisted and active motion exercises begin after the tendon has healed to the bone. Light strengthening exercises begin at about 10 to 12 weeks, although strengthening of the intact cuff in small tears early on is definitely recommended. Strengthening begins with isometric exercises controlled by the patient, progressing slowly to isotonic exercises. If the rotator cuff tear is small and repair is easily accomplished, strengthening begins at 6 weeks; if the rotator cuff tear is large or attrition of the tissues provides a precarious repair, strengthening begins at 12 weeks. At 3 months, the strengthening program is advanced as tolerated, while continuing to improve on pain-free range of motion. Adequate rehabilitation of a full-thickness rotator cuff repair requires a minimum of 6 months and may need up to 12 months following the surgery. The strength of the shoulder muscles and therefore the shoulder function substantially increases from 6 to 12 months following rotator cuff repair, supporting continued rehabilitation during this postoperative period.[144] If there is no further injury and the cuff remains intact, the results do not appear to deteriorate within the first 5 years.[50,53] The determination of maximal medical improvement is thus best performed at 1 year following surgery.

In terms of return to work, no significant use of the extremity is allowed for the first 3 months, as even writing or simple sedentary responsibilities that require the hand to be positioned slightly away from the person's side will aggravate the symptoms. At 3 months sedentary office-type work is allowed with gradual advancement to light physical activities. Medium-to-heavy physical labor may be initiated at approximately 6 months. Often, a work-hardening program helps bridge the gap from relatively short, intense exercise to the more long-term activities of a normal workday. Maximum heavy physical labor (such as a construction worker using a jackhammer) is not suggested until at least 1 year after surgery.

With these guidelines, one should consider job modifications or vocational rehabilitation in certain situations. The 55-year-old man who does heavy manual labor and develops the insidious onset of shoulder pain with confirmation of a rotator cuff tear is highly unlikely to return to his previous occupation without substantial restrictions, even after extended rehabilitation. The employer and employee often benefit from an early decision to change occupational responsibilities to a lighter physical activity with no above-shoulder responsibilities. The employee will have the potential to return to work at an earlier date, substantially decreasing the risk of longer-term disability.

Subacromial Abrasion

Subacromial abrasion is another subset of the frequently used diagnosis of impingement syndrome. The shoulder function is compromised due to roughness or a catching sensation experienced by the patient, usually in the intermediate positions of shoulder elevation.[83] The symptoms are generally localized to the anterior shoulder region. There may be a history of a previous injury or strain to shoulder area, without evidence of substantial weakness.

The examination is pathognomonic of this disorder. With the arm abducted 90°, internal and external rotation of the humerus demonstrates crepitation that the patient recognizes as the etiology of the shoulder's dysfunction. This finding is termed the abrasion sign.[83] Patients may also demonstrate tendon signs as seen with rotator cuff injuries. Posterior shoulder stiffness with decreased internal rotation and cross-body adduction is often present. Radiographs demonstrate a normal glenohumeral relationship. Special imaging of the rotator cuff is indicated if tendon signs are clearly evident on examination.

The initial management is similar to the management for partial-thickness cuff tears, including the RICE protocol, nonsteroidal anti-inflammatory medications, and occasionally a subacromial cortisone injection. However, if patients have reproducible crepitation or catching that is directly related to their initial symptoms, an acromioplasty may be recommended earlier than 6 months.

Postoperative rehabilitation is similar to surgery for partial-thickness cuff tears that do not require a repair of the tendon. Full use of the extremity for ADLs should be achieved by 3 months, with light physical labor allowed at 3 months, advancing as tolerated to heavy physical labor by 6 months.

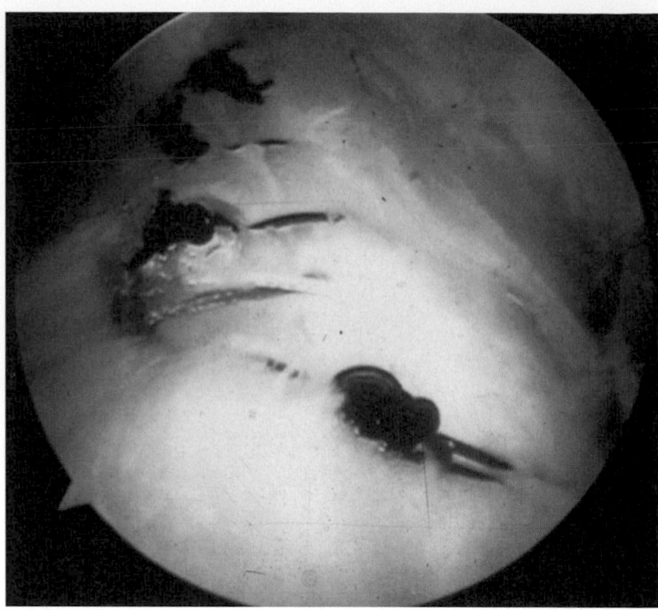

Figure 17–13. Arthroscopic stabilization of a Type IV SLAP lesion.

BICEPS TENDON DISORDERS

Proximal biceps tendon disorders can be divided into three categories: biceps tendonitis, biceps instability, and biceps/superior labrum lesions. The vast majority of biceps pathology is related to conditions of the rotator cuff.[100] Biceps tendonitis is seen rarely as a primary condition but, when present, demonstrates thickening of the tendon and stenosis at the bicipital groove.[31] Biceps instability occurs when the normal restraining mechanism, the transverse humeral ligament, is incompetent.[21] This is frequently associated with large rotator cuff tears that involve the subscapularis.[83] The treatment of these conditions is related to the primary pathology as discussed.

Biceps tendonitis can be effectively treated with the RICE protocol and anti-inflammatory medications. Patients may also be successfully treated with a subacromial injection with a combination of Xylocaine and a corticosteroid. In unresponsive cases of biceps tendonitis, direct injection into the bicipital groove may be required and is often very successful.

Lesions involving the superior labrum and biceps attachment site can be a source of persistent shoulder pain, although an actual reproducible functional deficit directly attributable to this lesion remains to be defined.[133] The superior labral injury generally involves the labrum from the anterior biceps attachment to the posterior superior aspect, hence the term SLAP lesion. Two mechanisms of injury have been described: the first is a fall on the outstretched hand where the humeral head is driven into the labrum and the biceps origin; the second involves a forceful contraction of the biceps as seen with certain overhead activities such as throwing, where during the deceleration phase, there is "traction and subsequent avulsion of the biceps and superior labral complex."[3,16] Most commonly, the patient will have discomfort with overhead activities.[3,117,133] Occasionally, a click or snap will be present with activities at shoulder level or above. This condition is often found coexisting with the other conditions such as partial-thickness rotator cuff tears and its significance remains unclear. However, when found on arthroscopic examination, this lesion should be stabilized because increasing evidence exists that patients respond favorably to arthroscopic stabilization of this condition (Fig. 17–13).[117]

Postoperatively, lifting is restricted for at least 6 weeks, although passive and active-assisted range of motion exercises are encouraged after the first few days. Most patients have good function but continued pain for 3 months. This dull, aching pain usually resolves by 6 months. Some patients will demonstrate objective findings of permanent impairment, primarily related to strenuous lifting and overhead activities. Maximum medical improvement is achieved at 6 months when this is an isolated condition.

ACROMIOCLAVICULAR JOINT DISEASE

Acromioclavicular joint pathology generally occurs secondary to trauma.[118] The traumatic event is frequently an injury to the stabilizing structures of the joint, acromioclavicular and coracoclavicular ligaments, and the intra-articular meniscus or fibrocartilage. Acute injuries to the acromioclavicular joint with compromise of the supporting ligaments and joint capsule represent the majority of acromioclavicular pathology in the non-physical labor population. However, early degenerative joint disease and distal clavicular osteolysis represent two conditions that commonly occur in the worker with heavy physical demands or frequent above-shoulder-level responsibilities.[118]

The acromioclavicular joint is a diarthrodial joint formed by the acromion and lateral clavicle, with the articular surfaces covered with fibrocartilage (Fig. 17–14). A fibrocartilaginous interarticular disc, meniscoid in shape, exists between the two articular surfaces. This tissue undergoes degeneration with age and is no longer functional by the fifth decade.[30] The acromioclavicular joint rotation is limited to approximately 5 to 8 degrees.[69,118]

Traumatic disruption of the acromioclavicular joint is usually the result of a fall on the elbow, particularly with the arm extended. In more severe cases, on inspection there is an obvious deformity of the lateral aspect of the shoulder. This is the result of the acromion and upper extremity being displaced downward, while the lateral end of the clavicle remains in its anatomic position. Acromioclavicular joint separation has been classified into six different types[118,122] based on the anatomic

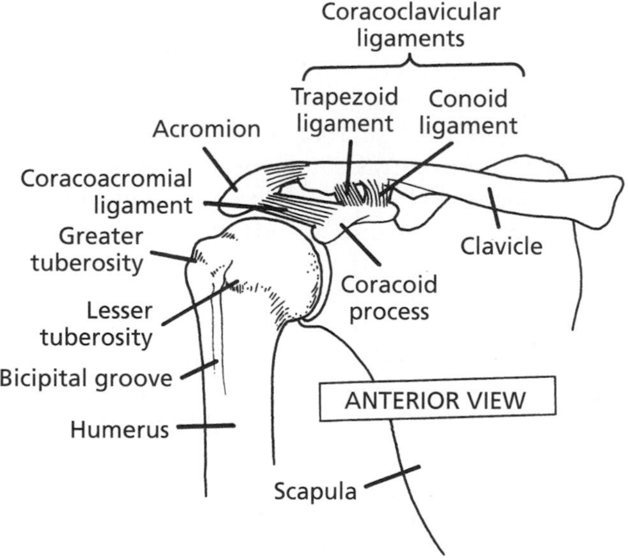

Figure 17–14. Normal anatomy of the acromioclavicular (ac) joint. The acromioclavicular ligaments are the primary horizontal stabilizers of the ac joint and they are more frequently involved in ac joint injuries. The coracoacromial ligaments are the primary vertical stabilizers of the ac joint. Substantial forces are required to rupture both the acromioclavicular ligaments as well as the coracoclavicular ligaments.

structures injured and the radiographic appearance of the clavicle and acromion relationship (Fig. 17–15). Type I is a sprain of the acromioclavicular ligaments. Type II involves a sprain with displacement, but the acromion and clavicle remain in a close relationship. Type III involves a complete separation of the acromion and clavicle, which occurs when the injury involves not only the acromioclavicular joint, but also the coracoclavicular ligaments. Types IV, V, and VI are indicative of severe displacement of the relationship between the acromion and clavicle, with complete disruption of the ligamentous attachments from the clavicle to the scapula.

Physical examination involves a careful inspection and palpation in the area of the acromioclavicular joint and the coracoclavicular ligaments. Deformity will be obvious in the more serious types of acromioclavicular separations but will be less recognizable in Type I and II injuries. Radiographic evaluation should include the standard trauma series as well as additional specialty views of the acromioclavicular joint. This is accomplished with a Zanca view, where the x-ray beam is projected with a ten to fifteen degree cephalad tilt during an anteriorposterior evaluation of the acromioclavicular joint.[118] Also, stress radiographs, where the patient has 10 to 15 pounds of weight hanging from each arm during an anteriorposterior view of the acromioclavicular joint, may help to distinguish between Type II and Type III injuries.[118]

Types I, II, and III injuries are generally treated nonoperatively with good results.[73,80,138] Treatment includes the RICE protocol plus anti-inflammatory medications, with immobilization in a sling to support the upper extremity. With Grade I injuries, range of motion can be started within 1 to 2 weeks following the injury, advancing to a strengthening program when a full range of pain-free motion has been achieved (4 to 6 weeks). With Grade II and III injuries, the extremity is supported for 1 to 2 weeks to allow the pain and swelling to subside. Range of motion activities are then initiated. A full range of pain-free motion is usually achieved by 6 weeks. At 6 weeks, strengthening exercises are added to the rehabilitation regimen. Recovery from this injury is approximately 3 months, although Grade I injuries heal more rapidly, while Grade II and III injuries may take longer.

Although most patients with Grade III acromioclavicular joint separations are appropriately treated nonoperatively, one exception may be laborers who are constantly required to lift heavy objects. These workers have symptoms of fatigue and/or paresthesias with repetitive heavy lifting. This is because the upper extremity work is being supported by soft tissues without the usual support of the acromioclavicular structures and coracoclavicular ligaments. On exami-

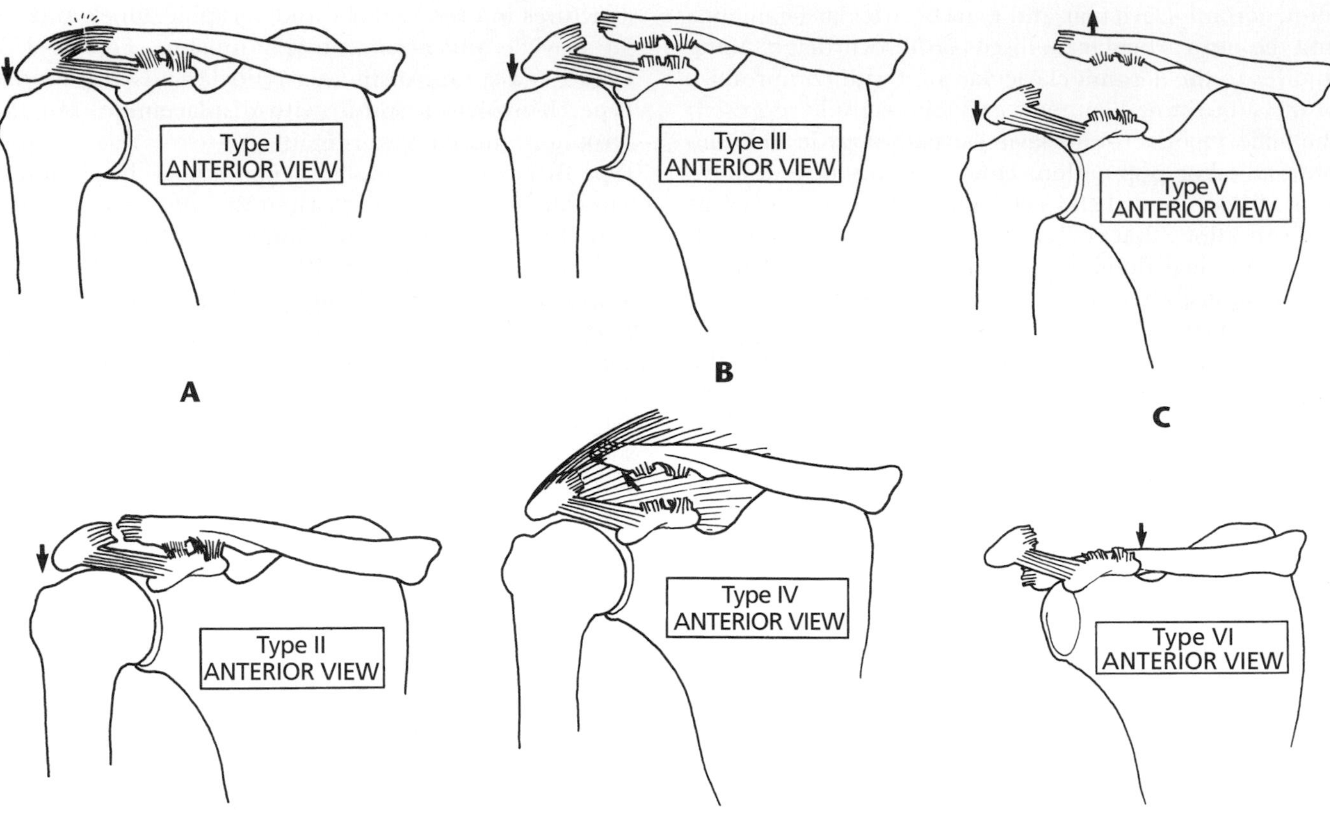

Figure 17–15. Classification of acromioclavicular joint injuries: A, Types I and II. B, Types III and IV. C, Types V and VI. Clinically, the most important differentiation is between Type III and Type V dislocations, because Type III dislocations are generally treated nonoperatively, whereas Type V dislocations are treated with stabilization. Types IV and VI are easily diagnosed with appropriate radiographs, and are also treated with surgical stabilization.

nation, the only objective finding may be the displacement of the acromioclavicular joint. Objective testing of the strength of the shoulder is usually noncontributory because the worker is able to demonstrate good strength during strenuous activities of short duration.[146] The surgical management, when indicated, involves reduction of the acromion back to the level of the clavicle, stabilization of the coracoclavicular junction, and commonly a resection of the distal clavicle.[122]

Types IV, V, and VI acromioclavicular separations are best managed operatively.[118,122,149] In these injuries, there is a disruption of the acromioclavicular joint as well as the coracoclavicular ligaments, with substantial injury to the remaining soft tissues. In essence, the supporting structure of the upper extremity and scapula are separated from the remainder of the torso. Weakness, paresthesias, and chronic discomfort are common. Stabilizing the scapula to the clavicle by reconstruction of the coracoclavicular ligaments is successful in relieving the symptoms and providing excellent functional results.[69,118,122,149] Postoperative management following surgical stabilization of the acromion back to level of the clavicle involves sling immobilization for 4 to 6 weeks. Patients can come out of their sling to perform gentle active, active assisted, and passive range of motion exercises. Direct abduction is avoided, and only light rotator cuff strengthening with the patient's arm at the side is performed during this early healing period. After 6 to 8 weeks, range of motion exercises are increased to include abduction. Strengthening of the rotator cuff as well as the scapular stabilizing musculature is also advanced when near normal ranges of motion are achieved. A return to labor intensive work responsibilities is restricted until strength and motion have approached preinjury levels, which is usually around the 3-month mark. Maximum medical improvement can be expected to be reached between 6 and 8 months in a well-motivated patient.

Chronic discomfort of the acromioclavicular joint secondary to degenerative arthritis may be related to occupational activities. However, the causal relationship is circumstantial. There is no study that documents a direct relationship between specific occupational activities and an increased risk of osteoarthritis of the acromioclavicular joint compared with the normal population. The acromioclavicular joint begins to deteriorate in the second decade with gradual loss of the fibrocartilaginous disc; by age 50, substantial narrowing of the joint space exists in the general population.[30,111,112]

An associated condition is osteolysis of the distal clavicle. This may be seen in workers who have occupational demands that include frequent strenuous use of their upper extremities.[17,118] It is also common in weight lifters. The proposed etiology is repetitive trauma across the acromioclavicular joint. Usually, pain begins insidiously and directly in the area of the acromioclavicular joint. On occasion, the worker remarks that a distinct pull or strain to the upper shoulder occurred. Examination demonstrates point tenderness at the acromioclavicular joint, which can be exacerbated by cross-body (horizontal) adduction. Glenohumeral joint motion is unaffected. Radiographs demonstrate osteopenia of the distal clavicle, often with tapering and cystic changes.[96]

Conservative management for acromioclavicular arthritis or distal clavicle osteolysis includes RICE, avoidance of strenuous upper-extremity activities, and nonsteroidal anti-inflammatory medication. An intra-articular injection of a corticosteroid is often very helpful for patients who present with significant discomfort in the area of the acromioclavicular joint or for patients who are unresponsive to conservative management. The acromioclavicular joint can be difficult to infiltrate with an injection. In order for the injection to work, the physician needs to be successful in delivering the medication intra-articularly. Using a 20-gauge needle, a gentle "pop" is felt as the joint is entered, and only a small volume of fluid (usually less than 2 cc, with a 1:1 ratio of a corticosteroid and Xylocaine) is accepted. A successful injection is accompanied by the patient experiencing an acute worsening of the presenting symptoms from the pressure in the joint; this is followed by complete relief of their symptoms within a few minutes. The injection can be repeated after 6 weeks if the patient's symptoms return, and is ideally suited for patients who demonstrated a good response following the initial injection.

Patients who have had symptoms for 6 months or more despite appropriate conservative treatment can be considered for distal claviclar resection. Distal claviclar resection is an effective treatment for both osteoarthritis of the acromioclavicular joint as well as distal clavicle osteolysis, resulting in decreased pain and return to precondition levels of function.[17,45,107,118] However, the return of normal strength takes much longer than 3 to 6 months. Even in well-motivated athletes, objective strength testing demonstrates a >10% deficit in side-to-side testing at 1 year following a distal claviclar resection.[24] Therefore, the postsurgical return-to-work guidelines must be modified based on the worker's upper-extremity (especially overhead) occupational demands. Light use of the extremity with the elbow by the side is possible at 6 to 12 weeks. Full use of the extremity for ADLs and light manual labor can be expected around 3 months. Medium labor activities will be possible between 4 to 6 months, and heavy labor, particularly overhead lifting, will be restricted for 6 to 12 months. Maximum medical improvement is achieved between 6 and 12 months, although strength may continue to improve beyond 1 year.

DEGENERATIVE ARTHRITIS OF THE GLENOHUMERAL JOINT

As with osteoarthritis of the acromioclavicular joint, the relationship between osteoarthritis of the glenohumeral joint and occupation remains vague. Occupations that require heavy labor with large forces occurring across the shoulder have been associated with a higher incidence of degenerative arthritis of the glenohumeral joint.[10,68,74] Typically, patients with osteoarthritis of the glenohumeral joint are between 54 and 74 years of age.[82] Functional symptoms often include difficulty sleeping and an inability to perform ADLs.

Patients with glenohumeral arthritis have pain as a result of their restricted motion. Reduced glenohumeral motion is present in all planes, but is particularly evident with rotation of the humerus with the arm by the patient's side. Internal rotation is usually the first motion which the patient notices to be limited and painful. Glenohumeral crepitance may be demonstrated with both active and passive shoulder motion. Plain radiographs are diagnostic, eliminating the need for advanced imaging studies. The required diagnostic views include a true anteroposterior view of the glenohumeral joint and an axillary lateral view.[119]

Initially, management includes avoidance of aggravating activities, anti-inflammatory medications, and occasionally an injection of cortisone. With increasing pain and decreasing function, a shoulder arthroplasty may be indicated.[151] After shoulder arthroplasty, patients usually have little or no pain and a functional range of motion. Lifetime restrictions for patients who require a glenoid resurfacing along with proximal humeral articular surface replacement include no lifting of more than 10 pounds on a regular basis, no impact-loading tasks such as shoveling, and no repetitive overhead activities. Light use of the extremity for occupational demands can begin between 6 and 12 weeks. ADLs are successfully achieved between 2 and 4 months, and patients achieve full use of their extremity with the above-mentioned restrictions at 4 to 6 months.

ELBOW DISORDERS

Acute injuries to the elbow primarily include contusions, muscular strains, and fractures. Aside from fractures, repetitive use can be a common etiology for these other elbow pathologies.[148] Early intervention is recommended, with the RICE protocol and an NSAID. The initial evaluation should include a careful history and physical examination, with supporting radiographs including an anteriorposterior and lateral view of the elbow joint. If there is concern of a ligamentous injury (ulnar collateral ligament), stress radiographs can also be obtained. Fractures involving the elbow are usually easily diagnosed on x-ray examination. Treatment techniques should focus on stable fracture fixation to allow early range of motion. Loss of elbow motion, especially terminal extension, is common with most elbow pathologies. Fortunately, loss of some elbow motion is well-tolerated because the vast majority of daily and occupational activities are possible with an extension-flexion arc of 30 to 130°.[92] Supervised therapy must be initiated early to maintain elbow motion. Most minor injuries resolve within 4 to 6 weeks. If symptoms persist, particularly mechanical symptoms, then consideration of specific elbow conditions should ensue.

Tendonitis: Lateral and Medial Epicondylitis

The elbow is susceptible to injury when substantial forces generated by the shoulder overwhelm the muscles of the elbow region, or alternatively, when the wrist and elbow are used in a chronic and repetitive manner. In addition to biomechanical constraints, "other factors such as psychosocial and personal factors play a role" in the incidence of lateral epicondylitis as well as other upper-limb disorders (carpal tunnel syndrome and wrist tendonitis).[76] Frequently, the lateral aspect of the elbow is involved and the term lateral epicondylitis (tennis elbow) is used to describe this condition. When the medial aspect of the elbow is involved, medial epicondylitis (golfer's elbow) is used. Lateral epicondylitis occurs at the origin of the extensor muscles of the forearm, primarily the extensor carpi radialis brevis (Fig. 17–16). Medial epicondylitis occurs at the origin of the flexor-pronator mass on the medial epicondyle of the distal humerus. Although the use of the term "epicondylitis" implies an inflammatory process, the histology of these conditions is more consistent with a chronic degenerative process,[19,67,116] suggesting that epicondylosis may be a more appropriate diagnostic designation.

Typically, epicondylitis of the elbow occurs in patients between the ages of 30 and 50, with a mean of 41 years.[105] Younger patients frequently report its association with sports participation such as tennis. Medial epicondylitis and ulnar nerve problems are commonly seen in throwers as a result of the increased valgus stress that the elbow experiences during the acceleration phase.[51] Usually, the dominant arm is affected, and there does not appear to be any correlation with gender. The condition is also commonly associated with repetitive eccentric wrist use, such as the activities of carpenters or welders. In addition, repetitive low-level activities such as typing or data entry may cause microtrauma to the involved tissues, resulting in epicondylitis.[20,33,105]

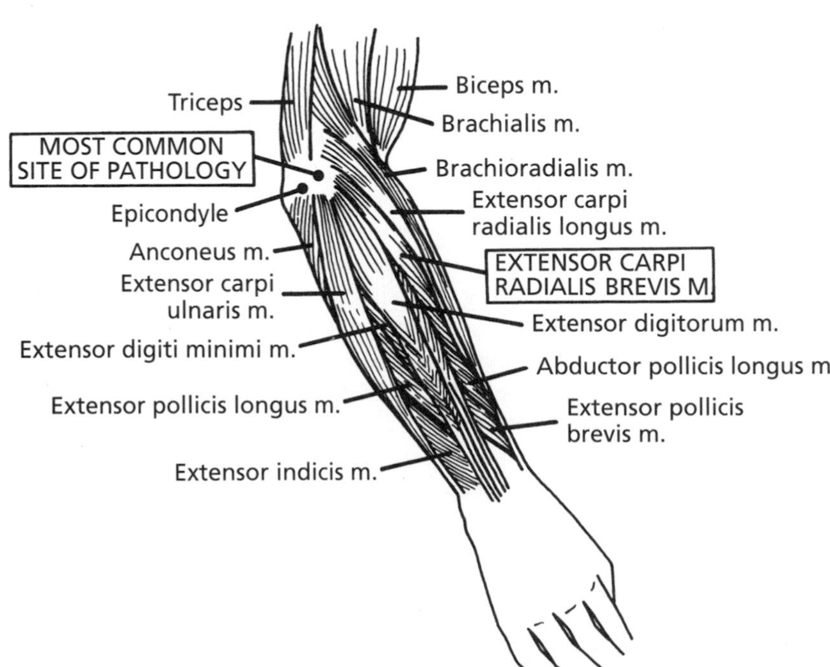

Figure 17–16. Anatomy of lateral epicondylitis. The extensor muscles of the forearm originate at the lateral epicondyle of the distal humerus. The structure most frequently involved in the condition of lateral epicondylitis is the origin of the extensor carpi radialis brevis, which originates at the lateral epicondyle and inserts at the base of the third metacarpal.

Although epicondylitis appears to be associated with work-related activities, the fact that this is a degenerative process histologically implies that work-related tendon degeneration may be superimposed on the normal aging process. The incidence of lateral epicondylitis is significantly correlated with increasing age.[33] It is also occupation dependent, with the estimated elbow stress directly proportional to the prevalence of epicondylitis.[33] The overall prevalence in a study of industrial workers was less than 10%, with one-third of the cases directly work-related, one-third due to sports or recreation, and one-third without a specific cause. Analyzing the reports of patients with lateral epicondylitis who were seen by a company physician shows that 50% of the patients claimed work-related causes.[32]

The diagnosis of epicondylitis is suspected after a careful history implicating an eccentric load or repetitive activity involving the wrist and elbow. Pain may be diffuse, but is commonly localized to a very specific area at the anterolateral (lateral epicondylitis) or anteromedial (medial epicondylitis) aspect of the distal humerus. Often, the worker will complain of pain radiating down the forearm, and decreased grip strength and dexterity. Resisted wrist extension may intensify the pain. Radiographs are usually normal, but up to 25% of patients may have soft-tissue calcifications involving the tendon origins, which have no prognostic value.[105]

The initial management of elbow epicondylitis is directed toward decreasing the stresses across the elbow and decreasing pain. The inciting activity must be avoided, or ideally, stopped until the acute phase has resolved. Cryotherapy is useful to decrease the discomfort. The benefits of nonsteroidal anti-inflammatory mediations are primarily pain relief; their role in the reparative process remains vague. The healing process may be facilitated by other modalities such as electrical stimulation or iontophoresis, but their efficacy is unproven.[13,25,135] A crucial component of rehabilitation is a consistent effort by the worker to stretch the affected area. Wrist extension with medial epicondylitis or wrist flexion with lateral epicondylitis should be performed three to five times per day. When the end-range of motion increases with decreasing pain at 2 to 4 weeks, then strengthening exercises can be initiated.

Counterforce bracing has been shown to improve wrist and grip strength as well as to decrease pain.[143] However, it has also been shown to increase the rate of fatigue in the wrist extensors in unimpaired individuals, which is believed to be a contributing factor in the development of lateral epicondylitis.[71] Bracing may be particularly useful in workers who continue with their occupational responsibilities. Unfortunately, a controlled, prospective study evaluating the effects of various modalities and medications has not been done.

If the worker does not respond to initial management, an injection of a corticosteroid may be considered. In some patients, a single injection may permanently relieve their problem, whereas in many patients, the pain relief is only transient.[114] In one follow-up study, surgery was avoided in 75% of cases of lateral epicondylitis following an injection, and in this population patients who responded to the first injection were twice as likely to avoid surgery than those who required multiple ones.[11] Injections for the treatment of medial epicondylitis have also been studied and seem to only provide short-term benefits for the treatment of this disorder, and in actuality may not affect the natural history of the disease process.[136] The detrimental effects of the steroid medication on the normal healing process of collagen and other tissues leads to the recommendation that corticosteroid injections should be used sparingly.[39]

Workers who are well-motivated, exercise (stretch) daily, avoid aggravating activities, and yet continue to suffer the effects of elbow epicondylitis after 6 to 12 months are considered for surgical intervention. This should represent around 10% of all patients who have symptoms of medial or lateral epicondylitis.[20,105,108] If surgery is not performed for a minimum of 12 months following the onset of symptoms, then less than 5% of all patients with lateral or medial epicondylitis would require surgery. Numerous surgical techniques have been described for the treatment of elbow epicondylitis.[13,25,65,103,105] As with any surgical procedure, the guiding principle should be a determination of the exact pathology preoperatively with an anatomic restoration of the tissues. However, with elbow epicondylitis, the technique most commonly used is an excision of pathologic tissue and release of any remaining affected tendon origin. The overlying fascia of the extensor communis (lateral epicondylitis) is usually repaired when closing the wound (Fig. 17–17) and the success rate is 90% or better. In patients with medical epicondylitis, results were significantly compromised in those who had coexistent ulnar nerve neuritis.[72] Success is primarily described in terms of pain relief, because other parameters such as objective measurements may demonstrate substantial deficits despite complete relief of pain.[65] Arthroscopic treatment for lateral epicondylitis has become an additional option to treat this problem. This approach is significantly less traumatic and allows the surgeon to diagnose and treat associated intra-articular pathology that would normally be missed during the open procedure. Early results indicate little change in grip strength (96% of unaffected limb)[4] and a expedited return to normal activities.[4,109]

Postoperatively, the elbow may be splinted briefly, but an early range of motion program should be instituted. After 4 weeks, a gradual strengthening program is started, initially with light resisted isometrics. This is

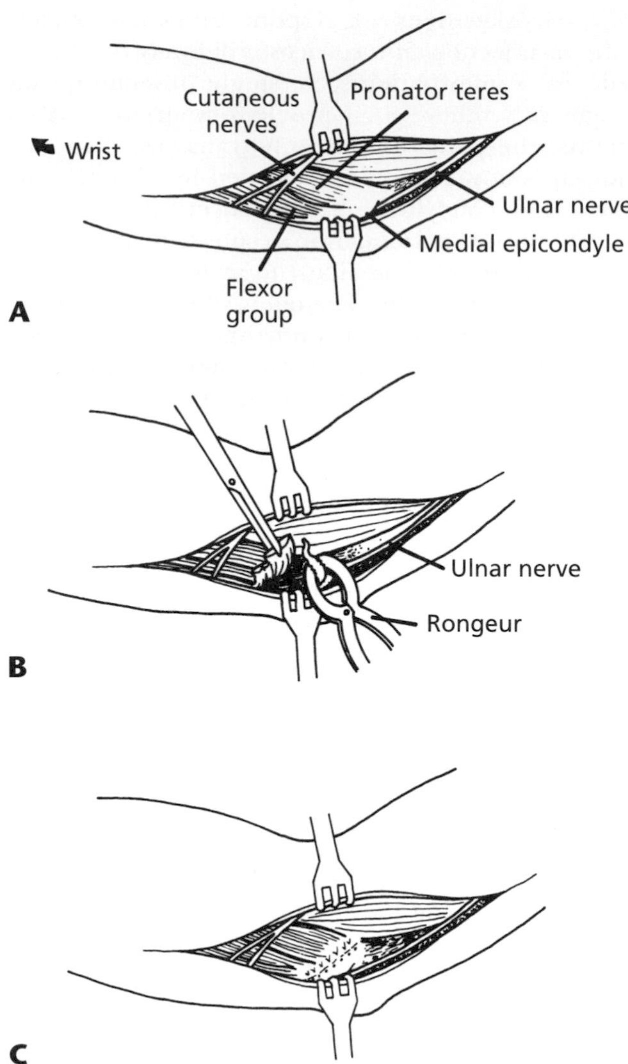

Figure 17–17. Surgical management of medial epicondylitis. The stages include the following: (A) exposure to the fascia of the common flexor-pronator group originating at the medial epicondyle; (B) reflection of the common flexor-pronator group origin and debridement of the involved tissue; and (C) repair of the fascia of the common flexor-pronator group.

advanced, as tolerated, at 6 weeks following surgery. Grip strengthening is gradually advanced. Stretching remains an essential component of the rehabilitation program, with the patient instructed to stretch three to five times per day, beginning with the elbow slightly flexed and advancing to stretching activities with the elbow fully extended. At 3 months following surgery, lifting activities and more athletic work responsibilities are permitted. For occupations that include high levels of elbow and wrist stress, full return to duty should occur between 4 and 6 months. If progress remains slow at 4 to 5 months, an intensive work-hardening program may be beneficial. Symptoms persisting beyond 6 months may indicate failure of the surgical procedure, often requiring advanced evaluation techniques to determine the cause of surgical failure.[90]

Olecranon Bursitis

Olecranon bursitis generally has a traumatic origin, although occasionally it may be related to an overuse of repetitive stress phenomenon, such as miner's elbow. Olecranon bursitis may also herald a systemic process such as gout or inflammatory arthropathies. A succinct history should determine the etiology. The differential diagnosis between nonseptic and septic bursitis can be challenging.[91] Septic bursitis predominantly affects young and middle-aged men involved in manual labor (e.g., plumbers, truck drivers, and auto mechanics).[115] The "superficial location of the olecranon bursa places it at a high risk for injury, possibly leading to the entry of bacteria into the bursal sac."[128] Predisposing medical conditions are evident in more than 70% of patients with septic olecranon bursitis.

Physical examination findings include a visible enlargement of the posterior aspect of the olecranon with a mobile, usually soft, mass. Traumatic olecranon bursitis is painful at the time of injury, but the pain quickly resolves. Septic bursitis is associated with a persistence or worsening of pain. Patient with septic bursitis have pain 80% of the time, whereas patients with aseptic bursitis have pain less than 20% of the time after the resolution of acute symptoms.[131] The skin temperature over a septic olecranon bursa is approximately 4° C warmer than the nonaffected side. Loss of motion, particularly flexion, may be present and more likely suggests a specific process.[91]

Treatment of acute olecranon bursitis without an associated systemic disease includes avoidance of the inciting activity and protection of the posterior elbow from recurrent trauma with a protective elbow sleeve. Anti-inflammatory medications usually provide pain relief. Aspiration may be indicated when the swollen bursa is painful and interferes with daily activities. However, a simple aspiration followed by the application of the compressive dressing is associated with a high rate of recurrence. Repeat aspirations cannot be recommended. Aspiration of the bursal fluid, instillation of methylprednisolone, and application of a compressive dressing may result in the lowest recurrence rate,[132] but the use of corticosteroids has been associated with a prohibitive risk of infection, that may be as high as 12%, and a 20% risk of subdermal atrophy.[151] If the bursitis persists despite conservative management, resection of the entire bursa through a midline incision is recommended. This procedure can have over a 90% success rate in patients with no concomitant comorbidities.[137] The patient is started on range of motion exercises after immobilizing the elbow in flexion for 1 to 2 weeks. Return to full activities is generally accomplished within 6 weeks.

For septic olecranon bursitis, the bursa must be drained. Drainage can be adequately accomplished through a small incision. Antibiotic therapy effective against Gram-positive organisms (e.g., staphylococci, streptococci) is started. Initially, antibiotics are adjusted according to the Gram stain, while definitive treatment is based on culture results at 48 hours. Recovery is generally complete within 2 to 3 weeks. Surgical removal of the bursa is rarely indicated in the acute phase of either septic or nonseptic olecranon bursitis.[91]

Surgical removal is considered if symptoms interfere with ADLs or occupational responsibilities. The entire bursa is removed through a longitudinal incision, a compressive dressing is applied, and the elbow is splinted for 10 to 14 days. After the wound has healed, an olecranon pad is used to protect this area and return to work is accomplished within 2 to 4 weeks.

Entrapment of the Ulnar Nerve at the Elbow: Cubital Tunnel Syndrome

Ulnar neuropathy at the elbow level is not uncommon, although the vast majority of compressive neuropathies involving the upper extremity are related to compression of the median nerve in the carpal tunnel. The ulnar nerve travels in a specific path, descending from the brachial plexus in the anterior compartment of the arm, passing through the intramuscular septum at the arcade of Struthers approximately 6 to 8 cm above the medial epicondyle, then continuing posterior to the medial epicondyle (Fig. 17–18). After passing the medial epicondyle, it enters into the flexor carpi ulnaris, underneath a connecting fibrous band. Compression or irritation of the nerve can occur at any of these three relatively fixed points. The term cubital tunnel syndrome initially referred to constriction of the nerve by the tunnel formed from the band crossing the ulnar nerve between the two heads of the flexor carpi ulnaris[40]; however, the term is now commonly used to describe most ulnar nerve conditions around the elbow.

Most commonly, symptoms begin with an insidious onset of intermittent paresthesias involving the ulnar nerve distribution into the little finger and ring finger. A vague discomfort at the posteromedial aspect of the elbow may be present. Symptoms are aggravated by repetitive or prolonged elbow flexion. Gradually, the paresthesia becomes more persistent, and loss of sensation, particularly in the ulnar aspect of the hand, can occur. Other complaints include loss of grip strength and decreased hand dexterity. Cubital tunnel syndrome can also begin with a single traumatic event from which the patient does not completely recover, although this mechanism is uncommon. Other disorders that may have similar associated symptoms include cervical radiculopathy and thoracic outlet syndrome.

On examination, light tapping with the index finger over the ulnar nerve distribution may elicit pain and paresthesias in the ulnar distribution of the hand

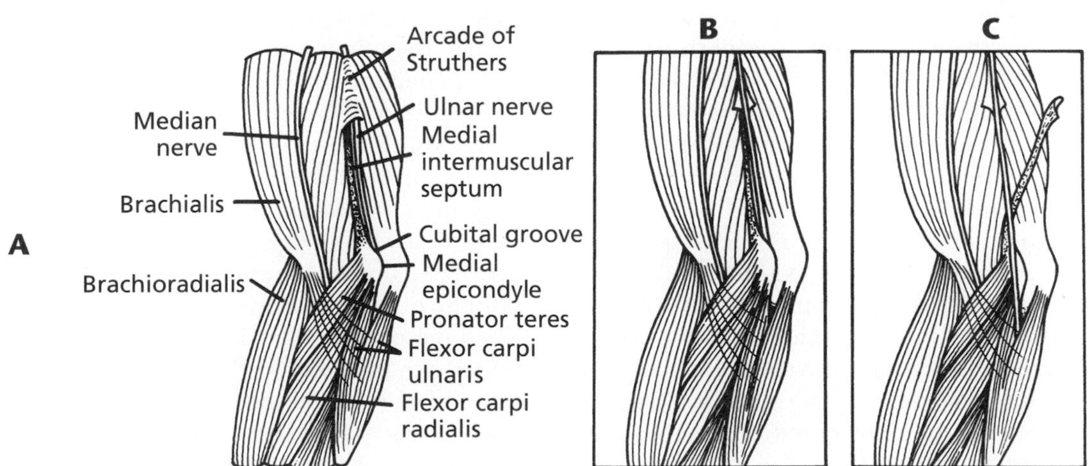

Figure 17–18. Cubital tunnel syndrome. Anatomy of the ulnar nerve. The normal dimensions of the ulnar nerve can be encroached upon at three important levels: (A) proximally, at the arcade of Struthers; (B) in the ulnar nerve groove at the posterior aspect of the medial epicondyle; and (C) distally by a fibrous band across the two heads of the flexor carpi ulnaris as the nerve enters into this muscle. Anterior transposition of the ulnar nerve requires release of the arcade and fibrous band at the flexor carpi ulnaris.

(positive Tinel sign). Another useful test is the elbow flexion test.[15] The elbow is held in flexion with the wrist in extension for up to 3 minutes. A positive test results in reproduction or worsening of the initial symptoms. Late findings include atrophy of the hypothenar eminence and the flexor carpi ulnaris, weakness of the intrinsic muscles of the hand, and gradual clawing of the small and ring fingers. Instability of the ulnar nerve (subluxation of the nerve out of the medial epicondylar groove with elbow flexion) is present in approximately 16% of the general population and therefore is not directly related to the development of ulnar neuropathy at the elbow level.[29] However, ulnar nerve instability may predispose patients to ulnar neuropathy if their occupation or recreation is associated with frequent flexion of the elbow beyond 90°.

Radiographs and electromyographic studies contribute to the evaluation of patients with cubital tunnel syndrome. The cubital tunnel is visualized on plain radiographs with the cubital tunnel view.[135] The elbow is fully flexed, placed on the radiographic plate, and the humerus is externally rotated 20°. The radiographic beam is directed perpendicular to the plate. This radiograph is particularly useful when the patient has a prior history of trauma. Osteophytes or a malunion in this area may encroach on the usual ulnar nerve pathway as it traverses along the medial edge of the trochlea. Electromyographic (EMG) studies can confirm the suspected clinical diagnosis, but occasionally they may be normal despite clinical findings.[27] Nerve conduction velocities are tested across the elbow with the intrinsic muscles of the hand used to determine the motor velocity. The little finger is tested for sensory deficits. The electromyographer must be skilled, the region to be tested should be clearly described, and the patient must be cooperative. The EMG may be unable to demonstrate the exact site of the ulnar nerve pathology in up to one-third of all cases.[34] EMG studies are particularly useful when the diagnosis of this condition remains uncertain based on clinical findings, because the results can assist in differentiating other conditions such as cervical radiculopathy or thoracic outlet syndrome.

Management includes avoiding the inciting activity. If a source of external trauma is evident, padding of the elbow is helpful. Modification of the work area, such as changing the height of the keyboard, may be helpful. Repetitive flexion activities can also be decreased by job restrictions or job rotation. A padded extension brace can be fabricated to prevent the elbow from flexing more than 30º during sleep. If an inflammatory component is recognized, an anti-inflammatory medication is prescribed. Treatment may last 3 to 9 months and is often successful. When only mild paresthesias are present, the likelihood of surgery over the following 6 years is 21%; however, if muscle atrophy is present on examination, the likelihood of surgery over the following 3 years is 62% despite conservative treatment.[29]

Surgery is reserved for patients with a clear clinical picture of cubital syndrome who do not respond to conservative management within 6 months. Subcutaneous, submuscular, or intramuscular transposition is recommended.[1,27,28,70,77] Other techniques, such as medial epicondylectomy, may also achieve good results.[1,43,48,70] However, a meta-analysis of the literature has revealed that in patients with moderate-stage cubital tunnel syndrome, submuscular transposition is the most efficcious.[95] After transposition of the nerve, the arm is rested with a splint for up to 2 weeks. Active range of motion can be started after removal of the splint. At 4 to 6 weeks, a strengthening program is instituted. Most patients will be able to resume full activities without restrictions by 8 to 12 weeks.

CONCLUSION

Occupational disorders of the upper extremities have a high incidence in the working population. Both laborers and nonlaborers are susceptible to overuse type injuries exacerbated by repetitive type motion activities. Traumatic injuries are more common in labor-intensive vocations, where treatment focuses on accident prevention. Regardless of the actual diagnosis, initial treatment focuses on the RICE protocol with the addition of a nonsteroidal anti-inflammatory medications. Early evaluation is recommended for traumatic injuries, and all assessments should include a thorough history, physical examinatio, and x-ray evaluation.

Symptomatic treatment may include a local injection with a combination of an anesthetic and a corticosteroid depending on the etiology. Injections should be used judiciously because of the potential negative effect that the medication may have on healing tissues. Surgical treatment is recommended in those patients who fail conservative management. Incorporation of a well-organized physical therapy program is an essential component of either conservative or operative treatment. The goal of treatment is to return the patient back to his or her previous work responsibilities in a safe and timely fashion. Utilization of work-conditioning programs is one way to help accomplish this goal effectively. There are some conditions (glenohumeral arthritis) where a patient may not be able to return to his or her previous activity level; in this situation, vocational re-education maybe required.

References

1. Adson AW: The surgical treatment of progressive ulnar paralysis. Minn Med 1:455–460, 1918.
2. Altchek DW, Warren RF, Wickiewicz TL, et al: Arthroscopic acromioplasty: Technique and results. J Bone Joint Surg 72A:1198–1207, 1990.
3. Andrews RJ, Carson WG, Mcleod WD: Glenoid labrum tears related to long head of the biceps. Am J Sports Med 13:337–341, 1985.
4. Baker CL Jr, Murphy KP, Gottlob CA, Curt DT: Arthroscopic classification and treatment of lateral epicondylitis: Two year clinical results. J Shoulder Elbow Surg 9:475–482, 2000
5. Bassett RW, Cofield RH: Acute tears of the rotator cuff: the timing of surgical repair. Clin Orthop 175:18–24, 1983.
6. Beltran J: The use of magnetic resonance imaging about the shoulder. J Shoulder Elbow Surg 1:321–332, 1993.
7. Bensen WG, Zhao SZ, Burke TA: Upper gastrointestinal tolerability of celecoxib, a COX-2 specific inhibitor, compared to naproxen and placebo. J Rheumatology 27:1876–1883, 2000.
8. Bigliani L, Cordasco F, McIlveen S, et al: Operative treatment of failed repairs of the rotator cuff. J Bone Joint Surg 74A:1505–1515, 1992.
9. Bokor DJ, Hawkins RJ, Huckell GH, et al: Results of nonoperative management of full-thickness tears of the rotator cuff. Clin Orthop 294:103–110, 1993.
10. Bovenzi M, Fiorito A, Volpe C: Bone and joint disorders in the upper extremities of chipping and grinding operators. Int Arch Occup Environ Health 59:189–198, 1987.
11. Bowen RE, Dorey FJ, Shapiro MS: Efficacy of nonoperative treatment for lateral epicondylitis. Am J Orthop 30:642–646, 2001.
12. Bowen MK, Warren RF: Ligamentous control of shoulder stability based on selective cutting and static translation experiments. Clin Sports Med 10:757–782, 1991.
13. Boyd HB, McLeod AC: Tennis elbow. J Bone Joint Surg 55A:1183, 1973.
14. Brems JJ: Digital muscle strength measurement in rotator cuff tears. Paper presented to American Shoulder and Elbow Surgeons, Third Open Meeting, San Francisco, 1987.
15. Buerhler MJ, Thayer DT: The elbow flexion test: a clinical test for the cubital tunnel syndrome. Clin Orthop 233:213–216, 1988.
16. Burkhead WZ Jr, Arcand MA, Zeman C, et al: The biceps tendon. In Rockwood CAJ, Matsen FA III (eds): The Shoulder. Philadelphia, WB Saunders, 1998, pp 1009–1063.
17. Cahill BR: Osteolysis of the distal part of the clavicle in athletes. J Bone Joint Surg 64A:1053–1058, 1982.
18. Caspari RB, Thal R: A technique for arthroscopic subacromial decompression. Arthroscopy 8:23–30, 1992.
19. Chard MD, Cawston TE, Riley GP, et al: Rotator cuff degeneration and lateral epicondylitis: A comparative histological study. Ann Rheum Dis 53:30–34, 1994.
20. Ciccotti MG, Lombardo SJ: Medial and lateral epicondylitis. In Jobe FW: Upper Extremity Injuries in Sports. St. Louis, CV Mosby, 1994.
21. Clark JM, Harryman DT II: Tendons, ligaments, and capsule of the rotator cuff. J Bone Joint Surg 74A:713–725, 1992.
22. Codman EA: The shoulder: rupture of the supraspinatus tendon and other lesions in or about the subacromial bursa. Boston, Thomas Todd, 1934.
23. Cole BJ, Warner JJP: Anatomy, biomechanics, and pathophysiology of glenohumeral instability. In Iannotti JP, Williams GR Jr (eds). Disorders of the Shoulder: Diagnosis and Management. Philadelphia, Lippincott Williams & Wilkins, 1999, pp 207–232.
24. Cook FF, Tibone JE: The Mumford procedure in athletes: an objective analysis of function. Am J Sports Med 16:97–100, 1988.
25. Coonrad RW, Hooper WR: Tennis elbow: Its course, natural history, conservative and surgical management. J Bone Joint Surg 55A:1177, 1973.
26. Craig EV: Continuous passive motion in the rehabilitation of the surgically reconstructed shoulder: A preliminary report. Orthop Trans 219, 1986.
27. Dawson DM: Entrapment neuropathies of the upper extremities. N Engl J Med 329:2013–2018, 1993.
28. Dellon AL: Review of treatment results for ulnar nerve compression at the elbow. J Hand Surg 14:688–699, 1989.
29. Dellon AL, Hament W, Gittelshon A: Nonoperative management of cubital tunnel syndrome: An 8-year prospective study. Neurology 43:1673–1677, 1993.
30. DePalma AF: The role of the disks of the sternoclavicular and acromioclavicular joints. Clin Orthop 13:7–12, 1959.
31. DePalma AF, Callery GE: Bicipital tenosynovitis. Clin Orthop 3:69–85, 1954.
32. Dimberg L: Lateral humeral epicondylitis (tennis elbow) among industrial workers. Swedish Work Environment Fund, 1983.
33. Dimberg L: The prevalence and causation of tennis elbow (lateral humeral epicondylitis) in a population of workers in an engineering industry. Ergonomics 30:573–580, 1987.
34. Eisen A: Early diagnosis of ulnar nerve palsy: An electrophysiologic study. Neurology 24:256–262, 1974.
35. Ellman H: Arthroscopic subacromial decompression: Analysis of 1–3 year results. Arthroscopy 3:173, 1987.
36. Ellman H: Diagnosis and treatment of incomplete rotator cuff tears. Clin Orthop 254:64–74, 1990.
37. Ellman H, Hanker G, Bayer M: Repair of the rotator cuff: End-result study of factors influencing reconstruction. J Bone Joint Surg 68A:1136–1144, 1986.
38. Ellman H, Kay SP, Wirth M: Arthroscopic treatment of full thickness rotator cuff tears: 2 to 7 year follow-up study. Arthroscopy 9:195–200, 1993.
39. Fadale PD, Wiggins ME: Corticosteroid injections: Their use and abuse. J Am Acad Orthop Surg 2:133–140, 1994.
40. Feindel W, Stratford J: The role of the cubital tunnel in tardy ulnar palsy. Can J Surg 38:287–300, 1958.
41. Flatow EL, Warner JJP: Instability of the shoulder: Complex problems and failed repairs. Part I. Relevant biomechanics, multidirectional instability, and severe loss of glenoid and humeral bone. J Bone Joint Surg 80A:122–140, 1998.
42. Flowers K: CPM for postop rotator cuff repair: A case history. Contin Care 1990.
43. Froimson AI, Zahrawi F: Treatment of compression neuropathy of the ulnar nerve at the elbow by epicondylectomy and neurolysis. J Hand Surg 5:391–395, 1980.
44. Gartsman GM: Arthroscopic acromioplasty for lesions of the rotator cuff. J Bone Joint Surg 72A:169–180, 1990.
45. Gartsman GM: Arthroscopic resection of the acromioclavicular joint. Am J Sports Med 21:71–77, 1993.
46. Gartsman GM, Brinker MR, Khan M: Early effectiveness of arthroscopic repair for full-thickness tears of the rotator cuff. J Bone Joint Surg 80A:33–40, 1998.
47. Gazielly DF, Gleyze P, Montagnon C: Functional and anatomical results after rotator cuff repair. Clin Orthop 304:43–53, 1994.
48. Goldberg BJ, Light TR, Blair SJ: Ulnar neuropathy at the elbow: results of medial epicondylectomy. J Hand Surg 14A:182–188, 1989.
49. Goldman AB, Ghelman B: The double-contrast shoulder arthrogram. Radiology 127:655–663, 1978.
50. Gore DR, Murray MP, Sepic SB, et al: Shoulder–muscle strength and range of motion following surgical repair of full-thickness rotator cuff tears. J Bone Joint Surg 68A:266–272, 1986.

51. Grana W: Medial epicondylitis and cubital tunnel syndrome in the throwing athlete. Clin Sports Med 20:541–548, 2001.
52. Ha'eri GB, Wiley AM: Shoulder impingement syndrome: results of operative release. Clin Orthop 168:128–134, 1982.
53. Harryman D II, Mack L, Wang K, et al: Repairs of the rotator cuff. J Bone Joint Surg 73A:982–989, 1991.
54. Harryman DT, Mack LA, Wang KY, et al: Repair of the rotator cuff: correlation of functional results with integrity of the cuff. J Bone Joint Surg 73A:982–989, 1991.
55. Hawkins RJ, Abrams JS: Impingement syndrome in the absence of rotator cuff tear (Stages 1 and 2). Orthop Clin North Am 18:373–382, 1987.
56. Hawkins RJ, Bokor DJ: Clinical evaluation of shoulder problems. In Rockwood CAJ, Matsen FA III: The Shoulder. Philadelphia, WB Saunders, 1998, pp 164–197.
57. Hawkins RJ, Brock RM, Abrams JS, Hobeika P: Acromioplasty for impingement with an intact rotator cuff. J Bone Joint Surg 70B:795–797, 1988.
58. Hawkins RJ, Chris T, Bokor MB, Kiefer G: Failed anterior acromioplasty. Clin Orthop 243:106–111, 1989.
59. Hawkins RJ, Kennedy JC: Impingement syndrome in athletes. Am J Sports Med 8:151–158, 1980.
60. Holder J, Fretz CJ, Terrier F, Gerber C: Rotator cuff tears: Correlation of sonographic and surgical findings. Radiology 182:431–436, 1988.
61. Holt R, Helms C, Steinbach L, et al: Magnetic resonance imaging of the shoulder: rationale and current applications. Skeletal Radiol 19:5–14, 1990.
62. Howell SM, Galinat BJ: The glenoid-labral socket. A constrained articular surface. Clin Orthop 243:122–125, 1989.
63. Iannotti J, Zlatkin M, Esterhai J, et al: Magnetic resonance imaging of the shoulder: Sensitivity, specificity, and predictive value. J Bone Joint Surg 73A:17–29, 1991.
64. Iannotti JP: Full-thickness rotator cuff tears: factors affecting surgical outcome. J Am Acad Orthop Surg 2:87–95, 1994.
65. Jobe FW, Ciccotti MG: Lateral and medial epicondylitis of the elbow. J Am Acad Orthop Surg 2:1–8, 1994.
66. Johnson DP: The effect of continuous passive motion on wound healing and joint mobility after knee arthroplasty. J Bone Joint Surg 72:1353–1358, 1990.
67. Kannus P, Jozsa L: Histopathological changes preceding spontaneous rupture of a tendon. J Bone Joint Surg 73A:1507–1525, 1991.
68. Katevuo K, Aitasalo K, Lehtinen R, et al: Skeletal changes in dentists and farmers in Finland. Commun Dent Oral Epidemiol 13:23–25, 1985.
69. Kennedy JC, Cameron H: Complete dislocation of the acromioclavicular joint. J Bone Joint Surg 36B:202–208, 1954.
70. Kleinman WB, Bishop AT: Anterior intramuscular transposition of the ulnar nerve. J Hand Surg 14A:972–979, 1989.
71. Knebel PT, Avery DW, Gebhardt TL, et al: Effects of the forearm support band on wrist extensor muscle fatigue. J Orthop Sports Phys Ther 29:677–685, 1999.
72. Kurvers H, Veehaar J: The results of operative treatment of medial epicondylitis. J Bone Joint Surg 77A:1374–1379, 1995.
73. Larsen E, Bjerg-Nielsen A, Christensen P: Conservative or surgical treatment of acromioclavicular dislocation. J Bone Joint Surg 68A:552–555, 1986.
74. Lawrence JS: Rheumatism in coal miners: Part III—Occupational factors. Br J Indust Med 12:249–261, 1955.
75. Leavitt F, Garron D, McNeill T, Whisler W: Organic status, psychological disturbance and pain report characteristics in low-back pain patients on compensation. Spine 7:398–402, 1982.
76. Leclere A, Landre MF, Chastang JF, et al: Upper-limb disorders in repetitive work. Scand J Work Environ Health 27:268–278, 2001.
77. Leffert RD: Anterior submuscular transposition of the ulnar nerve by the Learmonth technique. J Hand Surg 7:147–152, 1982.
78. Lirette R, Morin F, Kinnard P: The difficulties in assessment of results of anterior acromioplasty. Clin Orthop 278:14–16, 1992.
79. Liu SH: Arthroscopically assisted rotator-cuff repair. J Bone Joint Surg 76B:592–595, 1994.
80. MacDonald PB, Alexander MJ, Frejuk J, et al: Comprehensive functional analysis of shoulders following complete acromioclavicular separation. Am J Sports Med 16:475–480, 1988.
81. Mack LA, Matsen FA III, Kilcoyne JF, et al: Sonographic evaluation of the rotator cuff: accuracy in patients without prior surgery. Clin Orthop 234:21–28, 1988.
82. Matsen FA III: Subacromial impingement. In Rockwood CA, Matsen III FA (eds): The Shoulder. Philadelphia, WB Saunders, 1990, p 638.
83. Matsen FA III, Arntz C, Lippitt S: Rotator cuff. In Rockwood CA, Matsen III FA (eds): The Shoulder. Philadelphia, WB Saunders, 1998, pp 755–839.
84. Matsen FA III, Lippitt SB, Sidles JA, et al: Practical evaluation and management of the shoulder. Philadelphia, WB Saunders, 1994.
85. Melzack R, Katz J, Jeans ME: The role of compensation in chronic pain analysis using a new method of scoring, the McGill Pin Questionnaire. Pain 23:101–112, 1985.
86. Mendelson G: Compensation, pain complaints and psychological disturbance. Pain 20:169–177, 1984.
87. Milgrom C, Schaffler M, van Holsbeeck M: Rotator-cuff changes in asymptomatic adults: The effect of age, hand dominance and gender. J Bone Joint Surg 77B:296–298, 1995.
88. Miniaci A, Willits K, Vellet AD: Magnetic resonance imaging evaluation of the asymptomatic shoulder. Paper presented to the American Academy of Orthopaedic Surgeons, 61st Annual Meeting, New Orleans, 1994.
89. Mink JH, Harris E, Rappaport M: Rotator cuff tears: Evaluation using double-contrast shoulder arthrography. Radiology 153:621–623, 1985.
90. Morrey B: Reoperation for failed surgical treatment of refractory lateral epicondylitis. J Shoulder Elbow Surg 1:47–55, 1992.
91. Morrey BF: The Elbow and its Disorders, 2nd ed. Philadelphia, WB Saunders, 1993, pp 872–880.
92. Morrey BF, Askew LJ, An KN, et al: A biomechanical study of normal elbow motion. J Bone Joint Surg 63A:872, 1981.
93. Morrey BJ, Itoi E, An K: Biomechanics of the shoulder. In Rockwood CAJ, Matsen FA III (eds): The Shoulder. Philadelphia, WB Saunders, 1998, 233–276.
94. Morrison DS, Frogameni A, Woodworth P: Conservative management for subacromial impingement of the shoulder. Paper presented to the American Shoulder and Elbow Surgeons, Ninth Open Meeting, San Francisco, 1993.
95. Mowlavi A, Andrews K, Lille S, et al: The management of cubital tunnel syndrome: A meta-analysis of clinical studies. Plast Reconstr Surg 106:327–334, 2000.
96. Murphy OB, Bellamy R, Wheeler W, et al: Post-traumatic osteolysis of the distal clavicle. Clin Orthop 109:108–114, 1975.
97. National Health Interview Survey, Data tapes, 1988.
98. Neer CI: Anterior acromioplasty for the chronic impingement syndrome in the shoulder. J Bone Joint Surg 54A:41, 1972.
99. Neer CS II: Impingement lesions. Clin Orthop 173:70–77, 1983.
100. Neer CS II: Shoulder Reconstruction. Philadelphia, WB Saunders, 1990.
101. Neer CS, Welsh RP: The shoulder in sports. Orthop Clin North Am 8:583–591, 1977.
102. Nelson M, Leather G, Nirschl R, et al: Evaluation of the painful shoulder. J Bone Joint Surg 73A:707–716, 1991.
103. Neviaser TJ, Neviaser RJ, Neviaser JS, et al: Lateral epicondylitis: Results of outpatient surgery and immediate motion. Contemp Orthop 11:43, 1985.
104. Nicholson GG: The effects of passive joint mobilization on pain and hypomobility associated with adhesive capsulitis of the shoulder. J Orthop Sports Phys Ther 6, 1985.

105. Nirschl RP, Pettrone F: Tennis elbow: The surgical treatment of lateral epicondylitis. J Bone Joint Surg 61A:832, 1979.
106. Norberg FB, Field LD, Savoie FH III: Repair of the rotator cuff: Mini-open and arthroscopic repairs. Clin Sports Med 19:77–99, 2000.
107. Novak P, Romeo AA, Hager CA, et al: Open distal clavicle resection: an objective and subjective analysis of results. J Shoulder Elbow Surg 1994.
108. O'Dwyer KJ, Howie CR: Medial epicondylitis of the elbow. Int Orthop 19:69–71, 1995.
109. Owens BD, Murphy KP, Kuklo TR: Arthroscopic release for lateral epicondylitis. Arthroscopy 17:582–587, 2001.
110. Park JY, Levine WN, Marra G, et al: Portal-extension approach for the repair of small and medium rotator cuff tears. Am J Sports Med 28:312–316, 2000.
111. Peterson CJ: Degeneration of the acromioclavicular joint: A morphological study. Acta Orthop Scand 54:434–438, 1983.
112. Peterson CJ, Redlund-Johnell I: Radiographic joint space in normal acromioclavicular joints. Acta Orthop Scand 54:431–433, 1983.
113. Post M, Cohen J: Impingement syndrome: A review of late stage II and early stage III lesions. Clin Orthop 207:126–132, 1986.
114. Price R, Sinclair H, Heinrich I, et al: Local injection treatment of tennis elbow: Hydrocortisone, triamcinolone, and lidocaine compared. Br J Rheumatol 30:39–44, 1991.
115. Raddatz DA, Hoffman GS, Franck WA: Septic bursitis: Presentation, treatment and prognosis. J Rheumatol 14:1160–1163, 1987.
116. Regan W, Wold L, Coonrad R, et al: Microscopic histopathology of chronic refractory lateral epicondylitis. Am J Sports Med 20:746–749, 1992.
117. Resch H, Golser K, Thoeni H, et al: Arthroscopic repair of superior glenoid labral detachment. J Shoulder Elbow Surg 2:147–155, 1993.
118. Rockwood CA Jr, Williams GR Jr, Young DC: Disorders of the acromioclavicular joint. In Rockwood CAJ, Matsen FA III (eds): The Shoulder. Philadelphia, WB Saunders, 1998, pp 483–553.
119. Rockwood CAJ, Jensen KL: X-ray evaluation of shoulder problems. In Rockwood CAJ, Matsen FA III (eds): The Shoulder. Philadelphia, WB Saunders, 1998, pp 199–231.
120. Rockwood CAJ, Lyons FR: Shoulder impingement syndrome: Diagnosis, radiographic evaluation and treatment with a modified Neer acromioplasty. J Bone Joint Surg 75A:409–424, 1993.
121. Rockwood CAJ, Matsen FA III (eds): The Shoulder. Philadelphia, WB Saunders, 1990.
122. Rockwood CAJ, Williams GR, Young DC: Injuries to the acromioclavicular joint. In Rockwood CAJ, Green DP, Bucholz RW: Fractures in Adults. Philadelphia, JB Lippincott, 1984, pp 1181–1251.
123. Romeo AA, Cohen BS, Cole BJ: Arthroscopic repair of full-thickness rotator cuff tears: Surgical technique and instrumentation. Orthopedic Special Edition 7:25–30, 2001.
124. Romeo AA, Cohen BS, Primack S, Shott S: Arthroscopic rotator cuff repair: an evaluation of integrity, strength and functional outcome. Presented at the 8th International Congress on Surgery of the Shoulder, Cape Town, South Africa, April 2001.
125. Romeo AR, Hang DW, Bach BR Jr, Shott S: Repair of full thickness rotator cuff tears: Gender, age and other factors affecting outcome. Clin Orthop 367:243–255, 1999.
126. Sachs RA, Stone ML, Devine S: Open vs. arthroscopic acromioplasty: A prospective, randomized study. Arthroscopy 10:248–254, 1992.
127. Schmitt L, Snyder-Mackler L: Role of scapular stabilizers in etiology and treatment of impingement syndrome. J Orthop Sports Phys Ther 29:31–38, 1999.
128. Shell D, Perkins R, Cosgarea A: Septic olecranon bursitis: recognition and treatment. J Am Board Fam Pract 8:217–220, 1995.
129. Shelton GL: Comprehensive rehabilitation of the athlete. In Mellion MB, Walsh WM, Shelton GL: The Team Physician's Handbook. Philadelphia, Hanley & Belfus, 1997, pp 371–390.
130. Silverstein B, Welp E, Nelson N, Kalat J: Claims incidence of work-related disorders of the upper extremities: Washington State, 1987 through 1995. Am J Public Health 88:1827–1833, 1998.
131. Smith DL, McAfee JH, Lucas LM, et al: Septic and nonseptic olecranon bursitis: Utility of the surface temperature probe in the early differentiation of septic and nonseptic cases. Arch Intern Med 149:1581–1588, 1989.
132. Smith DL, McAfee JH, Lucas LM, et al: Treatment of nonseptic olecranon bursitis: a controlled, blinded prospective trial. Arch Intern Med 149:2527–2530, 1989.
133. Snyder SJ, Karzel RP, Del Pizzo W, et al: SLAP lesions of the shoulder. Arthroscopy 6:274–279, 1990.
134. Solomon PE, Prkachin KM: Bias in assessment of nonverbal pain in compensation patients: Does it exist? Physiotherapy Canada 47:181–184, 1995.
135. St John JN, Palmaz JC: The cubital tunnel in ulnar entrapment neuropathy. Radiology 158:119–121, 1986.
136. Stahl S, Kaufman T: The efficacy of an injection of steroids for medial epicondylitis. A prospective study of sixty elbows. J Bone Joint Surg 79A:1648–1652, 1997.
137. Stewart NJ, Manzanares JB, Morrey BF: Surgical treatment of aseptic olecranon bursitis. J Shoulder Elbow Surg 6:49–54, 1997.
138. Taft TN, Wilson FC, Oglesby JW: Dislocation of the acromioclavicular joint. J Bone Joint Surg 69A:1045–1051, 1987.
139. Tait R, Margolis R, Krause S, Liebowitz E: Compensation status and symptoms reported by patients with chronic pain. Arch Phys Med Rehabil 69:1027–1029, 1988.
140. Tauro JC: Arthroscopic rotator cuff repair: Analysis of technique and results of 2- and 3-year follow-up. Arthroscopy 14:45–51, 1998.
141. Teefey SA, Hasn SA, Middleton WD, et al: Ultrasonography of the rotator cuff: A comparison of ultrasonographic and arthroscopic findings in one hundred consecutive cases. J Bone Joint Surg 82A:498–504, 2000.
142. U.S. Department of Labor: Injury and Illness Data From 1987 Workers' Compensation Records. US Department of Labor, 1990.
143. Wadsworth CT, Nielson DH, Burns LT, et al: The effect of the counterforce armband on wrist extension and grip strength and pain in subjects with tennis elbow. J Orthop Sports Phys Ther 11:192–195, 1989.
144. Walker SW, Couch WH, Boester GA, et al: Isokinetic strength of the shoulder after repair of a torn rotator cuff. J Bone Joint Surg 69A:1041–1044, 1987.
145. Walsh WM, Hald RD, Peter LE, Mellion MB: Injury prevention, diagnosis, and treatment. In Mellion MB, Walsh WM, Shelton GL: The Team Physician's Handbook. Philadelphia, Hanley & Belfus, 1997, pp 361–369.
146. Walsh WM, Peterson DA, Shelton G, et al: Shoulder strength following acromioclavicular injury. Am J Sports Med 13:153–158, 1985.
147. Warner JJP, Flatow EL: Anatomy and biomechanics. In Bigliani LU (ed): The Unstable Shoulder. Rosemont, IL, American Academy of Orthopaedic Surgeons, 1996, pp 1–24
148. Watrous BG, Ho G Jr: Elbow pain. Primary Care 15:725–735, 1988.
149. Weaver JK, Dunn HK: Treatment of acromioclavicular injuries, especially complete acromioclavicular separation. J Bone Joint Surg 54A:1187–1197, 1972.

150. Weber SC: Arthroscopic versus open treatment of significant partial thickness rotator cuff tears. Paper presented to 13th Annual Meeting, Orlando, Fla, 1994.
151. Weinstein PS, Canoso JJ, Wohlgethan JR: Long-term follow-up of corticosteroid injection for traumatic olecranon bursitis. Ann Rheum Dis 43:44–49, 1984.
152. Yamanaka K, Matsumoto T: The joint side tear of the rotator cuff: A follow-up study by arthrography. Clin Orthop 304:68–73, 1994.
153. Zvijac JE, Levy HJ, Lemak LJ: Arthroscopic subacromial decompression in the treatment of full thickness rotator cuff tears: A 3 to 6 year follow-up. Arthroscopy 10:518–523, 1994.

CHAPTER

18

Joint Systems

Knee and Hip

JAMES V. LUCK, JR., MD ■ RANDALL D. LEA, MD

Early musculoskeletal impairment evaluation systems were mostly anatomic in orientation, focusing on range of motion (ROM) and amputation.[11,27] They were simple and reproducible but failed to cover most clinical situations adequately. A more comprehensive system is, of necessity, more complex, requiring more judgment and expertise. The fourth edition of the AMA Guides to the Evaluation of Permanent Impairment embodied major changes in the lower extremity section, enabling the evaluator to assess many more clinical situations accurately.[2] The fifth edition further clarified this system and made it more user friendly with instructions and sample worksheets on the appropriate use of the various lower extremity parameters.[4] This chapter applies this system to a broad range of pathology in the lower extremity and is intended to be used in conjunction with the fourth or fifth edition of the Guides.[2,4]

More than in the upper extremity or spine, the evaluation of lower extremity impairment lends itself to the utilization of all three general rating methodologies: anatomic, diagnostic, and functional (see Chapters 15 and 16 of the AMA Guides). The upper extremity utilizes all three but is primarily based on range of motion. The spine is predominately diagnostic but is anatomic for certain entities. Although most scholars agree that functional assessment, such as active range of motion (AROM), strength, and endurance measurement, is the ultimate method for impairment rating, it suffers from dependence on patient motivation and control. Its application will only progress when assessment techniques and equipment become more objective, valid, and reproducible. By including some of the simpler and more reproducible functional assessment methodologies, this section takes another step forward in that progression. The evaluating physician may utilize AROM and strength testing when the results are consistent between examinations and with the underlying pathology.

The principal advantage of utilizing all three methodologies is the flexibility that it gives the physician to match more closely the methodology to each patient's physical impairment and thus to more accurately, objectively, and appropriately rate each examinee. Some physical impairments are more accurately rated by alterations in ROM, whereas others fit best under diagnostic categories or functional assessment. In some cases, a combination of two or three methodologies will be required. However, using more than one rating methodology for a single anatomic lesion is only allowed under certain circumstances as described in this chapter and the AMA Guides.[2,4] Careful adherence to these principles will make it easier for the evaluating physician to select the best methodology and also ensure the highest degree of consistency between evaluators of the same examinee and between examinees with the same physical impairment. Combining the three methodologies requires medical knowledge, experience, and judgment as well as careful and thoughtful evaluation. It should only be undertaken by physicians who are adequately trained and experienced in examination techniques of the musculoskeletal system and musculoskeletal pathology.

LOWER EXTREMITY EVALUATION AND RATING PARAMETERS

In the fifth edition of the AMA Guides, lower extremity impairment evaluation includes all three basic methodologies through the use of 13 separate rating parameters, each with its own rating scale (Tables 18–1 and 18–2). Arriving at the correct impairment for a specific clinical situation requires a thorough history, careful

TABLE 18–1
Lower Extremity Impairment Parameters*

Parameter	Objectivity	Reliability	Specificity
Limb length discrepancy	1	1	1
Gait derangement	3	1	3
Muscle atrophy	1	3	2
Manual muscle testing	2	2	2
Range of motion	2	2	2
Ankylosis	1	1	1
Arthritic degeneration	1	1	1
Diagnosis-related estimates	1	2	1
Amputations	1	1	1
Peripheral nerve deficits	1	2	1
Skin deficits	1	1	1
Osteomyelitis	1	1	1
Chronic regional pain syndrome	3	3	3

*Scale: 1 = good; 2 = fair; 3 = poor.

physical examination, musculoskeletal specialty expertise, and thoughtful selection of the optimal parameter or combination of parameters. Certain parameters may be combined and others may not. The fifth edition of the AMA Guides contains a chart (Table 17–2) indicating possible combinations.[4] Where a choice exists between parameters, the one with the greatest objectivity, specificity, and reliability should be selected.

Objectivity relates to the successful elimination of confounding factors, such as motivation, that might influence the resulting impairment rating. Language barriers and other issues resulting in failure to understand instructions adequately are other examples of confounding factors. Active ROM and manual muscle testing for strength are dependent on cooperation and motivation. Electromyographic (EMG) and radiographic findings are highly objective. Reflex changes are much more objective than sensory changes.

Reliability refers to the consistency of results between two or more medical evaluators. Limb girth measurements may have a high variance between observers because of differences in technique, variations in local edema, and presence or absence of joint effusion. Limb-length measurement by teleroentgenograms is more reliable than by tape measure. For musculoskeletal disorders of the lower extremity, diagnosis-based estimates should be highly reliable.

Specificity refers to the accuracy with which a given parameter or combination of parameters describes a specific clinical situation. Amputation rating scales are highly specific. Radiographically measured arthritic degeneration of a joint is moderately specific. Muscle girth measurement, as an indicator of muscle strength and endurance, is objective but not specific or very consistent between examiners (reliability). Manual muscle testing is less objective but much more specific. In a cooperative and reliable examinee who is able to make a maximal effort, manual muscle testing should be utilized over girth measurements.

Few tests score high marks in all three areas (objectivity, reliability, and specificity), but in making decisions between choices, all of these factors must be considered.

The gait derangement scale is based on the use of assistive devices for ambulation. It is highly dependent on claimant integrity, reliability, and motivation and should rarely be used as a primary rating scale. Its greatest value is in serving as a general guide against which other lower extremity impairment values may be compared. The use of a cane or crutch for low back pain is generally inappropriate and would be a poor indicator for use of this scale. However, a person with superior gluteal nerve injury and no hip abductor function should use a cane on the opposite side and represents an appropriate use of this scale as a check against the other rating variables, such as manual muscle testing or peripheral nerve deficit rating scales. Of these, the peripheral nerve deficit scale is the most objective, reliable, and specific. Under no circumstances should the gait disturbance scale be added to other impairment values for the same extremity.

Diagnosis-based estimates are objective and specific. However, reliability is only fair because of occasional physician disagreement over the appropriate diagnostic value, especially when it relates to the outcome of surgery. For example, the operating surgeon may rate the result of an anterior cruciate ligament repair as good with no residual laxity (0% impairment), where an independent evaluating physician rates the same patient as fair with moderate residual laxity (17% lower extremity impairment).[3,4] This scale is designed to stand alone except where combination with another method is specifically permitted. A femoral neck fracture malunion, for example, is rated at a 30% lower extremity impairment, plus the value produced by ROM abnormalities.[3,4] These individuals will generally have significant restriction of motion. Those values would be added to the diagnostic values.

In a person with moderate to advanced degenerative arthritis, either ROM or radiographic measurement of cartilage interval can be utilized. In a person where the ROM was deemed reliable, the method giving the greatest value should be selected.

THE PELVIS

Work-related pelvic fractures are usually the consequence of motor vehicle–related injuries, falls, or crush injuries and are relatively uncommon. Subsequent musculoskeletal impairment evaluations and ratings may be divided into three areas: sacroiliac (SI) joint

TABLE 18–2

Parameter Prerequisites, Fifth Edition (Ready Review Checklist)

Parameter	Prerequisite	Table/page*
Limb length discrepancy	1. Absolute only—not relative (i.e., pelvic angulation, knee flexion contracture, indistinct landmarks)	Table 17–4, p 528
Gait disturbance	1. Must be on objective basis only. 2. Rarely appropriate for rating. 3. May be useful as check against other ratings.	Table 17–5, p 529
Muscle atrophy	Contralateral limb normal (i.e., no varicosities or swelling, etc.)	Table 17–6, p 530
Muscle weakness	1. Must have objective basis for weakness (non-neurologic) 2. Must have consistency of one grade or less between two examiners 3. Must be capable of maximal effort. Absence of fear of pain.	Tables 17–7, 17–8, p 531
Range of motion —ankylosis	1. Must have organic basis. 2. Must have a consistency level of one class or less between two examiners or one examiner on two different occasions.	Tables 17–9 thru 17–30, pp 533–543
Arthritis	X-ray must follow guidelines.	Table 17–31, p 544
Amputation	Total LE impairment cannot exceed rating for amputation at that level.	Table 17–32, p 545
Diagnosis-based estimates	See specific diagnosis. Some may be combined with other parameters.	Tables 17–33, 17–34, and 17–35, pp 545–549
Skin loss	Full-thickness skin loss required	Table 17–36, p 550
Peripheral nerve injury		Tables 16–10, 16–11, pp 482–484; Table 17–37, pp 550–552
Chronic regional pain syndrome	Subjective and very difficult to quantify	See Section 17.2m, p 553

*Tables and pages refer to Cocchiarella L, Andersson GBJ (eds): Guides to the Evaluation of Permanent Impairment, 5th ed. Chicago, American Medical Association, 2001.

injuries, acetabular fractures, and nonarticular fractures. Pelvic trauma is often associated with neurologic, vascular, and genitourinary injury, which requires additional evaluation and rating.

Sacroiliac Joint Injuries

Fractures that appear undisplaced on plain radiography may result in significant impairment if there is joint involvement or neuroforaminal encroachment on sacral roots. Computed tomography (CT) is essential to define these problems (Fig. 18–1). Isotopic bone scans will also identify an occult sacral fracture, but CT scans will still be necessary to define it clearly.[6,32] In most instances, CT alone is more cost-effective. Post-traumatic radiculopathy is associated with objective clinical findings and a positive EMG for the upper two sacral roots, but may only be manifest by perianal anesthesia for the lower roots. As long as the injury is unilateral, it is unlikely to result in the loss of bowel or bladder control. Radiculopathy caused by undisplaced fractures often improves. It is important not to rate the claimant until a permanent and stationary status is reached, which may take 12 to 18 months. Residual pain in the appropriate anatomic dermatome(s) should be rated the same as residual pain from a SI joint fracture (1% to 3% whole person).[2,4] Rarely, spinal root injuries from neuroforam-

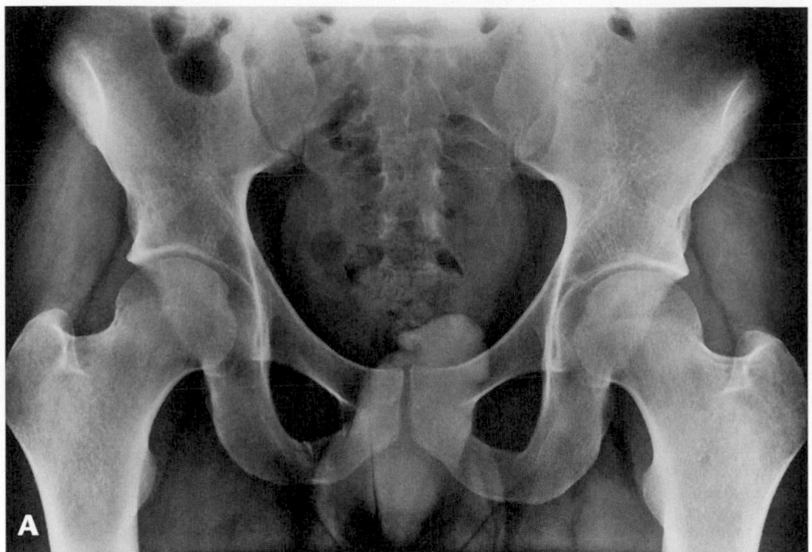

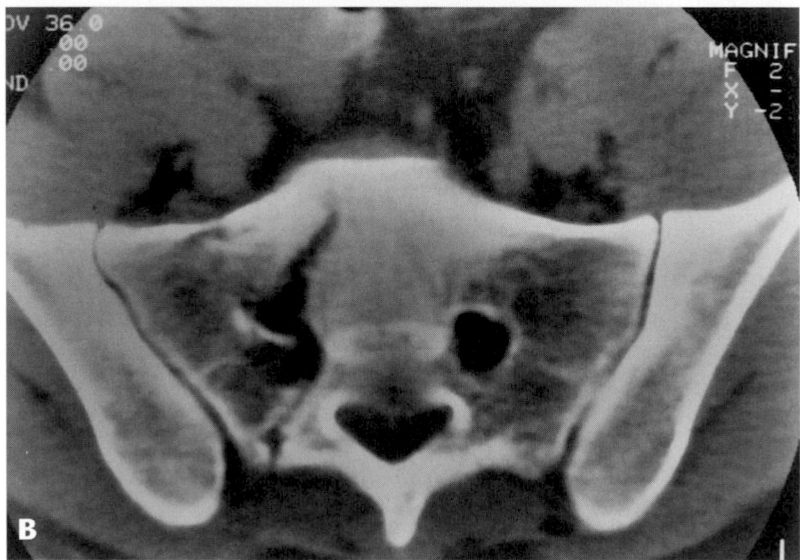

Figure 18–1. *A,* AP pelvis x-ray of a 29-year-old man who fell from a ladder. The x-ray shows some loss of definition of the right S1 foramen but, because of overlying bowel gas, fails to define the presence or absence of a fracture. This x-ray would usually be interpreted as normal. *B,* Computed tomography (CT) scan of the pelvis clearly demonstrating a displaced comminuted sacral fracture with significant involvement of the second sacral foramen. Other CT views demonstrated involvement of the first, second, and third sacral foramina. The patient clinically had weakness of plantar flexion of his right foot and ankle, which gradually recovered over a 6-month period.

inal fractures may result in residual causalgia that is impossible to measure and difficult to document. Rating musculoskeletal impairment on the basis of pain is highly controversial. The reader is referred to the Pain chapter (Chapter 18) of the AMA Guides, fifth edition.[4]

SI joint derangement from intraarticular fractures often results in some residual pain and limited ambulatory capacity, warranting an impairment rating. Objective findings include a positive flexion, abduction, external rotation (FABER) or Patrick test and a CT scan clearly indicative of joint surface abnormalities, since the plain x-ray may be deceptively negative. Undisplaced fractures with severe joint space narrowing merit a 3% whole person impairment rating.[3,4] Rarely, a degenerative SI joint is symptomatic enough to warrant arthrodesis. A fused SI joint would not warrant any permanent impairment unless there were associated physical findings such as loss of hip ROM or neurologic deficit.

Displaced SI joint fractures, such as a Malgaigne fracture that is associated with an anterior ring disruption, can rate as high as 10%.[2,4,34,36,41] Malgaigne fractures result in significant shortening of the lower extremity. In this case the pelvic fracture rating would be combined with the limb length discrepancy rating using the combined values table.[2] Furthermore, these injuries are frequently associated with sciatic nerve injury for which the nerve rating would be combined with the others, again using the combined values table. Patients with severe pelvic fractures often have associated lower extremity trauma, such as femoral fractures, with which any pelvic impairment values would be combined. An impairment estimate for loss of motion as a consequence of prolonged immobilization would also be combined if it were deemed substantial by the evaluating physician.

Acetabular Fractures

Truly undisplaced acetabular fractures are rare. All acetabular fractures should be evaluated with a CT scan to determine offset, separation, the presence of intra-articular fragments, and associated femoral head injury.[6,9,10,33,37,39,43] Many that appear undisplaced on plain radiographs will show separation or offset of a few millimeters on a CT scan (Fig. 18–2). Minor separation has a better prognosis than offset. Fractures that have only minor displacement should heal rapidly, within 6 to 12 weeks. When CT confirms union, muscle strengthening and activities can begin. Once permanent and stationary, the claimant and impairment can be rated by whichever scale is the most objective and best describes the impairment. The options include diagnostic values, ROM, radiographic cartilage interval, or manual muscle testing. The latter is difficult to perform objectivity and may vary between evaluators. A minimally displaced fracture should not change the cartilage interval until many years later, so the most appropriate rating methods are diagnostic or ROM. The fourth and fifth editions of the AMA Guides do not have a diagnostic value for acetabular fractures per se, and suggest that ROM be utilized and degenerative hip joint/SI joint changes.[2,4] If the range is not significant abnormal, the Trendelenburg test is clearly normal with no demonstrable abductor weakness, and if no narrowing of the cartilage interval is present, then there is no ratable permanent impairment. Potential future arthritic changes are not ratable. The forces necessary to cause an acetabular fracture can crush the articular cartilage, resulting in progressive post-traumatic degenerative arthritis over time, but, in this group of claimants with "undisplaced" acetabular fractures, it is difficult to predict in which cases this will occur. It is essential that the evaluating physician indicate that this possibility exists, so that if and when it does occur the claimant can be reassessed.

Nonarticular Pelvic Fractures

Minimally displaced pubic ramus fractures heal rapidly. Residual symptoms are often related to associated soft tissue trauma. Minimally displaced ramus fractures warrant no rating. Displaced ramus fractures may be assessed on the basis of limb-length discrepancy, associated nerve deficit, or loss of hip motion in the case of significant periarticular soft tissue injury with residual contracture. Fractures involving the sciatic notch may injure the sciatic nerve and the superior or inferior gluteal nerves. If permanent and complete, impairment from these nerve injuries is significant (superior gluteal = 25%, inferior gluteal = 15%, and sciatic = 30% whole person impairment).[2,4] The superior and inferior gluteal nerves are pure motor nerves and the muscles they supply (hip abductors and hip extensors, respectively) should be checked carefully. Residual weakness due to partial denervation may be difficult to determine on a routine office examination, but with extended walking the muscle fatigues, which results in an abnormal gait and limited ambulatory capacity. If this is suspected, an EMG can clarify the issue. If the EMG confirms partial denervation, rating can be on the basis of manual muscle testing by a physician or trained physical therapist.

THE HIP JOINT

Degenerative arthritis of the hip is rarely work-related unless it is the consequence of trauma either on the basis of intra-articular fracture or osteonecrosis of the femoral head. The latter condition may pose a difficult dilemma for the evaluating physician.[26] The relationship between osteonecrosis and a femoral neck fracture is clear. However, the more common situation is that of the claimant with osteonecrosis of nontraumatic etiology who claims the hip became symptomatic as a consequence of work-related activities, repetitive trauma, or a minor injury. These individuals present with Ficat stage IIb or III radiographic changes showing fracture of the subchondral cortex (Fig. 18–3).[13,35]

Although the hip may have become symptomatic at work, the etiology of the osteonecrosis is, with rare exception, not work related. The evaluating physician is often asked to determine if the subchondral fracture and onset of symptoms is in any way work-related. This is often an impossible question to answer with any certainty, but medical probability is the legal benchmark. If the evaluee is involved in heavy lifting or carrying, or if there was a specific injury, a partial relationship to work is usually established based on aggravation of a preexisting condition. Lacking a specific injury, and given work activities that are no more strenuous than routine activities of daily living, the progression of the osteonecrosis is probably unrelated to work. In most states, if the condition is even partially work-related, the workers' compensation system is responsible for covering medical expenses to correct the problem.

Two critical issues remain to be addressed by the evaluating physician: future medical coverage of the diseased hip and potential secondary disease in the opposite hip. Treatment of the osteonecrosis will depend on the stage, but in cases with fracture and collapse of the subchondral cortex, hip replacement is usually needed. Osteonecrosis is bilateral in up to 80% of cases depending on etiology and clinical series. It is

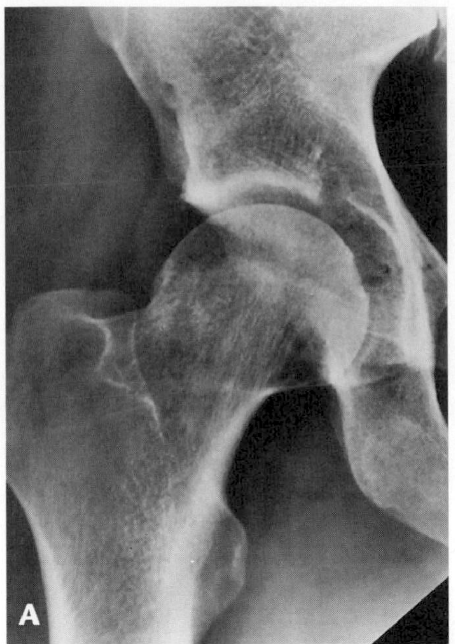

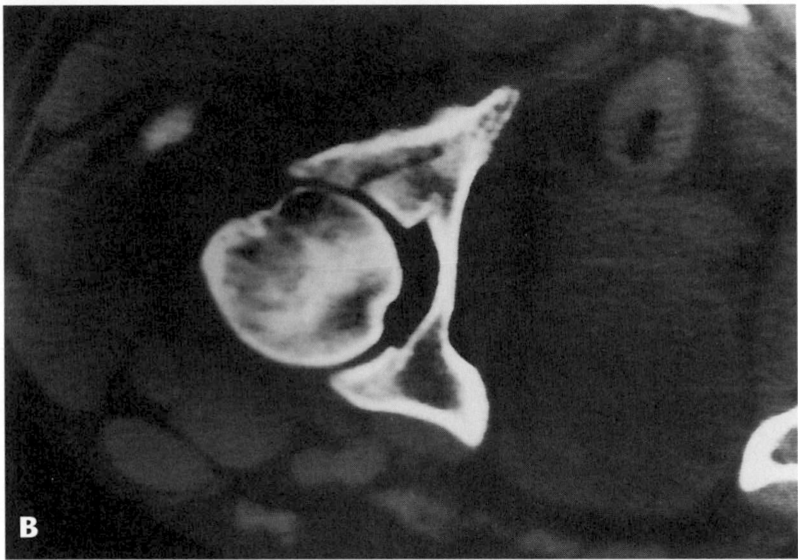

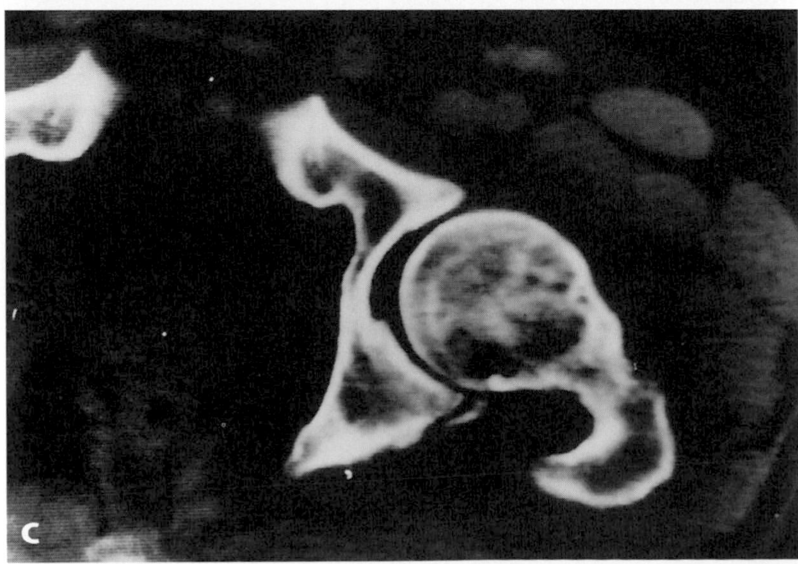

Figure 18–2. *A*, AP x-ray of the right hip shows a pelvic fracture involving the ischial spine but does not define the involvement of the acetabular articular surface. *B*, Computed tomography (CT) scan of the right hip demonstrates a 2-mm displacement of the articular surface. *C*, A more distal CT scan view shows displacement of the posterior rim and slight subluxation of the femoral head. There is a moderate probability that this patient will develop slowly progressive degenerative arthritis of the right hip.

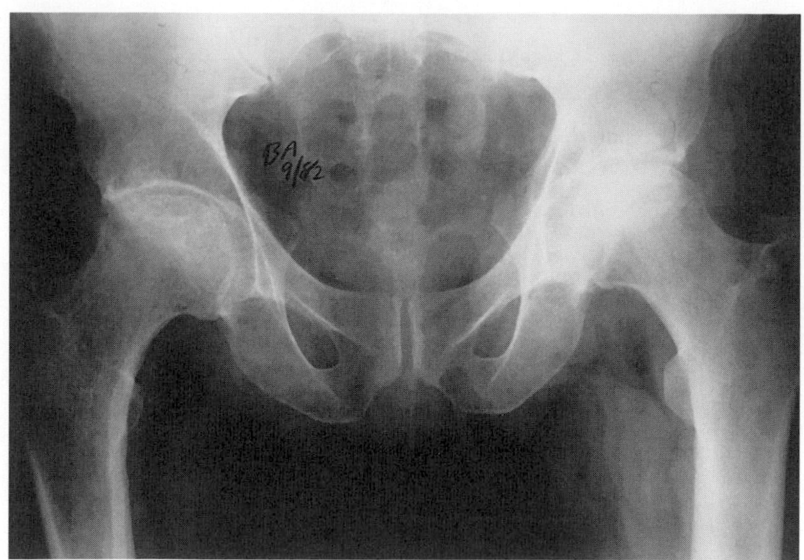

Figure 18–3. AP pelvis x-ray of a 52-year-old worker who complained of right hip pain after a twisting injury at work. The x-ray shows osteonecrosis of both hips, grade 2b on the right (with collapse of the subchondral cortex) and grade 2a on the left.

essential that the opposite hip be carefully evaluated by MRI and isotope scanning at the initial examination and that the evaluator comment on the likelihood of opposite side involvement.[30] If opposite side involvement later occurs, the claimant and representing attorney will commonly question whether the increased load borne during the convalescence of the first hip accelerated the progression of disease in the other hip. Medically this seems unlikely. However, a comment on this issue initially will often prevent a controversy later.

Degenerative arthritis that is not severe enough to warrant surgical intervention is best rated using either ROM or radiographically measured cartilage interval. The method of choice is the one that awards the highest value, consistent with objectivity. If ROM is difficult to assess owing to subjective factors, such as excessive pain behavior, the measured cartilage interval may be the preferred parameter. The cartilage interval, commonly referred to as the joint space, must be assessed by taking a radiograph with the source 36 inches from the cassette and directly over the involved joint with the hip in as close to neutral position as possible. Because the hip is a ball-and-socket joint, positioning is not as critical as it is in the knee and weight bearing is not required.

Patients will often have remarkable function with only 1 mm of cartilage interval, but when the last remnant of cartilage wears down, symptoms become severe and unrelenting, and require total hip replacement. Until the fourth edition of the AMA Guides, hip replacement was rated using a single diagnostic value recommended by the American Academy of Orthopedic Surgeons in its 1962 edition of the Manual for Orthopaedic Surgeons in Evaluating Permanent Physical Impairment.[1] This value was based on prophylactic work restrictions to protect the prosthetic joint. In this system, all hip replacement recipients would be rated the same. For many years, clinical research studies have utilized various scales to evaluate the results of hip replacement.[5,7] In the fourth and fifth editions of the AMA Guides, a modified Harris rating scale was utilized.[15] This allows the impairment rating to reflect the result of the hip replacement as measured by multiple parameters including pain, gait, activities of daily living, deformity, and ROM, and follows a widely used and widely accepted research instrument (Table 18–3).

Management of occupational injuries includes future medical care for the specific area involved. Joint replacements in a working-age population are likely to include the need for surgical revision. This raises significant apportionment issues in cases where the origin of the degenerative arthritis is nonindustrial but the condition was aggravated by occupational factors, and is often a source of controversy in claimants with osteonecrosis. If the occupational injury was only an aggravating factor and the joint replacement would have been needed in the relatively near future anyway, future medical care, after the claimant's condition is permanent and stationary, would seem to be nonindustrial. It is essential that the evaluating physician comment on the need for future revisions and the basis for apportionment.

THE THIGH AND FEMUR

Work-related injuries to the thigh may be divided into soft tissue trauma, boney fractures, or combined injuries. Lacerations of muscles often heal without impairment. Manual muscle testing is fairly accurate and reproducible for grades I to III if performed by a physical therapist or physician trained in these techniques.[38] Accuracy is also dependent on claimant cooperation and the ability to make a maximal effort, which

TABLE 18–3

Rating Hip Replacement Results*

	No. of Points
a. Pain	
None	44
Slight	40
Moderate, occasional	30
Moderate	20
Marked	10
b. Function	
Limp	
None	11
Slight	8
Moderate	5
Severe	0
Supportive device	
None	11
Cane for long walks	7
Cane	5
One crutch	3
Two canes	2
Two crutches	0
Distance walked	
Unlimited	11
Six blocks	8
Three blocks	5
Indoors	2
In bed or chair	0
c. Activities	
Stair climbing	
Normal	4
Using railing	2
Cannot climb readily	1
Unable to climb	0
Putting on shoes and socks	
With ease	4
With difficulty	2
Unable to do	0
Sitting	
Any chair, 1 hour	4
High chair	2
Unable to sit comfortably	0
Public transportation	
Able to use	1
Unable to use	0
d. Deformity	
Fixed adduction	
<10°	1
≥10°	0
Fixed internal rotation	
<10°	1
≥10°	0
Fixed external rotation	
<10°	1
≥10°	0
Flexion contracture	
<1.5 cm	1
≥1.5 cm	0
Leg length discrepancy	
<15°	1
≥15°	0
e. Range of motion	
Flexion	
>90°	1
≤90°	0
Abduction	
>15°	1
≤15°	0
Adduction	
>15°	1
≤15°	0
External rotation	
>30°	1
≤30°	0
Internal rotation	
>15°	1
≤15°	0

*Add the points from categories a, b, c, d and e to determine the total and characterize the result of replacement.
From Cocchiarella L, Andersson GBJ (eds): Guides to the Evaluation of Permanent Impairment, 5th ed. Chicago, American Medical Association, 2001, p 548.

may be inhibited by pain, fear of pain, or motivational factors. For this reason, two evaluators' results need to be consistent to use this parameter for impairment rating. In claimants who are unable to make a maximal effort, manual muscle testing should not be utilized.

Grades IV and V are difficult to differentiate on manual muscle testing. In the case of the quadriceps and hamstring muscle groups, isokinetic testing is well developed and can accurately differentiate between grades IV and V when the opposite side is normal for comparison.[23] The difference between grades IV and V is critical as it relates to endurance. Manual muscle testing is usually performed over a few minutes and does not take endurance into account. An individual with grade IV quadriceps may seem adequately strong for normal activities at the time of testing, but after working several hours, may be unable to climb stairs in a normal alternating fashion. Associated nerve injury, if complete, should be rated using peripheral nerve impairment scales.[2,4] Partial motor deficits should be rated using manual muscle testing. Sensory or dysesthesia components may be added from the table.

Proximal Femoral Fractures

Femoral neck fractures may heal without impairment but are subject to a variety of potential complications resulting in significant permanent impairment. Malunion and nonunion are rated under the diagnostic section, and a loss-of-motion impairment estimate would be added with the diagnostic impairment. Limb length or other impairments would be combined. Trochanteric bursitis following internal fixation of a femoral neck fracture, if chronic and associated with a positive Trendelenburg gait or abductor lurch, is rated in the diagnostic section of the AMA Guides at 3% whole person impairment and would be added to other ratings for the fracture.[2,4]

Intertrochanteric fractures rarely result in nonunion or osteonecrosis. Residual impairment estimates for these and femoral shaft fractures are based on examination findings, principally loss of motion and weakness, with a few exceptions. Malunion with angular deformity would be rated using specific values in Table 64 of the fourth edition[2] or Table 17–33 of the fifth edition[4] of the AMA Guides to which examination findings such as loss of motion or shortening are additive.[2] Tape measurements are highly variable owing to imprecise landmarks, especially in obese or edematous evaluees. Any hip or knee flexion will also invalidate the result. Standing measurements, using the iliac crest, are dependent on hip and knee position as well as the ability of the examiner to measure accurately the difference between the two sides in spite of the overlying soft tissues. The range of error with these two methods is 1 to 2 cm, whereas teleroentgenograms either with x-ray or CT are accurate to within less than 1 cm.[19] Evaluees with both joint flexion contracture of the hip or knee and structural shortening of the tibia or femur should be rated for the loss of joint motion and for the structural shortening of the long bone based on teleroentgenograms and independent of the joint position.

Distal Femoral Fractures

Values for angular deformity of supracondylar fractures are in the knee section of Table 64 of the fourth edition and Table 17–33 of the fifth edition of the AMA Guides, because that is the joint where the effect is manifest.[2,4] Loss of motion will be at this site as well. More severe angular deformities may result in gradually progressive degenerative arthritis of the adjacent joint. This effect will be accelerated if the joint has associated or preexisting damage. As in acetabular fractures, the evaluating physician should comment on potential future problems and apportion those problems between preexisting and work-related etiologies. Physicians appropriately view this task as onerous because there is no scientific basis that would allow quantification. Many decline to comment on these issues. Insurance administrators and legal representatives are equally frustrated and explain to the physicians that, even though a definitive scientific answer is impossible, a musculoskeletal specialist physician by virtue of training and experience can give a far better estimate than they. Medical probability is a legal construct that falls in the realm of opinion, not to be confused with medical science. These determinations are best made by physicians. To decline to comment is to relegate the responsibility to others less qualified (see Chapter 9).

THE KNEE JOINT

Intra-articular Fractures

Intra-articular fractures involving the knee may be divided into four categories (intercondylar, osteochondral, tibial plateau, and patellar), which have different prognoses and anticipated impairments. All of these fractures require a high level of examinee cooperation to obtain an optimal result.

Intercondylar fractures may heal with minimal impairment if the weight bearing articular surfaces are minimally involved. If the fracture is through the trochlea and is anatomically reduced with enough stability to allow early ROM, the end result may be excellent. At the opposite end of this spectrum is the comminuted, displaced, intraarticular fracture of the distal femur that, even if optimally reduced, will lead to progressive degenerative arthritis. The rate of progression is dependent on many factors but mostly on accuracy of reduction and the ability to initiate early ROM.

Isolated osteochondral fractures, involving weight bearing surfaces, have a guarded prognosis. If repaired early and anatomically, they may heal without significant impairment. However, the articular segment is avascular and may collapse at a later time, giving rise to degenerative arthritis.

Tibial plateau fractures are frequently comminuted and displaced, and analogous to displaced intercondylar femur fractures in their prognosis. Open reduction and some form of stabilization that will allow early ROM are required for any displaced tibial plateau fracture. Unlike intercondylar femoral fractures, these fractures are often associated with meniscal or ligament injury, which increases the degree of permanent impairment.

Patellar fractures, if minimally displaced and stable, may be treated nonoperatively. As in all intra-articular fractures, surface reduction is critical and offset adversely affects the prognosis. Unstable fractures, even if reducible, require internal fixation, which allows earlier ROM than casting alone, and minimizes loss of motion and maximizes muscle function.

Arthrofibrosis refers to the development of dense adhesions, fibrous pannus, and capsular hypertrophy.[25] It is common following intra-articular fractures that are immobilized and may result in severe loss of motion.

Early motion will help prevent this complication as well as maintain the health of the articular cartilage and muscle function.

Permanent impairment may be evaluated once the fracture is healed and the claimant has achieved maximum benefit from rehabilitation. Deformities including varus, valgus, or malrotation are rated using numerical values in Table 64 of the fourth edition or Table 17–33 of the fifth edition of the AMA Guides.[2,4] Loss of motion, loss of cartilage interval on standing x-ray, and shortening are combined. The examining physician must carefully evaluate ligament integrity because ligament injury may be associated with any intra-articular or periarticular fracture and may be overlooked owing to the more obvious fracture.

Ligament Injuries

Injuries of the collateral or cruciate knee ligaments are common and serious injuries of the lower extremity, and they often result in permanent impairment. This is especially true of the anterior cruciate ligament (ACL), which, because of its intra-articular location, is difficult to repair with a durable long-term result. These repairs may stretch out over 1 to 2 years, with recurrent problems of instability with twisting and pivoting activities. This results in joint subluxation and severe damage to the lateral meniscus and articular surface.[14] Because of uncertain results and the prolonged rehabilitation following anterior cruciate repair, individuals who do not engage in pivoting activities are often treated nonoperatively with quadriceps and hamstring strengthening and the use of an orthosis for sports. Some of these individuals will require a late reconstruction because of significant instability and progressive joint surface damage. In those people, an early repair might have prevented the joint damage and the result of repair before joint surface damage is better.

Posterior cruciate ligament (PCL) injuries are much less frequent and repairs, when indicated, are more predictable and successful. The principal impairment resulting from PCL instability is difficulty descending stairs and kneeling.

Isolated collateral sprains require repair only if they are associated with significant laxity. Mild to moderate sprains will often heal without problems, and mild laxity of the medical collateral ligament will usually diminish over 6 months.[16,18] All acute ligament injuries require magnetic resonance imaging or arthroscopy for evaluation because of the high incidence of associated injuries to menisci and the articular surfaces. Mild ligament sprains may be isolated but severe ones almost never are.

Impairment evaluation in claimants with ligament injuries requires the physician's ability to determine the degree of laxity (mild, moderate, or severe) on physical examination.[7] These examination techniques require significant experience and should only be performed by physicians who are trained to do this.[8] Instrumentation—a knee arthrometer—has been developed to quantify the amount of force used in the anterior drawer or Lochman tests, so that the amount of anterior tibial displacement will be more consistent among examiners.[28] This equipment was developed for clinical research but might be useful in impairment evaluations. The fifth edition of the Guides adds a rating for repair of the ACL without residual laxity because those ligaments tend to stretch over time and under significant stress are not as stable as a normal knee.[4] Repair without demonstratable laxity is rated the same as mild laxity. Muscle atrophy is common following these injuries and is included in the Guides impairment rating. Loss of motion impairment would be combined as would arthritic degeneration impairment demonstrated on standing radiographs. Discussion in the impairment report about prognosis and future medical care with special reference to arthritic degeneration is critical for evaluees with ligament and articular surface injury.

Meniscal Injuries

Small acute meniscal tears that are adequately symptomatic require arthroscopic debridement but usually do not result in any major permanent impairment.[21] Large acute tears, if simple, are best treated with repair, and this may result in some permanent loss of motion. Chronic tears are often associated with articular degeneration, especially in middle-aged and older patients.[17] This raises the issue of causation. Since the advent of magnetic resonance imaging, it has become apparent that most individuals have degenerative changes in the posterior horn of their medial menisci by early middle age if not sooner. In fact, the vast majority of tears in middle age and beyond are the result of minor trauma superimposed on meniscal degeneration.[42] This degeneration is slowly progressive and can eventually result in a full-thickness degenerative tear or horizontal cleavage lesion without specific trauma. Arthroscopy in individuals with degenerative tears usually reveals fairly extensive chondromalacia not limited to the area of the meniscal tear.

If the individual associates the onset of symptoms in his or her knee with work activity or a minor injury, the evaluating physician is asked to determine causation as well as to rate impairment. Often there is no clear answer, and each case must be decided on its specific merits. The need for future medical care and apportionment must also be determined. In the absence of a specific injury, the type of work is critical. If the person is involved in frequent squatting, twisting, carrying heavy objects, or climbing, his or her work probably played a role in the acceleration of the degenerative disorder. In this case, the need for acute care is work related. However, the degenerative arthritis will continue to progress. Eventually the worker may require further work restrictions and even a knee replacement.

The evaluator must determine if and how these further problems relate to work activities. Once the initial meniscal tear is accepted as work related, the future degenerative changes also are related, in part, because excision of a meniscus is believed to accelerate degenerative arthritis.

As mentioned, a degenerative tear of the lateral meniscus may follow anterior cruciate instability. For example, a worker with anterior cruciate laxity from a high school football injury later develops lateral meniscal pathology that he relates to his work as a plumber. The evaluating physician must decide if the lateral meniscal degeneration would have occurred within the same time frame absent this patient's work activities. If it is decided that the work played some role, then the same situation as described for degenerative tear of the posterior horn of the medial meniscus exists, with all of its ramifications for future medical care and apportionment issues.

With the substantial concurrent and future costs involved, the reader can readily appreciate why these cases result in the need for multiple expert opinions and may be highly contested. Under these circumstances, treatment is often delayed until financial responsibility can be resolved. Much of this may be avoided if these issues are addressed comprehensively and authoritatively by the initial impairment evaluator.

Impairment rating of meniscal injuries under the diagnostic section is divided into partial and complete lesions. Involvement of both menisci in the same knee is rated greater than double that for a single meniscus because of the significant decrease in function with both sides of the knee involved. Loss of motion, which is usually only present in meniscal lesions if there is associated degenerative arthritis, is combined using the combined values chart. Loss of cartilage interval on standing x-ray, if significant, is also combined using the combined values chart.[2,4]

Chondromalacia

Tibiofemoral chondromalacia in weight-bearing zones is progressive at a variable rate and has been discussed in the sections on fractures, and ligament and meniscal injuries. Patellofemoral chondromalacia is another issue.

Patellofemoral crepitation with active ROM is common in the general population from adolescence on and is usually asymptomatic. Patients commonly have a complaint of anterior knee pain that follows a minor contusion to the patella or state that the pain came on spontaneously after repetitive squatting or prolonged use of stairs. Physical examination reveals mild patellofemoral crepitation on the symptomatic side. Diagnostic studies, including magnetic resonance imaging, are usually negative except for degenerative changes within the meniscus without a tear. The physician is posed with a dilemma in determining if the symptoms are related to the mild patellofemoral chondromalacia if there is a work-related injury. Examination of the opposite, asymptomatic knee may help resolve this issue if there is similar mild patellofemoral crepitation. Often this is the case. Although it does not rule out an industrial aggravation of a preexisting problem, it adds credence to the assertion that some patellofemoral chondromalacia existed before the industrial injury. Furthermore, the presence of patellofemoral crepitation does not mean the latter is the source of symptoms.[22] Anterior knee pain has many causes including patellar tendinitis, inflammation of the iliotibial band insertion at Gerty tubercle, pes ancerina buristis, inflammation of the insertion of the anterior knee capsule or menisci, and fat pad syndrome. All of these should be self-limited and not result in permanent impairment. For all of these reasons, mild patellofemoral chondromalacia is not a ratable disorder. However, it is ratable if it is associated with narrowed cartilage interval on lateral radiographs, which indicates moderate to severe degeneration, or if there is associated loss of motion or measurable muscle atrophy.

The fifth edition of the Guides allows a rating for joint surface chondromalacia documented by arthroscopy. The defects must be full thickness and greater than 1 centimeter in diameter.[4]

Extensor Mechanism Injuries

These injuries may result from trauma to the quadriceps, fracture of the patella, or rupture or avulsion of the quadriceps or patellar tendons. Quadriceps lacerations or crush injuries will heal but often with some residual loss of function. This is best measured by manual muscle testing for strength grades I through III and by isokinetic testing for grades IV and V. There may also be significant residual fibrosis, contracture, and loss of motion. If the latter is significant, an impairment estimate for it may be combined. There is also atrophy, which is difficult to measure because of scar tissue and local swelling. Furthermore, if strength is used as the parameter, atrophy is not combined because it would be duplicative.

Patellar tendon ruptures, lacerations, and avulsions, if complete, require repair followed by immobilization for 3 to 6 weeks. If the tendon becomes infected as a consequence of severe open trauma and part of the substance is lost from necrosis, reconstruction is difficult and may require several procedures. The permanent impairment is significantly more than with closed injuries and simple primary repair.

Complete loss of knee extension is valued at 10% whole person impairment in addition to any loss of passive knee motion such as a fixed flexion contracture or loss of flexion range. An individual with complete loss of the extensor mechanism can walk normally on level surfaces by using the gluteus maximus and gastroc-soleus muscle groups to lock the knee. This is contingent on having full hip and knee extension. Only very strong individuals with loss of the extensor mechanism can climb stairs, alternating in a normal fashion. Descending hills or stairs is more difficult.

Degenerative Arthritis

Many causes of post-traumatic degenerative arthritis and the possible relationships to occupational factors have been described. According to the Framingham Study, the incidence of degenerative arthritis of the knee is clearly higher in certain occupations.[12] The rate of progression is variable, but ultimately knee replacement may be required. Osteonecrosis of the knee is less common than in the hip and is mostly seen in patients with systemic diseases such as sickle cell disease or systemic lupus erythematosus or in patients on high-dose steroids. Awareness of spontaneous osteonecrosis of the knee that sometimes follows meniscectomy is increasing.[44] Bilaterality is much less common than with osteonecrosis of the hip.

For younger patients with predominately unicompartmental degenerative arthritis, distal femoral or high tibial osteotomy may be performed to shift the weight to the healthier compartment, which may avoid the need for knee replacement for several years. The outcome of this procedure is less predictable than knee replacement. Poor results are rated using examination criteria including loss of motion and arthritic degeneration.

Knee replacements may be unicondylar or total condylar. They have various degrees of built-in constraint to compensate for loss of cruciate or collateral stability. Patellar resurfacing is usually included in a total knee replacement, although there is some debate about its indications. Isolated replacement of the patellofemoral joint is highly controversial and rarely performed. The results of knee replacement, once permanent and stationary, are rated using the Knee Society rating system, which is analogous to the methodology used for hip replacements (Table 18–4).[20] The longevity of knee replacements appears to exceed that of hip replacements, but future revisions may need to be addressed.

UPPER TIBIA AND FIBULA

Work-related injuries to the proximal and midshaft tibia and fibula and surrounding soft tissues are relatively common as a result of motor vehicle accidents, falls, and direct trauma from heavy equipment such as forklifts. Except for stress fractures, isolated fractures of the fibula are uncommon. Fractures of the tibia frequently require internal fixation except in the case of compound fractures, which may be stabilized with an external fixator, at

TABLE 18–4

Rating Knee Replacement Results*

	No. of Points
a. Pain	
None	50
Mild or occasional	45
Stairs only	40
Walking and stairs	30
Moderate	
Occasional	20
Continual	10
Severe	0
b. Range of motion	
Add 1 point per 5°	25
c. Stability (maximum movement in any position)	
Anteroposterior	
<5 mm	10
5–9 mm	5
>9 mm	0
Mediolateral	
5°	15
6°–9°	10
10°–14°	5
≥15°	0
Subtotal	
Deductions (minus) d,e,f	
d. Flexion contracture	
5°–9°	2
10°–15°	5
16°–20°	10
>20°	20
e. Extension lag	
<10°	5
10°–20°	10
>20°	15
f. Alignment	
0°–4°	0
5°–10°	3 points per degree
11°–15°	3 points per degree
>15°	20
Deductions subtotal	—

*The point total for estimating knee replacement results is the sum of the points in categories a, b, and c minus the sum of the points in categories d, e, and f.

From Cocchiarella L, Andersson GBJ (eds): Guides to the Evaluation of Permanent Impairment, 5th ed. Chicago, American Medical Association, 2001, p 549.

least until the wound is healed. Tibial fractures, especially those associated with soft tissue trauma, have a significant risk of anterior compartment syndrome that results in muscle ischemia.[29] If uncorrected by fasciotomy, this ischemia may result in permanent weakness of foot and ankle dorsiflexion.[31] Less commonly, the posterior compartment responsible for foot and ankle flexion may also be involved.

Intramuscular and peritendinous scarring following these high-energy injuries frequently results in contractures of the ankle, foot, and toes. The earlier motion can be restored the less severe these contractures will be. At the time of an impairment evaluation following lower leg injuries, attention must be focused on the foot and ankle to assess and identify carefully any fixed contractures, loss of motion, or weakness. These findings are in addition to the diagnostic ratings for the fractures that are based on malalignment including rotational, varus, or valgus deformities. A shortening impairment would be combined, as would peripheral nerve deficits.

Chronic osteomyelitis of the tibia is much less common today, but it can still follow major (type IV) tibial fractures with severe associated soft tissue trauma. If present when the patient's impairment is declared permanent and stationary, it warrants an additional impairment percent that is listed in the diagnostic section. Note, however that the total of the combined values may not exceed that for a below-the-knee amputation.

AMPUTATION

Amputations are rated using Table 63 of the fourth edition of the AMA Guides[2] or Table 17–32[4] of the fifth edition. Estimates for additional factors that limit prosthetic use would be combined. These include significant phantom pain, symptomatic neuromas, loss of protective sensation, chronic wound drainage, and recurrent skin breakdown. Skin breakdown can occur as a result of vascular insufficiency, infection, loss of protective sensation, and scarring or split-thickness skin grafts with limited durability. As indicated in the table, stump length in the thigh or leg must be greater than three inches to have adequate function, and a distal-thigh amputation is more favorable for the patient than a mid-thigh amputation. Post-traumatic amputation patients often have significant psychological problems and, as a group, do not function as well as patients in other amputation categories.[24,40]

CONCLUSION

The evaluation of musculoskeletal impairments has evolved from earlier systems that used only amputation and ankylosis as their primary assessment models. Diagnostic accuracy and rating flexibility are the hallmarks of present models.

Parameters vary in objectivity, reliability, and specificity. As the rating systems and diagnostic and therapeutic technologies continue to evolve, these factors will improve, resulting in increased accuracy that will make the job of the evaluating physician less judgmental and the ultimate awards more fair and consistent. The number of contested cases and the length of the contests will decrease, which will have a positive economic and rehabilitive impact. Furthermore, by reducing adversity, more injured workers will successfully return to work sooner. This evolution is not automatic but will require extensive research and diligence. Fortunately, there is an increasing interest in orthopaedic and other musculoskeletal academic programs that are studying and finding ways to improve these systems.

CLINICAL EXAMPLES

HIP, THIGH, KNEE AND LEG

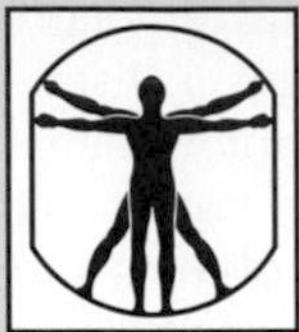

Editor's Note—Using the AMA Guides for the assessment of lower extremity impairment requires an awareness of the three methods of impairment evaluation—anatomic, diagnostic, and functional—as well as superb diagnostic skills and appropriate radiographs. In general, the highest award possible, based on the most appropriate of the three methods, is the preferred rating. Difficulties may arise when adequate medical records or radiographs are unavailable or when the physician is not skilled in the musculoskeletal examination.

The assessment of the lower extremities using the third edition of the Guides was based principally on the evaluation of range of motion (ROM), that is, a functional method. The fourth[3] and fifth[4] editions of the Guides follow more complex rules requiring evaluations and evaluators must be thoroughly familiar with the three methods of assessment.

EXAMPLE

Problem 1

A 24-year-old railroad worker fell between two rail cars, sustaining a valgus external rotation injury of the right lower extremity (knee). Physical examination revealed a large effusion, significant medial joint line discomfort, a 2+ anterior drawer sign, a 2+ pivot shift, and positive McMurray test along the medial joint line. A subsequent magnetic resonance imaging study showed an anterior cruciate ligament tear that was midsubstance, a large effusion, and a medial meniscal tear. Arthroscopic assisted anterior reconstruction using quadruple hamstring tendon was carried out, in addition to partial medial and lateral meniscectomies. He is now 18 months postop and has healed relatively well. He has returned to his previous job and does not require any type of bracing. He has approximately 1.5 cm of thigh and calf atrophy present in the affected extremity. Despite the atrophy, he has 5/5 strength in all muscle groups of the lower extremity tested. Range of motion testing reveals 0 to 128° of flexion on the injured side as compared to 0 to 136° of flexion on the contralateral side. He has 1+ drawer sign, but a negative pivot shift at this time. His gait is normal. His neurovascular status is intact distally.

Roentgenograms have been obtained that reveal that the tunnels have reossified and there are no visualized screws or hardware as bioabsorbable fixation was utilized. There are no other abnormalities seen on the anterior-posterior (AP), lateral, tunnel, and sunrise views of the right knee.

What is his impairment rating?

Questions for Consideration

What if this individual had a medial meniscus repair and a partial lateral meniscectomy?

What if this individual had a large osteochondral fracture of the medial femoral condyle, yet no degenerative changes on the follow-up x-ray?

What if the individual had significant degenerative joint disease in the knee prior to the time of the injury?

What if a brace was an absolute necessity in this individual's case?

Step	Right lower extremity (RLE)	Left lower extremity (LLE)
1. Establish diagnosis.	Anterior cruciate ligament tear with medial and lateral meniscal tears	
2. Maximal medical improvement (MMI)?	Yes	
3. List each lower extremity anatomic region with abnormalities that are related to the illness or injury in question. List potential methods.	*Thigh*—atrophy *Knee*—diagnosis-based estimate *Calf*—atrophy	
4. Calculate impairment according to text and tables for each applicable method.	*Thigh atrophy*—6% of the lower extremity (see Table 17–6) *Knee*—diagnosis-based estimate (see Table 17–33)–7% of the lower extremity for mild residual cruciate laxity should be combined with 10% of the lower extremity due to partial lateral and medial meniscectomy, which results in 16% of the lower extremity or 6% whole person (see Table 17–3) *Calf atrophy*—results in a rating of 6% of the lower extremity or 2% whole person (see Table 17–6)	
5. Identify and calculate illness/injury related to peripheral nerve system (PNS) impairment.	None	
6. Identify and calculate all illness/injury related to peripheral vascular system (PVS) impairment.	None	
7. Identify and calculate all injury/impairment related to complex regional pain syndrome (CRPS) impairment.	None	
8. If no other method available, determine impairment due to gait derangement if clinically applicable.	Not applicable	
9. Consult lower extremity cross-usage table (Table 17–2) to determine possible method groupings.	*Alternative 1*—Combine the thigh atrophy with the calf atrophy rating, which would result in an impairment rating of 12% of the lower extremity or 5% whole person. *Alternative 2*—Use the diagnosis-based methodology, which results in an impairment rating of 16% of the lower extremity or 6% whole person (see Step 4). Please note: atrophy cannot be used with a diagnosis-based estimate according to Table 17–2.	
10. Consider all medical data available and select the largest and most clinically appropriate method for each illness/injury; combine each parameter within each individual grouping in order to determine impairment for each leg. Figures should be in whole person units.	The largest and most appropriate method appears to be the diagnosis-based based estimate of 16% of the lower extremity or 6% whole person.	
11. Use the combined values (CV) chart to combine whole person impairment (WPI) from each regional impairment calculated in Step 10 of the same limb. The lower extremity impairment for each limb is then converted to WPI. If both lower extremities are involved, the impairment rating for each extremity is converted to WPI before being combined with WPI for the contralateral extremity.	Not applicable	

Table refers to Cocchiarella L, Andersson GBJ (eds): Guides to the Evaluation of Permanent Impairment, 5th ed. Chicago, American Medical Association, 2001, and this method of rating follows the principles set forth in Box 17–1 (pp 562–563) of the fifth edition.

CLINICAL EXAMPLES

HIP, THIGH, KNEE AND LEG

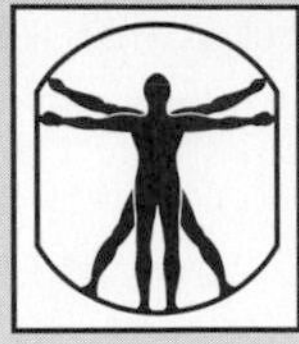

Problem 2

A 54-year-old career firefighter had a work-related dislocation of the right hip at age 32. He has continued working with the fire department, yet developed symptomatic avascular necrosis that was unresponsive to conservative measures and ultimately resulted in a successful, uncemented total hip arthroplasty. He is now approximately 2 years postop and has returned to a more sedentary type of work at his office. He has not had any significant complications and reports for an impairment evaluation. He continues to work daily, although his job is more sedentary now. He sits for approximately 6 hours per day and walks 2 hours a day. His office is on the first floor, but entry into his office necessitates that he ascend 12 stairs without any type of side railing. He does not use public transportation and drives his pick-up truck without any difficulty. He walks approximately 1.5 miles per day, 3 days a week, for exercise and swims approximately 1 day a week for diversification. He reports occasional discomfort, but only to a mild degree.

Physical examination today reveals that he has a mild short limb gait, but does not require any type of ambulatory assistive devices. The right limb is approximately 2.5 cm shorter than the left lower extremity. He has approximately 2 cm of thigh atrophy and 1 cm of calf atrophy. Strength is grossly intact about the hip and in the right lower extremity. Hip ROM testing reveals flexion of 100°, extension 15°, abduction 25°, adduction 10°, external rotation 25°, and internal rotation 20°. Neurovascularly, he is intact.

Roentgenograms today reveal an uncemented total hip arthroplasty in good position with no obvious loosening or lucency seen about the acetabular or femoral prosthesis.

Questions for Consideration

What if this individual had chronic draining osteomyelitis?

What if he refused to have any additional surgery in spite of this infection?

What if he had continued instability that necessitated using crutches on a full-time basis?

Step	RLE	LLE
1. Establish diagnosis.	Avascular necrosis/status post-right total hip arthroplasty	
2. MMI?	Yes	
3. List each lower extremity anatomic region with abnormalities that are related to the illness or injury in question. List potential methods.	*Right lower extremity*—limb length inequality (see Table 17–4) *Hip*—ROM and diagnosis-based estimate (see Tables 17–9 and 17–33) *Thigh*—atrophy (see Table 17–6) *Calf*—atrophy (see Table 17–6)	
4. Calculate impairment according to text and tables for each applicable method.	*Right lower extremity*—limb length inequality—6% of the lower extremity (see Table 17–4) *Hip*—ROM—abduction loss 5% LEI (lower extremity impairment); adduction loss 5% LEI; external rotation loss 5% LEI; internal rotation loss 5% LEI (see Table 17–9, p 537); these are additive and equal 20% lower extremity Diagnosis-based estimate—See Harris Hip Rating section—Table 17–34; results in overall numerical figure of 87 points—see Table 17–33 under hip section; results in impairment rating of 37% LEI *Thigh*—atrophy—8% LEI (see Table 17–6) *Calf*—atrophy—3% LEI (see Table 17–7)	
5. Identify and calculate illness/injury related to PNS impairment.	Not applicable	
6. Identify and calculate all illness/injury related to PVS impairment.	Not applicable	
7. Identify and calculate all injury/impairment related to CRPS impairment.	Not applicable	
8. If no other method available, then determine impairment due to gait derangement if clinically applicable.	Not applicable	
9. Consult lower extremity cross-usage table (Table 17–2) to determine possible method groupings.	Methods used—limb length inequality, ROM, diagnosis-based estimate, and atrophy Possible groupings—limb length inequality and ROM; limb length inequality and diagnosis-based estimate; limb length equality and atrophy	
10. Consider all medical data available and select largest and most clinically appropriate method for each illness/injury; combine each parameter within each individual grouping in order to determine impairment for each leg. Figures should be in whole person units.	Limb length inequality combined with ROM equals 25% LEI; limb length inequality combined with diagnosis-based estimate is 41% LEI; limb length inequality combined with atrophy is 16% LEI. The 41% lower extremity rating derived by combining the limb length inequality plus the diagnosis-based estimate is the most appropriate in this particular case. The overall whole person rating is 16% utilizing Table 17–3.	
11. Use CV chart to combine WPI impairments from each regional impairment calculated in Step 10 of the same limb. The lower extremity impairment for each limb is then converted to WPI. If both lower extremities are involved, impairment rating for each extremity is converted to WPI before being combined with WPI for the contralateral extremity.	Not applicable	

Table refers to Cocchiarella L, Andersson GBJ (eds): Guides to the Evaluation of Permanent Impairment, 5th ed. Chicago, American Medical Association, 2001, and this method of rating follows the principles set forth in Box 17–1 (pp 562–563) of the fifth edition.

CLINICAL EXAMPLES

HIP, THIGH, KNEE AND LEG

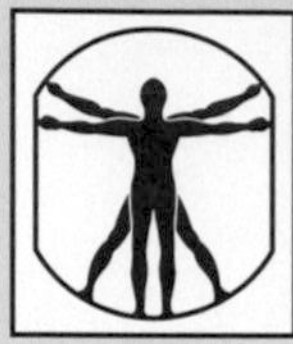

Problem 3

A 40-year-old man began working for a paint/sandblasting company approximately 1 week prior to the time of an injury/event. He inadvertently put the blaster near his foot, resulting in a water hydro-blast injury to the right foot. The water stream went through his boot and into the foot, resulting in an injection-type injury to the right foot region. He was brought to a local hospital where he underwent a fasciotomy of the forefoot and irrigation/debridement of a near amputation of the great toe through the MTP joint. Staged reconstruction of the right toe extensor tendon and fasciotomy closure with subsequent wound closures were done over a period of 10 days. His wounds healed approximately 3 weeks postinjury. He was immobilized for approximately 6 weeks. He was then started on physical therapy. He tolerated therapy well and progressed to the extent that, by 4 weeks of normal physical therapy, he was ready for work conditioning. He was in work conditioning for 3 weeks and was prepared to return to work the next week when he suddenly began to have increasing pain and swelling, according to his subjective report. This was unable to be verified by the therapist. It is also noteworthy that he was told at that time that he would be terminated as soon as he returned to work. He obtained the services of an attorney at that point in time. He returned to the treating physician, stating, "My foot is swollen and I cannot wear any type of shoe because of the swelling." No objective swelling was identified. Additional workup, including complete blood count and sedimentation rate, in addition to three-phase bone scanning, was accomplished; however, all studies returned within normal limits with no evidence of infection or complex regional pain syndrome.

A second medical opinion was obtained from a foot subspecialist at a local teaching hospital. His report suggested, "Patient may have mild medial sensory branch neuroma, but should be encouraged to increase activity as much as possible."

The patient reports for an impairment evaluation.

The physical examination today reveals that the individual is walking on crutches and is not wearing a shoe on the right lower extremity. He verbalizes pain immediately upon entering the examination suite. There is no measurable limb length inequality nor is there any measurable muscle atrophy. On palpation, he complains of significant discomfort not only over the MTP itself, but also over the incision just medial to the MTP with a "shocking" sensation with palpation of the incision over the MTP medially. Muscle strength testing reveals that he has "give-away weakness" and an unwillingness to perform even ankle plantar flexion/dorsiflexion strength testing, much less digital motion strength testing. Range of motion testing is met with a bit more success and reveals that MTP extension is approximately 10° and IP flexion is 10°. This is essentially the same amount of motion that on passively ROM. He also has decreased sensation from the distal portion of the MTP joint distally over the medial aspect of the great toe. There is no drainage or redness seen in the foot.

AP, lateral, and oblique x-rays of the foot do not show any obvious degenerative changes, osteopenia, or soft tissue abnormalities.

Step	RLE	LLE
1. Establish diagnosis.	Status post hydro-blast injury right foot with subsequent compartment syndrome—complex open wound. Healed with residual cutaneous nerve disruption medial aspect right great toe.	
2. MMI?	In all probability	
3. List each lower extremity anatomic region with abnormalities that are related to the illness or injury in question. List potential methods.	*Right lower extremity*—gait disturbance *Right ankle*—weakness *Right foot/toes*—weakness; ROM losses	
4. Calculate impairment according to text and tables for each applicable method.	*Right lower extremity*—gait disturbance—none (nonphysiologic) (see Table 17–5) *Ankle*—weakness—none (nonphysiologic) (see Table 17–7) *Foot/toe*—weakness—none (fear/pain/nonorganic?) (see Table 17–7) *Toe range of motion losses*—MTP extension loss 5% LEI; IP flexion loss 2% LEI (see Table 17–14)	
5. Identify and calculate illness/injury related to PNS impairment.	Right foot sensory branch of medial plantar nerve Motor—none (not applicable) Sensory—using Table 16–10 from the upper extremity section assume 100% sensory loss (as it does make medical sense as there was complete transection of the skin and nerve at that level). Therefore, his rating would be 100% of the sensory branch of the medial plantar nerve (5%), which equals 5% of the lower extremity.	
6. Identify and calculate all illness/injury related to PVS impairment.	None	
7. Identify and calculate all injury/impairment related to CRPS impairment.	None	
8. If no other method available, then determine impairment due to gait derangement if clinically applicable.	Not applicable	
9. Consult lower extremity cross-usage table (Table 17–2) to determine possible method groupings.	Right foot/great toe Methods used ROM and peripheral nerve system Possible grouping—peripheral nerve system combined with ROM losses—only one available	
10. Consider all medical data available and select largest and most clinically appropriate method for each illness/injury; combine each parameter within each individual grouping in order to determine impairment for each leg. Figures should be in whole person units.	ROM losses (7%) combined with PNS (5% lower extremity) equals 12% LEI or 5% WPI.	
11. Use CV chart to combine WPI from each regional impairment calculated in Step 10 of the same limb. The lower extremity impairment for each limb is then converted to WPI. If both lower extremities are involved, impairment rating for each extremity is converted to WPI before being combined with WPI for the contralateral extremity.		

Table refers to Cocchiarella L, Andersson GBJ (eds): Guides to the Evaluation of Permanent Impairment, 5th ed. Chicago, American Medical Association, 2001, and this method of rating follows the principles set forth in Box 17–1 (pp 562–563) of the fifth edition.

CLINICAL EXAMPLES

HIP, THIGH, KNEE AND LEG

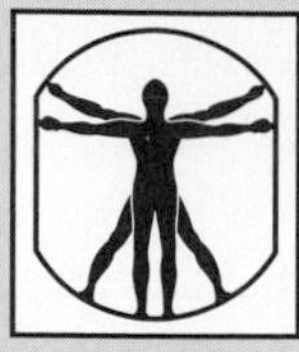

Problem 4

A 54-year-old man working in a foundry had a 1500-pound object fall on the dorsum of his right foot resulting in a severe crush injury to the forefoot. There was significant soft tissue disruption of all the toes and multiple distal open metatarsal fractures. He was brought to a local emergency room where he underwent debridement with delayed transmetatarsal amputation and secondary skin reconstruction with grafting. One year postinjury, the grafts have all healed with no residual infection. Unfortunately, he has had persistence of swelling from the mid-calf all the way to the tip of the residual limb. He has been seen by a neurologist, orthopedist, and physiatrist, and all three services have evaluated him extensively with various nuclear scans and even injection therapy, resulting in a definitive diagnosis of reflex sympathetic dystrophy (or CRPS [Complex Regional Pain Syndrome]) of the right lower extremity.

He presents at this time for an impairment evaluation.

The physical examination reveals no growth limb length discrepancy with the exception of a well-healed transmetatarsal amputation. His gait is such that he is wearing an extra-wide, extra-deep shoe with an appropriate insert. Unfortunately, he cannot wear this shoe more than approximately 4 hours a day. He is able to stand in the shoe, but he cannot ambulate in the shoe without using two crutches, at which time he essentially unloads the right lower extremity on the stance phase. The right lower extremity is approximately 1 cm larger at the distal calf, transmalleolar circumference, and transmetatarsal circumference on the right lower extremity as compared to the left lower extremity. Muscle strength testing of the hip and knee are 5/5 in all muscle groups tested; however, from the ankle distally muscle strength is unable to be assessed due to significant discomfort on even touching the skin of this area. ROM testing reveals hip and knee motion to be essentially normal in the right lower extremity. Ankle plantar flexion is limited to 10°, extension to 5°, inversion to 5°, and eversion to 5°. The vascular status appears to be intact distally and the neurologic status is unable to be fully assessed because he has hypersthesia on the dorsal and plantar aspects of the right residual limb from the ankle distally.

Roentgenograms reveal significant osteopenia in the residual metatarsal bones and in the tarsal bones. There is also osteopenia on the AP and lateral films taken of the distal tibia and ankle region.

Question for Consideration

What if the crush injury also amputated the left great toe and second toe at the MTP joints?

Step	RLE	LLE
1. Establish diagnosis.	1. CRPS right lower extremity 2. Status post right transmetatarsal amputation	
2. MMI?	Yes	
3. List each lower extremity anatomic region with abnormalities that are related to the illness or injury in question. List potential methods.	*Right lower extremity*—transmetatarsal amputation *Right ankle*—loss of ROM	
4. Calculate impairment according to text and tables for each applicable method.	*Transmetatarsal amputation*—40% of the lower extremity or 16% whole person (see Table 17–32) *Ankle ROM losses*—loss of plantar flexion 15% lower extremity; extension loss 7% lower extremity; inversion loss (see Table 17–11) 5% lower extremity; eversion loss (see Table 17–12) 2% lower extremity (all within same joint, therefore, additive and total figure is 29% LEI or 12% WPI)	
5. Identify and calculate illness/injury related to PNS impairment.	Not able to be done	
6. Identify and calculate all illness/injury related to PVS impairment.	Not able to be done	
7. Identify and calculate all injury/impairment related to CRPS impairment.	39% WPI (see Table 13–15)	
8. If no other method available, then determine impairment due to gait derangement if clinically applicable.	Not necessarily clinically applicable, but still can be done—40% WPI (see Table 17–5).	
9. Consult lower extremity cross-usage table (Table 17–2) to determine possible method groupings.	1. Gait derangement alone—40% WPI 2. ROM combined with amputation equals 26% WPI 3. CRPS combined with amputation equals 49% WPI	
10. Consider all medical data available and select largest and most clinically appropriate method for each illness/injury; combine each parameter within each individual grouping in order to determine impairment for each leg. Figures should be in whole person units.	Please note CRPS combined with amputation is the highest. However, the numerical rating of 49% WPI is worth more than value of the extremity, therefore, the rating will be decreased to value of the extremity (see Table 17–32), which equals 40% WPI	
11. Use CV chart to combine WPI impairments from each regional impairment calculated in Step 10 of the same limb. The LEI for each limb is then converted to WPI. If both lower extremities are involved, impairment rating for each extremity is converted to WPI before being combined with WPI for the contralateral extremity.		

Table refers to Cocchiarella L, Andersson GBJ (eds): Guides to the Evaluation of Permanent Impairment, 5th ed. Chicago, American Medical Association, 2001, and this method of rating follows the principles set forth in Box 17–1 (pp 562–563) of the fifth edition.

CLINICAL EXAMPLES

HIP, THIGH, KNEE AND LEG

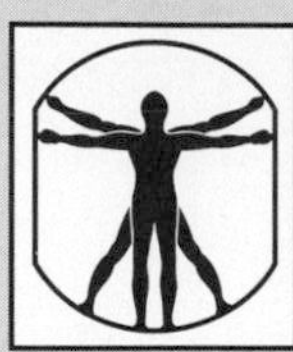

Problem 5

A 39-year-old man is now 3 years status post on-the-job injury. A 2500-pound winch fell and pinned his entire right lower extremity for an hour and a half, after which he was finally extracted and referred to a university-based hospital. He underwent three different surgeries: fasciotomy of the lower leg region, combined external/internal fixation of the medial tibial plateau of the right knee, and subsequent skin grafting of the fasciotomy wounds in the right lower extremity. He has seen multiple physicians and was diagnosed with a malunion of the right tibial plateau and chronic osteomyelitis at the healed fracture site. He has also developed significant degenerative joint disease—more in the medial than the lateral compartment of the same knee. He now has chronic pain, deformity, and instability of the right lower extremity. The physicians who have seen him in consultation have suggested major procedures aimed at stabilization/resolution of the infection, in addition to correction of his mechanical abnormalities, versus amputation. He states that he does not wish to have either one done and will live as he is now.

He reports for an impairment evaluation.

Physical examination reveals that he is a 6′2″, 436-pound man who uses a cane in his right hand for all activities. He has multiple scars and incisions over the right lower extremity; however, the most noteworthy incision is a 12 cm × 5 cm medial proximal tibial scar at the site of the fasciotomy and subsequent skin grafting which is now draining a yellow, purulent material. There is no one specific area of this scar where this purulence is coming from. It appears to be diffuse. There is an obvious varus deformity of the right lower extremity measured at 12 to 15° at the knee as compared to the left lower extremity, which is in 5° of valgus. Limb lengths are equal. Circumferential measurements of the upper legs are 81 cm on the right and 84 cm on the left, with right lower leg measurements of 61 cm on the right and 58 cm on the left. In other words, there is atrophy of the quadriceps area, but chronic swelling of the right lower leg area. Strength testing was attempted. His hip and ankle motion is intact at the level of 5/5; knee flexion and extension is difficult to assess secondary to discomfort at the fracture site. ROM testing has been accomplished and right knee extension is full; however, he is only able to accomplish 90° of flexion and has a roentgenographically measurable varus deformity of 15°. Surprisingly, the neurovascular status is intact.

Roentgenograms have been obtained that reveal a 15° varus deformity of the right knee secondary to a malunited tibial plateau fracture. There is a medial buttress plate in place with approximately six screws from medial to lateral, in addition to lateral to medial screws being identified. There is an irregular lucency in the tibial subchondral area just distal to the intercondylar notch measuring 3 cm × 4 cm.

Step	RLE	LLE
1. Establish diagnosis.	1. Compartment syndrome right lower extremity with subsequent fasciotomy and skin grafting—no residuals from compartment syndrome itself. 2. Status post-open reduction, internal fixation (ORIF)/external fixator left tibial plateau with subsequent infected malunion—residual varus deformity 15°.	
2. MMI?	Patient refuses any additional treatment—yes	
3. List each lower extremity anatomic region with abnormalities that are related to the illness or injury in question. List potential methods.	*Thigh*—atrophy *Knee*—ROM arthritis, diagnosis-based estimate *Calf*—skin loss	
4. Calculate impairment according to text and tables for each applicable method.	*Thigh*—atrophy—10% LEI (see Table 17–6) *Knee*—ROM—10% LEI plus 35% LEI (varus abnormality) equals 45% LEI (see Table 17–10) Degenerative joint disease—25% LEI (see Table 17–31) Diagnosis-based estimate—25% LEI (see Table 17–33) *Calf*—skin loss and chronic osteomyelitis 7% LEI (see Table 17–36)	
5. Identify and calculate illness/injury related to PNS impairment.	Not applicable	
6. Identify and calculate all illness/injury related to PVS impairment.	None	
7. Identify and calculate all injury impairment related to CRPS impairment.	None	
8. If no other method available, then determine impairment due to gait derangement if clinically applicable.	Has to use cane on a full-time basis —objective reason—20% LEI (see Table 17–5)	
9. Consult lower extremity cross-usage table (Table 17–2) to determine possible method groupings.	1. Gait derangement alone 2. Atrophy combined with skin loss 3. ROM combined with skin loss 4. Arthritis combined with diagnosis-based estimate combined with skin loss	
10. Consider all medical data available and select largest and most clinically appropriate method for each illness/injury; combine each parameter within each individual grouping in order to determine impairment for each leg. Figures should be in whole person units combined with the skin loss.	1. Gait derangement equals 20% WPI. 2. Thigh atrophy combined with skin loss equals 16% LEI equals 6% WPI. 3. Knee ROM loss combined with calf skin loss equals 35% LEI combined with 7%, which equals 40% LEI, which equals 16% WPI. 4. Arthritis combined with diagnosis-based estimate combined with skin loss: 25% LEI, combined with 25% LEI, then combined with 7% LEI, equaling 48% LEI or 19% WPI. The whole person rating of 20% is appropriate considering the severity of the individual's injury.	
11. Use CV chart to combine WPI impairments from each regional impairment calculated in Step 10 of the same limb. The LEI for each limb is then converted to WPI. If both lower extremities are involved, impairment rating for each extremity is converted to WPI before being combined with WPI for the contralateral extremity.		

Table refers to Cocchiarella L, Andersson GBJ (eds): Guides to the Evaluation of Permanent Impairment, 5th ed. Chicago, American Medical Association, 2001, and this method of rating follows the principles set forth in Box 17–1 (pp 562–563) of the fifth edition.

References

1. American Academy of Orthopaedic Surgeons: Manual for Orthopaedic Surgeons in Evaluating Permanent Physical Impairment. Chicago, American Academy of Orthopaedic Surgeons, 1962.
2. American Medical Association: Guides to the Evaluation of Permanent Impairment, 4th ed. Chicago, American Medical Association, 1993, pp 375–393.
3. American Medical Association: Guides to the Evaluation of Permanent Impairment, 4th ed. Chicago, American Medical Association, 1993, pp 385–386.
4. Cocchiarella L, Andersson GBJ (eds): Guides to the Evaluation of Permanent Impairment, 5th ed. Chicago, American Medical Association, 2001, pp 523–564.
5. Andersson G: Hip assessment: A comparison of nine different methods. J Bone Joint Surg 54B:621, 1972.
6. Burgess AR: Fractures of the pelvis. In Rockwood CA, Green DP, Bucholz RW (eds): Fractures, vol 2. New York, JB Lippincott, 1991, pp 1399–1441.
7. Callaghan JJ, Dysart SH, Savory CF, et al: Assessing the results of hip replacement. J Bone Joint Surg 72B:1008, 1990.
8. Daniel DM, Stone ML: Diagnosis of knee ligament injuries: Tests and measurement of knee motion limits. In Feagin JA Jr (ed): The Crucial Ligaments. New York, Churchill Livingston, 1994.
9. DeLee JC: Fractures and dislocations of the hip. In Rockwood CA, Green DP, Bucholz RW (eds): Fractures, vol 2. New York, JB Lippincott, 1991, pp 1481–1652.
10. Dunn EL, Berry PH, Connally JD: Computed tomography of the pelvis in patients with multiple injuries. J Trauma 23:378, 1983.
11. Esquemeling J: The Buchaners of America. New York, Dover, 1967.
12. Felson DT, Hannan MT, Naimark A, et al: Occupational physical demands, knee bending, and knee osteoarthritis: Results from the Framingham Study. J Rheumatol 18:10, 1587, 1991.
13. Ficat RP: Ideopathic bone necrosis of the femoral head. J Bone Joint Surg 67B:3–9, 1985.
14. Garth WP: Current concepts regarding the anterior cruciate ligament. Orthop Rev 5:565, 1992.
15. Harris WH: Traumatic arthritis of the hip after dislocation and acetabular fractures: Treatment by mold arthroplasty. J Bone Joint Surg 51A:737, 1969.
16. Hastings DE: The non-operative management of collateral ligament injuries of the knee joint. Clin Orthop 147:22, 1980.
17. Helfet AJ: Mechanism of derangements of the medial semilunar cartilage and their management. J Bone Joint Surg 41B:319–336, 1959.
18. Henning CE, Lynch MA, Glick KR Jr: Physical examination of the knee. In Nicholas JA, Hershman EB (eds): The Lower Extremity and the Spine in Sports Medicine, vol 1. St. Louis, Mosby, 1986, pp 765–800.
19. Hoikka V, Ylikoski M, Tallroth K: Leg-length inequality has poor correlation with lumbar scoliosis. Arch Orthop Trauma Surg 108:173, 1989.
20. Insall JN, Dorr LD, Scott RD, et al: Rationale of The Knee Society clinical rating system. Clin Orthop 248:13, 1989.
21. Katz JN, Harris TM, Larson MG, et al: Predictors of functional outcomes after arthroscopic partial menisectomy. J Rheumatol 19:1938, 1992.
22. LaBrier K, O'Neill DB: Patellofemoral stress syndrome: Current concepts. Sports Med 16:449, 1993.
23. Lord JP, Aitkins SG, McCrory MA, et al: Isometric and isokinetic measurement of hamstring and quadriceps strength. Arch Phys Med Rehabil 73:324–330, 1992.
24. Livingston DH, Keenan D, Kim D, et al: Extent of disability following traumatic extremity amputation. J Trauma 37:495, 1994.
25. Luck JV: Traumatic arthrofibrosis. Bull Hosp Joint Dis 12:394–403, 1951.
26. Luck JV Jr, Beardmore TD, Kaufman R: Disability evaluation in arthritis patients. Clin Orthop 221:59–67, 1987.
27. Luck JV Jr, Florence DW: A brief history and comparative analysis of disability systems and impairment rating guides. Orthop Clin North Am 19:839–844, 1988.
28. Markolf KL, Graff-Radford A, Amstutz HC: In vivo knee stability. J Bone Joint Surg 60A:664–674, 1978.
29. Matsen FA: Compartmental syndrome. Clin Orthop 113:8–13, 1975.
30. Mitchell DG, Steinberg ME, Dalinka MK, et al: Magnetic resonance imaging of the ischemic hip. Clin Orthop 244:60–77, 1989.
31. Mubarak SJ, Owen CA, Hargens AR, et al: Acute compartment syndrome: Diagnosis and treatment with the aid of the Wick catheter. J Bone Joint Surg 60A:1091–1095, 1978.
32. Nutton RW, Pinder IM, Williams D: Detection of sacroiliac injury by bone scanning in fractures of the pelvis and its clinical significance. Injury 13:473, 1982.
33. Olson SA, Matta JM: The computed tomography subchondral arc: A new method of assessing acetabular articular continuity after fracture (a preliminary report). J Orthop Trauma 7:402, 1993.
34. Peltier L: Joseph Malgaigne and Malgaigne's fracture. Surgery 44:777–784, 1958.
35. Schroer WC: Current concepts on the pathogenesis of osteonecrosis of the femoral head. Orthop Rev 23:487, 1994.
36. Semba RT, Yasukawa K, Gustilo RB: Critical analysis of results of 53 Malgaigne fractures of the pelvis. J Trauma 23:535, 1983.
37. Tile M: Fractures of the acetabulum. In Rockwood CA, Green DP, Bucholz RW (eds): Fractures, vol 2. New York, JB Lippincott, 1991, 1442–1479.
38. Tobis JS, Chang-Zern H: Muscle testing. In Kottke FJ, Lehman JF (eds): Krusen's Handbook of Physical Medicine and Rehabilitation, 4th ed. Philadelphia, WB Saunders, 1990, pp 33–60.
39. Walker RH, Burton DS: Computerized tomography in assessment of acetabular fractures. J Trauma 22:227, 1982.
40. Ward EGW, Bodiwala GG, Thomas PD: The importance of lower limb injuries in car crashes when cost and disability are considered. Accid Anal Prev 24:613, 1992.
41. Webb LX, Caldwell K: Disruption of the posterior pelvic ring caused by vertical shear. South Med J 81:1217, 1988.
42. Weber M: Die Beurteilung des Unfallzusammenhangs von Meniskusschaden. Orthopade 23:171, 1994.
43. White MSI: Three-dimensional computed tomography in the assessment of fractures of the acetabulum. Injury 22:13, 1991.
44. Yamamoto T, Bullough P: Spontaneous osteonecrosis of the knee: The result of subchondral insufficiency fracture. J Bone Joint Surg 82A:858–866, 2000.

CHAPTER

19

Joint Systems

Foot and Ankle

GEORGE B. HOLMES, JR., MD, MPH ■ LEE C. WOODS, MD

Impairment and disability evaluations of the foot and ankle are performed most frequently for work-related injuries. According to a recent survey, injuries to the foot and ankle account for approximately 7.5% of all occupational injuries.[8] Statistics from State Labor Departments in 1993 indicate that injuries of the foot and toes were responsible for 5% of work-related injuries and 3% of those that received compensation.[10] Injuries to the foot and ankle accounted for $3.4 to $8.7 billion of the estimated $115.9 billion in work accident costs in 1992.[8,10]

The worker with an injury to the foot or ankle is most typically a man, aged 30 to 40 years, who works in manual labor or vehicular operations jobs.[8] Most such work-related injuries (58.4%) are caused by a blow to the foot or ankle. In a study from the Rush–Presbyterian–St. Luke's Occupational Health Clinic, 22% of the foot and ankle injuries were fractures, sprains, or strains[8] and 5% of these injuries were caused by vehicles. The peak incidence of these injuries occurred in the summer months.

An appreciation of the nature of the injury and a description of the injury's cause and circumstance are helpful in the overall determination of the diagnosis, rehabilitation, time for recovery, temporary disability, permanent disability, and return-to-work status. Table 19–1, from a 1981 publication of the U.S. Department of Labor, categorizes foot injuries according to the description of the accident and the involved part of the foot.[12] The most common occurrence was when the foot was struck by a falling object. Injuries to the toes and metatarsal bones accounted for the vast majority of foot and ankle injuries. The most common specific injuries were contusions, lacerations (or punctures), fractures, and sprains.

CONTUSIONS, CRUSH INJURIES, AND BRUISES

The impact of contusion and crush injuries to the foot, as it relates to temporary or permanent impairment, is in large part based on the location and degree of soft tissue injury. The degree of injury can be assessed in part by the size and weight of the object striking the foot. However, in many instances the initial estimation of soft tissue damage is incorrect or misleading.

Significant crush injury can result in local or regional necrosis of skin and muscle. Large defects may require split thickness skin grafts or the grafting of one of several types of flaps. The possibility of compartment syndrome must always be considered in the presence of moderate to severe crush injury. Failure to appreciate the magnitude of the injury can lead to an inadequate awareness of a permanent sensory loss or loss of motor function. A lack of early intervention can lead to contractures or, possibly, the need for wider amputation. Regardless of the type of treatment, patients with severe crush injuries to the foot and ankle may be left with chronic pain and a limb that is unable to bear weight repetitively, a major disability particularly in an environment of manual labor and vehicular operation. Physical therapy and occupational therapy should stress the re-establishment of normal or near-normal range of motion, soft tissue mobilization, strengthening, and proprioception training. A return to normal function is predicated on the achievement of these goals. Recovery from minor bruises and contusions can be expected to occur within 3 to 6 weeks of the time of injury. Maximal medical improvement from more severe injuries can take 12 to 24 months. Not unexpectedly even following this period some patients may continue to have chronic pain, swelling, and functional deficits.

Contusions to the toes are common, especially if the worker is not wearing safety-tipped shoes at the time of the injury. Because of the lack of significant soft-tissue protection, the toes are particularly susceptible to chronic swelling after such injuries. This may result in chronic pain that is exacerbated by cold weather and constricting footwear. Adequate warmth and a shoe with an enlarged toebox are measures that will decrease symptoms and prolong weight-bearing tolerance. In nondiabetic patients partial- and multiple-toe amputations are usually well-tolerated without significant compromise of stability, balance, and energy expenditure. Multiple amputations and amputations of the great toe in diabetic patients will necessitate a significant reduction in the weight-bearing status or a significant modification in footwear. These modifications include use of an extra-depth shoe with a plastizoate liner and rocker bottom and change to a semisedentary status with lifting, climbing, and walking restrictions.

A common complication after direct impact trauma to the toes or metatarsals is the development of one or more interdigital (Morton) neuromas. Neuromas cause pain that increases with weight bearing, stair climbing, or the use of tight shoes. If metatarsal pads, a rigid shoe, or a wider shoe do not decrease the pain, the injured worker may require excision of the interdigital nerve. This will result in a satisfactory response in 80% of cases.[2,9] The remaining 20% may require a reduction in weight-bearing status along with various shoe modifications.

FRACTURES AND DISLOCATIONS

A specific discussion of every fracture and dislocation of the foot and ankle along with its treatment, rehabilitation, and impairment is beyond the scope of this text. A

TABLE 19–1

Foot Injuries by Description of Accident, Selected States, July–August, 1979[10]

Item	All Workers		Workers Wearing Safety Shoes	
	Number	Percent	Number	Percent
How did the accident occur?				
Total	1251	100	283	100
Stepped on sharp object	194	16	24	8
Struck by falling object	721	58	191	67
Object rolled onto or over foot	168	13	36	13
Squeezed between two surfaces	59	5	13	5
Struck foot against object	28	2	3	1
Occurred in another way	81	6	16	6
What part of your foot was injured?				
Total*	1251	*	283	*
Toes	719	57	118	42
Toes only	557	45	69	24
Toes and other part(s) of foot	162	13	49	17
Metatarsal	475	38	179	63
Metatarsal only	291	23	124	44
Metatarsal and other part(s) of foot	184	15	55	19
Sole	241	19	45	16
Sole only	153	12	19	7
Sole and other part(s) of foot	88	7	26	9
Heel	69	6	19	7
Heel only	28	2	4	1
Heel and other part(s) of foot	41	3	15	5
Ankle and other part(s) of foot	59	5	19	7
Were both feet injured?				
Total	1195	100	269	100
No	1176	98	266	99
Yes	19	2	3	1

*Because the categories listed are not mutually exclusive, the sum of the parts will exceed the total.

Note—Due to rounding, percentages may not add to 100. Because incomplete questionnaires were used, the total number of responses may vary by question.

Source—Survey questionnaire.

framework for the evaluation of fractures and their outcomes is presented within the context of impairment rating. In general, the treatment for a fracture or dislocation of the foot and ankle is the appropriate reduction and immobilization followed by rehabilitation and mobilization in order to achieve a return to optimal functioning. In specific instances, such as with intra-articular fractures treated with rigid internal fixation, early range of motion is initiated to enhance a more rapid and complete return to normal motion and function.

Permanent impairment is manifested by pain, loss of motion, decreased strength, or swelling. Loss of motion and pain occurs in the presence of arthritis, malunion, and soft tissue scarring along with associated nerve and muscle injury. Pain can be secondary to the presence of avascular necrosis, delayed union, nonunion, or chronic infection. These possibilities must be assessed thoroughly, because the status of temporary impairment versus permanent impairment depends in large part on establishment of the correct diagnosis. Obviously, in the absence of an early accurate diagnosis and treatment, the chances are increased for the development of a more protracted temporary disability and permanent impairment.

Lisfranc fracture dislocations and fractures of the calcaneus are common workplace injuries. A Lisfranc fracture dislocation can easily be overlooked, especially in a worker with multiple injuries. This is in sharp contrast to a calcaneus fracture, which usually exhibits a dramatic clinical and radiographic picture. The diagnosis and treatment of these two differing injuries is instructive in evaluation of temporary and permanent disability of the injured worker.

Prompt treatment of a Lisfranc fracture dislocation via open or closed reduction and internal fixation of the tarsometatarsal joints provides the injured worker with the greatest opportunity to return to pain-free weight bearing (Fig. 19–1). The recovery time is usually between 3 and 6 months. Commonly, when the fracture is subtle, the initial radiographs are normal. After a brief period on crutches, the worker attempts to return to regular duties and develops pain or swelling in the area of the midfoot. If this situation persists, arthritis can develop, which will later be observed on radiographs. The treatment becomes one of selective midfoot arthrodesis, which has a low rate of success in terms of relieving pain.[1] These patients may require the long-term use of a steel-shank rocker-bottom type of shoe and are often unable to return to an unrestricted level of activity. However, if diagnosed early and treated appropriately, most patients will be able to return to an unrestricted or minimally restricted weight-bearing status.

A fracture of the calcaneus is frequently a devastating, career-ending injury for the manual laborer. This is especially true when the fracture involves the posterior facet, when associated with a loss of the heel height, when there is comminution, and when the heel has undergone significant widening (Fig. 19–2). There is also a high association of injury to the posterior tibial nerve and its branches due to direct injury or concomitant swelling. The initial prognosis for return to unrestricted weight bearing is poor. However, several options can significantly improve the likelihood of return to a level of weight bearing that may allow the worker to return to his or her former employment. The prompt reduction of soft tissue swelling, accurate anatomic reconstruction of the posterior facet, narrowing of the heel, and restoration of heel height can improve the overall prognosis (Fig. 19–3). Maximal medical improvement is usually seen in 12 to 18 months. If the injured worker continues to have significant pain related to the subtalar joint of the hindfoot (as opposed to nerve injury), a subtalar fusion or triple arthrodesis offers an excellent chance for elimination of pain. However, if significant subtalar motion and flexibility are required

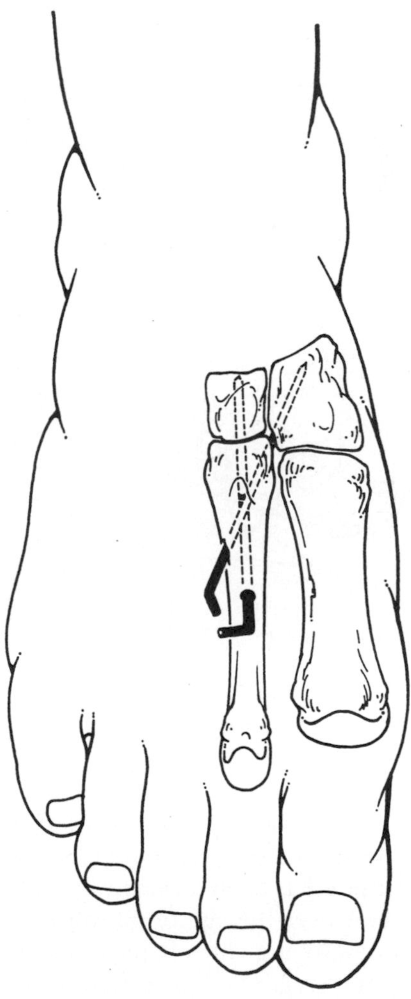

Figure 19–1. Internal fixation using smooth K-wires. (From Holmes GB: Surgical Approaches to the Foot and Ankle. New York, McGraw-Hill.)

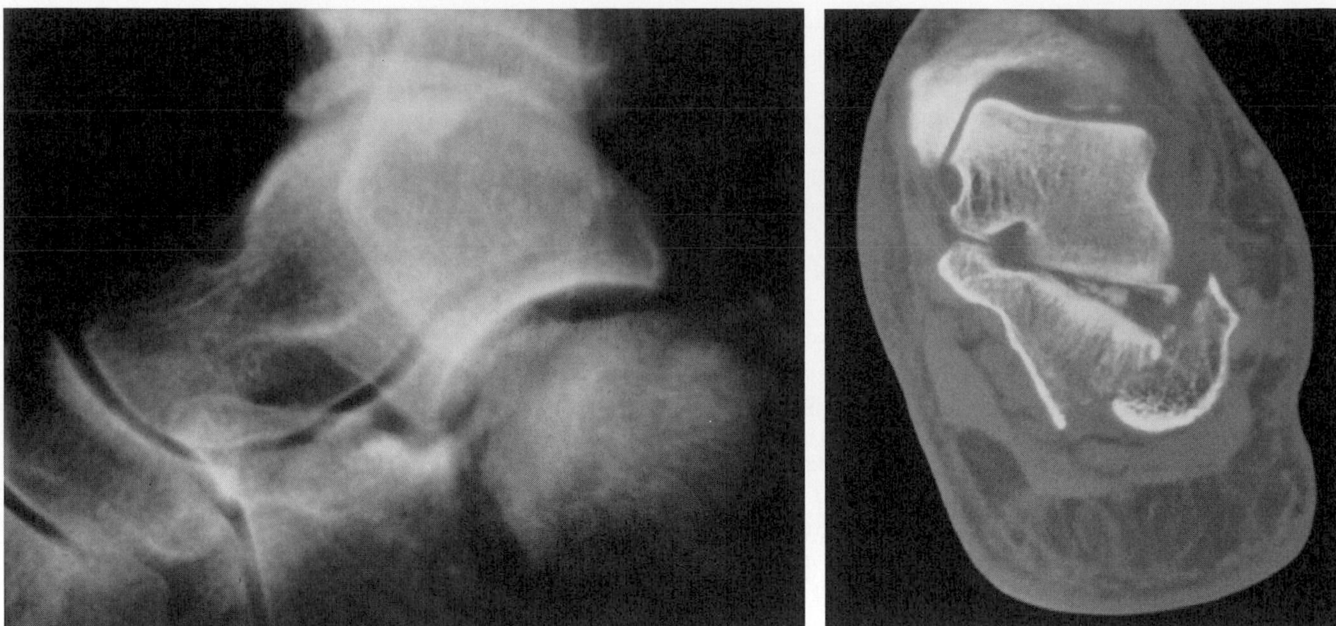

Figure 19–2. Fracture of the calcaneus.

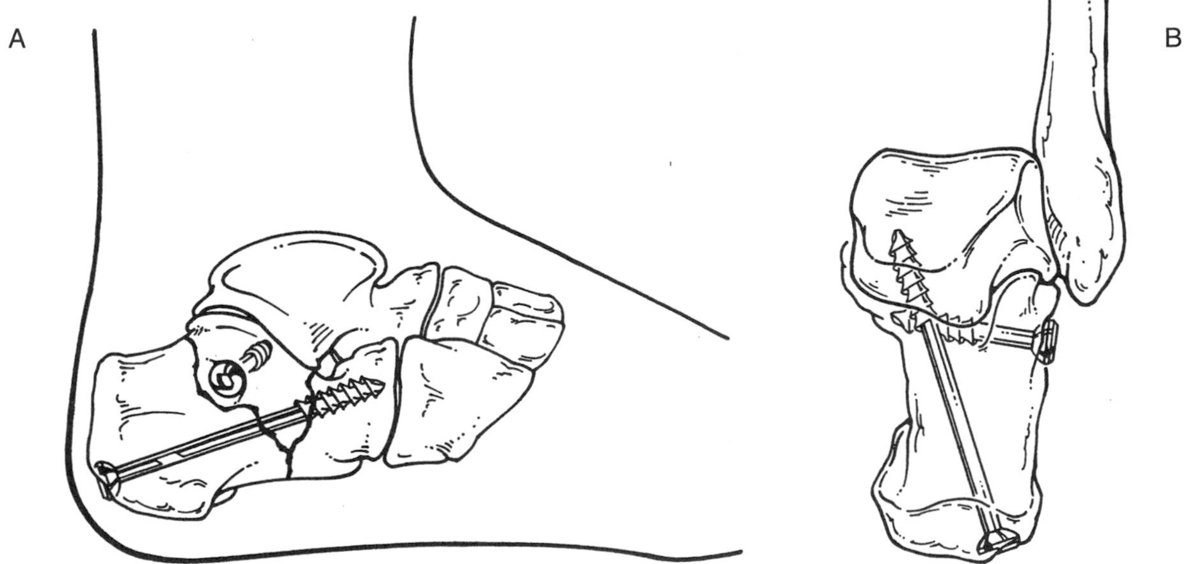

Figure 19–3. *A,* Lateral view after insertion of screws. *B,* Harris view: fixation for facet split and joint depression. (From Holmes GB: Surgical Approaches to the Foot and Ankle. New York, McGraw-Hill.)

to perform the worker's job (e.g., in the case of a roofer), significant activity restrictions may be essential even though there has been a reduction or elimination of pain. Workers over the age of 50 will have a greater likelihood of developing chronic postinjury pain after a calcaneus fracture regardless of the initial treatment.[11] Therefore, the overall prognosis for return to pain-free weight-bearing function is worst for the middle-aged or older worker.

CUTS, LACERATIONS, AND PUNCTURES

Simple cuts, lacerations, and punctures of the foot are usually easy to treat and carry a low propensity of long-term permanent impairment. However, because most structures of the foot and ankle are relatively superficial, careful assessment is necessary to ensure that vital structures have not been compromised by a seemingly minor injury.

A cut of the foot can result in injury to vessels, tendons, or ligaments. It may also penetrate a joint and lead to sepsis or an abscess. Cuts and lacerations associated with an adjacent fracture convert the injury to an open fracture that will require irrigation, exploration, and debridement.

Tendon injuries most frequently result from a worker stepping on, kicking, or dropping a sharp object on the foot or ankle. About 75% of these injuries occur in the forefoot.[4] Injuries to the lesser extensor and flexor tendons of the foot generally do not require surgical repair. These injuries lead to very little functional deficit. However, acute complete lacerations of the flexor hallucis longus, extensor hallucis longus, anterior tibial tendon, posterior tibial tendon, and peroneal tendons demand surgical repair. In most instances significant functional losses can be expected if there is no repair.

A laceration of the arteries and veins of the foot and ankle will cause injury in proportion to the importance of the vessel and the area supplied or drained by that vessel. If viability of the foot or even a portion of the foot is compromised, long-term functional losses may be anticipated.

Puncture wounds of the plantar aspect of the foot can be serious. Puncture wounds through a shoe or sneaker have a significant risk for the development of *Pseudomonas* infection of the soft tissue and adjacent bone. Prevention of complications calls for prompt irrigation, debridement, and appropriate antibiotic coverage.[3,7] Development of a chronic infection can lead to postinfection scarring, chronic pain, and chronic swelling.

SPRAINS AND STRAINS

Strains and sprains of the foot and ankle are common. They are frequently graded on a scale of 1 to 3, with the latter representing complete ligamentous disruption along with instability. In the most common instances of Grade 1 and Grade 2 injuries, early range of motion and rehabilitation will significantly reduce the period of total temporary impairment. The techniques of soft tissue mobilization, contrast baths, proprioception training, electrical stimulation, and dynamic support are crucial in the achievement of an early recovery. Slower recovery can be anticipated in middle-aged or older workers, workers with prior ligamentous injuries in the same location, or workers with associated injuries such as fractures or nerve damage.

The primary problem in the recovery from strains and sprains lies in the underdiagnosis of more serious problems. A seemingly simple strain or sprain may actually represent a posterior tibial tendon rupture, spring ligament injury, subluxation or rupture of a peroneal tendon, formation of an intra-articular loose body, turf toe, reflex sympathetic dystrophy, or Lisfranc fracture dislocation. This list could be expanded further, but the main point is to eliminate other diagnostic possibilities associated with strains and sprains, especially when the patient's recovery is unexpectedly prolonged.

NEUROLOGIC INJURIES

Neurologic injuries can be broadly categorized as being either local or diffuse. Local neurologic injuries of the foot and ankle usually result in one of several characteristic patterns of injury. There may be discrete pain at the site of injury to a somatic nerve. This may or may not be associated with a positive Tinel test over the proximal, and occasionally the distal, aspect of the nerve. With disruption of the nerve fibers there is also the possibility of a loss of sensation distal to the distribution of the nerve. This pattern of injury is typical of neuromas. In general, treatment options consist of desensitization techniques, relative immobilization (stiff shoe or orthosis), transcutaneous electrical nerve stimulation, local anesthetic injection (diagnostic purposes), lysis of adhesions, or surgical excision. It may take several months for the injured worker to experience decreased symptoms with the initial use of conservative and nonoperative techniques, but these techniques are generally successful.

Diffuse injuries will affect a wider area of the foot. The most common forms of injury include tarsal tunnel syndrome, the sequela of compartment syndrome, and reflex sympathetic dystrophy. The long-term prognosis for recovery, the success of nonoperative and operative modalities, and the avoidance of permanent impairment are less than would be expected for more discrete injuries such as neuromas. Injuries such as tarsal tunnel syndrome or reflex sympathetic dystrophy may require several months of examinations and tests before the diagnosis can be established by objective measures, such as electromyography, nerve conduction velocity, or bone scan.

Early diagnosis and intervention are important in reducing the short-term impairment and the probability of progression to long-term impairment associated with tarsal tunnel syndrome or reflex sympathetic dystrophy. From a rating standpoint these injuries pose a special problem in that patients may initially be seen with relatively well-maintained range of motion and normal motor function. However, they will have significant functional problems based on the presence of significant pain exacerbated by weight bearing.

CUMULATIVE INJURIES OF THE FOOT AND ANKLE

An important issue in the evaluation of the impaired foot and ankle is the role of chronic or cumulative trauma as the etiology of the injury. The central question is to what extent the job site or job duties contributed to the injured foot or ankle versus the contribution of activities of daily living. Job or occupational related injuries have been termed repetitive stress injury, cumulative stress disorder, or overuse syndrome.[5] Much focus regarding cumulative stress has been directed toward upper extremity injuries, particularly carpal tunnel syndrome. Until recently there has been little critical attention paid to reported cumulative injuries of the foot and ankle.

The recent analysis of Guyton et al has demonstrated an absence of the role of cumulative industrial trauma in the development of seven common disorders of the foot and ankle.[6] The standard of proof involved uses Koch postulates. The first postulate states that the etiologic agent must be found in each case of the disease or injury. Next, the etiologic agent must be able to be isolated. Finally, the etiologic agent should be able to cause disease if a normal human or animal is exposed to the agent. When applied to hallux valgus, lesser toe deformities, interdigital neuroma, tarsal tunnel syndrome, heel pain, adult acquired flatfoot, and foot and ankle osteoarthritis, not one of Koch's three postulates was satisfied in the analysis. The conclusion of the authors is that the requirements and mechanical stresses associated with industrial occupations represented normal manifestations of everyday environmental wear and tear for these seven common disorders.

TABLE 19–2

Temporary and Permanent Impairment

Injury	Projected Temporary Impairment	Risk of Long-Term Permanent Impairment
Minor/mild contusions		
Toe(s)	3–6 weeks	Low
Dorsum foot	3–6 weeks	Low
Severe contusions		
Toe(s)	6–12 weeks	Low
Dorsum foot	6–12 weeks	Mild-moderate
Ankle		
Avulsion	1–3 months	Low
Lateral malleolar	3–5 months	Low–mild
Bimalleolar	3–5 months	Low–mild
Trimalleolar	3–5 months	Low–mild
Plafond	3–6 months	Moderate
Hindfoot		
Extra-articular calcaneus	3–6 months	Low–mild
Intra-articular calcaneus	6–18 months	Moderate-high
Talus	6–18 months	Mild–high
Mid-foot		
Navicular	3–4 months	Mild–moderate
Cuboid	2–3 months	Low
Cuneiforms	2–3 months	Low
Lisfranc	3–6 months	Mild–moderate
Forefoot		
Metatarsals	1–3 months	Low–mild
Phalanges	1–2 months	Low
Sesamoids	2–6 months	Mild–moderate
Compartment syndrome	6–12 months	Moderate–high
Tarsal tunnel syndrome	3–6 months	Moderate–high
Sinus tarsi syndrome	3–6 months	Mild–moderate
Reflex sympathetic dystrophy	6–30 months	Moderate–high

CONCLUSION

The approach to determining temporary and permanent impairment (see Table 19–2) with respect to the foot and ankle is more efficient than those of other regions of the body such as the spine. Unlike other areas of the trunk, the anatomy of the foot and ankle is visible, which enhances its assessment by physical examination. Ancillary studies such as radiographs, bone scan, tomography, and magnetic resonance imaging are also enhanced by the relatively superficial nature of the anatomy. The key to a successful outcome of treatment and rehabilitation is early, accurate assessment of the problem, with the anatomy of the foot lending itself to the correct diagnosis.

References

1. Arntz CT, Veith RG, Hansen ST: Fractures and fracture-dislocations of the tarsometatarsal joint. J Bone Joint Surg 70A:173, 1988.
2. Bradley N, Miller WA, Evans JP: Plantar neuroma analysis of results following surgical excision in 145 patients. South Med J 69:853, 1976.
3. Fitzgerald RH, Cowan JDE: Puncture wounds of the foot. Orthop Clin North Am 6:965, 1975.
4. Floyd DW, Heckman JD, Rockwood CA Jr: Tendon lacerations in the foot. Foot Ankle 4:8, 1983.
5. Fry HJ: The treatment of overuse syndrome in musicians. Results in 175 patients. J R Soc Med 81:572–575, 1988.
6. Guyton GP, Mann RA, Krieger LE, et al: Cumulative industrial trauma as an etiology of seven common disorders in the foot and ankle: What is the evidence? Foot Ankle 21:1047–1056, 2000.
7. Johnson JE, Hall RL: Management of foot infections. In Gould JS (ed): Operative Foot Surgery. Philadelphia, WB Saunders, 1982, p 274.
8. Oleski DM, Hahn JJ, Leibold M: Work-related injuries to the foot. J Occup Med 34:650, 1992.
9. Mann RA, Reynolds JD: Interdigital neuroma: A critical clinical analysis. Foot Ankle 3:238, 1983.
10. National Safety Council: Accident Facts, 3rd ed. Itasca, IL, National Safety Council, 1993.
11. Paley D, Hall H: Intra-articular fractures of the calcaneus: A critical analysis of results and prognostic factors. J Bone Joint Surg 75A:342, 1993.
12. U.S. Department of Labor: Accidents Involving Foot Injuries (Report 626). Washington, DC, U.S. Department of Labor, 1981.

CHAPTER

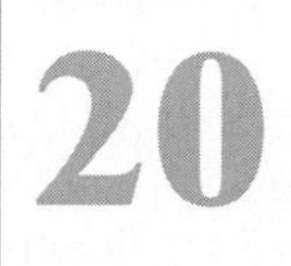

Joint Systems

Cervical Spine

CHOLL W. KIM, MD, PhD ■ JEFFREY D. KLEIN, MD ■ STEVEN R. GARFIN, MD

Symptoms related to degenerative conditions of the cervical spine can be divided into three categories: neck pain, arm pain, and myelopathy.[23] The clinical evaluation of patients with neck pain, arm pain, or myelopathy is based on the history, physical examination, and imaging studies. Electromyelographic assessment (electromyography [EMG], nerve conduction velocity [NCV], and evoked potentials) has an occasional role. This chapter describes the clinical presentation, physical examination findings, and radiographic imaging studies that distinguish the many causes of neck and arm pain.

Neck Pain

Cervical Spondylosis

The process of aging and degenerative change in the cervical spine involves all elements of the motion segment. Disc degeneration is accompanied by osteophyte formation around the degenerate disc and neurocentral joints, facet arthritis, and ligamentous thickening. Subluxation and disc herniation may also be present. Taken together, these changes are referred to as cervical spondylosis.

Cervical spondylosis is common in patients older than 40 years, and generally is asymptomatic or causes mild neck pain[3]; however, patients may initially be seen with significant neck pain, symptoms associated with nerve root compression (cervical spondylotic radiculopathy), symptoms associated with spinal cord compression (cervical spondylotic myelopathy [CSM]), or a combination of the above.

The neck pain associated with cervical spondylosis is generally gradual in onset, although it can be exacerbated by superimposed trauma. The pain varies in severity, is generally activity related, and is often accompanied by neck stiffness. The pain is commonly posterior in the midcervical spine, but referred pain to the shoulders and upper arms may be present. Headaches are not unusual and may be due to paraspinal muscle spasm secondary to nerve irritation, compression of the greater occipital nerve, or to many unknown, or nonspinal, causes.

The physical examination of patients with painful cervical spondylosis may demonstrate only limited range of motion. Extension is usually lost first. Passive extension by the examiner may be painful.[17] Paraspinal muscle spasm may be present, and tenderness may be elicited in the midsubstance of the trapezius muscle. Results of neurologic examination are generally normal.

Radiographs are useful for excluding potentially significant diseases such as tumor, infection, or trauma. Radiography is usually not required at the initial evaluation unless the clinical history suggests such diseases. Standard radiography begins with an anterior-posterior, odontoid, and lateral view. The lateral view may reveal disc space narrowing, loss of normal cervical lordosis, ankylosis, osteophytosis, and subluxation (Fig. 20–1*A*). Disease may be seen at one level or at many levels. The most mobile segments (C5-6, C6-7, and C4-5) are most commonly involved (in that order). Further radiographic studies include dynamic lateral (flexion and extension) films, which may demonstrate instability. The oblique views demonstrate the intervertebral foramen and may show osteophytes from the neurocentral joints projecting into the neuroforamen. However, the oblique views may be difficult to interpret owing to the variability in radiographic technique that is commonly encountered.

It is important to note that radiographs in asymptomatic individuals commonly reveal spondylotic changes.[5,33] Patients with radiographic findings of severe cervical spondylosis may be asymptomatic, whereas patients with minimal radiographic findings may have severe pain. Therefore, radiographs must be correlated with the clinical history and examination.

Compressive lesions of the nerve roots or spinal cord are better evaluated with advanced neurodiagnostic evaluation such as computed tomography (CT), usually with myelography, or magnetic resonance imaging (MRI) (Fig. 20–1*B*). Advanced imaging is warranted when there are specific signs of nerve root or spinal cord compression (discussed in the following), or when axial neck pain is unremitting or worsening. As is the case with radiography, clinical correlation is required, as MRI also has a high false positive rate. Boden et al reported that MRI evidence of disc degeneration, disc space narrowing, and nerve compression was seen in 25% of asymptomatic patients younger than 40 years and 60% of asymptomatic patients older than 40 years.[2]

Pathoanatomy

Progressive dehydration and fibrosis of the intervertebral disc results in loss of the normal disc architecture, and ultimately loss of the demarcation between the nucleus pulposus and the annulus fibrosus. There is a gradual loss of the gelatinous nucleus pulposus, coarsening of the annular lamellae, and later fissuring of the annulus.[11,12] Histologically, there is loss of the normal fibrillar structure of the nucleus accompanied by progressive cavitation, desiccation, fibroblastic proliferation, and calcium deposition. A decrease in overall proteoglycan content is also observed.[8] Proteoglycans are responsible for disc hydration by virtue of their osmotic properties.

Natural History

The morphologic changes of cervical spondylosis are progressive and not reversible. There is no correla-

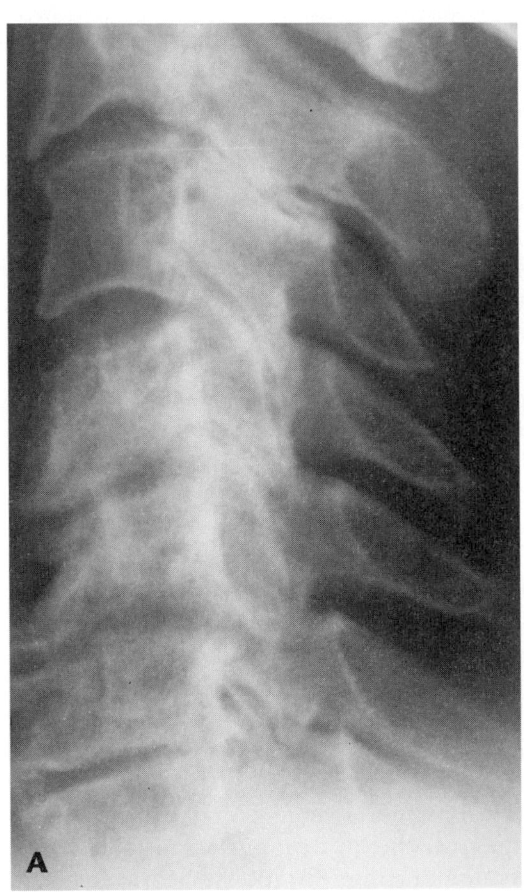

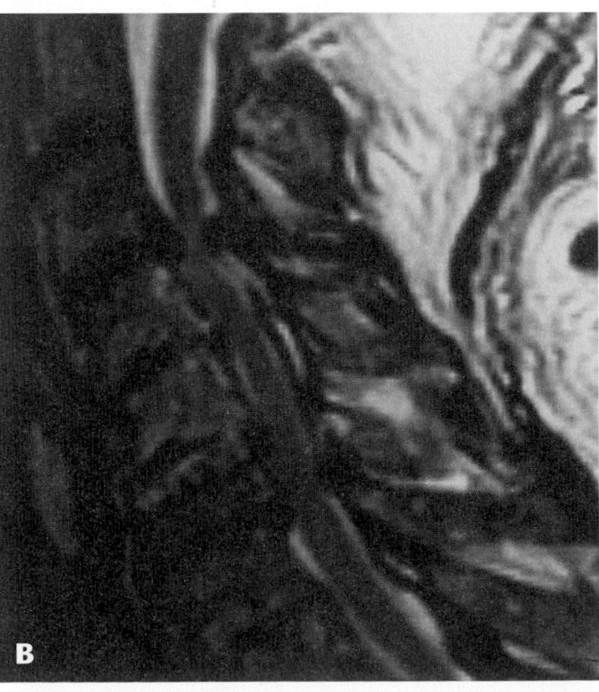

Figure 20–1. Cervical spondylosis.

tion, however, between the structural changes of disc degeneration and the clinical syndrome of pain without neurologic involvement.[45] Cervical spondylosis with isolated neck pain exhibits a variable course. Symptoms generally wax and wane. Short-term relief is quite common. DePalma et al reported that 21% of patients had complete relief, 49% had partial relief, and 22% had no relief after 3 months of conventional nonoperative care.[14] Gore et al reported that, at a 10-year follow-up, 79% of patients improved, with 43% pain-free; 32%, however, had severe residual symptoms.[24]

Treatment

A number of nonoperative modalities are available in the treatment of cervical spondylosis and are usually used in combination. Rest and immobilization are used to reduce irritation of inflamed structures. A soft cervical collar can be used to maintain the neck in a neutral or slightly flexed position. Hyperextension of the neck may aggravate the patient's symptoms.[24] Nonsteroidal anti-inflammatory drugs play a useful role in the treatment of these patients. Muscle relaxants can be used as well in patients with definite muscle spasm. They should be used for brief periods only. Their efficacy in reducing muscle spasm (if that is a cause of pain) has not been clearly demonstrated.

Physical therapy is used routinely in the treatment of pain related to cervical spondylosis. During acute episodes, exercise may make the pain worse, but should be performed as tolerated. Aerobic exercise should be encouraged. Patients should be instructed in isometric neck-strengthening activities and to avoid positions that provoke symptoms. Modifications at the workplace, such as telephone headsets and elevated workstations, are sometimes helpful. Other modalities, such as heat, cold, ultrasonography, and transcutaneous electrical stimulation may be helpful, but there are no good randomized, controlled studies that show these modalities provide long-term pain relief. After the acute episode has resolved, exercises should be used to strengthen the cervical musculature in an effort to decrease the frequency of future episodes.

The neck pain of cervical spondylosis is generally cyclical. The initial episode usually responds to simple nonoperative measures within 2 to 3 weeks. Episodes of pain are frequently associated with periods of increased physical activity and generally respond to modification of these activities. More chronic conditions respond with less certain results.

Surgical treatment is rarely indicated for neck pain in the absence of radiculopathy or myelopathy. Cervical spine fusion may be considered in very select patients with incapacitating mechanical neck pain, and preferably, one-level involvement in patients younger than 40 years. Provocative discograms may help to identify the symptomatic level. Such surgery, however, is controversial. Evidence of focal cervical instability in the setting of limited cervical spondylosis may also be an indication for one-level fusion. In the future, modalities such as intradiscal electrothermal treatment, which is being studied in the lumbar spine, may be useful in the cervical spine. Currently, however, this modality remains experimental.

Differential Diagnosis

Tumor

Although cervical spondylosis is the most common cause of neck pain, other diseases must be considered in the differential diagnosis. Neck pain is the most common complaint of patients with tumors, which cause significant bony destruction. The pain is classically constant and often worse at night. Night pain is often used to distinguish between pain caused by tumors from that caused by spondylosis. However, the specificity and sensitivity of this symptom has not been studied. Destruction of structures that render the spine unstable may cause the pain to be worse with neck motion and activity. Direct nerve-root compression may result in typical radicular findings. Compression of the spinal cord may result in signs and symptoms of myelopathy. Neural deficits may be due to collapse of bony structures or extension of the tumor mass.

Metastatic lesions constitute, by far, the largest group of malignant bone tumors. Common primary sites

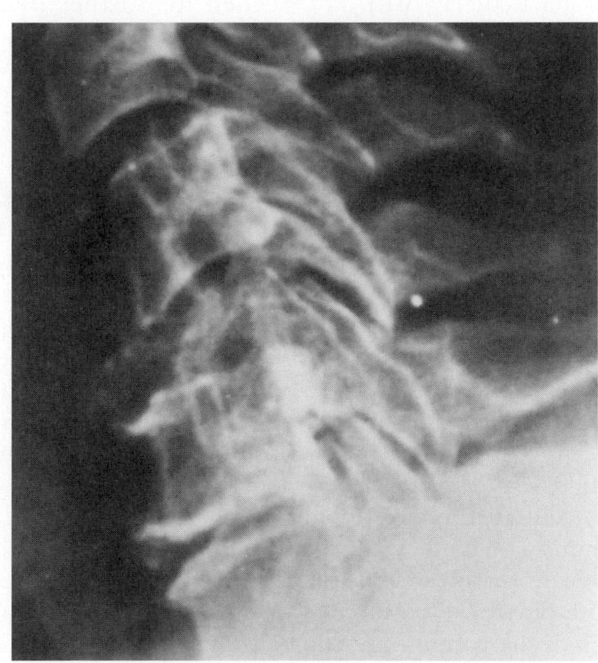

Figure 20–2. Metastatic lesion.

include the breast, prostate, lungs, thyroid, kidney, and parathyroid (Fig. 20–2). Primary bone tumors are rare in the cervical spine, accounting for only 1% of primary bone tumors. Primary malignant neoplasms of the cervical spine are extremely rare. Malignant tumors are frequently associated with large soft tissue masses and significant destruction. These often result in major neurologic deficits.

Tumors outside the cervical spine may mimic the signs and symptoms of spondylosis. Apical carcinomas of the lung (Pancoast tumors) may encroach upon the brachial plexus or subclavian vessels, causing shoulder pain, upper extremity weakness, and Horner syndrome. The classic sensory deficit is along the ulnar nerve distribution. These tumors are difficult to detect on routine chest film and frequently require apical lordotic views. Advanced imaging, such as CT and MRI, is often required.

Primary benign neoplasms include osteoid osteoma, osteoblastoma, and osteochondroma, all of which tend to occur in the posterior elements. Benign tumors of bone that occur in the vertebral body include hemangioma, fibrous dysplasia, eosinophilic granuloma, giant cell tumor, and aneurysmal bone cyst. Giant cell tumors and aneurysmal bone cysts may be associated with large soft tissue masses and significant lytic destruction.

Most symptomatic tumors of the cervical spine will be seen on radiographs, although bone scans may be positive earlier. Over 50% of bone mineral must be lost before a significant change is noted on plain films. Bone scans may useful to survey the remainder of the skeleton for metastatic lesions. It should be remembered that multiple myeloma is frequently cold on bone scan; CT, and particularly MRI, are needed for further delineation of these lesions. CT is helpful in the evaluation of the bony architecture. MRI best demonstrates an associated soft tissue mass, as well as the neural elements.

Infection

Patients with infection of the cervical spine present most commonly with neck pain. As with tumors, the pain is generally not relieved by rest. Often, the symptoms have persisted for several months or more. This is significant because 70% to 90% of patients with benign mechanical pain have resolution of their symptoms within a few months.[14,16,24] Concurrent symptoms may include fever, malaise, and weight loss. Vertebral osteomyelitis is seen more often in older, debilitated patients and intravenous drug users. A history of antecedent infection or immunologic compromise is common. The erythrocyte sedimentation rate and C-reactive protein are usually elevated, although the white blood cell count is often normal. Approximately 50% of the patients are clinically malnourished at presentation (albumin <3.5 g/dL, total lymphocyte count <1500/mm^3).[42]

Plain films are usually normal early in the course of the disease. This contributes to the delay in diagnosis, which unfortunately is common in osteomyelitis. Later, lytic lesions may be seen (Fig. 20–3*A*). These may span across the disc space, a finding that helps distinguish infection from tumor radiographically, as malignant lesions tend not to cross the disc space. Bone scans are positive early. Although CT scans are useful, MRI is now the study of choice in the evaluation of spinal infection, especially in the setting of concurrent neurologic findings (Fig. 20–3 *B* to *D*). Bony, as well as epidural, involvement is well seen, and the neural structures clearly identified.

Systemic Disorders

Inflammatory arthritides commonly involve the cervical spine and may lead to pain complaints, as well as focal, or generalized, stiffness. The pain and stiffness of the spondyloarthropathies is typically most severe in the morning and improves throughout the day. Cervical spine involvement is particularly common in patients with rheumatoid arthritis, especially those with longstanding polyarticular disease. Neck pain and occipital headaches are common complaints. These patients must be followed carefully for the development of myeloradiculopathy.

The bony changes in rheumatoid arthritis are destructive, rather than productive (as in osteoarthritis). Common radiographic findings include osteopenia and instability, both in the upper cervical spine and, to a lesser extent, in the subaxial cervical spine (Fig. 20–4*A*). Neurodiagnostic studies (CT myelography, MRI) are required when neurologic findings are present, or when significant instability is noted in the neurologically intact patient (Fig. 20–4*B*).

Neck pain can be a prominent symptom in metabolic diseases such as gout and renal osteodystrophy. Cervical spine involvement varies from minimal to severe destructive lesions. Treatment must be directed toward the cervical spine as well as correction of the underlying metabolic abnormality.

Fractures and Instabilities

The patient with acute cervical spine injury will have neck pain and tenderness, with or without associated neurologic deficit. Plain films should be obtained initially and include anterior-posterior, lateral, and odontoid views. Flexion-extension views are also recommended when static radiographs show no obvious fracture, dislocation, or subluxation. Dynamic radiographs may be difficult to obtain initially if the patient is in pain or is fearful of moving the neck. In most cases, dynamic radiographs in the acute setting should be done gently under the direct effort of the patient. No effort should be made to force a patient to move his or her neck if he or she is in considerable pain or is guarding the neck. Medical staff supervision is sometimes required. In the setting of a significant injury such as a motor vehicle accident or a fall from a height, bony injuries can be further defined by CT scan. Suspected disc herniation is evaluated by MRI. If the initial imaging studies are unrevealing, a hard collar can be worn for 7 to 14 days and repeat dynamic evaluation performed after the acute muscle spasm has resolved.

Patients presenting with neck pain long after the time of the injury also require plain films, including lateral flexion-extension views to assess for chronic instability (Fig. 20–5). An open-mouth odontoid view should be obtained, because nondisplaced odontoid fractures can be missed on initial evaluation. Advanced imaging should be considered if there are significant findings on clinical history or physical examination, or if pain is longstanding and unremitting.

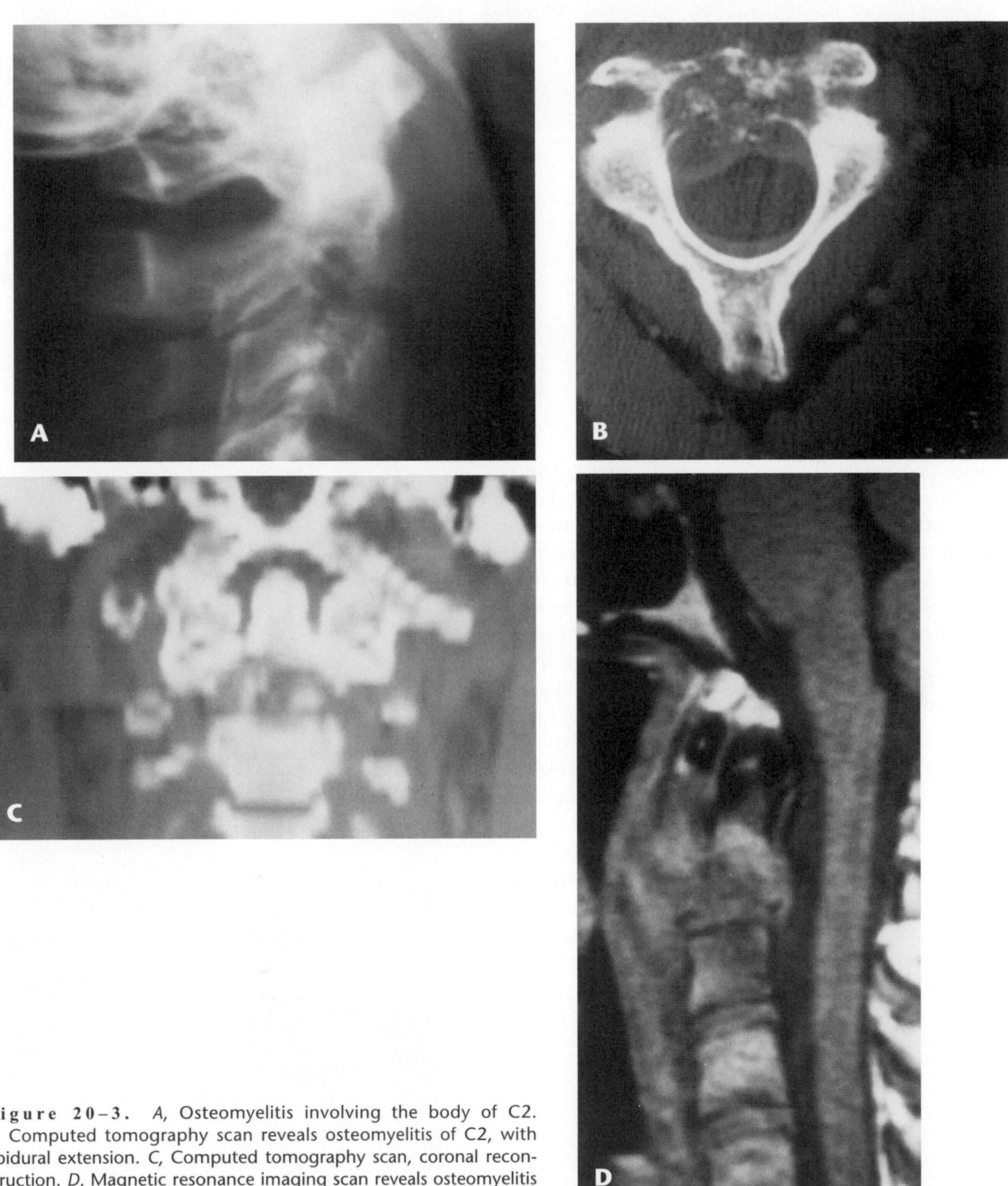

Figure 20–3. *A*, Osteomyelitis involving the body of C2. *B*, Computed tomography scan reveals osteomyelitis of C2, with epidural extension. *C*, Computed tomography scan, coronal reconstruction. *D*, Magnetic resonance imaging scan reveals osteomyelitis of C2, with epidural extension.

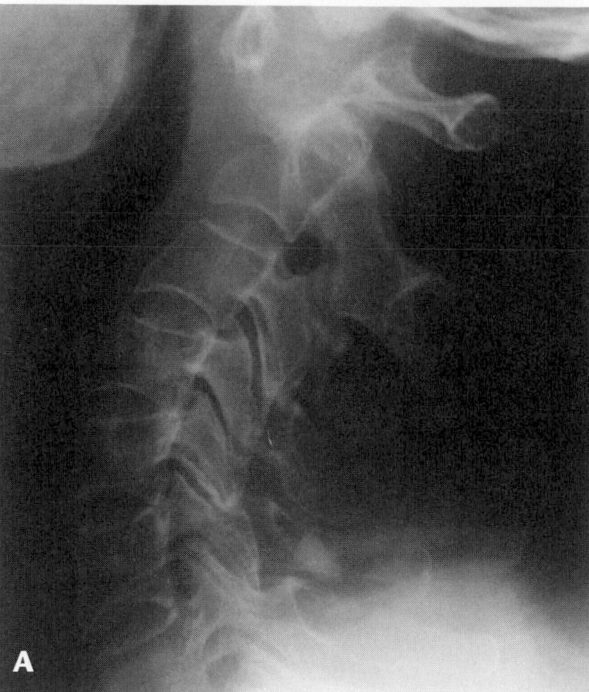

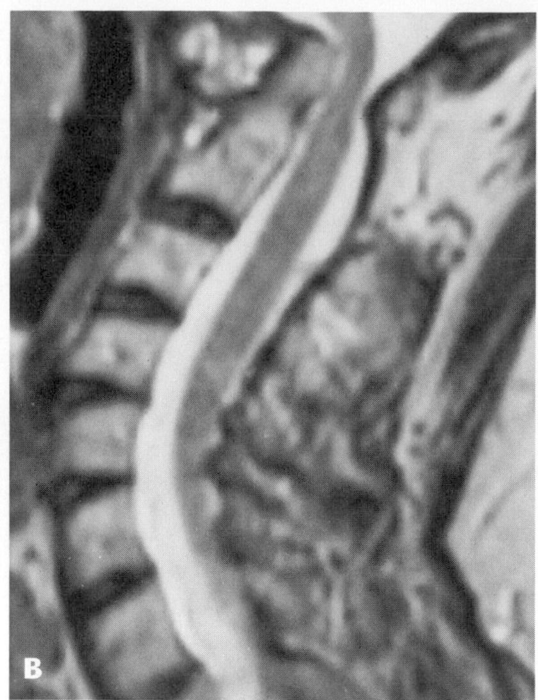

Figure 20–4. *A*, Rheumatoid arthritis, C1-2 instability. *B*, Rheumatoid pannus in the atlanto-dens interval; decreased space available for the cord at C1-2.

Arm Pain

The patient with cervical spondylosis may initially complain of arm pain. This can be referred pain secondary to degenerative joint disease, without evidence of nerve root involvement. It is, however, more commonly described as a shooting, radicular pain associated with numbness and paresthesias in a dermatomal distribution. Focal neurologic findings referable to a specific nerve root may be identified. Nerve root compression may be due to uncovertebral osteophytes (hard disc), herniation of degenerative discs (soft disc), spondylotic bars, or a combination of these. In cervical spondylosis, multiple nerve root involvement may occur.

Acute, isolated cervical disc herniation is a separate entity. This is usually a posterolateral herniation in patients younger than 50 years. There is usually a specific onset of the symptoms, regardless of whether a traumatic event is noted. In acute cervical disc herniation, single nerve root deficits are common. Each nerve root is associated with a specific set of symptoms and signs (Table 20–1).

Associated Tests

A number of provocative tests can be performed to elicit radicular symptoms (Table 20–2). The axial compression test is a provocative maneuver performed by applying axial pressure on the top of the patient's head. A positive response includes neck, and more importantly, arm pain. This is generally seen in the setting of disc herniation or neuroforaminal encroachment of the nerve root. The Spurling Maneuver consists of compression of the patient's head with the neck extended

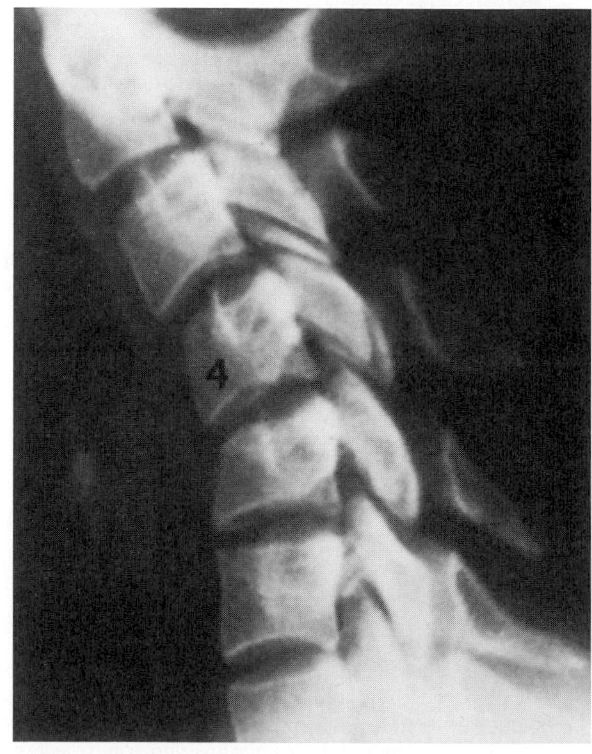

Figure 20–5. Posterior instability, C4-5.

TABLE 20–1
Cervical Root Findings

Root	Arm Distribution	Neck/Upper Trunk Distribution	Reflex	Motor
C4	None	Cape of neck/anterior chest	None	Diaphragm
C5	Shoulder/Upper lateral arm	Neck/shoulder junction	Some biceps	Deltoid
C6	Lateral forearm to thumb and index finger	Proximal portion of scapula	Biceps	Biceps, Wrist extension
C7	Forearm into Long finger	Midportion of scapula	Triceps	Elbow extenson Wrist extension
C8	Fprearm to ring and small fingers	Medical and inferior portion of scapula	None	finger flexion Grip strength
T1	Medial aspect of arm	Non-specific	None	Intrinsics

Adapted from Garfin SR: Cervical degenerative disorders: etiology, presentation and imaging studies. Instructional Course Lectures 49:335–338, 2000, with permission.

and rotated to the side of the radicular pain. A positive test produces radiating arm pain and suggests spinal nerve root entrapment in the neuroforamen. The cervical distraction test is performed by gradually distracting the patient's head. Patients with nerve root compression from herniated discs or neuroforaminal narrowing may note diminution of pain, because the distraction maneuver tends to enlarge the neuroforamen and decrease the load across the facet joints. The shoulder abduction relief test is performed by passively abducting the patient's involved arm. This reduces nerve root tension and relieves arm pain in many patients with cervical radiculopathy due to extradural compression.

Neurologic Evaluation

The examination of the upper extremity by neurologic levels is directly related to the physical examination of the cervical spine. Motor, sensory, and reflex activity, if appropriate, should be assessed at each root level. The critical importance of this examination warrants a review of these levels (Fig. 20–6).

The C5 nerve root innervates the deltoid muscle and, along with C6, the biceps muscle. It supplies sensation to the lateral arm (over the shoulder) and is primarily responsible for the biceps reflex. Patients with C5 radiculopathy may complain of shoulder pain and weakness. Loss of shoulder function creates a significant functional deficit. Some physicians recommend early (6 weeks) decompression for C5 radiculopathy with significant neurologic findings.

The C6 nerve root innervates the wrist extensors and, along with C5, the biceps muscle. The C6 sensory distribution includes the lateral forearm, the thumb, the index finger, and occasionally part of the middle finger. The posterior ramus of C6, as well as those of C7 and C8, supply sensation to the region overlying the scapula. The associated reflex at this level is the brachioradialis.

The C7 motor distribution includes the triceps muscle, the wrist flexors, and the finger extensors. C7 provides sensation to the middle finger and is primarily responsible for the triceps reflex.

The C8 neurologic level includes motor innervation of the middle finger flexors and the interossei. The sensory supply is to the ulnar side of the hand and the

TABLE 20–2
Tests Suggestive of Disk Herniation

Test	Maneuver
Spurling's sign	Neck axial compression with chin rotation toward the symptomatic side reproduces radiating arm pain
Axial compression test	Applying axial load through the examiner's hands on the head reproduces radicular pain
Shoulder abduction relief sign	Patient abducys the shoulder and flexes the elbow with hand behind head to relieve radicular symptoms

Adapted from Garfin SR: Cervical degenerative disorders: etiology, presentation and imaging studies. Instructional Course Lectures 49:335–338, 2000, with permission.

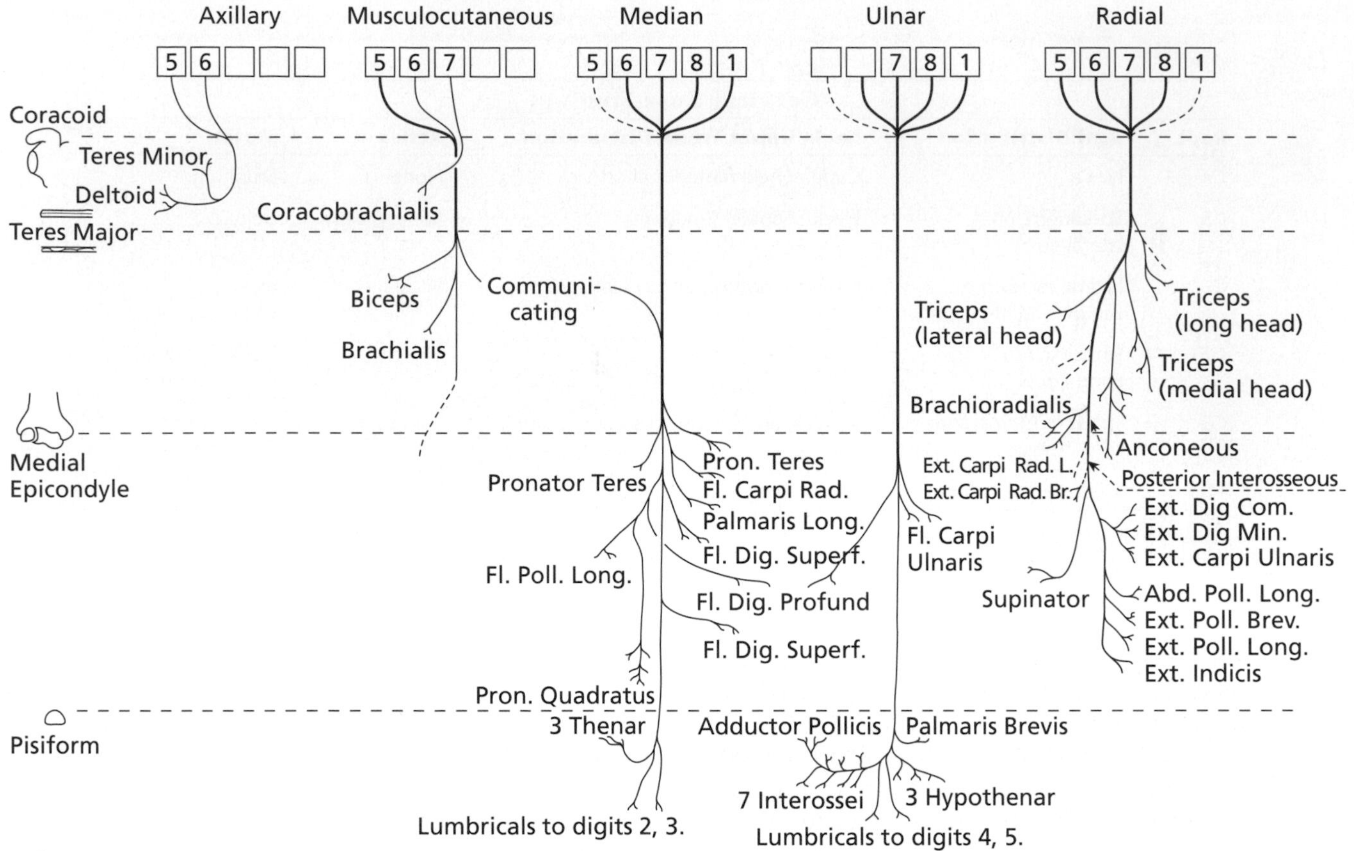

Figure 20–6. Motor innervation of the upper extremity (courtesy American Medical Association).

distal half of the ulnar aspect of the forearm. There is no reflex test for the C8 level.

The T1 level provides motor innervation of the interossei. Sensory supply is to the ulnar side of the proximal forearm and distal arm. There is no associated deep tendon reflex. Loss of intrinsic hand function creates a significant functional deficit, and many surgeons recommend early (6 weeks) decompression if marked neurologic deficit is present.

Natural History

Several studies on the natural history of cervical radiculopathy show that the majority of patients improve significantly over time. However, about one-third of patients have persistent or worsening pain. Lees and Turner reported in their classic article that 45% of patients had full resolution of their symptoms, 30% had mild continuing symptoms, and 25% had worsening of symptoms.[35] No patients progressed to myelopathy over 19 years of follow-up. DePalma and Subin reported a 5-year study of nonoperative management for cervical spondylosis and disc herniation in 311 patients. Overall, 29% of patients had resolution of symptoms, 49% had some improvement, and 22% had no improvement.[16] In a prospective study of 26 patients, nonoperative treatment consisting of traction, anti-inflammatory medication, physical therapy, and patient education led to a high success rate.[41] The majority of patients did not have surgery (24/26). Another series that reviewed nonoperatively treated athletes with acute cervical radiculopathy showed that 17 of 20 returned to full activity at an average of 17 weeks. Neurologic deficits took up to 5 months to improve.[40,43]

Diagnosis

Plain films are obtained initially (Fig. 20–7*A*). These are followed by either MRI or CT myelography, if surgery is being considered (Fig. 20–7*B*). MRI is superior for evaluating soft tissue structures, such as discs and the neural elements, and provides information on the intrinsic status of the spinal cord as well. The CT myelogram adds a dynamic quality, because the passage of dye can be followed. The CT scan also provides the best evaluation of the bony anatomy. Carefully performed EMG and NCV studies can be useful to confirm radiculopathy and rule out peripheral neuropathy or systemic illness such as amyotrophic lateral sclerosis. EMG/NCV should not be routinely performed, as the clinical history and examination often clarifies the diagnosis.

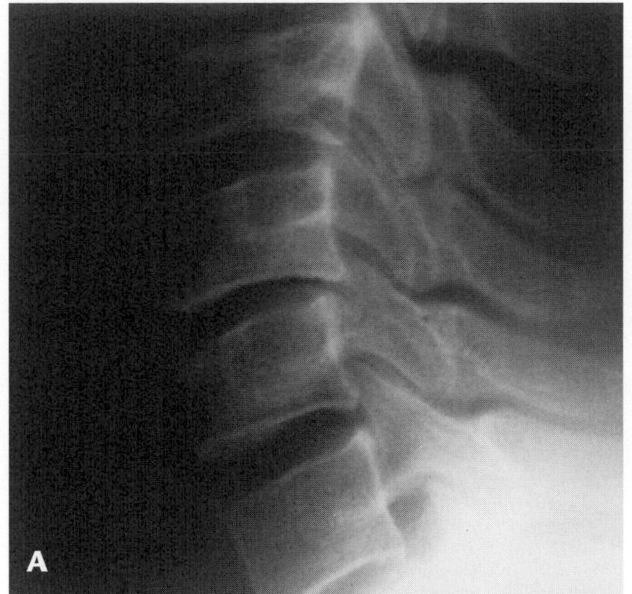

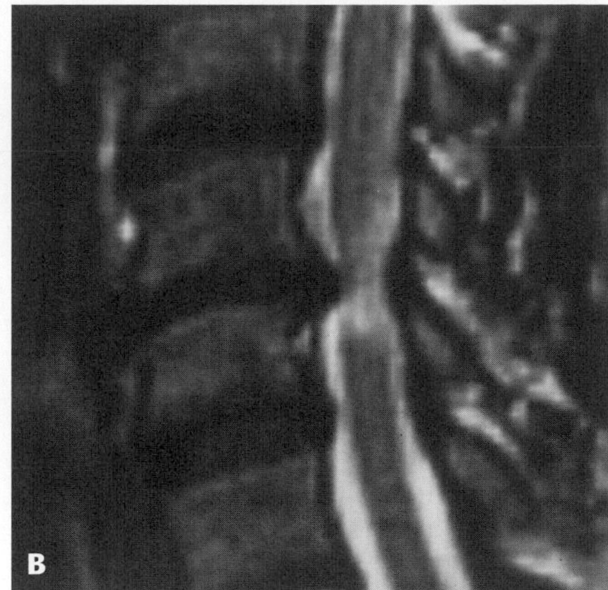

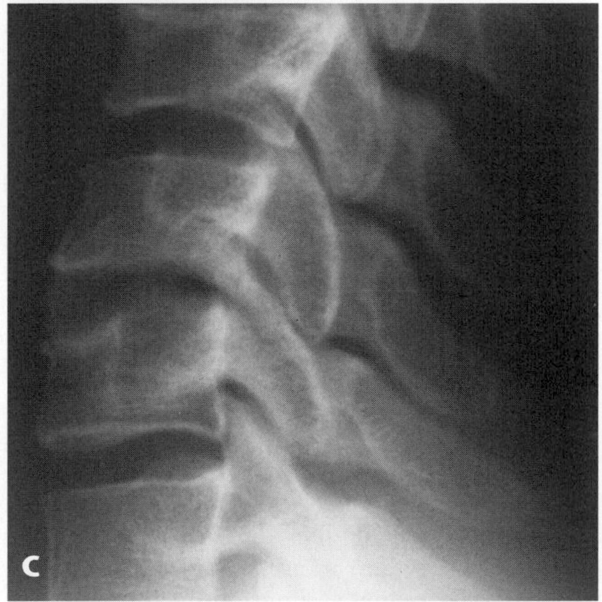

Figure 20–7. *A*, Decreased disc space, C5-6. *B*, Disc herniation, C5-6; myelomalacia of spinal cord. *C*, Status post C5-6 anterior discectomy and fusion.

Treatment

The nonoperative modalities used are the same as described for cervical spondylosis; namely, rest and immobilization, physical therapy after the acute episode has abated, anti-inflammatory medication, and time. The use of epidural steroid injections has been shown to be useful. Bush et al treated 68 patients with an average of 39 months of follow-up.[7] After an average of 2.5 injections, 76% had resolution of arm pain and the remainder had decreased pain. MRI evaluation of patients with herniated nucleus pulposus showed resorption of the disk bulge after epidural steroid injection.[6]

The primary indication for the surgical management of cervical spondylotic radiculopathy and cervical disc disease is nerve root compression with persistent radicular signs and symptoms that is not responsive to nonoperative measures. The findings on physical examination should correspond to the findings on neurodiagnostic studies. Early surgical intervention should be considered for more severe neurologic deficits, and certainly with progression of the neurologic deficit. Some recommend intervention at 6 weeks if the C5 and C8 nerve roots are involved, because of the significant loss of function associated with neurologic compromise at these levels.[27]

The surgical approaches for cervical radiculopathy include anterior discectomy and fusion and numerous posterior procedures. These include foraminotomy with or without lateral free fragment discectomy for single level disease and multilevel foraminotomy, laminectomy, and laminoplasty for multilevel involvement. Both approaches achieve excellent results when properly performed. To a certain extent, the choice depends on the

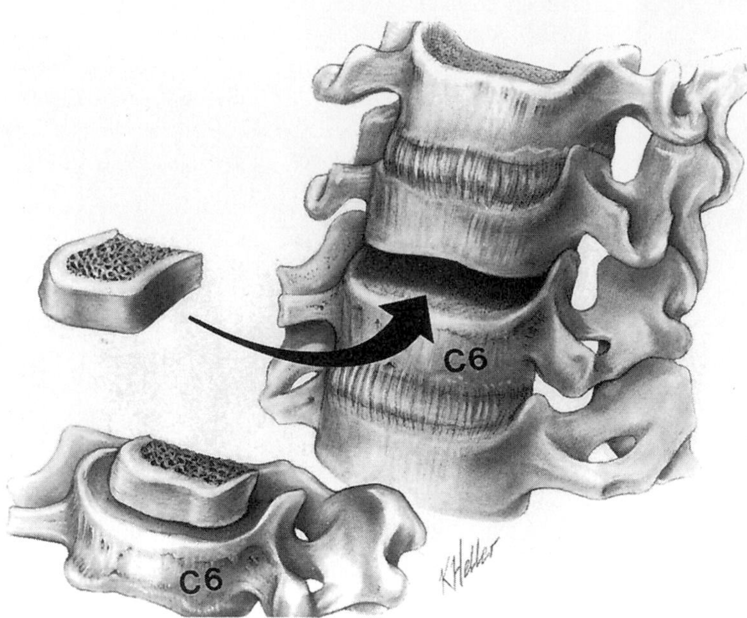

Figure 20–8. Anterior cervical discectomy and fusion. (From Abitbol JJ, Garfin SR: Semin Spine Surg 1:233, 1989.)

preference of the surgeon. If there is one level, unilateral involvement, with radiculopathy alone, and no associated neck pain or instability, the posterior foraminotomy approach may be chosen, particularly if the pathoanatomic compression is primarily posterolateral. The anterior approach is preferred if there is concurrent instability at the involved level that requires decompression and stabilization, associated neck pain, midline pathology, or bilateral involvement. The anterior approach has the added benefit of opening the neuroforamen by widening the disc space using a well-fashioned bone graft (Figs. 20–7*C* and 20–8).

Differential Diagnosis

Tumor and Infection

Cervical disc disease is the most common cause of cervical radiculopathy. Nonetheless, many other conditions can have similar findings. The spectrum of cervical spine tumors was reviewed in the discussion on neck pain. Bony collapse, extension of the tumor mass, and local inflammatory reaction can all cause nerve root compression, with subsequent radicular pain and neurologic findings.

Schwannomas and meningiomas are rarely seen in the cervical region, but when present, frequently occur with radicular symptoms. Schwannomas arise from the spinal nerve root and tend to compress the root at the level of the neuroforamen. Meningiomas, too, arise in the region of the dorsal root, and can be compressive in the neuroforamen. Both may cause bony foraminal enlargement seen on oblique radiographs, CT scan, or MRI.

Infection, like tumor, can cause nerve root compression on the basis of bony collapse or extension of disease into the epidural space. Primary epidural abscess can also result in radicular findings. Clinical suspicion must be high with any patient who has constant, unremitting neck pain associated with neurologic deficits.

Entrapment Syndromes

The peripheral nerves of the upper extremity may be compressed at specific sites along their course. This can produce sensory and motor findings in characteristic patterns. The median, ulnar, and radial nerves, and their branches, may all be involved at various levels. These syndromes can mimic cervical radiculopathy, but careful examination will reveal deficits referable to peripheral nerves and not nerve roots. The other peripheral nerves innervated by the nerve roots in question will be normal. Provocative testing, combined with EMG and NCV studies, will help distinguish between radiculopathy and peripheral compressive neuropathies.

Thoracic Outlet Syndrome

Thoracic outlet syndrome is an entity characterized by intermittent vascular or neurologic compromise in the upper extremity due to compression of the subclavian vessels or the lower two nerve roots (C8, T1) of the brachial plexus. Occasionally, a cervical rib may be palpable in the supraclavicular fossa. Compression of these neurovascular structures as they pass between the scalenus anticus and scalenus medius muscles can also cause this syndrome. Vasomotor symptoms usually affect the radial side of the hand, whereas neurologic symptoms usually involve the ulnar side of the hand. One maneuver to assess this compression is the Adson test. The patient's radial pulse is palpated and noted before and after the arm is passively abducted, extended, and externally rotated. The patient is then told to turn his or her head toward the arm in question. Diminution or loss of the pulse suggests compression of the subclavian artery and a possible diagnosis of thoracic outlet syndrome.

Brachial Neuritis

Patients with idiopathic brachial neuritis generally have unilateral neck and shoulder pain that, within 2 weeks, is followed by significant upper extremity weakness. The axillary, long thoracic, and suprascapular nerves are most often involved. Shoulder abductor weakness is common and often the brachial plexus is tender in either the supraclavicular fossa or axilla. Electrodiagnostic studies are helpful in establishing the diagnosis. The etiology is unknown (possibly viral). It often follows a systemic illness or a period of stress (e.g., surgery). The disease process is frequently self-limited over weeks to months. Anti-inflammatory medication may be helpful in reducing the symptoms. This is also called Parsonage-Turner syndrome.[37]

Shoulder Disease

Numerous disorders of the shoulder girdle cause local pain and weakness. These symptoms may mimic proximal cervical radiculopathy. The physical examination can usually help distinguish between shoulder and spine pathology, but it may be confusing, particularly if there are concurrent processes. Tenderness is usually present with rotator cuff tears, subacromial bursitis, impingement syndrome, and degenerative disease of the acromioclavicular and glenohumeral joints. Shoulder weakness is generally due to pain, spasm, or in the proper clinical setting, a large rotator cuff tear. Once again, electrodiagnostic or imaging studies may help distinguish cervical spine radiculopathy from primary shoulder pathology (see Chapter 21).

Myelopathy

The degenerative changes seen with advanced cervical spondylosis may be associated with compression of the spinal cord, causing CSM. CSM is the most common cause of spinal cord dysfunction in patients older than 55 years.[9,10,22,35,39] The spinal canal may be narrowed by degenerative disc bulges with or without herniation, transverse bony bars adjacent to the disc, osteophytes, or facet and ligamentum flavum hypertrophy. Subluxation also decreases the space available for the spinal cord. This pathology may occur at single or multiple levels.

CSM exhibits a protracted course with episodic progression.[9,10,22,35] There can be long periods without progression and even regression. Conversely, mild trauma, such as a minimal hyperextension injury, can produce a acute neurologic deterioration. In their classic article, Clarke and Robinson reported that 75% of patients had episodic symptoms, 20% had slow progression, and 5% had rapid deterioration.[10] Early diagnosis may be important because the results of treatment are related to the severity of the condition and the duration of findings.[31]

Generalized upper and lower extremity weakness, especially in concert with gait disturbance and bladder dysfunction, suggests myelopathy. Early findings may include neck pain; numb, cold, or painful hands; decreased fine motor skills; and subtle gait disturbances (broad-based). Some patients may exhibit a mild scissoring gait or describe a perceived loss of control. Others describe a foot drop, or slapping, when they walk, or an inability to internally or externally rotate a lower extremity smoothly. Radiculopathy and myelopathy may also coexist.

The findings on physical examination are those of cervical spondylosis in general, with the addition of pathologic upper motor neuron reflexes in both the upper and lower extremities. Neck range of motion is generally decreased, particularly in extension. Weakness may be present in the upper or lower extremities. Decreased vibratory sense and proprioception are subtle signs seen early in the course of myelopathy.

A number of physical examination findings assist in identifying hyperreflexia, which can be due to any upper motor neuron lesion including cervical myelopathy (Table 20–3). Clonus is a rhythmic, repetitive oscillation of the ankle in response to sudden, maintained dorsiflexion of the foot and stretching of the Achilles tendon. The Babinski test involves firmly stroking the plantar surface of the foot with a sharp instrument, starting from the heel and proceeding distally along the lateral aspect of the sole and then medially across the forefoot. The normal, or negative, response consists of no movement or downward motion of the toes. A positive response consists of extension of the great toe and spreading (fanning) of the lesser toes. The Hoffman sign is a pathologic reflex that is elicited in the upper extremity. The hand is held in a comfortable resting position, and the nail of the middle finger is "flicked." A positive reaction consists of flexion of the terminal phalanx of the thumb and index finger. The inverted radial reflex is elicited by hitting the radial

TABLE 20–3

Tests Suggestive of Myelopathy

Test	Maneuver
Clonus	Sudden dorsiflexion of foot produces sustained rhythmic beating of foot into plantar flexion
Babinski's test	Firm, irritating stroke with pointed instrument on the lateral base of foot across to the medial side of the forefoot. Negative test (normal) consists of no movement or downward movement of toes. A positive test (abnormal) consists of extension of the great toe and spreading (fanning) of the lesser toes.
Inverted radial reflex	With brachioradialis reflex examination, the fingers and thumbs flex
Hoffman's sign	With the patient's hand relaxed (as if gently grasping a can), the examiner flicks the distal inter-phalangeal joint of the long finger. A negative sign (normal) causes no movement of the fingers. A positive sign (abnormal) causes the index, ring, and thumb fingers to flex together.
finger escape sign	When the patient attempts to actively extend and abduct the fingers, the ring and small fingers flex and abduct.
L'Hermitte's sign	Neck flexion and axial compression through the examiner's hand leads to radiating pain the arms and or legs.

Adapted from Garfin SR: Cervical degenerative disorders: etiology, presentation and imaging studies. Instructional Course Lectures 49:335–338, 2000, with permission.

aspect of the forearm (brachioradialis muscle) and observing a grasp-type reaction of the hand. If pathologic reflexes are elicited in the lower extremity and the Hoffman sign is negative, this may suggest that the problem lies below the level of the cervical spinal cord. This would be further supported by hyperreflexia limited to the lower extremities.

Findings more specific for cervical myelopathy include the Lhermitte sign and the finger escape sign (Table 20–3). The Lhermitte sign is characterized by shock-like pains radiating down the arms or legs with passive flexion and compression of the neck. The Lhermitte sign is positive in 27% of patients with cervical myelopathy.[13] "Myelopathy Hand" refers to the loss of power of adduction and extension of the ulnar two or three fingers owing to weak intrinsics.[18,39] These fingers may spontaneously abduct, giving rise to the "finger escape sign." These findings, together with hyperreflexia, are suggestive of cervical myelopathy, usually above the C6-7 level.

Plain films, including flexion/extension views, are obtained initially (Fig. 20–9*A*). In the setting of myelopathy, neurodiagnostic evaluation with CT myelography or MRI is needed to search for sites of cord compression. MRI also provides information on the intrinsic status of the spinal cord (Fig. 20–9*B*).

Treatment

All of the nonoperative modalities discussed for cervical spondylosis can be used in these patients. Improvement of sensory and motor deficits has been reported in 33% to 50% of patients with CSM treated nonoperatively.[1,13,38] Such improvement, however, is generally mild to moderate. Furthermore, it is difficult to predict the pattern and timing of progression. Because the results of surgical treatment are related to the duration of myelopathic findings, there is general agreement that early surgical intervention is indicated for myelopathy, especially with documented neurologic progression.[31,33,35]

The decompression of CSM can be performed from the anterior or posterior approaches. Anterior procedures include decompressive discectomy and corpectomy, followed by fusion (Fig. 20–9*C* and *D*). Posterior procedures include laminectomy (with or without fusion) and laminoplasty. The side of maximal compression (anterior or posterior) should be determined on preoperative imaging studies. Generally, if the impingement is anterior, as it often is, an anterior approach should be utilized. If the impingement is posterior, as with hypertrophied ligamentum flavum or ossification of the posterior longitudinal ligament, a posterior approach should be used.

The posterior approach should be avoided, if possible, in the patient with a kyphotic cervical spine. In this situation, the spinal cord is draped over the spondylotic discs and vertebrae anteriorly, resulting in direct spinal cord compression, and possibly ischemic compromise as well. Posterior decompression cannot address this pathoanatomy. Additionally, with loss of the posterior elements, further progression of the deformity, as well as symptoms and signs, may occur.[26] Some authors reserve the posterior approach for patients with three

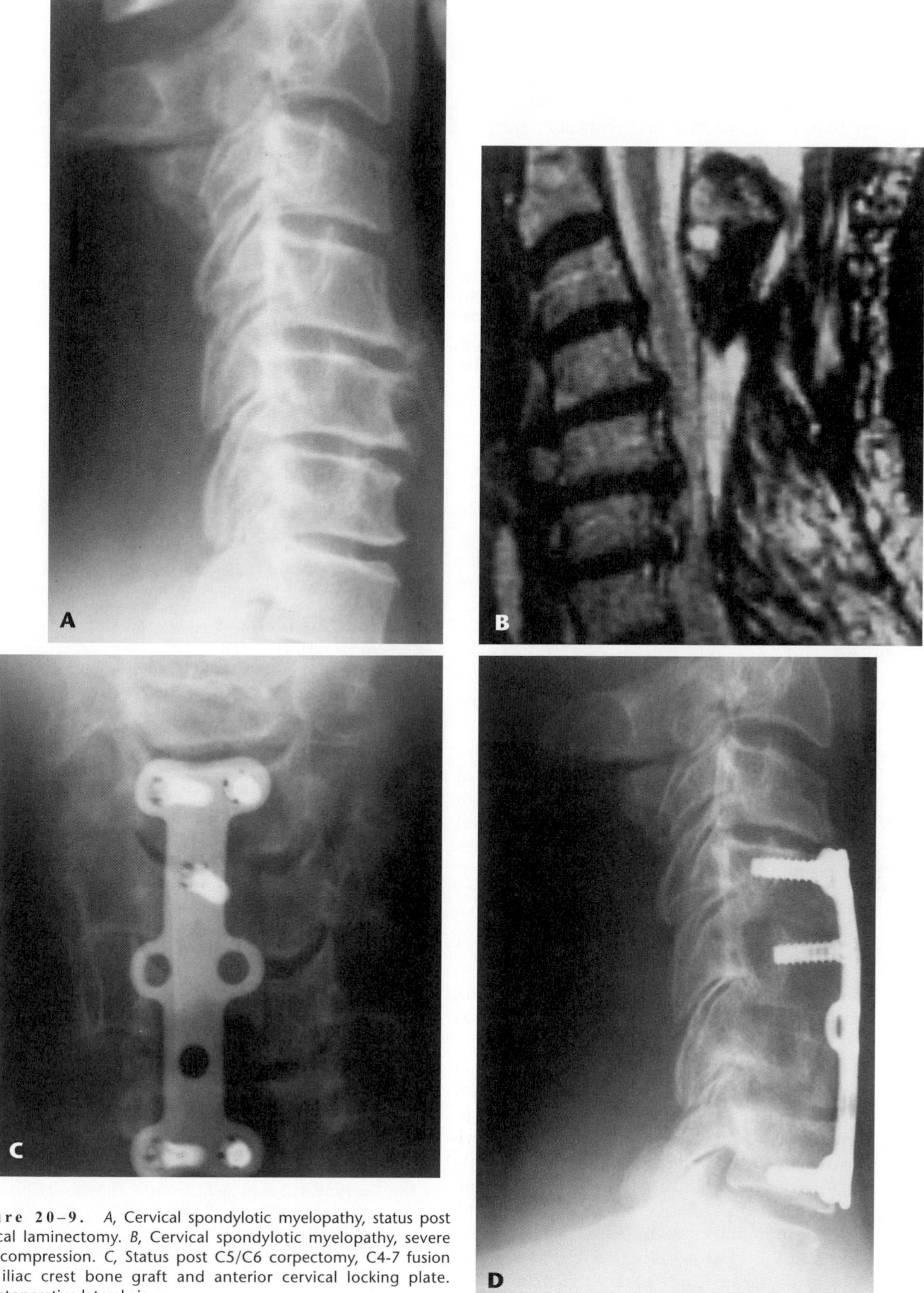

Figure 20–9. *A*, Cervical spondylotic myelopathy, status post cervical laminectomy. *B*, Cervical spondylotic myelopathy, severe cord compression. *C*, Status post C5/C6 corpectomy, C4-7 fusion with iliac crest bone graft and anterior cervical locking plate. *D*, Postoperative lateral view.

or more involved levels, particularly in stiff spines, and in elderly patients.[38]

The results of surgical decompression for CSM are generally good. Numerous reports document improvement in 70% to 90% of patients.[4,15,19,20,21,25,28–30,32,34,36] Neurologic return may be seen as late as 1 to 2 years after surgery. Anterior surgery tends to provide greater long-term relief than posterior decompression.[44] The primary goal, however, is to arrest the progressive myelopathic process.

Differential Diagnosis

As discussed in previous sections, tumor and infection, particularly epidural abscess, can cause acute or progressive myelopathy. These entities, however, are generally easily distinguished from CSM on imaging studies. One should always be alert to the possibility of concurrent tumor or infection in the patient with CSM, especially in the setting of an acute episode of pain and neurologic deficit in a previously stable patient.

The involvement of the cervical spine in rheumatoid arthritis was also discussed earlier. Owing to the instability that may develop in either the upper or subaxial cervical spine, myelopathy, with or without radiculopathy, is not an uncommon presentation. These patients are generally severely affected with polyarticular disease. Deformity of the extremities makes neurologic assessment difficult and unreliable. Nonetheless, distinguishing these patients from those with CSM is generally not difficult, based on clinical examination and diagnostic features on imaging studies.

Multiple sclerosis can present with acute sensory and motor loss in the extremities and can mimic cervical myelopathy. These patients are generally younger, with the average age at onset of 32 years. Frequent associated findings include central vision loss, diplopia, incoordination, and chronic fatigue.

Summary

Cervical disc disease and cervical spondylosis are the most common causes of neck and arm pain, as well as upper extremity radiculopathy and myelopathy. The diagnosis is based mainly on the clinical history and physical examination. There is often poor correlation between the clinical picture and radiographic findings. Imaging studies are useful only as confirmatory evidence of disease, for preoperative planning, and to rule out other causes of symptoms, such as tumor, infection, or trauma. Evaluation and treatment must be individualized. Reasonable outcomes can be expected generally, although certainly not uniformly. Early diagnosis of myelopathy is important because early surgical intervention enhances the likelihood of obtaining a good result, or at least preventing continued deterioration.

References

1. Boden S, Wiesel W: Conservative treatment for cervical disc disease. Semin Spine Surg 1:229–232, 1989.
2. Boden SD, McCowin PR, Davis DO, et al: Abnormal magnetic resonance imaging scans of the cervical spine in asymptomatic subjects. A prospective investigation [see comments]. J Bone Joint Surg Am 72:1178–1184, 1990.
3. Bradshaw P: Some aspects of cervical spondylosis. Q J Med 2:177–208, 1957.
4. Brigham CD, Tsahakis PJ: Anterior cervical foraminotomy and fusion. Surgical technique and results. Spine 20:766–770, 1995.
5. Buckwalter JA: Aging and degeneration of the human intervertebral disc. Spine 20:1307–1314, 1995.
6. Bush K, Chaudhuri R, Hillier S, Penny J: The pathomorphologic changes that accompany the resolution of cervical radiculopathy. A prospective study with repeat magnetic resonance imaging [see comments]. Spine 22:183–186; discussion 187, 1997.
7. Bush K, Hillier S: Outcome of cervical radiculopathy treated with periradicular/epidural corticosteroid injections: A prospective study with independent clinical review. Eur Spine J 5:319–325, 1996.
8. Campbell A, Phillips D: Cervical disc lesions with neurological disorder: Differential diagnosis, treatment, and prognosis. Br Med J 2:481–485, 1960.
9. Clark CR: Cervical spondylotic myelopathy: History and physical findings. Spine 13:847–849, 1988.
10. Clarke E, Robinson P: Cervical myelopathy: A complication of cervical spondylosis. Brain 79:483–510, 1956.
11. Coventry M, Ghormley R, Kernohan J: The intervertebral disc: Its microscopic anatomy and pathology: Part II—Changes in the interververtebral disc concomitant with age. J Bone Joint Surg Am 27A:233–247, 1945.
12. Coventry M, Ghormley R, Kernohan J: The intervertebral disc: Its microscopic anatomy and pathology: Part III—Pathologic changes in the intervertebral disc. J Bone Joint Surg Am 27A:460–474, 1945.
13. Crandall PH, Batzdorf U: Cervical spondylotic myelopathy. J Neurosurg 25:57–66, 1966.
14. DePalma AF, Rothman RH, Levitt RL, Hammond NL: The natural history of severe cervical disc degeneration. Acta Orthop Scand 43:392–396, 1972.
15. DePalma AF, Rothman RH, Lewinnek GE, Canale ST: Anterior interbody fusion for severe cervical disc degeneration. Surg Gynecol Obstet 134:755–758, 1972.
16. DePalma AF, Subin DK: Study of the cervical syndrome. Clin Orthop 38:1351–1342, 1965.
17. Dillane J, Fry J, Kaiton G: Acute back syndrome: A study from general practice. Br Med J 3:82–84, 1966.
18. Ebara S, Yonenobu K, Fujiwara K, et al: Myelopathy hand characterized by muscle wasting. A different type of myelopathy hand in patients with cervical spondylosis. Spine 13:785–791, 1988.
19. Emery S: Anterior approach for cervical myelopathy. In Clark C, Ducker T, Dvorak J, et al (eds): The Cervical Spine, 3rd ed. Philadelphia, Lippincott-Raven, 1998, pp 825–837.
20. Emery SE, Bohlman HH, Bolesta MJ, Jones PK: Anterior cervical decompression and arthrodesis for the treatment of cervical spondylotic myelopathy. Two to seventeen-year follow-up. J Bone Joint Surg Am 80:941–951, 1998.
21. Emery SE, Fisher JR, Bohlman HH: Three-level anterior cervical discectomy and fusion: Radiographic and clinical results. Spine 22:2622–2624; discussion 2625, 1997.
22. Epstein J, Epstein N: The surgical management of cervical spinal stenosis, spondylosis, and myeloradiculopathy by means of the posterior approach. In Sherk H, Dunn E, Eismont F (eds): The Cervical Spine, 2nd ed. Philadelphia, JB Lippincott, 1989, pp 625–643.

23. Garfin SR: Cervical degenerative disorders: Etiology, presentation, and imaging studies. Instructional Course Lectures 49:335–338, 2000.
24. Gore DR, Sepic SB, Gardner GM, Murray MP: Neck pain: A long-term follow-up of 205 patients. Spine 12:1–5, 1987.
25. Hanai K, Fujiyoshi F, Kamei K: Subtotal vertebrectomy and spinal fusion for cervical spondylotic myelopathy. Spine 11:310–315, 1986.
26. Herkowitz HN: A comparison of anterior cervical fusion, cervical laminectomy, and cervical laminoplasty for the surgical management of multiple level spondylotic radiculopathy. Spine 13:774–780, 1988.
27. Herkowitz HN: The surgical management of cervical spondylotic radiculopathy and myelopathy. Clin Orthop 239:94–108, 1989.
28. Hirabayashi K, Bohlman HH: Multilevel cervical spondylosis. Laminoplasty versus anterior decompression. Spine 20:1732–1734, 1995.
29. Hirabayashi K, Miyakawa J, Satomi K, et al: Operative results and postoperative progression of ossification among patients with ossification of cervical posterior longitudinal ligament. Spine 6:354–364, 1981.
30. Hirabayashi K, Watanabe K, Wakano K, et al: Expansive open-door laminoplasty for cervical spinal stenotic myelopathy. Spine 8:693–699, 1983.
31. Irvine D, Foster J, Newell D, Klukvin B: Prevalence of cervical spondylosis in a general practice. Lancet 1:1089–1092, 1965.
32. Kurz LT, Herkowitz HN: Surgical management of myelopathy. Orthop Clin North Am 23:495–504, 1992.
33. Lawrence JS: Disc degeneration. Its frequency and relationship to symptoms. Ann Rheum Dis 28:121–138, 1969.
34. Lee TT, Manzano GR, Green BA: Modified open-door cervical expansive laminoplasty for spondylotic myelopathy: Operative technique, outcome, and predictors for gait improvement. J Neurosurg 86:64–68, 1997.
35. Lees F, Turner J: Natural history and prognosis of cervical spondylosis. Br Med J 11:1607–1610, 1963.
36. Lunsford LD, Bissonette DJ, Zorub DS: Anterior surgery for cervical disc disease. Part 2: Treatment of cervical spondylotic myelopathy in 32 cases. J Neurosurg 53:12–19, 1980.
37. Misamore GW, Lehman DE: Parsonage-Turner syndrome (acute brachial neuritis). J Bone Joint Surg Am 78:1405–1408, 1996.
38. Nurick S: The natural history and the results of surgical treatment of the spinal cord disorder associated with cervical spondylosis. Brain 95:101–108, 1972.
39. Ono K, Ebara S, Fuji T, et al: Myelopathy hand. New clinical signs of cervical cord damage. J Bone Joint Surg Br 69:215–219, 1987.
40. Phillips DG: Surgical treatment of myelopathy with cervical spondylosis. J Neurol Neurosurg Psychiatry 36:879–884, 1973.
41. Saal JS, Saal JA, Yurth EF: Non-operative management of herniated cervical intervertebral disc with radiculopathy. Spine 21:1877–1883, 1996.
42. Simeone F: Surgical management of cervical disc disease: Posterior approach. Semin Spine Surg 1:239–244, 1989.
43. Simpson J, An H: Degenerative disc disease of the cervical spine. In An H, Simpson J (eds): Surgery of the Cervical Spine. London, Martin Dunitz, 1994, pp 181–194.
44. White AA, Southwick WO, Deponte RJ, et al: Relief of pain by anterior cervical-spine fusion for spondylosis. A report of sixty-five patients. J Bone Joint Surg Am 55:525–534, 1973.
45. Whitecloud T: Anterior surgery for cervical spondylitic myelopathy: Smith-Robinson, Cloward, and vertebrectomy. Spine 13:861–863, 1988.

CHAPTER

21

Joint Systems

Thoracic and Lumbosacral Spine

GUNNAR B.J. ANDERSSON, MD, PhD ■ JOHN W. FRYMOYER, MD, MS

Determining impairment in patients with painful conditions of the lumbar and thoracic spine is difficult not only because the actual impairment is difficult to assess, but also because there is no single universally accepted diagnostic classification system. Chapter 13 discussed the difficulties associated with range of motion (ROM) measurements when there is no healthy limb with which to compare a measurement. This chapter describes the two major classification approaches that can serve as a basis on which impairment and disability can be rated. The first approach is based on symptoms; the second, on pathoanatomic causation. Before describing these classification approaches, however, a brief review of how to evaluate patients with back pain is presented. This evaluation process is the foundation on which any classification system is based.

PATIENT EVALUATION

The evaluation of a patient with low back pain must always start with history and physical examination. Most patients with acute symptoms rapidly recover and do not require further tests. Others, with recurrent or chronic symptoms; more severe, unrelenting pain; or neurologic deficits may require imaging, electrodiagnostic, or laboratory studies. These tests should be based on specific indications derived from the history and physical examination, and the results must be correlated to the history and physical examination. Some patients with chronic symptoms may also need a psychologic evaluation, and attention may be diverted to psychosocial issues which can accompany work-related injury.

Clinical Examination

History

A complete history should contain information about present and previous symptoms, other significant medical diseases, and use of medications. The onset of the symptoms should be explored in detail, including the specific events when trauma is reported as the cause of the symptoms. Pain is the most important symptom. It should be evaluated in terms of its intensity, quality, localization, distribution, pattern, and factors that accentuate and relieve pain. Pain intensity is impossible to quantify, because of its subjective nature, but it is useful to use verbal descriptors, such as slight, moderate, or severe or to use visual analogue scales, usually calibrated from no pain to the worst possible pain. The quality of pain (sharp, stabbing, burning, or aching) is also helpful. Localization and distribution of pain can conveniently be recorded on a "pain drawing" (Fig. 21–1) and serves as a major determinant in symptom classification systems. A pain drawing can also be used to screen for inappropriate pain distribution, and thus can serve as one indicator of the need for further psychological evaluation. The duration of the painful episode is also important and is part of some classification systems. The natural history for recovery of most back conditions is excellent, but the chance of recovery lessens the longer the duration of a pain complaint (Fig. 21–2). The time of day when pain is most severe is valuable information. Worsening throughout the day suggests a mechanical etiology and is the most common pattern. Pain when

Parts of this chapter are based on previously published material by the authors, which appeared in Pope MH, Andersson GBJ, Frymoyer JW, et al: Occupational Low Back pain: Prevention, Diagnosis and Treatment. St. Louis, Mosby–Year Book, 1991.

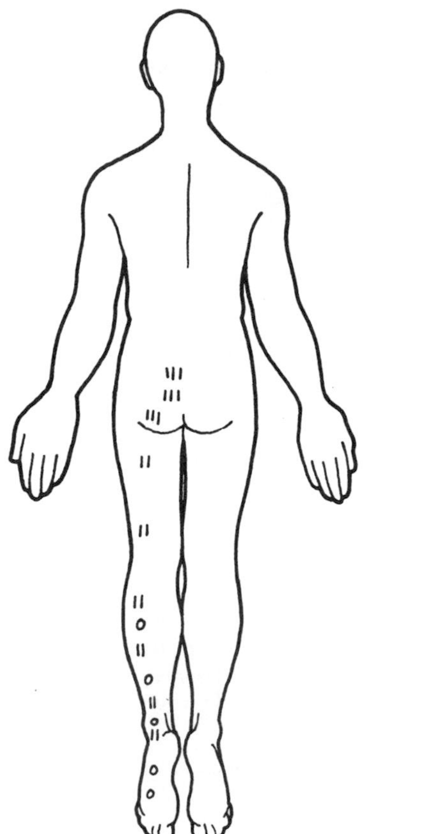

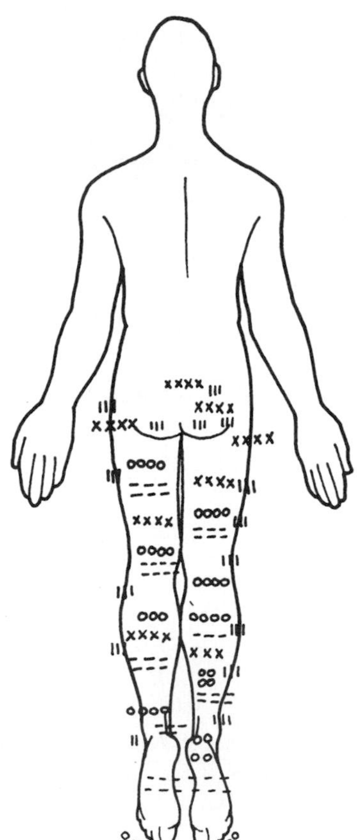

Figure 21–1. Example of a pain drawing from a patient with *an S1 root lesion and* a nonspecific nonorganic pain distribution. (From Pope MH, Andersson GBJ, Frymoyer JW, et al: Occupational Low-back Pain. St. Louis, Mosby–Year Book, 1991.)

the patient first arises in the morning with improvement during the day suggests the possibility of an inflammatory condition. Pain that is most severe at night and awakens the patient is unusual and is a sign of possible malignancy or infection. Factors that accentuate or relieve pain are also important indicators of its etiology (mechanical versus nonmechanical). Most types of back pain are aggravated by mechanical loading, such as lifting and bending, and are relieved by rest. Function is greatly influenced by pain and should therefore be analyzed, including the patient's ability to walk, sit, stand, lift, bend, drive, and work.

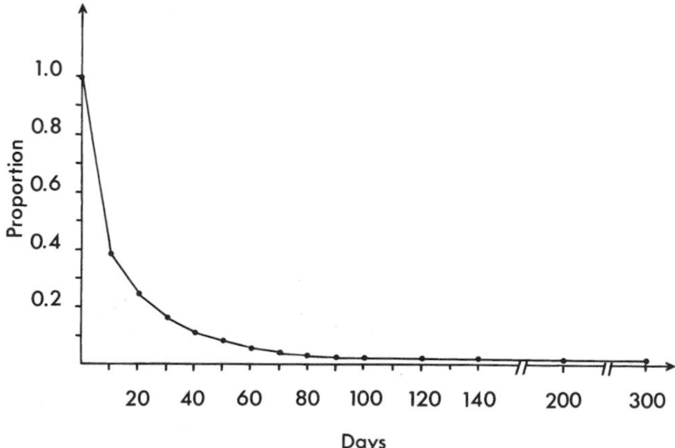

Figure 21–2. Proportion of subjects still absent from work as a function of time (in months). Based on 1588 sickness absence periods. (From Andersson GBJ, Svensson H-O, Oden A: The intensity of work recovery in low-back pain. Spine 8:880–884, 1983.)

Neurologic symptoms should be sought by specific questions regarding sensory changes (numbness and tingling), subjective sense of lower extremity weakness, and changes in bladder and bowel control or sexual function. Loss of ability to initiate voiding and loss of urinary or fecal control are symptoms of a cauda equina syndrome, which requires urgent evaluation. Progressive weakness and "foot drop" are other neurologic symptoms requiring further evaluation.

Information about previous painful episodes should include possible causative factors, as complete a pain description as possible, and associated disability. The success or failure of treatment, including surgery, is also important information. Significant other medical diseases such as diabetes or vascular disease, previous surgery, and previous or current use of medication should also be determined. Smoking and alcohol habits should be explored as well as any drug abuse.

A careful history will lead to plausible differential diagnoses that can be further evaluated during the physical examination. Serious conditions, such as tumors, infec-

TABLE 21–1
Performance Characteristics of the Medical History in the Diagnosis of Spine Diseases Causing Low Back Pain

Disease to Be Detected	Medical History	Sensitivity	Specificity	Group
Cancer care	Age ≥50 years	0.77	0.71	Unselected primary care
	Previous history of cancer	0.31	0.98	Unselected primary care
	Unexplained weight loss	0.15	0.94	Unselected primary care
	Failure to improve with a month of therapy	0.31	0.90	Unselected primary care
	No relief with bed rest	>0.90	0.46	Unselected primary care
	Duration of pain >1 month	0.50	0.81	Unselected primary care
Spinal stenosis	Pseudoclaudication	0.60–0.90	?	Surgical case series
	Age ≥50 years	0.90?	0.70	Surgical case series
Spinal osteomyelitis	Intravenous drug abuse, urinary tract infection, skin infection	0.40	?	Multiple case series
Herniated disc	Sciatica	0.98	0.88	Surgical cases series (sensitivity); population survey of patients with back pain (specificity)
Compression fracture*	Age ≥50 years	0.84	0.61	Primary care patients having x-ray
	Age ≥70 years	0.22	0.96	Primary care patients having x-ray
	Trauma	0.30	0.85	Unselected primary care
	Corticosteroid use	0.06	0.995	Unselected primary care

*Previously unpublished data from 833 patients with back pain at a walk-in clinic, all of whom received plain lumbar roentgenograms.

From Andersson GBJ, Deyo RA: Sensitivity, specificity, and predictive value: A general issue in screening for disease and in the interpretation of diagnostic studies in spinal disorders. In Frymoyer JF (ed): The Adult Spine, 2nd ed. Philadelphia, Lippincott, 1977.

tions, fractures, and cauda equina syndrome, are often indicated by the patient's history (Table 21–1).

Physical Examination

The physical examination includes inspection, palpation, ROM measurements, and neurologic tests. It is useful to develop a system for the examination because it reduces the time involved and ensures completeness (Table 21–2).

Inspection provides information about postural abnormalities such as kyphosis, lordosis, scoliosis, listing, asymmetry, and skin abnormalities. Body movements, gait, and posture provide information about the severity of symptoms and indicate functional limitations. Ability to walk on heels and toes suggests intact function of the L5 and S1 nerve roots. Quadriceps function, which tests the L2, 3, and 4 roots, can be assessed by asking the individual to squat and rise. The range of flexion-extension, lateral bending, and axial rotation are observed and measured.[2] The pattern of motion (rhythm) is important, as is any pain resulting from it. Although ROM is sometimes considered an objective test, it is greatly influenced by the patient. For those reasons it is important to evaluate ROM carefully and to use validation procedures described elsewhere in this book and in the fifth edition of the AMA Guides.[10]

The lower extremities are examined to determine the presence of significant joint deformities and to assess

TABLE 21–2
Physical Examination

Patient Position		
Standing	Posture	Scoliosis Lordosis/kyphosis
	Gait	
	Range of motion	Flexion Extension Lateral bend Axial rotation
	Screening muscle strength test	Heel-toe walk Squatting
Seated	Obversation	Seated posture
	Neurologic	Reflexes (ankle, knee) Straight leg raising
Recumbent (supine)	Measurements	Circumferences Leg length
	Neurologic examination	Reflexes (ankle, knee)
	Nerve tension sign	Posterior tibial Sensation Muscle strength
	Nerve tension sign	Straight leg raising
	Other tests	Abdominal examination Peripheral pulses Hip range of motion
Recumbent (prone)	Neurologic	Sensation Femoral stretch test
	Palpation	Muscle spasm Spinous process Interspinous spaces

neurologic function. Hip motion should also be evaluated, because hip conditions can sometimes produce leg pain that is difficult to distinguish from lumbar radiculopathies.

The evaluation of nerve root tension signs is one of the most important parts of the examination. The most common root tension test is the straight let raising test. When performing this test, the L-5 and S-1 nerve roots and, to a degree, the L-4 nerve root normally move 2 to 3 mm. This movement is restricted or painful when there is compression or inflammation of the nerve root. The straight leg raising (SLR) test is easiest to perform with the patient supine. The leg is elevated with the knee extended. The examining hand is placed on the pelvis to gauge pelvic motion. The test is positive when sciatica (posterior leg pain) is reproduced. The degree of elevation at which pain occurs is recorded. Often, the patient will complain of low back pain rather than sciatica. In this circumstance, the degree of elevation should be recorded, but the test is not positive for nerve-root tension. The SLR test should also be performed with the patient sitting, for reasons of consistency. The two positions should produce similar results. Straight leg raising may be restricted by tightness of the hamstring muscles. This should also be recorded but is not, again, a positive SLR test. Sometimes sciatic pain will occur in the opposite leg as the test is being performed. This finding, referred to as the contralateral or crossed positive SLR test, is highly specific for lumbar disk herniation.[21] A variety of other root tension tests have been described. They include the Lasegue test, where the hip and knee joints are flexed 90° and the knee extended to the point where sciatica is reproduced. The SLR and Lasegue tests can be further validated by dorsiflexing the foot or internally rotating the hip, which should both increase the leg pain.

The minimum testing of neurologic function of the lower extremities in patients with radicular symptoms includes the knee and ankle reflexes, the strength of the extensor hallucis longus, and the sensory function. Figure 21–3 illustrates the typical L4, L5, and S1 neurologic findings. About 95% of all lumbar herniations occur at those levels. Knee (quadriceps) and ankle (Achilles) reflexes should be obtained in the sitting and/or supine positions. The knee reflex is primarily a test of L4 nerve root function, whereas the ankle reflex is primarily mediated by the S1 nerve root. Sensation can be grossly evaluated by touch but, when indicated, is more precisely determined by means of a sterile, sharp object (pin prick), light touch, vibrating tuning fork, and the ability of the patient to feel position. Nonspecific loss of sensation must be differentiated from

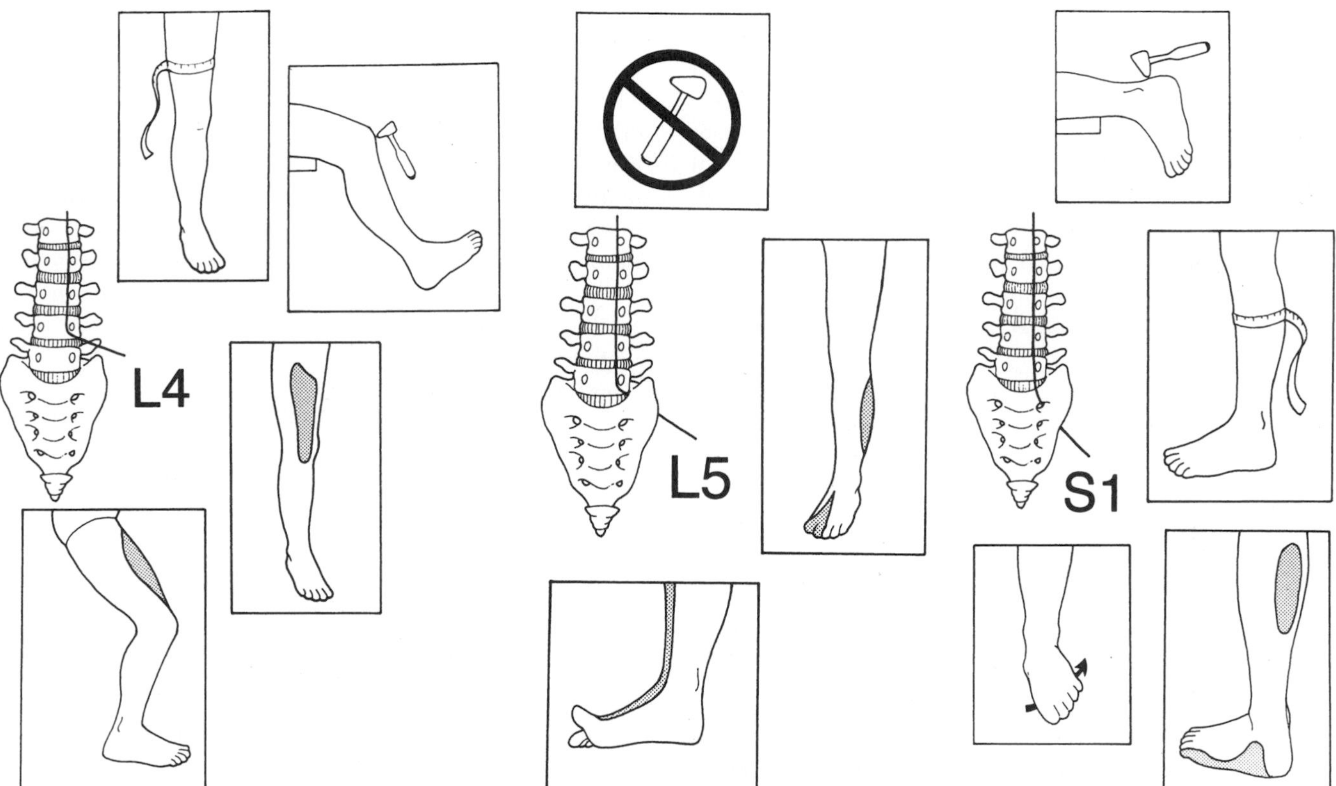

Figure 21–3. Typical findings in L4, L5, and S1 syndromes. L4 lesions are characterized by a loss of the knee reflex, *L5 by a weakness of the extensor hallucis longus, and S1 by a loss of the ankle reflex.* (From Pope MH, Andersson GBJ, Frymoyer JW, et al: Occupational Low-back Pain. St. Louis, Mosby–Year Book, 1991.)

TABLE 21–3

Lumbar Radicular Syndromes

Disc Level	Any Central Disc Herniation	L5/S1	L4/5	L3/4
Nerve root involved	Cauda equina (L4/5 > L5/S1)	S1	L5	L4
Pain referral pattern	Perineum Low back Buttocks Either or both legs	Unilateral Low back Buttocks Posterior leg	Unilateral Low back Buttocks Lateral leg and thigh	Unilateral Low back Buttocks Posterolateral leg
Motor deficit	Unilateral or bilateral leg weakness	Unilateral weakness; plantar flexion of foot; difficulty with toe walking	Unilateral weakness; dorsiflexion of foot; difficulty with heel walking	Unilateral quadriceps weakness
Sensory deficit	Perineum/buttocks, low back, thighs, legs, feet	Lateral foot, posterolateral lateral calf	Lateral calf; between first and second toes	Knee distal, anterior thigh
Reflexes compromised	Ankle jerk	Ankle jerk	0	Knee jerk

Modified from Andersson GBJ, McNeill TW: Lumbar Spine Syndromes: Evaluation and Treatment. Vienna, Springer-Verlag, 1989.

well-defined dermatomal loss. Strength of the extensor hallucis longus is typically affected by an L5 nerve root compression. The testing of muscle strength may also include ankle and toe dorsiflexors and ankle invertors (L4, L5 roots), ankle plantar flexors and evertors (S1, S2 roots), knee extensors and hip adductors (L2, L3, L4) and hip flexors (T12, L1, L2, L3). The Babinski sign and the presence of clonus are measures of upper motor neuron involvement. A summary of common lumbar radicular syndromes is provided in Table 21–3.

With the patient in the prone position, palpation of the spinous processes, interspinous spaces, paraspinal muscles, sacroiliac joint, and sciatic nerve is performed. Palpation should include the thoracic spine. A femoral stretch test, where the leg is extended at the hip joint, is sometimes performed to detect radicular pain from the L2, L3, and L4 nerve roots. A complete examination should include abdominal palpation and evaluation of the peripheral pulses. If ankylosing spondylitis is suspected, chest expansion should be measured. Normally there is a difference greater than 1.5 cm between expiration and inspiration.

A variety of tests have been developed to determine the reproducibility and consistency of patient responses. The best researched are those described by Waddell et al[49] (Table 21–4). These tests should alert the examiner to the possibility of psychologic distress and/or malingering, and may signify the need for psychological testing. A single positive Waddell test is of little significance, whereas several positive tests suggest a non-

TABLE 21–4

Nonorganic Physical Signs Indicating Illness Behavior

Symptoms or Signs	Physical Disease/Normal Illness Behavior	Abnormal Illness Behavior
Symptoms		
Pain	Anatomic distribution	Whole leg pain Tailbone pain
Numbness	Dermatomal	Whole leg numbness
Weakness	Myotomal	Whole leg giving way
Time pattern	Varies with time and activity	Never free of pain
Response to treatment	Variable benefit	Intolerance to treatments; emergency admissions to hospital
Signs		
Tenderness	Anatomic distribution	Superficial; widespread nonanatomic
Axial loading	No lumbar pain	Lumbar pain
Simulated rotation	No lumbar pain	Lumbar pain
Straight leg raising	Limited on distraction	Improves with distraction
Sensory	Dermatomal	Regional
Motor	Myotomal	Regional, jerky, giving way

Modified from Waddell G, Bircher M, Finlayson D, et al: Symptoms and signs: Physical disease or illness behavior? Br Med J 289:739, 1984.

organic component, particularly when other signs of illness behavior are present.

In addition to the tests included in the standard examination described, there are a number of other tests that are sometimes used. They include the Patric test, in which the hip is flexed, abducted, and externally rotated, and the pelvic rock test, where the pelvis is forcefully compressed by the examiner exerting force on both iliac tubercles. Both of these tests are done to determine sacroiliac joint involvement. Another test to the same purpose is the Gaenslen test. With the patient supine and the buttock over the edge of the table, the unsupported leg is allowed to drop down while the other leg is flexed and held to the chest. None of these tests has a high degree of specificity.

Other tests include the Milgram test, where the patient simultaneously lifts both legs off the table and holds for 30 seconds. This increases the intrathecal pressure and is used to rule out intrathecal pathology. The Naffziger test is another test aimed at increasing the intrathecal pressure. In this test, both jugular veins are compressed until the patient's face begins to flush, at which point the patient is asked to cough. The test is positive if radicular pain occurs. A large number of additional tests, some with eponyms, are also used. In general, their contribution to a specific diagnosis is small.

At the completion of the history and physical examination, a general formulation can be made of the patient's low back problem, including decisions regarding the need for any further diagnostic tests. An initial therapeutic plan can usually be initiated at this time as well.

Diagnostic Studies

For the majority of patients, further diagnostic studies are not required. If additional tests are indicated, two general categories are considered: those performed to detect physiologic abnormalities and those performed to detect anatomic abnormalities and provide anatomic definition. Physiologic tests include serologic studies, bone scans, and electrodiagnostic studies. Anatomic tests include x-rays and other imaging studies such computed tomography (CT) and magnetic resonance imaging (MRI). In select cases a psychological evaluation may also be required.

Serologic Studies

Serologic tests have limited value in the evaluation of patients with back pain but are indicated when there is clinical suspicion of systemic disease including infection, inflammation, and malignancy.

Spinal Radiography

Radiographs are commonly used and can reveal a variety of bony and structural abnormalities of which only a few are associated with back pain. For general diagnostic screening, spinal radiographs have limited value and findings correlate poorly with the presence of back pain.[13] Degenerative changes are common in patients with and without back problems, and are typically unrelated to the patient's pain. Spondylolisthesis, severe deformity, and severe degenerative changes are the main findings of clinical importance. Fractures, osseous tumors, and some infections can also be detected, but are rare. Thus plain film radiographs are indicated primarily in patients with recent trauma, suspicion of osteoporosis, a history of malignancy or recent infection, and when the clinical symptoms are suggestive of malignancy, infection, or fracture. Table 21–5 summarizes the most common indications from the history and physical examination that suggest pathologic changes requiring special attention (workup) are present. These are often referred to as red flags, and should heighten suspicion that a spine fracture, cancer, infection, or cauda equina syndrome is present. For many, the specificity and sensitivity are only moderate.

Flexion/extension radiographs are taken to detect abnormal motion between vertebrae (i.e., instability). However, this type of radiographic study is difficult to evaluate because of the inability to accurately identify bony landmarks. Abnormal motion can occur in the translational plane, rotational plane directions, or both. For the lumbar spine, an anteroposterior motion exceeding 4.5 mm is considered abnormal,[43] whereas greater than 2.5 mm movement is considered abnormal for the thoracic spine. Angular motion of the two adjacent vertebrae greater than 15 degrees at L1-2, L2-3, and L3-4; greater than 20 degrees at L4-5; and greater than 25 degrees at L5-S1 is considered abnormal.[10,51] Flexion/ extension views are also used to assess the integrity of a previously performed spinal fusion. Again, caution must be exerted in interpreting results. When instrumentation is used, flexion/extension films may show absence of movement even when the fusion has not healed. Figure 21–4 illustrates how these measures are made.

Other Imaging Techniques

A variety of other imaging techniques are available to assess patients with back pain and sciatica including CT scanning, MRI scanning, myelography, and discography (the uses of which are described in Chapter 14). These tests allow assessment of the anatomy of the spinal canal and its contents as well as of surrounding tissues. Estimates of the sensitivity and specificity of these tests are

TABLE 21–5

Red Flags in the History and Physical Examinations, With Associated Sensitivities and Specificities

Disease Category	Symptom or Sign	Sensitivity	Specificity
Cancer	Age ≥ 50 years	0.77	0.71
	History of cancer	0.31	0.98
	Unexplained weight loss	0.15	0.94
	Pain unrelieved by bed rest (night pain)	0.90	0.46
	Pain lasting > 1 month	0.50	0.81
	Failure to improve on therapy after 1 month	0.31	0.90
Infection	ESR ≥20 mm	0.78	0.67
	IV drug abuse, UTI		
	Skin infection	0.4	?
	Fever	0.27–0.83	0.98
Fracture	Age ≥ 50 years	0.84	0.61
	Age ≥ 70 years	0.22	0.96
	Trauma	0.30	0.85
	Steroid use	0.66	0.99

ESR, erythrocyte sedimentation rate; IV, intravenous; UTI, urinary tract infection.

Based on Nachemson AL, Jonsson E: Neck and Back Pain. Philadelphia, Lippincott, 2000.

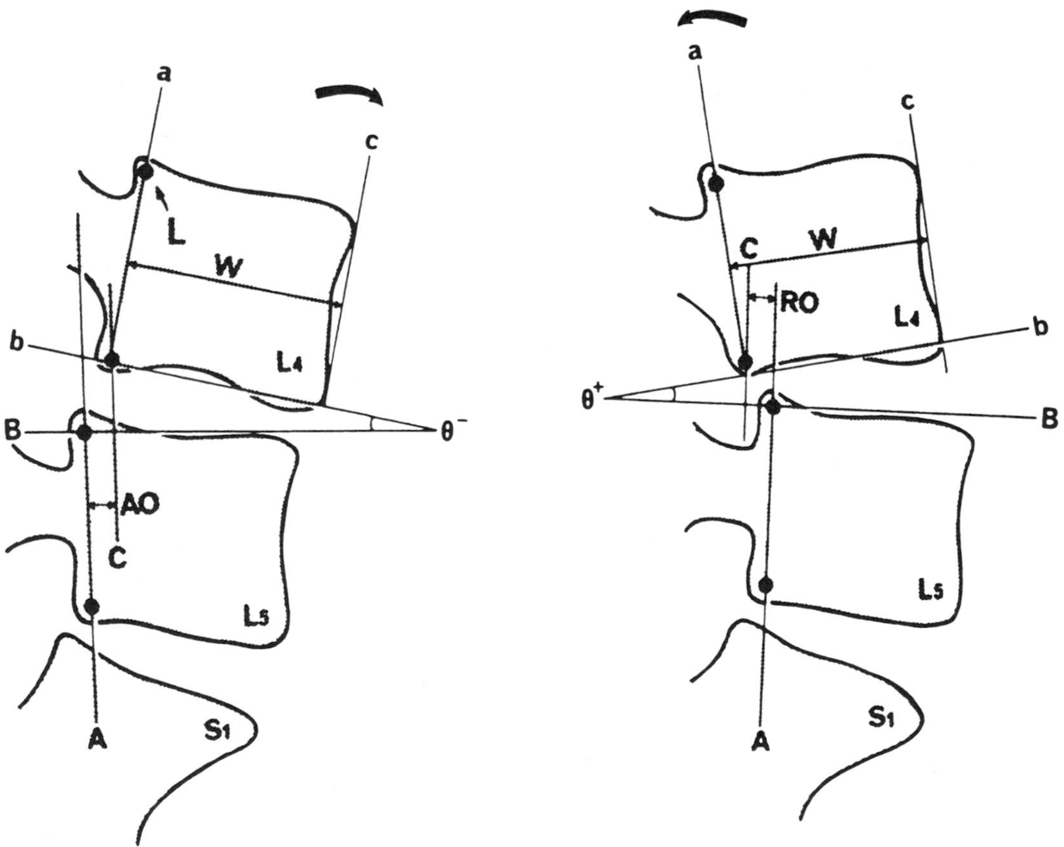

Figure 21–4. Measurements from flexion/extension views.

provided in Table 21–6 and further discussed in Chapter 14. Imaging should be used only when there is a clear indication based on the patient's history and physical examination. These studies are only valid when correlated with the clinical signs and symptoms. Imaging abnormalities are common in individuals who have never had low back symptoms or sciatica, occurring in about 25% of asymptomatic people with larger percentages in older populations.[9,23,24,28,50,52] Further, a number of other findings of questionable or unknown importance are commonly observed. These include disc bulging and disc degeneration, which are both nonspecific and present in the majority of the adult population.

Four imaging tests—CT, MRI, myelography, and myelo-CT—are used in similar clinical situations and often provide similar types of information.[25,26] Significant technologic advances in these imaging modalities are currently taking place. As a result, there has been a gradual shift from myelography toward CT and, more recently, from CT toward MRI. Discography and disc-CT are other tests used more specifically by some to determine severe degenerative changes of the disc. The use of discography to diagnose a painful degenerative disc remains controversial, yet it is the only available test for that purpose. A positive test requires concordant pain when the disc is injected under low pressure, and a pain-free injection of a normal (control) disc.

TABLE 21–6

Sensitivity and Specificity of Imaging Tests Used for the Diagnosis of Herniated Discs (HNP) and Spinal Stenosis (SS)

Condition and Test	Sensitivity	Specificity
HNP		
CT	0.90	0.70
MRI	0.90	0.70
CT myelography	0.90	0.70
SS		
CT	0.90	0.80–0.95
MRI	0.90	0.75–0.95
Myelography	0.77	0.70

CT, computed tomography; MRI, magnetic resonance imaging.

Modified from Andersson GBJ, McNeill TW: Lumbar Spine Syndromes Evaluation and Treatment. Vienna, Springer-Verlag, 1989.

Electrodiagnostic Studies

Electrodiagnostic studies are used to evaluate the physiologic function of the spinal cord, nerve roots, and peripheral nerves.[1] They include electromyography, reflex studies, somatosensory evoked potentials, and nerve conduction velocity studies. The use and value of these tests are further described in Chapter 33. They should only be used to confirm specific clinical suspicions.[40]

Psychological Assessment

Patients with chronic back pain occasionally require a psychological assessment. A variety of tests and techniques have been developed for that purpose.[29] They include personality and psychological test instruments, behavioral assessment methods, cognitive-behavioral assessment methods, and psychophysiologic measures. Some of these tests are the Minnesota Multiphasic Personality Inventory (MMPI) and the Million Behavioral Health Inventory (see Chapter 38). Chronic pain is sometimes associated with anger, irritability, and anxiety, and not infrequently with depression. Self-administered screens for depression include the Beck Depression Inventory and the Zung Depression Index (see Chapters 38 and 39).

CLASSIFICATION

As mentioned earlier, there is a lack of agreement on the classification of patients with back disorders. The two currently used approaches, symptoms-based classification and etiologic-based classification, are briefly discussed here. It will be apparent that none of the classification systems is pure, and that none fulfills all requirements for validity.

SYMPTOMS-BASED CLASSIFICATION

The most comprehensive system based on symptoms was developed by the Quebec Study Group.[45] Table 21–7 outlines the system, which is applicable to all anatomic regions of the spine. Broadly, it contains four symptom categories with diagnostic specificity, four categories based on pathoanatomic cause, two postsurgical categories, and one category that is unspecified.

Category 1 represents the majority of patients with low back disorders. These patients have pain that is typically aggravated by mechanical factors such as activity, worsens during the day, and is relieved by rest. Acute low back pain of this type can develop following single or repetitive loading events but can also develop from minor postural changes such as bending or twisting, from simple coughing, or, in the majority of cases, from an unknown event. Examination typically reveals loss of lumbar lordosis, varying degrees of back muscle tightness and spasm, and restriction of spinal motion. None of these signs has particular diagnostic significance. Neurologic signs and symptoms are absent. Commonly used diagnoses (International Classification of Diseases–9 codes) for this patient group include low back strain or sprain, implying a muscular or ligamentous injury. Unfortunately, these suspected diagnoses

TABLE 21-7

The Quebec Classification System

Classification	Symptoms	Duration of Symptoms From Onset	Working Status at Time of Evaluation
1	Pain without radiation		
2	Pain + radiation to extremity, distally	a (<7 days)	I (idle)
3	Pain + radiation to upper/lower limb, neurologic signs	b (>7 days to 7 weeks)	
		c (>7 weeks)	
4	Pain + radiation to upper/lower limb		
5	Presumptive compression of spinal nerve root		
6	Compression of a spinal nerve root confirmed by 1) specific imaging techniques (i.e., computed axial tomography, myelography, or magnetic resonance imaging) or 2) other diagnostic techniques (e.g., electromyography, venography)		
7	Spinal stenosis		
8	Postsurgical status, 1 to 6 months after intervention		
9	Postsurgical status, >6 months after intervention		
9.1	Asymptomatic		
9.2	Symptomatic		
10	Chronic pain syndrome		W (working)
11	Other diagnoses		I (idle)

From Spitzer WO, LeBlanc FE, Dupuis M, et al: Scientific approach to the assessment and management of activity-related spinal disorders: A monograph for clinicians. Report of the Quebec Task Force on Spinal Disorders. Spine 12(Suppl. 7):S1–S59, 1987.

are almost never verifiable; thus they are nonspecific terms. Imaging studies are not required to classify patients into this group, or indeed to develop an initial treatment plan, but if done, should be negative with respect to a specific diagnosis. Disc degeneration is often present on imaging studies of patients of Category 1.

Category 2 is characterized by proximal leg pain. Pain radiating into the proximal leg(s) can be induced experimentally by mechanical stimuli or injection of noxious substances, such as hypertonic saline, into back muscles, facet joints, ligaments, and bone.[22,30,35,37] Referred pain caused by stimulation of connective tissue structures is frequently referred to as sclerotomal. All of the structures that produce this type of pain derive their innervation from the posterior primary rami.

Category 3 includes patients with pain that radiates distally into the legs (below the knee). This pain may arise from three sources: by irritation of structures innervated by the posterior primary rami[38]; by increased tension, compression, or inflammation of an anterior primary rami; or by a reduction in the space available for the cauda and/or nerve roots. Mono- or polyradiculopathies are both included in this group, but are better defined in Categories 4, 6, and 7. Monoradiculopathies in Category 3 are typically called sciatica. Category 3 does not present with specific neurologic signs.

Category 4 increases the diagnostic specificity of mono- or polyradiculopathies by requiring neurologic signs, such as a positive nerve root tension sign (SLR) or loss (or reduction) of reflexes, sensation, or motor power. In the instance of a monoradiculopathy, the presence of these signs will accurately identify a lumbar disc herniation in a high proportion of patients affected.[21] When root tension signs such as a contralaterally positive straight leg raising test are present, the probability of lumbar disc herniation approaches 98%.[42] Confirmation of cause of root involvement by an imaging study transfers a patient in Category 4 to Category 6, because it identifies the pain source more specifically.

Category 5 includes spinal fractures that compromise the bony spinal canal, as well as the more subtle and controversial problem of segmental instability, which is discussed later in this chapter. In these patients, nerve root compromise can be present and is evaluated from clinical and radiographic presentation.

Category 6 is an extension of Category 4 in that it requires confirmation of nerve root compression by imaging techniques such as myelography, CT scans, and MRI, or by physiologic techniques such as electromyography.

Category 7 includes the most common cause of polyradiculopathy and neurogenic claudication (or spinal stenosis). If the patient has significant or advancing neurologic dysfunction, the diagnosis should be confirmed by the imaging techniques discussed above.

Categories 8 and 9 include patients who have undergone a surgical intervention for a spinal disorder. Dividing the postoperative period into two intervals, 1 to 6 months and greater than 6 months, is meaningful, because most patients with simple disc excisions should have recovered and returned to work within 6 months of the intervention. The separation of Category 9 into two classes (9.1 asymptomatic, 9.2 symptomatic) is important for impairment evaluation purposes and long-term prognosis.

Category 10, chronic pain syndrome, signifies a situation where acute pain has been transferred into a chronic pain syndrome and psychological and psychosocial factors gradually have become more important. Physical findings are inconclusive and often nonorganic, and "pain behavior" is common. There is no direct relationship between identifiable physical pathology and the patient's initial symptoms and disability. Determination of impairment in these patients should ideally not be made without psychological or psychiatric consultation.

A special group of patients who may belong in this last category have the so-called deconditioning syndrome. The deconditioning syndrome develops after injuries of unknown etiology suspected to involve the soft tissues. In these conditions the physiologic measurements of motion, strength, cardiovascular fitness, and lifting capacity are all significantly below normal. Determination of impairment should not be made until correction of this deconditioned state has been attempted.

Category 11 contains all other types of back pain not included in the 10 other categories. Although this list is extensive, including tumors, infections, metabolic, and inflammatory causes, it comprises only a small minority of patients with back disorders, and even fewer who need an impairment evaluation.

The Quebec classification introduces two other important parameters: duration of symptoms and working status. Based on duration, symptoms are divided into acute, subacute, or chronic. The Quebec Study Group suggests acute symptoms are 7 days or less in duration; subacute, 7 days to 7 weeks; and chronic, more than 7 weeks. Others use somewhat different time sequences: acute, less than 1 month; subacute, 1 to 3 months; and chronic, greater than 3 months.[19,39] Figure 21–2 demonstrates the normal recovery curve after an acute low back episode. About 90% of patients will recover within 3 months.[6] Failure to recover during that time increases the probability that a chronic pain syndrome will develop.

Another subset of patients not discussed in the Quebec classification system are those who have recurrent pain complaints. It is estimated that 60% of patients who have an acute low back episode and recover will have a recurrence, usually within the first 2 years.[8,46] Patients with sciatica have an increased risk of recurrence.

Subclassification by work status also has major implications to prognosis. As time passes, there is rapidly diminishing likelihood that the individual will ever return to work (see Fig. 21–2).

An alternative symptom-based classification system was developed by the Back Strategy Committee of the Australian Work Cover Corporation and has been endorsed by a variety of Australian medical associations and colleges (Table 21–8). It combines symptom diagnoses and anatomic diagnoses.[54] It is presented here to illustrate an even more simplified approach than the Quebec System. The Australian system has only three groups: two based on the patient's descriptions and one based on known etiology. It is anticipated that over 90% of work-related back pain will fall into Groups 1 and 2. It is also anticipated that classifications for a particular injury will change as more sophisticated diagnostic techniques become available. Interestingly, the classification system does not accept a diagnosis of back strain after 8 weeks, because of the normal healing time of muscle. After this, a different classification must be selected.

The American Medical Association has also included a symptom-based classification system in the fourth and fifth editions of its Guides to the Evaluation of Permanent Impairment.[2,10] This system, which applies to patients with traumatic injuries, assigns the patient to one of eight (fourth edition) or five (fifth edition) categories called diagnosis-related estimates (DREs). These estimates, which are listed in Table 21–9, are differentiated based on either clinical findings or structural changes (such as fractures and dislocations). The DRE classification does not include common developmental findings, such as spondylolysis and spondylolisthesis.[2] The DRE classification is applicable only to a small percentage of patients with spinal conditions because, to be included, there must be an injury. It is, however, applicable to the majority of individuals who are evaluated for impairment, as most will have an "injury-related" problem.

TABLE 21–8

Australian Work Cover Classification System

Group	Symptoms
One	Back pain (nonspecific)
Two	Back strain (diagnosis is not appropriate if 8 weeks or more have passed since the injury)
Three	Back pain with specific diagnosis. For all diagnoses in Group Three, it is stressed that the symptoms, signs, and investigatory findings must be in concordance. 1. Disc prolapse 2. Symptomatic disc or facet degeneration 3. Stenosis Central Subarticular Foraminal 4. Spondylolisthesis 5. Fracture and/or dislocation

* Relevant intercurrent medical conditions affecting the lumbosacral spine should be noted; for example, inflammatory arthritides.

TABLE 21–9

Lumbosacral Spine Impairments Described as Diagnosis-related Estimates (DRE) and Classified into Eight Categories

DRE Category	Complaints or Symptoms	Structural Inclusion
AMA Guides, 4th ed*		
I	No impairment	None
II	Minor impairment	Vertebral Fx
III	Radiculopathy	Vertebral Fx
IV	Loss of motor segment integrity (MSI)	Vertebral Fx or dislocation
V	Radiculopathy and loss of MSI	Structural compromise
VI	Cauda equina-like syndrome (without bowel or bladder paralysis)	None
VII	Cauda equina syndrome with bowel or bladder paralysis	None
VIII	Paraplegia, total loss of lumbosacral spinal cord function	None
AMA Guides, 5th ed†		
I	No clinical findings	None
II	Minor complaints and findings	Vertebral Fx
III	Radiculopathy	Vertebral Fx
IV	Loss of MSI	Vertebral Fx
V	Radiculopathy and loss of MSI	Vetebral Fx + neurologic compromise

* From American Medical Association: Guides to the Evaluation of Permanent Impairment, 4th ed. Chicago, American Medical Association, 1993.

† From Cocchiarella L, Andersson GBJ (eds): Guides to the Evaluation of Permanent Impairment, 5th ed. Chicago, American Medical Association, 2001.

Also included in the AMA Guides is a listing of specific spine disorders that are used in combination with range of motion measurements and neurologic changes when using the range of motion model. They fall into four categories: fractures; intervertebral discs or other soft tissue lesions; spondylolysis and spondylolisthesis, not operated on; and spinal stenosis, segmental instability, spondylolisthesis, fracture, or dislocation operated on.

PATHOANATOMIC CLASSIFICATION

The second main classification method is by pathoanatomic etiology. This system is presently applicable to only a few percent of all patients with low back pain, if degenerative changes are excluded, but has major significance in the treatment and prognosis of this small subset. The majority of patients with specific pathoanatomic causes for pain will fall into Quebec Categories 4 through 7. A small, but very important, minority will be classified as belonging in Category 11.

Degenerative Spinal Disorders

Degenerative spinal disorders are the bases for the most common pathoanatomic causes of low back pain, mono- and polyradiculopathies, and claudication. Although this is true, it is important not to assume that degeneration is synonymous with back pain and, indeed, is the cause of pain in an individual patient. Currently we cannot, with certainty, determine the difference between a disc that is degenerated and producing symptoms and one that is degenerated and asymptomatic. Nor can we, with certainty, determine if osteophytic spurs, facet osteoarthritis, or other degenerative conditions often seen on radiographs, CTs, and MRIs are producing symptoms.

It is critical to place normal, age-related spinal degeneration in perspective as a background when considering clinically significant degenerative syndromes, and to recognize that disc degeneration, as such, is usually not clinically significant. All human spines degenerate with time. Most autopsy specimens, and MRI studies in normal subjects, show the onset of gross and microscopic evidence of intervertebral disc degeneration by the third decade of life. These morphologic changes are accompanied by alterations in the biochemical composition of the disc, such as a decrease in water and proteoglycan content, and an increase in collagen.[16] The onset of changes occurs earlier in life in the male and affects the L4/5 and L5/S1 discs earlier and more frequently.

Radiographic changes such as disc-space narrowing, endplate sclerosis, and spinal osteophytes lag behind the histologic and chemical events. However, the prevalence of these degenerative changes is equivalent in patients with and without low back pain. The presence of a narrowed intervertebral disc is not correlated with the risk for, or the presence of, a disc herniation. In fact, disc space narrowing in one study was a negative predictor for lumbar disc herniation at that level.[21] Based on radiographs, disc degeneration has sometimes been divided into minimal, moderate, and severe. This division has no particular value to the determination of impairment.

The advent of MRI scanning allows earlier detection of disc degeneration, as discussed in Chapter 14, and has revealed that disc degeneration is present in many people in their twenties. Again, the presence of these so-called black discs on T2-weighted MR images does not imply clinical significance or impairment. Disc bulging, which is another common feature of disc degeneration, is also rarely of clinical significance, and is not equivalent to a disc herniation, as discussed subsequently.

Disc abnormalities on MRI in healthy individuals are common. Some studies indicate frequencies as high as 30% in individuals age 30 and younger.

Herniated Nucleus Pulposus

Clinically, the syndrome of a herniated nucleus pulposus (HNP) is characterized by radiculopathy, usually accompanied or preceded by low back pain. The physical examination usually reveals the presence of one or more objective neurologic changes such as reflex asymmetry, sensory change in the distribution of a nerve root, or muscle weakness (Fig. 21–3). The diagnosis of disc herniation requires a combination of an appropriate radicular pain distribution, a positive nerve root tension sign, objective neurologic abnormalities, and a positive confirmatory structural examination (CT, myelo, myelo-CT, MRI, discogram, disc-CT). For the straight leg raising test to be positive, sciatic pain should develop below the knee. Neurologic signs can be absent in the presence of a disc herniation. It is important to remember that reflex abnormalities, when present, can be a residual from a previous herniation, because a "lost" reflex usually does not return even after successful treatment. Although a positive structural examination is a requirement, the presence of a disc abnormality is not sufficient for diagnosis in the absence of clinical symptoms and signs, as more than 25% of healthy individuals have an abnormal imaging test (see Chapter 14). The structural examination should show a clear focal expansion of disc material posteriorly or posterolaterally, and displacement or indentation on the spinal cord if the lesion is above L1, or the thecal sac or one or both nerve roots at the affected level if below L1. Occasionally a free fragment, an extrusion, or even a sequestered disc fragment is found. An extraforamenal (far lateral) disc herniation can be present without obvious nerve root displacement. Diffuse disc bulging is not sufficient for diagnosis; nor is an abnormal EMG where there are no clinical or structural correlates (see Chapters 14 and 33).

It is important to emphasize that the majority of patients who fit the clinical criteria of HNP will recover from acute symptoms with conservative treatment and have minimal residual functional or work capacity impairment. However, patients who have had a known disc herniation are more likely to have a recurrent herniation. Surgical treatment is indicated in patients who do not respond to conservative treatment or who develop progressive motor deficits. A very small percent of patients who have lumbar disc herniations will have a massive extrusion of nuclear material sufficient to interfere with the neural control of bladder and bowel function.[34,44] This so-called cauda equina syndrome, which is also characterized by saddle anesthesia and weak or absent leg reflexes, is a true surgical emergency, because failure to decompress the lesion may result in permanent loss of bladder and bowel control.

Spinal Stenosis

Spinal stenosis is defined as a narrowing of the vertebral canal, lateral recesses, or vertebral foraminae.[4] Narrowing of the central lumbar spinal canal in its sagittal and/or coronal dimensions (central spinal stenosis) may occur at a single level or at many levels of the spine (Fig. 21–5). When multiple levels are involved, typical symptoms include recurrent or continued low back pain and leg symptoms aggravated by specific body postures and/or physical exertion. As stenosis increases, extension of the spine often becomes more painful, while flexion provides relief. Neurogenic claudication is a common symptom, but reflex, motor, and sensory

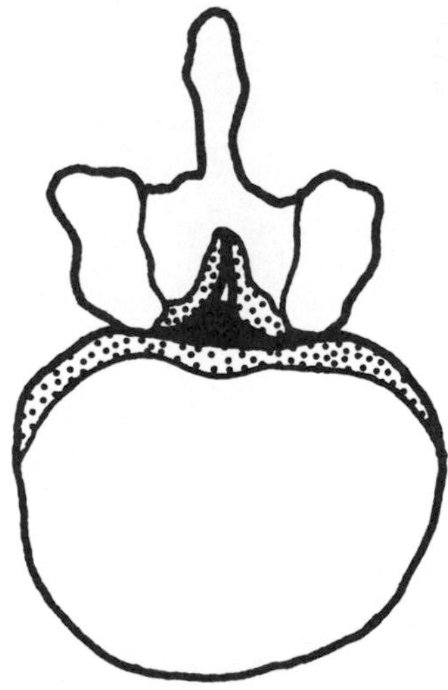

Figure 21–5. In central spinal stenosis, the spinal canal is narrowed. As seen in the Figure, ligamentous tissue often contributes to this narrowing. (From Andersson GBJ, McNeill TW: Lumbar Spinal Stenosis. St. Louis, Mosby–Year Book, 1992.)

changes are often confusing because of the involvement of multiple nerve roots. Because spinal stenosis is a slow and gradual narrowing of the spinal canal with gradually increasing pressure on nerve structures, neurologic findings also can be completely absent despite substantial neural encroachment. Unlike lumbar disc herniations, positive nerve root tension signs such as the straight leg raising test are usually absent. Diffuse narrowing of the spinal canal may be due to many causes, but most commonly the stenosis results from degeneration with disc bulging, posterior osteophytes projecting into the spinal canal, hypertrophy of the articular facets, and buckling of the ligamentum flavum.

A second group of stenotic lesions is associated with more focal degenerative disease. Degenerative spondylolisthesis is the most common of these and typically affects women in the fifth and sixth decades of life (Fig. 21–6). It occurs most commonly at the L4/L5 level. Radiographic surveys have shown that as many as 9.1% of females and 5.8% of males have this deformity, although many have no symptoms.[47] In other patients, disc space collapse leads to backward displacement (retrospondylolisthesis), which may less frequently lead to compromise of the nerve root canals or central spinal stenosis.

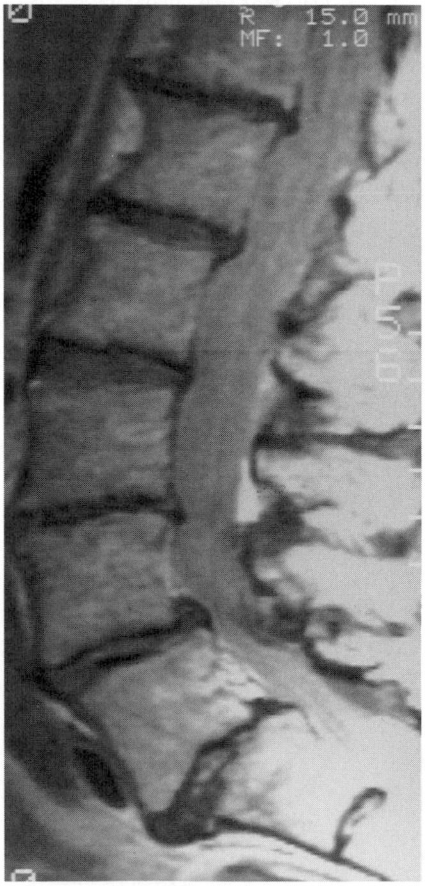

Another group of patients has predominantly lateral (nerve root canal) stenosis (Fig. 21–7). In this situation, a combination of facet hypertrophy and varying degrees of disc bulging reduces the lateral recess and/or foraminal space available at the affected disc level(s) and compromises the nerve root(s). Lateral spinal stenosis may present as a mono- or polyradiculopathy, but the characteristic complaints of neurogenic claudication are less likely to be present. Yong-Hing and Kirkaldy-Willis[55] have emphasized the interrelationships between spinal stenosis and disc herniations. When the spinal canal and lateral nerve root canal are narrowed, a relatively small disc herniation can produce clinically significant symptoms such as sciatica, which would not have occurred if the canal had been of adequate dimensions. This exemplifies how a pre-existing condition can contribute to the development of symptoms.

Spinal stenosis can be classified etiologically as well as anatomically (Table 21–10). Impairment evaluations, however, are based on symptoms, not on classification and diagnoses are not purely clinical, but require positive imaging tests.

Figure 21–6. Magnetic resonance scan of a patient with degenerative lumbar spine changes and a degenerative spondylolisthesis at L4/L5.

Other Degenerative Changes

Two peculiar types of degenerative changes of minor clinical importance are idiopathic vertebrogenic sclerosis and diffuse idiopathic spinal hyperostosis (DISH).

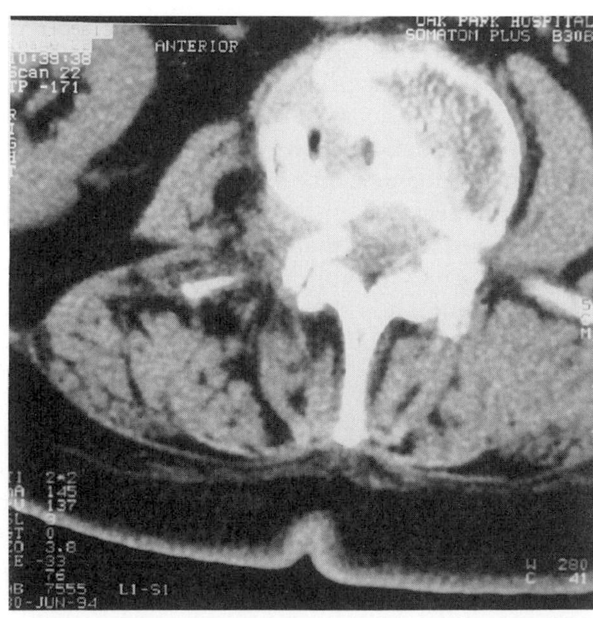

Figure 21–7. Computed tomography scan of a patient with lateral spinal stenosis. Note the large osteophytes at the facet joints.

TABLE 21-10

Classification of Spinal Stenosis

Etiologic classification*

I. Congenital—Developmental stenosis
   A. Idiopathic (hereditary)
   B. Achondroplastic
II. Acquired stenosis
   A. Degenerative
   B. Combined congenital and degenerative stenosis
   C. Spondylolytic/spondylolisthetic
   D. Iatrogenic
      1. Postlaminectomy
      2. Postfusion
      3. Postchemonucleolysis
   E. Post-traumatic
   F. Metabolic
      1. Paget's disease
      2. Fluorosis

Anatomic classification

I. Central stenosis—The central canal is narrowed in the sagittal or coronal plane or in both planes
II. Lateral stenosis—The nerve root canal is narrowed in the lateral recess or in the nerve root canal or both

* Etiologic classification after Arnoldi CC, Brodsky AE, Cauchoix J, et al: Lumbar spinal stenosis and nerve root entrapment syndromes: Definition and classification. Clin Orthop 115:4, 1976.

The former is characterized by severe low back pain, focal severe disc space narrowing, and diffuse sclerosis of the vertebral body adjacent to the disc. Most commonly the L4 vertebral body is affected. Women are affected four to five times more often than men. In contrast, DISH affects multiple vertebrae, is more common in men, and is characterized radiographically by diffuse flowing osteophytes, which bridge over a minimum of three vertebral levels. Patients commonly have associated metabolic conditions such as diabetes and gout, and may also have other joints affected.

Degenerative Conditions of Less Certain Significance

Three additional conditions are commonly considered as causes of low back pain, with or without radiculopathies: segmental instability, facet syndrome, and disc disruption syndrome.

Segmental Instability

Many patients with low back pain have recurring episodes of increasing severity, sometimes transiently, associated with nerve root irritation, and usually triggered by minor mechanical overloads.[19,32] Radiographic criteria associated with this diagnosis have included the presence of disc space narrowing and spinal osteophytes projecting away from the disc space, the so-called traction spur.[36] The most important criterion is abnormal shifts in the alignment of vertebrae observed on lateral spinal radiographs taken with the patient in a flexed and extended position, so-called flexion/extension views.[15,33] Friberg[18] proposed a different method whereby the spine is overloaded by a backpack and then placed in traction (traction/compression films). Attempts to classify segmental instability associated with spinal degeneration have not been uniformly accepted.[20] Despite the absence of certain clinical and radiographic criteria, segmental instability remains one of the most common indications for lumbar spinal fusion. The diagnosis should require translation of at least 4.5 mm in the lumbar spine as measured from dynamic radiographs. Rarely, there is instead abnormal angular rotational movement of the vertebrae. Rotation occurs normally at each motion segment. An angular change of greater than 15° at L1-2, L2-3, and L3-4, greater than 20° at L4-5, and greater than 25° at L5-S1 is considered abnormal. Figure 21–4 illustrates how to measure flexion/extension films.

Facet Syndrome

Sixty years ago, it was proposed that many causes of low back pain originated from the facet joints. Mooney and Robertson[38] repopularized this diagnosis. They described a group of patients who had pain mainly in spinal extension or rotation, often accompanied by referred pain to the upper buttocks, posterolateral thigh, and sometimes even into the calf. Spinal radiographs were often normal. Provocative injections with saline into the facet joints resulted in referred pain, whereas relief of pain followed injection of the facet with local anesthetic. In other patients, radiographic evidence of degeneration of the facets was present, and this group was given the diagnosis of facet arthritis. Treatment with antiinflammatory medications, and, in some instances, local steroid injection into the affected joint, was associated with symptom relief. Denervation has also been attempted. Since this original description, there have been a number of attempts to characterize precisely the clinical syndrome and develop rational therapy. A comprehensive analysis of over 400 patients led to the conclusion that facet syndrome cannot be classified with any certainty.[27] A small subset of patients have facet pathology associated with a degenerative cyst. If this cyst projects into the spinal canal and affects the nerve root, it can produce symptoms indistinguishable from lumbar disc herniation.

Disc Disruption Syndrome

Crock[11] described the disc disruption syndrome as characterized by severe, unrelenting, mechanical low back pain following a suspected compression injury. He reported that spinal radiographs were usually normal and the diagnosis was dependent on discography whereby injection of the radiopaque contrast media into the disc must faithfully reproduce the patient's pain and also demonstrate the disruption of the normal disc architecture. Disc disruption syndrome is a source of controversy and uncertainty, as is the use of discography.

Congenital Abnormalities

In the normal development of the spine, defects in the formation of spinal structures may occur. The majority of these abnormalities have minimal significance but are often erroneously believed to cause low back pain. Most of the common congenital abnormalities occur equally in populations with and without back pain. The most common are spina bifida occulta and segmentation abnormalities such as lumbarization and sacralization.

Spina Bifida Occulta

As the neural arch forms, incomplete closure may occur, accompanied by partial or complete absence of the spinous process. In a small subgroup (1/100,000), the bony defect is accompanied by a herniation of the neural elements through the defect. This condition is termed meningomyelocele and is associated with a variety of neurologic defects usually apparent at birth. For the vast majority of patients, spina bifida occulta is a finding of no significance.

Segmentation Abnormalities

There are wide variations in the number and shape of lumbar vertebrae. Lumbarization occurs when the first sacral segment has the appearance of a lumbar vertebra and, thus, there are six rather than five lumbar segments. Conversely, the fifth lumbar vertebra may be incorporated into the sacrum (sacralization), resulting in only four mobile lumbar vertebrae (Fig. 21–8). Sometimes the incorporation occurs only on one side (hemisacralization), and, infrequently, may be associated with the development of a false joint between the ilium and the elongated transverse process of the fifth lumbar vertebrae. In general, segmentation abnormalities are not associated with an increased risk of back pain and are not the cause of back pain per se. A few patients with hemisacralization may have pain arising from the false joint, and there is some evidence of increased susceptibility to L4/5 disc herniations in this group, the so-called Bertelocci syndrome. Segmentation abnormalities are important sources of confusion in determining the level of a herniated disc or stenosis.

Conjoined Nerve Roots

Anatomic variants may also occur in neural structures. For example, nerve roots may be conjoined. This condition has minimal significance except as a possible cause of sciatica, but it may pose technical problems in surgical interventions. It can also confuse the interpretation of an imaging examination, particularly a myelogram, as the conjoint root can produce a picture resembling a disc herniation.

Spondylolysis and Spondylolisthesis

Spondylolisthesis is broadly defined as forward displacement of one vertebra relative to the next lower vertebra (Fig. 21–9). This condition can arise from numerous causes.[53] The most common form is isthmic spondylolisthesis, which involves an acquired or, more rarely, congenital defect in the neural arch at the pars interarticularis. The defect is termed spondylolysis and may be unilateral or bilateral. The presence of the defect varies widely in the population and ranges from 1 to 10%. Isthmic spondylolisthesis is less common, affecting 1 to 4% of the population. The most common site of isthmic spondylolisthesis is at L5 which slips forward on S1. This lesion is far more common in males than females. Importantly, although L5/S1 slippage may increase in childhood and adolescence, continuation of the forward slippage ceases with adulthood and, thus, adult patients with the common L5/S1 lesion do not

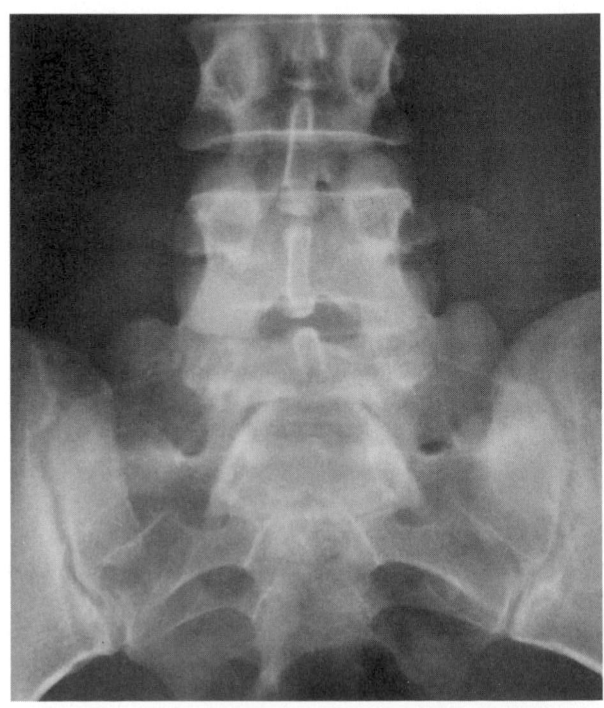

Figure 21–8. Sacralization of the fifth lumbar vertebrae (L5).

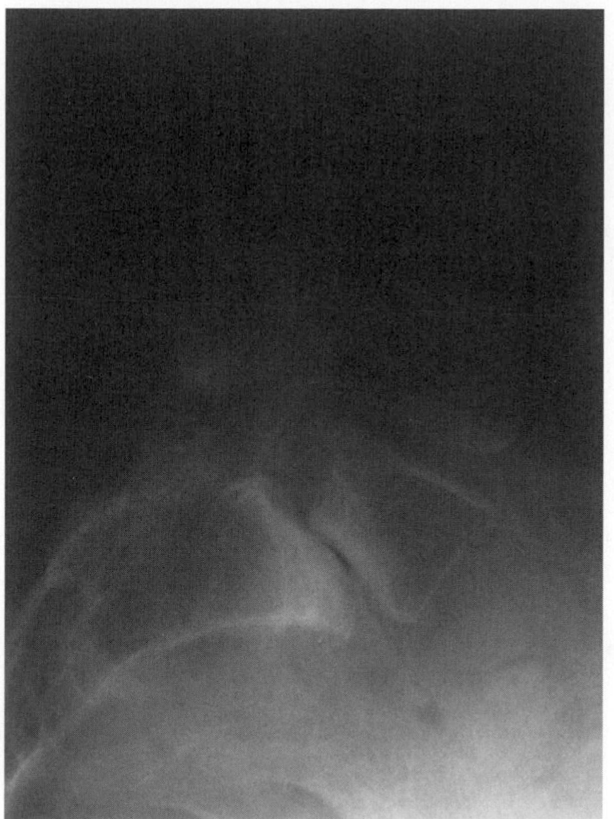

Figure 21–9. Grade 2 spondylolisthesis (L5/S1).

have an unstable spine.[17] When the isthmic lesion occurs at L4/5, there is evidence that slippage may continue during adulthood, unlike the L5/S1 lesion.

The development of spondylolysis and subsequent isthmic spondylolisthesis is thought to be due to a fatigue failure of the neural arch in many patients rather than being a congenital abnormality. Typically, this occurs in childhood or adolescence and, when recognized on radiographs later in life, has no appearance or signs of an overt fracture. In a few patients, the fracture is recent. This can only be identified by the presence of increased radioisotope uptake within the neural arch, and usually no bony defect is observed on routine spinal radiographs. In these patients, bracing may resolve the symptoms and the actual defect may never develop (i.e., the fracture heals). Because spondylolysis is more common in certain athletes, such as football linemen and female gymnasts, repetitive flexion-extension forces have been thought to be the mechanism of injury. Spondylolysis is equally common in populations with and without pack pain. However, workers with advanced spondylolisthesis are somewhat more susceptible to low back pain, particularly if the slip is Grade 2 or higher.

The type of spondylolisthesis should be described etiologically and anatomically. The following list (modified from reference 53) presents an etiologic classification of spondylolysis[7]:

I. Dysplastic (congenital)
II. Isthmic (pars lesion)
    A. Lytic (fatigue fracture)
    B. Elongated (with intact pars)
    C. Acute fracture
III. Degenerative
IV. Traumatic
V. Pathologic (bone disease)

The anatomic classification describes the degree of slip, as illustrated in Figure 21–10. In Grades 3 and 4 spondylolisthesis, additional features may have prognostic value. The level at which spondylolisthesis is present should be specified, because patients with L4/5 spondylolisthesis have more clinical symptoms than patients with an equivalent spondylolisthesis at L5/S1. The diagnosis should be based on radiographs, and the grade of slippage should be measured on true lateral views (Chapter 14).

Spine Trauma

Acute fractures and fracture dislocations develop when an external load exceeds the strength of the tissues. The resulting type of injury is a function of the magnitude and velocity and direction of the applied loads. A variety of classifications have been devised (Fig. 21–11).[12] The most common fracture is the result of a fall with the patient landing on the buttocks and is termed a compression fracture. Compression fractures are usually quantified by the degree of vertebral body collapse that has occurred; for example, a 25% compression. Because of the structure of the trabecular network, the anterior part of the body is usually more compressed than the posterior. If the force magnitude is greater, the same type of trauma can result in a burst fracture of the vertebral body where bony fragments may be displaced into the spinal canal, sometimes resulting in neurologic compromise.

With the exception of very severe (greater than 50% of vertebral body height) compression fractures, burst fractures, and fracture-dislocations, the majority of these injuries do not require operative treatment, heal uneventfully, and are compatible with the resumption of normal activities after healing is complete. Neurologic dysfunction associated with more severe injuries has major functional implications, including paraplegia.

Spinal Infections

Acute or chronic bacterial infections of the spine are uncommon. Acute infections are the result of

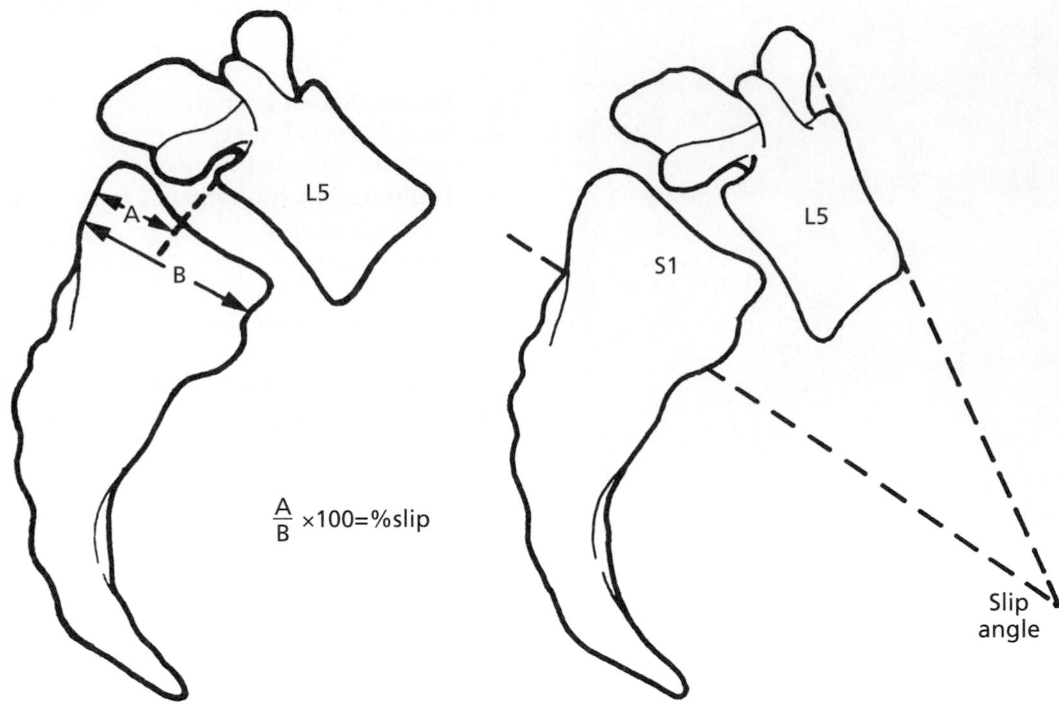

Figure 21–10. Measurements in spondylolisthesis. The degree of slip is measured as a percentage obtained by dividing the amount of displacement *by the a-p (anterio-posterior) diameter of the inferior vertebra (here sacrum)* and multiplying by 100. Commonly, the olisthesis is classified as Grade 1 (0 to 25%), 2 (25 to 50%), 3 (50 to 75%), or 4 (75 to 100%). The slip angle is a measure of the angular relationship of L5 and S1. A higher slip angle is associated with a greater potential for progressive slip.

hematogenous spread of bacteria to the vertebrae and are rare in individuals who are otherwise healthy. Predispositions include diabetes, the use of corticosteroids or other immunosuppressive drugs, and recent genitourinary surgery. Intravenous drug abusers and patients with acquired immunodeficiency syndrome are also at risk. Staphylococci are the most commonly cultured bacteria, but a variety of other organisms are seen with increasing frequency. Tubercular infections are common in underdeveloped countries, still exist in the United States, and are increasing in drug-abusing populations. Postoperative infections occur after disc surgery in about 0.25% of patients, almost always in the form of discitis.

The history of patients with spinal infections is variable, ranging from a very acute, severe systemic illness with pain and fever to an insidious onset with minimal, if any, systemic symptoms. An acute onset is most common with blood-borne bacterial infections, whereas an insidious onset is typical of tuberculosis. A distinctive characteristic is the complaint of pain at night. The physical examination varies widely, ranging from restricted spinal motion and muscle spasm to excruciating pain. In the small subset of patients with epidural abscesses, neurologic dysfunction may be rapidly progressive and constitute a surgical emergency.

Early in the course of these infections, the spinal radiographs may be normal. Radioisotope scans and MRIs are often necessary for diagnosis. Later, destruction of the vertebral bodies with collapse and obliteration of the disc space may occur, occasionally with the development of an epidural abscess. The outcome of these patients and their ability to return to their occupation depends on the underlying disease that may have predisposed to the condition, and the successful eradication of the infection by appropriate antibiotics. The need for surgical intervention depends on the infecting organism, the response to antibiotics, and the development of neurologic symptoms and signs. Many of the patients ultimately resume fairly normal activities, particularly those with postoperative disc space infections.

Inflammatory Spinal Conditions

Inflammatory lesions affecting the lumbar spine are termed spondyloarthropathies, of which ankylosing spondylitis is most prevalent, affecting 2% of the popu-

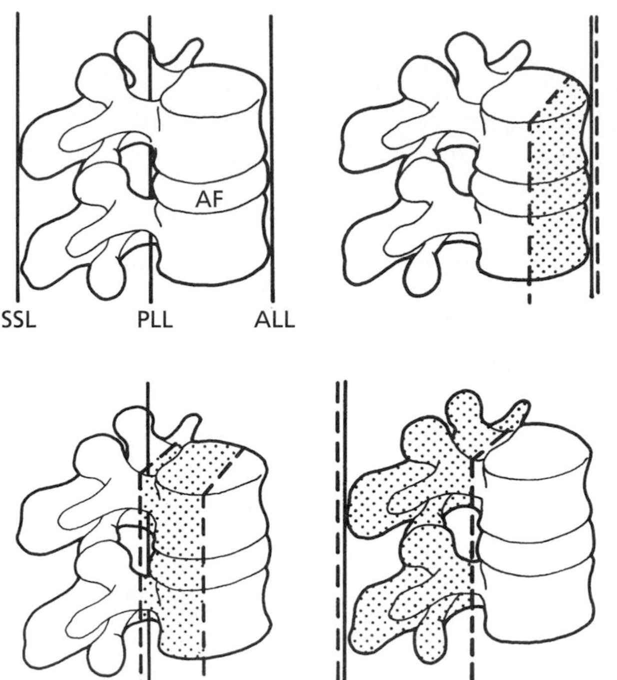

Figure 21–11. The three-column concept divides the spine into an anterior column (the anterior longitudinal ligament, anterior disc, and anterior vertebral body), a middle column (the posterior disc, posterior vertebral body, and posterior longitudinal ligament), and a posterior column (posterior bony complex and ligamentous complex). Failure of two columns results in an unstable spine. (From Denis F: The three-column spine and its significance in the classification of acute thoraco-lumbar spinal injuries. Spine 8:817, 1983.)

lation. The patient is typically a man, younger than 40 years of age. The onset of back pain is insidious. The patients often describe early awakening and spinal stiffness, particularly in the morning. These symptoms often improve as the day progresses. The physical examination reveals decreased chest expansion and reduced spinal mobility. Early radiographic studies are often normal but eventually demonstrate erosive changes at the sacroiliac joints. In severe cases, complete ankylosis (fusion) of the sacroiliac joints and spine may occur. Laboratory studies can be normal, but more commonly there are mild elevations of the erythrocyte sedimentation rate, and in 95% of patients, a specific serum antigen, the human leukocyte antigen (HLA)-27B, is present. However, a positive HLA-27B test alone is not diagnostic because 5 to 12% of the population has this finding, most of whom do not have the disease.

Other types of spondyloarthropathies include Reiter's syndrome (a disease characterized by the triad of genitourinary inflammation [urethritis], eye inflammation [uveitis], and sacroiliitis) and spondylitides associated with psoriasis or inflammatory bowel disease such as ulcerative colitis (Table 21–11).

The majority of patients with inflammatory spinal conditions are able to carry on normal physical activities. In the most severely affected individuals, limitation of spinal mobility or involvement of other joints, such as the hips, may preclude all but sedentary occupations.

Fibromyalgia

Fibromyalgia and myofascial pain syndrome are conditions that are thought to be caused by muscle inflammation. These controversial diagnoses are characterized by nonspecific, chronic low back pain, sometimes radiating into the upper parts of the lower legs. Three major criteria that are required for the diagnosis include chronic generalized aches, pains, or stiffness (involving at least three musculoskeletal regions for at least 3 months); absence of other systemic conditions to account for these symptoms; and multiple tender points at characteristic locations (trigger points). With the exception of trigger points, these major criteria are similar to those symptoms reported by patients with nonspecific chronic low back pain. A number of minor criteria (disturbed sleep, generalized fatigue, subjective swelling or numbness of extremities, pain in neck or shoulders, chronic headache, and irritable bowel symptoms) strengthen the diagnosis but are not absolutely required. The most

TABLE 21–11

Differential Diagnoses of Seronegative Spondyloarthropathies

Characteristic	Ankylosing Spondylitis	Reiter's Syndrome	Inflammatory Bowel Disease	Psoriasis
Sacroiliitis	100%, Early symmetric	20%, Late symmetric	20%, Symmetric	20%, Late asymmetric
Peripheral arthritis	Hips and shoulders	Lower extremity	Hips and shoulders	Upper extremity
Calcaneous periostitis	Frequent	Very frequent	Occurs	No
Extra-articular	Occurs	Frequent (eye/skin)	Occurs	Frequent (skin)
Sex	M > F	M > F	F = M	F > M
Age at onset	>20	>20	Any	Any
Onset	Gradual	Sudden	Variable	Gradual

Modified from Andersson GBJ, McNeill TW: Lumbar Spine Syndrome: Evaluation and Treatment. Vienna, Springer-Verlag, 1989.

important diagnostic criterion is the presence of trigger points, which are localized tender areas of tissue within the muscle and the fascia. Relief of symptoms by anesthetic injections into these trigger points is thought to be diagnostic. Sleep disturbances are common. Almost half of the patients report that they are awakened during the night and fatigue is often a significant functional problem. Whereas some physicians are strong proponents of fibromyalgia and myofascial pain as distinct disease entities, others believe they are simply variants of idiopathic chronic low back pain.

Treatment of fibromyalgia is nonspecific and includes muscle relaxants, heat, stretching, aerobic exercises, and education. Prognosis is generally good but symptoms may persist for a long period. These patients are sometimes unnecessarily subjected to expensive and sometimes invasive diagnostic tests (see also Chapter 42).

Metabolic Disorders

The most important spinal metabolic disorder is osteoporosis. It most commonly affects women after the age of 50. Other risk factors include northern European descent, small stature, early menopause, positive family history on the female side, inactive lifestyle, smoking, and chronic treatment with corticosteroids. The major consequence of osteoporosis is weakening of the bone, which makes the individual more susceptible to compression fractures. Awareness of this problem is important because osteoporosis can be treated medically. It may be necessary to reduce the affected individual's lifting and bending requirements to protect the weaker spine.

Neoplasms

Tumors can involve osseous or neural structures, producing pain or neurologic dysfunction. They are rare in patients younger than 50. The most common tumors result from metastatic spread from some other primary site, most commonly breast cancer in the female, prostate cancer in the male, and lung, kidney, and thyroid cancer in both sexes (Fig. 21–12). Multiple myeloma is the most common primary malignant bone tumor, but a variety of other, rarer, primary bone or neural tumors may cause low back pain or sciatica. Bony malignant tumors often present with the insidious onset of pain, although acute pain may occur if structural weakening causes a compression fracture. The characteristic pain complaint is night pain, awakening the patient. The spinal radiograph is often diagnostic, but early in the development of a tumor, bone scan, CT scan, or MRI may be required for definitive diagnosis.

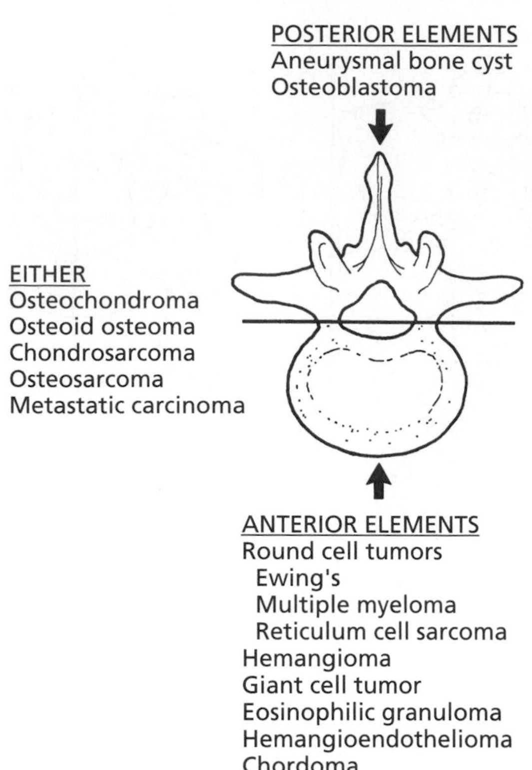

Figure 21–12. Frequent location of spinal tumors. (From Andersson GBJ, McNeill TW: Lumbar Spine Syndromes: Evaluation and Treatment. Vienna, Springer-Verlag, 1989.)

SUMMARY

The lumbar spine is susceptible to a variety of pathologic conditions, but the majority of patients do not have a definable pathoanatomic cause for their pain, if strict diagnostic criteria are used. The Quebec Classification overcomes the reliance on the more classic, pathoanatomic classification systems and has the important attributes that, not only is the pain pattern characterized, but the duration and effect on work status are incorporated. These factors are more important in defining treatment and employability than is the actual diagnosis in the majority of patients. However, the examiner must remember that there is a smaller subgroup of patients who have a clear diagnosis for their symptoms, which is more likely when sciatica or claudication accompany the complaint. The patient's complaint of pain must be carefully evaluated and may give important clues to the causation. Because radiographic abnormalities are so common in asymptomatic individuals, the most important lesson in the clinical diagnosis and impairment evaluation is to correlate the radiographic studies with the patient's/claimant's clinical complaint, rather than to define or rate impairment solely on a radiographic diagnosis of spinal degeneration or disk degeneration.

References

1. Aiello I, Serra G, Tugnoli V, et al: Electrophysiological findings in patients with lumbar prolapse. Electromyogr Clin Neurophysiol 24:313–320, 1984.
2. American Medical Association: Guides to the Evaluation of Permanent Impairment, 4th ed. Chicago, American Medical Association, 1993.
3. Andersson GBJ, Deyo RA: Sensitivity, specificity, and predictive value: A general issue in screening for disease and in the interpretation of diagnostic studies in spinal disorders. In Frymoyer JF (ed): The Adult Spine, 2nd ed. Philadelphia, Lippincott, 1977, pp 93–141.
4. Andersson GBJ, McNeill TW: Lumbar Spinal Stenosis. St. Louis, Mosby–Year Book, 1992.
5. Andersson GBJ, McNeill TW: Lumbar Spine Syndromes: Evaluation and Treatment. Vienna, Springer-Verlag, 1989.
6. Andersson GBJ, Svensson H-O, Oden A: The intensity of work recovery in low-back pain. Spine 8:880–884, 1983.
7. Arnoldi CC, Brodsky AE, Cauchoix J, et al: Lumbar spinal stenosis and nerve root entrapment syndromes: Definition and classification. Clin Orthop 115:4, 1976.
8. Bergquist-Ullman M, Larsson U: Acute low back pain in industry. Acta Orthop Scand 170(Suppl.):1, 1977.
9. Boden S, Davis DO, Dina TS, et al: Abnormal magnetic resonance scans of the lumbar spine in asymptomatic subjects. J Bone Joint Surg (Am) 72:403–408, 1990.
10. Cocchiarella L, Andersson GBJ (eds): Guides to the Evaluation of Permanent Impairment, 5th ed. Chicago, American Medical Association, 2001.
11. Crock HV: Internal disc disruption: A challenge to disc prolapse fifty years on. Spine 11:650, 1986.
12. Denis F: The three-column spine and its significance in the classification of acute thoraco-lumbar spinal injuries. Spine 8:817, 1983.
13. Deyo RA, Diehl AK: Lumbar spine films in primary care: Current use and effects of selective ordering criteria. J Gen Intern Med 1:20–25, 1986.
14. Deyo RA, Rainville J, Dent DL: What can the history and physical examination tell us about low-back pain? JAMA 268:760–765, 1992.
15. Dupuis PR, Yong-Hing K, Cassidy JD, et al: Radiologic diagnosis of degenerative lumbar spinal instability. Spine 10:262, 1985
16. Eyre D, Buckwalter J, et al: The intervertebral disk: Part B—Basic science perspective. In Frymoyer JW, Gordon SL (eds): New Perspectives on Low-Back Pain. Park Ridge, Ill, American Academy of Orthopaedic Surgeons, 1989, pp 147–207.
17. Fredrickson BE, Baker D, McHolick WJ, et al: The natural history of spondylolysis and spondylolisthesis. J Bone Joint Surg 66A:699, 1984.
18. Friberg O: Lumbar instability: A dynamic approach by traction-compression radiography. Spine 12:119, 1987.
19. Frymoyer JW: Back pain and sciatica. N Engl J Med 318:291, 1988.
20. Frymoyer JW, Selby DK: Segmental instability: Rationale for treatment. Spine 10:280, 1985.
21. Hakelius A, Hindmarsh J: The significance of neurological signs and myelographic findings in the diagnosis of lumbar root compression. Acta Orthop Scand 43:239, 1972.
22. Hirsch C, Inglemark B-E, Miller M: The anatomical basis for low back pain: Studies on the presence of sensory nerve endings in ligamentous, capsular and intervertebral disc structures in the human lumbar spine. Acta Orthop Scand 33:1, 1963.
23. Hitselberger WE, Witten RM: Abnormal myelograms in asymptomatic patients. J Neurosurg 28:204–208, 1968.
24. Holt EP: The question of lumbar discography. J Bone Joint Surg (Am) 50:720–726, 1968.
25. Jackson RP, Cain JE, Jacobs RR, et al: The neuroradiographic diagnosis of lumbar herniated nucleus pulposus: I—A comparison of computed tomography (CT), myelography discography, and CT-discography. Spine 14:1356–1360, 1989.
26. Jackson RP, Cain JE, Jacobs RR, et al: Neuroradiographic diagnosis of lumbar herniated nucleus pulposus: II—A comparison of computed tomography (CT), myelography, CT-myelography, and magnetic resonance imaging. Spine 14:1362–1367, 1989.
27. Jackson RP, Jacobs RR, Montesano PX: Facet joint injection in low-back pain, a prospective statistical study. Spine 13:966, 1988.
28. Jensen MC, Brant-Zawdzki MN, Obuchowki N, et al: Magnetic resonance imaging of the lumbar spine in people without back pain. N Engl J Med 331:69–73, 1994.
29. Keefe FJ, Beckham JC, Fillingim RB: The psychology of chronic back pain. In Frymoyer JW (ed): The Adult Spine: Principles and Practice. New York, Raven Press, 1991, pp 185–197.
30. Kellgren JH: The anatomical source of back pain. Rheumatol Rehabil 16:3, 1977.
31. Kent DL, Haynor DR, Larson EB, et al: Diagnosis of lumbar spinal stenosis in adults: A meta-analysis of the accuracy of CT, MR, and myelography. Am J Roentgenol 158:1135–1144, 1992.
32. Kirkaldy-Willis WH, Farfan HF: Instability of the lumbar spine. Clin Orthop 165:110, 1982.
33. Knutsson F: The instability associated with disk degeneration in the lumbar spine. Acta Radiol 25:593, 1944.
34. Kostuik JP, Harrington I, Alexander D, et al: Cauda equina syndrome and lumbar disc herniation. J Bone Joint Surg 68A:386, 1986.
35. Lewis T, Kellgren JH: Observations relating to referred pain, visceromotor reflexes, and other associated phenomena. Clin Sci 4:47, 1939.
36. Macnab I: The traction spur: an indicator of segmental instability. J Bone Joint Surg 53A:663, 1971.
37. McCall IW, Park WM, O'Brien JP: Induced pain referral from posterior lumbar elements in normal subjects. Spine 4:441, 1979.
38. Mooney V, Robertson J: The facet syndrome. Clin Orthop 115:149, 1976.
39. Nachemson AL, Andersson GBJ: Classification of low-back pain. Scand J Work Environ Health 8:134, 1982.
40. Nachemson AL, Jonsson E: Neck and Back Pain. Philadelphia, Lippincott, 2000.
41. Pope MH, Andersson GBJ, Frymoyer JW, et al: Occupational Low-back Pain. St. Louis, Mosby–Year Book, 1991.
42. Scham SM, Taylor TKF: Tension signs in lumbar disc prolapse. Clin Orthop 75:195, 1971.
43. Shaffer W, Spratt K, Weinstein J, et al: The consistency and accuracy of roentgenograms for measuring sagittal translation in the lumbar vertebral motion segment. Spine 15:741–750, 1990.
44. Spangfort EV: The lumbar disc herniation: A computer aided analysis of 2504 operations. Acta Orthop Scand 142(Suppl.):1, 1972.
45. Spitzer WO, LeBlanc FE, Dupuis M, et al: Scientific approach to the assessment and management of activity-related spinal disorders: A monograph for clinicians. Report of the Quebec Task Force on Spinal Disorders. Spine 12(Suppl. 7):S1–S59, 1987.
46. Troup JDG, Martin JW, Lloyd DCEF: Back pain in industry: A prospective survey. Spine 6:61, 1981.
47. Valkenburg HA, Haanen HCM: The epidemiology of low-back pain. In White AA, Gordon SL (eds): American Academy of Orthopaedic Surgeons Symposium on Idiopathic Low-back Pain. St. Louis, CV Mosby, 1982.
48. Waddell G, Bircher M, Finlayson D, et al: Symptoms and signs: Physical disease or illness behavior? Br Med J 289:739, 1984.
49. Waddell G, McCulloch JA, Kummel E, et al: Nonorganic physical signs in low-back pain. Spine 5:117, 1979.

50. Walsh TR, Weinstein JN, Spratt KF, et al: Lumbar discography in normal subjects: A controlled, prospective study. J Bone Joint Surg (Am) 72:1081–1088, 1990.
51. White AW, Punjabi MM: Clinical Biomechanics of the Spine, 2nd ed. Philadelphia, Lippincott, 1990.
52. Wiesel SW, Tsourmas N, Feffer HL, et al: A study of computer-assisted tomography: I—The incidence of positive CAT scans in an asymptomatic group of patients. Spine 9:549–551, 1984.
53. Wiltse LL, Newman PH, Macnab I: Classification of spondylolysis and spondylolisthesis. Clin Orthop 117:23, 1976.
54. Work Cover Corporation: Work Cover Guidelines for the Management of Back-injured Employees. Adelaide, South Australia, Work Cover Corporation, 1993.
55. Yong-Hing K, Kirkaldy-Willis WH: The pathophysiology of degenerative disease of the lumbar spine. Orthop Clin North Am 14:491, 1983.

SECTION

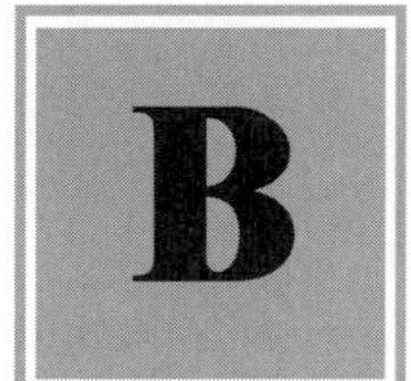

Internal Medicine Impairment Assessment

CHAPTER

22

Pulmonary Diagnostic Techniques

STEPHEN L. DEMETER, MD, MPH

In the investigation of pulmonary impairment and disability, greater reliance is given on pulmonary function tests (PFTs) than on the history and physical examination. Reasons for this include the following:

1. These tests provide quantifiable discriminations between degrees of pulmonary function/ dysfunction.
2. PFTs are reliable and historically valid.
3. Compared to the history and physical examination, these tests are generally more accurate, more reliable, and more readily reproduced.

This chapter on pulmonary tests is separated into sections covering the history and physical examination, pulmonary function studies, exercise testing, radiography, serologic testing and biopsies, and sleep studies. One very important PFT, the integrated cardiopulmonary exercise stress test, is covered briefly in this chapter but is discussed more fully in Chapter 24.

The History and Physical Examination

As discussed in Chapter 11, the history and physical examination are extremely important in the standard medical examination. Although they are also important in impairment and disability examinations, there are some major differences. For a pulmonary impairment or disability examination, greater reliance is placed on physiologic testing than on the physical examination or the historical interview.

A careful review of medical records serves to establish the historical basis behind a person's claim and gives important clues about the reliability of the history taken during the impairment or disability evaluation. Nevertheless, a properly performed history and physical examination gives the examiner important information, especially when the examiner is able to independently affirm many of the historical aspects from the record review.

The history provides information regarding the incidents of the claim, the work history, present job requirements, and other issues addressed in Chapters 12 and 43. It is not the intention of the current chapter to review these points. Rather, a few key issues peculiar to the pulmonary history and physical examination are presented.

Dyspnea

The AMA Guides state: "Dyspnea is the most common symptom noted on initial examination of individuals with any type of pulmonary impairment. Despite its importance, dyspnea is nonspecific; it is often caused by cardiac, hematologic, metabolic, or neurologic disease, or by anxiety or physical deconditioning."[26(p89)] A table entitled "Classification of Dyspnea" is reprinted here from the fifth edition of the Guides (Table 22–1).[26] The

TABLE 22–1

Classification of Dyspnea

Severity	Definition and Question
Mild	Do you have to walk more slowly on the level than people of your age because of breathlessness?
Moderate	Do you have to stop for breath when walking at your own pace on the level?
Severe	Do you ever have to stop for breath after walking about 100 yards or for a few minutes on the level?
Very severe	Are you too breathless to leave the house, or breathless after dressing or undressing?

From Cocchiarella L, Andersson GBJ (eds): Guides to the Evaluation of Permanent Impairment, 5th ed. Chicago, American Medical Association, 2001, p 89, with permission.

footnote in the Guides explains that "(T)he person's lowest level of physical activity and exertion that produces breathlessness denotes the severity of dyspnea."[26(p89)] The Guides notes that when "a disparity is found between subjective complaints of dyspnea and findings on respiratory testing, consider a nonrespiratory dyspnea component."[26(p89)]

Besides these statements and this table, no further mention is made of dyspnea in the Guides. It seems that the dyspnea classification scale can be used when determining where, on a spectrum, an examinee's final impairment rating is placed (although this is not directly stated in the Guides). For example, if a person is in a Class 4 impairment category, how should the examiner arrive at a final number? Should the impairment percent be 51%, 100%, or somewhere in between? The impairment rating is chosen based upon the severity of the condition (e.g., using pulmonary function parameters and a dyspnea) and the impact on activities of daily living. For example, to be in a Class 4, the forced vital capacity (FVC) needs to be <50% of predicted, or the forced expiratory volume in 1 second (FEV_1) <40% of predicted, or the DCO <40% of predicted. If the actual values are FVC = 60%, FEV_1 = 35%, and DCO = 60%, then an impairment rating closer to 51 to 55% may be more appropriate than a rating of 61 to 65%. The same would hold true for any other imagined numbers—the lower the global values, the higher the rating. The other way is to weigh the physiologic values with the dyspnea score.

When using dyspnea as a discriminator on impairment or disability examination, the examiner must feel comfortable with its reliability. That claimants can and do exaggerate symptoms comes as no surprise to anyone with any experience in this field. A historically corroborated history of dyspnea can be very powerful information; however, even when reliable, how valid is that information?

The sensation of dyspnea is multifactorial in origin.[24,81] The physiologic need of the body to increase the minute ventilation (respiratory rate x tidal volume) is perceived by the brain as the sensation of dyspnea. The list of causations of dyspnea is quite large. As pointed out previously, perturbations in many organ systems can cause this sensation.[26,78,81] An increase in minute ventilation can be caused by insufficient oxygen transport to metabolizing tissues. This may be a result of pulmonary disease (poor air exchange, diminished gas diffusion), cardiac disease (decreased cardiac output), anemia, or peripheral vascular disease. These organ-specific abnormalities produce dyspnea as a reflection of disturbed physiology. When mild, the sensation is perceived only with strenuous exertion. As the physiology becomes more disturbed, the sensation is perceived closer and closer to the resting state. Obesity can cause dyspnea owing to altered breathing mechanics and a greater need for oxygen delivery for a given amount of work owing to the need to move a greater body bulk. Being out of shape also produces a level of exertional dyspnea greater than that found during exercise in a fit person. As seen in Chapter 24, muscles of trained athletes utilize a lower amount of oxygen ($\dot{V}O_2$) to produce the same degree of work as do the muscles of out of shape individuals, reflecting a different degree of dyspnea. Psychological causes are also important (see the section on hyperventilation syndrome in Chapter 25). Other causes include neuromuscular disorders, skeletal deformities, hyperthyroidism, and pregnancy.[68]

However, as Mahler et al point out, "(D)yspnea begs a precise definition."[80] Perhaps the best way to define this term is a sensation of abnormal shortness of breath. Thus, shortness of breath that occurs after exercise would not be categorized as dyspnea unless the exerciser considered it to be inappropriate for the level of exercise. A number of variables affect the perception of dyspnea, including age, sex, socioeconomic status, social learning, verbal acuity, tolerance levels, and others.[80]

How useful, then, is the sensation of dyspnea in an impairment rating or disability determination? Is this symptom akin to the perception of pain when testing the musculoskeletal system? In other words, is it a limiting factor with a high degree of correlation with functional capacity or is it an independent factor? If it is independent of functional capacity, which factor more reliably predicts impairment (or a deviation from normality) or disability (an inability to perform at a certain exercise level)—physiology (or functional capacity) or symptomatology?

Dyspnea has been studied in a number of ways in patients with pulmonary diseases. Some of these include dyspnea in the patient with chronic obstructive pulmonary disease (COPD), rehabilitation of patients with dyspnea and COPD, dyspnea as a reflection of quality of life in patients with pulmonary diseases, and the relationship of dyspnea to physiologic parameters. Each of these issues is discussed in the following; its place in the impairment or disability evaluation will be determined from these parameters.

Dyspnea in COPD

A useful model is the symptom of dyspnea in patients with COPD (a disease encompassing various mixes of emphysema and chronic bronchitis or obstructive lung disease [OLD]). Patients with COPD have symptoms that include dyspnea, altered physiology, abnormalities on physical examination, and abnormal chest radiographs. The degree of physiologic alteration is directly linked to both morbidity and mortality. In individuals aged <60 years with FEV_1 >50%, the predicted mortality is 10% in 3 years; for patients aged >60 years with FEV_1 >50%, the predicted 3-year mortality is 20%; and for patients aged >60 years with FEV_1 40 to 49%, the 3-year mortality is 25%.[99] The normal person has a decline in FEV_1 of 20 to 30 cc per year.[65] In patients with COPD who decrease their FEV_1 by 70 cc per year, the 10-year mortality is 70%.[99] In patients with FEV_1 <0.75 L, the approximate mortality at 1 year is 30% and at 10 years it is 95%.[22]

The British Thoracic Society (BTS) stated that "an individual patient's perception of breathlessness varies considerably for the same degree of airflow limitation and this may be particularly poor in old age"[99(ps8)] and concluded that the "presence of symptoms can be extremely variable in patients with COPD; a firm diagnosis can only be made by objective measurement of airways obstruction with spirometric tests."[99(ps7)] Wolkove et al noted: "intuitively, it would appear that those patients with the most severe airway obstruction should be the most dyspneic. However, clinical experience teaches that this is not always the case ... the relationship between airway obstruction and dyspnea is complex, and it is unclear to what extent measures of each correlate in patients with OLD."[131(p1247)] They performed a study in 93 patients with OLD, or COPD, and measured dyspnea on the Borg Scale Dyspnea Index (BSDI) before and after a bronchodilator administration. In those patients there was a concordance of findings in only 43% of patients (improvement in both the BSDI and the FEV_1), whereas 17% had an improvement in physiology but not symptomatology, 26% had an improvement in symptomatology but not physiology, and 14% had improvement in neither parameter.[131]

Dyspnea in Rehabilitation Programs for Patients with COPD

Pulmonary rehabilitation does not improve pulmonary physiology.[22] It is used and recommended, however, because it improves strength and endurance, improves a sense of well being, and decreases dyspnea, cough, and sputum production.[22,99,115,129] It also improves a patient's sense of control over the disease. However, there appears to be a disparity in patients with COPD based on their degree of dyspnea. In 126 patients studied by Wedzicha et al, only those with a moderate intensity of dyspnea (using an MRC [Medical Research Council] scale) improved their exercise capacity and health status (measured by a variety of scales), whereas those with more severe dyspnea had no significant improvement in either their exercise capacity or health status. However, there were no significant differences in FEV_1 between these two groups.[129] Nevertheless, the dyspnea rating correlates better than the physiologic parameters (e.g., FEV_1) in the anticipated outcome of a rehabilitation program for a patient with pulmonary disease.[22,99,115,129]

TABLE 22–2

FEV_1 (% Predicted) and the Classification of COPD Severity

Source	Mild	Moderate	Severe
ATS[22]	≥50%	35–49%	<35%
BTS[99]	60–79%	40–59%	<40%
ERS[115]	≥70%	50–69%	<50%

FEV_1, forced expiratory volume in 1 second; COPD, chronic obstructive pulmonary disease; ATS, American Thoracic Society; BTS, British Thoracic Society; ERS, European Respiratory Society.

Dyspnea and Health-Related Quality of Life

Health-related quality of life (HRQOL) can be measured in patients with COPD using a variety of scales (as seen in the above section). The Guides state in Chapters 1 and 2 that interference with activities of daily living (ADL) is the fulcrum upon which all impairment determinations rest.[26] Thus considering the HRQOL would seem to be an appropriate way of assessing pulmonary impairment and is in keeping with the general philosophy of the Guides.

Measurements of quality of health and life in patients with COPD are categorized by physiology and symptomatology. When addressing the physiologic parameters of COPD, the American Thoracic Society (ATS),[22] the BTS,[99] and the European Respiratory Society (ERS)[115] have various cutoff criteria for rating the severity of this disease. As seen in Table 22–2, there are large variations among these three societies in their categorization of COPD based on physiology alone. It should be noted that the articles from which Table 22–2 was derived represent consensus statements by these three societies. As stated by the ERS, "such grading is inevitably arbitrary, however."[115(p1400)]

Dyspnea can be classified as mild, moderate, or severe. As noted in the previous sections, dyspnea categorization correlates poorly with physiology (FEV_1) but correlates better then physiology in anticipated improvements in rehabilitation programs. How, then, do dyspnea and physiology correlate with HRQOL?

Various scales have been used to assess dyspnea and HRQOL (for specifics, see references in this section and reference 79; also, reference 73 provides a useful section on various direct and indirect methods of measurement). In general, HRQOL correlates more closely with dyspnea scales than with scales of altered physiology. The sensitivity and specificity of any given study will depend on a variety of factors, including which scale was used. Hajiro et al found that "the HRQOL of patients with COPD was more clearly separated by the level of dyspnea than by the ATS disease staging"[59(p1632)] when dyspnea was measured by the St. George's Respiratory Questionnaire and HRQOL by the Medical Outcomes Study Short Form 36-item questionnaire method. Ferrer et al addressed the same issue but found that the ATS criteria for FEV_1 correlated better with the HRQOL than the criteria proposed by the ERS.[50]

Curtis et al reviewed published studies that defined the concept of HRQOL and the various tests used for this type of assessment.[34,35] HRQOL reflects that subcomponent of quality of life that is affected by the health status of the individual that is influenced by his or her "functional status" (the person's ability to function physically, socially, and emotionally). The reliability (a measurement of internal consistency), validity (or accuracy of a test), and responsiveness (the ability of a test to distinguish small, but clinically important, changes in health status over time) of various HRQOL tests (especially COPD and asthma-specific tests) were also reviewed. Values for r^2 (correlation coefficients) are provided in Table 22–3. As can be seen, the best index of HRQOL is the sensation of dyspnea. The authors state that "in summary, several studies have shown that health status measures correlate with physiologic measures of chronic lung disease and that they correlate in the expected direction. The correlation is not strong, suggesting that the physiological parameters do not accurately predict health status (and vice versa). These studies also suggest that dyspnea ratings and exercise tolerance are better predictors of health status than FEV_1 or oxygenation."[35(p1035)] Similar remarks were made regarding the effects of treatment (oxygen, bronchodilators [salmeterol, ipratropium, theophylline], and pulmonary rehabilitation) demonstrating disparities between changes in physiology (FEV_1 and exercise capacity) and HRQOL; the authors noted, "if investigators are concerned about health status, they must measure it rather than assuming that it will change with a physiologic parameter such as FEV_1."[35(p1036)] On the other hand, Mahler and Wells found a reasonable correlation between the FVC and FEV_1 and three tests of dyspnea (MRC, Baseline Dyspnea Index [BDI], and oxygen-cost diagram [OCD]). The r^2 for FVC was –0.41 for the MRC, 0.16 for the OCD, and 0.41 for the BDI. The values for FEV_1 were –0.42, 0.16, and 0.43, respectively. There were a total of 153 patients: 91 had COPD, 23 interstitial lung disease (ILD), 17 asthma, 9 heart disease, 6 obesity, and 7 miscellaneous.[82] This subject is also reviewed in reference 86, which describes many such tests and includes comments on the validity and reliability of each test.

TABLE 22-3

Values for r^2 for various parameters in patients with COPD

Parameter	HRQOL	Dyspnea	FEV_1	Exercise Tolerance
Dyspnea	0.44			
FEV_1	0.26	0.17		
Exercise tolerance	0.27	0.34	0.12	
Pao_2	0.01	0.02	—	0.0

COPD, chronic obstructive pulmonary disease; HRQOL, health-related quality of life; FEV_1, forced expiratory volume in 1 second.
From Curtis JR, Martin DP, Martin TR: Patient-assessed health outcomes in chronic lung disease. What are they, how do they help us, and where do we go from here? Am J Respir Crit Care Med 156:1032–1039, 1997.

Dyspnea Scales versus Physiologic Testing for Pulmonary Impairment or Disability

If dyspnea scales correlate better ($r^2 = 0.44$) with HRQOL than do FEV_1 ($r^2 = 0.26$) or exercise testing ($r^2 = 0.27$) in patients with COPD, which, then, is the better parameter for evaluating the pulmonary claimant for impairment or disability—the history or the physiologic examination?

First, it must be remembered that the above studies and conclusions dealt with, for the most part, patients with COPD. Are they applicable for all patients with pulmonary disorders? The correlation coefficient for dyspnea with FEV_1 in one study[82] was 0.32 in patients with COPD, but it was 0.78 for patients with asthma and 0.37 for patients with ILD. Thus the dyspnea score may not be homogenous in its relationship with HRQOL in all patients with different types of lung disease. Second, these measurements, although showing a better correlation between a dyspnea scale and HRQOL than between physiologic tests and HRQOL, found a correlation that was only 0.44 (a "perfect correlation" yields a r^2 value of 1.0; see Appendix A). Finally, these studies were performed on patients, not claimants. In these studies, patients would not be expected to have secondary gain issues impacting upon the validity of the study, whereas claimants might. Whether these secondary gain issues affect the reliability and validity of the perception of dyspnea and HRQOL has yet to be determined.

Summary and Recommendations

Although the symptom of dyspnea can be a valuable tool in clinical medicine, its place in disability medicine is yet to be determined. The sensation of dyspnea should not be used in impairment ratings or disability determinations until further research is performed on pulmonary claimants. Physiologic testing is reliable, valid, and reproducible, and although more imperfect than the dyspnea scale in clinical medicine, should be considered the only valid method of assessment of impairment. However, because impairment is defined as a deviation from normality, the issue of whether physiologic tests can measure function needs to be established before adapting them as criteria. The crux of the issue here is what should be measured. Should it be the amount of physiologic deviation from normality or the amount of deviation from health (or at least the perception of health)? If it is the latter, then perhaps the dyspnea scales should be reconsidered.

Physical Examination

Wheeze

"All that wheezes is not asthma and not all asthmatics wheeze." This is an old saw that most physicians first heard in medical school.

Wheezing is heard in most asthmatics and is dependent on the presence of disease activity. Because asthma can be intermittent, wheezes may not be heard in the patient with mild or moderate asthma, and their presence is also a reflection of the adequacy of treatment. A partial list of differential diagnoses producing wheezing in the nonasthmatic is found in the following list (this list is neither complete nor exhaustive; textbooks of pulmonary medicine should be perused for additional diagnoses):

- Asthma
- Infections
  - Acute bronchitis
  - Bronchiolitis
- Upper airway disorders
  - Tumor
  - Abscess
  - Infection (epiglottitis)
  - Extrinsic compression
  - Laryngeal edema
  - Bilateral vocal cord paralysis
  - Stricture
- Functional vocal cord adduction
- Carcinoid syndrome
- Hypersensitivity pneumonitis
- Chronic obstructing diseases
  - Chronic bronchitis
  - Emphysema
  - Bronchiectasis
  - Cystic fibrosis
  - Immunoglobulin deficiency
  - Bronchiolitis obliterans
- Left heart failure
- Pulmonary embolus
- Drug side effects
- Large airway obstruction
  - Tumor
  - Foreign body
  - Extrinsic compression
  - Strictures

Vocal cord adduction can produce a noise that is often confused with wheezing. It is a voluntary maneuver created by exhaling against partially closed vocal cords. It produces a "wheeze" (actually stridor—an upper airway noise that sounds like a wheeze) on physical examination. Stridor is a particularly troublesome physical finding. This is usually differentiated from wheezing by the location of the most intense noise on physical examination. It is also differentiated by its timing. Stridor caused by vocal cord adduction is inspiratory, whereas wheezing caused by asthma is usually expiratory or both inspiratory and expiratory or, if heard in only one phase, it is expiratory. Stridor should also be heard best, or localized, over the site of the obstruction, which in this case is the larynx. Wheezing, on the other hand, is a lower airway noise and should be heard more loudly over the lungs. The problem occurs in the patient with severe asthma in whom intense, severe wheezing may be reflected into the upper airways, producing a noise that is virtually indistinguishable from stridor on a routine physical examination.[84,92,116]

Functional vocal cord adduction is best identified by direct visualization using fiberoptic laryngoscopy.[84,92,116] The usual finding is adduction (or partial closure of the laryngeal opening) of the vocal cords during the time when the upper airway noise is heard. This disorder, termed Functional Vocal Cord Adduction Syndrome, is a somatization disorder and should be considered as such during an impairment evaluation or disability determination (see also Chapter 42).

Rales

The precise mechanism behind rales is still open to debate. The predominant theory is that it reflects the opening of small airways. Rales are found in a variety of disease states, especially ILD. The frequency of rales in ILD differs among the various causes of ILD (currently there are approximately 150 causes including various pneumoconioses and types of hypersensitivity pneumonitis) and not all patients with ILD will have rales.[113] Therefore, their absence in a patient who has ILD on a radiograph should not be taken as proof of absence of the disease.

Pulmonary Function Testing

Specific to impairment evaluation, the goal of PFTs is to determine the degree of an impairment or deviation from normality in a person with a breathing disorder. Various impairment rating systems specify different tests and different endpoints that reflect the peculiarities of that system (for example, the Guides use different tests and different endpoints than do the Social Security System or the Black Lung Law—see following). In addition, the ATS has published criteria for the machine used,[9,10] performance of the test,[9,10] selection of reference values for normal,[7] testing for asthma,[6,7,33] tests of diffusing capacity,[8] use of computers,[52] quality assurance in the pulmonary function laboratory,[53] and persons performing the test.[54,55,61] In addition, the National Institute of Occupational Safety and Health provides both guidelines and training seminars for the personnel who provide these tests.[61] More recently (in 2000), the American College of Occupational and Environmental Medicine published its own position statement on many of these issues.[124]

Tests of lung function include tests of lung volumes, expiratory flow rates, and gas exchange. In impairment evaluations, tests of lung volumes are rarely used, but these measurements can provide important background information regarding disease states. Impairment rating systems emphasize tests of flow rates and gas exchange. Flow rates relate to the ability to breathe and, therefore, to perform work on a sustained basis; they are also used for asthma testing. Gas exchange tests include the diffusing capacity and arterial blood gas levels and culminate in the cardiopulmonary exercise stress test (see Chapter 24), which combines the elements of breathing ability and gas exchange in the lungs and various organs of the body.

Many variables can influence pulmonary function testing, including height, age, weight, sex, race, posture, altitude at which the test is done, the ambient environment on the day of testing, presence of disease, presence of training (for example, in a wind instrument player), recent exposure to inhaled irritants, diurnal rhythms (including time of day or year or time in menstrual cycle for women), motivation, and prior testing.[7,14,25]

There are many tables of "normal" values (see reference 7) and the values derived by Crapo et al[31] were selected for use by the second through the fifth editions of the AMA Guides.[2,3,26,45,47] (From a historical perspective, the first edition of the Guides[27] and the JAMA article from which it was taken[28] used tables adapted from a Veterans Administration Army Cooperative Study for men, with no mention of the source used for the tables for women.)

Several points need to be made regarding the "normal" values:

1. **These values were developed and expected to be used for the interpretation of pulmonary function tests**. They were never developed to be used as instruments of or cutoff values for impairment ratings, although the ATS stated that the severity scores "are most appropriately derived from studies that relate pulmonary function test values to independent indices of performance such as ability to work and function in daily life, morbidity, and prognosis. ... In clinical practice, predicted values are also used to grade severity. The severity of the spirometric abnormality is usually based on the actual or percent predicted FEV_1 in the case of obstructive disorders or on FVC in nonobstructive disorders." At this point, the article describes a suggested algorithm suggesting cutoff points and concludes with the comment that this algorithm "is based as much on clinical impression as on objective data. Although clinical experience has always played a major role in assessing severity, it can be enhanced by more exact methods, and physicians should probably view arbitrary severity scoring systems with caution. Comments of the severity or significance of any abnormality depend on the circumstances under which a test is obtained."[7(p1212)] The Guides (probably for lack of any other better method for rating impairment) adapted the ATS cutoff values of normal, mild, moderate, and severe physiologic abnormalities as their cutoff points for Classes 1 through 4 pulmonary impairment.[2,3,26,45,47] Other than the statement regarding the above severity scoring as a reflection of a variety of variables, there appears to be no apparent support for whether these cutoff points actually reflect no, mild, moderate, or severe interferences in ADL (which is the goal of the impairment rating).
2. **The values are not "normal"—they are** ***average*** values. These values are derived from population studies and the population chosen reflects the values that were measured. As noted above, these values depend on age, height, sex, weight, race, posture, and other factors. Posture is ignored in the tables of "normal" results as all patients are expected to be tested in the same manner.[7] Factors such as altitude, ambient environment, presence of training, diurnal rhythms, and prior testing are also ignored because their inclusion would present too many variables for analysis. Motivation is discussed in the following in the section on the flow volume loop and examinees with poor performance are excluded from statistical analyses. Finally, all recent tables of "normal" spirometric values have been prepared from healthy subjects, but this was not always the case (especially in the 1950s).

Having ignored all these variables, are these values, then, "normal" values? The answer is no. They are *average* values with a fifth percentile cutoff being used. Thus, 95% of all healthy people, adjusted for age, height, and other anthropomorphic data, will have values above this cutoff. More importantly, 5% (1.65 standard deviations) of all healthy people will have a value below this figure. The ≥80% value for normality of the FVC and FEV_1 comes from the approximate averages of the coefficients of variation for these two tests which were performed on many normal subjects and are derived from regression equations. Pennock et al addressed this issue.[100] Three regression studies were chosen. The range of coefficients of variation for the FVC was 12.1 to 14.5 with a mean of 13; for the FEV_1 it was 13.0 to 13.7 with an average of 13; 13 x 1.65 = 21.5%; hence the 80% cutoff. They also looked at coefficients of variation in three other studies and found that an individual's coefficient of variation was, on the average, 3% on a single day for the FVC (the 3% was for normal controls; higher values were found in individuals with obstructive or restrictive disease). When the coefficient of variation was addressed on a week-to-week (not within a day) basis, it was found to be 5 to 11%. For the FEV_1, the values were 3 to 11% (within a day) and 7 to 14.2% (week-to-week) for normal controls versus patients, respectively.

In 1991, the ATS addressed this issue and found that, although regression formulae were valuable for values centered around the mean, the expected Gaussian distribution did not work well for values at the extremes. Therefore they recommended using a separate reference table for the lower limits of normal individuals.[7] The second and fifth editions of the Guides followed these principles; the first, third, third (revised), and fourth editions did not.[2,3,26,27,45,47] The values for the lower limit of normal in the second and fifth editions of the Guides are identical. They are the predicted normal value minus the 95% confidence interval for the variable chosen. Those variables are the FVC, FEV_1, and DLCO with a separate confidence interval for men and women for each of these variables.

Thus, although it appears as though the numbers derived in a single testing session are completely reliable and indicative of true performance or health status, there is a great deal of variation that can occur. Similar findings were found by Enright et al.[48] A more accurate reflection of a pulmonary perturbation would be a change in a given individual's PFT values when adjusted for effort and time. Thus a claimant who had FEV_1 drop by 27% of predicted (110% to 80%) due to a toxic inhalation would have suffered a significant loss of lung function, yet still be within the "normal" range. This important issue was addressed in the Guides for the first time in the fifth edition: "(i)n individuals where the preinjury or preillness values differ from the population-listed values, the examiner may depart from the population-listed values for determining an impairment rating, using the preinjury and preillness 'normal' value, and explain the reason for the departure"[26(p107)] (see also Chapter 25).

Variables Used in Deriving Regression Formulae

There are a variety of factors that can affect the "normal" values for a given PFT. As noted previously, these can include factors that relate to the individual and factors that are external to the individual. Examples of the latter include the posture at which the test is performed (standing, sitting, or lying), altitude of the testing facility, the barometric pressure on the day of the test, the humidity of the testing facility, and others. As a rule, most testing facilities use the seated position as the norm. However, these "external" variables are not used or taken into consideration when regression formulae were developed.

When a researcher attempts to derive a regression formula for a given PFT variable, that person will need to stratify the individuals tested by certain anthropomorphic considerations (the "internal variables"). A large person is expected to have a greater lung volume than a smaller person. A middle-aged person is expected to have better lung function than an older person. The major inter-person variables that are accounted for in the regression formulae for PFTs are:

1. Age
2. Sex
3. Height

These are the three variables that are found in all prediction formulae and account for the greatest differences between people. These three variables are reflected in the tables of all the editions of the Guides.[2,3,26,27,45,47] The Social Security Administration (SSA), however, uses only one of these variables (height).[117] These factors can be described mathematically and will vary slightly depending on the reference system. The variation based on these variables is, roughly, 30% for sex and 20% for height.[44] The effect of age is discussed separately later.

4. Weight—weight will affect the spirometric values. A 2% intersubject variation in the FVC has been estimated to be due to weight alone and, therefore, this value is usually ignored under standard tables of normality. However, the severely obese individual will have alterations in some tests of pulmonary function, most notably the FVC, owing to upward displacement of the diaphragm causing a restricted (or lowered total lung capacity) pattern. Some tests mitigate this abnormality (for example, the FEV_1/FVC or the DLCO/VA [alveolar volume]—see following).
5. Race—tables of "normal" values of PFTs have been obtained for a variety of races.[7,11,30,44,56,63,64] North American blacks have values for the FVC and FEV_1 from 5 to 30% below those of Caucasians, although this difference was found to be greatest in 25-year-olds and much less in 55-year-olds.[11,14,64] Additionally, not all blacks are homogenous. Nigerian men (west coast of Africa), after standardization, have an FVC one liter lower than that of Ethiopian men (east coast Africans).[14] Asian adults have values more closely resembling those of Caucasians, although some reports state that

they are slightly lower.[14,30] Mexican Americans have values similar to or slightly lower then those of Caucasians when adjusted for height.[30,64] Native American values are also slightly lower than those of Caucasians.[30]

The fourth and fifth editions of the Guides recommended a 12% reduction in the FVC and FEV_1 and a 7% reduction in the DLCO for black examinees.[26(p94),45(p160)] (From an historical perspective, the first and second editions did not address this issue[2,27] and the third and third [revised] editions used a correction factor of 0.9 for the FVC and FEV_1 but not for the DCO[3,47]).

For other racial groups, the fifth edition of the Guides states, "reliable population data are not yet available for other ethnic groups, such as Hispanics, Native Americans, and Asians. For these ethnic groups, the values for North American whites may be used."[26(p94)] These populations were not addressed in the first, second, or fourth editions of the Guides.[2,27,45] The third and third (revised) editions used a correction factor of 0.9 for the FVC and FEV_1 in Asians but not for the DCO (these were the same correction factors used for blacks in these editions).[3,47]

The American College of Occupational and Environmental Medicine (ACOEM) has recently recommended that a 12% reduction from Caucasian values be applied to the FVC and FEV_1 not only for people of African ancestry but also for Asians.[124] Additionally, they stated that it "is important to use a subject's self-declared race or ethnic group as a basis for deciding whether or not to race-adjust Caucasian predicted values."[124(pp236–237)]

Another commonly raised issue concerns examinees of mixed racial heritage. The ACOEM statement noted previously addresses this concern. The 1991 ATS position paper stated that "people of mixed race usually have intermittent values,"[7(p1204)] but did not comment further on how to derive those values. One solution entails using the examinee's self-reported race or, for a person whose heritage is 50% African and 50% Caucasian, using a correction factor of 50% that suggested by the Guides.

Implicit in the above discussion is that there are many variables that will affect the normal or predicted value of a person's expected pulmonary performance. There are many reference tables. These have been derived from diverse groups of people who had spirometries performed according to established principles. From these data, prediction equations were established for a variety of endpoints (e.g., FVC, FEV_1, $FEF_{25\text{-}75}$, DLCO) and linear regression formulae were developed to explore the effects of some of the variables (e.g., height, age, race). Additionally, all these people were presumed to be healthy from a cardiopulmonary perspective.

Which reference table is the best is difficult to determine. The AMA Guides in the second through fifth editions[2,3,26,45,47] and the ATS[7] use Crapo et al's formulae.[31] Other groups and sources use other formulae (see following).

Tests of Flow Rates

A flow-volume loop is the standard measurement performed in most pulmonary function laboratories. It measures flow (liters per second) versus volume and uses a computer for the resulting calculations. These measurements, once limited to expensive and comprehensive laboratories, are now done with simpler machines and are performed frequently in private offices.

The flow-volume loop (Fig. 22–1) graphically presents the flow rates, makes the peak expiratory flow (PEF) easily discernible, and produces a shape that yields important information (Fig. 22–2 demonstrates several poor flow-volume loops that convey information regarding consistency of effort).

Spirometers can also produce a volume-time curve from which FVC is measured and various flow rates calculated. The SSA requires volume-time curves (not flow-volume loops) during pulmonary function testing.[117]

The classic flow rates measured include the FEV_1, which is the total volume of exhaled air in the first second of exhalation; the forced expiratory flow between 200 and 1200 cc ($FEF_{200\text{-}1200}$ or $FEF_{0.2\text{–}1.2}$), which reflects the rate of airflow between the points on the volume axis representing the first 200 cc and the next 1 L of air exhaled; and the forced expiratory flow between 25% and 75% of the total exhaled volume ($FEF_{25\text{-}75}$) (see Fig. 22–1).

FEV_1

A low FEV_1 value can result from airway obstruction, poor effort, or restrictive lung diseases. Because it is a volume (and not a flow rate), any disease that seriously restricts the total volume will have a parallel change in the FEV_1. For this reason, the FEV_1/FVC is believed to be a more sensitive measurement of airflow than the FEV_1 alone in the determination of true obstructive phenomena.[7] Generally, the FEV_1/FVC is about 75% to 80%, meaning that the normal individual exhales 75% to 80% of his or her total exhaled volume in the first second when done as a forceful maneuver. Thus if the FVC is 4.0 L, then the FEV_1 is expected to be approximately 3.0 L. If the FVC diminishes (for whatever reason), then the FEV_1 must also decrease. For example, if a person has had a pneumonectomy, the vital capacity (see following) as well as the FVC must be diminished. To make the example simple, allow

Name: 000 ID: 08-03-1994 12:32:48
Age: 44 Height: 66.0 in. Sex: M Ethnic: C Normal: Knudson/IMTS
Medications:
Test #1 lasted 5.4 s
Last calibration: 08-03-1994

Expiratory	Actual	Pred.	%Pred.
FVC	4.19 L	4.47 L	93.8%
$FEV_{0.5}$	3.08 L	2.90 L	106.1%
FEV_1	3.68 L	3.68 L	100.1%
FEV_3	4.19 L	4.27 L	98.2%
$FEV_{0.5}$/FVC	73.5%	65.0%	113.1%
FEV_1/FVC	87.9%	82.4%	106.7%
FEV_3/FVC	100.0%	95.5%	104.7%
PEF	13.05 L/s	8.24 L/s	158.3%
FEF 25-75%	4.65 L/s	3.59 L/s	129.5%
FEF 75-85%	1.40 L/s	1.06 L/s	132.2%
FEF 50%	5.73 L/s	4.44 L/s	128.9%
FEF 75%	1.88 L/s	1.70 L/s	110.6%
$FEF_{0.2-1.2}$	12.50 L/s	7.14 L/s	175.2%

Inspiratory		
IVC	4.17 L	4.17 L
FIV1	3.78 L	3.78 L
PIF	4.34 L/s	
FIF 50%	3.84 L/s	
FEF_{50}/FEF_{50}	1.49	

Analysis

Test is within NORMAL limits

Current BEST test

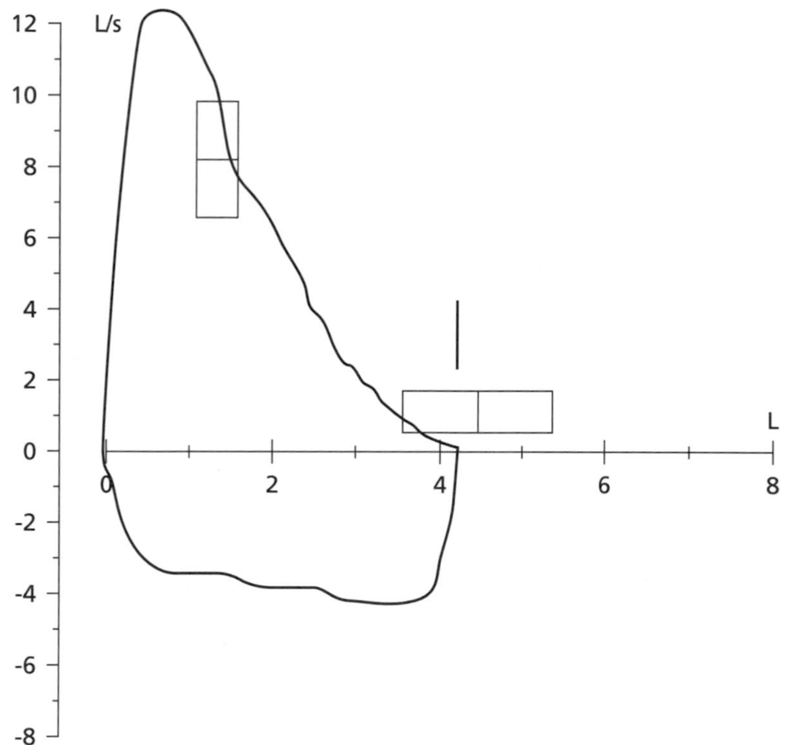

Figure 22–1. Flow volume loop with subdivisions. See text for explanation. Note the calibrations for age, height, sex, and race. Also note the date of the last calibration of the spirometer.

the volume of lung removed to represent 50% of the total lung volume; the FVC then is reduced by 50%. If the normal FEV_1/FVC ratio is to be held, the FEV_1 must also be reduced by 50%. Yet by itself, an FEV_1 of 50% reflects moderate airflow obstruction. Thus it can be appreciated that the FEV_1/FVC ratio is a more reliable prediction of airflow rates and obstruction than the FEV_1 alone.

The FEV_1 is traditionally considered to be a reflection of airflow obstruction in the "large" airways (as opposed to the $FEF_{25\text{-}75}$, which is considered to be a reflection on small airflow obstruction). Although it is not as useful as the FEV_1/FVC ratio, it has such a long-established traditional role in the medical literature that, despite its flaws, it is used as the principal value when referring to

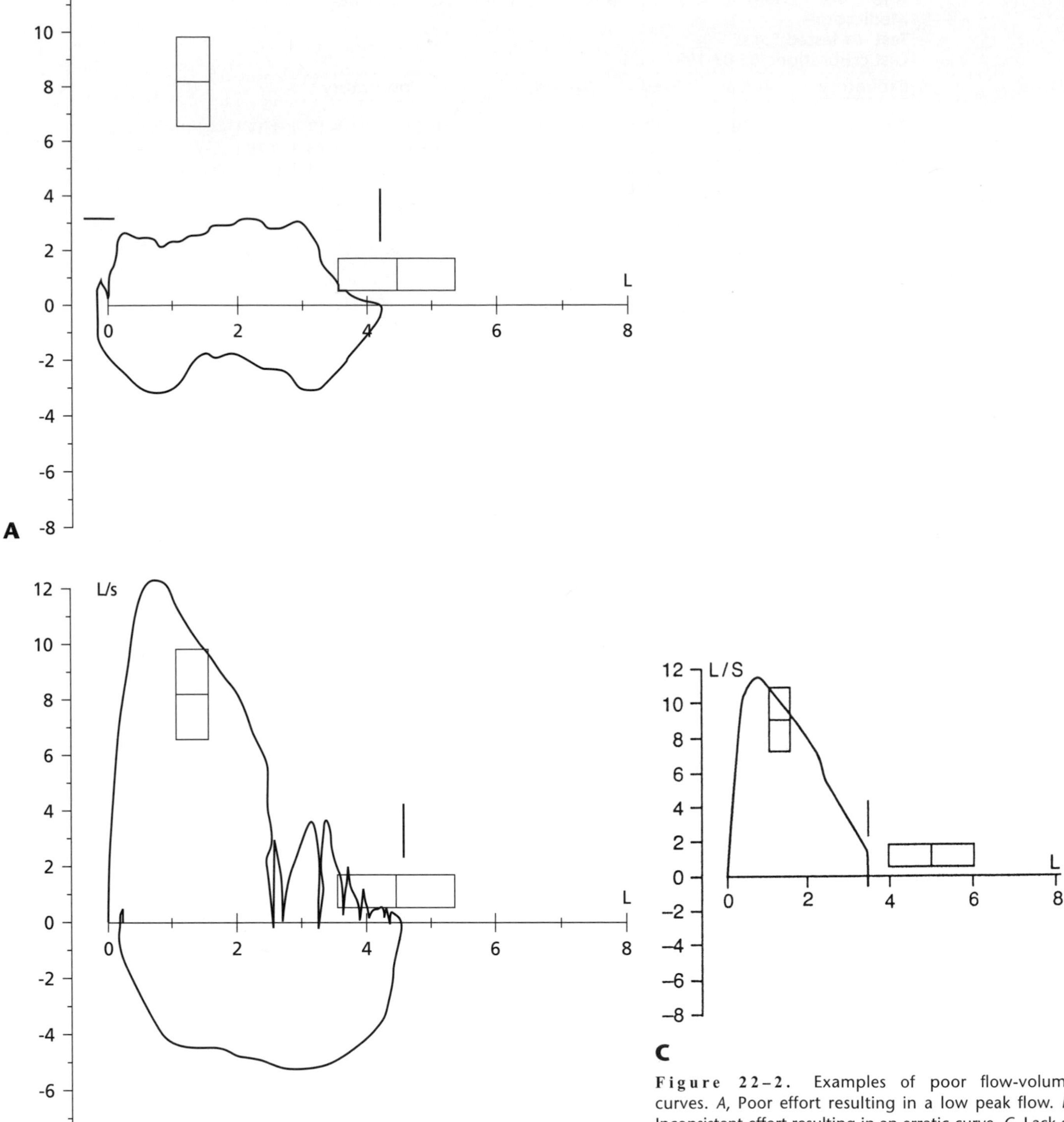

Figure 22–2. Examples of poor flow-volume curves. *A*, Poor effort resulting in a low peak flow. *B*, Inconsistent effort resulting in an erratic curve. *C*, Lack of complete effort producing a "cut-off" at the end of the flow-volume curve.

airflow obstruction. There are a number of variables that can influence the FEV_1, including the following:

1. Age
2. Height
3. Weight
4. Sex
5. Race
6. Medications
7. Disease states
8. Smoking—current, past, never
9. Accelerated decline in 10 to 20% of smokers
10. Accelerated decline in some patients with COPD
11. Occupational exposures
12. Environmental exposures

Peak Expiratory Flow

The PEF rate represents the greatest flow rate achievable during a forceful exhalation. Thus it is highly effort-dependent. In contrast, small airflow rates, such as the $FEF_{25\text{-}75}$, are considered effort-independent. The PEF represents the highest point on the flow-volume curve.

The four major differential diagnoses in a patient with a decreased PEF are as follows:

1. Moderate or severe airflow obstruction
2. Neuromuscular disease
3. Poor effort
4. Upper airway obstruction (for example, tracheal stenosis, endobronchial foreign bodies or tumors, or laryngeal obstructions)

Although the PEF is not used as a criterion of impairment, it may be useful in asthma testing where variable degrees of airflow obstruction can be found when measured over time. This simple test can provide evidence of obstructive phenomena occurring at variable times and with variable exposures, provided that the effects of variable effort are eliminated (see Chapter 25 for a more complete discussion).

$FEF_{25\text{-}75}$

The $FEF_{25\text{-}75}$ (also termed the mid-maximal expiratory flow or MMEF) is considered an excellent test of small airway flow rates. However, it is not used in impairment ratings, where preference is given to the FEV_1.

Maximum Voluntary Ventilation

The maximum voluntary ventilation (MVV) is a special test measuring an individual's maximal ability to breathe in and out during a 60-second period. The test is actually conducted over 12 to 15 seconds and is extrapolated to the full 60 seconds owing to the difficulty in actually performing this type of maneuver for a full 60 seconds. The waveforms during a "good" test are uniform and give a classic "sawtooth" appearance (Fig. 22–3). This test is used during cardiopulmonary exercise testing to determine breathing reserve (see Chapter 24) and for Social Security disability determinations.[117]

The Effects of Aging and Other Variables on Spirometric Values

One of the major philosophical changes in the pulmonary chapter of the fifth edition of the Guides from prior editions is the concept of using a person's premorbid spirometric values for a baseline rather than the population norms found in the tables. This concept is also introduced twice in the introductory chapter that discusses the general philosophy of the Guides[26] (see Chapter 25).

As can be seen from a quick perusal of the table of normal values in the pulmonary chapter of the Guides, the FVC, FEV_1, and DCO all diminish with age. However, the effects of age are not as simple as the regression formulae derived by Crapo et al[31] and others would suggest. Many other factors enter into the regression over time for these values. Thus one cannot simply state that the FEV_1 was 3.4 L 2 years ago and now it is 2.8 L and therefore the disease process accounted for a loss of 0.6 L minus a correction factor (e.g., 2 years times × cc per year). Reference 7 provides a table of some of these regression factors and several prediction formulae. Crapo et al's formula is linear and uses a value of –0.024 L per year. The spread of the linear regression coefficients is –0.023 to –0.032 with a mean of –0.028; three other regression coefficients are provided, but their equations are nonlinear. Thus in Crapo et al's formula, the FEV_1 declines by 24 cc per year and it is linear.

A traditional statement is that the FEV_1 declines by approximately 20 to 30 cc per year after the age of 30 to 35, with the effects on the FVC not as well accepted.[22,65,115] As noted previously, there are many variables found in the predictive formulae for the spirometric values, including height, race, sex, and others. It is not surprising that these same variables also confound a simplistic approach to a correction for the spirometric values based solely on time.

Hankinson and Wagner found that the normal FEV_1 declined by 13, 23, and 29 cc per year in Caucasian, African American, and Mexican American men, respectively, when measured at ages greater than 18. For women, the FEV_1 values declined by 4, 13, and 12 cc per year in similar groups. The FVC declined by 0.6, 18, and 9 cc per year for men and 19, 5, and 3 cc per year for women, aged 18 or older, in the same three respective racial groups.[65]

In addition to age and race, there are other factors that will cause the FEV_1 to decline with time. These factors include disease states, smoking, body weight, and others. Additionally, these factors are not homogenous. In other words, one smoker may decline minimally and another will have a much greater rate of decline. In one study, there was a 20-cc per year loss in the FEV_1 in nonsmokers but a 45-cc per year loss in smokers (63% of the referent population were men and 96% were Caucasian). However, in smokers, there is a subset (approximately 10 to 20%) that develops COPD and has an accelerated decline in the FEV_1, by as much as 150 cc per year.[48,115] Some nonsmoking patients with COPD can also have an accelerated decline, with values ranging from 50 to 90 cc per year.[115]

Patients who quit smoking appear to lose their accelerated decline in the annual FEV_1 quickly, with their new rates reflecting those found in the nonsmoker. Camilli et al found that in subjects younger than 35 years, quitting smoking increased the FEV_1 over the pre-quit value. They also found that there was a decline in the FEV_1, especially in men, that accelerated between the ages of 50 to 70 compared to ages 20 to 50.[19] Others have found similar differentials of decline although different rates and different age cutoffs were cited.[18,128] The latter two studies also found that height was a factor, with greater rates of decline per year for taller individuals. (This subject was also reviewed in reference 64). In 2000, Morgan and Reger published a report stating: "While age and smoking play an important role in determining the rate of decline in the ventilatory capacity, it is clear that body weight plays a significant role and needs to be taken into account in all epidemiologic studies of the ventilatory capacity."[89(p1639)] Their study principally looked at the FEV_1. They also cited references showing that the FEV_1 in nonsmokers usually increases up to the age of 30, is stable until 35, and decreases thereafter. However, they found that in

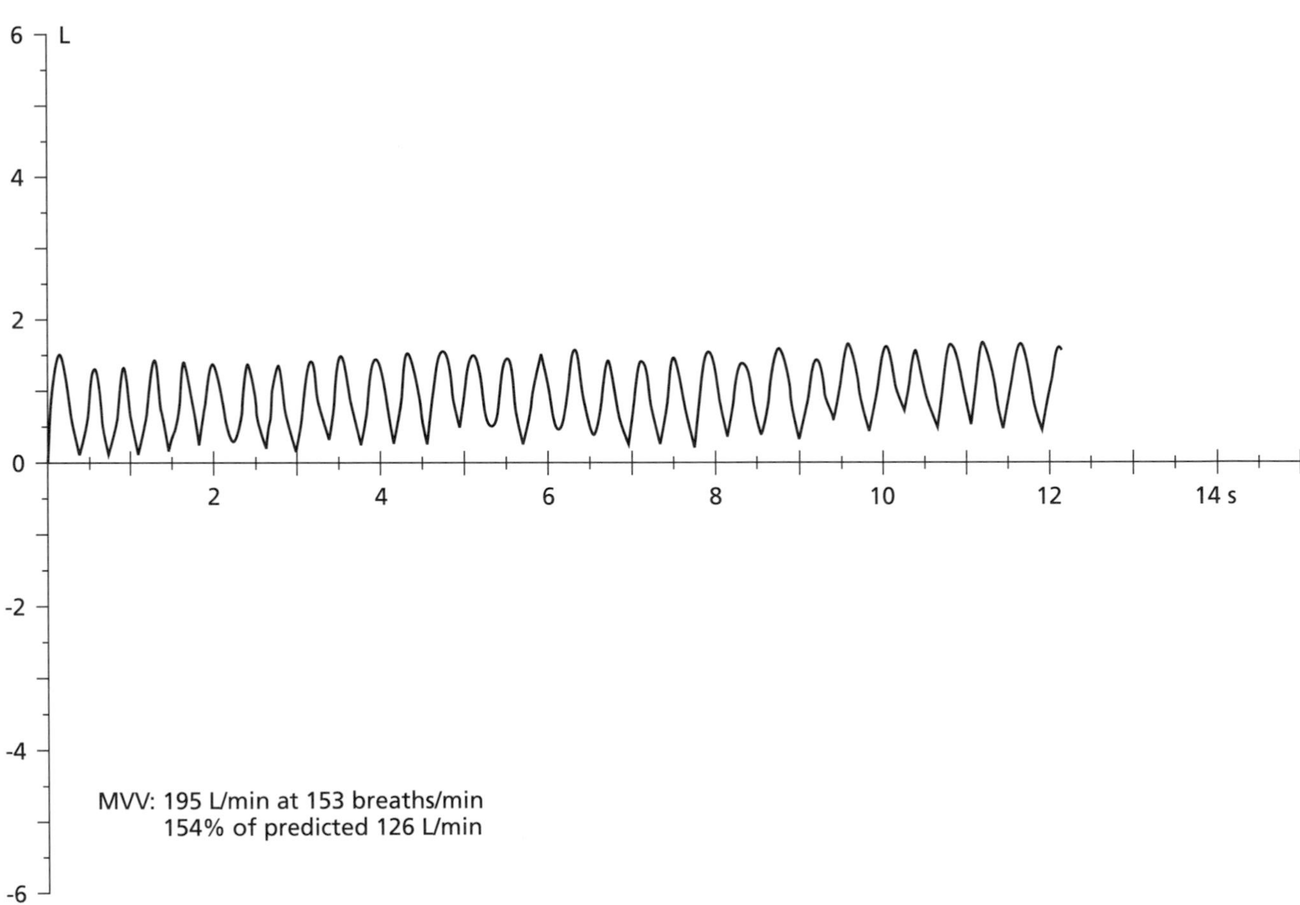

Figure 22–3. Maximum voluntary ventilation curves. *A*, Good curve. Note "sawtooth" pattern with high respiratory rate. *B*, Unacceptable curve. Note good "sawtooth" but low rate. *C*, Unacceptable curve. Note erratic effort, moderate rate.

Figure continued on opposite page

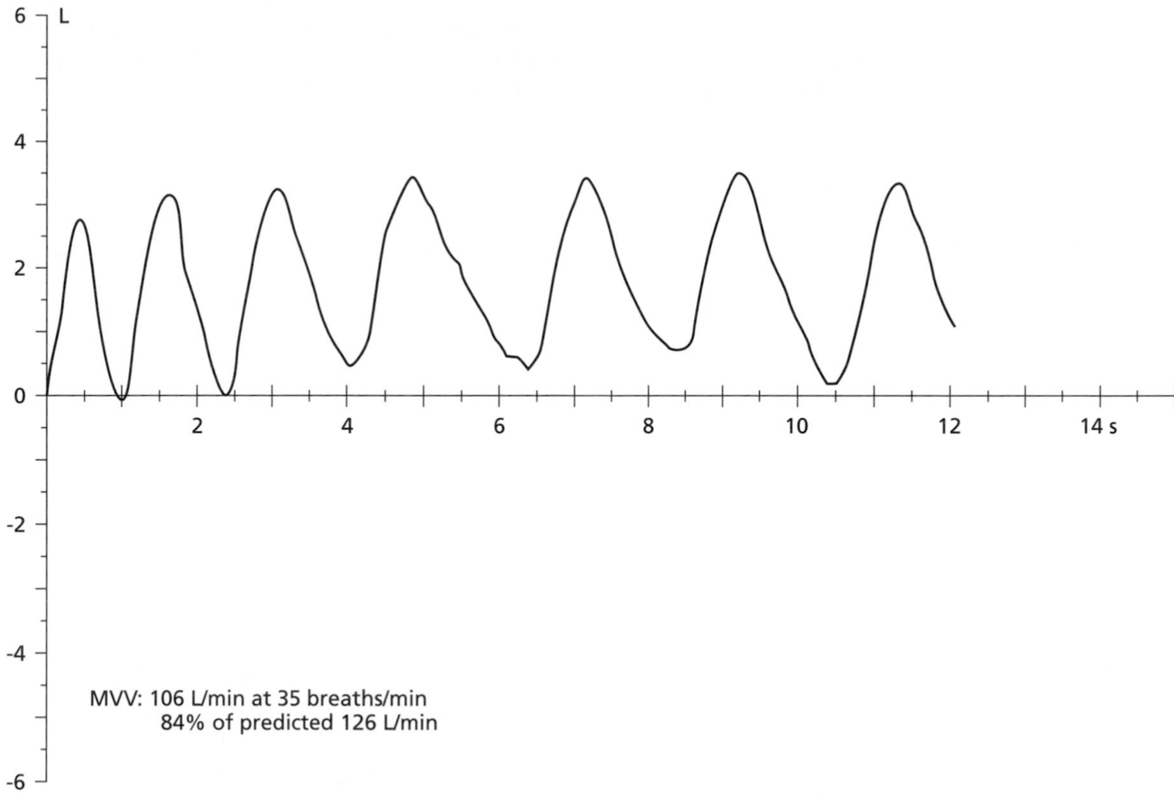
MVV test lasted 12.0 s at 35 breaths/min
MVV = 106 L/min or 84% of predicted 126 L/min
L
6
4
2
0
-2
-4
-6
2
4
6
8
10
12
14 s
MVV: 106 L/min at 35 breaths/min
84% of predicted 126 L/min

B

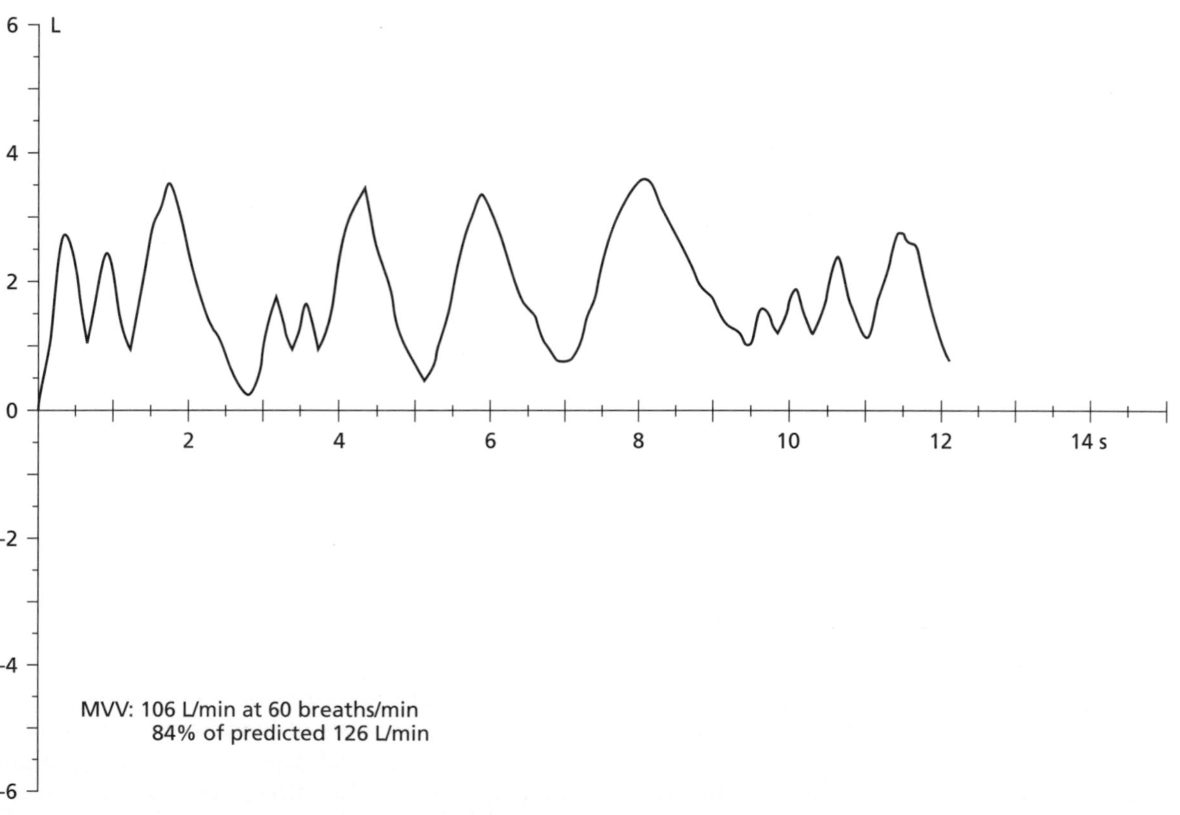
MVV test lasted 12.0 s at 60 breaths/min
MVV = 106 L/min or 84% of predicted 126 L/min
L
6
4
2
0
-2
-4
-6
2
4
6
8
10
12
14 s
MVV: 106 L/min at 60 breaths/min
84% of predicted 126 L/min

C

smokers between the ages of 25 and 30, the FEV_1 either remains constant or increases more slowly than that in the nonsmoker, and that the FEV_1 starts its decline at the age of 30 rather than 35.[89]

The ACOEM, in its position statement on spirometric testing in the workplace, also reviewed this subject and recommended that there be at least 4 to 6 years between successive tests before the effects created by the occupational setting can be considered valid.[124] Other protocols have been developed for assessing the loss of lung function due to the workplace using the expected age-related declines in FEV_1.[43,65,127]

As can be seen, although all authorities agree that the FEV_1 and FVC decline with age, there is a great deal of controversy over how much. The simplistic approach is to state that the FEV_1 declines by 20 to 30 cc per year and ignore the effects of smoking, the precise age when the premorbid value was obtained, changes in body weight, and other variables. This approach may not necessarily be the most accurate. For the FVC, there is no simplistic approach, with most authorities not even addressing the subject owing to its wide variation with age.

These changes assume importance when the examiner is attempting to extrapolate premorbid spirometric values into current losses. How should one proceed? If the examiner can be assured that there have been no substantial biasing factors, and if the premorbid FEV_1 was measured after the individual was 30 years old (but not before), the FEV_1 may be reduced by a factor of 25 cc per year. Any further reduction would be the effect of the impairing process. To derive the impairment rating, one would take the baseline FEV_1, subtract a value of 25 cc per year from the study date to the present, and calculate an FEV_1 percent predicted using the calculated FEV_1 value as the baseline (numerator) rather than the value found in Tables 5–4A and 5–4B or 5–5A and 5–5B in the AMA Guides.[26(pp97–98)] If any of the confounding factors are present, this concept may be reconsidered and the impairment rating may be derived from the tables and methods found in the Guides as if the premorbid values did not exist (see also Chapter 25).

Application of Air Flow Rates in Impairment Evaluations

For impairment evaluations, the only airflow rate values considered in any of the rating systems are the FEV_1, the FEV_1/FVC, and the MVV. Only in very special and unusual circumstances will the PEF be considered. The FEV_1 and FEV_1/FVC values are easily derived from volume-time curves and flow-volume curves.

In an ideal spirometry, there should be no variation between tests in an individual when the repeated tests are performed at the same time. The coefficient of variation, however, is accepted at 3 to 5% owing to an inconsistency either in inhaling to the same total lung capacity (TLC) or producing the same effort.[9,11,44] Some authorities accept variations of 5% or 100 cc in the FVC and FEV_1, whichever is greater.[99] It should also be remembered that forceful inspiratory/expiratory maneuvers might cause bronchospasm and thus create decrements in lung function as more tests are performed in the asthmatic.[14]

This concept of low variation is what makes pulmonary function testing so useful in impairment and disability evaluations. Less than full cooperation on effort can usually be detected using these tests. There are several ways of identifying the examinee who does not produce maximum effort:

1. Inconsistency of effort (the variation is greater than 5%)
2. Abnormal flow-volume curves or MVV curves (see Figures 22–2 and 22–3 and reference 9)
3. A lowered PEF, especially if the PEF percent is significantly lower than the FEV_1 percent

It must be remembered, however, that no test is foolproof. Additionally, factors other than noncompliance may produce changes similar to those listed. For example, the examinee with a fractured rib will produce inconsistent and submaximal effort owing to pain. Also, people with smaller lung volumes (either owing to short stature[56] or poor health[62,75]) may have a greater degree of difficulty in meeting the reproducibility standards.

Perhaps the largest problem with the use of spirometric tests (FVC, FEV_1, FEV_1/FVC) in the evaluation of impairment or disability is determining whether they truly and accurately predict impaired lung function. When a percentage of normal is produced from direct measurements, the "normal" only refers to population averages and not to what is normal for that individual (see previous). Thus, unless the premorbid physiology is known, this type of testing is inherently flawed. The larger consideration, however, is whether resting tests accurately predict exercise impairment or disturbances in ADL.

For example, if a person has a paralyzed arm, one could approach the impairment or disability evaluation by simple inspection. The arm is present and its resting function is normal. This is an example of a "static" test, much like spirometry, resting DLCO, and arterial blood gases (ABGs). All impairment and disability systems require a demonstration of function, not merely appearance. Thus the person who has a paralyzed arm will have markedly abnormal findings on a dynamic test. To follow the analogy, are tests of resting pulmonary function adequate assessors of the pulmonary system or should dynamic tests of lung function (exercise studies that measure the full capacity of the lung to permit air ingress or egress [air flow], gas exchange, and proper distribution of pulmonary blood flow) be used? This issue is discussed later in this chapter.

Another problem when using static tests of pulmonary function to assess impairment or disability is the choice of reference values and regression formulae. The ATS uses Crapo et al's values as its norm.[7] The ACOEM noted that Crapo et al's values were also recommended by the AMA Guides[26] but stated that Knudson's values were more widely used in occupational settings because the Occupational Safety and Health Administration Cotton Dust Standard of 1978 mandated them.[124] They also noted that, in the occupational setting, the ATS recommends picking reference values based on testing 20 to 40 local, nonsmoking, healthy subjects and determining which set of regression equations best fit that locality. However, ACOEM recommended using the data developed by the third National Health and Nutrition Examination Survey,[2] considering them the best values for use in an occupational setting. One of the reasons was that race was more clearly separated in the prediction formulas. Therefore, concerns exist within the medical community about which reference value to use and in which circumstance, as reflected in the previous examples.

Tests of Gas Exchange

The primary function of the lungs is gas exchange; specifically, oxygen acquisition and carbon dioxide release. The one alveolus–one capillary model shown in Figure 22–4 illustrates the basic elements necessary for gas exchange: an intact airway, a functional alveolus, a normal interstitial compartment, a normal capillary, and hemoglobin. If any of these elements is abnormal or missing, gas exchange will be abnormal. However, the lungs are not made up of a single alveolus/single capillary, but many such units—about 350 million. Because many units do not participate in respiration on a normal basis, there exists a large reserve under resting conditions. Thus tests of gas exchange under resting conditions rarely show abnormalities until at least a moderate amount of disease is present. Diseases of the airways, alveoli, interstitium, or blood supply are detectable in lesser degrees of lung disease tested only during exercise. (Exercise testing is discussed in Chapter 24.) The two principal tests of gas exchange are the diffusing capacity and arterial blood gases.

Diffusing Capacity

The diffusing capacity (DLCO—the diffusion [D] across the lung [L] by carbon monoxide [CO]—or the $DLCO_{sb}$—the single breath DLCO; the Guides use the designation DCO) measures gas transfer from the alveolus to the capillary. Carbon monoxide represents the best gas for testing the diffusing capacity because it is readily diffusible, it is normally not present either in the inhaled air or in the blood, and it readily attaches to the hemoglobin molecule so that as soon as it transfers across the membrane, it is immediately removed from the lung. Any existing CO in the blood creates problems with diffusion measurements (as is seen in cigarette smokers).

Figure 22–5 serves as an example of how the DLCO is measured. In this example, the reservoir for inhaled air

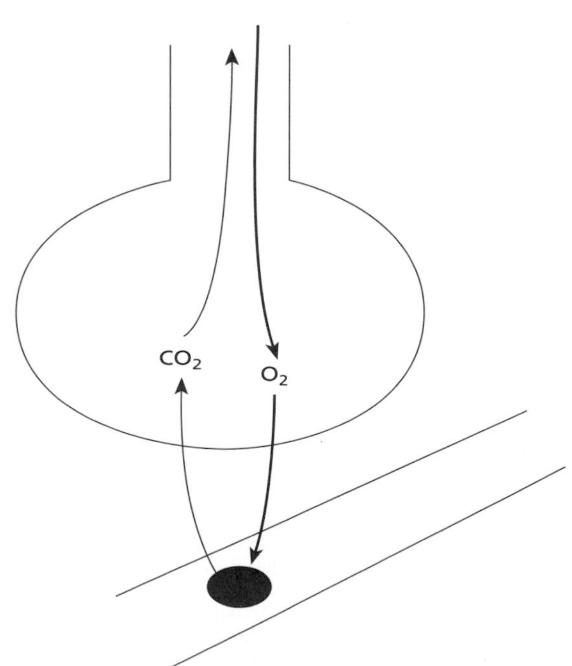

Figure 22–4. One alveolus/one capillary model.

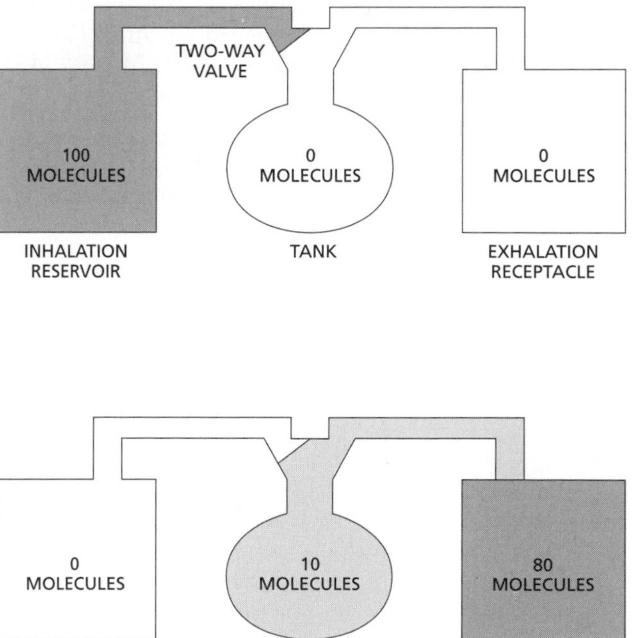

Figure 22–5. Gas diffusion model.

contains 100 molecules of CO. Boyle's Law states that $P_1 \times V_1 = P_2 \times V_2$ in a freely movable situation (or, the pressure of a gas in the first volume times that volume is equal to the pressure of the gas in the second container times that volume if the gas molecules are allowed to freely interchange between the two containers). This relationship can be used if the total lung capacity is known (by direct measurement). All the CO molecules are drawn into the lungs, and the number of molecules in the exhaled air is counted. If only 80 are present and the amount of residual air in the lungs would be expected to contain 10 molecules (after complete mixing of the gases), then the 10 missing molecules are assumed to have diffused across the alveolar–capillary membrane, yielding a DLCO of 10%. If the blood perfusing the alveoli already contains CO, extra CO is found in the exhaled air as a result of back-diffusion (blood to alveolus to airway). This would result in a drop in the measured DLCO.

The major factors influencing the DLCO include elevated levels of carbon monoxide preexistent in the blood (HgCO), reduced hemoglobin content, and abnormal lung volumes. These confounding factors can be addressed during complete pulmonary function testing. It should be noted that the fourth and fifth editions of the Guides recommend that the patient should be instructed not to smoke for at least 8 hours before the test because of the issue of back-diffusion of carbon monoxide creating a falsely depressed DLCO.[26(p94),45(p161)] This issue was not addressed in the second or the two third editions of the Guides.[2,3,47] The first edition did not use the DLCO as a criterion of impairment.[27]

Arterial Blood Gases

ABGs are infrequently used for the determination of impairment. The FEV_1 is preferred in the AMA Guides.[26] The Social Security System uses ABGs but cites three important qualifiers with respect to the oxygen level:

1. The altitude must be specified. Because the amount of oxygen presented to the alveolus is a function of the number of oxygen molecules in the air (the partial pressure of oxygen [PO_2]) and, because this is a function of altitude or barometric pressure, then the expected PaO_2 should then be adjusted for the altitude.
2. The arterial partial pressure of carbon dioxide ($PaCO_2$) must be known. Hyperventilation (reflected as a low $PaCO_2$) increases PaO_2 and hypoventilation (reflected as a high $PaCO_2$) depresses the PaO_2 in a predictable fashion by the alveolar gas equation.
3. The PaO_2 must be tested after exercise, not in the resting state. This depicts the functional capability of the lungs more accurately.[117]

In addition, the Social Security System provides tables of expected PaO_2 levels in obese individuals.[117(pp78–79)]

The Black Lung Benefits Law uses the $PaO_2/PaCO_2$ levels at rest or at exercise.[41]

Lung Volumes

TLC is defined as the total amount of air the lung can hold at the end of a full inhalation (Fig. 22–6). The TLC can be considered to comprise the respirable air of the lung as well as the structural air (some air must remain within the lungs at the end of a full exhalation or the work of breathing would become so excessive that the body would spend a disproportionate amount of its energy simply breathing). This volume of air remaining in the lungs at the end of a complete exhalation is the residual volume (RV). The difference between the TLC and the RV is called the vital capacity (VC).

Other lung volumes and capacities are expressed as follows:

1. Tidal volume (TV): the volume of a normal breath
2. Functional residual capacity (FRC): FRC = expiratory reserve volume (ERV) + RV
3. Inspiratory capacity (IC): IC = TLC – FRC
4. Inspiratory reserve volume (IRV): IRV = TLC – (FRC + TV)

Except for TV, these are rarely used in impairment or disability evaluations. TV is usually small (approximately 250 to 350 cc). During exercise, however, it increases as the demands for oxygen acquisition and carbon dioxide

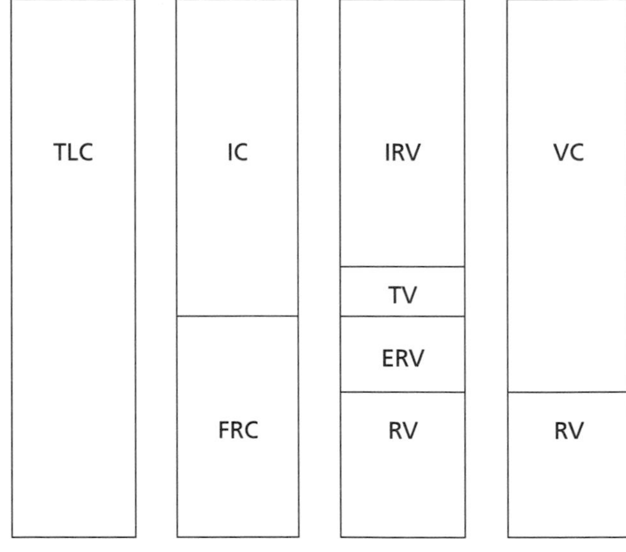

Figure 22–6. Lung compartments. TLC = total lung capacity, IC = inspiratory capacity, FRC = functional residual capacity, VC = vital capacity, IRV = inspiratory reserve volume, ERV = expiratory reserve volume, TV = tidal volume, RV = residual volume.

removal increase. This is the only time that the TV is used and is part of the complete cardiopulmonary exercise stress test.

Residual Volume

The RV reflects the size of the lungs, which itself reflects the size of the body. Prediction formulae for the RV include the variables of height, sex, age, and race.

If the size of the alveoli could increase, the RV would increase. Although this does not happen, it is mimicked by four conditions: aging, emphysema, air trapping, and cysts or blebs. During the aging process, the integrity of the elastic tissue of the lung diminishes. In emphysema, lung tissue is destroyed. Thus, where alveoli, respiratory bronchioles, and connecting tissue surrounding these alveoli once existed, a large "mega-alveolus" exists. In air-trapping states (such as mucous plugs or asthma), the air is not allowed to escape, so the individual cannot empty the lungs completely. Therefore, the air at the end of a forceful exhalation (the definition of RV) increases. Finally, abnormalities such as cysts, blebs, or bronchopleural fistulas can increase the RV by a similar mechanism.

Vital Capacity

The VC may be measured either as a long, slow breath from TLC to RV (also called the slow vital capacity [SVC]) or as a quick, forceful breath from TLC to RV (known as FVC or forced vital capacity). Diseases causing air trapping can cause a discrepancy between these two values. The FVC is the measurement found in most rating systems of pulmonary impairment or disability. The advantages of using the FVC are ease of measurement, low cost, and reproducibility of findings. Depending on the skill of the technician, spirometric machines produce accurate and reproducible FVCs using a quick test, usually lasting less than 3 to 5 minutes and costing approximately $100 (total fee for the test and interpretation; costs vary by testing facility).

The four major differential diagnoses of a low FVC are emphysema, ILD, severe airflow obstruction with or without air trapping, and poor effort. Emphysema can decrease the FVC by producing a reciprocal increase in the RV (Fig. 22–7). Restrictive or interstitial lung diseases decrease the air-occupying spaces of the lung. They replace or collapse the alveoli by increasing the solid tissue of the lungs with inflammatory cells, collagen, or tumor cells. Obliteration or filling of the air spaces can cause a similar physiologic change and occurs in pneumonias, pulmonary edema, and alveolar proteinosis, among other diseases. If air trapping exists (for example, a mucous plug or an endobronchial tumor), less total air is expelled during a complete exhalation. Severe airway obstructive states also diminish total exhaled volume. Finally, poor effort (either voluntarily or involuntarily as in a patient with a fractured rib or neuromuscular disorder) diminishes the FVC. Repeated testing helps discriminate between these two conditions; the individual giving less than optimal effort voluntarily will have erratic flow-volume loops and variable volumes in the FVC. The individual with involuntary, incomplete effort-induced reductions in the FVC often has characteristic flow-volume loops and a relatively constant volume of air (see previous).

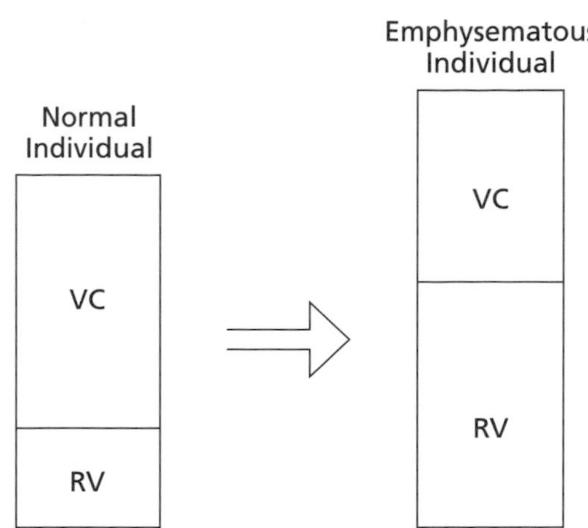

Figure 22–7. Changes with emphysema-increased RV causing a decreased VC.

As shown in Figure 22–6, if the TLC remains constant, a reciprocal relationship exists between the RV and the VC. Disease states increasing the RV diminish the VC. Because the VC is much easier and cheaper to obtain than the RV and the TLC, the VC is used as a surrogate measurement for diseases producing major alterations in the RV or TLC. For the purposes of an impairment rating, individuals with severe emphysema can be adequately assessed using this simpler test.

Disease states producing emphysema or air trapping often increase the TLC (Fig. 22–7), as seen by the "barrel-chest" in patients with emphysema or the "low diaphragms" seen on the chest x-rays (CXRs) of patients with emphysema or status asthmaticus (an example of air trapping). Emphysematous and air-trapping diseases often have coexistent abnormalities in either airflow rates or gas exchange systems. These latter two areas have proven more sensitive in determining the ability to work and, hence, disability, than the measurement of the RV.

For these reasons, tests of lung volumes are not used in the impairment or disability arenas. The FVC can provide most of the information needed to properly assess most patients with structural lung abnormalities. As noted in the section on flow rates, the FVC is reproducible and can often be used to assess maximal effort, thus identifying examinees who produce less than their true capabilities in order to inflate an impairment rating. Therefore, it is used as the surrogate for abnormalities in these compartments.

Validity of the Use of Resting PFTs in Impairment or Disability Evaluations

Historical Perspective

The tests that are and have been used by the AMA Guides[2,3,26–28,45,47] for measuring pulmonary impairment are the FVC, FEV_1, FEV_1/FVC, DLCO, and $\dot{V}O_2$ (the latter value is the maximum oxygen uptake, measured during an integrated cardiopulmonary exercise stress test; this test is covered briefly in this chapter and extensively in Chapter 24). The values for and categories of impairment were those published as an "official ATS statement" in 1986.[5] This statement was based on an earlier statement published in 1982,[4] although that statement only discussed the concepts of normal and severe impairment without establishing gradations of impairment.

The authors of the second ATS statement recommended that the FVC, FEV_1, FEV_1/FVC ratio, and DLCO be used as a first step in the determination of respiratory impairment: "With these results, the majority of subjects will be appropriately categorized as to their degree of impairment."[5(p1206)] The only difference between their cutoff values for normal and mild, moderate, or severe impairment and those of the AMA Guides is the cutoff for the DLCO for normal/mild impairment. (Normal is defined as ≥80% in the DLCO or DCO in the ATS statement paper,[5] ≥80% in the third and third revised editions,[3,47] ≥70% in the fourth edition,[45] and ≥ a lower limit of normal in the second and fifth editions [a correction factor for the DCO was given in the second edition[2] and a separate table using an identical correction factor in the fifth edition[26]].) The cutoff between mild/moderate impairment is the same in each of these sources—<60%). The first edition did not use the DCO as a criterion of impairment.[27] The MVV was not recommended owing to its effort dependency and its fixed relationship to the FEV_1[5(p1206)] and has not been used by the Guides since the first edition.[27] The FEF_{25-75} was not recommended because it added "nothing of clinical significance to the determination of functional impairment"[5(p1206)] and has not been used by any of the editions of the Guides.[2,3,26,27,45,47] Exercise testing was recommended "only when there are grounds for believing that the routine tests may have underestimated the impairment."[5(p1207)] The stated reason for this was as follows: "(B)ecause there is a well documented relationship between the FEV_1 and $DLCO_{sb}$ and oxygen consumption and work capacity, it can confidently be predicted that the majority of patients being evaluated for respiratory impairment will not require exercise testing."[5(p1207)]

The second through fifth editions of the Guides use this test with the same cutoff points as the ATS.[2,3,26,45,47] The spirometric values derived by Crapo et al were adapted as the ones used by the ATS[31] and, as noted previously, by the second through fifth editions of the Guides.[2,3,26,45,47]

The ATS separated impairment, based on the $\dot{V}O_2$ max, into three categories:

1. $\dot{V}O_2$ max ≥25 mL/kg/min: "the subject will be capable of continuous heavy exertion throughout an 8-hour shift and of all but the most physically demanding of jobs"[5(p1207)]
2. $\dot{V}O_2$ max between 15 and 25 mL/kg/min: the ATS recommended that the subject be matched with the $\dot{V}O_2$ requirements of the job
3. $\dot{V}O_2$ max ≤15 mL/kg/min: "the subjects will be unlikely to perform most jobs because they would be uncomfortable in traveling back and forth to their place of employment"[5(p1207)]

Although the ATS called this a rating of impairment, there was no categorization of these values from mild to severe. Nevertheless, the AMA Guides[2,3,26,45,47] use these values for categorizing impairment. Normal function in the Guides is a $\dot{V}O_2$ max ≥25 mL/kg/min, mild impairment is between 20 and 25 mL/kg/min, moderate is between 15 and 20 mL/kg/min, and severe is <15 mL/kg/min. However, the ATS, in a position paper, recommended matching the $\dot{V}O_2$ max in the area between normal and severe impairment with the job requirements,[5] a position not taken by the Guides. The ATS stated (supported by others[83,106]): "A worker involved in manual labor who is more or less free to set the work pace can work comfortably at approximately 40% of his maximal aerobic power ($\dot{V}O_2$ max). During shorter periods of time an individual can work without fatigue at about 50% of his $\dot{V}O_2$ max."[5(p1207)] With respect to Category 2, the ATS states: "If the subject's oxygen consumption is between 15 and 25 mL/kg/min, and 40% of his observed $\dot{V}O_2$ max is greater than or equal to the average metabolic work requirement of his job, then the subject should be able to perform that job comfortably. ... An exception would be a job which demands frequent and extended periods (>5 min) of exertion requiring substantially greater than 40% of the $\dot{V}O_2$ max."[5(p1207)]

Several very important points need to be raised concerning the ATS position paper (and by inference the AMA Guides):

1. Are the reference "normal" values the best?
2. How were the various cutoff points for the FVC, FEV_1, FEV_1/FVC, and DLCO chosen?
3. Are the ATS $\dot{V}O_2$ max positions similar to those found in the Guides?
4. Are those positions valid?

Are the Reference "Normal" Values the Best?

Again, Crapo et al's values for "normal" FVC, FEV_1, and DLCO[31] were chosen as opposed to other prediction formulae by both the ATS and the Guides.[2,3,5,26,45,47] In Crapo et al's database, 311 subjects were screened. All were lifetime nonsmokers with no signs of cardiopulmonary disease. More than 90% were Mormons and, presumably, white. A total of 126 were women and 125 were men with an equal age distribution. In the 25- to 34-year-old group, only 18 men were studied (two men were studied in the 85 to 91 group). The tests were performed at 1400 meters. No mention was made of weight, race, or other variables (see previous). Regression formulae were then developed.[31] The obvious shortcomings include the small number of subjects, lack of racial groups other than white, and altitude. Indeed, Crapo et al stated that their prediction formulae "can be recommended for the prediction of reference values for rural or urban whites of northern and middle European extraction..."[31]

The reason for the concern is easily seen in an example. For a 48-year-old man, 178 cm tall, the Crapo et al estimate of the FVC is 5.0 L. If the measured FVC is 2.70 L, the subject has an FVC of 54% predicted. Using the AMA Guides (the fifth edition will be used at this point exclusively; as noted, the other editions are similar in cutoff points), a 54% FVC is a Class 3 impairment level (for the FVC, a Class 1 is if the FVC is ≥ lower limit of normal, a Class 2 [10–25% whole person impairment {WPI}] is for the FVC ≥ 60% predicted and < lower limit of normal, a Class 3 [26–50% WPI] is for the FVC ≥ 51% and ≤ 59% of predicted, and a Class 4 [51–100% WPI] is for the FVC ≤ 50% of predicted).[26(p107)] If the Crapo et al formula is given a 10% variation (+10% = 5.5 L; –10% = 4.5 L), then the percent predicted becomes either 49 or 60%. This gives either a Class 4 impairment rating or a Class 2 rating.

This point is obviously of some concern but if one consistently uses the same "normal value" table, there will be no variability among examinees, with all people being treated equally by using the same tables. Of greater concern, however, are the other issues described previously, most importantly the race issue. As noted before, Nigerian blacks have a substantially lower FVC than do Ethiopians. The correction factors used in the AMA assume homogeneity of pulmonary function in all black patients. The correction for Asians is uneven, as are the corrections for black patients between editions, as noted. In none of the editions is the issue of mixed ancestry discussed. As can be seen from the example, a 10% variation in the "normal" value can make a great deal of difference in an impairment rating (see reference 32 for a discussion of various prediction formulae for the diffusing capacity).

This concept was reviewed by Harber et al, who examined four variables in establishing a disability determination[66]:

1. Choice of prediction equation
2. Choice of adjustment factors (e.g., height, race, sex, age)
3. Method of comparison of measured to predicted values
4. Choice of cutoff points

Of the four variables, the choice of prediction equation had the least influence. Nevertheless, not all groups endorse the Crapo et al prediction formula, as noted previously. Major factors in Harber et al's paper included the remaining three issues, especially the influence of sex, race, and cutoff points. "It is much 'easier' to meet the criteria of the new Black Lung regulations than those of the Social Security Administration."[66(p417)] This subject is also addressed by Becklake, who looked at the sources of variations in lung function testing.[12]

These comments are best exemplified by looking at the SSA's method of determining impairment/disability.[117] The criteria for pulmonary impairment, based on spirometric results, are very simplistic, with only height used as an adjustment factor. Because, as previously discussed, lung volumes are predictably higher for men and whites (addressing only two of the many variables), the SSA listings are inherently biased against these two groups. As an example, see Table 22–4, which uses the AMA Guides reference tables as the source of predicted values[26] and presents the percent predicted values for various groups in order to qualify for SSA benefits. Height was chosen as a constant. A 30-year-old white man meets the SSA criteria for disability if his FVC is 36% of predicted or his FEV_1 is 34% of predicted. A 50-year-old black woman only needs values of 50% of the FVC and 52% of the FEV_1 to be accepted (remember, the higher the value, the closer the person is to normal). Although the bias against Caucasians and men is presumed to be unintentional, it is present and it

TABLE 22–4

Differences in % predicted for FVC and FEV_1 in men/women and Caucasian/African American patients for meeting the SSA requirements for disability (for a man 5′11″ [180cm] tall or a woman 5′4″ [162cm] tall)

FVC or FEV_1	Male		Female	
FVC				
Age, y	30	50	30	50
Caucasian	31%	34%	40%	44%
African American	36%	39%	44%	50%
FEV_1				
Age, y	30	50	30	50
Caucasian	34%	38%	39%	46%
African American	38%	43%	44%	52%

FVC, forced vital capacity; FEV_1, forced expiratory volume in 1 second; SSA, Social Security Administration.

is striking. The bias makes it less likely that a young Caucasian man, as opposed to an older black woman, will be accepted. The same could be said for a nonsmoker as opposed to a smoker with similar declines in lung function created by occupational or other types of lung disease (e.g., pneumoconiosis). The same holds true for the person who is compliant with medications as opposed to the person who decides not to take them. These latter two biases are present not only in the SSA listings but also in the AMA Guides.

As mentioned previously, there are many tables of "normal" values and the ACOEM uses different "normal" values than do the Guides when assessing occupational issues.

How Were the Various Cutoff Points Chosen?

Other than the issue of the validity in the predicted values, there are other concerns. As mentioned previously, the ATS used a number of variables in deciding the cutoff values for the FVC, FEV_1, and DLCO, "such as the ability to work and function in daily life, morbidity, and prognosis."[7(p1212)] However, they also caution that these values should be used based on the disease status of the individual, and state, "physicians should probably view arbitrary severity scoring systems with caution." [7(p1212)] Although there is probably some rationale behind the cutoffs, the rounded numbers (e.g., 60–80, 40–60) most likely represent more personal selection than a reliance on science.

When interpreting a PFT, an FVC of 70% is a mild restrictive abnormality. It is also a mild impairment. The ATS defined mild impairment as "usually not correlated with diminished ability to perform most jobs"; moderate impairment as "progressively lower levels of lung function correlated with diminishing ability to meet the physical demands of many jobs"; and severe impairment as "unable to meet the physical demands of most jobs including travel to work,"[5(p1206)] with no supporting statements.

Cotes et al[29] examined the ATS hypothesis[5] that the combination of the FEV_1, FVC, and DLCO could accurately assess a loss of exercise capacity; in other words, they assessed the validity of the ATS's position. As noted, the ATS stated that "there is a well documented relationship between FEV_1 and $DLCO_{sb}$ and oxygen consumption and work capacity, it can confidently be predicted that the majority of patients being evaluated for respiratory impairment will not require exercise testing."[5(p1207)] Tables 22–5 and 22–6 are taken from the Cotes et al study[29(p1091)] and summarize their findings. Their conclusion was that "loss of exercise capacity cannot be predicted with acceptable accuracy from the 4 commonly used lung function indices alone or in combination."[29(p1093)] The four tests are the FVC, FEV_1, FEV_1/FVC, and DLCO.

Ortega et al found r values (correlation coefficient) of 0.37 for the FVC, 0.52 for the FEV_1, and 0.39 for the FEV_1/FVC in 78 patients with COPD when these variables were correlated with the peak $\dot{V}O_2$.[95] Carleson et al found r values of 0.56 for the FVC, 0.70 for the FEV_1, and 0.53 for the FEV_1/FVC.[20] Similar results have been found by other authors[103,107,109,120] (see also Appendix A; the degree of association between variables is weak for r values of 0.2 to 0.5 and only moderate for r values between 0.5 and 0.8).

Similar values are found in patients with restrictive (interstitial) lung diseases. In a very early study, Fulmer et al correlated physiology and pathology in idiopathic pulmonary fibrosis.[51] Resting values correlated very poorly with the morphologic assessment of the degree of fibrosis or cellularity. The r value for the

TABLE 22–5

Cross-correlation Matrix Giving Simple Correlations Between the Several Indices of Lung Function and Exercise Performance (n = 157, $P < 0.05$)

	FEV_1	FVC	IVC	FEV_1/FVC	IAO	TL^1	TLCO	KCO	VE
FVC	0.78								
IVC	0.54	0.85							
FEV_1/FVC	0.72	0.17	NS						
IAO	−0.78	−0.44	−0.23	−0.79					
TL^1	0.51	0.50	0.43	0.24	−0.28				
TLCO	0.28	0.33	0.31	NS	NS	0.92			
KCO	0.21	NS	−0.19	0.36	−0.29	0.70	0.67		
VE	0.27	0.16	NS	0.27	−0.23	NS	−0.14	−0.18	
$\dot{V}O_2$max	0.45	0.39	0.34	0.29	−0.39	0.50	0.36	0.35	−0.44

FEV_1, forced expiratory volume in 1 second; FVC, forced vital capacity; IVC, inspiratory vital capacity; IAO, index of airway obstruction; TL^1, single-breath lung transfer factor (DLCO); TLCO, transfer factor measured using a multibreath estimate of residual volume; KCO, the rate of CO uptake from alveolar gas/time (DLCO = VA × KCO, or the diffusion of a gas is defined by the number of contributing units times the efficiency of each unit for the transfer of the gas [carbon monoxide]); VE = ventilation at an oxygen consumption of 1.0 L/min.

From Cotes JE, Zejda J, King B: Lung function impairment as a guide to exercise limitation in work-related lung disorders. Am Rev Respir Dis 137:1091, 1998, with permission from the American Journal of Respiratory and Critical Care Medicine.

TABLE 22–6

Percentages of the Variance in Maximal Oxygen Uptake in Absolute Units or as % Predicted, Described by Different Physiologic Indices. The Latter Were Expressed in Absolute Units or, in the Case of Lung Function Indices Used to Describe % $\dot{V}O_2$max, as Percentages of the Reference Values

	Percentage of Variance Explained		
Dependent Variable	**$\dot{V}O_2$max* (n = 157)**	**% $\dot{V}O_2$max (n = 157)**	**% $\dot{V}O_2$ max (n = 35)†**
Single lung function indices			
FEV_1, FVC, TL^1, TLCO	15–25	11–14	23–31
Combination of lung function indices			
FEV_1 (or FVC and FEV_1/FVC) and TL^1 (or TLCO)	29	12–14	42
IVC and FEV_1/FVC	19.5	17	‡
Lung function and exercise indices			
FEV_1 (or FVC and FEV_1/FVC) and VE	54	44	68
FEV_1, TL^1 (or TLCO), and VE	54	44	71

*See text of reference 29.
† Subgroup of men with lung disease caused by asbestos.
‡ No improvement over IVC alone.
FEV_1, forced expiratory volume in 1 second; FVC, forced vital capacity; TL^1, single-breath lung transfer factor (DLCO); TLCO, transfer factor measured using a multibreath estimate of residual volume; IVC, inspiratory vital capacity; VE, ventilation at an oxygen consumption of 1.0 L/min.
From Cotes JE, Zejda J, King B: Lung function impairment as a guide to exercise limitation in work-related lung disorders. Am Rev Respir Dis 137:1089–1093, 1988, with permission.

vital capacity was 0.422 with an r^2 of 0.168. The r for the resting PaO_2 was –0.231 for the degree of fibrosis and –0.238 for the degree of cellularity. Demeter and others found similar results for the resting PaO_2 and DLCO.[37,38,94] Violante et al derived correlation coefficients (r) for a number of variables in 45 patients with simple silicosis (11 were 1/0, 13 were 1/1, 9 were 1/2, 7 were 2/1, and 5 were 2/2; the values 1/0, 1/1, etc., refer to the degree or amount of pneumoconiosis or interstitial abnormalities on the CXR; see radiography section). They also divided their data into smoking/nonsmoking groups (see Table 22–7). None of the values was significant.[126]

TABLE 22–7

Correlation Coefficients for a Number of Variables and $\dot{V}O_2$

Variable	r For All Patients	r For Smokers	r For Nonsmokers
FVC (% predicted)	–0.036	0.083	–0.236
FEV_1 (% predicted)	0.050	0.007	0.059
DLCO (% predicted)	0.133	0.270	–0.127
PaO_2 (resting)	–0.108	–0.047	–0.180
Dyspnea	–0.202	–0.079	–0.205

From Violante B, Brusasco V, Buccheri G: Exercise testing in radiologically limited, simple pulmonary silicosis. Chest 90:411–415, 1986, with permission.

Additionally, there are internal, even fatal inconsistencies in the resting PFTs. In a study by Aaron et al, the positive predictive value for the FVC in predicting restriction (confirmed by direct volume measurements either by body plethysmography or helium dilution method) was only 41%. The negative predictive value (normal FVC in the absence of restriction) was 2.4%.[1]

If the resting spirometric indices have such a poor correlation with the $\dot{V}O_2$ max, does the exercise test become the better test for impairment? (See the above discussion about the paralyzed arm.) The major limitation when using the cardiopulmonary exercise stress test is that it does not measure only pulmonary limitations. This test also measures cardiac performance but the differential list of problems identified by the test is even broader.[120] Additionally, the test is terminated for a variety of reasons. Rampulla et al[107] tested 66 patients with COPD. The patients stopped exercising owing to dyspnea only 42% of the time. The other causes were fatigue (41%), cardiac limitations (12%), and other reasons. Sue studied 138 men with asbestosis.[120] The primary cause of exercise limitation was cardiovascular, in 69%. Other causes were obstructive lung disease (15%), restrictive lung problems (4%), musculoskeletal problems (11%), and obesity (2%).

This concern regarding the lack of precision based on diagnosis represents the major weakness of the cardiopulmonary exercise stress test for use in an impairment examination. Although the $\dot{V}O_2$ can be measured and a variety of causations (either a single disease state or multiple variations involving various organ systems) can be ascertained, impairment evaluations are interested, usually, in only one variable, not the totality of a person's health. Thus an impairment evaluation might address the issue of how much WPI was created by the COPD or the coronary artery disease in order to produce a financial settlement for the effects of a single disease. The cardiopulmonary exercise stress test will not allow for this discrimination. It provides the whole person's energy producing capability without defining the contribution created by a perturbation in a single variable (disease state) unless that variable is the sole abnormality creating the lowered $\dot{V}O_2$.

Wiedemann et al stated, "In summary, some conclusions about an individual's working capacity can be made from resting pulmonary function data. If resting lung function is either severely impaired or normal, exercise testing probably is unnecessary. However, in the range of mild to moderate resting lung function abnormality, exercise testing may provide objective information to help evaluate work capacity."[130(p161)] Their article also summarizes various cutoffs from various authors and countries for "severe impairment" based on the $\dot{V}O_2$ max.

To return to the original question of how cutoff values were determined, then, it appears to have been arbitrary and unsupported by exercise (hence work capability) data. Although not directly addressing impairment or disability, it is helpful to look at the cutoff values in patients with COPD. In 1995, the ATS graded COPD by the FEV_1 and correlated this with the impact on HRQOL.[22] The ERS and BTS published similar tables.[99,115] Table 22–2 provides the various cutoffs. As can be seen, there is a great variation in the FEV_1 among the three societies. Yet all three were essentially studying and addressing the same issue. No justifications were given for the cutoff values. As the BTS stated, "precise demarcation remains arbitrary."[99] It appears that the "precise demarcations" for the cutoff values in the FVC, FEV_1, DLCO, and $\dot{V}O_2$ max might also have been arbitrary. Despite their long usage and wide acceptance, they may not be giving the information that is asked of them; namely, the extent of impairment or disability in an individual.

Are the ATS $\dot{V}O_2$ max Positions Similar to Those Found in the Guides and Are They Valid?

The cutoffs for normal (≥25 mL/kg/min) and severe impairment (<15 mL/kg/min), as noted, were identical in the AMA Guides and the ATS position paper. The categories for mild and moderate pulmonary impairment in the AMA Guides deviate from the position taken by the ATS, which described, in its category 2, the concept of matching the worker and the metabolic requirements of the job (see previous).[5] The second through fifth editions of the AMA Guides use cutoff values of 20 to 25 and 15 to 20 mL/kg/min for mild and moderate impairment.[2,3,26,45,47]

In the "normal" category, it is stated that "if the $\dot{V}O_2$ max is greater than or equal to 25 mL/kg/min (7.1 METS), the subject will be capable of continuous heavy exertion throughout an 8-h shift and of all but the most physically demanding of jobs."[5(p1207)] However, this is at odds with various references that contain tables of $\dot{V}O_2$.[74,106]

When applying the $\dot{V}O_2$ max to sustainable work, a 40% rule is usually applied.[5,106] The ATS states that an individual can comfortably sustain work at 40% of the $\dot{V}O_2$ max or at 50% of $\dot{V}O_2$ max for shorter periods of time without fatigue. This places the sustainable $\dot{V}O_2$ at 10 mL/kg/min. This is in the range of moderate manual labor (approximately 8 to 15 mL/kg/min), with heavy manual labor being higher. (For examples, refer to Table 22–8.) As can be seen, this value is at the lower end of manual labor.

Sedentary activities have a $\dot{V}O_2$ of less than 6 to 8 mL/kg/min. The ATS chose a level of 15 mL/kg/min as their lower cutoff point. Below this, "subjects will be unable to perform most jobs because they would be uncomfortable in traveling back and forth to their place of employment."[5(p1207)] Again, this value is the one chosen for a Class 4 impairment level (51 to 100% WPI) by the AMA Guides.[26] Forty percent of 15 mL/kg/min is 6.0 mL/kg/min. It is doubtful that a person capable of sustaining 4 to 6 mL/kg/min will have difficulty in traveling to and from his or her job. In fact, he or she should be capable of sustainable employment at a sedentary to light normal labor level.[74,106] It needs to be appreciated, however, that the ATS cutoff values were published in 1982 and 1986.[4,5] Despite the important work that has been done in this field in the last 20 years, neither the ATS statement nor the AMA Guides have been updated.

TABLE 22–8

Estimated $\dot{V}O_2$ During Various Activities

Activity	Estimated $\dot{V}O_2$
Resting	3.5
Sitting at desk and writing	4.25
Driving a car	4.25
Using a riding mower	8.75
Light assembly, standing, slow pace	8.75
Light welding	10.5
Playing pool	10.5
Standing at assembly line with brief lifting (less than 45 lb)	12.25
Standing at assembly line with brief lifting (greater than 45 lb)	14.0
Lifting and carrying 20–44 lbs	15.75
45–64 lbs	21.0
65–84 lbs	26.25
85–100 lbs	29.75
Pushing objects >75 lb (e.g., desk)	28
Swimming	28–33
Basketball game	42

From Wasserman K, Hansen JE, Sue DY, et al (eds): Principles of Exercise Testing and Interpretation. Philadelphia, Lippincott Williams & Wilkins, 1999; and Jones NL, Campbell EJM: Clinical Exercise Testing, 4th ed. Philadelphia, WB Saunders, 1997.

Thus it appears as though the ATS may have been generous when assigning levels of impairment to various $\dot{V}O_2$ levels. Additionally, there appears to be little support for subdividing the values between 15 and 25 mL/kg/min. (However, the concept of matching the worker's capability and the job demands [point 2] appears to have a great deal of merit.) It appears as though both references could stand an update.

Summary and Recommendations

Measurements of resting pulmonary function testing will produce values that can be applied in one of two ways. They can be assessed according to population norms or they can be compared with prior values when modified by the effects of time. The latter will give a more accurate value for any discrepancy created by a disease process but is rarely measured owing to the lack of premorbid pulmonary function testing. Thus, by default, values reflecting a percentage of population norms are normally used to measure impairment. The premorbid value should take precedence over the one derived from population norms whenever possible (see Chapter 25). In most circumstances, however, population norms will be used, using static PFTs as the state of the art despite serious flaws and drawbacks and despite improvements that have been seen in the past 20 years.

Measurements of resting PFTs are valuable in the diagnosis and quantification of various pulmonary diseases. It remains to be validated whether they can be used to assess impairment or disability. Because disability is defined as the inability to perform a specific task owing to a medical impairment and because the $\dot{V}O_2$ for various tasks are known, then measuring an individual's $\dot{V}O_2$ appears to be a more appropriate means of determining disability than using resting PFTs. Additionally, the philosophical approach of the Guides is to assess impairment based on disturbances in ADL. Because the $\dot{V}O_2$ of many of these activities is known, the $\dot{V}O_2$ would appear to be a more appropriate means of determining impairment than the resting PFT if the issue of selectivity of diagnosis can be overcome.

When measuring impairment (the loss of physiologic function), resting PFTs, as noted, will give numbers that reflect the deviation from normality (either population derived or person-specific). However, loss of function, not loss of a physiologic parameter, is the more important issue to be measured when assessing impairment. The resting PFT does not provide this measure of function. Therefore, a better system of measuring pulmonary impairment must be devised for assessing the impact of a pulmonary disease on an individual's health or performance of ADL. As was seen in the beginning of this chapter, dyspnea scales best reflected this disturbance in ADL. Exercise studies correlated less well, and static PFTs poorly.

Many of these issues were raised in a National Heart, Lung and Blood Institute Workshop Summary published in 1988.[13] These issues remain unresolved.

Asthma Testing

Asthma is characterized by reversible airflow rates. This factor and the need to test the individual in the absence of wheezing make it difficult to assess impairment or disability from asthma using the FVC, the FEV_1, the FEV_1/FVC, the FEF_{25-75}, or the MVV alone.

Two principal tests address the issue of the variability in airflow rates: bronchodilation studies and bronchoconstriction studies. In these studies, a simple, baseline spirometric test is performed and the FVC and the flow rates are contrasted after a (broncho)dilator or (broncho)constrictor agent is inhaled. Many controversies exist concerning which test is better, how much change is needed, and the sensitivity and specificity of each in diagnosing asthma (see following).[16,114]

When wheezing is heard or when the flow rates on the screening spirometry are low, asthmatic testing using a bronchodilator substance is generally chosen. The expected result in asthma is an increase in airflow rates with diminished wheezing. When the airflow rates are normal and wheezing is not heard, a constrictor agent is used. The expected result in an asthmatic is decreased airflow rates and wheezing. When wheezing is heard or airflow rates are low, constrictor

TABLE 22–9
Inhalation Challenge Tests

Variable	Methacholine	Histamine	Antigen	Exercise	Cold Air	Osmotic
Clinical usefulness	High	High	Low	Moderate	High	High
Sensitivity	High	High	Moderate	Moderate	High	High
Specificity	Moderate	Moderate	High	High	High	High
Reproducibility	High	High	Moderate	Moderate	High	High
Adverse effects	Low	Low	Potent; high	Potent; high	Low	—
Cost	High	High	High to very high	Moderate	High	—

agents may precipitate an asthmatic reaction that can be severe, may be delayed, and possibly require hospitalization (and rarely death).

Because constrictor agents provoke an asthmatic or bronchospastic response, they are also called bronchoprovocative agents and the test may be termed a bronchoprovocative test or maneuver. It can be performed with a variety of agents, each with its own sensitivity and specificity (see Table 22–9). Examples include histamine, acetylcholine (acetylcholine is liberated from nerve endings in the lungs causing smooth muscle contraction in the airways or bronchospasm), methacholine, cold air, dry air, exercise, hyperventilation, inhaled hypo-osmolar substances, and even ice cubes applied to the face. Theoretically, the most sensitive test would use a substance to which an individual has a suspected reaction. The following conditions are associated with a false positive bronchoprovocative asthma test:

Allergic rhinitis
Chronic bronchitis
Congestive heart failure
Viral upper or lower respiratory tract infection (within 8 weeks of testing)
Cystic fibrosis
COPD
Hypersensitivity pneumonitis
Adult respiratory distress syndrome
Sarcoidosis

Normal subjects also may experience a false positive result.

The following factors may increase, decrease, or have no effect on airway hyperresponsiveness (see also references 16 and 23; reference 6 provides some of the expected durations of the effects noted)[39]:

Factors That Enhance Hyperresponsiveness
- Aeroallergens (late phase response)
- Chemical sensitizers (e.g., toluene diisocyanate, western red cedar dust)
- Noxious gases (e.g., ozone, So_3, No_2)
- Cigarette smoke (chronic exposure)
- Viral respiratory infections (up to 8 weeks)
- Influenza vaccination
- Air pollutants

Factors That Do Not Enhance Hyperresponsiveness
- Aeroallergens (early phase response)
- Pharmacologic agents (histamine, methacholine)
- Cold air
- Exercise and hyperventilation
- Cigarette smoke (acute exposure)

Factors That Decrease Hyperresponsiveness
- Bronchodilators
- Antihistamines (during a histamine challenge test)
- Anticholinergics (during a methacholine challenge test)
- Pulmonary anti-inflammatory medications (chronic usage of corticosteroids, cromolyns, leukotriene modifiers)
- Substances containing caffeine (coffee, colas, chocolate) or theobromine (tea)

The following is a list of some substances causing asthma in the workplace (see reference 39 for a more complete list):

Animal origin
- Allergens from hair, scales, urine, serum, and remains of arthropods

Vegetable origin
- Wood, roots, leaves, flowers, cereals, grains, green coffee beans, castor beans, vegetable gums (arabic, adragante, karaya)

Textiles
- Cotton, jute, flax, hemp

Chemical products
- Pharmaceuticals (penicillin, ampicillin, cephalosporin powder, macrolides, tetracyclines)

Metals
- Chromium, nickel, platinum, vanadium, mercury

Plastic materials
- Isocyanates (toluene diisocyanate, diphenyl methane diisocyanate, hexamethylene diisocyanate), phthalic anhydrides, trimellitic anhydride

Formaldehyde

The major indications and contraindications for bronchoprovocative asthma testing are as follows:

Indications
- Proof that an individual has a hyperreactive response to a special agent
- Proof that a previously unreported agent is capable of causing an asthmatic reaction
- Research purposes

Contraindications
- Lack of experienced personnel who can recognize and assess the occurrence of clinical changes that will require therapeutic intervention
- Lack of emergency facilities (must be done in a hospital where facilities for emergency respiratory care are immediately available)
- Medication interference, including sustained-release theophyllines, beta-adrenergic agents, antihistamines, and mast cell stabilizers; mast cell stabilizers should be avoided for 24 hours, antihistamines for 48 hours, and beta-adrenergic agents and short-term theophylline compounds for 8 hours (all these agents will inhibit or block the response to chemical challenge)
- Moderate to marked abnormalities in the baseline pulmonary function test; because severe reductions in pulmonary function can occur with

bronchoprovocation testing (especially if baseline values are less than 65% to 70% of predicted), it is best to avoid this procedure in these circumstances; however, if an intermediate-type reaction is expected, the test can usually be performed, as treatment with a beta-antagonist reverses the constrictive effect quickly (late-type responses usually require corticosteroids[39])

Note that there are no specific values for sensitivity or specificity in Table 22–9. There is a major problem when attempting to define these values—how does one accurately diagnose asthma? Is it defined by the response to a test or by the history and physical examination or a combination of the two? This issue is further developed by the "rheostat model" of asthma (which is discussed in detail in Chapter 52).

This subject was studied by Toren et al, who performed a literature review of a variety of studies that correlated the results of various asthma questionnaires (self-reported asthma), physician-diagnosed asthma, presence of wheezing, and a positive bronchoprovocative test. The mean sensitivity of the self-reported asthma questionnaires was 36% (range of 7 to 80%) with a mean specificity of 94% (range 74 to 100%) when correlated with the pulmonary function test. When the self-reported asthma questionnaires were correlated with a clinical diagnosis, the mean sensitivity was 68% (range 48 to 100%) and the mean specificity was 94% (range 78 to 100%).[122]

Perpina et al performed a Bayesian analysis on the degree of bronchial hyperactivity as demonstrated in a methacholine test. They found that the cutoff value of 15 mg/mL for a 20% drop in the FEV_1 was the best discriminating point in making this diagnosis. When the pretest probability of the presence of asthma was 0.50, the probability of having asthma when the test was positive (sensitivity) was 86% and the probability of excluding asthma when the test was negative (specificity) was 84%.[102] As can be seen, there is obvious overlap, so that disease-positive individuals can have a negative test. The opposite is also true, exemplifying the point made by the rheostat model. A list of diseases or conditions associated with a false positive bronchoprovocative maneuver was provided previously. References 93, 97, 98, 104, 105, 110, 121, and 123 provide more background and discussion for the interested reader. Reference 6 is the position paper presented by the ATS for asthma testing using methacholine or exercise as the provoking agent.

The ATS recommends that asthma challenge testing be interpreted based on both the degree of hyperresponsiveness and the clinical condition. They state that if the probability of asthma is 30 to 70% and if the cutoff of the test is exceeded, then there is a high degree of certainty that asthma is not present. If the same patient has a strongly positive test, then the presence of asthma is confirmed. For any test result between these two points, "one must be more cautious about stating whether or not the patient has asthma."[6(p318)]

Peak Flow Measurements in Asthma Testing

As noted previously, the PEF is the highest point on the flow volume curve. As such, it is routinely measured when airflow rates are assessed. It can also be measured using a peak flow meter. These devices are inexpensive, small, and portable. They can be used easily after simple training and do not require supervision. These are their strong points. The last issue also represents its weakest point. The lack of supervision makes it difficult to verify the results.

PEF monitors are useful in occupational settings when a worker is being assessed for occupational asthma. In this setting, a person may have normal pulmonary function testing and yet allege breathing difficulties in the workplace. As noted previously, bronchoprovocative tests, including those using methacholine or histamine, are not 100% sensitive in the diagnosis of asthma and bronchoprovocative tests using occupational agents are not always possible or desirable (see reference 39). As a portable device, peak flow monitors can be used by an examinee while at work and at varying times of the day.

Asthma can present with diminished airflow rates (including the PEF) after exposure to an offending agent. Pepys describes four separate times for an asthmatic to have a reaction following an exposure[101]:

1. Immediate (within minutes, rapidly maximal, and lasting 1.5 to 2 hours)
2. Delayed (starting about 1 hour after exposure and lasting about 5 hours)
3. Delayed (starting several hours after exposure and lasting about a day)
4. Delayed (starting in the early morning hours on the day after the exposure and recurring at the same time of the night for several nights thereafter without repeat exposure)

The dual concepts of random asthmogenic exposures and variability in the timing of the asthmatic reaction make the peak flow monitor a useful tool. Because it is portable, it can be taken into the workplace. Because it is used without supervision, the worker can test his or her PEF before, during, and after (frequently and repeatedly) a workplace exposure. It is a useful test for establishing a diagnosis of occupational asthma and very useful in disability determinations (see Chapter 52). That the accuracy of the peak flow monitor will never approach that of a bronchoprovocative test with workplace agents is established; the remaining question is whether it is reliable in this setting.

The absolute value obtained from the peak flow monitor varies considerably from that measured on a spirometer and is dependent on the meter used. Thus the absolute values are not quite as important as the trends.[46] There are a variety of factors, other than asthmogenic factors, that are known to affect airflow rates (especially the PEF), including medications and diurnal variations.[36] Finally, and perhaps most importantly, the lack of supervision makes it easy for the informed and intelligent worker to create a false positive test. Various protocols have addressed this issue.[17,36,90,124] However, when properly used, these tests are quite sensitive and specific in diagnosing asthma when compared with more traditional methods of testing with values ranging from 74 to 100% for each.[36,91,124]

Exercise Testing

Exercise testing is done in pulmonary diseases to assess three issues: the variability of airflow rates that can be produced by exercise, the adequacy of gas transfer, and the functional capability/capacity.

Airflow rates change with exercise. The expected change is a slight drop in airway resistance resulting in a slight increase in flow rates. These changes are caused by either neural or hormonal (e.g., circulating epinephrine) changes that occur during exercise. Certain individuals, however, can have diminished airflow rates and are diagnosed with exercise-induced asthma. Thus, exercise testing can represent an adjunctive test for the presence or degree of asthma (see section on asthma testing) although bronchoprovocative or bronchodilator testing is usually preferred owing to reliability, ease of testing, and cost.

As noted previously, the lung, on the average and in good health, is made up of approximately 350,000,000 alveolar–capillary units. Only a fraction of these are used at rest. It is for this reason that ABG analysis is useful under resting conditions only when the lungs are moderately to severely abnormal. The exercise state maximizes both ventilation in and blood perfusion of the lungs. Thus, loss of alveoli, loss of pulmonary capillaries, mismatching of the remaining alveolar–capillary units, or a thickened interstitial membrane will affect the gas transfer during exercise. This subject is more fully covered in Chapter 24 on cardiopulmonary exercise testing.

As can be inferred from the previous discussion, exercise testing can be important in making a determination of impairment (the AMA Guides use the $\dot{V}O_2$ max—the maximum oxygen uptake during exercise—as one of its major criteria for classification of impairment). It is useful and important, but other types of tests are generally easier to obtain and less costly. However, in a disability evaluation (i.e., determining an individual's functional capacity or how much work a person can do) or in establishing a cause for dyspnea during exertion, exercise testing is ideal. The subject is covered fully in Chapter 24.

Oxygen Saturation Measurements

Hemoglobin can reversibly attach oxygen and carbon dioxide molecules. This provides metabolizing tissues with a renewable oxygen delivery and carbon dioxide removal mechanism via the circulatory system. Normal hemoglobin attaches oxygen molecules to its binding sites. The normal saturation of arterial blood is close to 100%. Physiologic shunting causes the slight decrease. The normal venous saturation is 75% but this is tissue specific with some organs removing more oxygen (a lower $S\bar{v}O_2$) and some less. During exercise, greater amounts of oxygen are extracted due to increased utilization by muscle cells. However, there is a simultaneous increase in both lung perfusion and ventilation with better matching of the ventilation and perfusion (decreased shunt) causing the SaO_2 to increase as the mixed venous oxygen saturation ($S\bar{v}O_2$) decreases.

Aging is associated with a predictable decrease in PaO_2 in healthy individuals. Thus, the SaO_2 also must decline. Further, the effects of disease (especially pulmonary) also decrease the PaO_2 and the SaO_2.

ABG analyses are obtained invasively. Either a needle is inserted into an artery for blood withdrawal or a catheter is placed into the artery for repeated sampling. These procedures are not only invasive but also costly, painful, and liable to have potential complications. For this reason, a noninvasive method of measuring the PaO_2/SaO_2 would be a preferred method of analysis, if the correlation between the PaO_2/SaO_2 and noninvasive SaO_2 were sufficiently high. Further, this correlation needs to hold true not only for normal individuals but also for individuals with disease and during exercise for both healthy and diseased individuals.

The theory of using the light absorbing properties of hemoglobin was first proposed in the 1930s.[72] The first oxygen saturation monitor was developed in 1936 and has been refined through the years. Clinical use began in the 1980s and oxygen saturation monitors are now routinely used in a variety of settings such as during surgery or in an intensive care unit setting.[72] These monitors rely on the differential absorption of light between oxygenated and reduced hemoglobin. Capillarized blood is used as the sample. The first clinically used devices were ear oximeters that slightly warmed the earlobe to provide a more constant supply of capillarized blood. Current oximeters are either ear probes or (more commonly) finger probes that use the capillarized blood found in the nail beds. These monitors are very accurate for an SaO_2 >70% but can be influenced by a variety of factors that can decrease their accuracy and utility (Table 22–10). The designation Spo_2 is given for the oxygen saturation detected by a pulse or peripheral monitor.

In impairment or disability determinations, the Spo_2 can be used in one of two circumstances. The Spo_2 can be measured in a resting state. Medicare guidelines call for payment of oxygen if the Pao_2 is <55 mm Hg or the Sao_2 <89%.[40] The AMA Guides state that a Pao_2 of <60 mm Hg (if certain coexisting criteria are met) or <55 mm Hg by itself are evidence for severe impairment.[26(p101)] The Social Security Listings[117] also use the Pao_2 as a criterion for disability but do not use the Sao_2 (or Spo_2): "Oximetry and capillary gas analysis are not acceptable substitutes for the measurement of arterial blood gas."[117(p40)] The fifth edition of the Guides states that the Spo_2 "often provides an adequate estimate of hypoxia. Arterial blood gases, although more invasive, provide a more accurate measurement of hypoxia. Physicians should use their clinical judgment as to which measurement is needed, based on individual assessment."[26(p101)] (Interestingly, the first edition of the Guides uses the Sao_2, but this should not be considered as the Spo_2 as this technology was not commonplace when the original JAMA article or the first edition was written.[27,28] The second through fourth editions do not mention the use of the Sao_2.[2,3,45,47])

TABLE 22–10

Factors Affecting the Spo_2

Condition	Cause
Underestimate Sao_2	
Methylene blue, indocyanine green	Light absorption similar to reduced hemoglobin
Excessive skin pigmentation (possible)	Signal loss
Reduced perfusion	Signal loss
Reduced pulsations	Intermittent to complete loss of readings
Sensor malposition	Change in calibration curve
Anemia (<5 g/dL)	Photon scattering
Motion artifact	Signal loss
Ambient light on sensor probe	Signal loss
Intravenous dyes	
Nail polish	Signal loss
Excessive venous pulsations	Measure venous blood
Overestimate Sao_2	
Carboxyhemoglobinemia	Light absorption similar to oxyhemoglobin
Methemoglobinemia	
Hyperbilirubinemia (Sao_2 < 90%)	
Severe hypoxemia	Magnifies error

Modified from Jensen LA, Onyskiw JE, Prasad NGN: Meta-analysis of arterial oxygen saturation monitoring by pulse oximetry in adults. Heart Lung 27: 387–408, 1998; and Department of Health and Human Services Medicare Program: Coverage of oxygen for use in a patient's home. Final Notice. Fed Reg 50:13742–13750, 1985.

The SSA criteria for hypoxemia take into account the altitude at which the test is performed, the effects of obesity, and the effects of hyperventilation (simplistically, the lower the $Paco_2$, the higher the Pao_2). Further, the Pao_2 is obtained in a two-step process. It is performed on room air at rest. If it is low, it is repeated later to ensure validity. If it does not meet the cutoff criteria, it is performed after exercise.[117] The AMA Guides do not address the issue of requiring the Pao_2 to be performed during or after exercise testing as one of the conditions for using the Pao_2 cutoff values of <60 or 55 mm Hg as a criterion of severe impairment.

Oxygen saturation monitors are used extensively during impairment or disability examinations as a part of exercise testing protocols (see Chapter 24). However, as mentioned, it is not a stand-alone test for these determinations and needs to be combined with other data.

In early reports of Spo_2 monitors, divergent results were seen between the Pao_2 and the Spo_2, especially during exercise or at lower levels of Pao_2/Sao_2, with r values between 0.52 and 0.99.[49,87,88,112] However, by the 1990s, the correlation became tighter, with r values usually exceeding 96% (depending on the oximeter used[72]) except with low levels of oxygen (e.g., exercising at altitude), with the cutoff value being an Spo_2 <75%.[15,21,85,88] Reference 72 provides r values for 21 pulse oximeters and was published in 1998. Currently, the expectation is a 2% accuracy range (–1 SD) or 5% (–2 SD) of the simultaneous Sao_2.[72] This level of accuracy applies to healthy individuals with the proviso that the conditions in Table 22–10 be eliminated. The Spo_2 is also a bit lower in patients with sickle cell disease but not sufficiently to exclude its use (underestimating the Sao_2 by approximately 3.4 percentage points).[96]

The Spo_2 overestimates the Sao_2 consistently in the presence of an elevated carbon monoxide level in a proportional fashion[60] and examinees may need to have their carboxyhemoglobin levels checked under certain circumstances during an evaluation. The normal carboxyhemoglobin concentration is <0.5%. Smokers have levels between 5 and 10% and occasionally higher.[57] Greater concern should be expressed for those individuals who have traveled to the testing facility on freeways (especially those below ground level), who were "stuck in traffic," or who traveled through tunnels. This is even more important if the examinee smoked during this drive. Symptoms of CO poisoning do not typically develop until the carboxyhemoglobin saturation is over 20%.[57] The excretion of CO is due to the pressure gradient between the blood and the alveolus (appreciating the fact that CO is over 200 times more avidly held by hemoglobin than is O_2). The excretion is logrithmic with 50% excreted within 320 minutes or within 80 minutes if 100% oxygen is breathed.[77]

Radiography

The fifth edition of the Guides states that "chest roentgenographic findings often correlate poorly with physiological findings"[26(p91)] and, as such, are not used in quantifying impairment. Similar statements are found in previous editions and none use the CXR as a criterion for impairment.[2,3,27,28,45,47] CXRs are very important in diagnosing the reasons for abnormal physiology or establishing a diagnosis, but, by themselves, rarely alter a person's functional classification. The SSA has a similar attitude on radiographic testing.[117]

As technology advances, newer radiographic tests have been devised, yet they are similarly poorly applicable to impairment ratings. They assume a more important role, however, in disability determination. As discussed in Chapter 1, disability is the inability to participate in a workplace environment owing to a medical impairment. This is discussed more fully in Chapter 59 on pulmonary disability. It is in these determinations that radiographic tests can assume an important role, specifically in the individual with ILD or hypersensitivity pneumonitis (HP).

ILD is caused by a variety of factors. Approximately 150 causes have been identified at last count. Some of these factors or causes are specific to a work environment. In addition to diagnosing and suggesting causation (a biopsy is necessary in some circumstances), radiographs can assist the physician in recommending that an individual not be allowed to participate in certain job settings owing to the progressive nature of some diseases with continued exposure. Thus diseases such as pneumoconioses (asbestosis, silicosis, coal worker's pneumoconiosis, and others) or HP can be assessed using radiographic means. During impairment evaluations, physiologic deviations from normality are more important than a precise diagnosis. In a disability evaluation, however, both assume equal importance. Physiologic capabilities can define a persons work capacity for manual labor or even for certain jobs. The diagnosis may also create job restrictions in and by itself (see above).

Radiographic testing for the presence of pneumoconiosis or other type of work-related ILD is best performed with a computed axial tomography (CAT) scan. High-resolution CAT (HRCT) scanning is different from normal CAT scanning; the slices of lung being averaged drop from 10 mm to 1 to 2 mm and are imaged using a high spatial frequency reconstruction algorithm. Thus the interstitial tissue is more clearly imaged. HRCT is the preferred method of diagnosing various work-related lung diseases although it is performed infrequently owing to cost.[70] CAT scans are also of importance in determining the presence or absence of other abnormalities that are disease and exposure specific including pleural abnormalities (asbestosis, silicosis), hilar lymphadenopathy (coal workers' pneumoconiosis), and lung cancers.

When CXRs are interpreted for the presence or absence of a pneumoconiosis they are interpreted using the International Labour Organization/University of Cincinnati (ILO/UC) classification that was originally devised in the 1950s for reading CXRs of workers with suspected coal workers' pneumoconiosis (the most recent update of this classification was in 1980).[58] Its application has been extended to use in silicosis and asbestosis. It can be used, however, for any pneumoconiosis or even any ILD. This classification allows different observers to understand what others are referring to in the interpretation of ILD. This classification is a verbal attempt to describe the type, location, and amount of the interstitial abnormality. It also describes the presence (or absence) of other types of abnormalities on the CXR (see Table 22–11).

It should be noted that the designations upper lobe (UL), middle lobe (ML), and lower lobe (LL) do not refer to anatomic regions of the lung but to the upper, middle, and lower thirds of the CXR without attempting to distinguish the lobes (for example, the right upper lobe occupies the RUL zone; the right middle lobe, the RML and RLL lung zones; and the right lower lobe, the RUL, RML, and RLL lung zones). Additionally, when the CXR is interpreted using this scheme, the profusion (the number of abnormalities) is expressed as two numbers. Thus a radiograph with a profusion of 1

TABLE 22–11

International Labour Organization/ University of Cincinnati Classification of Interstitial Lung Disease

Term	Meaning
p	Small, rounded opacities up to 1.5 mm in diameter
q	Medium, rounded opacities with a diameter >1.5 mm but <3 mm
r	Larger, rounded opacities with a diameter >3 mm but <10 mm
s	Thin, linear or irregular opacities with a width up to 1.5 mm
t	Thicker, linear or irregular opacities with a width >1.5 mm but <3 mm
u	More thick, linear or irregular opacities with a width >3 mm but <10 mm
0	Complete absence of any interstitial abnormalities
1	Presence of slight interstitial abnormalities
2	Presence of medium interstitial abnormalities
3	Presence of large amounts of interstitial abnormalities (0–3 are defined by matching to a set of reference radiographs)
R	Right lung
L	Left lung
UL	Upper lung zone
ML	Middle lung zone
LL	Lower lung zone

From Guidelines for the Use of ILO International Classification of Radiographs of Pneumoconiosis. Occupational Safety and Health Series No. 22, ref. Geneva: International Labour Office, 1980.

(minimal amount of interstitial abnormalities) can be read as 0/1, 1/0, or 1/1. The first number reflects the first look by the reader and the second number reflects the second look by the same reader.[58]

Unfortunately, the vast majority of CXRs demonstrating ILD will belong in the category of grade 1 profusion.[42,76] The sensitivity and specificity of the ILO/UC system in interpreting a grade 1 CXR is dramatically lower then those showing profusion levels of 2 or 3.[70] Various other causes of low profusion opacities exist, creating problems with this examination. The concepts of "increased bronchovascular markings" or "dirty lungs" in the patient with chronic bronchitis are well known examples.[42]

Small irregular opacities can also be influenced by variables such as radiographic technique, age, obesity, and influence of smoking. Poor inhalation, underpenetration, and body habitus (especially obesity) can all create, what appears to be, increased interstitial markings.[42] CXRs taken at two thirds of TLC are frequently interpreted as showing profusion scores from 1/0 to 1/2.[76] Cigarette smoking frequently produces small, irregular opacities with a profusion of 0/1 to 1/1 in the lower lung zones.[42,76]

Several other problems exist in the interpretation of the CXR using the ILO/UC criteria or CAT scan to assess for the presence or degree of ILD. First, there is a significant inter- and intraobserver variation, especially with small, irregular opacities, on the order of 18%.[111] Secondly, the correlation among CAT scans, CXRs read by the ILO classification, physiology, and pathology have been reported to be from good to poor.[111] Finally, not all cases of ILD will show up on the CXR or even a CAT scan.[67] It is estimated that approximately 10 to 20% of patients with biopsy-proven asbestosis will have normal CXRs.[111] In a study by Staples et al of 169 asbestos-exposed workers who had normal CXRs (ILO <1), HRCT was normal or near normal in 76 (Group 1), intermediate in 36, and abnormal and suggestive of asbestosis in 57 (Group 2; 34% of the total study population). The latter group (Group 2) had a significantly lower VC and DLCO than did Group 1. Although a biopsy was not performed, these workers were presumed to have asbestosis. Additionally, 77% of workers in Group 2 had pleural disease, providing inferential evidence of asbestosis.[118]

The plain chest radiograph is a less sensitive instrument than the HRCT in identifying the above abnormalities but is the preferred screening examination because of availability, ease, and cost. It is of particular importance, however, in HP, where transient radiographic findings are common. Even though CAT scanning better assesses the interstitial abnormalities found in HP, the transient nature of those infiltrates are often identified more easily on serial chest radiographs.

Serology and Biopsy

There are a few serologic tests for lung diseases but many of these are useful in occupationally induced lung diseases. Examples include tests for occupational asthma and HP.[39,71] By themselves, they are merely an indication of an immune response by the body to an external agent. However, when combined with abnormal physiologic or radiographic testing and the appropriate history, they provide compelling evidence of not only causation but also a need for workplace restrictions.

Biopsies have a similar role. They are rarely performed yet when done are diagnostic in terms of causation and provide evidence for workplace restrictions.[70,71]

Polysomnography

A polysomnogram is a sleep test performed for the evaluation of obstructive sleep apnea (OSA). This test has become commonplace since the early 1990s as physicians have become more aware of the frequency of OSA. Numerous variables are tested during a sleep study including frequency of ventilation, ventilatory efforts with or without air exchange (measured by surface electromyography), oxygen saturation, eye movements, electrocardiogram, and electroencephalogram. Ideally, all patients should be referred to a facility that specializes in this disorder (and is accredited by the American Sleep Disorders Society) and interpreted by an individual possessing the knowledge and experience necessary to interpret the results correctly (and usually certified by the American Board of Sleep Medicine).

The typical history obtained in a patient with OSA is one of daytime fatigue or drowsiness, snoring, and breathing cessation during sleep (the latter two symptoms are more reliably obtained by asking the bed partner). Various methods have been proposed to predict OSA. However, history is an unreliable indication of the presence of OSA. OSA is found in 2 to 4% of the population, yet in a population wherein 46% had OSA, the history obtained by a specialist was only 50 to 60% sensitive and 63 to 70% specific in diagnosing OSA.[119]

The results of the sleep study are expressed in one of two terms—the respiratory disturbance index (RDI) or the apnea/hypopnea index (AHI). These two terms mean the same thing and are used synonymously. Apnea is defined as a cessation of air movement lasting longer than 10 seconds. A hypopnea is a significant slowing of either the rate or the depth of respiration with a drop in the Spo_2. The RDI or AHI is the number of apneas and hypopneas per hour of recorded sleep. Apneas can be either central (no neural input to the respiratory muscles) or, more commonly, peripheral (neural input to and contraction of the respiratory muscles without the presence of air flow owing to upper airway obstruction). Other variables that are measured during polysomnography include the number of awakenings or arousals, periodic limb movements, and the quality of sleep (e.g., the total amount of rapid eye movement sleep). Any significant abnormalities of the above variables can produce disordered and inefficient sleep. If the AHI or RDI is excessive, there is an increased risk of hypertension, pulmonary hypertension, congestive heart failure, cardiac arrhythmias, and stroke. Conversely, successful treatment of OSA has been found to decrease the morbidity and mortality caused by those conditions (see Chapter 25).

An overnight oxygen saturation test (the Spo_2 measured with a continuous recorder) cannot be used as a substitute for a full polysomnogram for establishing the diagnosis of OSA. First, it does not measure all the variables measured in a full study. Second, it is not a sensitive test for the presence of OSA. In 102 consecutive patients (40 had OSA defined by an RDI >15), the sensitivity and specificity of the mean Spo_2 was 48% and 80% (threshold 85%), and for the CT_{80} (amount of time with an Spo_2 <80 and with a threshold of 5%), 63% and 66%.[69] Clinical methods are also incapable of arriving at the diagnosis with sufficient reliability to positively diagnose individuals and are probably better used when deciding not to perform sleep studies.[69,125] For example, disruptive snoring alone has a sensitivity and specificity of 71% and 32%; disruptive snoring plus reported apnea 23% and 94%; snoring, observed choking, sleepiness while driving, body mass index, sex, and age had values of 50% to 70% and 60% to 80%; observed apneas, body mass index, age, and diastolic hypertension had 92% and 51%; and neck size, hypertension, snoring, and choking or gasping had values of 50% to 85% and 30% to 70%, respectively.[108]

From an impairment or disability perspective, OSA is both an impairing and a disabling condition. Not only associated with and causative of many adverse cardiovascular problems and neurocognitive consequences, OSA can produce significant daytime somnolence. The degree of drowsiness or sleeping during the daytime is a factor of both the AHI and the individual. Diminished intellectual performance and personality disturbances are seen at the lower end of the spectrum with frequent, inappropriate, and uncontrollable sleeping at the higher end. These individuals can have significant problems in carrying out the essential components of their job and can be at risk while traveling to and from work. These issues are covered in greater detail in Chapters 25 and 59.

References

1. Aaron SD, Dales RE, Cardinal P: How accurate is spirometry at predicting restrictive pulmonary impairment? Chest 115: 869–873, 1999.
2. American Medical Association: Guides to the Evaluation of Permanent Impairment, 2nd ed. Chicago, American Medical Association, 1984.
3. American Medical Association: Guides to the Evaluation of Permanent Impairment, 2nd ed, rev. Chicago, American Medical Association, 1990.
4. American Thoracic Society: Evaluation of impairment/disability secondary to respiratory disease. Am Rev Respir Dis 126: 945–951, 1982.
5. American Thoracic Society: Evaluation of impairment/disability secondary to respiratory disorders. Am Rev Respir Dis 133:1205–1209, 1986.
6. American Thoracic Society: Guidelines for methacholine and exercise challenge testing—1999. Am J Respir Crit Care Med 161:309–329, 2000.
7. American Thoracic Society: Lung function testing: Selection of reference values and interpretative strategies. Am Rev Respir Dis 144:1202–1218, 1991.
8. American Thoracic Society: Single-breath carbon monoxide diffusing capacity (transfer factor): Recommendations for a standard technique. Am Rev Respir Dis 136:1299–1307, 1987.
9. American Thoracic Society: Standardization of spirometry. Am J Respir Crit Care Med 152:1107–1136, 1995.
10. American Thoracic Society: Standardization of spirometry—1987 update. Am Rev Respir Dis 136:1285–1298, 1987.
11. Bates DV: Normal pulmonary function. In Bates DV (ed): Respiratory Function in Disease, 3rd ed. Philadelphia, WB Saunders, 1989, pp 106–151.
12. Becklake MR: Concepts of normality applied to the measurement of lung function. Am J Med 80:1158–1164, 1986.
13. Becklake MR, Rodarte JR, Kalica AR: NHLBI workshop summary. Scientific issues in the assessment of respiratory impairment. Am Rev Respir Dis 137:1505–1510, 1988.
14. Becklake MR, White N: Sources of variation in spirometric measurement: Identifying the signal and dealing with noise. In Eisen EA (ed): Occupational Medicine: State of the Art Reviews. Philadelphia, Hanley & Belfus, 1993:8, pp 241–264.
15. Benoit H, Costes F, Feasson L, et al: Accuracy of pulse oximetry during intense exercise under severe hypoxic conditions. Eur J Appl Physiol 76:260–263, 1997.
16. Braman SS, Corrao WM: Bronchoprovocation testing. In Mahler DA (ed): Clinics in Chest Medicine. Philadelphia, WB Saunders, 1989:10, pp 165–176.
17. Burge PS: Use of serial measurements of peak flow in the diagnosis of occupational asthma. In Eisen EA (ed): Occupational Medicine: State of the Art Reviews. Philadelphia, Hanley & Belfus, 1993:8, pp 279–302.
18. Burrows B, Lebowitz MD, Camilli A, et al: Longitudinal changes in the forced expiratory volume in one second in adults. Methodologic considerations and findings in healthy nonsmokers. Am Rev Respir Dis 133:974–980, 1986.
19. Camilli AE, Burrows B, Knudson RJ, et al: Longitudinal changes in the forced expiratory volume in one second in adults. Effects of smoking and smoking cessation. Am Rev Respir Dis 135: 794–799, 1987.

20. Carleson DJ, Ries AL, Kaplan RM: Prediction of maximum exercise tolerance in patients with COPD. Chest 100:307–311, 1991.
21. Carter BG, Carlin JB, Tibballs J, et al: Accuracy of two pulse oximeters at low arterial hemoglobin-oxygen saturation. Crit Care Med 26:1128–1133, 1998.
22. Celli BA, Snider GL, Heffner J, et al: Standards for the diagnosis and care of patients with chronicobstructive pulmonary disease. Am J Respir Crit Care Med 152(Suppl.):s77–s120, 1995.
23. Chan-Yeung M: Assessment of asthma in the workplace. Chest 108:1084–1117, 1995.
24. Cherniak NS, Altose MD: Mechanisms of dyspnea. In Braman SS (ed): Clinics in Chest Medicine. Philadelphia, WB Saunders, 1987:8, pp 207–214.
25. Clausen JL: Prediction of normal values in pulmonary function testing. In Mahler DA (ed): Clinics in Chest Medicine. Philadelphia, WB Saunders, 1989:10, pp 135–143.
26. Cocchiarella L, Andersson GBJ (eds): Guides to the Evaluation of Permanent Impairment, 5th ed. Chicago, American Medical Association, 2001.
27. Committee on Rating of Mental and Physical Impairment: Guides to the Evaluation of Permanent Impairment. Chicago, American Medical Association, 1977.
28. Committee on Rating of Mental and Physical Impairment: The respiratory system. JAMA 194:913–932, 1965.
29. Cotes JE, Zejda J, King B: Lung function impairment as a guide to exercise limitation in work-related lung disorders. Am Rev Respir Dis 137:1089–1093, 1988.
30. Coultas DB, Gong H, Grad R, et al: Respiratory diseases in minorities of the United States. Am J Respir Crit Care Med 149:s93–s131, 1993.
31. Crapo RD, Morris AH, Gardner RN: Reference spirometric values using techniques and equipment that meet ATS recommendations. Am Rev Respir Dis 123:659–664, 1981.
32. Crapo RD, Forster RE: Carbon monoxide diffusing capacity. In Mahler DA (ed): Clinics in Chest Medicine. Philadelphia, WB Saunders, 1989:10, pp 189–198.
33. Cropp GJA, Bernstein IL, Boushey HA, et al: Guidelines for bronchial inhalation challenges with pharmacologic and antigenic agents. Am Thoracic Society News 11–19, 1980.
34. Curtis JR, Deyo RA, Hudson LD: Health-related quality of life among patients with chronic obstructive pulmonary disease. Thorax 49:162–170, 1994.
35. Curtis JR, Martin DP, Martin TR: Patient-assessed health outcomes in chronic lung disease. What are they, how do they help us, and where do we go from here? Am J Respir Crit Care Med 156:1032–1039, 1997.
36. Dahlqvist M, Eisen EA, Wegman DH, et al: Reproducibility of peak expiratory flow measurements. In Eisen EA (ed): Occupational Medicine: State of the Art Reviews. Philadelphia, Hanley & Belfus, 1993:8, pp 295–302.
37. Demeter SL: Gas exchange across abnormal interstitial tissue in pulmonary sarcoidosis—results of therapy. Angiology 38:256–267, 1987.
38. Demeter SL: Interstitial vasculitis—interstitial lung disease; case studies. Angiology 37:325–328, 1986.
39. Demeter SL, Cordasco EM: Occupational asthma. In Zenz C, Dickerson OB, Horvath EP (eds): Occupational Medicine, 3rd ed. St. Louis, Mosby, 1994, pp 213–228.
40. Department of Health and Human Services Medicare Program: Coverage of oxygen for use in a patient's home. Final notice. Fed Reg 50:13742–13750, April 5, 1985.
41. Department of Labor, Employment Standards Administration: Standards for determining coal miners' total disability or death due to pneumoconiosis. Fed Reg 45:13678–13712, 1980.
42. Dick JA, Morgan WKC, Muir DFC, et al: The significance of irregular opacities on the chest roentgenogram. Chest 102:251–260, 1992.
43. Dockery DW: Percentile curves for evaluation of repeated measures of lung function. In Eisen EA (ed): Occupational Medicine: State of the Art Reviews. Philadelphia, Hanley & Belfus, 1993:8, pp 323–338.
44. Dockery DW: Percentile curves for evaluation of repeated measures of lung function. In Eisen EA (ed): Spirometry—Occupational Medicine: State of the Art Reviews. Philadelphia, Hanley & Belfus, 1993:8, pp 323–338.
45. Doege TC, Houston TP: Guides to the Evaluation of Permanent Impairment, 4th ed. Chicago, American Medical Association, 1993.
46. Eisen EA, Wegman DH, Kriebel D: Application of peak expiratory flow in epidemiologic studies of occupation. In Eisen EA (ed): Occupational Medicine: State of the Art Reviews. Philadelphia, Hanley & Belfus, 1993:8, pp 265–277.
47. Engelberg AL: Guides to the Evaluation of Permanent Impairment, 3rd ed. Chicago, American Medical Association, 1988.
48. Enright PL, Johnson LR, Connett JE: Spirometry in the Lung Health Study. Methods and quality control. Am Rev Respir Dis 143:1215–1223, 1991.
49. Escourrou PJL, Delaperche MF, Visseaux A: Reliability of pulse oximetry during exercise in pulmonary patients. Chest 97:635–638, 1990.
50. Ferrer M, Alonso J, Morera J, et al: Chronic obstructive pulmonary disease and health-related quality of life. Ann Intern Med 127:1072–1079, 1997.
51. Fulmer JD, Roberts WC, vonGal ER, et al: Morphologic-physiologic correlates of the severity of fibrosis and degree of cellularity in idiopathic pulmonary fibrosis. J Clin Invest 63:665–676, 1979.
52. Gardner RM, Clausen JL, Cotton DJ, et al: Computer guidelines for pulmonary laboratories. Am Rev Respir Dis 134:628–629, 1986.
53. Gardner RM, Clausen JL, Crapo RO, et al: Quality assurance in pulmonary function laboratories. Am Rev Respir Dis 134:625–627, 1986.
54. Gardner RM, Clausen JL, Epler G, et al: Pulmonary function laboratory personnel qualifications. Am Rev Respir Dis 134:623–624, 1986.
55. Gardner RM, Crapo RO, Nelson SB: Spirometry and flow-volume curves. In Mahler DA (ed): Clinics in Chest Medicine. Philadelphia, WB Saunders, 1989:10, pp 145–154.
56. Glindmeyer HW, Lefante JJ, McColloster C: Blue-collar normative spirometric values for Caucasian and African–American men and women aged 18 to 65. Am J Respir Crit Care Med 151:412–422, 1995.
57. Graham DR: Noxious gases and fumes. In Baum GL, Crapo JD, Celli BR, et al (eds): Textbook of Pulmonary Diseases, 6th ed. Philadelphia, Lippincott-Raven, 1998, pp 741–753.
58. Guidelines for the Use of ILO International Classification of Radiographs of Pneumoconiosis: Occupational Safety and Health Series No. 22, rev. Geneva: International Labour Office, 1980.
59. Hajiro T, Nishimura K, Tsukino M, et al: A comparison of the level of dyspnea vs. disease severity in indicating the health-related quality of life of patients with COPD. Chest 116:1632–1637, 1999.
60. Hampson NB: Pulse oximetry in severe carbon monoxide poisoning. Chest 114:1036–1041, 1998.
61. Hankinson JL: Instrumentation for spirometry. In Eisen EA (ed): Occupational Medicine: State of the Art Reviews. Philadelphia, Hanley & Belfus, 1993:8, pp 397–407.
62. Hankinson JL, Bang KM: Acceptability and reproducibility criteria of the American Thoracic Society as observed in a sample of the general population. Am Rev Respir Dis 143:516–521, 1991.

63. Hankinson JL, Kinsley KB, Wagner GR: Comparison of spirometric reference values for Caucasian and African American blue-collar workers. J Occup Environ Med 38:137–143, 1996.
64. Hankinson JL, Odencrantz JR, Fedan KB: Spirometric reference values from a sample of the general U.S. population. Am J Respir Crit Care Med 159:179–187, 1999.
65. Hankinson JL, Wagner GR: Medical screening using periodic spirometry for detection of chronic lung disease. In Eisen EA (ed): Occupational Medicine: State of the Art Reviews. Philadelphia, Hanley & Belfus, 1993:8, pp 353–361.
66. Harber P, Schnur R, Emery J, et al: Statistical "biases" in respiratory disability determinations. Am Rev Respir Dis 128:413–418, 1983.
67. Harkin TJ, McGuinness G, Goldring R, et al: Differentiation of the ILD boundary chest roentgenograph (0/1 to 1/0) in asbestosis by high-resolution computed tomography scan, alveolitis, and respiratory impairment. J Occup Environ Med 38:46–52, 1996.
68. Harver A, Mahler DA: The symptoms of dyspnea. In Mahler DA (ed): Dyspnea. Mount Kisco, NY, Futura Publishing, 1990, pp 1–53.
69. Herer B, Roche N, Carton M, et al: Value of clinical, functional, and oximetric data for the prediction of obstructive sleep apnea in obese patients. Chest 116:1537–1544, 1999.
70. Inhalation of inorganic dust (pneumoconiosis). In Fraser RS, Mullen NL, Colman N, et al (eds): Diagnosis of Diseases of the Chest, 4th ed. Philadelphia, WB Saunders, 1999, pp 2386–2484.
71. Inhalation of organic dust. In Fraser RS, Mullen NL, Colman N, et al (eds): Diagnosis of Diseases of the Chest, 4th ed. Philadelphia, WB Saunders, 1999, pp 2361–2385.
72. Jensen LA, Onyskiw JE, Prasad NGN: Meta-analysis of arterial oxygen saturation monitoring by pulse oximetry in adults. Heart Lung 27:387–408, 1998.
73. Jones PW: Measurement of breathlessness. In Hughes JMB, Pride NB (eds): Lung Function Tests: Physiological Principles and Clinical Applications. London, WB Saunders, 1999, pp 121–131.
74. Jones NL, Campbell EJM: Clinical Exercise Testing, 4th ed. Philadelphia, WB Saunders, 1997.
75. Kellie SE, Attfield MD, Hankinson JL, et al: Spirometry variability criteria—association with respiratory morbidity and mortality in a cohort of coal miners. Am J Epidemiol 125:437–444, 1987.
76. Kilburn KH, Warshaw RH: Severity of pulmonary asbestosis as classified by International Labour Organization profusion of irregular opacities in 8749 asbestos-exposed American workers. Those who never smoked compared with those who ever smoked. Arch Intern Med 152:325–327, 1992.
77. Kindwall EP: Carbon monoxide. In Zenz C, Dickerson OB, Horvath EP (eds): Occupational Medicine, 3rd ed. St Louis, Mosby, 1994, pp 447–452.
78. Mahler DA: Dyspnea: diagnosis and management. In Braman SS (ed): Clinics in Chest Medicine. Philadelphia, WB Saunders, 1987:8, pp 215–230.
79 Mahler DA: How should health-related quality of life be assessed in patients with COPD? Chest 117:54s–57s, 2000.
80 Mahler DA, Harvon A: Clinical measurement of dyspnea. In Mahler DA (ed): Dyspnea. Mount Kisco, NY, Futura Publishing, 1990, pp 75–126.
81. Mahler DA, Horowitz MB: Clinical evaluation of exertional dyspnea. In Weisman IM, Zeballos RJ (eds): Clinics in Chest Medicine. Philadelphia, WB Saunders, 1994:15, pp 259–269.
82. Mahler DA, Wells CK: Evaluation of clinical methods for rating dyspnea. Chest 93:580–586, 1988.
83. Manual on Exercise Testing: A Training Handbook, 3rd ed. Zavala DC. Iowa City, Press of the University of Iowa, 1993.
84. Marsh CB, Trudeau MD, Weiland JE: Recurrent asthma despite corticosteroid therapy in a 35-year-old woman. Chest 105:1855–1857, 1994.
85. Martin D, Powers S, Cicale M, et al: Validity of pulse oximetry during exercise in elite endurance athletes. J Appl Physiol 72:455–458, 1992.
86. McDowell I, Newell C: Measuring Health. A Guide to Rating Scales and Questionnaires, 2nd ed. New York, Oxford University Press, 1996.
87. McDowell JW, Thiede WH: Usefulness of the transcutaneous Po_2 monitor during exercise testing in adults. Chest 78:853–855, 1980.
88. Mengelkoch LJ, Martin D, Lawler J: A review of the principles of pulse oximetry and accuracy of pulse oximeter estimates during exercise. Phys Ther 74:40–49, 1994.
89. Morgan WK, Reger RB: Rise and fall of the FEV_1. Chest 118:1639–1644, 2000.
90. Moscato G, Gudnic-Cvar J, Maestelli P: Statement of self-monitoring of peak expiratory flows in the investigation of occupational asthma. Eur Respir J 8:1605–1610, 1995.
91. Neukirch F, Liard R, Segala C, et al: Peak expiratory flow variability and bronchial responsiveness to methacholine. An epidemiologic study in 117 workers. Am Rev Respir Dis 146:71–75, 1992.
92. Newman KB, Mason UG, Schmaling KB: Clinical features of vocal cord dysfunction. Am J Respir Crit Care Med 152:1382–1386, 1995.
93. O'Connor G, Sparrow D, Taylor D, et al: Analysis of dose–response curves to methacholine. An approach suitable for population studies. Am Rev Respir Dis 136:1412–1417, 1987.
94. Oren A, Sue DY, Hansen JE, et al: The role of exercise testing in impairment evaluation. Am Rev Respir Dis 135:230–235, 1987.
95. Ortega F, Montemayor T, Sanchez A, et al: Role of cardiopulmonary exercise testing and the criteria used to determine disability in patients with severe chronic obstructive pulmonary disease. Am J Respir Crit Care Med 150:747–751, 1994.
96. Ortiz FO, Aldrich TK, Nagel RL, et al: Accuracy of pulse oximetry in sickle cell disease. Am J Respir Crit Care Med 159:447–451, 1999.
97. Palmeiro EM, Hopp RJ, Biven RE, et al: Probability of asthma based on methacholine challenge. Chest 101:630–633, 1992.
98. Pattemore PK, Asher MI, Harrison AC, et al: The interrelationship among bronchial hyperresponsiveness, the diagnosis of asthma, and asthma symptoms. Am Rev Respir Dis 142:549–554, 1990.
99. Pearson MG, Bellamy D, Calverly PMA, et al: BTS guidelines for the management of chronic obstructive pulmonary disease. Thorax 52(Suppl.):s1–s28, 1997.
100. Pennock BE, Rogers RM, McCaffree DR: Changes in measured spirometric indices. What is significant? Chest 80:97–99, 1981.
101. Pepys J: Occupational asthma: An overview. J Occup Med 24:534–538, 1982.
102. Perpina M, Pellicer C, deDiego A, et al: Diagnostic value of the bronchial provocation test with methacholine in asthma. A Baysian analysis approach. Chest 104:149–154, 1993.
103. Pineda H, Haas F, Axen K, et al: Accuracy of pulmonary function tests in predicting exercise tolerance in chronic obstructive pulmonary disease. Chest 86:564–567, 1984.
104. Popa V, Singleton J: Provocation dose and discriminant analysis in histamine bronchoprovocation. Are the current predictive data satisfactory? Chest 94:466–475, 1988.
105. Pratter MR, Irwin RS: The clinical value of pharmacologic bronchoprovocation challenge. Chest 85:260–265, 1984.
106. Principles of Exercise Testing and Interpretation, 3rd ed: Wasserman K, Hansen JE, Sue DY, et al (eds). Philadelphia, Lippincott Williams & Wilkins, 1999.
107. Rampulla C, Baiocchi S, Dacosto E, et al: Dyspnea on exercise. Pathophysiologic mechanisms. Chest 101(Suppl.):248s–252s, 1992.

108. Redline S, Strohl KP: Recognition and consequences of obstructive sleep apnea hypopnea syndrome. In Strollo PJ, Sanders MH (eds): Clinics in Chest Medicine. Philadelphia, WB Saunders, 19:1–19, 1998.
109. Ries AL, Farrow JT, Clausen JL: Pulmonary function tests cannot predict exercise-induced hypoxemia in chronic obstructive pulmonary disease. Chest 93:454–459, 1988.
110. Rijcken B, Schouten JP, Weiss ST, et al: The distribution of bronchial responsiveness to histamine in symptomatic and in asymptomatic subjects. A population-based analysis of various indices of responsiveness. Am Rev Respir Dis 140:615–623, 1989.
111. Rockoff SD, Schwartz A: Roentgenographic underestimation of early asbestosis by International Labour Organization classification. Analysis of data and probabilities. Chest 93:1088–1091, 1988.
112. Schonfeld T, Sargent CW, Bautista D, et al: Transcutaneous oxygen monitoring during exercise stress testing. Am Rev Respir Dis 121:457–462, 1980.
113. Schwarz MI: Clinical overview of interstitial lung disease. In Schwarz MI, King TE (eds): Interstitial Lung Disease, 2nd ed. St Louis, Mosby Year Book, 1993, pp 1–22.
114. Shin C: Response to bronchodilators. In Mahler DA (ed): Clinics in Chest Medicine. Philadelphia, WB Saunders, 1989:10, pp 155–164.
115. Siafakas NM, Vermeire P, Pride NB, et al: Optimal assessment and management of chronic obstructive pulmonary disease (COPD). Eur Respir J 8:1398–1420, 1995.
116. Sim TC, McClean SP, Naranjo MS, et al: Functional laryngeal obstruction: A somatization disorder. Am J Med 88:293–295, 1990.
117. Social Security Administration, US Department of Health and Human Services: Disability Evaluation Under Social Security (Social Security Administration publication #64-039/ICN # 468600). Washington, DC, Social Security Administration, 1998.
118. Staples CA, Gamsu G, Ray CS, et al: High resolution computed tomography and lung function in asbestos-exposed workers with normal chest radiographs. Chest 139:1502–1508, pp 1989.
119. Strohl KP, Redline S: Recognition of obstructive sleep apnea. Am J Respir Crit Care Med 154:279–289, 1996.
120. Sue DY: Exercise testing in the evaluation of impairment and disability. In Weisman IM, Zeballos RJ (eds): Clinics in Chest Medicine. Philadelphia, WB Saunders, 1994:15, pp 369–387.
121. The International Clinical Respiratory Group: Assessment of therapeutic benefit in asthmatic patients. Chest 103:914–916, 1993.
122. Toren K, Brisman J, Jarvholm B: Asthma and asthma-like symptoms in adults assessed by questionnaires. A literature review. Chest 104:600–608, 1993.
123. Townley RG, Bewtra AK, Nair NM, et al: Methacholine inhalation challenge studies. J Allergy Clin Immunol 64:569–574, 1979.
124. Townsend MC: ACOEM position statement. Spirometry in the occupational setting. J Occup Environ Med 42:228–245, 2000.
125. Viner S, Szalai JP, Huffstein V: Are history and physical examinations a good screening test for sleep apnea? Ann Intern Med 115:356–359, 1991.
126. Violante B, Brusasco V, Buccheri G: Exercise testing in radiologically limited, simple pulmonary silicosis. Chest 90:411–415, 1986.
127. Volmer WM: Reconciling cross-sectional with longitudinal observations on annual decline. In Eisen EA (ed): Occupational Medicine: State of the Art Reviews. Philadelphia, Hanley & Belfus, 1993:8, pp 339–351.
128. Ware JH, Dockery DW, Louis TA, et al: Longitudinal and cross-sectional estimates of pulmonary function decline in never-smoking adults. Am J Epidemiol 132:685–700, 1990.
129. Wedzicha JA, Bestall JC, Garrod R, et al: Randomized controlled trial of pulmonary rehabilitation in severe chronic obstructive pulmonary disease patients, stratified with the MRC dyspnea scale. Eur Respir J 12:363–369, 1998.
130. Wiedemann HP, Gee BL, Balmes JR, et al: Exercise testing in occupational lung diseases. In Loke J (ed): Clinics in Chest Medicine. Philadelphia, WB Saunders, 1984:5, pp 157–171.
131. Wolkove N, Dajczman E, Colacone A, et al: The relationship between pulmonary function and dyspnea in obstructive lung disease. Chest 96:1247–1251, pp 1989.

CHAPTER

23

Cardiac Diagnostic Techniques

CHRISTOPHER T. BAJZER, MD, FACC

The presence of cardiac disease can impose functional limits on an individual. Cardiac disease can be divided into categories of coronary insufficiency, cardiac muscle dysfunction (both systolic and diastolic), cardiac valvular dysfunction, and cardiac arrhythmia. The severity of the functional limitations imposed by cardiac disease defines the severity of an individual's cardiac disability. Several tests are available to the physician to establish the diagnosis of cardiac disease and determine its severity for a given individual. The tests range from qualitative to semiquantitative to quantitative and vary in accuracy and reliability of determining the presence and severity of cardiac disease. The purpose of this chapter is to review the accuracy and reliability of selected tests used to assess cardiac disease. The accuracy and reliability of cardiac testing is directly reflected in the accuracy and reliability of the assessment of an individual's impairment or cardiac disability.

Diagnosis of Atherosclerotic Coronary Artery Disease and Assessment of Cardiac Ischemia

Exercise Electrocardiography

Exercise electrocardiography with blood pressure monitoring is a widely available and frequently utilized test to screen for the presence of coronary insufficiency. Exercise electrocardiography is performed at a relatively low cost in comparison to other screening tests for coronary disease. The type and pattern of exercise utilized for testing is widely variable to allow testing in individuals with preexisting, functional limitations. Historically, repetitive step climbing was used to perform exercise electrocardiography. Graded treadmill and leg or arm cycle ergometer devices are presently used for exercise electrocardiography. Graded treadmill is the most common means of performing exercise electrocardiography in the United States and this form of exercise has the largest body of reported literature on its usage. There are several prescribed exercise protocols for both exercise devices used to establish the uniformity and reproducibility of the results.[36] National guidelines on the use and performance of exercise electrocardiography exist to maximize the usefulness of the test in specific clinical situations.[12,14,33] The accuracy and reliability of exercise electrocardiography in diagnosing coronary insufficiency is dependent on the competence and experience of the professional and technical staff performing and interpreting the test, as well as on the compliance of the test subject with the prescribed exercise protocol.

As with any test, the diagnostic outcome of exercise electrocardiography is subject to Bayesian probability. The probability of a subject having coronary insufficiency is the product of the pretest probability of disease and the probability that the test provided a true result. Exercise electrocardiography is most valuable to the clinician in subjects with an intermediate pretest probability of having coronary insufficiency. The pretest probability of disease is conventionally determined clinically from variables acquired from a thorough history and physical examination of a subject. According to Bayes' theorem, the probability of coronary insufficiency in subjects with either low or high pretest probability is minimally altered by performing exercise electrocardiography.[14]

The ability of a test to discriminate between subjects with disease and those without disease can be described by using statistics (see Appendix A). All tests used in the diagnosis of coronary insufficiency and cardiac disease in general have some degree of overlap in the values of measured variables for subjects with disease and subjects without disease. Sensitivity is the measure of patients with disease who will have an abnormal test. Specificity is the measure of patients free from disease who will have a normal test. The measures of sensitivity and specificity are inversely related. The predictive value of a test is dependent on the prevalence of disease in the population tested. The positive predictive value is the percentage of individuals with an abnormal test result who have disease. The negative predictive value is the percentage of individuals with a normal rest result who do not have disease. A certain discriminating value in a measured variable determined by a test is used to separate the population tested into one group described as having disease and a second group described as not having disease. For example, defining 2 mm of ST segment depression as the discriminant value for determining the presence of coronary insufficiency has higher specificity and lower sensitivity compared with 1 mm ST segment depression.[14]

Meta-analyses of previous studies have been performed to evaluate the accuracy and reliability of exercise electrocardiography.[7,13] The meta-analyses revealed wide variability in both the sensitivity and specificity of exercise electrocardiography (Table 23–1). Meta-analysis of 24,074 patients who underwent both exercise electrocardiography and coronary angiography demonstrated a mean sensitivity of 68% (range 23% to 100%, standard deviation 16%) and a mean specificity of 77% (range 17% to 100%, standard deviation 17%). The sensitivity of exercise electrocardiography is generally less than the sensitivity of imaging procedures.[5,38] Classifying upward sloping ST segment depression as abnormal increases the sensitivity and decreases the specificity in exercise electrocardiography.[14,37,42]

Several comorbid conditions are known, based on pooled data, to have an adverse effect on the accuracy of exercise electrocardiography.[14] The presence of electrocardiographic findings of left ventricular hypertrophy results in a mean sensitivity of 68% and a mean specificity of 69% for exercise electrocardiography versus 72% and 77% in patients without such findings. Baseline ST segment depression on the resting electrocardiogram results in a mean sensitivity of 69% and a mean specificity of 70% for exercise electrocardiography compared with 67% and 84% in patients without resting ST segment depression. The presence of electrocardiographic findings of digitalis therapy results in a mean sensitivity of 68% and a mean specificity of 74% for exercise electrocardiography compared with 72% and 69% for patients without evidence of digitalis therapy on electrocardiogram.[14]

Other baseline electrocardiographic findings or use of certain medications exert effects on the accuracy of exercise electrocardiography. Beta blocker therapy does not affect the accuracy of exercise electrocardiography, but does decrease its diagnostic value by limiting a subject's ability to reach the target heart rate response. The use of nitroglycerin reduces the sensitivity of exercise electrocardiography. The presence of a right or left bundle branch block on resting electrocardiography significantly decreases the specificity of exercise electrocardiography. The use of computer analyses of ST segment depressions can increase the rate of false positive exercise electrocardiograms.[25]

The results of exercise electrocardiography help to define a subject's diagnosis and prognosis and monitor the effects of therapy. The simple determination of exercise capacity as expressed in metabolic equivalents (METs) or in duration of exercise is also a defining element of functional capacity and prognosis. One MET is equal to the amount of oxygen per minute consumed by the body at rest (1 MET = 3.5 millimeter oxygen/kilogram body weight/minute). The inability to achieve at least five METs during exercise electrocardiography after myocardial infarction is associated with a poor prognosis. In comparison, most occupational activities, including domestic chores, require less than five METs of energy expenditure.[14] Conversely, higher levels of physical fitness as determined by exercise capacity are associated with reduced risk of mortality post myocardial infarction and this provides a compelling argument for the utilization of cardiac rehabilitation post myocardial infarction. Risk scoring has been used to provide individual patients an estimate of survival based on larger population statistics. An example of a risk scoring system is the Duke nomogram, which provides an estimate of 5-year survival and average annual mortality as a function of the following: ST segment deviation during exercise, symptoms of ischemia during exercise, and maximal METs achieved.[45]

TABLE 23–1

Factors Affecting the Sensitivity and Specificity of Treadmill Electrocardiography

Factor	Sensitivity	Specificity
Nitroglycerine	↓	—
Beta-blocker	↓	↑
Digitalis	↓	↑
Left ventricular hypertrophy	↓	↓
Bundle branch block	↓	—

Exercise Stress Electrocardiography With Nuclear Imaging

Nuclear perfusion imaging is a useful adjunct to exercise electrocardiography in the detection of significant coronary artery disease. Nuclear perfusion imaging provides functional and physiologic information that is both quantifiable and reproducible. Perfusion imaging provides an assessment of the physiologic importance of suspected and known coronary artery disease. The information obtained from nuclear perfusion imaging also provides a basis for risk stratification among patients with chest pain syndromes or coronary artery disease.

Several techniques are currently employed to perform nuclear perfusion imaging. The quality and accuracy of the image output is a function of the patient's body habitus and compliance with protocol, the specific radiopharmaceutical employed, and the imaging equipment used to produce the raw data. The quality and accuracy of the interpretation of the test is a product of the quality and accuracy of the image output and the experience of the person interpreting the test. A detailed discussion of the equipment, radiopharmaceuticals, mechanics, and techniques used to perform nuclear perfusion imaging are beyond the scope of this chapter. The most prevalent types of nuclear perfusion imaging are planar thallium-201 imaging, single photon emission computerized tomographic (SPECT) thallium-201 imaging, and dual isotope imaging such as thallium-201 in combination with technecium-99m.

The sensitivity of both planar and SPECT perfusion imaging has repeatedly been reported in the 90% and greater range for the detection of coronary disease. However, the number of vessels that are diseased affects the sensitivity of perfusion imaging. Single vessel disease has a higher likelihood of producing a false negative scan result as compared to two- or three-vessel disease. False negative scans are potentially caused by the following: inadequate stress, the use of anti-ischemic medications, the presence of less than severe (< 70%) stenoses, the presence of collateral circulation or balanced ischemia, or problems with image quality or interpretation (Table 23–2). The following potentially cause false positive scans: attenuation defect owing to body habitus, the presence of anomalous coronary circulation, coronary vasospasm, conduction defects, or cardiomyopathy. The specificity of planar imaging has been reported to be greater than 80%. The specificity of SPECT imaging has been reported to be in the 60% to 80% range.[14,45,46]

TABLE 23–2
Potential Etiologies for Inaccurate Cardiac Stress Nuclear Perfusion Results

Increases False Positive Rate	Increases False Negative Rate
Attenuation (body habitus)	Inadequate stress
Anomalous coronary artery anatomy	Antianginal therapy
Vasospasm	<70% Stenosis
Conduction abnormality	Collateral circulation
Cardiomyopathy	Balanced ischemia
Poor image quality	Poor image quality

TABLE 23–3
Common Radioisotopes Utilized for Cardiac Nuclear Stress Testing

SPECT		PET	
Single Isotope	**Dual Isotope**	**Perfusion**	**Metabolic**
Tl201	Tl201 + Tc^{99m}	Rb82	F18
Tc99m		Cu62	C11
		N13	
		O15	

SPECT, single photon emission computed tomography; PET, positron emission tomography.

In general, the choice of a single radiopharmaceutical to perform a nuclear perfusion imaging test does not significantly affect the accuracy of the test. The exception to this general rule is the use of a positron emitting radiopharmaceutical for positron emission tomography (PET), which has been reported to improve accuracy of nuclear perfusion imaging by as much as 10% over standard SPECT imaging. The sensitivity and specificity of PET's ability to detect significant (>70% stenosis) coronary artery disease is 93% for both. The increase in accuracy is accomplished in part by the ability of PET imaging to make allowances for noncardiac sources of radioactivity (using subtraction techniques) that otherwise act as interference to the desired detection of cardiac source radioactivity. The radiopharmaceuticals rubidium-82, copper-62, nitrogen-13, and oxygen-15 are used for PET perfusion studies and fluorine-18 or carbon-11 for metabolic activity studies (Table 23–3).

PET perfusion studies are used to detect coronary artery disease. PET metabolic studies are used to differentiate infarcted myocardial tissue from severely ischemic and viable myocardium. The use of dual isotope imaging (e.g., thallium-201 and technetium-99m) SPECT will reduce the time needed to obtain images (as will multicrystal cameras and digitized detectors). Dual isotope imaging has been shown to be comparable to conventional SPECT imaging with sensitivities in the 90% range and specificity in the >75% range.[14,45]

Data obtained from nuclear perfusion imaging can be used as independent predictors of risk of future adverse clinical events (Table 23–4). For example, a patient with an uncomplicated myocardial infarction and a single fixed defect on thallium-201 imaging has a 6% cardiac event rate in 1 year. In the same study, a patient with an uncomplicated myocardial infarction and a reversible defect on thallium-201 imaging has a 51% cardiac event rate in 1 year. This is in contrast to a patient without a myocardial infarction and a normal thallium-201 imaging stress test who has less than a 1% cardiac event rate in 1 year. Other high-risk features in a perfusion scan include increased radiopharmaceutical uptake in the lung, transient left ven-

TABLE 23-4

Prognosis Based on Results of Tl201 Cardiac Testing After Myocardial Infarction

Tl201 Interpretation	Major Cardiac Event Rate/Year
Normal	<1%
Fixed defect	6%
Reversible defect	51%

TABLE 23-5

Sensitivity and Specificity Associated with the Assessment of Severe Ischemia with Viability

	Tl201 Reinjection	FDG PET	Tc^{99m} mibi
Sensitivity	86%	88%	81%
Specificity	47%	73%	60%

FDG, fluorodeoxyglucose; PET, positron emission tomography.

tricular cavity dilatation, and perfusion defects in more than one vascular distribution. In general, the greater the number of perfusion defects identified on nuclear perfusion imaging, the greater the incidence of morbidity and mortality in 1 year.[45]

Assessment of Myocardial Viability Using Nuclear Imaging

Myocardium that is dysfunctional owing to decreased perfusion and has the potential for recovery of function if perfusion is re-established is considered viable myocardium. Assessment of myocardial viability is useful in identifying patients both with and without apparent ischemia who are likely to have improvement in ventricular function if the supplying coronary vessel is revascularized by either surgical or percutaneous methods. PET nuclear imaging is considered the best means available for assessment of myocardial viability (Table 23–5). In a meta-analysis of 12 studies, the sensitivity of 18-fluorodexyglucose PET in identifying viable myocardium was 88% (range 71% to 100%) and the specificity was 73% (range 38% to 91%). Thallium-201 stress nuclear imaging with reinjection techniques is also used to assess for myocardial viability. This technique has a sensitivity of 86% (range 80% to 100%) and a specificity of 47% (range 38% to 80%). There is an 88% concordance rate between thallium-201 stress nuclear imaging with reinjection techniques and 18-fluorodexyglucose PET in identifying viable myocardium. Despite potential advantages of technecium-99m radiolabeled tracers in evaluating myocardial perfusion, it has inferior accuracy when used for detection of myocardial viability. The sensitivity of technecium-99m radiolabeled tracers is on average 81% (range 73% to 100%) with a specificity of 60% (range 35% to 86%).[14,45,46]

Stress Electrocardiography With Echocardiographic Imaging

Stress electrocardiography with echocardiographic imaging is an effective method for detecting the presence of hemodynamically significant coronary flow insufficiency commonly caused by atherosclerosis.[10] The stress modalities common in clinical use are exercise treadmill or bicycle, cardiac pacing, or pharmacologic agents such as dobutamine or arbutamine with atropine, dipyridamole, or adenosine. Stress echocardiography is based on the detection of new wall motion abnormalities or the deterioration of baseline wall motion abnormalities with stress. The normal response to stress as seen with echocardiography is a global increase in contractility with an improved ventricular ejection fraction owing to hyperdynamic wall motion. An abnormal response to stress on echocardiography is a global decrease in contractility or a deterioration or lack of improvement in segmental wall contraction. The prognosis for a patient with an intermediate pretest probability of coronary disease and a normal stress echocardiogram is a 1-year cardiac event (myocardial infarction, surgical or percutaneous revascularization, or death) rate in the range of 5% to 10%. The prognosis for a patient with an abnormal stress echocardiogram in 1-year is a cardiac event rate in the range of 26% to 50%.[21,39]

The interpretation of stress echocardiographic data is more subjective as compared to interpreting stress nuclear imaging data. It has been demonstrated that experienced readers have better interpretive accuracy compared to readers without experience. The learning curve for reader experience appears to be 100 studies. After proper instruction and supervised interpretation of 100 studies, the difference in accuracy between expert readers and less experienced readers is not significant.[31] As with other diagnostic testing, stress echocardiography is prone to false positive and false negative interpretive results (Table 23–6). Recognized causes of false negative stress echocardiogram results include single vessel coronary artery disease (sensitivity decreases with decreasing number of diseased vessels), moderate coronary stenosis (<60% diameter reduction), inadequate stress achieve (<85% maximal predicted heart rate), prolonged delay between time of maximum stress and imaging, obliteration of the ventricular cavity with stress, and poor image quality. Recognized causes of false positive stress echocardiogram results include the presence of abnormal septal motion (postoperative patients, bundle branch block, or septal hypertrophy), nonischemic cardiomyopathy and hypertensive response to exercise (both can develop wall motion abnormalities unrelated to coronary insufficiency), overinterpretation by the reader, and poor image quality.[23]

TABLE 23-6

Potential Etiologies for Inaccurate Cardiac Stress Echocardiogram Results

Increases False Positive Rate	Increases False Negative Rate
Abnormal septal motion	Single vessel disease
Bundle branch block	<60% Stenosis
Post open chest operation	Inadequate stress
Septal hypertrophy	Delayed stress imaging
Nonischemic cardiomyopathy	Ventricular cavity obliteration with stress
Hypertension	
Poor image quality	Poor image quality
Reader inexperience	Reader inexperience

TABLE 23-7

Comparison of Stress Echocardiogram and Stress Nuclear Perfusion Cardiac Testing

Test	Sensitivity	Specificity
Stress nuclear	>90%	60–80%
Stress echocardiogram	80–85%	85–90%
Inotrope stress echocardiogram	68–96%	80–85%
Vasodilator stress echocardiogram	40–91%	87–100%

Exercise echocardiography, compared with cardiac catheterization as the gold standard, has a sensitivity of 80% to 85% and a specificity of 85% to 90%. Stress echocardiography has, in general, comparable sensitivity and superior specificity compared to stress nuclear imaging (Table 23–7). Stress echocardiography is able to provide more information about cardiac structure and function than stress nuclear imaging. Stress nuclear imaging provides a quantitative assessment of perfusion abnormalities and allows for a more objective interpretation of data.[22] Dobutamine echocardiography has a sensitivity of 68% to 96% and a specificity of 80% to 85%. Arbutamine echocardiography has similar sensitivities and specificities.[1,34] Adenosine echocardiography has a sensitivity of 40% to 91% and a specificity of 87% to 100%. Dipyridamole echocardiography has a sensitivity of 52% to 92% and a specificity of 80% to 100%. The wide range of reported sensitivities and specificities reflects the qualitative nature of the test, the quality of the stress echocardiography laboratory, and the experience of the reader.[45]

Catheterization Laboratory Evaluation

Coronary arteriography is considered the reference standard for the assessment of luminal obstruction of coronary arteries. Using contemporary imaging equipment, coronary arteriography is limited in resolution to arteries greater than 0.2 mm in diameter. The finding of luminal narrowing on coronary arteriography, regardless of severity and in the absence of coronary vasospasm, almost uniformly correlates to atherosclerotic disease on pathologic study. Visual assessment of coronary stenoses has significant interobserver and intraobserver variability ranging from 7.5% to 50%.[3,11,24,40] This variability can be reduced, but not eliminated, by the use of either electronic calipers or computer based quantitative coronary angiography (QCA). Electronic calipers can reduce interobserver and intraobserver variability down to the range of 5.9% to 9%.[40] QCA uses videodensitometric edge detection algorithms and calibration methods to calculate coronary dimensions and report percent stenoses.[8] QCA provides the lowest interobserver and intraobserver variability in the range of 3.5% to 7.3%. QCA's determination of >50% stenosis has a positive predictive value of 79% for a positive dobutamine stress echocardiogram. Conversely, a QCA determination of >50% stenosis has a negative predictive value of 80% for a positive dobutamine stress echocardiogram.[2] Use of QCA to determine a minimal luminal diameter <1.0 mm has a positive predictive value of 81% and a negative predictive value of 90% for a positive dobutamine stress echocardiogram.[2]

Coronary arteriography has a high positive predictive value for the presence of atherosclerotic coronary artery disease when luminal narrowing is observed. However, the absence of luminal narrowing does not exclude the presence of clinically relevant atherosclerotic coronary artery disease. This is due to several factors that limit the accuracy of coronary arteriography to exclude disease. Examples of limiting factors include but are not limited to complex morphology of atherosclerotic plaques, vessels overlapping and constraints of imaging geometry, reference indexed sizing and quantification of coronary stenoses, and adaptive coronary remodeling.[40]

The use of digital technology to acquire, analyze, and display coronary angiographic images is rapidly becoming the norm in most catheterization laboratories. The adoption of the Digital Imaging and Communication (DICOM) standard insures compatibility of image handling among the manufacturers of image handling equipment for cardiac catheterization laboratories. Archiving digital images is often a problem for many high volume cardiac catheterization laboratories. Archiving digital images on either analog super video head system (VHS) tape or analog optical disk can result in up to 50% degradation of image quality. The use of various digital compression algorithms to store a coronary angiogram on media with limited digital capacity can result in image degradation to a degree dependent on the individual compression algorithm. The effect of this image degradation on clinical use is not known at present.

Intravascular ultrasound (IVUS) is both an adjunct and an alternative to coronary arteriography for invasive visualization of coronary anatomy. Coronary angiography is limited to the display of a silhouette of the coronary lumen in a two-dimensional projection. IVUS displays cross-sectional anatomy in two dimensions, with the ability to display three-dimensional topographic anatomy using tomographic constructions. The resolution of IVUS is dependent on the operating frequency of the ultrasound transducer. In general, IVUS has a resolution superior to coronary angiography. IVUS is considered the reference standard for precision measurement of arterial dimensions (i.e., luminal diameter and cross-sectional area). Unfortunately, IVUS is unable to visualize the entire coronary tree owing to limits on the ability to place the imaging transducer in small diameter arteries. The ability of IVUS to contrast different types of tissue based on echodensity and reflectance allows the detection of many structural features of coronary anatomy not detected by other imaging modalities. IVUS imaging is also limited by "shadowing" produced by the presence of calcification in the wall of diseased arteries.[40] Several imaging artifacts potentially limit the accuracy of IVUS imaging in the absence of corrective action. A mechanical rotating transducer can show cyclical oscillations in rotational speed, which produces nonuniform rotational distortion (NURD) in imaging. Transducer ring-down is a result of acoustic oscillations in the transducer material resulting in high amplitude signals that can distort near-field imaging. Geometric image distortion is produced when the transducer ultrasound beam interrogates the vessel in an oblique plane to the vessel wall. The reproducibility of ultrasound imaging can be unreliable owing to the inability to place the transducer in the exact same location on re-imaging.[40]

Fractional flow reserve (FFR) is the ratio of the mean pressure distal to a coronary stenosis to the mean pressure proximal to a coronary stenosis. Pressure data is measured with a pressure transducer and a fluid-filled coronary catheter or with a coronary guide-wire with a pressure transducer at its tip. The FFR is typically measured under the condition of maximal coronary vasodilatation as can be pharmacologically induced by either adenosine or papaverine. If the FFR falls below 0.75 there is 88% sensitivity and 84% specificity for predicting a subsequent abnormal exercise cardiac stress test.[6,32]

Coronary flow reserve (CFR) is the ratio of hyperemic coronary flow to basal coronary flow as assessed using a Doppler flow wire. The Doppler flow wire actually mea sures flow velocity rather than a volumetric flow rate. For all clinical purposes, coronary velocity reserve is equivalent to coronary flow reserve. Nondiseased coronary arteries have a CFR of 2.4 ± 0.7 and diseased coronary arteries have a CFR of 1.1 ± 0.2.[29] Several authors have set a discriminating threshold dividing diseased and nondiseased coronary arteries at 1.8.[27] A data comparison between CFR and diameter and area stenosis as determined by IVUS demonstrates that single tomographic IVUS data do not correlate well with the coronary physiologic response characterized by CFR. CFR and IVUS data have been used simultaneously to assess the relative contributions of agonist-mediated and flow-mediated coronary vessel responses.[18] CFR has been shown to be higher in patients with eccentric atherosclerotic lesions as compared to concentric lesions.[41] Nicotine or other substances in tobacco smoke have been demonstrated to have an adverse effect on CFR.[44] The physiologic data provided by measurements of CFR are complementary to anatomic data provided by IVUS.[27]

Coronary vasospasm (>50% reduction in coronary lumen) can occur with the clinical sequelae of myocardial ischemia with angina and potentially can progress to myocardial infarction. The diagnosis of coronary vasospasm is evident in a patient with a normal coronary angiogram and with ST segment elevation during episodes of anginal chest pain. The diagnosis of coronary vasospasm can be confirmed by pharmacologic provocation of vasospasm during coronary angiography evaluation (Table 23–8). Several pharmacologic agents have been used for intracoronary administration to provoke coronary vasospasm. Intracoronary administration of methylergonovine (5 to 10 microgram increments, not to exceed a total of 50 micrograms) is safe in select populations, and is reported to have a sensitivity ranging from 53% to 90% and specificity ranging from 88% to 100% for the detection of coronary vasospasm.[4,16,19] Intracoronary administration of acetylcholine (10 to 25 microgram increments, not to exceed 100 micrograms per dose per 5 minutes) is also safe in select populations and has a reported sensitivity ranging from 6% to 100% and specificity greater than 90%.[26,30] Intracoronary administration of nitroglycerin (100 to 200 micrograms per dose) or verapamil (100 to 200 micrograms per dose) can be used to reverse the coronary vasospasm and relieve angina that is a result of provocative testing.[40] A hyperventilation protocol is an effective provocative test for coronary vasospasm but is rarely used for coronary vasospasm in the patient population experiencing more than one daily episode of angina.[35] Current clinical practice often utilizes a therapeutic trial with a calcium channel blocker to arrive at a presumptive diagnosis of coronary vasospasm in patients with suspected coronary vasospasm. The use of a therapeutic trial often obviates the use of provocative testing.

TABLE 23–8
Intracoronary Administration of Provocative Agents to Detect Coronary Vasospasm

Agent	Sensitivity	Specificity
Methylergonovine	53–90%	88–100%
Acetylcholine	6–100%	>90%

Cardiac Valvular Dysfunction and Assessment of Circulatory Flow Impairment

Echocardiographic Assessment of Valvular Dysfunction

The use of echocardiography (two-dimensional, three-dimensional constructs, M-mode, and continuous wave, pulse wave, and color flow map Doppler methods) is, in general, considered the gold standard for assessment of cardiac valvular structure and function. Transthoracic and transesophageal echocardiography techniques are used in order to obtain the desired imaging data. Stenotic valve areas can be determined with planimetry using two-dimensional imaging. Other means of assessing the severity of valvular stenoses utilize physics equations such as the Bernoulli equation and the conservation of mass to derive valve areas. The accuracy of echocardiographic means of evaluating valvular stenoses is dependent upon two major factors: the hemodynamic loading conditions at the time of assessment and the quality of imaging data obtained. Any errors in precision in the input echocardiographic imaging data will be propagated and potentially magnified by the mathematical analysis. The assessment of valvular regurgitation is qualitative to semiquantitative. The most useful means of assessing valvular regurgitation is color flow mapped Doppler data. The imaging data are used to assign the degree of valvular regurgitation—a score based on a five-category index scale (0 = no regurgitation to 4 = severe regurgitation). Inaccuracies and variability in the assessment of valuable regurgitation are caused by hemodynamic loading conditions and the subjective assessment of the person interpreting the data. Characterizations of constrictive versus restrictive physiology is also possible with the use of Doppler data.[9,28]

Right Heart Catheterization in Evaluation of Valvular Dysfunction

Right heart catheterization with the placement of a pulmonary artery (Swan-Ganz) catheter is considered the gold standard for the determination of key clinically relevant hemodynamic data. Precise pressure measurements are made using an electronic pressure transducer. In the assessment of cardiac performance, either thermodilution or Fick methods can determine cardiac output. The thermodilution technique for determining cardiac output is dependent on the proper placement of the catheter and proper calibration of the pressure transducer. Right heart catheterization has good utility in the differentiation of shock states. Evaluation of the severity of mitral regurgitation, tricuspid regurgitation, and the presence or absence of cardiac tamponade can be made by analyzing the pressure waveform data available from the pulmonary artery catheter. Characterization of constrictive versus restrictive physiology is possible with pulmonary artery catheter data. Data collected from the performance of both left and right heart catheterization can closely characterize the severity of mitral and aortic stenosis using the Gorlin formula or one of its derivatives. The clinical data obtained from hemodynamic calculations have been validated in both in vitro and in vivo models.[43]

Cardiac Pump Failure and Assessment of Circulatory Flow Impairment

Echocardiographic Assessment of Myocardial Pump Function

Transthoracic and transesophageal echocardiography are both frequently used to assess both the global ejection fraction and segmental myocardial function. The left ventricular ejection fraction can be semiquantitatively assessed by extrapolation of two-dimensional data to three dimensions using some assumptions with regards to ventricular cavity geometry. These semiquantitative ejection fractions correlate well with assessments using gold standard nuclear imaging techniques ($r > 0.9$). Additional mathematical analysis of the data can provide an assessment of cardiac output. Such information has been found to have reasonable correlation to the same data derived from measurements taken during right heart catheterization. Recently marketed continuous bedside noninvasive hemodynamic monitoring devices take advantage of the application of physics equations to echocardiographic data in order to provide clinically relevant information. Echocardiography can also provide detailed information on segmental wall motion and wall thickening as additional assessments of ventricular function. In general, echocardiographic data on segmental wall function are equal to or superior to similar data that can be obtained using nuclear imaging. As with other echocardiographic imaging data, information on segmental wall function is highly dependent on image quality and the skill of the person interpreting the imaging data.[45]

Nuclear Imaging Assessment of Myocardial Pump Function

In addition to quantifying myocardial perfusion, radiopharmaceutical imaging can also be used to quantify cardiac pump performance. Techniques of radiopharmaceutical based assessment of ventricular function include first pass ventriculography and gated blood pool ventricular imaging. First pass ventriculography uses detection of the passage and ultimate distribution of a radiopharmaceutical (frequently technetium-99m) through the central circulation of the ventricle (commonly the right ventricle) after a rapid intravenous bolus administration to calculate a measure of ventricular ejection fraction. Gated blood-pool imaging or multigated acquisition (MUGA) uses electrocardiographic gating to analyze a series of images of the cardiac blood pool tagged with a radiopharmaceutical acquired in specific phases of the cardiac cycle. A MUGA derived ejection fraction is based on averaged volumes and is generally accepted as the gold standard for calculation of the ejection fraction. However, owing to volume averaging over many cardiac cycles, MUGA may be inferior to two-dimensional echocardiography for accuracy in the evaluation of regional wall motion. Perfusion imaging also provides data on regional myocardial wall motion. Perfusion imaging data with technetium-99m labeled tracers have sufficient count density to be able to evaluate regional wall motion when electrocardiographic gating is used. Electrocardiogram-gated perfusion imaging provides regional wall motion data that correlate well ($r > 0.9$) with echocardiography.[45,46]

Cardiac Arrhythmias and the Assessment of Syncope

Fixed period continuous electrocardiographic monitoring, otherwise known as Holter monitoring, is used primarily to detect the frequency, duration, and symptomatology of arrhythmias. Episodic electrocardiographic monitoring (loop recorder, event monitor) is used to detect arrhythmias that have a frequency of less than one episode every 48 hours and can be external or a component of an implantable device. Holter monitoring is one of the most commonly utilized tests in the evaluation of syncope or near-syncope. The duration of Holter monitoring correlates with the negative predictive value of the test. Holter monitoring for 48 hours is a useful balance between the practicalities of monitoring and maximizing the negative predictive value. Only 2% to 4% of patients with symptoms of syncope or near-syncope have an arrhythmia detected on Holter monitoring that correlates with symptoms. A normal Holter monitor in the presence of symptoms effectively eliminates an arrhythmia as the etiology for symptoms.[15] The sensitivity and specificity of Holter monitoring in the evaluation of syncope are not known owing to the lack of a gold standard that is independent of arrhythmia detected by monitoring.[45] Holter monitoring is useful in the identification of both atrial and ventricular arrhythmias. However, the combination of the presence of coronary disease, a left ventricular ejection fraction less than 30%, and syncope has a better positive predictive value for detection of inducible sustained ventricular tachycardia compared with Holter monitoring.

Holter monitoring can be used to detect coronary disease using ST segment analysis. In one study, Holter monitoring in patients with fixed threshold angina had a diagnostic accuracy of 80%, equal to that of bicycle stress electrocardiography, for predicting the presence of coronary artery disease by angiography. In the same study, Holter monitoring was superior to bicycle stress electrocardiography in the accuracy (68% versus 55%) of predicting the presence of coronary artery disease by angiography.[17]

Invasive electrophysiologic testing is indicated in the diagnosis and treatment of ventricular tachyarrhythmias, suspected cardiac syncope, and the investigation and treatment of late potentials on signal averaged electrocardiogram or impaired left ventricular function. The sensitivity and specificity of sustained monomorphic ventricular tachycardia is greater than 90% as compared with findings on Holter monitoring. The sensitivity of a prolonged sinus node recovery time (indicating sino-atrial node dysfunction) is low at 69% and the specificity is reported as high as 100% compared with Holter monitoring.[45]

The etiology for a single episode of syncope or recurrent syncope remains unknown for 50% or more of patients who experience these symptoms despite the best scrutiny. Neurocardiogenic (or vasovagal) syncope is thought to be the cause for up to 40% of the cases of syncope depending on the age range of the population studied. Heads-up tilt table testing is an accepted means of providing supporting evidence to implicate a suspected neurocardiogenic etiology of syncope. In general, patients without a history suggestive of neurocardiogenic syncope should not undergo heads-up tilt table testing. As with any diagnostic test, the indiscriminant use of heads-up tilt table testing will have a low diagnostic yield and is cost ineffective. Heads-up tilt table testing, performed at tilts of 60 to 70 degrees without pharmacologic provocation, has a sensitivity of 32% to 85% and a specificity of 80% to 90%. The addition of an isoproterenol will increase the sensitivity with a decreased specificity. The reproducibility of heads-up tilt table testing is in the range of 65% to 85%.[20,45]

Conclusion

Many diagnostic tests are available to the physician to both establish a diagnosis and provide a prognosis for a number of cardiac disease entities. The incidence and prevalence of a specific cardiac disease entity varies according to the population of interest. This corresponds to variation in the sensitivity, specificity, positive and negative predictive values, and overall accuracy of a particular diagnostic test in providing needed clinical data. The severity of the clinical impact of a particular cardiac disease entity, otherwise known as cardiac impairment, varies according to the severity of the disease process as it affects an individual. The ability to define cardiac impairment in an individual is subject to

TABLE 23-9

Fractional Impairment due to Cardiac Disability

1 → 20%	21 → 40%	41 → 60%	61 → 80%	81 → 100%
Criteria	Criteria	Criteria	Criteria	Criteria
1	1	1	1	1
|	|	|	|	|
n	n	n	n	n

the serial variations in the precision of cardiac diagnostic testing, and the variation in the impact of a disease entity on a specific individual. Knowledge of the various precisions of cardiac diagnostic tests can be correlated, in part, to the precision of a clinician's assessment of cardiac impairment.

Cardiac impairment, as it applies to a specific individual, is a point on a continuum that varies over time. Attempts to quantify the severity of cardiac impairment in an individual have resulted in the formation of impairment classification schema that categorizes the continuous spectrum of cardiac impairments into discrete quartiles or quintiles. These discrete categories are defined by assigning them a sequential range of fractional impairment (Table 23–9) of the whole persons. The specific criteria that are used by specific outcomes of specific cardiac diagnostic testing. The validity and accuracy of the results of a specific cardiac diagnostic test gains importance in the greater scheme of defining cardiac disability. Knowledge of the accuracy and limitations of cardiac testing remains important to the assessment of cardiac impairment and disability (see Chapters 26 and 60).

References

1. Afridi I, Quinones M, Zoghbi W: Dobutamine stress echocardiography: Sensitivity, specificity, and predictive value for future cardiac events. Am Heart J 127:1510–1515, 1994.
2. Baptista J, Arnese M, Roelandt J: Quantitative coronary angiography in the estimation of the functional significance of coronary stenosis: Correlations with dobutamine-atropine stress test. J Am Coll Cardiol 23:1434–1439, 1994.
3. Beauman G, Vogel R: Accuracy of individual and panel visual interpretations of coronary arteriograms: Implications for clinical decisions. J Am Coll Cardiol 16:108–113, 1990.
4. Bertrand M, Rousseau M, Lablanche J, et al: [Detection of coronary artery spasm by the methylergometrin test. Technic. Results. Indications]. Arch Mal Coeur Vaiss 72:123–129, 1979.
5. Cheitlin M, Alpert J, Armstrong W, et al: ACC/AHA guidelines for the clinical application of echocardiography: executive summary. A report of the American College of Cardiology/American Heart Association Task Force on Practice Guidelines (Committee on Clinical Application of Echocardiography). J Am Coll Cardiol 29:862–879, 1997.
6. De Bruyne B, Baudhuin T, Melin J: Coronary flow reserve calculated from pressure measurements in humans: Validation with positron emission tomography. Circulation 89:1013–1022, 1994.
7. Detrano R, Froelicher V, Gianrossi R: The diagnostic accuracy of the exercise electrocardiogram: A meta-analysis of 22 years of research. Prog Cardiovasc Dis 32:173–206, 1989.
8. Escaned J, Foley D, Haase J: Quantitative angiography during coronary angioplasty with a single angiographic view: A comparison of automated edge detection and videodensitometric techniques. Am Heart J 126:1326–1333, 1993.
9. Feigenbaum H: Echocardiography. Philadelphia, Lea & Febiger, 1993.
10. Feigenbaum H: Exercise echocardiography. J Am Soc Echocardiography 1:161–166, 1988.
11. Fisher L, Judkins M, Lesperance J: Reproducibility of coronary arteriographic reading in the coronary artery surgery study (CASS). Cathet Cardiovasc Diagn 8:565–575, 1982.
12. Fletcher G, Balady G, Froelicher V, et al: Exercise standards: A statement for healthcare professionals from the American Heart Association writing group. Special report. Circulation 91:580–615, 1995.
13. Gianrossi R, Mulvihill D, Detrano R, et al: Exercise-induced ST depression in the diagnosis of coronary artery disease: A meta-analysis. Circulation 80:87–98, 1989.
14. Gibbons R, Balady G, Beasley J, et al: ACC/AHA Guidelines for Exercise Testing: A report of the American College of Cardiology/American Heart Association Task Force on Practice Guidelines (Committee on Exercise Testing). J Am Coll Cardiol 30:260–315, 1997.
15. Gibson T, Heitzman M: Diagnostic efficacy of 24-hour electrocardiographic monitoring for syncope. Am J Cardiol 53:1013–1017, 1984.
16. Hackett D, Larkin S, Chierchia S, et al: Induction of coronary artery spasm by a direct local action of ergonovine. Circulation 75:577–582, 1987.
17. Hoberg E, Kunze B, Rausch S, et al: Diagnostic value of ambulatory Holter monitoring for the detection of coronary artery disease in patients with variable threshold angina pectoris. Am J Cardiol 65:1078–1083, 1990.
18. Hollenberg S, Tamburro P, Johnson M, et al: Simultaneous intracoronary ultrasound and Doppler flow studies distinguish flow-mediated from receptor-mediated endothelial responses. Cathet Cardiovasc Intervent 46:282–288, 1999.
19. Igarashi Y, Yamazoe M, Shibata A: Effect of direct intracoronary administration of methylergonovine in patients with and without variant angina. Am Heart J 21:1094–1100, 1991.
20. Kapoor W, Smith M, Miller N: Upright tilt testing in evaluating syncope: A comprehensive literature review. Am J Med 97:78–88, 1994.
21. Krivokapich J, Child J, Gerber R: Prognostic usefulness of positive or negative exercise stress echocardiography for predicting coronary events in ensuing twelve months. Am J Cardiol 71:646–651, 1993.
22. Marwick T, Brunken R, Meland N: Accuracy and feasibility of contrast echocardiography for detection of perfusion defects in routine practice: Comparison with wall motion and technetium-99m sestamibi single-photon emission computed tomography. J Am Coll Cardiol 32:1260–1269, 1998.
23. Marwick T, Nemec J, Pashkow F: Accuracy and limitations of exercise echocardiography in a routine clinical setting. J Am Coll Cardiol 19:74–81, 1992.
24. Meier B, Gruentzig A, Goebel N, et al: Assessment of stenoses in coronary angioplasty: Inter- and intraobserver variability. Int J Cardiol 3:159–169, 1983.
25. Milliken J, Abdollah H, Burggraf G: False-positive treadmill exercise tests due to computer signal averaging. Am J Cardiol 65:946–948, 1990.
26. Miwa K, Fujita M, Ejiri M, Sasayama S: Comparative sensitivity of intracoronary injection of acetylcholine for the induction of coronary spasm in patients with various types of angina pectoris. Circ Res 66:18–27, 1990.

27. Moses J, Undermir C, Strain J, et al: Relation between single tomographic intravascular ultrasound image parameters and intracoronary Doppler flow velocity in patients with intermediately severe coronary stenoses. Am Heart J 135:988–994, 1998.
28. Nishimura R, Tajik A: Quantitative hemodynamics by Doppler echocardiography: A noninvasive alternative to cardiac catheterization. Prog Cardiovasc Dis 36:309–342, 1994.
29. Ofili E, Labovitz A, Kern M: Coronary flow velocity dynamics in normal and diseased arteries. Am J Cardiol 71:3D–9D, 1993.
30. Okumura K, Yasue H, Matsuyama K, et al: Sensitivity and specificity of intracoronary injection of acetylcholine for the induction of coronary artery spasm. J Am Coll Cardiol 12:883–888, 1988.
31. Picano E, Lattanzi F, Orlandini A: Stress echocardiography and the human factor: The importance of being expert. J Am Coll Cardiol 17:666–669, 1991.
32. Pijls N, Van Gelder B, Van der Voort P: Fractional flow reserve: A useful index to evaluate the influence of an epicardial coronary stenosis on myocardial blood flow. Circulation 92:3183–3193, 1995.
33. Pina I, Balady G, Hanson P, et al: Guidelines for clinical exercise testing laboratories: A statement for healthcare professionals from the Committee on Exercise And Cardiac Rehabilitation, American Heart Association. Circulation 91:912–921, 1995.
34. Poldermans D, Fioretti P, Boersma E: Dobutamine-atropine stress echocardiography and clinical data for predicting late cardiac events in patients with suspected coronary artery disease. Am J Med 97:119–125, 1994.
35. Previtali M, Ardissino D, Storti C, et al: Hyperventilation and ergonovine tests in Prinzmetal's variant angina: Comparative sensitivity and relation with the activity of the disease. Eur Heart J 10:F101–F104, 1989.
36. Reid M, Lachs M, Feinstein A: Use of methodological standards in diagnostic test research: Getting better but still not good. JAMA 274:645–651, 1995.
37. Rijneke R, Ascoop C, Talmon J: Clinical significance of upsloping ST segments in exercise electrocardiography. Circulation 61:671–678, 1980.
38. Ritchie J, Bateman T, Bonow R, et al: Guidelines for clinical use of cardiac radionuclide imaging: Report of the American College of Cardiology/American Heart Association Task Force on Assessment of Diagnostic and Therapeutic Cardiovascular Procedures (Committee on Radionuclide Imaging), developed in collaboration with the American Society of Nuclear Cardiology. J Am Coll Cardiol 25:521–527, 1995.
39. Sawada S, Ryan T, Conley M: Prognostic value of a normal exercise echocardiogram. Am Heart J 120:49–55, 1990.
40. Scanlon P, Faxon D, Audet A, et al: ACC/AHA guidelines for coronary angiography: A report of the American College of Cardiology/American Heart Association Task Force on Practice Guidelines (Committee on Coronary Angiography). J Am Coll Cardiol 33:1756–1824, 1999.
41. Schwarzacher S, Uren N, Ward M, et al: Determinants of coronary remodeling in transplant coronary disease: A simultaneous intravascular ultrasound and Doppler flow study. Circulation 101:1384–1389, 2000.
42. Stuart R, Ellestad M: Upsloping S-T segments in exercise stress testing: Six-year follow-up study of 438 patients and correlation with 248 angiograms. Am J Cardiol 37:19–22, 1976.
43. Swan H, Ganz W, Forrester J: Catheterization of the heart in man with use of a flow-directed balloon-tipped catheter. N Engl J Med 283:447–451, 1970.
44. Tanaka T, Oka Y, Tawara I, et al: Acute effects of nicotine content in cigarettes on coronary flow velocity and coronary flow reserve in men. Am J Cardiol 82:1275–1278, 1998.
45. Topol E, Marso S, Griffin B: Manual of Cardiovascular Medicine. Philadelphia, Lippincott Williams & Wilkins, 2000:836.
46. Zaret B, Wackers F: Nuclear cardiology. N Engl J Med 12:385–389, 1994.

CHAPTER

24

The Integrated Cardiopulmonary Exercise Stress Test

JAMES E. HANSEN, MD, FACP, FCCP ■ KARLMAN WASSERMAN, MD, PhD

The objective of this chapter is to inform physicians who evaluate individuals for impairment and disability about the importance, value, indications, economy, and safety of integrated cardiopulmonary exercise testing using gas exchange measurements. The authors briefly review the basic physiology of exercise to show why measures of O_2 uptake ($\dot{V}O_2$) and CO_2 output ($\dot{V}CO_2$) provide important data for an informed assessment of work capacity. The authors also review how exercise testing equipment, methods, measures, and protocols can be used to clarify how they discriminate among diseases involving the respiratory, circulatory, and musculoskeletal systems. Such testing assists in identifying the dominant disorder when multiple disorders coexist, and helps exclude or quantitate impairment. Further reading[5,66,72] and training are required before testing patients.

Essentials of Exercise Physiology

Bioenergetics of Muscle Contraction

In brief, muscle contraction and relaxation depend upon the immediate availability of high-energy phosphates in the form of adenosine triphosphate (ATP) and creatine phosphate (CP).[45] At the start of exercise there are ample stores of ATP, CP, and O_2 in the muscle. In the muscle cell mitochondria, O_2 is utilized to regenerate ATP in the energy-yielding electron-transport process, keeping the level of ATP relatively constant while the CP decreases in proportion to the work rate, and CO_2 and water are produced predominantly in the tricarboxylic acid cycle.[41] If exercise continues, cellular respiration (CO_2 production and O_2 consumption) continues at a rate proportional to the power output and substrate respiratory quotient (RQ).[66]

Coupling of External Exchange With the Atmosphere to Cellular Respiration

As depicted in Figure 24–1, the delivery of O_2 to the muscle and removal of CO_2 from the muscle depends on several processes: the effectiveness of the heart and blood in transporting O_2 and CO_2, the ability of the peripheral and pulmonary circulations to exchange O_2 and CO_2 at the muscle and pulmonary capillaries, and the effectiveness of the lungs and ventilatory apparatus in transporting O_2 and CO_2 from and to the atmosphere.[62]

The Mechanism and Consequences of Exercise Lactic Acidosis

If O_2 delivery to the exercising muscles is adequate, the catabolism of glycogen or glucose, fatty acid, ethanol, or (rarely) amino acids through the tricarboxylic acid cycle and O_2 transport chain results in the production of H_2O and CO_2 plus large amounts of ATP (36 ATP from six molecules of O_2 and one molecule of glucose).[41] When adequate O_2 is not delivered to the cell, there is a major decrease in the efficiency of production of ATP (i.e., one molecule of glucose produces only two ATP molecules). This is accompanied by the obligate conversion of two molecules of pyruvate to two molecules of lactate with two accompanying hydrogen ions.[41]

When metabolism is partially anaerobic, the lactic acid produced must be immediately buffered in the cells because its pH is 3.9 whereas the cell pH is about 7.0. The hydrogen ion reacts immediately with the bicarbonate, resulting in the immediate production of carbonic acid, which dissociates into water and CO_2.[63] This CO_2 can be considered "excess" because it did not come directly from aerobic metabolism. On a molar basis, the decrease in bicarbonate approximately equals the increase in lactate; 22 mL of CO_2 are produced for each mEq of lactate formed (Fig. 24–2).[66] With mild anaerobiasis, the normal respiratory tract eliminates this excess CO_2 promptly. With increasing anaerobiasis and lactic acid production, the blood becomes more acid and ventilation is further stimulated, thereby enhancing CO_2 output. This decreases the alveolar P_{CO_2} (P_{ACO_2}) and arterial P_{CO_2} (P_{aCO_2}) in those who are not limited in ventilatory capability.[70] While anaerobiasis in some muscular sites produces lactate from pyruvate, lactate can be concurrently reconverted to pyruvate in other body sites where oxygenation is adequate.[68]

Fuel Utilization and the RQ

The ratio of CO_2 production to the O_2 consumption at the cellular level is identified as the RQ and is partially dependent on the substrate metabolized.[20] The metabolism of 1 gram of fatty acid yields 9 kcal of energy: for each 4.7 kcal of energy, approximately 1.0 L of O_2 is used and 0.7 L of CO_2 is produced ($\dot{V}CO_2/\dot{V}O_2$ or RQ = 0.7 for fat). The metabolism of 1 gram of carbohydrate yields 4 kcal of energy: for each 5.1 kcal of energy, approximately 1 L of O_2 is used and 1 L of CO_2 is produced ($\dot{V}CO_2/\dot{V}O_2$ or RQ = 1.0 for carbohydrate). Because of the small differences in O_2 requirements per liter of O_2 (4.7 kcal versus 5.1 kcal) and the fact that a mixture of substrates is usually utilized, energy requirements expressed as kcal/L O_2 are relatively insensitive to the dietary source. Thus $\dot{V}O_2$ has a high correlation with power output during aerobic work. The respiratory exchange ratio (RER or R), which is the instantaneous ratio of $\dot{V}CO_2/\dot{V}O_2$, needs to be contrasted with the RQ. The R is dependent not only on the RQ, but also on transient hyperventilation or hypoventilation or changes in body stores of O_2 and CO_2.

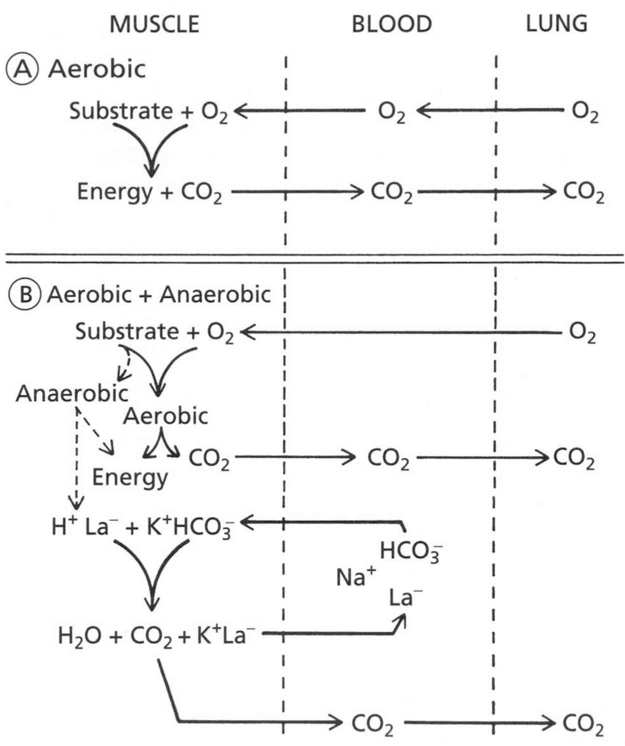

Figure 24–2. Gas exchange during aerobic (A) and aerobic plus anaerobic (B) exercise. In the former situation, O_2 is used and CO_2 is produced in approximately equal volumes. In the latter situation, cell lactic acid is produced, which must be immediately buffered at the pH of cell water, primarily by bicarbonate. The buffering reaction increases CO_2 production by 22 mL for each mEq of bicarbonate buffering lactic acid. This excess CO_2 must be eliminated through the lungs. (From Wasserman K, Hansen JE, Sue DY, et al: Principles of Exercise Testing and Interpretation, 2nd ed. Philadelphia, Lea & Febiger, 1994, with permission.)

Metabolic Requirements to Perform Work: Effects of Body Size, Work Efficiency, and Work Intensity

Total metabolic requirements depend on body size and the external work performed, which are directly related to kcal or $\dot{V}O_2$ measurements. Resting metabolism increases with body size, fever, and many illnesses. Although the ease or difficulty of performing an external task depends in part on the intelligence, skill, and

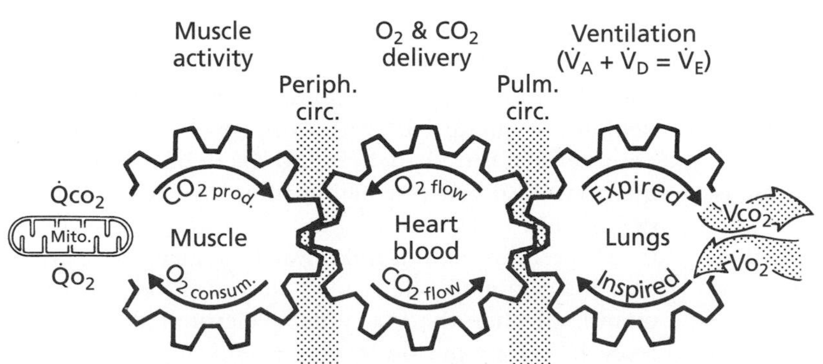

Figure 24–1. Schematic representation of O_2 and CO_2 transport between atmospheric air and muscle mitochondria during exercise. External and internal (cellular) respiration are linked through the circulatory system. (From Wasserman K: Breathing during exercise. N Engl J Med 298:780, 1978, with permission.)

agility of the worker, its metabolic requirement is primarily based on the action of the musculoskeletal system in overcoming resistance and gravity.[5]

Work efficiency, however, is reasonably similar for all persons. It is defined as the $\dot{V}O_2$ required to perform external work above the $\dot{V}O_2$ cost of moving the body without external load.[74] Several studies have shown that below the lactic acidosis threshold (LAT) the $\dot{V}O_2$ requirement to perform 1 W of external cycling work (after subtracting the $\dot{V}O_2$ of unloaded cycling at the same frequency) is 10 ± 1 mL of O_2 per minute, regardless of age, sex, or body size.[30,31,69]

The ability of the musculoskeletal system to perform work depends on the ability of the circulatory and respiratory systems to transport O_2 from the atmosphere to the working muscles and remove CO_2 and lactic acid from them, as work is rarely limited by the availability of water, carbohydrate, or fatty acids.[66] The ability to increase $\dot{V}O_2$ also depends on the quantity of muscle involved in the task performed; the more muscle involved the higher the possible $\dot{V}O_2$. For example, the peak $\dot{V}O_2$ is less for arm cycling than for leg cycling because of the greater muscle mass in the legs than in the arms. It is still higher for treadmill walking or running or other exercise that combines the use of both arms and legs.[66] The ambulatory peak $\dot{V}O_2$ for normal, sedentary, middle-aged adults is about 10 times that at rest.

The amount of work that an individual is capable of performing depends on the relative ease of increasing the $\dot{V}O_2$ compared to the $\dot{V}O_2$ required to perform that task and the task duration.

For the approximate relationships among activity, metabolic rate (expressed as $\dot{V}O_2$ in L/min), and work intensity (from minimal to extreme) in several individuals differing in body size and health,[1,5,10,20] the key points are as follows:

1. For a given age, sex, and height, the peak $\dot{V}O_2$ usually depends on the capability of the weakest link in the cardiovascular, respiratory, and musculoskeletal systems of the individual.
2. Individuals differ little in work efficiency, once the differences between individual metabolic requirements to perform activity without an external load and the learned ability to perform motor skills are accounted for.
3. Despite similar work efficiency, the energy (and $\dot{V}O_2$) requirements for a given task are higher in larger individuals, especially when movement of the body or large body parts are involved, because they must use more energy to move a larger mass. Tasks that require lifting the person's body weight, as in climbing (rather than just moving the legs, as in cycling), cause even greater differences in the $\dot{V}O_2$ requirements between smaller and larger individuals.
4. The intensity of a task increases as the ratio of the task $\dot{V}O_2$ to the individual's peak $\dot{V}O_2$ approaches 1.0.
5. Tasks of very heavy intensity can be performed for only brief periods.

The Steady State, Gas Exchange Kinetics, O_2 Deficit, and O_2 Debt

A person can be considered to be in a "steady state" when metabolism is constant. In such a state variables such as heart rate (HR), blood pressure, expired ventilation ($\dot{V}E$), $\dot{V}O_2$, $\dot{V}CO_2$, and blood chemistry also remain constant, and the metabolic rate ($\dot{V}O_2$) can be maintained indefinitely. During this state the work task is being performed without anaerobic metabolism or increasing O_2 debt, and there is no lactic acidosis (i.e., the work rate is below the subject's LAT).[66] Commonly, work tasks fluctuate, so the above variables change with time delays related to changes in the body stores of O_2, CO_2, ATP, and CP. Figure 24–3 shows the changes in $\dot{V}O_2$, $\dot{V}CO_2$, R (respiratory exchange ratio or $\dot{V}CO_2/\dot{V}O_2$), and $\dot{V}E$ in a normal person during a 12-minute test: rest for 2 minutes, loaded cycling at a work rate of 100 W, and a recovery period of 4 minutes. During exercise a steady state is reached well before 6 minutes with a $\dot{V}O_2$ of 1.50 L/min. After the onset of exercise, $\dot{V}O_2$, $\dot{V}CO_2$, $\dot{V}E$, and HR abruptly rise, with the $\dot{V}O_2$ increasing more rapidly than the $\dot{V}CO_2$, which in turn increases more rapidly than the $\dot{V}E$.[15,18] The $\dot{V}O_2$ reaches a plateau by 3 minutes and the $\dot{V}CO_2$ and the $\dot{V}E$ reach a plateau by 4 minutes.

The mean response time (MRT) (the time to reach 63% of the way between the original and new steady state) is used as a measure of the response kinetics for each variable. It assumes a first order (single exponential) response from the start of exercise despite the fact that the response may have several components that distort the response curve from that of a single exponential function.[66]

The terms O_2 deficit and O_2 debt (Fig. 24–3) identify the differences in O_2 volume consumed and O_2 volume required at the onset and offset of exercise, respectively.[5,73] The O_2 deficit is the difference between the $\dot{V}O_2$ metabolically required to perform the work rate and the actual $\dot{V}O_2$ during this time. The O_2 debt is the quantity or volume of $\dot{V}O_2$ during recovery in excess of that required during rest (i.e., the amount that was repaid to replete body O_2 stores and regenerate ATP and CP). In the example shown, both O_2 deficit and O_2 debt approximate 1 L. With exercise of mild to moderate intensity, the O_2 deficit and O_2 debt are similar in quantity. With heavy or higher intensity exercise, the O_2 deficit may not be quantified accurately because the true O_2 requirement is unknown (a plateau in $\dot{V}O_2$ is not reached); the O_2 debt also may not be accurately quantified when the $\dot{V}O_2$ remains elevated above resting levels for a long period (even hours).[5]

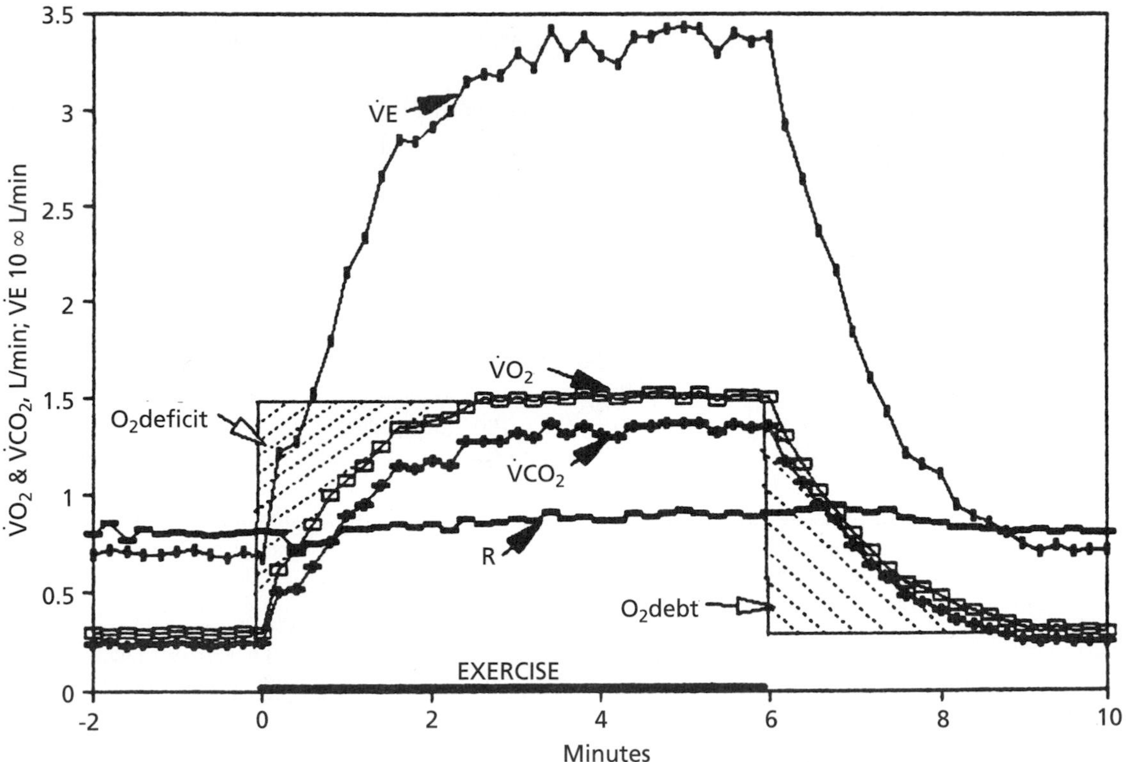

Figure 24–3. Gas exchange values for 6 minutes of exercise on a cycle ergometer at 100 W in a healthy subject. O_2 uptake ($\dot{V}O_2$), CO_2 output ($\dot{V}CO_2$), minute ventilation ($\dot{V}E$), and respiratory exchange ratio (R) values are plotted. The exercise is preceded by 2 minutes of rest and followed by 4 minutes of recovery. Note the more rapid rise in $\dot{V}O_2$ than in $\dot{V}CO_2$ or $\dot{V}E$, the decline in R immediately after the onset of exercise (due to the increasing stores of CO_2 in the body), and the plateau of these values after 3 minutes of exercise. The latter indicates that the work rate is below the lactic acidosis threshold of the subject and that a steady state has been reached. The O_2 deficit and O_2 debt (crosshatched areas) are equal in size. (From Hansen JE, Tierney DF [eds]: Current Pulmonology, Vol 14. St. Louis, Mosby-Year Book, 1993, p 43, with permission.)

Responses to Constant Work of Differing Intensities

Figure 24–4 shows the changes in the $\dot{V}O_2$, the $\dot{V}CO_2$, and the $\dot{V}E$ from unloaded cycling to loaded cycling at seven exercise levels from mild to very heavy.[15] At the four lower work rates (29, 59, 88, and 117 W) this person could work for several hours without resting, if needed, because the work is supported completely by atmospheric O_2. At the three higher work rates (146, 176, and 205 W) this person cannot support the work rate totally by aerobic sources. This exercise is above the anaerobic threshold (AT) or LAT (lactic acidosis develops at the $\dot{V}O_2$ above which metabolism cannot be fully supported aerobically for a long period of time. This is referred to as the LAT. It is also referred to as the AT, because the lactic acidosis develops when anaerobic energy-producing mechanisms supplement the aerobic energy-producing mechanisms. These terms, therefore, identify the same $\dot{V}O_2$ [i.e., they are equivalent]). Blood lactate levels, $\dot{V}E$, HR, and blood pressure also continue to rise during work levels above the LAT. Work rates higher than 205 W cannot be sustained for even 6 minutes.

At work rates above the LAT, many variables demonstrate characteristic changes. The $\dot{V}CO_2$ exceeds the $\dot{V}O_2$ owing to the production of excess CO_2 resulting from the dissociation of bicarbonate as it buffers the intracellularly accumulating lactic acid.[64,65] Initially the ventilatory response is isocapnic (i.e., the $PaCO_2$ remains relatively constant) as the $\dot{V}E$ is tightly linked to the $\dot{V}CO_2$.[71] As exercise continues so that lactic acid accumulation increases, the arterial bicarbonate and pH decrease. The latter stimulates the carotid body chemoreceptors to increase ventilation even more than that predicted from the CO_2 load to the lung. The disproportionate decrease in $PACO_2$ and $PaCO_2$ minimizes the decrease in blood pH. The disproportionate increase in the $\dot{V}E$ to the $\dot{V}O_2$ raises the alveolar PO_2 (PAO_2).[50] Thus, despite an increase in the difference between PAO_2 and PaO_2 ([P(A–a)O_2]) commonly found with very heavy exercise in normal persons, the PaO_2 does not usually decrease below resting levels.[32] Except for occasional elite athletes with high cardiac outputs and high tolerance for discomfort, the arterial oxygen saturation (SaO_2) rarely declines with exercise in normal persons.[23]

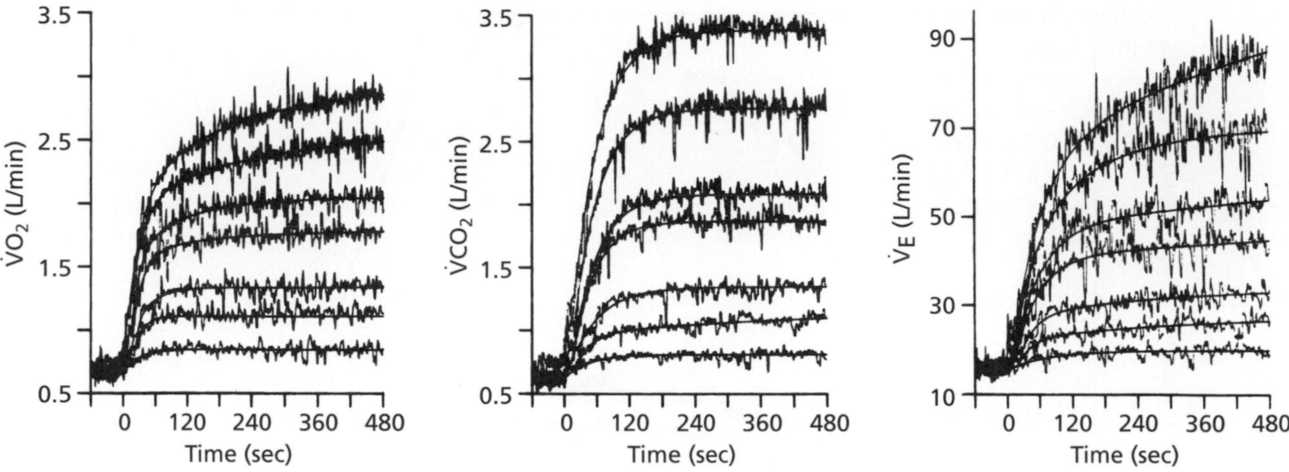

Figure 24–4. Gas exchange values, second-by-second, with curve fitting, showing the transition from unloaded pedaling to seven levels of work rate sustained for 6 minutes. *A*, O_2 uptake ($\dot{V}O_2$). *B*, CO_2 output ($\dot{V}CO_2$). *C*, Ventilation ($\dot{V}E$). The 32-year-old male subject was 180 cm tall and weighed 80 kg. The work levels were 29, 59, 88, 117, 146, 176, and 205 W. Venous blood lactate values 1 minute after cessation of exercise were 1.2, 1.4, 1.4, 1.7, 3.2, 4.3, and 8.7 mEq/L, respectively. At the three highest work rates $\dot{V}O_2$ and $\dot{V}E$ continued to rise, indicating the absence of a steady state and that these work rates were above the subject's lactic acidosis threshold for leg cycling. (From Casaburi R, Barstow TJ, Robinson T, et al: Influence of work rate on ventilatory and gas exchange kinetics. J Appl Physiol 67:547, 1989, with permission.)

What Is Integrated Cardiopulmonary Exercise Testing (CPET)?

Definition

Integrated cardiopulmonary exercise testing assesses the physiologic mechanisms that couple external to cellular respiration.[66] As such, it measures not only the electrocardiogram (ECG), but also evaluates the functional status of the heart, peripheral and pulmonary circulations, lungs, and the matching of ventilation to pulmonary blood flow as they relate to the changing metabolic rate. Exercise testing can be performed using a cycle or treadmill ergometer. The collected data should be accurately measured and displayed in such a manner that an informed decision can be made about the subject's functional capacity (including that for all daily activities) and the components limiting gas transport. The latter often reduces the need for further more costly or invasive investigations.[66]

How Measurements Are Made

After a preliminary history, physical, and laboratory examination (including chest roentgenogram, resting ECG, and spirometry), multiple noninvasive measures of cardiopulmonary variables are obtained in 20 minutes or less (i.e., during rest, constant low-intensity exercise, incremental exercise to tolerance, and recovery). After preliminary evaluations, the patient is introduced to the general laboratory environment and ergometer (cycle or treadmill) and familiarized with the mouthpiece or tightly fitting face mask, breathing valve, and instrumentation (flow or volume meters and rapidly responding CO_2 and O_2 analyzers).[9,35,56,72] Informed consent is obtained and electrodes are placed for recording the 12-lead ECG, from which HR and ECG pattern can be determined. Together, the simultaneous gas exchange and ECG recordings allow repetitive measurement of HR, $\dot{V}E$, breathing frequency (f), tidal volume (VT), $\dot{V}CO_2$, $\dot{V}O_2$, end-tidal CO_2 pressure ($PETCO_2$), and end-tidal O_2 pressure ($PETO_2$). With appropriate analyzers and computer software, gas exchange data can be measured and displayed breath by breath or averaged over any interval. Additionally, the external work rate can be computer controlled and estimated in the case of the treadmill or quite accurately measured in the case of the cycle. If an arterial line is used, samples can be taken for measurement of PaO_2, $PaCO_2$, pH, and lactate values and arterial blood pressure tracings can be recorded. If not, blood pressure is measured by auscultation, arterial blood can be sampled once or twice during exercise, and ear or finger oximetry values can be obtained. Either an incremental or constant work rate protocol may be used. A dedicated microcomputer is commonly used to calculate, tabulate, and display the results graphically. The latter is particularly important in order to interrelate the multiple ventilatory, circulatory, blood, and work rate variables. A nine-panel plot (Fig. 24–5) of these variables displays the most amount of information,[66] but a four-panel plot, as shown in Figure 24–6, illustrates the major findings.[28]

Ergometry Methods

For impairment and clinical evaluations, leg cycling or treadmill exercise are most commonly used. The cycle can be used for upper-extremity exercise if leg exercises on the cycle or treadmill are unsuitable. Table 24–1 lists some of the advantages and disadvantages of each of these ergometers. Because persons on the treadmill can be "dragged along" without actually climbing or propelling themselves, any connection other than that between the exercising person's feet and the treadmill belt can reduce the external work performed. The ability to quantitate the relationship of $\dot{V}O_2$ to work rate (e.g., panel 3 of Fig. 24–5) accurately is a major advantage of cycle ergometry.[66]

Exercise Protocols

Incremental Work

Usually increasing work rate to tolerance gives all the necessary information for an impairment evaluation with the least effort on the part of the patient. On the cycle ergometer, a useful protocol includes data collection during 2 to 3 minutes of rest, 3 to 4 minutes of unloaded pedaling at a rate of 60 rpm, 7 to 10 minutes of continued pedaling while work rate is increased in

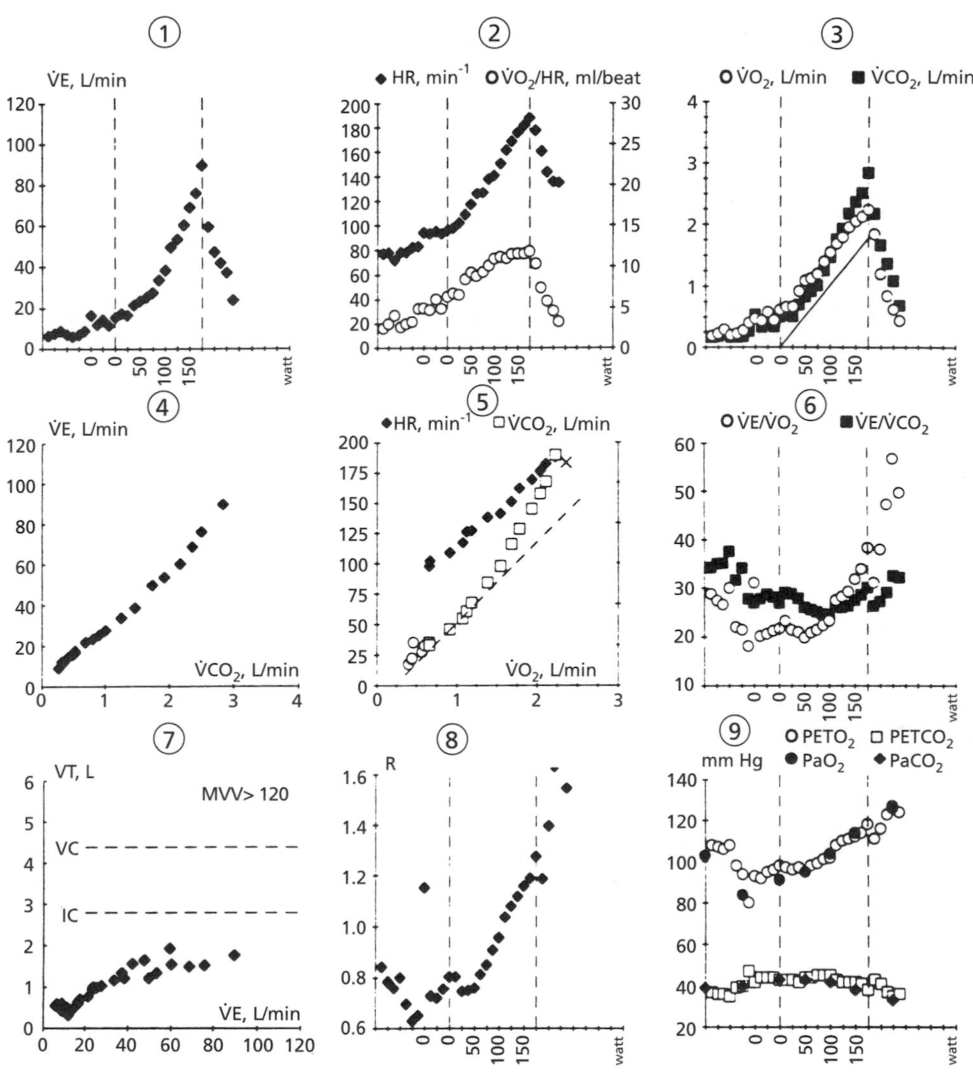

Figure 24–5. A nine-panel plot of a cycle exercise study in a 37-year-old shipyard machinist complaining of dyspnea. After 3 minutes of rest, the evaluee pedaled at 60 rpm for 3 minutes. The workload was then increased 25 W/min to his symptom-limited tolerance. Intra-arterial blood was obtained from a brachial catheter. He stopped exercise because of fatigue. Resting and exercise electrocardiograms (ECGs) were normal. Values are measured breath by breath and plotted every 30 seconds. Abbreviations are: ventilation ($\dot{V}E$), heart rate (HR), O_2 pulse ($\dot{V}O_2$/HR), O_2 uptake ($\dot{V}O_2$), CO_2 output ($\dot{V}CO_2$), ventilatory equivalents for O_2 and CO_2 ($\dot{V}E/\dot{V}O_2$ and $\dot{V}E/\dot{V}CO_2$), tidal volume (VT), vital capacity (VC), inspiratory capacity (IC), maximal voluntary ventilation (MVV), respiratory exchange ratio (R), arterial and end-tidal PO_2 (PaO_2 and $PETO_2$), and arterial and end-tidal PCO_2 ($PaCO_2$ and $PETCO_2$). The vertical dashed lines in several panels indicate the beginning and end of the incremental work period. The solid line in the right upper panel indicates a $\dot{V}O_2$/work rate relationship ($\Delta\dot{V}O_2/\Delta WR$) of 10 mL/min of o_2/W). The "X" in the center panel indicates the predicted peak $\dot{V}O_2$ and peak HR; the diagonal dashed line has a slope of 1.0. The exercise findings shown in this figure are normal. (From Wasserman K, Hansen JE, Sue DY, et al: Principles of Exercise Testing and Interpretation, 3rd ed. Baltimore, Lippincott, Williams and Wilkins, 1999, with permission.)

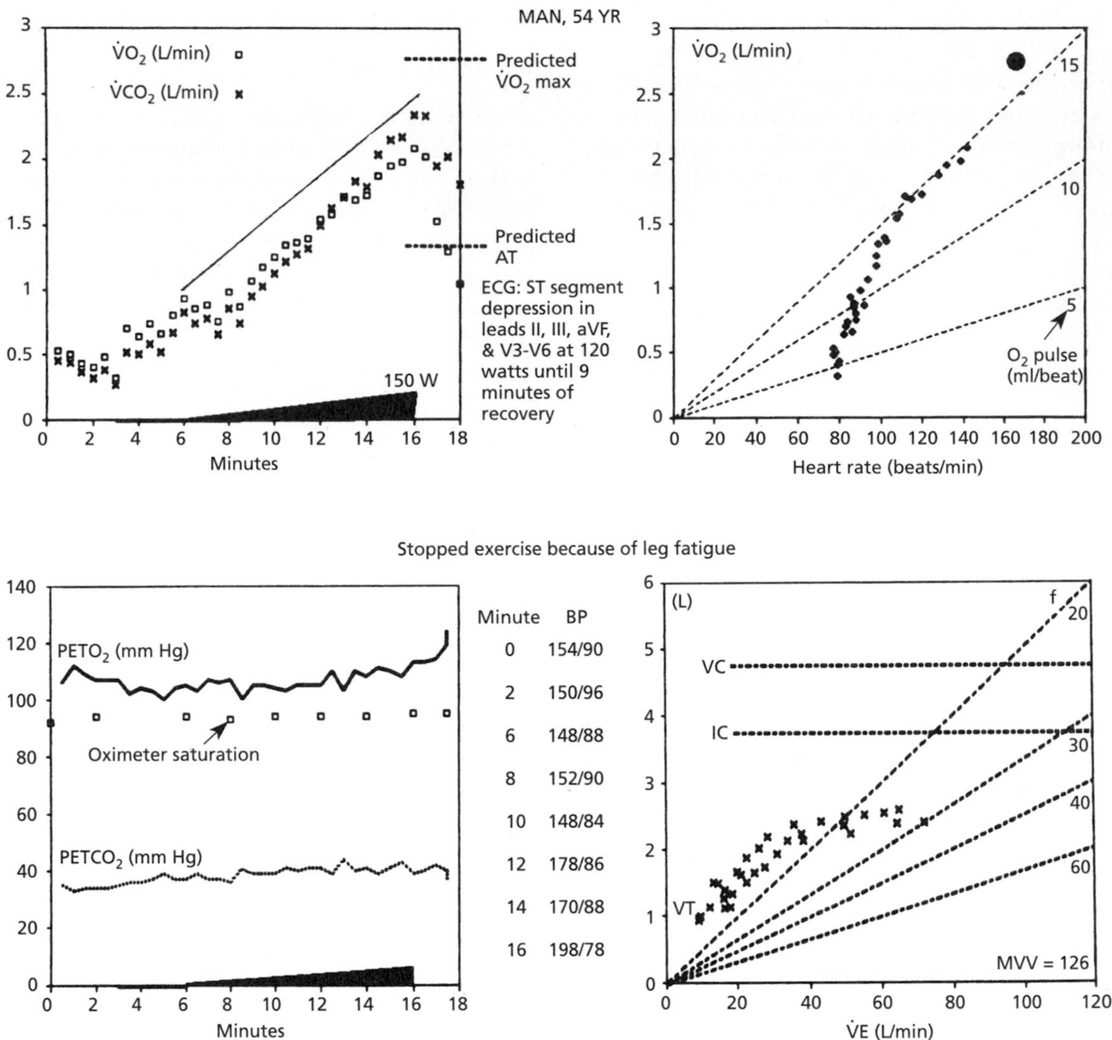

Figure 24–6. A four-panel plot of a cycle exercise study in a 54-year-old asbestos-exposed worker (191 cm and 98 kg) referred by a government agency for disability evaluation because of 15 years of work exposure to asbestos. He was an ex-smoker. He noted leg numbness after walking 20 minutes. Crackles were heard at the left lung base and linear scarring was seen on roentgenograms. Heart sounds and resting electrocardiogram (ECG) were normal. The vital capacity (VC) and diffusing capacity for carbon monoxide (DLCO) were normal, but the FEV_1/VC of 64% was reduced. The exercise protocol included 3 minutes of rest, 3 minutes of unloaded pedaling at 60 rpm, and work increments of 15 W/min until the patient stopped at 16 minutes (150 W) with leg fatigue. Values of O_2 uptake ($\dot{V}O_2$), CO_2 output ($\dot{V}CO_2$), ventilation ($\dot{V}E$), and heart rate (HR) were measured breath by breath but plotted every 30 seconds. The black circle in the upper right panel indicates the predicted peak HR, peak $\dot{V}O_2$, and peak O_2 pulse. The solid line in the left upper panel slope is a $\Delta\dot{V}O_2/\Delta WR$ of 10 mL/W. Significant downsloping ST segment depressions were noted in the inferior and lateral ECG leads from 14 minutes of exercise until they resolved completely by 9 minutes of recovery. The evaluee denied chest pain or pressure or shortness of breath during or after exercise. The peak $\dot{V}O_2$ and peak HR were reduced. The anaerobic threshold (AT) and the $\Delta\dot{V}O_2/\Delta WR$ were normal, but the O_2 pulse did not increase for the last 3 minutes of exercise. The abnormal exercise ECG and the concurrent failure of the O_2 pulse and diastolic pressure to increase during late exercise indicate the likelihood of a significant cardiovascular problem as the cause of the abnormal O_2 transport. Breathing reserve was ample. The ventilatory equivalents for O_2 and CO_2 (not graphed) and ear oximeter values were normal, all indicating that significant ventilation/perfusion mismatching was unlikely. Other abbreviations are: end-tidal PO_2 and PCO_2 ($PETO_2$ and $PETCO_2$), inspiratory capacity (IC), and maximum voluntary ventilation (MVV). Although this evaluee had evidence for obstructive and interstitial lung disease at rest, he was limited in his exercise tolerance by a cardiovascular problem, likely previously unsuspected coronary artery disease. Further workup was recommended.

TABLE 24–1
Treadmill and Cycle Ergometer Comparisons

Attribute	Treadmill	Cycle
Quantify external work	Fair	Excellent
Highest HR and $\dot{V}E$	Equal	Equal
Highest $\dot{V}O_2$ and O_2 pulse	Yes	
Familiarity of exercise	Yes	
Fewer artifacts in physiologic measurement		Yes
Can be used supine		Yes
Ease of obtaining arterial blood specimens		Yes

HR, heart rate; $\dot{V}E$, expired ventilation; $\dot{V}O_2$, O_2 uptake.

equal increments to tolerance, and 2 minutes of recovery. Work can be increased in a ramp fashion or in 1-minute steps. If a treadmill is used, the unloaded cycling is replaced by walking at an easy pace for 3 to 4 minutes at zero grade, followed by increasing the grade the same amount (1% to 3%) every minute to tolerance.

Usually a work rate increment can be selected (considering the evaluee's age, sex, body size, usual activity level, and known illnesses) so that the incremental work rate period lasts 6 to 14 minutes. Too short a period (under 6 minutes) may prevent the investigator from obtaining enough data for an accurate interpretation. Too long a period (over 14 minutes) leads to boredom or physical discomfort at a submaximal work rates.[12,66]

As evaluees cannot speak while on the mouthpiece or be understood clearly while wearing a face mask during the exercise test, they are taught to signal discomfort by pointing to the site of discomfort and to quantitate severity by extending one, two, or three digits or pointing to a scale (Borg or visual analog) displaying the degree of distress.

The evaluee and the monitors are closely observed during exercise. Exercise is not stopped because the evaluee reaches some predetermined percentage of the predicted peak HR or maximal voluntary ventilation (MVV), but is continued as long as safely tolerated. The development of a significant arrhythmia, substernal pressure or discomfort of more than mild severity, hypotension, hypertension greater than 260 mm Hg systolic or 130 mm Hg diastolic, pallor, or lightheadedness is sufficient to stop the study. After the mouthpiece has been removed, the evaluee should be asked in a nonleading fashion to explain exactly why he or she stopped exercise. If, after the exercise test, the investigator considers that the evaluee stopped prematurely, the study can be repeated after a short rest period.[66]

Constant Work

Occasionally evaluees are so infirm that they can perform only unloaded pedaling or walking at a slow pace. For that reason it would be impractical to use an increasing work rate protocol. At other times, constant work protocols can be used to evaluate the efficacy of O_2 breathing or drug therapy in relieving symptoms or for an accurate measure of the LAT or $\dot{V}O_2$ kinetics.[52]

Measurements Describing Physiologic Impairments

Presentation of Data

Because of the large number of important variables that can be measured and displayed during incremental exercise and later graphed or tabulated, it is easy to overwhelm the interpreter or viewer with information. For over a decade, a group at the Harbor–UCLA Medical Center has reported the results of exercise testing using a format that includes a brief history of the evaluee and a description of the protocol, a figure of nine panels displaying key variables plotted either versus time and work rate or versus each other (Fig. 24–5), a large table listing 10 to 20 variables every half minute, a small table listing key predicted and measured parameters, and an interpretation of the study with recommendations.[66] Table 24–2 lists the more important predicted values for sedentary adult men; Table 24–3 gives exercise data for a typical adult man.

A simpler, but less complete, graphical method of visual presentation of exercise data in another impairment evaluee is shown in Figure 24–6.[28] The two panels on the left illustrate the patterns of $\dot{V}O_2$ and $\dot{V}CO_2$ (upper left) and $PETO_2$, $PETCO_2$, and related blood values (lower left) during rest, three minutes of unloaded cycling exercise, incremental cycling exercise, and recovery. The two panels on the right show the relationships of $\dot{V}O_2$, HR, and O_2 pulse (upper right) and the interrelationships of exercise $\dot{V}E$, VT, and f to the preliminary measures of VC, inspiratory capacity (IC), and MVV (lower right). The center space gives additional information.

Cardiovascular Peak $\dot{V}O_2$

A person's ability to increase $\dot{V}O_2$ (measured in L/min or mL/min/kg) to its highest values depends not only on the circulatory system, but also on the quantity of muscle involved in the task being performed: the more muscle involved, the higher the possible $\dot{V}O_2$. For example, in untrained individuals, the peak $\dot{V}O_2$ reached will be least for arm cycling (approximately 50% to 60% of treadmill exercise), much greater for upright leg cycling (approximately 90% of treadmill exercise), and highest for treadmill walking or running (uphill rather than on the level) or tasks that include arm and leg exercise (such as cross-country skiing or combined arm and leg cycling).

Multiple studies have shown that an individual's peak $\dot{V}O_2$ for a given task is similar whether determined by a series of constant work rate tasks repeated at progressively higher intensities (the classical approach, which takes 1 or more days) or continuous incremental exercise to exhaustion (the practical approach), as long as the incremental work period lasts for a reasonable period of time (e.g., 6 to 14 minutes).[27,66]

Predicted or "normal" peak $\dot{V}O_2$ values for a given age, weight, sex, and degree of fitness differ slightly between reported series, primarily because of the different attributes of the population selected to be tested.[11,32,34,36] Values derived primarily from nonobese athletes, faculty, graduate students, or military personnel may be inappropriate to use for an impairment evaluation. Additionally, peak $\dot{V}O_2$ values derived from Japanese and European populations tend to be higher than values from Canadian or American populations. This is probably due to a lower level of physical activity and physical fitness in North American inhabitants.[34] For disability testing, the authors usually select peak $\dot{V}O_2$ reference values from a sedentary, working, blue-collar population rather than a population oriented to regular leisure sports.[32,66] Readers should refer to Table 24–2 for predicted values and to the references for more complete information.[35,66]

Peak $\dot{V}O_2$ values are usually expressed in units of mL/min/kg of body weight for athletes and competitors, with predicted values based on sex, age, and fitness. It is reasonable to express cardiovascular performance this way in nonobese individuals, as peak $\dot{V}O_2$ has a high correlation with lean body mass (which is primarily muscle). Peak $\dot{V}O_2$ values (in L/min) tend to be higher in early adult life, in larger and taller individuals, in men than women of the same age and size, and most importantly, in those engaged in endurance training and more active lifestyles.

TABLE 24–2

Predicted Cycle Exercise Values for Sedentary Middle-Aged Men

Measure and Units	Approximate Mean Value
Peak $\dot{V}O_2$, mL/min	(Height in cm – age in y) × 21
LAT, mL/min	(Height in cm – age in y) × 11
Peak heart rate, beats/min	220 – age in y
Peak O_2 pulse, mL/beat	Peak $\dot{V}O_2$/Peak heart rate
$\Delta\dot{V}O_2/\Delta WR$, mL/min/W	10
Brachial artery blood pressure, mm Hg	205/95
Exercise breathing reserve, L/min	35
Breathing frequency, end-exercise, breaths/min	40
VT/IC, end-exercise	0.6
$\dot{V}E/\dot{V}CO_2$ at LAT	29
$\dot{V}E/\dot{V}O_2$ at LAT	27
PaO_2, end-exercise, mm Hg	90
$P(A–a)O_2$, end-exercise, mm Hg	20
$P(a–ET)CO_2$, end-exercise, mm Hg	–3
VD/VT, end-exercise	0.20
Bicarbonate, arterial, end-exercise, mEq/L	20
pH, arterial, end-exercise	7.35
Respiratory exchange ratio (*R*), end-exercise	1.2

$\dot{V}O_2$, O_2 uptake; LAT, lactic acidosis threshold; WR, work rate; VT, tidal volume; IC, inspiratory capacity; $\dot{V}E$, expired ventilation; $\dot{V}CO_2$, CO_2 output; $\dot{V}O_2$, O_2 uptake; PaO_2, arterial O_2 pressure; $P(A-a)O_2$, alveolar – aterial O_2 pressure difference; $P(a-ET)CO_2$, arterial – end tidal CO_2 pressure difference; VD, dead space.

TABLE 24–3

Cycle Exercise Values for a Typical Sedentary 50-Year-Old Man (170 cm and 70 kg)

Measure and Units	Resting	Peak
$\dot{V}O_2$, mL/min	300	2300
Heart rate, beats/min	74	170
O_2 pulse, mL/beat	4.2	15
Brachial artery blood pressure, mm Hg	120/72	206/95
$\dot{V}E$, L/min	8	102
Breathing frequency, breaths/min	14	42
VT, L	0.5	1.8
$\dot{V}E/\dot{V}CO_2$	35	29*
$\dot{V}E/\dot{V}O_2$	30	27*
PaO_2, mm Hg	88	96
$P(A-a)O_2$, mm Hg	14	24
$P(a-ET)CO_2$, mm Hg	3	–3
VD/VT	0.40	0.20
Bicarbonate, arterial, mEq/L	24	17
pH, arterial	7.40	7.34
Respiratory exchange (*R*)	0.85	1.15

At lactic acidosis threshold (LAT) rather than at peak exercise.

Note – Resting values: $\dot{V}C$ = 4.3 L; IC =2.8 L; FEV_1 = 3.3 L; MVV = 135 L/min. Other values: LAT = 1.2 L/min; breathing reserve =33 L/min; heart rate reserve = 0 beats/min; $\Delta\dot{V}O_2/\Delta WR$ = 10 mL/W.

$\dot{V}O_2$, O_2 uptake; $\dot{V}E$, expired ventilation; VT, tidal volume; $\dot{V}CO_2$, CO_2, output; PaO_2, arterial O_2 pressure; $P(A-a)O_2$, alveolar–arterial O_2 pressure difference; $P(a-ET)CO_2$, arterial–end tidal CO_2 pressure difference; VD/VT, dead space/tidal volume ratio.

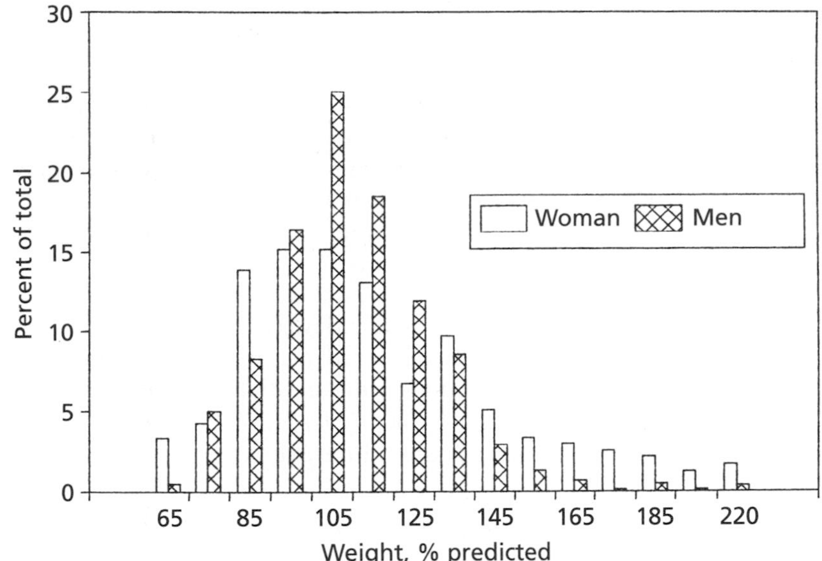

Figure 24–7. Relationship of actual to predicted weight in approximately 1000 men and women evaluated at the authors' exercise laboratory. Predicted weight for men is 0.79 kg, height is 60.7 cm. Predicted weight for women is 0.65 kg, height is 42.8 cm. Each column indicates the percentage of the total of each sex by decile of predicted weight (e.g., 65 = 60 to 69.9% of predicted weight), continuing until the last column, which indicates those with a mean value of 220% of predicted weight. Values are skewed to the right, indicating more corpulence than a normal population. Less than 1% of the men are less than 70% of their predicted weights, whereas 14.6% exceed 130% of their predicted weights; 3.4% of the women are less than 70% of their predicted weights, whereas 28.7% exceed 130% of their predicted weights.

On the other hand, peak $\dot{V}O_2$ values for patients or impairment evaluees should (nearly always) be related to predicted values based primarily on age, sex, and body height rather than age, sex, and body weight.[66] This is not a minor distinction considering the high percentage of overweight evaluees and patients who are referred for exercise testing. Figure 24–7 shows the high incidence of obesity in men and women sent to the authors for exercise testing. On average, 60% of the referred men were 19% overweight, whereas 63% of the referred women were 33% overweight. If predicted values for peak $\dot{V}O_2$ (and consequently peak O_2 pulse and LAT) in these overweight patients had been based on weight and age rather than height and age, about two-thirds of the healthy men would have had a reduced peak $\dot{V}O_2$, peak O_2 pulse, and LAT (81% or less of predicted) and about two-thirds of the healthy women would have had a measured peak $\dot{V}O_2$, peak O_2 pulse, and LAT of 67% or less than predicted solely on the basis of excess body weight.

In nonathletes, changes in body weight are much more often due to increased body fat than muscle. Consequently, in comparing two individuals of the same height, age, and sex, one should not expect an otherwise healthy individual with 40% body fat to have a peak $\dot{V}O_2$ 20% higher than another person with 20% body fat.

When predicted values for $\dot{V}O_2$, O_2 pulse, and LAT are based on weight rather than height (as is done in some laboratories), the obese person with normal cardiovascular function and normal peak $\dot{V}O_2$, O_2 pulse, and LAT for height, sex, and age may be deemed to have abnormal cardiovascular function because his or her measured values will be below the predicted values for peak $\dot{V}O_2$, O_2 pulse, and LAT. Indeed, such a person likely has a decreased ability to perform external work, but this decreased work ability is due to obesity rather than cardiovascular disease. Thus it is of great importance to select appropriate predicted values in an impairment evaluation.[66]

Lactic Acidosis Threshold

Tasks that require an energy expenditure above the LAT require rest periods for recovery. Energy expenditure requiring $\dot{V}O_2$ below the LAT should be considered as moderate or of lesser intensity, whereas $\dot{V}O_2$ above the LAT is considered as heavy, very heavy, or extreme intensity exercise.[64,67]

In the average young person, the LAT occurs at a $\dot{V}O_2$ value that is approximately 45% to 60% of the peak $\dot{V}O_2$.[66] The LAT does not necessarily occur synchronously with the respiratory compensation point (ventilatory threshold) or when the respiratory exchange ratio exceeds 1.0. It can be detected with repeated arterial blood lactate measurements. It is easiest, however, to recognize the LAT using noninvasive gas exchange measurements with a graphical display of $\dot{V}CO_2$ versus $\dot{V}O_2$ values (center panel, Fig. 24–5) during a progressively increasing work rate test of less than 12 minutes duration.[8,58] The LAT value should be expressed in units of $\dot{V}O_2$ rather than work rate. Regardless of age, sex, or body size, a LAT that is less than 40% of the predicted (not the measured) peak $\dot{V}O_2$ is abnormal (below the 95% confidence limits) and is indicative of circulatory dysfunction.[66] With physical training, both the LAT and the peak $\dot{V}O_2$ increase. Generally the LAT/peak $\dot{V}O_2$ ratio also increases, to as high as 0.85 in some highly trained endurance athletes. With maintenance of good health, the LAT/peak $\dot{V}O_2$ ratio also increases with age, probably more in women than men.[66]

Oxygen Uptake/Work Rate ($\Delta\dot{V}O_2/\Delta WR$) Relationships

The ability to quantify the $\Delta\dot{V}O_2/\Delta WR$ is an important advantage of cycle ergometry.[30,31] When a steady state is reached during multiple constant work-rate-cycle ergometry tests below the LAT, the steady state $\dot{V}O_2$ increases by approximately 10 mL/min/W, regardless of age, sex, or body size.[15] Similarly, during incremental cycle ergometry to exhaustion of reasonable duration (5 to 20 minutes), the $\dot{V}O_2$ also increases in healthy persons (after a delay of about 3 to 4 minutes) by approximately 10 mL/min/W.[30] A smaller increase in $\dot{V}O_2$ per watt increase in work rate (low $\Delta\dot{V}O_2/\Delta WR$) during an incremental test reflects a reduced rate of aerobic metabolism and an increased rate of anaerobic metabolism; i.e., a decreased ratio of aerobic to total work. Possible causes include failure of the lung to oxygenate the pulmonary blood at an appropriate rate, an inability of the circulatory system to transport O_2 effectively, a high resistance to diffusion at the capillary level, or a defect in aerobic enzymes or the electron transport chain in muscle mitochondria.[31] Although not everyone with these disorders has a statistically significant decrease in $\Delta\dot{V}O_2/\Delta WR$, the finding of a low $\Delta\dot{V}O_2/\Delta WR$ indicates a reduced use of atmospheric O_2 and a higher than normal use of anaerobic metabolism to support muscle bioenergetics.

Oxygen Pulse ($\dot{V}O_2$/HR)

Regardless of age, sex, or body size, a near-linear relationship between $\dot{V}O_2$ and HR from rest to exhaustive exercise is noted in every healthy person.[66] The $\dot{V}O_2$ in mL/min divided by the HR in beats/min equals the $\dot{V}O_2$/HR in mL/beat and is identified as the O_2 pulse. Graphically, these relationships can be observed in Figures 24–5 and 24–6. Note that the linear intercept of HR versus $\dot{V}O_2$ intersects the HR axis well above zero.

The predicted peak O_2 pulse for normal individuals can be calculated by dividing their predicted peak $\dot{V}O_2$ (based on age, sex, and height) by their predicted peak HR (220 minus age). From the Fick principle, which relates cardiac output to $\dot{V}O_2$, it can be shown that the O_2 pulse is the product of effective ventricular stroke volume and the difference between the arterial and mixed-venous O_2 contents. Any process that decreases maximal stroke volume (e.g., valvular heart disease, cardiomyopathy, coronary artery disease, pulmonary vascular disease, or peripheral vascular disease), decreases arterial O_2 content (anemia, hypoxemia, or carboxyhemoglobinemia), or increases mixed-venous O_2 content (poor peripheral O_2 extraction or inability to increase exercise to higher levels because of the presence of other systemic disease) will reduce the peak O_2 pulse.[66]

During incremental exercise the O_2 pulse normally increases in a curvilinear fashion from rest to exhaustion (Fig. 24–5, top center panel). A change from this pattern during an incremental exercise test indicates dysfunction in O_2 transport. A smaller than appropriate increase of the O_2 pulse during increasing exertion indicates that the product of stroke volume and O_2 extraction has prematurely reached its maximal value. In many persons with coronary artery disease who have myocardial ischemia during exercise without angina, the O_2 pulse abruptly stops increasing concurrent with the development of significant ST segment or T wave abnormalities, indicating ventricular dysfunction.[66] (See reference 66 for case examples of this functional impairment of cardiac output detected noninvasively when ECG changes consistent with myocardial ischemia develop.) This finding is important because the ECG changes alone may be difficult to interpret. (See also Fig. 24–6.)

$\dot{V}O_2$ Kinetics: MRT and Change in $\dot{V}O_2$ From 3 to 6 Minutes [$\Delta\dot{V}O_2$(6–3)]

In the transition from a low metabolic steady state (sitting or cycle exercise with unloaded pedaling at 60 cycles per minute) to a moderate-intensity exercise in normal persons, it takes 2 to 3 minutes for the $\dot{V}O_2$ to reach a steady state. The normal $\dot{V}O_2$ MRT (63% of the steady-state response) is approximately ½ minutes. Longer values indicate O_2 delivery or utilization problems, such as primary cardiac disease, pulmonary vascular disease, or peripheral vascular disease.[53] In the latter illness, the MRT is much improved following surgical correction of the vascular obstructions and reestablishment of better O_2 delivery to the exercising leg muscles.[6]

During exercise at a constant work rate above the LAT, the $\dot{V}O_2$ does not reach a constant value in 3 minutes but continues to rise. The higher the intensity of the exercise, the more obvious is the lack of a steady state. In such constant work tests, the difference in the $\dot{V}O_2$ between 3 and 6 minutes can be quantitated.[15,52] The finding of a positive $\Delta\dot{V}O_2$(6–3) identifies exercise above the LAT. The $\Delta\dot{V}O_2$(6–3) is proportional to lactate in normal subjects and patients with heart disease.[66]

Blood Pressure

Both systolic and diastolic pressures continue to rise as work rate increases with the systolic rising much more than the diastolic. Commonly, systolic pressure reaches values over 200 mm Hg whereas intra-arterially recorded diastolic pressure reaches about 100 mm Hg. By auscultation, fifth phase diastolic pressures may rise, but usually remain stable or decline minimally.[51]

Electrocardiogram

The development of downsloping ST segment depression is suggestive, but not diagnostic, of myocardial ischemia. The development or increase in the number of premature ventricular contractions or a significant atrial arrhythmia during exercise also suggests myocardial ischemia.

Respiratory Mechanics

When resting respiratory function testing does not reveal severe abnormalities in respiratory mechanics, exercise tests are needed to determine impairment. In evaluees with moderate airway obstruction or restriction, exercise studies are needed to evaluate ventilation/perfusion mismatching and whether hypoxemia develops. For example, the comparison of integrated cardiopulmonary exercise tests with resting respiratory function tests is helpful in deciding whether a person is limited in ventilatory ability during exercise. Preliminarily, it is preferable to measure the MVV directly; if this is not done, it should be estimated by multiplying the forced expiratory volume in 1 second (FEV_1) times 40.[13] Initially, as exercise begins, $\dot{V}E$ rises primarily by increasing VT; as the work rate increases, ventilatory frequency (f) also increases. Ventilation is likely to be limiting exercise if the maximum exercise ventilation ($\dot{V}E_{max}$) closely approaches (i.e., within 10 to 15 L/min) the MVV measured prior to exercise (identified as a low exercise breathing reserve); the exercise VT approaches to within 10% of the resting IC; or the f exceeds 50 per minute.[66]

There are two other findings suggestive of ventilatory limitation. One is a rise in $Paco_2$ during heavy exercise. With normal ventilatory control, the development of a lactic acidosis during heavy exercise stimulates ventilation, causing $PAco_2$ and $Paco_2$ to decline, which in turn tends to minimize the acidemia. If ventilation is mechanically limited, it fails to increase appropriately in response to the exercise lactic acidosis. The resulting increase in $Paco_2$ late in the exercise test aggravates the metabolically induced acidemia so that arterial pH decreases more than normal. Such a respiratory acidosis is sometimes seen in patients with severe obstructive or (less commonly) restrictive lung disease who are limited in ventilatory ability. A mild respiratory acidosis is tolerated by some elite athletes who have learned to reduce their ventilatory requirements at very high work levels.[66]

The other evidence for ventilatory limitation, which can be recognized without blood gas measures, is a lack of the normal prompt decrease in VE early during recovery accompanying the prompt decrease in HR early in recovery.

Ventilation/Perfusion Mismatching

Ventilatory Equivalents for O_2 ($\dot{V}E/\dot{V}o_2$) and CO_2 ($\dot{V}E/\dot{V}co_2$) and slope of ratio of $\dot{V}E$ versus $\dot{V}co_2$ ($\dot{V}E$ versus $\dot{V}co_2$)

Ventilatory equivalents express the efficiency of ventilation related to metabolism. They are defined as the liters of $\dot{V}E$; body temperature and pressure, saturated (BTPS) required per liter of $\dot{V}o_2$ or $\dot{V}co_2$; and standard temperature and pressure, dry (STPD). Normally, the $\dot{V}E/\dot{V}co_2$ and the $\dot{V}E/\dot{V}o_2$ decline from resting values of 35 to 60 to values of 30 or less near the LAT for $\dot{V}E/\dot{V}co_2$ and 27 or less for $\dot{V}E/\dot{V}o_2$. They then increase considerably as metabolic acidosis develops. If the $\dot{V}E/\dot{V}o_2$ and $\dot{V}E/\dot{V}co_2$ do not decline appropriately at the LAT, a high VD/VT (dead space volume/tidal volume ratio) is likely to be the cause. However, elevated ventilatory equivalents can also be due to an unusually low $Paco_2$ (as with acute hyperventilation, chronic respiratory alkalosis, or chronic metabolic acidosis).[66] In evaluees with elevated ventilatory equivalents at the LAT, arterial blood gas measurements should be made and matched to concurrent expired gas measurements during moderate or high intensity exercise. These simultaneous measurements should clarify the cause of the high $\dot{V}E/\dot{V}o_2$. A measure now commonly used in the evaluation of patients with heart disease is the slope of the ratio of $\dot{V}E$ versus $\dot{V}co_2$. The slope is normally linear during work except near the end of exercise when lactic acidosis increases the slope slightly. An increase in slope with heart disease and especially heart failure is due to relatively poor perfusion of ventilated lung.

End-tidal pressures of O_2 and CO_2 ($PETo_2$ and $PETco_2$), which are easy to obtain noninvasively, give indications of mean alveolar values of O_2 and CO_2 and their trends in normal persons but cannot reliably predict alveolar or arterial Pco_2 or Po_2 values in patients or evaluees.

Dead Space/Tidal Volume Ratio (VD/VT)

The evaluee's physiologic VD/VT is calculated from knowing the mixed expired CO_2, the $Paco_2$, the VT, and the dead space of the breathing valve and mouthpiece or face mask. The physiologic VD/VT cannot be validly measured noninvasively without measures of $Paco_2$ (in contrast to statements made by some commercial exercise systems). These purported VD/VT values should never be utilized or reported. Normally the VD/VT decreases from rest to exercise as the VT increases and perfusion of the airspaces with high CO_2-laden blood increases. In normal older men, the VD/VT falls to 0.30 or less at maximal exercise; in younger men the decrease is even greater.[32,37,38,55,66,68] In persons with primary or secondary pulmonary vascular disease or severe maldistribution of ventilation to perfusion, the VD/VT does not decline appropriately and may be increased at rest and markedly increased with exercise.

Arterial–End Tidal Carbon Dioxide Pressure Difference [$P(a–ET)co_2$]

The $Paco_2$ at rest, which reflects the ideal $PAco_2$, is slightly higher than the $PETco_2$.[37] As exercise progresses, the $PETCO_2$ normally becomes higher than the $PaCO_2$. This finding is so consistent that a positive $P(a\text{–}ET)CO_2$ at the end of exercise is equivalent to a pathologic increase in physiologic VD/VT (over 0.30) (i.e., evidence for uneven ventilation/perfusion relationships due to lung or pulmonary vascular disease).[55,66]

Alveolar–Arterial O_2 Pressure Difference [$P(A\text{–}a)O_2$]

The $P(A\text{–}a)O_2$ may remain constant but usually increases during exercise, even to as high as 30 to 35 mm Hg.[66] Greater increases are usually due to ventilation/perfusion mismatching but may also be due to diffusion abnormalities or blood shunting through a patent foramen ovale.

Other Measurements

Normally there is a few percentage increase in hematocrit and hemoglobin during incremental exercise. With heavy exercise, the SaO_2 remains relatively constant despite a decrease in pH (rightward shift in oxyhemoglobin dissociation curve) due to a small increase in the PaO_2. Values found with ear or finger oximetry during exercise often, but not invariably, parallel simultaneous directly measured arterial oxyhemoglobin saturation.[19] The discrepancies between directly measured and peripherally estimated blood saturations are likely to be greater during intense exercise, when perfusion of the ear or finger may be compromised (see Chapter 22).[29]

With low intensity exercise the arterial and mixed venous values for both PCO_2 and bicarbonate rise slightly. With moderate intensity exercise the arterial bicarbonate falls while the mixed venous PCO_2 and bicarbonate increase. With high intensity exercise the mixed venous PCO_2 rises strikingly to nearly double its resting value, the bicarbonate declines to near-resting levels, and the mixed venous oxyhemoglobin saturation, O_2 content and pH all decline strikingly.[16,28] Throughout this time, arterial bicarbonate decreases approximately equimolar to the increase in arterial lactate concentration.[7,59]

The respiratory exchange ratio (R) rises with the production and elimination of excess CO_2 during exercise. During early recovery, R increases further, reflecting the abrupt decrease in $\dot{V}O_2$ and elimination of tissue CO_2 stores that had increased during exercise and further hyperventilation secondary to the arterial acidemia. If R does not increase to over 1.05 during recovery, it is likely that the maximal exercise level was below the LAT.[32,55,66]

Pathophysiology of Work Intolerance and Disease

For a comprehensive presentation of pathophysiology, readers should refer to Reference 66 for actual case reports that are partially illustrated here in the form of a nine-panel plots (Fig. 24–5). That reference includes the following case conditions and many of the more than 80 cases have more than one disorder:

Normal men and women
Normal athlete
Cycle and treadmill compared
Air and O_2 breathing compared
Effect of acute cigarette smoking
Pre-β and post-β adrenergic blockade
Poor effort
Acute hyperventilation
Psychogenic dyspnea
Coronary artery disease
Cardiomyopathy
Valvular heart disease
Congestive heart failure
Diastolic dysfunction
Heart disease with oscillatory gas exchange
Congenital heart disease
Vasoregulatory asthenia
Patent ductus arteriosus
Pulmonary arteriovenous fistulae
Peripheral vascular disease
Anemia
Carboxyhemoglobinemia
Primary pulmonary hypertension
Pulmonary hypertension with patent foramen ovale
Thromboembolic pulmonary vascular disease
Pulmonary vasculitis
Mica pneumoconiosis
Pulmonary microlithiasis
Idiopathic interstitial lung disease, before and after corticosteroids
Alveolar proteinosis, before and after lavage
Sarcoidosis
Asbestosis
Mixed connective tissue disease
Lung cancer with preoperative evaluation
Bullous emphysema
Emphysema
Chronic bronchitis
Asthma
Obstructive lung disease, before and after rehabilitation
Obstructive lung disease, room air and oxygen
Extreme obesity

Obesity

Obesity is an important factor in work intolerance for many reasons. Obese persons have higher $\dot{V}O_2$ requirements at all work rates than their leaner counterparts.[62] The effect of obesity on the $\dot{V}O_2$ requirement for work depends on how overweight the subject is and whether the body is supported or ambulatory when performing the work tasks. Ambulatory work, especially, has higher $\dot{V}O_2$ requirements in the obese. It should be stressed that the $\dot{V}O_2$ requirement for unloaded cycling (no external work accomplished) is primarily dependent on the weight of the legs. The efficiency in performing external work while cycling in normal obese subjects is normal (i.e., $\Delta\dot{V}O_2/\Delta WR = 10$ mL/min/W).

It is preferable to discriminate between cardiovascular disease and obesity by basing predicted peak $\dot{V}O_2$ values on height rather than on weight.[32,66] Resting hypoxemia is common in obese persons and may suggest that an evaluee has primary lung disease. The relief of hypoxemia during mild to moderate exercise, however, indicates that the resting hypoxemia was due to obesity-induced atelectasis at the lung bases, which cleared as tidal volume increased.[66] Thus obesity is a significant disadvantage, even without considering accompanying complicating illnesses such as atherosclerosis, hypertension, and diabetes mellitus.

Heart, Pulmonary Vascular, and Peripheral Vascular Disease

Many persons with cardiovascular disorders have normal electrocardiographic, hemodynamic, and gas exchange findings at rest but have distinctly abnormal findings during integrative cardiopulmonary exercise testing. Any of these disorders may manifest a reduced ability to transport O_2 from the lungs to the cells, as evidenced by a low peak $\dot{V}O_2$, low LAT, low or abnormal O_2 pulse, or low $\Delta\dot{V}O_2/\Delta WR$. In the case of coronary artery disease, these abnormalities plus electrocardiographic abnormalities may be evident only at high work intensities.

In contrast, patients with cardiomyopathy, valvular heart disease, or heart failure from any cause often evidence the above dysfunctions at lower work rates.[66] The change in $\dot{V}E/\dot{V}CO_2$, or the more easily graphed slope of the $\dot{V}E$ versus $\dot{V}CO_2$ during work, is a useful parameter to evaluate patients, as the $\dot{V}E$ versus $\dot{V}CO_2$ slope changes concurrently and in opposite directions to improvements or worsening of heart failure.[39]

Cardiac output increase in response to exercise may also be severely limited by pulmonary vascular disease, whether embolic, secondary to destruction of the pulmonary vascular bed (e.g., interstitial lung disease or emphysema), or idiopathic (e.g., primary pulmonary hypertension). An increase in pulmonary vascular resistance impedes blood flow from the right ventricle to the left ventricle. The low cardiac output response causes a low work rate lactic acidosis that stimulates ventilation. Additionally, with pulmonary vascular disease, the VD/VT is increased (which increases the ventilatory requirement) while hypoxemia (a potent ventilatory stimulus) commonly develops during exercise. Thus dyspnea is a common feature of pulmonary vascular disease.

With peripheral vascular disease, sclerotic vessels may restrict blood flow to the exercising extremities. In addition to low peak $\dot{V}O_2$, LAT, O_2 pulse, and $\Delta\dot{V}O_2/\Delta WR$, the MRT is elevated and systemic blood pressure usually rises more than expected for the level of exercise performed. Commonly, pain in the affected leg or legs is given as the reason for stopping exercise.

Obstructive Lung Disease

Resting pulmonary function tests are usually abnormal in persons with asthma, chronic bronchitis, or emphysema except for those with only exercise-induced asthma. Exercise limitation may be due to airway obstruction (with reduced ability to increase ventilation) or ventilation/perfusion mismatching (which increases the ventilatory requirement). When ventilation is limited, the exercise breathing reserve (resting MVV – $\dot{V}E_{max}$) is low (usually in the range of –5 to +15 L/min). Patients with predominantly obstructive disease rarely have exercise ventilatory frequencies higher than 45/min. When exercise is ventilatorily limited, it is common for the peak $\dot{V}O_2$ to be reduced, the HR reserve to be high, and the subject to complain of dyspnea as the limiting factor during the exercise test. With well-motivated persons with obstructive lung disease, the $PaCO_2$ may rise near the end of incremental exercise, indicating that a respiratory acidosis is accompanying the exercise-induced metabolic acidosis. If exercise is chronically limited by obstructive lung disease, then the LAT may be also reduced because of the inactivity of the patient.[66]

Restrictive Lung Disease

Some interstitial diseases are subtle and difficult to diagnose even after thorough laboratory and radiologic investigation at rest. In such individuals, exercise testing may be critically important because hypoxemia during heavy exercise may be the only conclusive evidence, short of open lung biopsy, of otherwise latent interstitial lung disease.[25] Other patients with restrictive disease have obvious abnormalities at rest and exercise. In patients with severe interstitial lung disease, the breathing reserve tends to be low, breathing frequency high, and the VT/IC approaches 1.0, while the blood gases, $P(a-ET)CO_2$, and VD/VT may be clearly abnormal.[66]

With either obstructive or restrictive lung disease, an accompanying pulmonary vascular disease (which may be evidenced by a low gas transfer index or diffusing capacity for carbon monoxide [DLCO] at rest) commonly causes a reduction in maximal stroke volume and maximal cardiac output so that the peak $\dot{V}O_2$, LAT, O_2 pulse, and $\Delta\dot{V}O_2/\Delta WR$ may also be abnormal, causing more impairment than is evident from resting pulmonary function studies.[66] Similarly, measurements of VD/VT, $P(a-ET)CO_2$, PaO_2, and $P(A-a)O_2$ during exercise are often more useful than resting measurements for the purpose of defining ventilation-perfusion mismatching.

Anemia, Carboxyhemoglobinemia, and Cigarette Smoking

Any mechanism that reduces the capacity of blood to take up O_2 in the lungs also reduces the ability of the circulatory system to deliver O_2.[40] Even if the $Pa{O_2}$ and $Sa{O_2}$ are normal, the O_2 content of arterial blood ($Ca{O_2}$) is reduced in proportion to the reduction in available hemoglobin. At rest and at low activity levels, such a reduction in $Ca{O_2}$ may be compensated for by an increased extraction of O_2 from the peripheral blood (a lower mixed-venous O_2 content) or by an increase in cardiac output. Because of the reduced O_2 transport, lactic acidosis develops at a reduced work rate and the LAT and peak $\dot{V}{O_2}$ are reduced in proportion to the reduction in available hemoglobin.[40] The same work rate, consequently, is less well tolerated than in an individual not so affected. A reduction in available hemoglobin due to carboxyhemoglobinemia increases the work of the heart more than a reduction due to anemia because the carboxyhemoglobin must be circulated. Acute cigarette, cigar, or pipe smoking not only causes carboxyhemoglobinemia, but also increases HR and blood pressure and may decrease ventilation/perfusion matching.[33] The adverse effects of chronic tobacco abuse on the respiratory and circulatory systems are too numerous to enumerate here.

β-Adrenergic Blockade

Patients on β-adrenergic blocking drugs are frequently referred for an impairment or a disability evaluation. The normal practice is to evaluate and exercise such persons without modifying their drug intake. If the β-blockade is high, the expected changes from predicted exercise values (in persons with otherwise normal cardiovascular systems) are likely to be a large reduction in peak HR, a mild to moderate reduction in peak $\dot{V}{O_2}$, and a moderate increase in the peak O_2 pulse.[66] The high O_2 pulse reflects an increased time for ventricular filling and a resultant increase in effective stroke volume. Whether the person should be retested after reducing β-blockade depends on whether β-blockade can be safely decreased and the desire to increase his or her exercise tolerance.

Defects in Bioenergetics

Rarely, persons are found to have deficiencies in O_2 utilization by the exercising muscle due to enzymatic or metabolic disorders, usually genetic. Because O_2 is not extracted from the capillary blood and metabolized normally by individuals with these disorders, the muscle end-capillary and mixed-venous O_2 contents do not decline to low levels during intense exercise as they do in normal subjects and those with the usual circulatory disorders.[42,66] Individuals with these defects usually demonstrate a high peak HR, low peak $\dot{V}{O_2}$, and low O_2 pulse during exercise testing. In persons with McArdle's syndrome, for example, there is considerable muscle pain during maximal exercise without elevation of blood lactate values.[42] The HR response is high and O_2 extraction is low, indicating the failure of the muscles to utilize O_2 normally. In other individuals, muscle biopsy and enzymatic analysis or measurements of mixed-venous blood may be necessary to establish a diagnosis.

Secondary Gain and Anxiety

In some individuals, the secondary gain associated with an impairment or disability evaluation makes testing more difficult. All evaluees are encouraged to perform as well as possible during all pre-exercise and exercise tests so that the evaluation will provide a conclusive diagnosis to which the evaluees' symptoms can be attributed. When behavior and test results are erratic, the evaluees are told that such findings are not advantageous for them. If an exercise test shows a low peak $\dot{V}{O_2}$, a high HR reserve, a high breathing reserve, no suggestion of gas exchange abnormality, a normal LAT, a low recovery R, or no local musculoskeletal cause for cessation of exercise and the reason the evaluee stopped exercise is not clear and logical, then there is no choice but to attribute the limited performance to poor effort. The evaluee is encouraged to repeat the exercise test. If the ventilatory equivalents are high or if the oximetry is not entirely normal, a second test with an arterial line is helpful.[66]

Evidences for high anxiety are a bizarre or irregular ventilatory pattern with intermittent and episodic breathing, especially at rest and early in exercise; a high R during rest and early exercise (hyperventilation); and a high resting HR. Ordinarily, the physiologic requirements of increasing work rate soon override the manifestations of anxiety, and the circulatory and ventilatory response approach normal.[66]

Applications of Cardiopulmonary Exercise Testing (CPET) for Disability Evaluation And Follow-up

Reproducibility of Measurements and Utility in Disease States

Equipment must be properly maintained and calibrated before each use. Experience from several laboratories[3,22,43] confirms that unless there is a change in an individual's fitness or health status or environmental conditions surrounding the tests, measurements on the same individual whether healthy or ill should be highly reproducible, both in the peak values and the pattern of changes of the multiple variables from rest to maximal exercise. Recent studies also confirm the utility of CPET with gas exchange measurements in assessing individuals with occupational asthma and reactive airways dysfunction, systemic lupus erythematosus, hypertrophic cardiomyopathy, chronic obstructive pulmonary disease, and heart failure.[26,36,43,46]

The O_2 Cost of Various Activities

In the early and mid 20th century, many investigators in Europe, Africa, and the Americas measured energy expenditure during rest or during common recreational or work activities.[2,3,44,48,49] Their original data have frequently been reported in review articles and tables. Unfortunately, for current use, their subjects often performed tasks not commonly required in modern industrial settings. The investigators rarely compared individuals with marked differences in body size performing similar tasks. Considering the small size, portability, and current availability of modern equipment, which can measure and transmit data in a wireless mode for up to hours at a time, it should now be relatively easy to quantify energy expenditure for a wide variety of current recreational or industrial tasks.

Table 24–4, listing $\dot{V}O_2$ requirements for different activities and body sizes, should be used and interpreted cautiously, following the suggestions in the footnote, repeated here. Some compilations of data, which were obtained primarily from workers 65 to 70 kg in weight, incorrectly calculate caloric or $\dot{V}O_2$ values for individuals heavier or lighter than 70 kg by assuming that the energy expenditure is directly proportional to body weight. For example, the assumption that a 100-kg person requires twice as much $\dot{V}O_2$ to accomplish the same task as a 50-kg person is invariably an overestimate. Table 24–4 is based on $\dot{V}O_2$ values for a 70-kg person with a height of 170 cm. Doubling or halving this weight modifies sitting or standing $\dot{V}O_2$ values by about 35%. Extreme heat, altitude, or cold stress can also increase energy requirements but differences in body height are of much lesser importance. For activities that are carried out in the sitting or standing position without change in body position, each 10% change in body weight changes $\dot{V}O_2$ requirements by about 3%. For activities during which the body moves consistently horizontally, each 10% change in body weight changes $\dot{V}O_2$ requirements by about 4%. For activities during which the body moves primarily vertically, each 10% change in body weight changes $\dot{V}O_2$ requirements by about 6% to 7%.

TABLE 24–4

Oxygen Uptake Requirements for Various Activities for a 70-kg 170-cm Person

Activity	$\dot{V}O_2$, mL/min
Sitting or lying, resting	250
Desk work: calculating, typing, reading	300–350
Standing quietly	300
Standing with small movements	400
Personal grooming	300–600
Bartending, washing dishes by hand	400–800
Making beds	400–800
Washing windows; painting walls	400–1000
Scrubbing floors, kneeling	600–800
Standing cashier or clerking	400–600
Upright gardening	500–1000
Light industry, sitting	300–500
Light industry, standing	400–600
Medium industry	500–1000
Heavy industry	1000–1500 +
Pick and shovel work/digging trenches	1200–2000
Underground mining	600–1800
Lumbering	1200–2400
Walking, good surface	
2.5 mph	750
3.5 mph	1000
4.5 mph	1500
Walking, bad surface	
2.5 mph	900 +
3.5 mph	1300 +
4.5 mph	2000 +
Running, good surface	
5 mph	1600
7 mph	2700
10 mph	4000
Climbing stairs 40 feet/min	1200
Climbing 15% grade at 2.5 mph	1700
Climbing 10% grade at 3.5 mph	1800

These values are for a 70-kg person wearing normal attire. Extreme heat, altitude, or cold stress can also increase energy requirements but differences in body height are of minimal importance. For activities that are carried out in the sitting or standing position without change in body position, each 10% change in body weight changes $\dot{V}O_2$ requirements by about 3%. For activities during which the body moves consistently horizontally, each 10% change in body weight changes $\dot{V}O_2$ requirements by about 4%. For activities during which the body moves primarily vertically, each 10% change in body weight changes $\dot{V}O_2$ requirements by about 6% to 7%.

The Risk in Relying on Resting Studies Alone

In a 1971 study of 14 patients with extremely severe obstructive lung disease (mean FEV_1 29% of predicted), Vyas et al[60] found that 80% of the variance of peak $\dot{V}O_2$ was explained by the FEV_1. Thus it is tempting to rely on the American Thoracic Society statement[4] hypothesis that exercise limitation and peak $\dot{V}O_2$ can be correctly predicted by regression analysis using resting respiratory function tests alone in impairment evaluees with a diversity of lung diseases.

Sue has recently summarized and pointed out several problems in the use of this hypothesis.[54] First, in individuals with demonstrated reduced ventilatory capacity at rest (FEV_1 or MVV), ventilatory requirements during exercise are dependent not only on ventilatory capacity but also on the ventilatory requirement. The latter depends on the efficiency of gas exchange (ventilation/perfusion matching or mismatching), the ventilatory set point ($PaCO_2$), ventilatory drive (lung receptors, hypoxemia, metabolically induced acidemia), and the respiratory exchange ratio. Second, data from a recent larger study did not validate the hypothesis that exercise limitation can be quantified by resting pulmonary function testing. Cotes and coworkers,[21] in examining 157 referred men with a variety of lung diseases and abnormal resting studies (low FEV_1, FVC, FEV_1/FVC, or DLCO) who stopped exercise because of dyspnea (rather than other causes), found that the best combination of resting pulmonary function tests could account for only 29% of the variance of peak $\dot{V}O_2$ and 14% of the peak $\dot{V}O_2$ in percent predicted. As might be expected, both Cotes et al[21] and Carlson,[14] with 110 patients, found that adding values obtained during exercise appreciably improved their ability to predict peak $\dot{V}O_2$ or peak work rate using multiple regression analyses, but that the high variability of the prediction limited its usefulness in individual patients. Dillard[24] points out the difficulty in transferring such prediction formulae from one laboratory to the other. Third, ventilatory limitation is frequently not the factor limiting exercise in patients with known lung disease.[66] Finally, the finding of abnormal blood gases during exercise is poorly predicted from resting studies (see also Chapter 22).[57]

Differential Diagnosis

Many potential evaluees have symptoms and findings at rest that are suggestive of either heart or lung disease, or both. Exercise testing with exchange measurements is a logical early step in deciding which organ system is most limiting to evaluees in their work.

Consider an obese 53-year-old, cigarette-smoking, male foundry worker who has dyspnea, a daily cough, infrequent wheezing, and complains of vague epigastric discomfort with exertion or emotional upset. Routine examination discloses systemic hypertension, normal heart and breath sounds, a normal 12-lead ECG, and chest roentgenogram suggestive of interstitial lung disease. Respiratory function studies show a mildly reduced VC and a moderately reduced FEV_1, MVV, and DLCO. Resting arterial blood shows mild hypoxemia, mild hypercarbia, and a carboxyhemoglobin of 6%. It is unclear whether the evaluee's dyspnea is due primarily to obesity, obstructive or interstitial lung disease, or coronary artery disease. On incremental cycle ergometry with gas exchange, arterial blood, and ECG measurements, one of the following scenarios might occur:

1. At a moderate work rate the ECG shows 2-mm ST segment depression in the lateral chest leads, while the $\dot{V}O_2$ increases more slowly and the O_2 pulse does not increase appropriately as exercise is continued beyond this work rate. This strongly suggests that coronary artery disease is limiting cardiac output and O_2 transport increase when the ECG changes. Thus coronary artery disease is likely the dominant disorder.
2. The evaluee's exercise ventilation reaches his MVV with a ventilatory frequency of 55. The evaluee's peak $\dot{V}O_2$ nearly reaches his predicted peak $\dot{V}O_2$. However, he also becomes progressively hypoxemic and has an elevated VD/VT. The ECG remains normal. The finding of progressive hypoxemia, increased VD/VT, and tachypnea during exercise suggests that interstitial lung disease is his dominant disorder.
3. The resting hypoxemia resolves with exercise and the ECG remains normal. This indicates that the resting hypoxemia is due to obesity atelectasis rather than intrinsic lung disease.
4. The evaluee remains minimally hypoxemic and stops exercise close to his MVV with a ventilatory frequency of 35, a peak HR of 140, and a normal ECG. This indicates that the disorder limiting the evaluee's exercise tolerance is his obstructive lung disease.

In patients with known obstructive or restrictive lung disease, exercise testing may clarify not only whether impairment exists but also whether the limitation is primarily ventilatory or whether the impairment is secondary to accompanying pulmonary vascular disease and its effect on cardiac output.

Severity of Impairment

Exercise testing also assists in quantitating the severity of the impairment. This is one of the many sources of data that helps the examiners, both medical and nonmedical, in deciding the extent of impairment and whether a person is disabled. In the example given previously, the exercise findings would assist not only in establishing a diagnosis, but also in planning the most effective therapy and follow-up.

Neder et al,[47] in a study of 75 silicotic claimants, found that reduction in aerobic capacity (peak $\dot{V}O_2$), expressed as a percent of the predicted value for peak $\dot{V}O_2$ should be used for rating dysfunction rather than using the more traditional approach of normalizing impairment on the basis of mL/min/kg of $\dot{V}O_2$ body weight.

Assessment of Therapy

Exercise studies are often more useful than resting measures in assessing the results of therapy, whether pharmacotherapy (e.g., β-blockers for heart disease or β-agonists for obstructive lung disease); vessel repair of coronary artery or peripheral vascular disease; physical therapy for rehabilitation of patients with ventilatory limitation,[17] obesity, or coronary artery disease; O_2 therapy for interstitial, obstructive, or pulmonary vascular disease; or adjustment of cardiac pacemakers.

References

1. Ainsworth BE, Haskell WL, Leon AS, et al: Compendium of physical activities: Classification of energy costs of human physical activities. Med Sci Sports Exerc 25:71, 1993.
2. Altman PL, Gibson JF Jr, Wang CC: Handbook of Respiration. Dayton, Ohio, Wright-Patterson AFB, 1958.
3. American Heart Association Science Advisory: Assessment of functional capacity in clinical and research application. Circulation 102:1591, 2000.
4. American Thoracic Society: Evaluation of impairment/disability secondary to respiratory disorders. Am Rev Respir Dis 133:1205, 1986.
5. Astrand P-O, Rodahl K: Textbook of Work Physiology: Physiological Bases of Exercise, 3rd ed. New York, McGraw-Hill, 1986.
6. Auchincloss JH Jr, Ashoutosh K, Rana S, et al: Effect of cardiac, pulmonary, and vascular disease on one-minute oxygen uptake. Chest 70:486, 1976.
7. Beaver WL, Wasserman K, Whipp BJ: A new method for detecting the anaerobic threshold by gas exchange. J Appl Physiol 60:2020, 1986.
8. Beaver WL, Wasserman K, Whipp BJ: Bicarbonate buffering of lactic acid generated during exercise. J Appl Physiol 60:472, 1986.
9. Beaver WL, Wasserman K, Whipp BJ: On-line computer analysis and breath-by-breath graphical display of exercise function tests. J Appl Physiol 34:128, 1973.
10. Brooks GA, Fahey TD: Exercise Physiology: Human Bioenergetics and its Applications. New York, Wiley, 1984.
11. Bruce RA, Kusimi F, Hosmer D: Maximal oxygen uptake and nomographic assessment of functional aerobic impairment in cardiovascular disease. Am Heart J 85:546, 1973.
12. Buchfuhrer MJ, Hansen JE, Robinson TE, et al: Optimizing the exercise protocol for cardiopulmonary assessment. J Appl Physiol 55:1558, 1983.
13. Campbell SC: A comparison of the maximal voluntary ventilation with forced expiratory volume in one second: An assessment of patient cooperation. J Occup Med 24:531, 1982.
14. Carlson TA: Exercise capacity in patients with chronic obstructive lung disease. Chest 100:297, 1991.
15. Casaburi R, Barstow TJ, Robinson T, et al: Influence of work rate on ventilatory and gas exchange kinetics. J Appl Physiol 67:547, 1989.
16. Casaburi R, Daly J, Hansen JE, et al: Abrupt changes in mixed venous blood gas composition after the onset of exercise. J Appl Physiol 67:1106, 1989.
17. Casaburi R, Patessio A, Ioli F, et al: Reduction in exercise lactic acidosis and ventilation as a result of exercise training in patients with obstructive lung disease. Am Rev Respir Dis 143:9, 1991.
18. Casaburi R, Weissman ML, Huntsman DJ, et al: Determinants of gas exchange kinetics during exercise in the dog. J Appl Physiol 46:1054, 1979.
19. Clark JS, Votteri B, Ariagno RL, et al: Noninvasive assessment of blood gases. Am Rev Respir Dis 145:220, 1992.
20. Consolazio CF, Johnson RE, Pecora LJ: Physiological Measurements of Metabolic Functions in Man. New York, McGraw-Hill, 1963.
21. Cotes JE, Zejda J, King B: Lung function impairment as a guide to exercise limitation in work-related lung disorders. Am Rev Respir Dis 137:1089, 1988.
22. Covey MK, Larson JL, Alex CG, et al. Test-retest reliability of symptom-limited cycle ergometer tests in patients with chronic obstructive pulmonary disease. Nurs Res 48:9, 1999.
23. Dempsey JA, Hansen PG, Henderson KS: Exercise-induced arterial hypoxemia in healthy persons at sea level. J Physiol (Lond) 355:161, 1984.
24. Dillard TA: Exercise capacity in patients with chronic obstructive pulmonary disease. Chest 100:297, 1991.
25. Epler GR, McLoud TC, Gaensler EA, et al: Normal chest roentgenograms in chronic diffuse infiltrative lung disease. N Engl J Med 298:934, 1978.
26. Forte S, Carlone S, Vaccaro R, et al: Pulmonary gas exchange and exercise capacity in patients with systemic lupus erythematosus. J Rheumatol 12:2591, 1999.
27. Hansen JE: Exercise instruments, schemes, and protocols for evaluating the dyspneic patient. Am Rev Respir Dis 129:S25, 1984.
28. Hansen JE: Exercise testing for the pulmonologist. In Tierney DF (ed): Current Pulmonology. St Louis, Mosby-Year Book, 1993:14, pp 43–72.
29. Hansen JE, Casaburi R: Validity of ear oximetry in clinical exercise testing. Chest 91:333, 1987.
30. Hansen JE, Casaburi R, Cooper DM, et al: Oxygen uptake as related to work rate increment during cycle ergometer exercise. Eur J Appl Physiol 57:140, 1988.
31. Hansen JE, Sue DY, Oren A, et al: Relation of oxygen uptake to work rate in normal men and men with circulatory disorders. Am J Cardiol 59:669, 1987.
32. Hansen JE, Sue DY, Wasserman K: Predicted values for clinical exercise testing. Am Rev Respir Dis 129:S49–S55, 1984.
33. Hirsch GL, Sue DY, Wasserman K, et al: Immediate effects of cigarette smoking on cardiorespiratory responses to exercise. J Appl Physiol 58:1975, 1985.
34. Itoh H, Tanaguchi K, Koike A, et al: Evaluation of severity of heart failure using ventilatory gas analysis. Circulation 81(Suppl. 2):31, 1990.
35. Jones NL, Campbell EJM: Clinical Exercise Testing, 3rd ed. Philadelphia, WB Saunders, 1988.
36. Jones S, Elliott PM, Sharma S, et al: Cardiopulmonary responses to exercise in patients with hypertrophic cardiomyopathy. Heart 80:60, 1998.
37. Jones NL, Makrides L, Hitchcock C, et al: Normal standards for an incremental progressive cycle ergometer test. Am Rev Respir Dis 131:700, 1985.
38. Jones NL, McHardy GJR, Naimark A, et al: Physiological dead space and alveolar-arterial gas pressure differences during exercise. Clin Sci 31:19, 1966.
39. Kleber FX, Vietzke G, Wernecke KD, et al: Impairment of ventilatory efficiency in heart failure. Prognostic impact. Circulation 101:2803, 2000.
40. Koike A, Weiler-Ravell D, McKenzie DK, et al: Evidence that the metabolic acidosis threshold is the anaerobic threshold. J Appl Physiol 68:2521, 1990.
41. Lehninger AL: Biochemistry. New York, Worth, 1971.
42. Lewis SF, Haller RG: The pathophysiology of McArdle's disease: Clues to regulation in exercise and fatigue. J Appl Physiol 61:391, 1986.
43. Mannix ET, Dresser KS, Aukley D, et al: Cardiopulmonary exercise testing in the evaluation of patients with occupational asthma and reactive airways dysfunction syndrome. J Invest Med 46:236, 1998.
44. McArdle WD, Katch FI, Katch VL: Exercise Physiology: Energy, Nutrition, and Human Perfomance. Philadelphia, Lea & Febiger, 1981.
45. McGilvery RW: Biochemistry: A Functional Approach. Philadelphia, WB Saunders, 1970.
46. Meyer K, Westbrook S, Schwaibold M, et al: Short term reproducibility of cardiopulmonary measurements during exercise testing in patients with severe heart failure. Am Heart J 134:20, 1997.
47. Neder JA, Nery LE, Bagatin E, et al: Differences between remaining ability and loss of capacity in maximum aerobic impairment. Braz J Med Biol Res 31:639, 1998.
48. Passmore R, Durnin JVGA: Human energy expenditure. Physiol Rev 35:801, 1955.

49. Physician's Handbook for Evaluation of Cardiovascular and Physical Fitness. Nashville, Tennessee Heart Association, 1972.
50. Rahn H, Fenn WO: A graphical analysis of the respiratory gas exchange: The O_2–CO_2 diagram. Washington, DC, American Physiological Society, 1955.
51. Robinson TE, Sue DY, Huszczuk A, et al: Intra-arterial and cuff blood pressure responses during incremental cycle ergometry. Med Sci Sports Exerc 20:142, 1988.
52. Roston WL, Whipp BJ, Davis JA, et al: Oxygen uptake kinetics and lactate concentration during exercise in man. Am Rev Respir Dis 135:1080, 1987.
53. Sietsema KE: Oxygen uptake kinetics in response to exercise in patients with pulmonary vascular disease. Am Rev Respir Dis 145:1052, 1992.
54. Sue DY: Exercise testing in the evaluation of impairment and disability. Clin Chest Med 15:369, 1994.
55. Sue DY, Hansen JE: Normal values in adults during exercise testing. Clin Chest Med 5:89, 1984.
56. Sue DY, Hansen JE, Blais M, et al: Measurement and analysis of gas exchange during exercise using a programmable calculator. J Appl Physiol 49:456, 1980.
57. Sue DY, Oren A, Hansen JE, et al: Single breath diffusing capacity for carbon monoxide as a predictor of lung function and exercise gas exchange. N Engl J Med 316:1301, 1987.
58. Sue DY, Wasserman K, Moricca RB, et al: Metabolic acidosis during exercise in chronic obstructive pulmonary disease. Chest 94:931, 1988.
59. Sun X-G, Hansen JE, Stringer WW, et al: Carbon dioxide pressure–concentration relationship in arterial and mixed venous blood during exercise. J Appl Physiol 90:1798, 2001.
60. Vyas MN, Banister EW, Morton JW, et al: Response to exercise in patients with airways obstruction. Am Rev Respir Dis 103:410, 1971.
61. Wasserman K: Breathing during exercise. N Engl J Med 298:780, 1978.
62. Wasserman K: Dyspnea on exertion. JAMA 248:2093, 1982.
63. Wasserman K: The anaerobic threshold measurement to evaluate exercise performance. Am Rev Respir Dis 129(Suppl.):35, 1984.
64. Wasserman K, Beaver WL, Whipp BJ: Gas exchange theory and the lactic acidosis (anaerobic) threshold. Circulation 81(Suppl. 2):4, 1990.
65. Wasserman K, Hansen JE, Sue DY: Facilitation of oxygen consumption by lactic acidosis during exercise. News Physiol Sci 6:29, 1991.
66. Wasserman K, Hansen JE, Sue DY, et al: Principles of Exercise Testing and Interpretation, 3rd ed. Baltimore, Lippincott, Williams and Wilkins, 1999.
67. Wasserman K, McIlroy MB: Detecting the threshold of anaerobic metabolism in cardiac patients during exercise. Am J Cardiol 14:844, 1964.
68. Wasserman K, Van Kessel AL, Burton GG: Interaction of physiological mechanisms during exercise. J Appl Physiol 22:71, 1967.
69. Wasserman K, Whipp BJ: Exercise physiology in health and disease. Am Rev Respir Dis 112:219, 1975.
70. Wasserman K, Whipp BJ, Koyal SN, et al: Anaerobic threshold and respiratory gas exchange during exercise. J Appl Physiol 35:236, 1973.
71. Wasserman K, Whipp BJ, Koyal SN, et al: Effect of carotid body resection on ventilatory and acid-base control during exercise. J Appl Physiol 39:354, 1975.
72. Weber KT, Janicki JS (eds): Cardiopulmonary Exercise Testing: Physiologic Principles and Clinical Applications. Philadelphia, WB Saunders, 1986.
73. Whipp BJ, Seard C, Wasserman K: Oxygen deficit–oxygen debt relationships and efficiency of anaerobic work. J Appl Physiol 28:452, 1970.
74. Whipp BJ, Wasserman K: Efficiency of muscular work. J Appl Physiol 26:644, 1969.

CHAPTER

25

Pulmonary Impairment

STEPHEN L. DEMETER, MD, MPH

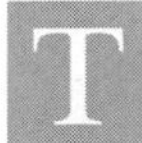he introduction of the fifth edition of the AMA Guides states:

> The Guides was first published in book form in 1971 in response to a public need for a standardized, objective approach to evaluating medical impairments ... The purpose of this fifth edition of the Guides is to update the diagnostic criteria and evaluation process used in impairment assessment, incorporating scientific evidence and prevailing medical opinion. Chapter authors were encouraged to 'use the latest scientific evidence from their specialty and, where evidence was lacking, develop a consensus view.'[11(p1)]

Toward these ends, the authors of the pulmonary chapter(s) have provided major revisions in the sections dealing with asthma and obstructive sleep apnea (OSA). A third major area of revision deals with the lower limits of normal used for forced vital capacity (FVC), forced expiratory volume in 1 second (FEV_1), and the diffusing capacity for carbon monoxide (DCO).

"The Guides continues to define impairment as a loss, loss of use, or derangement of any body part, organ system, or organ function."[11(p2)] Additionally, "(T)he term impairment in the Guides refers to permanent impairment ... "[11(p2)] Finally, impairment ratings are "consensus-derived estimates that reflect the severity of the medical condition and the degree to which the impairment decreases an individual's ability to perform common activities of daily living (ADL), excluding work. Impairment ratings were designed to reflect functional limitations and not disability."[11(p4)]

The chapter on respiration (Chapter 5) in the fifth edition of the Guides follows this philosophy. Although tables are provided reflecting the physiologic deviation from population-derived norms, for the FVC, FEV_1, DCO, and other variables, the concept of a decrease in a person's ability to perform ADL is well represented. The major emphasis of that chapter is on deviation from physiologic normality, as reflected in the FVC, FEV_1, DCO, or $\dot{V}O_2$ as opposed to functional limitations as measured either by cardiopulmonary exercise stress testing (see Chapter 24) or by work restrictions. Some pulmonary diseases, either by definition (e.g., occupational asthma) or by the predominant site of exposure (e.g., pneumoconiosis or hypersensitivity pneumonitis), by necessity cross the theoretical line separating impairment from disability; these distinctions are well explained in the respiratory chapter of the fifth edition of the Guides.

This chapter (25 on Pulmonary Impairment) concentrates on various diseases, explains how they are measured using the fifth edition of the Guides, and, in some circumstances, offers alternative means of arriving at an impairment rating. The last statement is not a criticism of the AMA Guides. The Guides provides for alternative methods of deriving impairment and this chapter works with the Guides to offer specific guidance in arriving at these values. Specific examples in this chapter include asthma, bronchiectasis, and OSA. Additionally:

> (S)ymptomatic assessment of individuals with respiratory disease is diagnostically useful, but it provides limited quantitative information and should not serve as the sole criterion upon which to make decisions about impairment. Rather, the examiner should obtain objective data about the extent of the limitation and integrate those findings with the subjective data to estimate the degree of permanent impairment.[11(p88)]

This chapter will also make comments on the fourth edition of the Guides because it is still widely used in many jurisdictions. Significant changes from the fourth to the fifth editions are discussed. The rules for impairment or disability under the Social Security system are included as the last section of this chapter.

This chapter has two foci: impairment rating by disease status and impairment rating by specific tests. Before an analysis of the disease status and tests can be performed, however, an important concept, especially in pulmonary disease—maximum medical improvement (MMI)—needs to be discussed.

MAXIMAL MEDICAL IMPROVEMENT

The fourth edition of the Guides defines impairment as "an alteration of an individual's health status."[15(p1)] It defines a permanent impairment as "one that has become static or stabilized during a period of time sufficient to allow optimal tissue repair, and one that is unlikely to change in spite of further medical or surgical therapy."[15(p1)] In the section "Rules for Evaluations," the fourth edition of the Guides state the following:

> (T)he treatment of an illness may result in apparently total remission of the patient's signs and symptoms. In these instances, the physicians may choose to increase the impairment by a small percentage (e.g., 1% to 3%) ... A patient may decline treatment of an impairment with a surgical procedure, a pharmacologic agent, or other therapeutic approach. The view of the Guides contributors is that if a patient declines therapy for a permanent impairment, that decision should neither decrease nor increase the estimated percentage of the patient's impairment. However, the physician may wish to make a written comment in the medical evaluation report about the suitability of the therapeutic approach and describe the basis of the patient's refusal.[15(pp8,9)]

The fifth edition uses the same philosophical approach but provides a number of recommendations that can modify the previous statements to allow for greater latitude when providing the final impairment rating:

> An impairment should not be considered permanent until the clinical findings indicate that the medical condition is static and well stabilized, often termed the date of Maximal Medical Improvement (MMI). It is understood that an individual's condition is dynamic. Maximal Medical Improvement refers to a date from which further recovery or deterioration is not anticipated, although over time there may be some expected change.[11(p9)]

The statements used in the Guides regarding a patient declining treatment still stand (see previous) but the fifth edition adds the following: "The physician may also need to address whether the impairment is at maximal medical improvement without treatment and the degree of anticipated improvement that could be expected with treatment."[11(p20)] Further, " (I)f, in spite of an observation or test result, the medical evidence appears insufficient to verify that an impairment of a certain magnitude exists, the physician may modify the impairment rating accordingly and then describe and explain the reason for the modification in writing."[11(p19)]

Consider the following three cases and the impact that the fifth edition makes upon the fourth. A 55-year-old man was seen for an impairment evaluation. He is a never-smoker. He had significant asbestos exposures in his early twenties and now has evidence of asbestosis on a chest x-ray. On physical examination, no wheezes were heard. His FVC is 70% of predicted and FEV_1 is 65% of predicted. The diffusing capacity (DLCO) is 70% of predicted. The second example is a 55-year-old never-smoker who was exposed to toxic fumes during the course of employment. He developed severe asthma. A review of his medical records showed that he had had a full pulmonary work-up in the past, after his toxic inhalation. His PC_{20} (see following) was 0.25 and his percent FEV_1 change was 12%, although he was on some breathing medications at the time of that evaluation. He now receives a beta-sympathomimetic (two puffs five times a day), an anticholinergic (two puffs five times a day), an inhaled steroid (beclamethasone equivalent of >1000 mcg), a theophylline (200 mg five times a day), a leukotriene antagonist, cromolyn (two puffs five times a day), and alternate day steroids (40 mg prednisone). On these medications, and with strict environmental and occupational restrictions, he is stable, experiencing an exacerbation only once or twice a year, on the average. On the day of the examination, no wheezing was heard. His FVC was 70% of predicted, FEV_1 was 65% of predicted, and DLCO was 70% of predicted. The third example is a 55-year-old man. He has smoked two packs per day since he was 18. He has mild dyspnea on exertion, frequent episodes of "bronchitis," and a daily productive cough. On the day of examination, he was so nervous that he smoked a full pack of cigarettes prior to seeing the examining physician, even though his appointment was at 11:30 AM. On examination, diffuse rhonchi and wheezing were heard. He takes no medications. A pre- and post-bronchodilator pulmonary function test was performed. After the bronchodilator, he stated that he felt better. The physical examination, while documenting improved airflow rates, was still positive for diffuse wheezing and rhonchi, although to a lesser degree. His spirometric values revealed an FVC of 70% of predicted, an FEV_1 of 65% of predicted, and a DLCO of 70% of predicted.

The above three examples, using the fourth edition, may have led the impairment examiner to produce identical impairment ratings. The asthma section of the fourth edition provided little direction for rating physicians when arriving at a whole person impairment (WPI) value. Using the fifth edition, Examinees 1 and 3 could still have been given the same rating (Class 2, 10% to 25% WPI)[11(p107)] but there are now new, discrete methods for rating asthmatics that would have resulted in a WPI percent of 26% to 50% (Class 3) for the second examinee.[11(p104)] Further, the smoker might receive a 0% rating based on the near-normal physiologic parameters and the expected changes that would occur after 6 months of smoking cessation and the possible use of minimal amounts of medications. These changes from the fourth to the fifth edition have allowed for a more equitable method of rating various claimants with different diseases and different levels of treatment.

Impairment by Disease Category

Chronic Obstructive Pulmonary Disease

There exist many discrete pulmonary diseases. Therefore, any simple categorization scheme will not and cannot cover each disease perfectly. However, the vast majority of pulmonary diseases, especially the more common ones, can be assorted relatively easily. Chronic obstructive pulmonary disease (COPD) could easily refer to the majority of respiratory diseases excluding acute infections but by common usage, it refers to a disease state characterized by varying degrees of emphysema and chronic bronchitis (Fig. 25–1). "Pure emphysema" is best exemplified in the never-smoking patient with alpha-1-antitrypsin deficiency. The pathologic changes are those of centri- and panacinar emphysema. Pulmonary function testing (PFT) abnormalities include hyperinflation (increased residual volume), small airflow obstruction (due to loss of elastic recoil), and disturbances in gas exchange. The "pink puffer" is a good example of a patient with COPD with emphysema predominating (Fig. 25–1, left).

Chronic bronchitis can be defined in several ways (Table 25–1). The "blue bloater" is a good example of the smoker with "chronic bronchitis" (Fig. 25–1, right) and is the clinical example used in this chapter as well as standard textbooks of internal and pulmonary medicine. The physiologic findings include airflow obstruction; there may be some improvement with bronchodilators but there is still airflow obstruction even after maximum bronchodilation. A reduced FVC is found, usually in overweight patients or caused by atelectasis from mucus plugging. It is always found in the presence of airflow obstruction that is of a greater degree than the amount

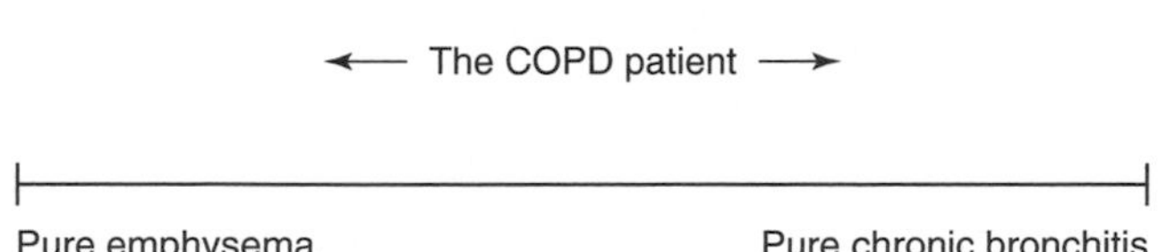

Figure 25–1. Distribution of patients with chronic obstructive pulmonary disease.

TABLE 25–1
Definitions of Chronic Bronchitis

Discipline	Definition
Epidemiologist	Cough and mucus secretion, at least 3 months per year, for 2 consecutive years
Radiologist	Excessive "bronchovascular markings" especially at the lung bases; "dirty lung"
Physiologist	Any nonreversible element of airflow obstruction
Pathologist	Hyperplasia of mucus secreting cells, smooth muscle hypertrophy, increased numbers of inflammatory cells
Clinician	A patient, usually a smoker, who presents with symptoms of cough, mucus hypersecretion, and some degree of shortness of breath; excludes asthmatics

of restriction, resulting in a decreased FEV_1/ FVC. The diffusion of gas is usually normalized when modified by the restriction although it can still be mildly abnormal (DLCO/VA; the diffusing capacity divided by the alveolar volume).

In the impairment evaluation of chronic bronchitis, measurement of the FVC or FEV_1 usually are adequate for assessment. There is usually some degree of improvement in the FVC, FEV_1, and FEV_1/ FVC with bronchodilator treatment although, as noted, these values never normalize. Thus many of the principles used in the assessment of asthma (see following) can be applied to patients with chronic bronchitis because these patients will generally display some degree of hyperresponsiveness on pulmonary function testing, although not to the same degree as the asthmatic, and usually require airway medications such as bronchodilators and anti-inflammatories.

The impairment evaluation of pure emphysema is more problematic. As discussed in Chapter 22, when the severity of the hyperinflation reaches a certain degree, a diminished VC will be found, although this is only in the presence of very severe hyperinflation. Thus, a reduction in the FVC will tend to underestimate the degree of pulmonary impairment because it does not change significantly in mild, moderate, or even mildly severe cases. As noted, the airflow obstruction in emphysema is in the small airways. Thus the $FEF_{25\text{-}75}$ (see Chapter 22) will reflect the changes in airflow in the emphysema patient better than the FEV_1, which reflects airflow obstruction in the larger airways. In the patient with emphysema, the decreases in FEV_1 follow the reductions in the $FEF_{25\text{-}75}$ but always to a lesser degree. The DLCO is a test of gas diffusion and is a reflection of V/Q (ventilation/perfusion) matching. It may or may not adequately express the pulmonary impairment in emphysema. As an example, imagine a lung composed of three alveolar-capillary units (Fig. 25–2*A*). If one of the alveoli is collapsed, a

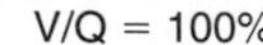

V/Q = 100%

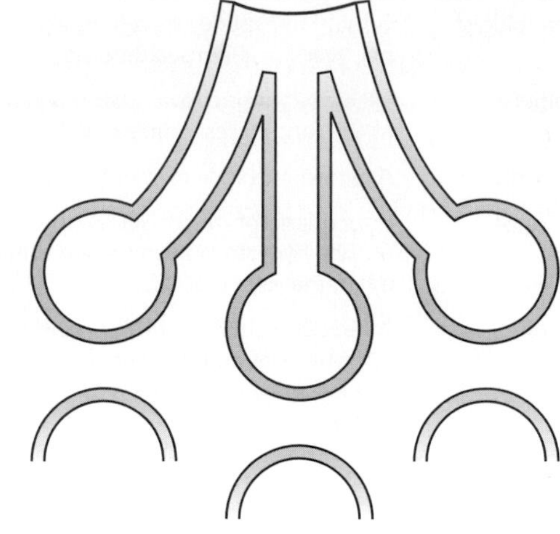

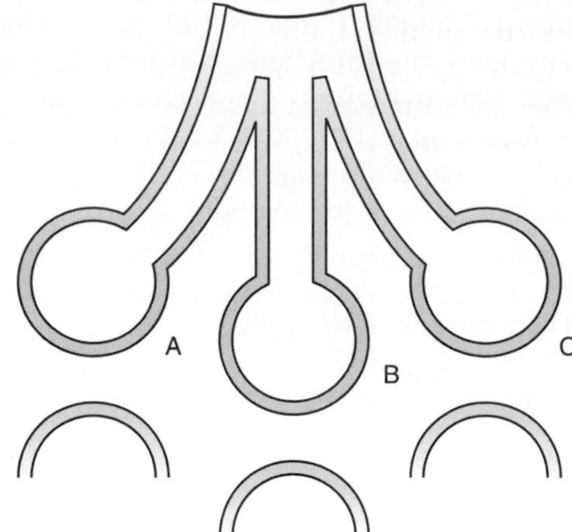

A

V/Q = .67%

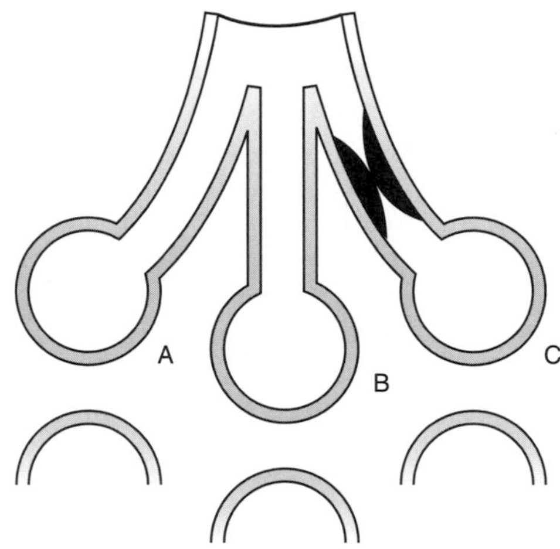

B

Figure 25–2. Ventilation/perfusion relationships. *A,* All alveoli are ventilating. All capillaries are perfusing. *B,* V/Q mismatch. Three alveoli are ventilating. Two capillaries are perfusing. *C,* V/Q mismatch. Two alveoli are ventilating. Two capillaries are perfusing.

V/Q = .33%

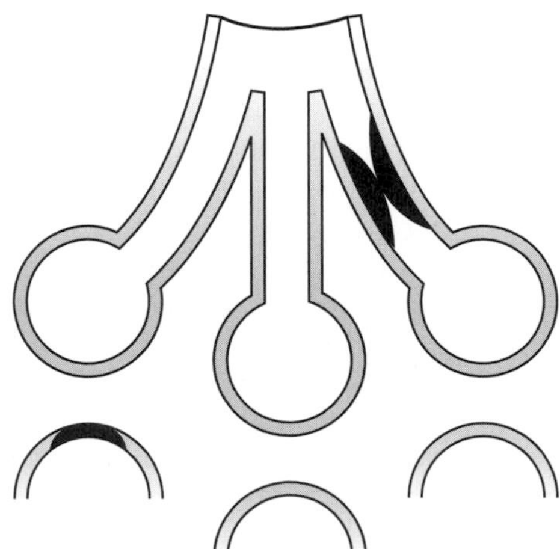

V/Q = .67%

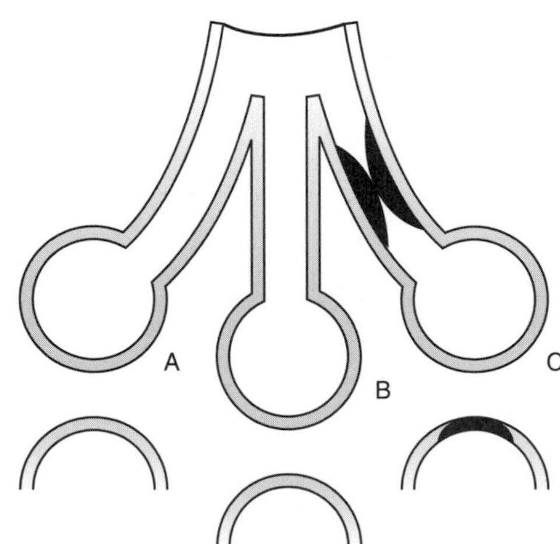

C

V/Q mismatch occurs. The same holds true if one of the capillaries is destroyed. If alveolus C is nonfunctional and if capillary A is nonfunctional, then the V/Q matching is only 33% (Fig. 25–2*C*). On the other hand, if only alveolus C is nonfunctional, then the V/Q matching is 66% of the total that would have been expected if all three alveoli and all three capillaries had been functional (Fig. 25–2*B*). If, in the resting condition, one relies on 50% of the total lung capacity for air exchange, then there is a sufficiently high disparity (V/Q = 33%) in the third example (Fig. 25–2*C*) to create a diminished DLCO at rest (which is how the test is performed in accordance with the rules expressed in the Guides[11(p94)]). The gas exchange abnormality in the second example (Fig. 25–2*B*; V/Q = 67%) is not sufficiently high to produce an abnormality at rest but an abnormality will be expressed when all the alveoli and all the capillaries are asked to function, as in maximal exercise. Therefore, the abnormality in the second example will be seen only during an exercise test. The normal lung is composed of varying degrees of V/Q mismatching. Thus, there is a potential to seriously underestimate the true impairment in emphysema when using a resting DLCO. The same potential, for reasons cited, exists when using the decrease in the FVC as a surrogate of the increased RV.

Recommendations

In a patient with COPD, the greater to the right in Figure 25–1 the examinee is, the greater can be the reliance on the resting FVC and FEV_1 (especially the post-bronchodilator value). The DLCO may well be superfluous because it is usually normalized by the reduction in the VC in these patients (a normalized DLCO/VA—or the diffusing capacity divided by the alveolar volume). Therefore, measurement of the FVC and FEV_1 will usually suffice to arrive at an impairment rating. Whereas the fifth edition of the Guides does not specifically address the issue of medication usage in these individuals, the examiner may wish to use a modification of the principles found in the asthma section when assessing these patients. As noted, a written explanation must be given if one wishes to make this type of modification. Further, the greater to the right that a person is on the graph in Figure 25–1, the more applicable these modifications become.

The greater to the left the examinee is (signifying more parenchymal and less pure airway problems), the greater the need for exercise testing becomes. The greater to the left the examinee is, the more the measurements of the resting FVC, FEV_1, and DLCO inaccurately assess the degree of impairment. Therefore, the examiner should, by physical examination, radiography, or analysis of more complete pulmonary function testing (see Chapter 22), determine if the examinee is sufficiently close to the pure emphysema model. In that circumstance, exercise testing should be used as the sole test for an adequate assessment of pulmonary impairment.

The fifth edition of the Guides provides for this change in rating procedure when it states that a complete cardiopulmonary stress test (CPEST) "can be helpful when the results of pulmonary function tests do not correlate with the individual's symptoms or when additional information is needed to clarify the nature and severity of an impairment."[11(p161)] (See the example of impairment due to emphysema.[11(p111)])

The fourth and fifth editions of the Guides provide for impairment when a persons' PaO_2 is <55 mm Hg or when it is <60 mm Hg with certain associated qualifying conditions and when the PaO_2 is assessed twice, 4 weeks apart, to ensure validity. Neither edition uses the SpO_2 value although the fifth edition states that it "often provides an adequate estimate of hypoxia."[11(p101)] The reliability of the SpO_2 was discussed in Chapter 22. Therefore, a simple method of assessment for the claimant with severe emphysema would be exercising while wearing an oxygen monitor (for example, walking to tolerance on the level or climbing stairs provided the history and physical examinations preclude angina as the exercise limiting factor). This should be done without oxygen and assumes that the resting SpO_2 was >89% (if it were less, the examination is over and the physician should rate the claimant as having severe impairment, in accordance with the rules set forth in the Guides; the patient with severe emphysema, however, usually has near normal resting values that quickly fall with exercise). If the SpO_2 does not fall below 89%, then a CPEST can be performed.

Asthma and Chronic Bronchitis

The major problem in the assessment and rating of pulmonary impairment due to obstructive airway disease is the reversible nature of these diseases. The examples given at the beginning of this chapter suffice to demonstrate the difficulty in these assessments. Problems encountered by the nature of the disease include the following:

1. Is the patient stable and at baseline or temporarily worsened?
2. What medication(s) is/are the person taking (including type, number, and dosages)?
3. Is the person receiving the medications in an optimal fashion?
4. How should impairment be assessed when a patient is treated by a family practitioner versus a pulmonary or allergy specialist?

A corollary problem is the concept of MMI.

As noted, the fourth edition of the Guides states, "(A) patient may decline treatment of an impairment with a surgical procedure, a pharmacologic agent, or other therapeutic approach. The view of the Guides contributors is that if a patient declines therapy for a permanent impairment, that decision should neither decrease nor increase the estimated percentage of the patient's impairment."[15(p9)] Further, the fourth edition of the Guides defined permanent impairment as "one that has become static or stabilized during a period of time sufficient to allow optimal tissue repair, and one that is unlikely to change in spite of further medical or surgical therapy."[15(p1)] The marked disparity in these two statements is obvious.

In 1987, Chan-Yeung addressed this problem during impairment evaluations in patients with asthma by recommending impairment values that take into account the degree of hyper-responsiveness, the amount of medication given (as a surrogate of the degree of hyper-responsiveness, especially if those studies were not available), and an impairment grade based on both factors.[9] In 1993, Dr. Chan-Yeung and others sitting on an ad hoc committee of the American Thoracic Society (ATS) published a formal set of rules based on several variables including the degree of hyper-responsiveness, the postbronchodilator FEV_1, and the minimum medication needed to maintain control of the asthma. Point criteria were developed and asthma was divided into five rating classes.[3] Dr. Chan-Yeung and her co-chair, Dr. Harber, extended these criteria for the first edition of this book.[22] These papers become the basis for the changes in the asthma section of the fifth edition of the Guides.

Table 5–9 in the fifth edition of the Guides[11(p104)] (reprinted as Table 25–2) and Table 2 in the ATS guidelines[3(p1059)] both address the issue of airway hyperresponsiveness as reflected by improvement in FEV_1 following the use of a bronchodilator or by the PC_{20}. Both sources give the rules for which of the two to use. It is important for the examiner to use one or the other, not both. This concept can be overlooked easily on casual reading.

Table 5–9 of the Guides and Table 2 of the ATS paper both develop scores based on 3 variables: the postbronchodilator FEV_1, the % change of the FEV_1 *or* the PC_{20}, and the minimum medication need. The score of these 3 variables are then added and the WPI for asthma is determined by that total score (Table 5–10 of the Guides; reprinted here as Table 25–3) or an impairment class is derived (Table 4 of the ATS guideline paper).[3(p1060)]

TABLE 25–2

Asthma Impairment Scoring: Impairment Classification for Asthma*

Score	Postbronchodilator FEV_1	% of FEV_1 Change (Reversibility) or	PC_{20} mg/mL or Equivalent (Degree of Airway Hyperresponsiveness)†	Minimum Medication‡
0	≥ lower limit of normal	<10%	>8 mg/mL	No medication
1	≥ 70% of predicted	10% to 19%	8 mg/mL to >0.6 mg/mL	Occasional but not daily bronchodilator and/or occasional but not daily cromolyn
2	60% to 69% of predicted	20% to 29%	0.6 mg/mL to >0.125 mg/mL	Daily bronchodilator and/or daily cromolyn and/or daily low-dose inhaled corticosteroid (≤800 μg of beclomethasone or equivalent)
3	50% to 59% of predicted	≥30%	≤0.125 mg/mL	Bronchodilator on demand and daily high-dose inhaled corticosteroid (>800 μg of beclomethasone or equivalent) or occasional course (one to three courses a year) of systemic corticosteroid
4	<50% of predicted	. . .	. . .	Bronchodilator on demand and daily high-dose inhaled corticosteroid (>1000 μg of beclomethasone or equivalent) and daily or every other day systemic corticosteroid

* FEV_1 indicates forced expiratory volume in the first second; PC_{20} is the provocative concentration that causes a 20% fall in FEV_1. Add the scores for postbronchodilator FEV_1, reversibility of FEV_1 (or PC_{20}), and medication use to obtain a summary severity score for rating respiratory impairment.

†When FEV_1 is greater than the lower limit of normal, PC_{20} should be determined and used for rating of impairment; when FEV_1 is less than 70% of the predicted, the degree of reversibility should be used; and when FEV_1 is between 70% of the predicted and the lower limit of normal, either reversibility or PC_{20} can be used. The score for minimum medication use is added to the appropriate measurement criteria outlined above.

‡Need for minimum medication should be demonstrated by the treating physician, for example, through previous records of exacerbation when medications have been reduced.

From Cocchiarella L, Andersson GBJ (eds): Guides to the Evaluation of permanent Impairment, 5th ed. Chicago, American Medical Association, 2001, p 104, with permission.

TABLE 25-3

Asthma Impairment Scoring: Impairment Rating for Asthma*

Total Asthma Score	% Impairment Class	Whole Person Impairment
0	1	0%
1–5	2	10% to 25%
6–9	3	26% to 50%
10–11 or asthma not controlled despite maximal treatment, i.e., FEV_1 remaining <50% despite use of >20 mg/day of prednisone	4	51% to 100%

* The impairment rating is calculated as the sum of the individual's scores from Table 25-2. FEV_1 indicates forced expiratory volume in the first second. From Cocchiarella L, Andersson GBJ (eds): Guides to the Evaluation of permanent Impairment, 5th ed. Chicago, American Medical Association, 2001, p 104, with permission.

Despite the improvement in asthma assessment found in the fifth edition, there are still some areas of concern. Table 1 of the ATS Guidelines discusses the postbronchodilator FEV_1.[3] This table is similar but not identical to the postbronchodilator FEV_1 section in Table 5–9 of the fifth edition.[11(p104)] A score of 1 is given by the ATS when the postbronchodilator FEV_1 is between 70% of predicted and the lower limit of normal. A score of 0 is given if it is greater than the lower limit of normal. The Guides gives a score of 1 if it is ≥70% of predicted but less than the lower limit of normal and 0 if it is greater than or equal to the lower limit of normal. The other scores (2 through 4) are the same. However, more importantly, the ATS recommends that:

> (S)pirometric measurements should be made, if possible, after withholding inhaled bronchodilators for 6 h and long-acting bronchodilators (e.g., long-acting theophylline preparations) for 24 h. However, if it is not possible to withhold bronchodilators for this period of time, they can be used, but the time these medications are taken before the test should be noted. Antiinflammatory preparations such as cromolyn, inhaled or systemic corticosteroid should not be withheld.[3(p1056)]

These restrictions are not mentioned in the Guides.

The concept of the postbronchodilator FEV_1 is confusing. There is a separate table/section assessing bronchial hyper-responsiveness as determined either by the % change in the FEV_1 after the administration of a bronchodilator or by the PC_{20}. There is also a table/section reflecting medications. In an asthmatic or suspected asthmatic, obtain the prebronchodilator FEV_1 and use this value if it is normal or above. Use the post bronchodilator FEV_1 if the prebronchodilator FEV_1 is below the lower limit of normal (pg 103).

It seems that this FEV_1 should be the value measured at MMI—i.e., when the claimant is stable, on full treatment, and with no medications held. It should be measured before and after the administration of a bronchodilator. This value would then represent the FEV_1 at MMI, which, unfortunately, is not the population "normal" for all patients with asthma owing to a variety of factors including airways remodeling (a condition recognized recently; it is characterized by permanent airway obstruction caused by fibrosis of small airways due to persistent, unrelieved inflammation).

Another problematic area concerns the ATS testing protocol. The ATS guidelines mention certain testing requirements.[3] As noted, inhaled bronchodilators should be held for 6 hours and long-acting bronchodilators for 24 hours. The ATS guidelines do not recommend that anti-inflammatory medications (such as cromolyn or inhaled or systemic steroids) be held.[3(p1056)] However, as discussed in Chapter 22, these medications can diminish the degree of bronchial hyper-responsiveness and, therefore, depress an individual's overall score, thus penalizing the claimant who is compliant with medication.

When determining the PC_{20}, if the bronchoconstrictor chosen is methacholine, the ATS guidelines recommend holding the short-acting beta-sympathomimetic or ipratropium for 6 hours and the long-acting beta-sympathomimetic or theophylline for 24 hours.[3(p1057)] Ipratropium is an anticholinergic medication and, therefore, an antagonist of methacholine. It will cause a falsely increased PC_{20} when administered within 6 hours of the methacholine challenge. Beta-sympathomimetics can also falsely increase the PC_{20}. Therefore, instead of "or," the guidelines should have said "and." If the bronchoconstrictor chosen is histamine, "short-acting antihistamines should be withheld for 48 hours and astemizole for 1 or 2 months."[3(p1057)]

The ATS recommends the following: "subjects should be asked to refrain from smoking and exposure to cold air for two hours before the test."[3(p1057)] The implications of this last statement are obvious. However, if the authors of the guidelines wished to have the examinee avoid asthmogenic precipitators prior to the test, other precipitators such as exercise, secondhand smoke, and fumes (including perfumes and hair sprays) should also have been mentioned.

As seen, there are a variety of rules in the testing protocol developed by the ATS although some are incomplete. No rules or protocols are found in the Guides.[11] This deficiency is covered by the following statement: "(T)he AMA recommends that the examinee follow ATS guidelines when assessing asthma impairment and include measurements of pulmonary mechanics, airway hyper-responsiveness, and medication requirements,"[11(p103)] with a reference to the ATS guidelines.[3] Nevertheless, it would have been helpful for the Guides to list the ATS protocol in this section.

Another area of concern is the table of minimum medication need. The Guides and the ATS use an identical scoring scheme in this section. The medications listed are bronchodilators (not defined, although the ATS guidelines mention both short- and long-acting beta-sympathomimetics and theophylline as bronchodilators; ipratropium is also a bronchodilator and, although mentioned, it was not afforded this status in the ATS guidelines), cromolyn, and inhaled or systemic corticosteroids. Medication usage was meant to be a reflection of the medication recommendations found in the Expert Panel Report published by the National Heart, Lung, and Blood Institute (NHLBI). This consensus report was first published in 1991 (the only version available to the ATS when it published its guidelines in 1993)[17] and updated in 1997.[18] These guidelines recommend an escalating usage of medications based on their general properties (i.e., short- or long-acting bronchodilators or anti-inflammatories) and the clinical severity of the asthma, ranging from mild and intermittent to severe and persistent.[17,18]

The concept of minimal medication need is well defined in both the Guides and the ATS paper.[3,11] The ATS defines it as the "minimum required to maintain control (or the best results) in a subject and that reduction in medications leads to exacerbations of symptoms and reduced lung functions."[3(p1060)] This is the same concept used in the Guides.[11(pp103–104)]

This raises the next problem. First, is the minimum amount of medication needed to prevent exacerbations also the same amount needed to produce the "best overall results"? (This is a term found in the ATS guidelines and the AMA Guides. It is defined as the medications needed to produce the "least symptoms, least need for β-adrenergic agonist when taken only if required, best expiratory flow rates, least diurnal variation of flow rates and least side-effects from medication."[3[p1059]]) It would seem intuitively obvious that the best results would be achieved with a level of medication above that necessary only to prevent acute exacerbations. If the minimum medication need is defined as that amount needed to prevent an acute exacerbation ("[T]he need for minimum medication should be demonstrated by the treating physician, e.g., previous records of exacerbation when medications have been reduced,"[3[p1059]] with a similar remark found in the Guides[11[p104]]), how should the evaluating physician make this assessment? As suggested by both sources, this task can only be performed by the treating physician, but only if that physician had liberally "experimented" on his or her patient, using various medications in varying dosages, and while completely documenting every change based on the history of asthma symptoms, the physical examination, and spirometric indices. Without such "experimentation" and documentation and without a prolonged follow-up period to demonstrate the efficacy of this prescription package, the evaluating physician cannot be assured that the minimum medication need requirement of these protocols has been fulfilled.

Further, the ATS states the following:

> (E)valuation for permanent impairment/disability should be done after the objectives of optimal treatment of asthma have been attained ... If the objectives of treatment are not achieved, the following should be done: 1. Give rating for temporary impairment (see tables 1 through 4). 2. Recommend specific treatment, or give referral to a specialist experienced in the management of asthma (e.g., pulmonary physician or allergist). 3. State when to reevaluate (when the objectives of treatment have been achieved or in 6 months, whichever is shorter).[3(p1059)]

The shortcomings of this protocol are less obvious for the treating physician than for the impairment evaluator. There is no evidence to suggest that the 6-month interval will fulfill the anticipated objectives. However, if one is the impairment evaluator, there are two major problems: if one does as suggested above, then the impairment evaluator has crossed over the threshold of becoming a "treating physician" (a role that most impairment evaluators scrupulously avoid); and the protocol introduces a time factor that most impairment evaluators and most referring sources would find difficult.

Asthma medications are listed in Table 3 of the ATS paper and Table 5–9 in the Guides (they are identical) and are limited to bronchodilators (not defined), cromolyn, and inhaled or systemic steroids. The inhaled steroid is beclomethasone or "equivalent." Currently, there are six recognized, major medication groups for the treatment of asthma: sympathomimetics, anticholinergics, theophyllines, corticosteroids, cromolyns, and leukotriene modifiers. There are a number of other medications that are used, albeit very infrequently, that modify the asthmatic response by diminishing the bronchial inflammatory response, including methotrexate, gold compounds, tetracyclines, and others. Antihistamines are commonly used for the treatment of asthma in Europe but have not been commonly used in the United States.

The last problem encountered concerns the inhaled steroids used in asthma treatment. Table 3 of the ATS guidelines[3(p1059)] and Table 5–9 of the fifth edition of the Guides[11(p104)] define low/high dose inhaled corticosteroids as being ≤800 mg/>800 mg and >1000 mg of beclomethasone or equivalent. Neither source defines the concept of a beclamethasone equivalent. To define a beclomethasone equivalent from a review of the medical literature is a study fraught with difficulty. Some of the variables encountered, which make direct comparisons difficult, are found in Table 25–4. Despite the diffi-

TABLE 25-4

Some Variables Affecting the "Head-to-head" Comparison Between Various Inhaled Corticosteroids

1. Means of determining therapeutic index (TI = efficacy/side effects)
   a. Therapeutic benefit as measured in changes in the FEV_1 or (peak expiratory flow rate)
   b. Side effect profile as assessed by:
      i. Disturbances in the hypothalamic-pituitary axis
      ii. Growth retardation in children
      iii. Development of osteoporosis
      iv. Development of cataracts
      v. 24-Hour urinary cortisol excretion
   c. Binding affinity for human lung glucocorticoid receptors
   d. Topical blanching potency in human skin
   e. Pharmacokinetics including:
      i. Plasma half-life
      ii. Volume of distribution
      iii. Clearance
      iv. First pass metabolism
      v. Bioavailability
2. Dosing
   a. Number of doses
   b. TI equivalents
   c. mg Content
3. Preparation
   a. Aerosol
   b. Dry powder
4. Delivery system
   a. Metered dose inhaler
   b. Aerosol
   c. Spinhaler
   d. Tubohaler
   e. Twisthaler
   f. Diskus device
5. Frequency of administration (difference in the TI existing between qd, bid, tid, and qid dosing)
6. Time of administration (difference between AM and PM dosing)
7. Speed of inhalation
8. Use of spacer device
9. Propellant
   a. Chlorofluorocarbon
   b. Hydrofluoralkane
10. Hygroscopic nature of the inhaled formulation
11. Systemic levels
   a. Site of absorption
   b. Efficacy of metabolism
12. Technique

qd = once a day; bid = twice a day; tid = three times a day; qid = four times a day.

TABLE 25-5

"Beclomethasone Equivilants" Conversion Formulae

Generic Name	Brand Name	Equivalent Dose*	Conversion Formula
Beclomethasone	Vanceril	20	1:1
Dipropionate	Vanceril DS	10	1:2
	Beclovent	20	1:1
	Q Var 40	10	1:2
	Q Var 80	5	1:4
Triamcinolone Acetinide	Azmacort	10	1:2
Budesonide	Pulmicort	5	1:4
Flunisolide	Aerobid	8	1:3
Fluticasone†	Flovent 44	6.6	1:3
Propionate	Flovent 110	3.3	1:6
	Flovent 220	1.7	1:12

800 μg Beclomethasome = 20 puffs; 1,000 μg beclomethasone = 25 puffs.
*Equivalent doses are based on 20 puffs of beclomethasone.
† Flovent DPI (diskus) μg—50, 100, and 250—use the values for the metered dose inhaler of 44, 110, and 220, respectively.

culties, a suggested comparison scheme is found in Table 25–5. This table was developed by the author and reflects references 7, 8, 14, 18, 26, 27, 31, and 33, a general perusal of the medical literature, product information from various manufacturers, and personal communications. Because of the problems noted in Table 3, this table represents a "gestalt" of the author's opinions, based on experience and the various sources noted previously, and is offered as a suggested comparison between various preparations.

A final problem, not necessarily germane to the asthma section of the Guides or to the ATS guidelines, is other reactive airways diseases. Hyper-reactivity or asthmogenicity is seen with a variety of other conditions and diseases (see Tables 22–12 and 22–13). The example of chronic bronchitis was given previously. Because these diseases are predominantly diseases of the airways, should an application of the tables and philosophy found in the asthma section of the Guides be applicable to these diseases as well? Chapter 5 in the fifth edition does not address this issue.[11] Indeed, the example used for chronic bronchitis (5–4, page 109[11]) does not mention the use of medications.

Table 25–6*A–C* represent this author's recommendation for assessing impairment due to respiratory diseases. Parts A, B, and C address the issues of air flow obstruction, reversibility, hyper-responsiveness, and medication usage germane to patients with asthma or chronic bronchitis. Of note, the PC_{20} is not used in this scheme, as opposed to the ATS criteria[3] or the Guides.[11] This deletion was intentional as it is believed that the degree of responsiveness, as reflected in the final FEV_1 and the amount of medication used, are adequate surrogates for the degree of hyper-responsiveness. It is intuitively obvious that the greater the degree of hyper-responsiveness, as reflected by a low PC_{20}, the greater the need for higher levels of treatment (see Chapter 59 on the "rheostat" model of asthma). Further, if a person with severe hyper-responsiveness is not on sufficient medication to maximally treat his or her airways disease, then a lower FEV_1 will be found on the day of testing.

TABLE 25–6 A

Whole Person Impairment WPI due to Medication Usage in Pulmonary Conditions

Medications[a,b,c]	WPI (%)
1	3
2	6
3	9
4	12
5	15
6	18
7[d]	21

To use Table A, the claimant must demonstrate his or her metered dose inhaler (MDI) technique if he or she is on this type of medication. If, in the opinion of the evaluator, little or no medication is actually being inhaled, then the WPI% should be downgraded appropriately. It should be recognized that there is buccal absorption of sympathomimetics and anticholinergics. Therefore, rate the improper use of these medications at ½ the value that would have had if were being used appropriately. Poorly administered steroids or cromolyns receive a value as if they were not being used. See reference 18 for various inhalational techniques for MDIs.

[a] Medication for 1–6 include B_2 sympathomimetics (inhaled or oral), anticholinergics, theophyllines, cromolyns, inhaled steroids, and leukotriene modifiers.

[b] Does not include herbal preparations, "alternative" medicines, nonmedical prescriptions (e.g., biofeedback, hypnosis), or allergy desensitization preparations.

[c] The above medications are expected to be used at therapeutic doses and on a daily basis. As needed medication usage only is rated at a 1% level.

[d] Alternative medicines in 7 include gold salts, methotrexate, minocycline, and other immune modulators.

Table 25–6*A–C* shares the goals and objectives of the ATS guidelines[3] and the Guides.[11] It also uses medication need/usage as a surrogate for the severity of a person's asthma. It differs in some respects. Less reliance is placed on asthma tests. Table 25–6*A–C* anticipates that the treating physician uses airway medications appropriately (e.g., the patient with "pure emphysema" is not receiving large numbers and doses of airway medications). It uses a larger number of medications, better reflecting the NHLBI guidelines. The table is meant to be used for all pulmonary diseases that encompass airway pathology, not just asthma. Finally, it was not meant to replace the Guides. Rather, it is to be used for determining impairment where difficulties arise when using the Guides. Its philosophical and physiologic approach is entirely consistent with that developed by the Guides and differs only in methodology.

Lung Cancer

Lung cancer is covered well within section 5.9 of the fifth edition[11(p106)] and will not be further commented on. The approach used in the fourth edition is consistent with the fifth.[15]

Chronic Cough

Chronic cough can be caused by a variety of pathologic entities and is a symptom or sign of the disease rather than a distinct pathologic entity. It can be thought of in the same fashion as chronic pain in a patient with a musculoskeletal problem. Common pulmonary causes of chronic cough include asthma and chronic bronchi-

TABLE 25–6 B

WPI due to Altered Physiology

FEV_1 or FVC[a]	Decreased From Prior FEV_1%[c,d,e,f]	WPI (%)	Extrapolation Value[b]
>80	0–10	0	0
70–80	10–15	1–5	2
60–70	16–20	6–10	2
50–60	20–30	11–15	2
40–50	30–40	16–25	1
30–40	40–50	26–35	2
20–30	50–60	36–50	2
<20	>60	51–100	1

To use Table B, the following criteria must be met:

1. No smoking on the day of the examination.
2. No exposure to asthmogenic stimulants on the day of the examination.
3. Absence of active respiratory infection for at least 6 weeks.
4. Fulfill criteria in Table A. Further, the claimant must be taking medication on his or her routine schedule and on the day of testing.
5. This test can be done before or after an inhaled bronchodilator is used. If done after, add one point to the medications in Part A if there is ≥10% change in the FEV_1.

[a] Use the forced vital capacity FVC or forced expiralory volume in 2 second FEV_1, not both

[b] Use the extrapolation value for an FVC or FEV_1 e.g., 72% = 4% WPI (70–80% = 10% spread; 1–5% = 5% spread; 5/10> = 0.5% WPI for each 1% change in the FEV_1; therefore, a 72% FEV_1 = 3% WPI as the FEV_1 is decreased by 8% and 8% 0.5=4%)

[c] When corrected for time, FEV_1 only

[d] Is preferred over the % predicted FEV_1 or FVC

[e] Must be done while the claimant is on similar medications; otherwise there is no meaningful comparison

[f] See also Chapter 22.

TABLE 25-6 C

WPI due to Usage of Oral Corticosteriods*

Medication	WPI
Low dose alternate day	5%
Low dose daily	10%
High dose alternate day	10%
High dose daily	20%

To use Table C, the following criteria must be met:
1. Use of oral steroids for at least 6 months
2. Anticipation of chronic use
3. Fulfill criteria in Tables A and B
4. Require oral doses greater than or equal to 10 mg in the absence of adrenal failure; with adrenal failure, subtract replacement dose from total daily dose (est. 5–10 mg/day of prednisone
5. Cutoff between low and high dose in prednisone equivalent is 25 mg

* If the examinee is Cushingoid while on inhaled corticosteroids and is not currently receiving oral corticosteroids (within 2 weeks of the examination) and if in the examiner's opinion the Cushingoid features are believed to be caused solely by the systemic absorption of the inhaled corticosteroids, add 10% to the WPI and subtract one medication in Table A.

tis. Less common pulmonary causes include interstitial lung disease, bronchiectasis, bronchiolitis obliterans, and endobronchial lesions (including tumors). As a rule, rating the pulmonary disorder adequately assesses impairment caused by chronic cough. However, there are other causes of chronic cough that are not solely due to pulmonary disease, including gastroesophageal reflux disease and chronic rhinosinusitis. These two syndromes can create impairment due to the chronic cough alone or due to a worsening of underlying asthma. As such, assessing impairment for these diseases should be done by rating the asthma or for the primary organ system disease, and then combining the two values.

Occasionally, chronic cough can be the principal cause of impairment. As noted, chronic cough is a symptom of a disease rather than a disease itself and can be considered, during the course of an impairment evaluation, in a fashion similar to pain. Pain presenting from an orthopedic problem is included in the impairment rating given for the restricted function of the joint. Yet separate guidelines exist when pain is the principal problem or when the degree of pain is out of proportion to the degree of functional loss. The same problem may hold true for a chronic cough. The Guides mention, indirectly, this type of issue when addressing impairment due to bronchiectasis.[11(p107)]

Indeed, chronic cough can be severe and frequent (occurring every several minutes) with frequent paroxysms (lasting several minutes) causing near or true syncope, vomiting, urinary/fecal incontinence, chest pain, sleep disruptions, hoarseness, and headache. Thus there can be significant disturbances in ADL. Following the example of chronic pain as a cause of impairment, if chronic cough is to be assessed as the principal problem, regardless of cause (except for lung cancer), then the assessment and rating should be given for its impact on ADL and not added to or combined with the disturbance created by the underlying physiologic abnormalities.

When assessing impairment created by a chronic cough, an exhaustive search should be performed to identify the underlying pathologic cause. These causes, as mentioned above, can be created by both pulmonary and nonpulmonary diseases and may or may not create pulmonary physiologic disturbances. Nonpulmonary causes that are devoid of pulmonary disturbances are rare but can occur and include problems such as vagal nerve stimulation caused by a lesion in the left hilar area (aortic aneurysm, hilar lymphadenopathy) or other causes of vagal stimulations such as gastroesophageal reflux disease (stimulation of the vagus nerve due to irritation of the distal esophagus) or foreign material (such as a hair) on the tympanic membrane. Textbooks of pulmonary disease can assist with the list of differential causes.

If no underlying pathology is found, a fictitious or functional cough should be considered. Signs and symptoms suggesting a functional cough include a harsh, brassy cough; lack of cough during sleep; and symptoms suggesting secondary gain or psychological disturbances. If one were to assess impairment due to a functional cough, the rating would be based on the disturbance of ADL. This is the same approach as used in the assessment of psychological diseases and the overlap is obvious. It is best, however, to address this as a symptom of a psychological disturbance and assess the chronic cough from that perspective or to refer the claimant to a psychologist or psychiatrist for a more thorough psychological examination.

Cysts, Cavities, Blebs, and Bullae

The above pathologic entities are discovered radiographically and may or may not be associated with emphysema. As isolated entities, they rarely produce pulmonary impairment until they are large enough to restrict the functional capacity of the lung. Therefore, the VC (or FVC) becomes the primary method of analysis on the static PFTs, with the exercise test being a more accurate reflection of the degree of reduction in maximal lung function. The amount of pulmonary impairment in these disorders is a direct reflection of the amount of the total lung capacity (TLC) that is reduced by these areas of nonfunctioning lung.

Hyperventilation Syndrome

Hyperventilation syndrome (HVS) refers to the constellation of symptoms that occur in response to hyperventilation. Hyperventilation is physiologically expressed as an increase in the alveolar minute ventilation (a product of the tidal volume times the respiratory rate times the proportion of air actually reaching the alveoli [represented by the dead space/tidal volume ratio (VD/VT); the lower the ratio, the greater the alveolar respiration; the greater the depth of an inhalation, all things being equal, the lower the VD/VT, as the VD will remain constant at any given point in time for any given disease process]). It is reflected by the following equation:

$$\dot{V}A = \frac{TV \times RR}{VD/VT}$$

A higher alveolar minute ventilation can be caused by an increase in the tidal volume, a decrease in the dead space/tidal volume ratio, or an increase in the respiratory rate. Any of the three variables, singly or in combination, may cause a sufficient change in the $PaCO_2$ and pH to produce the symptoms of HVS. Another frequent respiratory pattern associated with HVS is frequent "sighing." A sigh ventilatory effort may easily produce a VT (or tidal volume [TV]) that is 5 to 10 times higher than a normal TV. Because the VD (dead space volume) is constant, the VD/VT decreases and the $\dot{V}A$ increases substantially during that minute. Patients with HVS have been observed to sigh as frequently as once every 1 to 3 minutes, thus creating an increase in $\dot{V}A$ sufficient to cause the syndrome.

A useful test to confirm the presence of HVS is to ask the examinee to hyperventilate for 30 to 60 seconds. In the author's experience, this will reproduce the symptoms in at least 80% of individuals with this syndrome. The only test cited in traditional medical literature for this syndrome is an arterial blood gas analysis performed during a symptomatic period. The classic finding is a respiratory alkalosis and is quite helpful in emergency ward settings. Unfortunately, it is less useful in the patient with chronic, intermittent symptomatology. If this approach is used (hyperventilation for 30 to 60 seconds), the examiner should be cautious. Hyperventilation may produce coronary vasospasm, thus precipitating a myocardial infarction in a patient with significant coronary artery blockage.[14] Some individuals with HVS have underlying asthma and testing for this condition should also be considered.[14]

Interstitial Lung Diseases (Including Hypersensitivity Pneumonitis)

There are at least 150 different causes of interstitial lung disease (ILD). All are characterized by pathology in the interstitial compartment. The ultimate physiologic expression of abnormality in ILDs will be V/Q mismatching (see previous and Chapter 22).

The first through fourth editions of the Guides were basically silent on these disorders. The fourth edition described the physical examination findings[15(pp156–157)] and radiographic abnormalities[15(pp157–158)] and discussed impairment rating for pneumoconioses and hypersensitivity pneumonitis in Table 10.[15(p164)] When rating impairment caused by ILD, the fourth edition of the Guides stated: "(I)mpairments in persons with these conditions should be evaluated by physicians with expertise in lung disease, and the impairment estimate should be left to the physician's judgment."[15(p164)] The fourth edition also provided an example (an examinee with asbestosis) and used the values for the FVC, FEV_1, and DLCO for impairment assessment, although it also provided the exercise $\dot{V}O_2$ max and stated that the "oxygen uptake was decreased, probably because of pulmonary dysfunction."[15(pp165–166)]

The fifth edition[11] has a separate section for hypersensitivity pneumonitis (section 5.7, pp 105–106) and pneumoconioses (section 5.8, p 106) and offers several examples. It suggests using Table 5–12 (reprinted as Table 25–8) when assessing impairment using the variables of FVC, FEV_1, DCO, and $\dot{V}O_2$.

Because the primary alteration in ILDs is a V/Q mismatch, exercise testing should be the preferred method of impairment assessment. A chest x-ray or, better, high-resolution computed axial tomography scan of the lung, is required for confirmation of the presence of ILD. A pathologic specimen is an alternative and may be necessary in x-ray negative disease (see Chapter 22). Many ILDs are characterized by disease progression with little expectation of reversal, stabilization, or even slowing of the rate of progression with medication (e.g., asbestosis). Therefore, by definition, these diseases are frequently never "static or well stabilized." The report by the examining physician should address this issue, when appropriate, and make recommendations for future testing and reporting. Some ILDs (e.g., hypersensitivity pneumonitis) may respond to treatment, either partially or completely. It is therefore reasonable to suggest that when these types of diseases are present, the examination be deferred for up to 6 months after withdrawal from the precipitating agent or after the disease is treated.

Should radiographic abnormalities alone be used as a method of impairment rating, either in place of or in addition to physiologic testing methods? The Guides do not address this as an issue. The fourth edition of the Guides stated, "the correlation of interpretations and reading with physiologic measures of impairment is poor."[15(p158)] Yet impairment is a deviation from normality. ILD on a chest x-ray represents a deviation from normality. The Guides state that the goal of an impairment rating is to determine the effect of that deviation on ADL. A person with an ILD on a radiograph may or may not have disturbed physiology, even during maximal exercise. Therefore, should a person with only radiographic abnormalities have an impairment rating? (By way of comparison, a person without a fifth digit has a 5% WPI rating, although this may produce no impact on his or her ADL.) The concern is the possibility that subtle disturbances in pulmonary physiology exist that may not be accurately measured. For example, the claimant who was previously capable of working at a level of 12 to 15 metabolic equivalents (METS) and is currently capable of 10 METS has developed a physiologically important deviation from his or her prior health status. Yet using Table 5–12 (fifth edition)[11(p107)] or Table 8 (fourth edition)[15(p162)] of the Guides (see Table 25–6), this person would have a 0% impairment rating unless one were to use the concept of a decrease from prior exercise levels as defined in the fifth edition. However, if the amount of deviation from the prior health status is less marked than in the above example, then such extrapolations become extremely difficult. Table 25–9 reflects this author's recommendations on the use of radiographs as a means of determining WPI caused by ILD.

How Should Impairment Caused by ILDs Be Assessed?

As a rule, by using Table 8 of the fourth edition of the Guides (Table 25–7) or Table 5–12 of the fifth edition of the Guides (Table 25–8), one can adequately assess the claimant with an ILD by using the $\dot{V}O_2$ section. When the examiner believes that this table does not adequately express the deviation from premorbid health, then it is recommended that the examiner extrapolate to determine the estimated premorbid $\dot{V}O_2$ max by perusing appropriate reference tables and matching these values with the examinee's stated premorbid capabilities, either occupational or recreational. This estimated value would then be the "normal" for this individual and the impairment rating would be assessed using the principles found in Chapter 5 of the Guides and Table 5–12 (e.g., a person who was capable of playing full court basketball prior to the development of an ILD would have needed to produce, on the average, 12 METS. If the examinee is a currently capable of performing only at an 8-MET level, then there is a current discrepancy of 4 METS. Admittedly, there is no clear-cut way to use Table 5–12 in this fashion, but a 33% decline in lung function would place a person in Class 2 [10% to 25% WPI] using the spirometric portion of the chart). However, one must be cognizant that other variables can also create this discrepancy, including the effects of aging, other organ system disease, and deconditioning. For these reasons, these types of extrapolations are best left within the hands of specialists skilled in this type of physiologic assessment. Any opinion should be supported in writing so that the goal of a 10% deviation between two experts may be achieved (see Chapter 2 of the fifth edition[11]).

It is also recommended that an impairment rating be given for the presence of ILD on a radiograph or biopsy in those cases where the physiologic changes are minor or impossible to calculate (see Table 25–9).

Masses

The same comments that apply to cysts and bullae can be applied to masses because the same general physiologic abnormalities will be found, albeit for a different reason.

Sleep Apnea Syndrome

OSA syndrome is a frequent problem affecting an estimated 2% to 4% of the adult U.S. population.[31] As discussed in Chapters 22 and 59, OSA can cause both morbidity and mortality. Untreated OSA is associated

TABLE 25–7

Classes of Respiratory Impairment*

	Class 1: 0%, no impairment of the whole person	**Class 2: 10–25%, mild impairment of the whole person**	**Class 3: 26–50%, moderate impairment of the whole person**	**Class 4: 51–90%, severe impairment of the whole person**
FVC FEV_1 FEV_1/FVC (%) Dco	FVC ≥ 80% of predicted; and FEV_1 ≥ 80% of predicted; and FEV_1/FVC ≥ 70%; and Dco ≥ 70% of predicted or	FVC between 60% and 79% of predicted; or FEV_1 between 60% and 79% of predicted; or Dco between 60% and 69% of predicted or	FVC between 51% and 59% of predicted; or FEV_1 between 41% and 59% of predicted; or Dco between 41% and 59% of predicted or	FVC ≤ 50% of predicted; or FEV_1 ≤ 40% of predicted; Dco ≤ 40% of predicted. or
$\dot{V}O_2$ max	>25 mL/(kg·min); or >7.1 METS	Between 20 and 25 mL/(kg·min); or 5.7–7.1 METS	Between 15 and 20 mL/(kg·min); or 4.3–5.7 METS	< 15 mL/(kg·min); or < 1.05 L/min; or <4.3 METS

* FVC, forced vital capacity; FEV_1, forced expiratory volume in the first second; Dco, diffusing capacity of carbon monoxide. The Dco is primarily of value for persons with restrictive lung disease. In Classes 2 and 3, if the FVC, FEV_1, and FEV_1/FVC ratio are normal and the Dco is between 41% and 79%, then an exercise test is required.

$\dot{V}O_2$max, or measured exercise capacity, is useful in assessing whether a person's complaint of dyspnea is a result of respiratory or other conditions. A person's cardiac and conditioning status must be considered in performing the test and in interpreting the results.

From Doege T, Houston TP (eds): Guides to the Evaluation of Permanent Impairment, 4th ed. Chicago, American Medical Association, 1993, p 162, with permission.

TABLE 25–8

Impairment Classification for Respiratory Disorders Using Pulmonary Function and Exercise Test Results*

Pulmonary Function Test	Class 1: 0% Impairment of the Whole Person	Class 2: 10%–25% Impairment of the Whole Person	Class 3: 26%–50% Impairment of the Whole Person	Class 4: 51%–100% Impairment of the Whole Person
FVC	Measured FVC ≥ lower limit of normal (see Tables 5–2b and 5–3b) *and*	≥ 60% of predicted and < lower limit of normal *or*	≥ 51% and ≤ 59% of predicted *or*	≤ 50% of predicted *or*
FEV_1	Measured FEV_1 ≥ lower limit of normal (see Tables 5–4b and 5–5b) *and*	≥ 60% of predicted and < lower limit of normal *or*	≥ 41% and ≤ 59% of predicted *or*	≤ 40% of predicted *or*
FEV_1/FVC	FEV_1/FVC ≥ lower limit of normal *and*			
Dco	Dco ≥ lower limit of normal (see Tables 5–6b and 5–7b) *or*	≥ 60% of predicted and < lower limit of normal *or*	≥ 41% and ≤ 59% of predicted *or*	≤ 40% of predicted *or*
$\dot{V}o_2$ max	$\dot{V}o_2$ max ≥ 25 mL/(kg·min) *or* > 7.1 METS	≥ 20 and < 25 mL/(kg·min) *or* 5.7–7.1 METS	≥ 15 and < 20 mL/(kg·min) *or* 4.3 to < 5.7 METS	< 15 mL/(kg·min) *or* < 1.05 L/min *or* < 4.3 METS

* FVC indicates forced vital capacity; FEV_1, forced expiratory volume in the first second; Dco, diffusing capacity for carbon monoxide; $\dot{V}o_2$max, maximum oxygen consumption; and METS, metabolic equivalents (multiples of resting oxygen uptake). Dco is primarily of value for persons with restrictive lung disease. In Classes 2 and 3, if FVC, FEV_1, and FEV_1/FVC are normal and Dco is between 41% and 79%, then an exercise test is required to determine level of impairment.
From Cocchiarella L, Andersson GBJ (eds): Guides to the Evaluation of Permanent Impairment, 5th ed. Chicago, American Medical Association, 2001, p 107, with permission.

with the risk of developing a variety of cardiovascular complications including stroke, hypertension, cardiac arrhythmias, and congestive heart failure. Untreated OSA is associated with daytime somnolence, occasionally of a severe degree. Patients with untreated OSA can have intellectual dulling that can affect not only work performance but also ADLs. Occasionally, patients with OSA will have daytime somnolence severe enough to cause sleeping while driving or during other significant or risky activities. These patients obviously pose a risk to themselves and to others. This also poses a problem with traveling to and from the workplace. OSA is treated in a variety of ways (see Chapter 59) with variable degrees of success.

TABLE 25–9

Interstitial Lung Disease (ILD) Impairment Based on Abnormal Radiographs or Biopsy[a,b,c]

Variable	Percent
Presence of ILD with no physiologic disturbances	5%
Presence of ILD with physiologic disturbances creating 1–10% WPI	5%
Presence of ILD with physiologic disturbances greater than 10% WPI	0%

[a] ILO/UC classification 1/1 or greater for the CXR (see Table 22–11)
[b] This category requires that the interstitial fibrosis makes up most of a single lobe, at the minimum
[c] ILDs creating >10% WPI are not assessed by this method as this section is reserved for those individuals with trivial physiologic disturbances or disturbances impossible to measure (see text)
[d] Extrapolate to find the value. The maximum value in this category is 10%. The physiologic WPI is divided by 0.5 and then added to the impairment based on the value provided by the radiographic or biopsy value. For example, a 6% value based on the $\dot{V}o_2$ yields an 8% WPI (6 × 0.5 = 3; 3 + 5 = 8)
WPI, whole person impairment; CXR, chest x-ray.

The diagnosis of OSA depends on the sleep study (polysomnogram). The history and physical examination, although providing important clues, are insufficient in making this diagnosis (see Chapters 22 and 59). Likewise, an overnight oxygen desaturation recording, although providing evidence of need for oxygen treatment and identifying cardiovascular risk, is insufficient when making a diagnosis of OSA (see Chapters 22 and 59). Finally, OSA is a clinical syndrome. It is a combination of significant symptoms and OSA. The amount of sleep apneas a person has is expressed as a number referred to as the apnea/hypopnea index (AHI) or respiratory disturbance index (RDI); the two terms are synonymous. An AHI of 5 or less is considered normal. An AHI greater than 30 is graded as moderate to severe OSA. OSA is graded into four levels of severity based primarily on the degree of daytime symptoms (Table 25–10).

The fourth edition of the Guides provided little direction for assessing impairment in OSA. In the introduction to the pulmonary chapter in the fifth edition,[11(p87)] the authors state that "the section on sleep apnea has been updated to reflect current assessment and practice." Section 5.6 covers OSA.[11(p145)]

TABLE 25-10

Obstructive Sleep Apnea Syndrome Severity Index

Severity	AHI	Symptoms
Asymptomatic	5–15	Observed apneas or incidental finding of apneic activity (elevated from age-adjusted AHI values)
Mild	5–15	Passive sleepiness with apneic activity and cardiovascular risk
Moderate	15–30	Active sleepiness, breathing-disturbed sleep, and cardiovascular risk
Severe	>30	Disabling sleepiness and cardio-pulmonary failure, neurocognitive deficits, and increased apneic activity

AHI, apnea/hypopnea index.
From Nieto FJ, Young TB, Lind BK, et al: Association of sleep-disordered breathing, sleep apnea, and hypertension in a large communitity-based study. JAMA 283:1829–1836, 2000; and Strohl KP, Redline S: Recognition of obstructive sleep apnea. Am J Respir Crit Care Med 154:279–289, 1996, with permission.

From an historical perspective, the first edition of the Guides[12] did not mention OSA. The second edition, however, devoted a whole section to it (Appendix C, pp 229–239) and provided several examples of how to rate impairment based on OSA and narcolepsy.[1] The third and third revised editions recommended using criteria found in the chapters on neurology, cardiovascular disease, and mental and behavioral problems.[2,16] The fourth edition spends a full page of text (pp 163–164) describing OSA and recommends that "(P)atients with documented sleep apnea who have received effective therapy should be reevaluated by polysomnography before they are judged to be severely impaired."[15(p164)]

Causes of Medical Impairment

OSA is linked with a variety of cardiovascular complications. Hypertension was one of the first recognized comorbid conditions and it appears to be about twice as frequent in patients with OSA as in the general population.[24,29] Daytime hypertension is estimated to occur in 50% to 90% of OSA patients, with OSA being found in approximately 20% to 60% of all hypertensive patients.[19,29,30] OSA is an independent risk factor for the development of hypertension and the chances of developing hypertension are linked to the AHI. One study found that the odds ratio for developing hypertension with an AHI of 0 to 4.9 was 1.42; for an AHI of 5 to 14.9, it was 2.03; and it was 2.89 with an AHI of >15.[25] In another study, there was an odds ratio of 2.0 for an RDI of 5 and 5.0 for an RDI of 25.[37] Reductions in the degree of hypertension are seen with control of the OSA.[19,29,30]

A variety of arrhythmias have been reported in patients with OSA, including sinus arrhythmias, extreme sinus bradycardia (<30 beats per minute), asystoles (up to 6.3 seconds), second-degree atrio-ventricular (AV) block, premature ventricular contractions, and ventricular tachycardia.[10,23,32] These arrhythmias are more frequent during sleep and are diminished with successful treatment of the sleep apnea.[10,32] However, atrial arrhythmias (atrial flutter, atrial fibrillation, paroxysmal atrial tachycardia), first and second degree AV block, and bradyarrhythmias (with sinus arrest of 2.9 seconds) can all be found during rapid eye movement sleep in young, healthy adults.[13] Thus the implications of arrhythmias in patients with OSA are currently unknown.[13,23] Nevertheless, serious arrhythmias can occur, are related to RDI, and can be successfully treated in most circumstances with nasal continuous positive airway pressure (NCPAP) therapy.[10]

Most of the data linking OSA and ischemic heart disease are found in reports of patients who snore or in patients who are studied after a myocardial infarction. Prospective studies are lacking to suggest a relationship between OSA and the development/causation of myocardial ischemia/coronary artery disease.[23] Two other issues further confound the problem. Myocardial infarctions tend to occur more commonly in the early morning hours, regardless of the presence of OSA. Nocturnal desaturations and hormonal changes are believed to be the causative factors.[6] Both right and left ventricular dysfunction is found in patients with acute myocardial infarction. OSA is more frequently found in patients with pulmonary edema/left-sided congestive heart failure.[13,23] Thus, an effect/cause rather than a cause/effect relationship is more likely to be present. Cheyne-Stokes breathing is seen in approximately 40% of patients with a left ventricular ejection fraction less than 40% and Cheyne-Stokes breathing may present as OSA.[13] OSA has been diagnosed with an odds ratio of 23.3 in these circumstances.[13] OSA, however, is a likely cause of nocturnal angina in patients with coronary artery disease created by ischemic events caused by oxygen desaturation during the anemic episode.[6]

Both right and left ventricular dysfunction, with frequencies of 71% and 31%, respectively, have been described in patients with severe OSA. Obstructed breathing that creates increased negative intrathoracic pressures and a decrease in the cardiac output causes these abnormalities. Whereas improved physiology has been demonstrated in treated patients, the overall frequency of congestive heart failure in all patients with OSA is yet to be defined.[23]

Articles linking OSA to stroke make similar comments to those made regarding myocardial ischemic events. Strokes occur more commonly between the hours of 6:00 AM and noon and are caused by diminished blood flow and oxygen carrying capacity to areas of the brain with arterial obstructions. Strokes are seen more commonly in snorers and patients with other features of OSA. Sleep disturbances are seen following strokes. However, again, the implications of OSA, from a prospective point of view, are yet unclear.[6,23]

Weiss et al reviewed the medical literature regarding the link between OSA and cardiovascular physiology and pathophysiology.[39] They found a direct relationship between OSA and systemic hypertension but, owing to numerous confounding variables, could not establish a direct cause and effect relationship for OSA and myocardial infarction, stroke, meaningful atrial or ventricular arrhythmias, pulmonary hypertension, or left ventricular hypertrophy.[39]

From a neuropsychiatric viewpoint, OSA is associated with abnormalities in mood and affect including depression, anxiety, irritability, and diminished quality of life.[23] The neurocognitive impairment of OSA appears to be correlated with the RDI with changes in general intellectual ability, learning and memory, sustained and focused attention, executive functions, information processing efficiency, visual and psychomotor performance, bilateral motor speed, and reaction times.[23,29] Improvement is seen in treated patients.[35,36]

The daytime drowsiness and neurocognitive disturbances help to explain the increased risk of traffic accidents in patients with OSA. The risk of a traffic accident is correlated with the RDI and also the concomitant use of alcohol (independently).[5] In 1994, the Board of Directors of the ATS produced an official policy statement on OSA and driving risk. It summarized the risk to the patient, the risk to the physician, and legal issues.[4]

Impairment Assessment in OSA

As noted, untreated OSA is associated with a variety of medical conditions that either enhance or create both morbidity and mortality. A suggested scheme for rating impairment combines Tables 25–11*A* and 25–11*B*. This table incorporates Table 13–4 from the neurology chapter of the 5th edition of the Guides (Table 25–11*A*).[11(p317)] Chapter 5 (the Pulmonary chapter of the fifth edition of the Guides) provides no clear direction on rating OSA. "For purposes of impairment rating as discussed in this chapter, refer to the judgment of a sleep specialist."[11(p105)] The fourth edition does not even offer this statement on rating.

The difference between Tables 25–11*A* and *B* and the fifth edition of the Guides is the addition of impairment for the use of CPAP or bilevel CPAP mask or oral-facial appliances. This impairment rating is added owing to the interference in ADL created by wearing these devices (without which the symptoms and risks recur). Additionally, as noted, Table 13–4 (Table 25–11*A*) is incorporated into the recommendations for impairment rating. This table is preferred over Table 6 of the fourth edition[15(p143)] because it more accurately reflects disturbances in ADL in these individuals. When the two tables are compared, it is seen that there are marked differences in the impairment ratings for Classes 2 through 4. In the fifth edition, Class 2 has a rating value of 10% to 29% as opposed to 10% to 19% in the fourth edition; for Class 3 it is 30% to 69% versus 20% to 39%; and for Class 4 it is 70% to 90% versus 40% to 60%. The descriptions are not the same but are close enough not to make too much difference. Class 4, for example, refers to a person who has such severe problems that he or she is "unable to care for self in any situation or manner."[11(p317)] A 70% to 90% rating is more appropriate for these individuals than a 40% to 60% rating.

As described in Chapter 59 and above, successful treatment of OSA can reduce its impact on both the cardiovascular and neurocognitive sequelae of the syndrome. However, not all patients can be successfully treated. Also, in many circumstances, the full clinical implications of lowering the RDI and diminishing daytime somnolence are unknown. Nevertheless, a WPI is considered appropriate owing to the excessive rates of morbidity and mortality. Additionally, OSA treatment effects should be considered when addressing the cardiac or psychiatric patient.

TABLE 25–11 A

Impairment due to Sleep Apnea Syndrome (Combine Tables A and B)

A: Criteria for Rating Impairment Due to Sleep and Arousal Disorders

Class 1: 1%–9% Impairment of the Whole Person	**Class 2: 10%–29% Impairment of the Whole Person**	**Class 3: 30%–69% Impairment of the Whole Person**	**Class 4: 70%–90% Impairment of the Whole Person**
Reduced daytime alertness; sleep pattern such that individual can perform most activities of daily living	Reduced daytime alertness; interferes with ability to perform some activities of daily living	Reduced daytime alertness; ability to perform activities of daily living significantly limited	Severe reduction of daytime alertness; individual unable to care for self in any situation or manner

From Cocchiarella L, Andersson GBJ (eds): Guides to the Evaluation of Permanent Impairment, 5th ed. Chicago, American Medical Association, 2001, p 317, with permission.

TABLE 25-11B

Sleep Apnea Syndrome

Presence and Compliance with Treatment

Treatment	WPI%
NCPAP/BiPAP	10
Appliances	10

NCPAP, nasal continuous positive airway pressure; BiPAP, bilevel positive airway pressure.

Criteria have been proposed for the treatment of OSA.[4,28,33] A consensus statement by the ATS recommended treatment with CPAP for "all OSA patients with an RDI ≥30 events per hour, regardless of symptoms, based upon the increased risk of hypertension" and "patients with an RDI of 5 to 30 events per hour accompanied by symptoms of excessive daytime sleepiness, impaired cognition, mood disorders, insomnia, or documented cardiovascular diseases to include hypertension, ischemic heart disease, or stroke."[28(pp864–865)]

As discussed above, this author recommends an approach departing from the Guides rating impairment based on OSA by adding Tables 25–11*A* and 25–11*B*. There are two sources of WPI created by OSA. The first deals with interruption of ADLs created by daytime somnolence. The second deals with the interference in ADLs created by the treatment of OSA. The WPI rating for claimants with OSA should also be assessed from a cardiovascular and neurocognitive perspective, using the appropriate chapters of the Guides. This value should then be combined with the rating from Table 25–11*B*. Several examples are given in the following to demonstrate the author's approach to rating for OSA (without mentioning comorbid disease states) using the combination of Tables 25–11*A* and 25–11*B*.

■ Example 1: A 45-year-old woman with documented OSA presents for an impairment evaluation. Her RDI is 35 and she has symptoms of daytime somnolence. NCPAP treatment is recommended and she is compliant with it. On treatment, her RDI is 8 and she is asymptomatic. Her impairment rating is 10% (0% from Table 25–11*A* and 10% from Table 25–11*B*). ■

■ Example 2: The same patient as in Example 1 except that she cannot tolerate the CPAP mask or appliances. Surgery was not considered to be an effective form of treatment for her and was not offered. Her only real complaint caused by the OSA is excessive fatigue. Her husband tells you that she goes to work but can rarely go out at night. She goes to bed at 8:30 PM and awakens at 6:30 AM during the week and 10:00 AM on weekends. Her impairment rating is 9% (she is in Class 1 = 9%; 9% from Table 25–11*A* and 0% from Table 25–11*B*). ■

■ Example 3: The same patient as in Example 1 except that her pretreatment RDI was 65 and her post-treatment RDI is 45. Her daytime symptoms are the same as in Example 2. Her impairment is now 18% (9% from Table 25–11*A* combined with 10% from Table 25–11*B* = 19% WPI). ■

■ Example 4: Same as in Example 3 except that the patient continues to have excessive daytime somnolence as witnessed by her husband. She no longer falls asleep while driving or eating but cannot do her housework efficiently because of fatigue. She no longer works outside of the home for the same reason. Her impairment is now 55% (she is now in Class 3 = 50% from Table 25–11*A*, combined with 10% from Table 25–11*B* = 55% WPI. Of course, the 50% from Table 25–11*A* was arbitrary, but it reflects the disturbance in her ADL). ■

■ Example 5: A 40-year-old man weighs 350 pounds. He is not capable of sustaining wakefulness for more than 1 hour at a time although his episodes of sleep may be brief (5 minutes). He is noncompliant with treatment. His impairment rating is 90% (he is in Class 4 = 90% from Table 25–11*A* and 0% from Table 25–11*B*. (The Guides state "a 90% to 100% WP impairment indicates a very severe organ or body system impairment requiring the individual to be fully dependent on others for self-care, approaching death."[11(p5)]) ■

Other Airway Obstructive Diseases

Asthma will be the predominant problem in all examinees with obstructive airways diseases. However, other diseases fall into this category, including bronchiectasis and bronchiolitis obliterans. The approach to these diseases is similar to that seen in the COPD section. As with chronic bronchitis, airway diseases other than asthma will share ventilation (or airways) abnormalities with perfusion problems. The approach to an impairment assessment for these diseases should be considered as a spectrum, similar to the approach used in the COPD examinee. The greater the ventilation problem, the greater the reliance on the FVC and FEV_1. In these cases, assessing for the amount of medications used (as a surrogate of the amount of airways disease or hyperresponsiveness) will be of value. At the other end of the spectrum, the perfusion end, the greater the reliance on the arterial blood gases, SpO_2, and CPEST. Which of these two approaches is used initially depends on the clinical skill and judgment of the evaluator. Ultimately, both approaches may be needed in these patients and the choices are, again, left to the impairment evaluator.

TABLE 25–12

Criteria for Rating Permanent Impairment Due to Pulmonary Hypertension

Class 1: 0%–9% Impairment of the Whole Person	Class 2: 10%–29% Impairment of the Whole Person	Class 3: 30%–49% Impairment of the Whole Person	Class 4: 50%–100% Impairment of the Whole Person
No symptoms or signs of right HF and mild pulmonary hypertension (PAP 40–50 mm Hg) or a Doppler echocardiography-derived peak tricuspid velocity of 3.0–3.5 m/sec	No symptoms or signs of right HF and moderate PA hypertension (PAP 51–75 mm Hg)	Moderate pulmonary hypertension (PAP > 75 mm Hg) **and** signs and symptoms of right HF **or** symptoms of mild limitation (Class 2) with any degree of pulmonary hypertension	Severe pulmonary hypertension (PAP > 75 mm Hg) **or** symptoms of severe limitation (Class 3 or 4) with any degree of pulmonary hypertension

From Cocchiarella L, Andersson GBJ (eds): Guides to the Evaluation of Permanent Impairment, 5th ed. Chicago, American Medical Association, 2001, p 79, with permission.

Pulmonary Vascular Disease

The most common pulmonary vascular disorder is pulmonary hypertension. Most patients with pulmonary hypertension have secondary causes that are created by a variety of diseases including those that cause a loss of the pulmonary vasculature, especially the pulmonary capillaries (e.g., emphysema, ILD, bronchiectasis, chronic pulmonary emboli); hypoxemic pulmonary vascular constriction ("blue bloater" chronic bronchitis, OSA); or increased pulmonary vascular resistance caused by an elevated left heart pressure (congestive heart failure, cardiomyopathies, and aortic and mitral stenoses). Less frequently, pulmonary vascular disease can be a pri-mary event (e.g., primary pulmonary hypertension, pulmonary vasculitides) or the major problem in other disease states (e.g., Churg-Strauss syndrome, scleroderma).[20] When the principal pathophysiologic cause of symptoms is pulmonary vascular disease, the CPEST should be used as the sole means of assessment. If the pulmonary vascular disease is an independent, comorbid problem, it may be combined with other problems (e.g., scleroderma where the pulmonary impairment is combined with impairment due to skin problems, neuropathy, peripheral vascular disease, or arthritis; or Churg-Strauss syndrome, where the pulmonary vascular impairment is combined with the asthma impairment). In other circumstances, the impairment from the pulmonary vascular disease is ignored such as in primary cardiac diseases where the cardiac impairment value covers peripheral issues such as the pulmonary vascular changes or in pulmonary diseases such as emphysema, ILD, or bronchiectasis, where the CPEST includes the vascular component as a part of the diminished exercise capability.

The fifth edition of the Guides has a new section devoted to the vascular system (Chapter 4). Section 4.4 specifically addresses pulmonary hypertension. Table 4–6 (reprinted as Table 25–12) provides the criteria for class selection and impairment rating for this disorder. It utilizes the pulmonary pressure, signs of congestive heart failure (right sided), and New York Heart Association classification for discriminating between the classes of impairment. It may be used as an alternative to the CPEST for deriving an impairment rating.

ASSESSMENT OF PULMONARY IMPAIRMENT

Choice of Tests

As noted in Chapter 22, and in keeping with the philosophy of the fifth edition of the Guides, the assessment of pulmonary impairment is based on disturbances in the ADL. ADL disturbances, from a pulmonary perspective, are highly subjective. There are some patients who have extremely poor lung function yet, owing to personal motivation, are capable of performing most ADLs. Thus, the assessment of pulmonary impairment based on disturbances in the ADL, while correlating with physiologic deviations, is also a reflection of factors other than just the abnormal physiology. Many of these factors are highly subjective and individualistic.

The ideal test is not available to merge the two concepts of impaired pulmonary function and motivation when defining deviations from normality or impairments in the ADL. As described in Chapter 22, the test that most closely produces this result is the complete CPEST. Tables exist that define the energy requirements of various activities including those that comprise ordinary ADLs. The CPEST measures an individual's energy-producing capabilities. If optimum levels of exercise are produced during the test, then the examinee's energy-producing capabilities can be matched to the energy requirements of a variety of tasks, including occupational demands and those that comprise the ADL. It further defines the causation for the restricted ability—whether it is due to pulmonary disease, cardiac or vascular disease, or the effects of deconditioning. Finally, it identifies whether suboptimal performance was given by the examinee; if so, the test can be repeated.

Static PFTs are not as capable of defining physiologic ADL capabilities nor does it come as close to matching a person's subjective concept of ADL capabilities, as does the CPEST (see Chapter 22). Why then do the Guides prefer to use static PFTs as its principal method of deriving pulmonary impairment? There are three simple answers: tradition, an inherent belief that deviations from normality can adequately measure impairment, and economics.

Static PFTs were the first to be developed and continue to be the assessment test of choice when arriving at physiologic or clinical diagnoses of various types of lung diseases as well as quantifying the degree of abnormality in those diseases. The frequency of performing PFTs outnumbers the frequency of pulmonary exercise tests by at least a thousandfold. There are many tables of population norms. For all these reasons, the static PFT is a conventional test. When the issue of impairment is raised, and using the Guides definition or that found in this book, a static PFT would appear to be an ideal test for deriving a deviation from a population norm if not a personal norm. Unfortunately, as noted previously and within Chapter 22, it does not adequately express disturbances in the ADL.

There are also significant problems with the CPEST, as discussed in Chapter 22. First, it is costly. A screening spirometry, with interpretation, costs approximately $60 to $200. A DLCO, with interpretation, costs approximately $100 to $400. A CPEST, with interpretation, costs approximately $800 to $1500. Second, it is invasive (the arterial puncture[s], arterial line, and, rarely, a Swan-Ganz catheter). Third, and most importantly, when multiple abnormalities exist, this test cannot discriminate between different disease states well enough to apportion the abnormal results for a single, defined condition. Therefore, the claimant with a recognized condition of COPD who also has peripheral vascular and coronary artery disease will have an abnormal CPEST. However, the results will be expressed as the global impairment that the claimant possesses and it will be impossible to select out the amount being tested for; i.e., the claim allowance for the COPD, absent the comorbid conditions.

The assessment of pulmonary impairment, using the fourth and fifth editions of the Guides, relies heavily on static PFTs. Alternative tests that are suggested include the CPEST and arterial blood gases or Spo_2 (before and after exercise). Other tests mentioned in the pulmonary chapters of the Guides are used primarily as diagnostic aids rather than for impairment assessment. An example is the chest radiograph.

A major problem for impairment evaluators is the concept of MMI, as seen in the following example:

■ A 55-year-old man was admitted to the hospital for an acute myocardial infarction. He was a heavy smoker (two packs per day since the age of 18). Following the myocardial infarction, PFTs were performed. His static PFTs yielded an FVC of 80%, FEV_1 of 30%, and Dco of 68% of predicted. He was referred to a pulmonary specialist. After stabilization on medications, the PFTs were FVC 94%, FEV_1 72%, and Dco 75% of predicted. One year later, he became depressed and refused to take his medications. He resumed smoking. On the day of his impairment evaluation, he smoked a pack of cigarettes. His Hbco level (blood carbon monoxide) was 10.2%. His static PFTs were FVC 64%, FEV_1 21%, and Dco 40%. A repeat spirometry after the administration of a bronchodilator yielded an FVC of 71% and an FEV_1 of 28%. ■

Was this person at MMI on the day of the test? Clearly not. Yet the Guides state that the use of a medication should neither increase nor decrease a person's rating although the physician may make comment on it.[11,15] At the three measured points in the example, this person would have had WPI ratings of 51% (post myocardial infarction), 15% (following treatment), and 70% on the day of examination. If the first two PFTs had not been performed, the rating physician would have, appropriately, given a 70% WPI rating. Even with knowledge of the first two tests, the rating physician would probably be forced to recommend the 70% rating value owing to the ambiguities involved in the definition of MMI. If one rigidly holds to the position that all claimants need to refrain from the inhalation of irritants for several months prior to examination and that they be on optimum medications, then very few claimants would ever be examined or given an impairment rating. Yet to do less, using the current and past editions of the Guides, creates marked disparities, with the compliant patient being penalized.

The last problem with the assessment of pulmonary impairment deals with a problem with the entire approach that the AMA Guides uses. This problem is best exemplified in the musculoskeletal portion of the book. An amputation of the tip of the fifth digit (at the distal interphalageal [DIP] joint) is a 50% impairment of the digit or a 3% impairment of the whole person. This value reflects impairment as opposed to interference in ADL. Realistically, how much interference does this amputation cause in a person's ability to perform self-care such as urinating, defecating, brushing teeth, combing hair, bathing, dressing, and eating (to use examples from Table 1–2 of the Guides[11[p4]])? These issues are primarily functional applications of the medical impairment and come closer to the definition of disability, as opposed to impairment, even though they do not relate specifically to occupational restrictions. The static PFTs are a reflection of deviation from normality (impairment) and are similar to the amputation values or restricted range of motion abnormalities in the musculoskeletal section. The CPEST describes the functionality of the medical impairment created by the abnormal PFT and derives the limitations placed upon ADL (for example, how much energy is needed to perform the above mentioned aspects of self care?). Thus the confusion is created by the concept of exactly what one is measuring—deviations from normality or disability created by those deviations in the ADLs.

The Effect of Aging on Spirometric Values

One of the major changes in the pulmonary chapter of the fifth edition of the Guides from prior editions is the concept of using a person's premorbid spirometric values for a baseline rather than the population norms found in the tables. This concept is mentioned twice in the first chapter that introduces the general philosophy of the Guides:

> When evaluating an individual, a physician has two options: consider the individual's healthy preinjury or preillness state of the condition of the unaffected side as "normal" for the individual if this is known, or compare that individual to a normal value defined by population averages of healthy people. The Guides uses both approaches. Accepted population values for conditions such as extremity range-of-motion or lung function are listed in the Guides; it is recommended that the physician use those values as detailed in the Guides when applicable. In other circumstances, for instance, where population values are not available, the physician should use clinical judgment regarding normal structure and function and estimate what is normal for the individual based on the physician's knowledge or estimate of the individual's preinjury or preillness condition.[11(p2)]
>
> If an individual had previous measurements of function that were below or above average population values, the physician may discuss that prior value and any subsequent loss for the individual, as well as compare it to the population normal. For example, a highly functioning athlete with documented, above-normal lung function, who has sustained an injury and now has decreased lung function that is nonetheless similar to population averages, has experienced a loss in his or her lung function and has sustained an impairment. Based only on a population comparison, the athlete would be given a 0% impairment rating. However, it would be more appropriate in this instance for the physician to assign an impairment rating based on the degree of change from the athlete's preinjury to postinjury state.[11(p4)]

In the pulmonary chapter, the fifth edition states: "As discussed in Chapter 1, in individuals where the preinjury or preillness values differ from the population-listed values, the examiner may depart from the population-listed values for determining an impairment stating, using the preinjury and preillness 'normal' value, and explain the reason for the departure."[11(p107)]

Chapter 22 describes the complexities of extrapolating the current FVC, FEV_1, and DCO from premorbid values. The Guides provide no clear direction on how to perform these extrapolations. Whereas any recommendation will be empirical, a suggested approach is found in Table 25–13. (See also the section on the effects of aging in Chapter 22.) This approach appears to be physiologically valid based on literature sources (see Chapter 22). However, it is fairly difficult to use and, especially in the smoker, introduces variables that tend to limit the application of this method. Nevertheless, it is presented as the preferred approach for the extrapolation of FEV_1 based on time.

An alternative method is to determine the percent deviation from the premorbid normal value and apply that percent change to the current, measured value. For example, if a person's FEV_1 were 5.00l when measured at a time prior to the development of a disease process and if the population predicted norm were 4.00l, then the individual would have a "personal norm" 25% higher than the predicted norm. This extrapolation factor (either higher or lower) can then be applied to the population norm.

■ Example: A 38-year-old man, 172 cm tall, has a predicted FEV_1 of 4.00l. (All the values used in this example are taken from Table 5–4a found on page 97 of the fifth edition of the Guides[11] and are used with permission.) However, at that age, he had a spirometry performed as part of a respiratory protection screening. His FEV_1 was measured at 5.00l. At the age of 51, he had a toxic inhalation and is being assessed for impairment. His population predicted normal value is 3.66l and the lower limit of normal is 3.158l. Using the 25% "correction factor," the predicted normal values would now be 4.575l and 3.948l, respectively. The measured FEV_1 could then be applied to these values with a class assortment and WPI percent derived in the usual fashion using Table 5–12. The same principle would hold if the examinee's personal norm were lower than the population-predicted norm. For example, if the population norm were 4.00l and the measured value were 3.00l, then the present (age-specific value) would be reduced by a factor of 33%. ■

This method has the advantage of simplicity and can also be used for the FVC and DCO, not just the FEV_1. As noted previously, the first and preferred approach is valid only for the FEV_1. The second (alternative approach) would appear to be valid if one assumes a linear relationship in the regression formulae for these values (FVC, FEV_1, and DLCO). Unfortunately, not enough is known, from a physiologic viewpoint, to attest to the validity and reliability of this method. Therefore,

TABLE 25–13

Rules When Deriving the Predicted FEV_1 Based on Known Premorbid Values

1. Not to be used for the FVC or DLCO
2. The premorbid FEV_1 must have been obtained when the claimant was at least 30 years old
3. There must have been no change in smoking status
4. There must have been no change in medication usage
5. Decrease the FEV_1 by 25 cc per year
6. Take the premorbid value, subtract 25 times the number of years that have elapsed = predicted current FEV_1
7. Use this value as the predicted FEV_1 rather than the values found in Table 5–4a or 5–5a
8. To find the lower limit of normal value (Tables 5–4b and 5–5b), subtract 0.842 from the derived FEV_1 for men and 0.561 for women
9. Proceed as normal, using Table 5–12 to arrive at the WPI

FEV_1, forced expiratory volume in 1 second; FVC, forced vital capacity; WPI, whole person impairment.

it is recommended that when using personal norms as a prediction of current, expected lung function, the age regression for the FEV_1 be derived using the approach found in Table 25–13 when the only variable is time (age). When other variables are introduced (such as age younger than 30 when the measured FEV_1 was obtained or a history of smoking), then the second (alternative) approach is suggested.

CONCLUSIONS

Over the years, the Guides have refined their approach to WPI assessment. When the third edition was used, a low-back claimant could have increased his or her WPI by performing a very limited range of motion during the examination. Yet the examining physician who saw the person walk out to the parking lot, pick up his or her keys from the ground, and then climb into his or her sports car with no obvious difficulty could only make comment on the disparity of the formal examination and the observed activities. The fourth edition tried to resolve this problem with the introduction of the diagnosis-related estimate. This concept has been extended in the fifth edition in a variety of chapters.

In the pulmonary chapter, the authors of the fifth edition have added a major section on asthma and offered tables reflecting the lower limits of normal in order to be in compliance with recommendations made by the ATS. However, principally owing to the lack of scientific evidence, several problematic areas remain. The remainder of this section provides the examining physician a method of impairment rating that extends but does not supplant the pulmonary chapter of the fifth edition (or prior editions). Of note are the same parameters and the same values. The recommendations offered are provided as an attempt to make the impairment values more equitable, especially in those claimants with airway diseases. Those sections recommend a method of impairment assessment that utilizes the principles found in the asthma assessment section of the fifth edition. These methods attempt to minimize the effects of compliance or noncompliance with prescribed medications, unevenness in physician prescribing patterns, and proscriptions for the examinee to avoid inhaled airway irritants. Much of the explanations underlying the offered tables are found either in this chapter or in Chapter 22.

Table 25–6*A–C* offers a method of arriving at a WPI rating for pulmonary diseases. It is divided into three subtables. It addresses the same issues that are found in the pulmonary chapter of the present and prior editions of the Guides but it adds several layers of refinement. Hopefully, if those levels of refinement are used, different evaluating physicians will be able to arrive at similar levels of WPI reflecting the stated goal of no greater than a 10% difference between evaluators, as expressed under the philosophical goals of the first chapter of not only the fifth edition but also previous editions. Hopefully, its use will preclude the marked variations in WPI created by the issues of compliance/noncompliance, smoking, and others.

Tables 25–6*A* and 25–6*B* are to be used for all obstructive diseases, not just asthma. Medication usage is used as a surrogate for the intensity of the disease. The values were arbitrary and only application can validate them. A rather low WPI value was chosen in this table as it was meant to be added to other values. For example, a patient with asthma who has an FEV_1 of 85% of predicted while taking four medications would have a WPI of 12%. On only three medications, the FEV_1 might be 78%. (Class 1 using the Guides: 0% to 10% WPI; 10% to 14% using this example). Of note, there is a change of 1% WPI for each 2% change in the FEV_1 and FVC; therefore, by extrapolation, this person has a WPI of 10% [9% for the three medications and 1% for the 78% FEV_1] using this table. On two medications the FEV_1 might be 65% (Class 2 using the Guides: 10% to 25% WPI; 14% using this table—6% for the two medications and 8% for the 65% FEV_1). On one medication, the FEV_1 might be 54% (Class 3 using the Guides: 25% to 50% WPI; 16% using this table—3% for the one medication and 13% for the 54% FEV_1). On no medications the FEV_1 might be 46% (Class 4 using the Guides: 50% to 100% WPI; 20% using this table—0% for the medication use and 20% for the 46% FEV_1). Thus, using the Guides alone, this individual would have had a range of WPI from 0% to 100% (or more realistically, 10% to 60%) and a range of 10% to 20% using this table. Again, these tables were developed to minimize the compliance and medication usage issues. The restriction of no respiratory irritants on the day of the exposure may also not be ideal but is more realistic, although difficult to prove.

Table 25–6*C* was added because many practitioners still rely on these medications (oral corticosteroids) rather than adhering to the NHLIB guidelines.[18] By themselves, oral steroids work so well that they will obviate the need for one and potentially more classes of other medications (Table 25–6*A*), depending on dosage. Thus the amount of WPI given for the use of this class of medications was higher.

Table 25–9 was developed to address radiographic or pathologic abnormalities that are devoid of measurable changes in the vital capacity or gas exchange. ILD found on a chest radiograph or computed axial tomography scan is, by definition, a deviation from both personal and population norms. It is never normal. Some ILDs, either by their nature (nonprogressive) or etiology (e.g., siderosis), do not produce significant physiologic abnormality but represent true pathology. Therefore, an impairment rating is assigned. The minimum cutoff for the chest x-ray abnormalities is an ILO/UC classification of 1/1 (see Chapter 22). The minimum need for diffuse disease in at least one lobe was recommended to eliminate WPI for "focal fibrosis" that can be found after an inflammatory condition (e.g., pneumonia, aspiration, and others) but, owing to its limited extent, would be expected to produce little to no physiologic changes in lung function owing to the large number of intact, functioning alveolar-capillary units in the remaining lobes.

Tables 25–11*A* and *B* address the issue of impairment created by sleep apnea. The fifth edition develops the concept of impairment created by OSA. Tables 25–11*A* (which is taken directly from the Neurology chapter of the Guides) and 25–11*B* assist the examiner in rating all the disturbances in ADL created by OSA.

The WPI ratings for pulmonary diseases assessed by Tables 25–6*A–C*, 25–9, and 25–11*A*,*B* should be combined rather than added in keeping with the philosophy established in the Guides.

IMPAIRMENT/DISABILITY UNDER SOCIAL SECURITY

Impairment and disability are synonymous under the Social Security system. Disability for pulmonary diseases is categorized into seven areas, often reflecting certain pathologic conditions. The Social Security system has rules and regulations that differ quite markedly from those used in the Guides. These rules and regulations are found on pages 32 through 47 of the Social Security Listings[38] and include issues such as which tests are recommended and paid for, specific criteria for the performance of certain tests (especially spirometries, measurements of the diffusing capacity, and exercise testing), rationales for the selection of these tests, and definitional concepts for disease categorizations. Some of the diseases included in the listings require adherence to a prescribed medical regimen prior to testing, most notably asthma. Some pulmonary conditions (asthma, cystic fibrosis, and bronchiectasis) require a certain amount of hospitalizations per year as a surrogate of the intensity of the disease. Each of the seven disease categories is briefly presented in this section.

Chronic Pulmonary Insufficiency

Included in this operational concept are diverse diseases such as COPD and restrictive lung diseases. For the claimant to be awarded disability in this area, he or she must fulfill certain testing criteria. There is a ranking of tests so that if the claimant qualifies with a certain level of testing then no more tests are necessary; if not, then he or she proceeds to the next level. These tests start with a simple spirometry. The tested variables are the FVC and the FEV_1. The only discriminator is height (see the discussion on the methods used by the Guides for comparison where sex, age, and race are also used; see also Chapter 22 for a complete discussion of the effect of these variables on the predicted values). As discussed in Chapter 22, the use of only one discriminator gives rise to inequities in this system.

If the claimant's spirometric values are above the cutoff values, then a diffusing capacity measurement if performed. There are no listed predicted values for the DLCO in the listings and the SSA relies on its own table of predicted values while allowing the evaluator to rely on the values established at the PFT laboratory where the test is performed. If the claimant has a value less than 10.5 mL/min/mm Hg or less than 40% of predicted, then he or she qualifies and no further testing is performed. Corrections are made for altitude, anemia, and elevated levels of carboxyhemoglobin.

If the claimant still does not qualify, a resting ABG is performed. The PaO_2 is corrected for the $PaCO_2$ and the altitude. There is a separate section in the listings for disability caused by obesity (9.09) that also lists ABGs as a method of assessing disability. However, the PaO_2 values found in this section are identical to those found in the respiratory section (3.00). The ABGs need to be performed when the claimant is stable, on at least two occasions, and 2 to 3 weeks apart within a 6-month period. Cutoff values are listed.

If the claimant still does not qualify, the ABGs are repeated during an exercise test with the same rules applicable regarding the altitude and $PaCO_2$ and with the same cutoff values as in the resting state.

Asthma

As noted, the patient with asthma must be compliant with a prescribed medical regimen.[38(p35)] Various definitional concepts for "episodic respiratory disease" are given in section 3.00-C, which covers asthma and other diseases.[38(p34)] If the asthma is part of a COPD complex, the claimant should be assessed using spirometry. For the "pure" asthmatic, the frequency of exacerbations requiring physician visits or hospitalizations serves as the surrogate for the intensity of the disease. Unfortunately, this discriminates against the person who receives medical attention from a physician skilled in the management of asthma. In its paper on the assessment of impairment/disability in patients with asthma, the ATS stated:

> (T)he frequency of acute exacerbations requiring emergency room treatment or hospitalization has been used in previous attempts to rate impairment. ... Given the efficacy of currently recommended antiinflammatory preparations in the treatment of asthma, frequent emergency room visits or hospitalizations generally reflect inadequate treatment and failure to achieve the objectives of treatment. The nature and frequency of medications required to maintain asthma under control (or the best results) give a better reflection of the severity of the disease and are more useful for the purpose of impairment assessment.[3(p1060)]

Cystic Fibrosis

This disease has specific rules for the diagnosis (3.00-D).[38(p35)] It is evaluated in one of three ways: by simple spirometry, by a method similar to that for asthma, or because of persistent respiratory infections. There is a table for the FEV_1 that is similar to the one for chronic pulmonary insufficiency except the values for FEV_1 are higher.

Pneumoconiosis

This needs to be demonstrated radiographically and is assessed similarly to chronic respiratory insufficiency.

Bronchiectasis

This disease is assessed in a fashion similar to that of pneumoconiosis or asthma.

Persistent Infections

This section includes mycobacterial, mycotic, and other chronic persistent infections. The listings state, in the introduction, that only those medical conditions that are expected to last at least 12 months (or less if death is expected) are ratable. Certain rules cover these diseases (3.00-B[38[p34]]) and disability is assessed either by the persistence and severity of the disease or by its residuals in a fashion similar to that for chronic respiratory insufficiency.

Cor Pulmonale

Section 3.00-G[38(pp41–42)] gives definitional and operative concepts underlying Social Security's views on cor pulmonale as well as describing diagnostic testing. It is evaluated either by the documentation of a pulmonary artery pressure >40 mm Hg or by the ABG or spirometric criteria used for chronic respiratory insufficiency.

Obstructive Sleep Apnea

The rules and regulations for OSA are found in section 3.00-H. This section states that the evaluation for OSA be performed under 3.09 (chronic cor pulmonale), 9.09 (obesity), or 12.02 (organic mental disorders).[38(p42)]

References

1. American Medical Association: Guides to the Evaluation of Permanent Impairment, 2nd ed. Chicago, American Medical Association, 1984.
2. American Medical Association: Guides to the Evaluation of Permanent Impairment, 3rd ed, rev. Chicago, American Medical Association, 1990.
3. American Thoracic Society: Guidelines for the evaluation of impairment/disability in patients with asthma. Am Rev Respir Dis 147:1056–1061, 1993.
4. American Thoracic Society: Indications and standards for use of nasal continuous airway pressure (CPAP) in sleep apnea syndrome. Am J Respir Crit Care Med 150:1738–1745, 1994.
5. American Thoracic Society: Sleep apnea, sleepiness, and driving risk. Am J Respir Crit Care Med 150:1463–1473, 1994.
6. Bahammam A, Kryger M: Decision making in obstructive sleep-disordered breathing. Putting it all together. In Strollo PJ, Sanders MH (eds): Clinics in Chest Medicine: Sleep Disorders 19. Philadelphia, WB Saunders, 1998, pp 87–97.
7. Barnes PJ: Inhaled corticosteroids for asthma. N Engl J Med 332:868–875, 1995.
8. Chan-Yeung M: Evaluation of impairment/disability in patients with occupational asthma. Am Rev Respir Dis 135:950–951, 1987.
9. Barnes PJ, Pedersen D: Efficacy and safety of inhaled corticosteroids in asthma. Am Rev Respir Dis 148:s1–s26, 1993.
10. Chokroverty S: Sleep disturbances in other medical disorders. In Chokroverty S, Daroff RE (eds): Sleep Disorders Medicine: Basic Science, Technical Considerations, and Clinical Aspects, 2nd ed. Boston, Butterworth-Heinemann, 1999, pp 587–617.
11. Cocchiarella L, Andersson GBJ (eds): Guides to the Evaluation of Permanent Impairment, 5th ed. Chicago, American Medical Association, 2001.
12. Committee on Rating Mental and Physical Impairment: Guides to the Evaluation of Permanent Impairment. Chicago, American Medical Association, 1977.
13. Culebras A: Clinical Handbook of Sleep Disorders. Boston, Butterworth-Heinemann, 1996, pp 233–281.
14. Demeter SL, Cordasco EM: Hyperventilation syndrome and asthma. Am J Med 81:989–994, 1986.

15. Doege T, Houston TP (eds): Guides to the Evaluation of Permanent Impairment, 4th ed. Chicago, American Medical Association, 1993.
16. Engelberg AL (ed): Guides to the Evaluation of Permanent Impairment, 3rd ed. Chicago, American Medical Association, 1988.
17. Expert Panel Report: Guidelines for the Diagnosis and Management of Asthma (National Institutes of Health publication 92-3042A). Bethesda, Md, National Asthma Education Program, National Heart, Lung, and Blood Institute, 1991.
18. Expert Panel Report 2: Guidelines for the Diagnosis and Management of Asthma (NIH publication 97-405). Bethesda, Md, National Institutes of Health, 1997.
19. Fletchon, EC, DeBehnke RD, Lovoi MS, et al: Undiagnosed sleep apnea in patients with essential hypertension. Ann Intern Med 103:190–195, 1985.
20. Gaine S: Pulmonary hypertension. JAMA 284:3160–3168, 2000. In Kryger MH, Roth T, Dement WC (eds): Principles and Practice of Sleep Medicine, 3rd ed. Philadelphia, WB Saunders, 2000, pp 859–868.
21. Grunstein R, Sullivan C: Continuous positive airway pressure for sleep breathing disorders. In Kryger MH, Roth T, Dement WC (eds): Principles and Practice of Sleep Medicine, 3rd ed. Philadelphia, WB Saunders, 2000, pp 894–912.
22. Harber P, Chan-Yeung M: Assessment of respiratory impairment and disability. In Demeter SL, Andersson GBJ, Smith GM (eds): Disability Evaluation. St. Louis, Mosby; Chicago, American Medical Association, 1996, pp 338–354.
23. Harbison J, O'Reilly P, McNicholas WT: Cardiac rhythm disturbances in the obstructive sleep apnea syndrome. Effects of nasal continuous positive airway pressure therapy. Chest 118:591–595, 2000.
24. Hla KM, Young TB, Bidwell T, et al: Sleep apnea and hypertension. A population-based study. Ann Intern Med 120:382–388, 1994.
25. Hoffstein V, Chan CK, Slutsky AS: Sleep apnea and systemic hypertension: A causal association review. Am J Med 91:190–196, 1991.
26. Kamada AK, Szefler SJ, Martin RJ, et al: Issues in the use of inhaled corticosteroids. Am J Respir Crit Care Med 153:1739–1748, 1996.
27. Kampa AK, Szefler SJ: Mechanisms of action of glucocorticoids in asthma and rhinitis. In Busse WW, Holgate ST (eds): Asthma and Rhinitis. Cambridge, Blackwell Science, 1995, pp 1255–1266.
28. Loube DL, Gay PC, Strohl KP, et al: Indications for positive airway pressure treatment of adult obstructive sleep apnea patients. A consensus statement. Chest 115:863–866, 1999.
29. Nieto FJ, Young TB, Lind BK, et al: Association of sleep-disordered breathing, sleep apnea, and hypertension in a large community-based study. JAMA 283:1829–1836, 2000.
30. Peppard P, Young T, Palta M, et al: Prospective study of the association between sleep-disordered breathing and hypertension. N Engl J Med 342:1378–1384, 2000.
31. Piccicillo JF, Duntley S, Schotland H: Obstructive sleep apnea. JAMA 284:1492–1494, 2000.
32. Redline S, Strohl KP: Recognitive and consequences of obstructive sleep apnea syndrome. In Stroll PJ, Sanders MH (eds): Clinics in Chest Medicine: Sleep Disorders, 9. Philadelphia, WB Saunders, 1998, pp 1–19.
33. Respiratory Inhalant Products: In Drug Facts and Comparisons 2001, 55th ed. St. Louis, Wolters Kluwer, 2000, pp 677–682.
34. Riley RW, Powell NB, Li KK, Guilleminault C: Surgical therapy for obstructive sleep apnea-hypopnea syndrome. In Kryger MH, Roth T, Dement WC (eds): Principles and Practice of Sleep Medicine, 3rd ed. Philadelphia, WB Saunders, 2000, pp 913–928.
35. Strohl KP, Redline S: Recognition of obstructive sleep apnea. Am J Respir Crit Care Med 154:279–289, 1996.
36. Teran-Santos J, Jimenez-Gomez A, Cordero-Guevera J: The association between sleep apnea and the risk of traffic accidents. N Engl J Med 340:847–851, 1999.
37. Tilkian, AG, Guilleminault C, Schroeder JS, et al: Sleep-induced syndrome. Prevalence of cardiac arrhythmias and their reversal after tracheostomy. Am J Med 63:348–358, 1977.
38. U.S. Department of Health and Human Services/Social Security Administration: SSA Publication No.64-039. Washington, DC, U.S. Department of Health and Human Services/Social Security Administration, 1994.
39. Weiss JW, Launois SH, Anand A: Cardiorespiratory changes in sleep-disordered breathing. In Kryger MH, Roth T, Dement WC (eds): Principles and Practice of Sleep Medicine, 3rd ed. Philadelphia, WB Saunders, 2000, pp 859–868.

CHAPTER

26

Cardiac Impairment

HARVEY L. ALPERN, MD

Cardiac impairment evaluation is challenging because it involves an often difficult assessment of subjective complaints. Of the array of objective diagnostic modalities that can be utilized in support of an evaluation, many are expensive and some are more reliable than others. An examiner must rely most significantly on his or her judgment in making a final assessment of impairment in light of all the subjective and objective facts of a given case.

Impairment ratings will be based on objective measurements and use of various scales, including those adapted from the AMA Guides to the Evaluation of Permanent Impairment.[3] Estimating the degree of a person's impairment is the physician's responsibility. In general, physicians do not judge disability.[3] The physician's role in cardiac disability is discussed in Chapter 60.

The impairment ratings for each of the cardiovascular conditions assume that the condition is being rated when the individual has reached maximum medical improvement (MMI). If a condition is stable but a surgical procedure may alter the impairment rating, but the individual declines surgery, for practical purposes the individual is permanent and stationary for rating the impairment and may be considered to be at MMI. The physician may indicate that if a certain treatment is given then a different impairment level may be expected, but nonetheless, the rating may still be given at the time that the individual is stable even if surgery or other therapy has been refused.

This chapter focuses on the AMA Guides. In general, the fifth edition has extended the concept of measuring cardiac impairment using exercise studies with multiples of energy expended (MET) levels initially given in the fourth edition of the Guides which were expanded in the fifth edition.

CORONARY ARTERY DISEASE

Numerous risk factors are associated with coronary artery disease. Impairment examinations should include a careful history to determine which are applicable. Sex, age, and a family history of coronary artery disease are factors that cannot be controlled; however, hypertension, hyperlipidemia, cigarette smoking, diabetes mellitus, obesity, sedentary lifestyle, and psychological stress are risk factors that can be modified to prevent coronary artery disease.

A history should provide details as to the duration and severity of risk factors identified in a given case. How long has the hypertension been present? When did treatment commence? Describe the degree and type of hyperlipidemia. Report the length of time of cigarette smoking and the number of cigarettes per day. If smoking has stopped, when did this occur? This is an important detail given the direct relationship between the number of cigarettes smoked and the incidence of cardiac events, and that this risk returns to near normal approximately 1 year after smoking is discontinued. Diabetes mellitus must be noted because it contributes to an increased incidence of atherosclerosis and small vessel disease. Obesity greater than 30% of ideal body weight is a notable risk factor. Lesser degrees of obesity do not contribute to coronary artery disease and need not be reported. Exercise abstinence is a risk factor to document.

Psychological stress, a potent risk factor, can precipitate a cardiac event. Shoveling snow or moving a stalled car are examples of physical stress that may precipitate a cardiac event. Severe emotional stressors, such as the 1994 earthquake in Southern California, result in a significant increase in myocardial infarctions. Another precipitating emotional stressor could be the death of a spouse, which has been shown to result in a marked increase in cardiac events in the subsequent 24 hours.

Studies have focused on chronic stress as it contributes to the development of coronary artery disease; some are now attempting to identify the subcomponents of Type A behavior that may lead to coronary disease. An association has been suggested between hostility and anger and cardiac morbidity and mortality.[9,19,23] High levels of chronic stress, social isolation, and an inability to control, alter, or avoid stress are all associated with the risk of a cardiac event. The situation of high demand and low control is considered to be a cause of stress leading to coronary artery disease and hypertension.[11,22,25]

Damage to the epithelium of the coronary vessel due to the effects of associated risk factors provides the catalyst for the gradual development of coronary artery disease and myocardial infarction. In response to the damage, macrophages in the form of foam cells enter the area to promote healing of the epithelium, bringing with them lipid particles from the bloodstream. Platelets accumulate and calcification begins to occur. The foam cells and platelets release a substance that stimulates the growth of fibrous tissues in the blood vessel. The cumulative effect is the progressive development of atherosclerotic plaque. Myocardial infarction occurs when a plaque ruptures, a thrombus forms, and vessel occlusion occurs. Emotional and physical stresses are additionally linked to myocardial infarction because such stresses tend to increase the coagulability of blood causing platelet aggregation and may also cause spasm of a vessel.

DIAGNOSIS OF CORONARY ARTERY DISEASE

A careful history and a physical examination are crucial to any diagnostic procedure. All applicable risk factors should be documented. Note the initial onset of symptoms, the frequency of their occurrence, and their relationship to any physical or emotional activity. The notation of anginal symptoms should include a detailed description of a person's own perception of the pain and a description of any precipitating activity.

The physical examination should include the vital signs and a description of the eye grounds, jugular venous pressure, carotid pulse with a description of duration and upstroke, and evidence of bruits. Pulmonary findings should be noted. The heart examination should include a description of cardiac impulse felt in the left lateral decubitus position. Heart tones, extra heart sounds, and murmurs are reported according to standard procedures. The abdominal examination should include the presence or absence of bruits. Describe venous abnormalities and the quality of arterial supply as found during an examination of the extremities.

Diagnostic studies are not indicated if these have been done recently and the results are available, unless their accuracy is in question. A complete blood cell count, renal function studies, liver function studies, and lipid concentrations are usually appropriate. Thyroid function studies are indicated when suggested by the history or on examination.

Magnetic resonance angiography is still in the experimental stages. Tests to evaluate coronary artery disease and coronary artery impairment are detailed in the chapter on cardiac diagnostic testing.

A resting electrocardiogram and chest x-ray are appropriate if these have not been done recently. Based on the extent of information needed for a thorough diagnosis, a standard stress test, a pharmacologic stress test, or a stress test associated with an echocardiogram or radionuclide material might be indicated. If coronary artery disease is suspected and there is a history of hypertension, a stress echocardiogram to determine the level of cardiac impairment from heart disease and simultaneously diagnose any enlargement from hypertension is a cost-effective test. If the diagnosis of coronary artery disease is at issue and there is an equivocal standard treadmill test available, then a radionuclear stress test using thallium or a combination of thallium and technetium-99 sestamibi can provide information about wall motion function and the area of ischemia to the heart.

In individuals with intermittent chest pain or palpitations, a Holter monitor worn during a 24-hour period of normal activity may provide information useful for an evaluation of arrhythmias or angina. Patients with chest pain may have electrocardiographic evidence of st segment changes indicating evidence of spasm or ischemic heart disease. A Holter monitor used for this purpose should have a high frequency response to ensure that the st segment evaluation is reliable.

Treadmill exercise time can be used to predict the $\dot{V}O_2max$ (maximum oxygen consumption). If oxygen consumption can be directly measured during the treadmill test, this is ideal; but if not logistically feasible, one may estimate $\dot{V}O_2max$ by the time of exercise on the treadmill.[21] Tables and nomograms are available for this purpose.[14] A variance in the results up to 30% has been suggested when direct oxygen consumption cannot be measured.[16] The results of treadmill testing should be expressed in metabolic units called METs (Table 26–1).[13] Each MET represents 3.5 cc of oxygen consumption per kilogram per minute. One MET refers to the oxygen uptake at rest. Because protocols vary with regard to exercise testing, this method of reporting provides a common ground for physicians when communicating the degree of exercise accomplished. The peak level in METs should always be stated. When exercise is stopped, note the reason, including any symptoms and signs that occurred. Note any arrhythmias, describe the degree of st segment

TABLE 26–1

Relationships of METS and Functional Class According to Five Treadmill Protocols

METS	1.6	2	3	4	5	6	7	8	9	10	11	12	13	14	15	16
Treadmill tests																
Ellested																
Miles per hour					1.7	3.0			4.0						5.0	
% grade					10	10			10						10	
Bruce																
Miles per hour					1.7		2.5		3.4				4.2			
% grade					10		12		14				16			
Balke																
Miles per hour				3.4	3.4	3.4	3.4	3.4	3.4	3.4	3.4	3.4	3.4	3.4	3.4	3.4
% grade				2	4	6	8	10	12	14	16	18	20	22	24	26
Balke																
Miles per hour			3.0	3.0	3.0	3.0	3.0	3.0	3.0	3.0	3.0	3.0				
% grade			0	2.5	5	7.5	10	12.5	15	17.5	20	22.5				
Naughton																
Miles per hour	1.0	2.0	2.0	2.0	2.0	2.0	2.0									
% grade	0	0	3.5	7	10.5	14	17.5									
METS	**1.6**	**2**	**3**	**4**	**5**	**6**	**7**	**8**	**9**	**10**	**11**	**12**	**13**	**14**	**15**	**16**
Clinical status																
Symptomatic patients	←						→									
Diseased, recovered		←					→									
Sedentary healthy				←						→						
Physically active					←											→
Functional class	IV	←	III →	←	II →	←				I and Normal						→

From Cocchiarella L, Andersson GBJ (eds): Guides to the Evaluation of Permanent Impairment, 5th ed. Chicago, American Medical Association, 2001, p 27, with permission.

depression (horizontal or downsloping) and report the blood pressure response to exercise.

Discontinue exercise testing if the individual is limited by chest pain, dyspnea, or orthopedic problems. Testing should be stopped subsequent to the onset of supraventricular tachycardia or runs of three or more ventricular ectopies. Unifocal ectopic beats generally are not a reason to stop exercise. Blood pressure changes with systolic values greater than 250 mm Hg signal the need to stop exercise but lesser levels do not. The diastolic blood pressure normally increases mildly with exercise. A 10 mm Hg drop in systolic blood pressure with exercise may indicate ventricular dysfunction and is an indication to stop exercise.

Thallium, once the standard radionuclide used to measure areas of death of tissue of the myocardium and reversible ischemia, has been generally replaced by single-photon emission computed tomography (SPECT) thallium-201 or SPECT technetium-99 sestamibi. SPECT increases quantification of the extent of left ventricular dysfunction. Use of Tc-99 sestamibi, one of several newer radioactive agents, allows for better imaging and simultaneous assessment of the first-pass ejection fraction and wall motion.

CT angiography may soon be available for noninvasive imaging of the coronary arteries.

Pharmacologic stress testing is indicated when debility or musculoskeletal problems preclude exercise. Dipyridamole or adenosine is commonly used. Dobutamine is frequently used with stress echocardiogram studies.

Echocardiography with stress testing, either pharmacologic with dobutamine or treadmill, gives comparable results to radionuclear studies. The relative sensitivity and specificity of these modalities are shown in Table 26–2.[7]

Positron emission tomography (PET) gives information about the metabolic viability of the myocardium. There are usually fewer artifacts with this technique and the sensitivity and specificity is >90%. The test is infrequently used owing to its expense, although it is becoming cheaper owing to less expensive radionuclides.

Electron beam CT scans or helical CT scans are now being used to screen for calcium in the coronary arteries. A positive result does not imply impairment or disability but usually requires further study as outlined previously. Risk factor modification may be indicated even if no significant obstruction is subsequently found.

The ejection fraction, obtained from echocardiograms, multigated radionuclide studies, or cardiac catheterization, is a useful figure because a reduced value of less than 50% is associated with a risk of higher mortality over 5 years.

TABLE 26–2

Sensitivity and Specificity of Exercise Tests

Test	Sensitivity	Specificity
Stress ECG	68%	77%
Thallium-201	84%	87%
Quantified thallium	89%	89%
SPECT thallium	90%	89%
Tc-99 sestamibi	89%	90%
SPECT Tc-99 sestamibi	90%	93%
Dipyridamole thallium-201	85%	87%
Stress echo	80%	90%
During exercise	93%	86%
Dobutamine	89%	85%
PET scan	95%	95%
History and physical examination	79%	83%

From Beller GA: New Stress Testing Methods. Presented at the ACC Lake Louise Cardiologists' Conference. March 1994.

When exercise is discontinued owing to dyspnea, one should consider a cardiopulmonary exercise test where oxygen consumption is measured to differentiate between cardiac and pulmonary causes of dyspnea (see Chapter 24).

Cardiac catheterization provides valuable information, although this study is seldom ordered in conjunction with an impairment evaluation. Data regarding ventricular function, wall motion, pressures in the ventricle, valvular abnormalities, and the anatomy of the coronary arteries are obtained; coronary artery vasospasm can be seen.

Coronary artery vasospasm is frequently implicated as a cause of chest pain at rest; however, most of these chest pains are not of cardiac etiology. Coronary artery vasospasm of the Prinzmetal variant type occurs in a normal coronary artery during the nocturnal hours generally, and is usually associated with st segment elevation. Fixed coronary artery lesions are also associated with coronary artery spasm. These lesions may be seen on angiography if ergonovine is given, or if a mental stress test is given simultaneously. Lesions of this type are often responsive to a stimulus of emotional stress.

A mental stress test can be administered during a standard electrocardiogram, Holter monitor testing, or studies measuring cardiac ischemia through other methods. Public speaking is a potent stimulus for mental stress testing. Engaging the individual in word recognition games, arithmetic, or computer games is another technique.[23,26]

The choice of the appropriate diagnostic test requires matching the best test to a particular individual. Many evaluees will require no testing because studies have been done in the recent past. If the tests were done in the past 6 months and there are no historical clinical changes, no further testing is likely needed. If the question is not diagnosis but detection of symptoms at a measured exercise level, then a simple stress test is reasonable. If the diagnosis of chest pain is required and past studies have not been done or were not diagnostic, then a radionuclear stress study or stress echocardiogram would be the tests of choice. If both the evaluation of wall thickness due to hypertension and the diagnosis of coronary artery disease is the goal, then a stress echocardiogram would be the cost-effective choice. If risk stratification for future mortality is needed, an ejection fraction could be estimated from a Tc-99 sestamibi or echocardiogram study.

If no diagnostic studies are available and only the history and physical examination were done, the diagnosis of coronary artery disease could be made with about the same sensitivity and specificity as the standard treadmill test, but less than that of a radionuclear exercise study or a stress echocardiogram. Regardless of the quoted sensitivity and specificity of the history and physical examination, standard treadmill tests are usually ordered and performed to accommodate the requirements of various impairment schemes including the AMA Guides and the Social Security system.[3,32]

IMPAIRMENT RATINGS

In the past, occupational tables were used to categorize impairment. The energy used to accomplish a particular job was calculated in METs.[15] If during testing, an individual could achieve a level of METs greater than the number on the work table associated with a particular occupation, then that individual was deemed able to do the job. The problem with categories is that they are based on averages of energy needed, and peak energies are often much higher. Also, healthy individuals, not those with coronary artery disease, participated in the studies that determined the categories (see Chapter 24).

Haskell et al have devised a simple classification of work based on MET level achieved that ranges from very heavy work to sedentary work (Table 26–3).[15] Individuals who can do more than 7 METs of work, or greater than a $\dot{V}O_2$max of 25, are said to have no impairment; those with a $\dot{V}O_2$max of less than 12 are totally impaired (Table 26–4). Graphs that correlate exercise capacity for normal individuals, both active and inactive men and women, can be used as a reference.

Another method of expressing cardiac impairment is to take the current measurement of work or exercise capability in METs, compare it with preinjury or preillness level of METs (either previously measured or estimated), and then calculate the percentage of impairment as a result of the injury or illness[17]:

$$\text{Percentage impairment} = \frac{1 - \text{current MET level}}{\text{prior MET level}} \times 100\%$$

TABLE 26–3
Haskell Work Classification

Classification	Peak METS	Activity
Very heavy	>6	Climb stairs
Medium	4–6	Carry 50 pounds
Light	2–4	Carry 20 pounds
Sedentary	<2	Sit/carry 10 pounds

From Haskell W, et al: Task Force II: Determination of occupational working capacity in patients with ischemic heart disease. JACC 14:1027, 1989.

TABLE 26–4
Impairment Rating

$\dot{V}o_2$ max	Peak METS	Activity
>25	>7	None
20–25	5–7	Mild to moderate
15–20	2.5–5	Severe
<15	<2.5	Total

Adapted from Fox SM, Naughton JP, Haskill WL: Physical activity and prevention of coronary artery disease. Ann Clin Res 3:404, 1971.

The New York Heart Association (NYHA) Functional Classification has been in use since 1964 (Table 26–5). This classification is based entirely on subjective evaluation. The AMA impairment classification of Classes 1 through 4 is based on subjective and objective evaluations,[3] where the objective in METs are measured as described previously (Table 26–6).

The most common cardiac problem seen by an impairment rating physician is chest pain. The claimant may be referred for consultation or sent for an independent medical evaluation. One of the most common causes of chest pain is chest wall pain where there is association of stress with the appearance of chest pain. In this case, the physical examination is most important with the finding of tenderness somewhere in the chest wall or, more commonly, in the paracervical muscles where there is spasm and tenderness. Thus the impairment rating would be based on the finding of chest pain as a result of muscle spasm. No cardiovascular impairment rating would be given. In this type of case, the diagnostic study that would be done, in addition to the standard history, physical examination, chest x-ray, and electrocardiogram, would be some type of exercise study with a standard treadmill test probably sufficing. A radionucleotide or echocardiographic study could also be done at a slightly higher cost but slightly higher sensitivity and specificity, as described in Chapter 23.

The impairment rating of chest pain without a cardiovascular diagnosis is addressed in some states' workers' compensation system as requiring a work restriction from undue emotional stress. The fifth edition AMA Guides stresses chronic pain on page 566 under the general discussions of chronic pain.[3]

HYPERTENSIVE HEART DISEASE

The most common form of hypertension is essential hypertension. An evaluation for hypertension must address a history of any factor that may reveal a primary cause for hypertension other than essential. Questions should focus on a history of renal disease and symptoms suggestive of paroxysmal elevations such as those associated with pheochromocytoma. The history should expose any secondary effects of the hypertension on other organ systems including neurologic symptoms and visual changes. The complete physical examination, in addition to determining the blood pressure in both upper extremities in the supine and standing positions, allows the physician to look for evidence of neurologic

TABLE 26–5
NYHA Functional Classification of Cardiac Disease

Class	Description
I	Individual has cardiac disease but no resulting limitation or physical activity; ordinary physical does not cause undue fatigue, palpitation, dyspnea, or anginal pain.
II	Individual has cardiac disease resulting in slight limitation of physical activity; is comfortable at rest and in the performance of ordinary, light, daily activities; greater than ordinary physical activity, such as heavy physical exertion, results in fatigue, palpitation, dyspnea, or anginal pain.
III	Individual has cardiac disease resulting in marked limitation of physical activity; is comfortable at rest; ordinary physical activity results in fatigue, palpitation, dyspnea, or anginal pain.
IV	Individual has cardiac disease resulting in inability to carry on any physical activity without discomfort; symptoms of inadequate cardiac output, pulmonary congestion, systemic congestion, or anginal syndrome may be present, even at rest; if any physical activity is undertaken, discomfort is increased.

From Cocchiarella L, Andersson GBJ (eds): Guides to the Evaluation of Permanent Impairment, 5th ed. Chicago, American Medical Association, 2001, p 26, with permission.

abnormalities or cardiac enlargement (best done by feeling for left ventricular sustained impulse in the left lateral decubitus position) as well as listening for a fourth heart sound and abdominal bruits.

In addition to the physical examination, certain diagnostic studies are required. A chest x-ray will indicate if there is cardiac enlargement and the Social Security Administration requires the specific finding of cardiac enlargement on chest x-ray.[32] However, chest x-rays sometimes are unreliable in diagnosing cardiac enlargement and echocardiogram is considered superior.

Some institutions use impedance cardiography to determine cardiac output and peripheral vascular resistance in relation to changes in blood pressure with stimuli such as emotional stress. These findings are utilized in the usual impairment ratings but information may support the conclusion based on altered physiology.

A urinalysis to determine if proteinuria is present is important in patients with hypertension as well as those with diabetes. However, it is usually not the role of the evaluating physician to do extensive laboratory studies to determine underlying etiologies unless indicated. These studies would include electrolytes, renal function, and occasionally testing for adrenal hormone levels.

Research by Eliot has shown that stress is a major and often overlooked component of illness.[10,12] Studies by Barker and Schnall et al show that job strain is a potential risk factor for hypertension and structural changes in the heart, leading to an increased left ventricular mass index.[6,27,28] Impairment evaluations must include a

TABLE 26-6

Criteria for Rating Permanent Impairment Due to Coronary Heart Disease

Class 1: 0% to 9% Impairment of the Whole Person	Class 2: 10% to 29% Impairment of the Whole Person	Class 3: 30% to 49% Impairment of the Whole Person	Class 4: 50% to 100% Impairment of the Whole Person
Because of serious implications of reduced coronary blood flow, it is not reasonable to classify degree of impairment as 0% through 9% in anyone who has symptoms of CHD corroborated by physical examination or laboratory tests; this class of impairment should be reserved for individuals with equivocal histories of angina pectoris on whom coronary angiography is performed, or for those on whom coronary angiography is performed for other reasons and in whom less than 50% reduction in cross-sectional area of coronary artery is found with a normal EF; METS determination is not applicable	History of MI or angina pectoris documented by appropriate laboratory studies, but at time of evaluation, no symptoms while performing ordinary daily activities or even moderately heavy physical exertion (functional class I) **and** may require moderate dietary adjustment or medication to prevent angina or to remain free of signs and symptoms of CHF **and** able to walk on treadmill or bicycie ergometer and obtain HR of 90% of predicted maximum HR (see Table 3–6B) without developing significant ST-segment shift, VT, or hypotension; if uncooperative or unable to exercise because of disease affecting another organ system, this requirement may be omitted; METS >7 **or** has recovered from coronary artery surgery or angioplasty, remains asymptomatic during ordinary daily activities, and able to exercise as outlined above; if taking a beta-adrenergic blocking agent, should be able to walk on treadmill to level estimated to cause energy expenditure of at least 7 METS as substitute for HR target	History of MI documented by appropriate laboratory studies, or angina pectoris documented by changes on resting or exercise ECG or radioisotope study suggestive of ischemia **or** either fixed or dynamic focal obstruction of at least 50% of coronary artery, angiography and function testing **and** requires moderate dietary adjustment or drugs to prevent frequent angina or to remain free of symptoms and signs of CHF, but may develop angina pectoris after moderately heavy physical exertion (function class II); METS >5 but <7 **or** has recovered from coronary artery surgery or angioplasty, continues to require treatment, and has symptoms described above	History of MI documented by appropriate laboratory studies, or angina pectoris documented by changes on resting ECG or radioisotope study highly suggestive of myocardial ischemia **or** either fixed or dynamic focal obstruction of at least 50% of one or more coronary arteries, demonstrated by angiography and function testing **and** requires moderate dietary adjustment or drugs to prevent angina or to remain free of symptoms and signs of CHF, but continues to develop symptoms or angina pectoris or CHF during ordinary daily activities (functional class III or IV); METS <5 **or** has recovered from coronary artery bypass surgery or angioplasty and continues to require treatment and have symptoms as described above

From Cocchiarella L, Andersson GBJ (eds): Guides to the Evaluation of Permanent Impairment, 5th ed. Chicago, American Medical Association, 2001, p 36, with permission.

TABLE 26–7
Classification of Hypertension in Adults

	Blood Pressure Categories			Hypertension Categories		
Blood Pressure	**Optimal**	**Normal**	**High-normal**	**Stage I**	**Stage II**	**Stage III**
Systolic	<120	<130	130–139	140–159	160–179	≥180
	and	and	or	or	or	or
Diastolic	<80	<85	85–89	90–99	100–109	≥110

From Cocchiarella L, Andersson GBJ (eds): Guides to the Evaluation of Permanent Impairment, 5th ed. Chicago, American Medical Association, 2001, p 66, with permission.

careful history of stress, if stress is relevant to the case.[26] Of particular concern is any pattern of continuous, unrelenting stress where the individual is in a trapped position with no options for avoiding or altering the stress.[20,25] One should evaluate for the possible presence of a "hot reactor"—an individual who has a normal blood pressure at rest and may appear calm, but with mental stress has marked increase in blood pressure. This increase in blood pressure may be due to increased cardiac contraction, increased peripheral resistance, or both. Eliot has described a method for identifying a "hot reactor" by determining the blood pressure and, through noninvasive techniques, peripheral vascular resistance so as to individualize therapy (pharmacologic and nonpharmacologic).[11] When a cerebrovascular accident (CVA) occurs in a hypertensive individual, and the CVA is not believed to be embolic, a history of any stress that might have elevated blood pressure immediately proximal to the event should be noted, as such stress may precipitate either a hemorrhage or thrombosis of the cerebral vessel.

CLASSIFICATION OF HYPERTENSION

The classification of hypertension in adults is described in Table 26–7. The stages listed are used in impairment criteria in the AMA Guides fifth edition. Impairment as a result of hypertension is related to end-organ damage. An individual should be considered temporarily impaired until the hypertension is controlled with medication, then rated as to his or her level of impairment based on pathological manifestations in other organs such as the brain, eye, heart, and kidneys. Progressive doses or additions of medications are considered an additional impairment. The AMA Guides fifth edition define as Class 1 those individuals who are normotensive with medication and have no end-organ damage (Table 26–8). A Class 2 individual is stage 1 or 2 and shows abnormalities in the urinalysis without evidence of renal impairment or a history of a cerebrovascular episode or retinal changes. There may be no symptoms. Class 3 individuals are asymptomatic and still may be

TABLE 26–8
Criteria for Rating Permanent Impairment Due to Hypertensive Cardiovascular Disease

Class 1: 0% to 9% Impairment of the Whole Person	Class 2: 10% to 29% Impairment of the Whole Person	Class 3: 30% to 49% Impairment of the Whole Person	Class 4: 50% to 100% Impairment of the Whole Person
Asymptomatic; stage 1 or 2 hypertension without medications **or** normal blood pressure on antihypertensive medication **and** no evidence of end-organ damage	Asymptomatic; stage 1 or 2 hypertension despite multiple medications **or** antihypertensive medication with any of the following: (1) proteinuria, urinary sediment abnormalities, no renal function impairment as measured by the blood urea nitrogen (BUN) and serum creatinine; (2) definite hypertensive changes on funduscopic examination in arterioles, e.g., "copper" or "silver wiring," or arteriovenous crossing changes with or without hemorrhages and exudates; either abnormality suggests end-organ damage	Asymptomatic; stage 3 hypertension despite multiple medications **or** antihypertensive medication with any of the following: (1) proteinuria, urinary sediment abnormalities, renal function impairment as measured by the BUN and serum creatinine, and a decreased creatinine clearance of 20% to 50% normal; (2) LV hypertrophy by ECG or echocardiography but no symptoms of HF; either abnormality suggests more extensive end-organ damage	Antihypertensive medication with stages 1–3 and any of the following abnormalities: (1) proteinuria, urinary sediment abnormalities, renal function impairment as measured by the BUN and serum creatinine, and a creatinine clearance < 20% normal; (2) hypertensive cerebrovascular damage or episodic hypertensive encephalopathy; (3) LV hypertrophy, systolic dysfunction, and/or signs and symptoms of HF due to hypertension

From Cocchiarella L, Andersson GBJ (eds): Guides to the Evaluation of Permanent Impairment, 5th ed. Chicago, American Medical Association, 2001, p 66, with permission.

stage 3 in spite of multiple medications or having renal insufficiency, a history of stroke, left ventricular hypertrophy, or retinopathy. An individual whose high blood pressure cannot be controlled belongs in this category. Individuals who have more than one of the Class 3 complications or have cardiac decompensation belong in the Class 4 category.[3]

VALVULAR HEART DISEASE

Any history suggestive of rheumatic fever should be noted. The progression of dyspnea on exertion should be documented by an estimation of prior and current tolerance to exercise. Obtain a history of the number of stairs the individual could climb in past years as compared to present time, for example, and any history of treadmill testing. Slowly progressive cardiac decompensation is seen most often in conditions such as mitral stenosis or aortic stenosis. Aortic regurgitation may not be symptomatic unless there is relatively rapid decompensation. These conditions are not known to be related to work phenomena; however, an impairment evaluation and the rating for such an impairment are necessary first steps in a disability evaluation to determine a feasible work assignment for the individual.

Rating the level of impairment for an individual with valvular heart disease is especially important when there are coexisting conditions, such as coronary artery disease. Coexisting conditions may also impair the individual. An attempt must be made to distinguish the level of impairment for all existing conditions so that the impairment classification may be appropriately judged (Table 26–9).

Testing for valvular heart disease when the diagnosis is known may only require a history to determine activity level or a treadmill study to document this level in METs. A chest x-ray for the evaluation of heart size and pulmonary vasculature is another objective measure of

TABLE 26–9

Criteria for Rating Permanent Impairment Due to Valvular Heart Disease

Class 1: 0% to 9% Impairment of the Whole Person	**Class 2: 10% to 29% Impairment of the Whole Person**	**Class 3: 30% to 49% Impairment of the Whole Person**	**Class 4: 50% to 100% Impairment of the Whole Person**
Evidence by physical examination or laboratory studies of valvular heart disease **and** no symptoms in the performance of ordinary daily activities (functional class I; 5 METS; Table 3–2) or with moderately heavy exertion (7 to 10 METS) **and** does not require continuous treatment, except for intermittent prophylactic antibiotics for surgical or dental procedure to reduce risk of bacterial endocarditis **and** no evidence of CHF **and** no signs of ventricular dysfunction or dilation, and severity of stenosis or regurgitation estimated to be mild (METS >7; TMET [Bruce protocol] >6 min) **and** in the individual who has recovered from valvular heart surgery, all above criteria are met	Evidence by physical examination or laboratory studies of valvular heart disease, and no symptoms in performance of daily activities, but symptoms develop on moderately heavy physical exertion (functional class II) **or** requires moderate dietary adjustment or drugs to prevent symptoms or to remain free of signs of CHF or other consequences of valvular heart disease, such as syncope, chest pain, and emboli **or** signs or laboratory evidence of cardiac chamber dysfunction and/or dilation, severity of stenosis or regurgitation estimated to be moderate, and surgery correction not feasible or advisable; METS >5 but <7; TMET (Bruce protocol) >3 min **or** has recovered from valvular heart surgery and meets criteria for functional class II	Signs of valvular heart disease and slight to moderate symptomatic discomfort during performance of ordinary daily activities (functional class III) **and** dietary therapy of drugs do not completely control symptoms or prevent CHF **and** signs or laboratory evidence of cardiac chamber dysfunction of dilation, severity of stenosis or regurgitation estimated to be moderate or severe, and surgical correction not feasible; METS >2 but <5; TMET (Bruce protocol) >1 min but <3 min **or** has recovered from heart valve surgery but continues to meet criteria for functional class III	Signs by physical examination of valvular heart disease, and symptoms at rest or in performance of less than ordinary daily activities (functional class IV) **and** dietary therapy and drugs cannot control symptoms or prevent signs of CHF **and** signs or laboratory evidence of cardiac chamber dysfunction or dilation, severity of stenosis or regurgitation estimated to be moderate or severe, and surgical correction not feasible; METS <2; TMET (Bruce protocol) <1 min **or** recovered from valvular heart surgery but continues to meet criteria for functional class IV

CHF, congestive heart failure; METS, metabolic equivalents.
From Cocchiarella L, Andersson GBJ (eds): Guides to the Evaluation of Permanent Impairment, 5th ed. Chicago, American Medical Association, 2001, p 30, with permission.

the effect of valvular heart disease. An echocardiogram to determine chamber size and estimate valve area is usually required. Valve area is usually estimated from echocardiographic measurement, but the information may also be derived from catheterization data if available. Cardiac catheterization is usually not required for an impairment rating but would usually be done before surgery to determine if coronary or other cardiac abnormalities are present. If coronary artery disease and valvular disease co-exist, the physician should indicate whether the exercise test was terminated due to angina. Fatigue or dyspnea could result from either condition.

Existing tables that measure the severity of valve disease are based on valve diameter and exercise tolerance (Table 26–10). The AMA guidelines are dependent on the number of METs achieved and the necessity of therapy for heart failure.

TABLE 26–10

Severity of Valve Stenosis

Severity of Stenosis	Mean Valve Gradient (mm Hg)	Valve Area (cm^2)
Aortic valve		
Mild	<25	>1.5
Moderate	25–50	1.0–1.5
Severe	>50	<1.0
Mitral valve		
Mild	<5	>1.5
Moderate	5–10	1.0–1.5
Severe	>10	<1.0

From Cocchiarella L, Andersson GBJ (eds): Guides to the Evaluation of Permanent Impairment, 5th ed. Chicago, American Medical Association, 2001, p 29, with permission.

CARDIAC ARRHYTHMIAS

A complete physical examination is necessary for the impairment evaluation and should focus on symptoms and signs of cardiac abnormality. The history of an individual with cardiac arrhythmias should include the onset of symptoms of palpitations, whether they start or stop suddenly, and whether they are associated with any neurologic symptoms. Any factors that may have caused the onset of the arrhythmia should be explored in the history. Questions should be asked concerning the history of a possible thyroid condition and symptoms of hyperthyrodism. If the patient is taking thyroid medication, note the dosage.

Impairment in patients with arrhythmias is the result of decreased blood flow during the arrhythmia, resulting in dizziness or syncope. There are other subjective complaints in addition to dizziness such as palpitations, dyspnea, and chest pain. Objective findings are the recording of the arrhythmia, such as on a Holter monitor recording, and associating this finding with ischemic st change, syncope, or seizures. Emboli from the left atrium in atrial fibrillation may result in dysfunction in a variety of different organs (e.g., brain, gut, extremities) and hence impairment of any target body part.

In situations of cardiac arrhythmia, laboratory studies are a reasonable part of the impairment evaluation in order to diagnose anemia, check levels of potassium and other electrolytes, and assess thyroid function.

Sometimes a simple electrocardiogram and rhythm strip will suffice as an analysis of cardiac arrhythmias; however, a 24-hour Holter monitor may be necessary at least once. As noted in Chapter 23, 48 hours gives a higher sensitivity and specificity to the results of the Holter monitor. If symptoms recur less frequently, an event monitor recording is indicated. The Holter monitor records every heartbeat over 24 hours and is analyzed both visually and by computer to determine the frequency of ectopic beats and the type. If symptoms are rare, an event monitor with fixed leads or a chest contact box monitor may be used. The usual event monitor records when an individual presses a button to activate the recording when symptoms occur. This device can be carried for weeks at a time. An attempt should be made to uncover and document in the history any emotional stress that may relate to the onset of arrythmias.[1]

The AMA Guides are clear in delineating the four classes of arrhythmias. Class 1 distinguishes an individual who is asymptomatic, does not have a complex arrhythmia, and has no evidence of organic heart disease. A Class 2 individual may be symptomatic; a person in this category is undergoing treatment for symptoms, or has been diagnosed with organic disease. A Class 3 individual is one under treatment whose symptoms from arrhythmia continue infrequently. A Class 4 type is functionally a NYHA Class 3 or 4 and has palpitations or syncope, even though on treatment.[3]

If arrhythmias occur during exercise, the MET level attained would establish the impairment level. Supraventricular arrhythmias may result in impairment related to the extent of subjective symptoms. It should be noted that ventricular arrhythmias in the presence of ventricular dysfunction are associated with increased mortality.[7]

Heart block or any slow arrhythmia resulting in symptoms is generally treated with pacemaker implantation. Impairment rating would be as described in the section of the AMA Guides[33] on cardiac arrhythmias if further arrhythmias or symptoms were present after pacemaker insertion. The table for the impairment of rating arrhythmias is found in the fifth edition on page 56.[33]

CARDIOMYOPATHY

Cardiomyopathy is frequently the result of an unknown condition. Congenital or hereditary factors may lead to a cardiomyopathy or it may be secondary to infections of many types, usually viral. Amyloid or thyroid disease, parasitic conditions, or alcohol abuse can all result in a cardiomyopathy. There is no evidence that the illness is related to emotional stress. The history and physical examination is similar to that indicated for patients with coronary and valvular disease. A myocardial biopsy may be done for diagnosis or research, but is unnecessary for an impairment evaluation. A treadmill exercise test would give the level of impairment by noting the MET level where exercise is stopped due to fatigue or dyspnea. A stress echocardiogram would also give this information along with the ejection fraction. Given that the diagnosis was previously made, radionuclear exercise testing would not be needed.

The impairment rating for cardiomyopathies is a function of the person's ability to exercise as determined by a treadmill test. When symptoms are present, the impairment rating is also based on the NYHA guidelines. Arrhythmia may add to the impairment by causing dizziness and palpitations. Some individuals will need surgery for hypertrophic cardiomyopathy or even a heart transplant, but overall ratings would depend on measured impairment in an exercise study after recovery from surgery.

Guidelines for impairment rating of cardiomyopathy are given in Table 3–9 of AMA Guides fifth edition and are based on findings of congestive heart failure (CHF) and symptoms when the individual has reached maximum medical improvement.[33(p47)]

CONGESTIVE HEART FAILURE

When CHF complicates any cardiac condition, treatment is undertaken; only when maximal medical therapy has been given is an impairment rating considered. The impairment rating guides outlined for coronary heart disease may be used to determine the impairment rating for CHF. It would be expected that the limiting factor on exercise testing would be dyspnea or fatigue rather than angina. A cardiopulmonary exercise test using peak $\dot{V}O_2$ and ventilatory threshold are highly reproducible and thus recommended for this population by the American Health Association Science Advisory. If exercise cannot be done, an ejection fraction measured by echocardiogram or by angiogram—either radionuclear or at catheterization—may be used to estimate impairment. An ejection fraction of greater than 50% is generally considered as normal indicating no impairment. However, a normal ejection fraction at rest may be seen when there is significant coronary or other heart disease and may be lower with exercise. An ejection fraction of less than 25% indicates severe impairment, with moderate impairment for ejection fractions between 25% and 50%.

CONGENITAL CARDIAC DISEASE

Congenital heart abnormalities may be rated by exercise capability as outlined in the sections on coronary disease and congestive heart failure. Chapter 3.4 of the AMA Guides fifth edition also rates impairment based not only on symptoms and exercise tolerance but also on chamber size, valve dysfunction, systemic-pulmonary shunting, and pulmonary vascular resistance.[33(pp42–46)]

PULMONARY HYPERTENSION

Pulmonary hypertension may be primary and due to narrowing of the pulmonary arteriolar bed of unknown etiology, pulmonary emboli, primary pulmonary disease, or CHF. Classically it is associated with dyspnea, finding of right ventricular lift, accentuated P2, and elevated pulmonary artery pressure (on echocardiogram or right heart catheterization). Impairment is by functional status and pulmonary artery pressure as listed in Table 4–6 of the AMA Guides, fifth edition.[33(p79)] Treadmill exercise testing will be of value as the level where symptoms occur will also be reflective of the functional status of the evaluee and is more objective in measurement.

PERICARDIAL DISEASE

Pericardial disease is usually an acute inflammatory condition associated with a systemic immune disorder such as lupus erythematosis, trauma to the chest, cardiac surgery (postmyocardotomy syndrome), or infection, or can be idiopathic. Pericardial disease is usually an acute problem with temporary total impairment. It would not be rated for impairment until maximum medical improvement occurs which could take months. If there were continuing symptoms and findings, the AMA Guides fifth edition allows for rating on Table 3–10, taking into consideration continuing symptoms (functional classification) and findings of abnormal hemodynamics and recovery from surgery. Echocardiography or CT scanning are used to document pericardial abnormality.[33(p52)]

Chronic pericardial disease with constrictive pericarditis occurs and frequently requires surgery. An echocardiogram or a CT scan can document the pericardial thickening. Hemodynamic studies can document whether significant restriction is present. Impairment rating should be done after recovery from surgery and is based on symptoms, functional class, and evidence of residual disease.

References

1. Allen R, et al: Is coronary heart disease a lifestyle disorder? A review of psychologic and behavioral factors. CVR & R 1992.
2. Alpern HL: Cardiac disability: An overview. J Disabil 1:2, 1990.
3. American Medical Association: Guides to the Evaluation of Permanent Impairment, 4th ed. Chicago, American Medical Association, 1993.
4. Astrand I: Aerobic work capacity in men and women with special reference to age. Acta Physiol Scand 49 (Suppl. 169):1–92, 1960.
5. Astrand I: Degree of strain during building work as related to individual aerobic work capacity. Ergonomics 10:293–303, 1967.
6. Barker S: High-strain jobs' role in hypertension. Cardiology World News, 1993.
7. Beller GA: New Stress Testing Methods. Presented at the ACC Lake Louise Cardiologists' Conference. March 1994.
8. Clark WL, Alpern HL, et al: Suggested guidelines for rating cardiac disability on workers' compensation. West J Med 158:263–267, 1993.
9. Denollet J, et al: Coping subtypes for men with coronary heart disease: Relationship to well-being, stress, and Type-A behaviour. Biol Psychol 34:1–4, 1992.
10. Eliot RS: Stress and the Heart. New York, Futura, 1988.
11. Eliot RS: The dynamics of hypertension—an overview. Present practices, new possibilities, and new approaches. Am Heart J 116:2, 1988.
12. Eliot RS: Psychophysiologic stress testing as a predictor of mean daily blood pressure. Am Heart J 116:2, 1988.
13. Fletcher GF, et al: Exercise standards. Circulation 82:6, 1990.
14. Froelicher VF, et al: Nomogram for exercise capacity using METs and age. Highlights 8:2, 1992.
15. Haskell WL, et al: Task Force II: Determination of occupational working capacity in patients with ischemic heart disease. J Am Coll Cardiol 14:1016–1042, 1989.
16. Higginbotham MB (ed): Cardiopulmonary Exercise Testing. St. Paul. Medical Graphics Corporation, 1993.
17. Industrial Medical Council: State of California Guidelines for Evaluation of Cardiac Disability. 1994.
18. Johnson JV, et al: Combined effects of job strain and social isolation on cardiovascular disease, morbidity and mortality in a random sample of the Swedish male working population. Scand J Work Environ Health 15:271–279, 1989.
19. Lachar EL: Coronary-prone behavior: Type A behavior revisited. Tex Heart Inst J 20:3, 1993.
20. Markovitz JH, et al: Psychological predictors of hypertension in the Framingham study: Is there tension in hypertension? JAMA 270:20, 1993.
21. McConnell TR, et al: Prediction of maximal oxygen consumption during handrail-supported treadmill exercise. J Cardiol Rehab 7:324–331, 1987.
22. McEwen BS, et al: Stress and the individual. Arch Intern Med 153:2093–2101, 1993.
23. Merz CNB, et al: Mental stress and myocardial ischemia: Correlates and potential interventions. Tex Heart Inst J 20:3, 1993.
24. National Institutes of Health, National Heart, Lung, and Blood Institute: The Fifth Report of the Joint National Committee on Detection, Evaluation, and Treatment of High Blood Pressure. National Institutes of Health, 1994.
25. Rosengren A, et al: Self-perceived psychological stress and incidence of coronary artery disease in middle-aged men. Am J Cardiol 68:1171–1175, 1991.
26. Rozanski A, et al: Impact of psychological factors on the pathogenesis of cardiovascular disease and implications for therapy. Circulation 99:2192–2217, 1999.
27. Schnall PL, et al: The workplace and cardiovascular disease. Occup Med 15:307–321, 2000.
28. Schnall PL, et al: The relationship between "job strain," workplace diastolic blood pressure, and left ventricular mass index. JAMA 263:14, 1990.
29. Shaw LK, Pryor DB, et al: Sensitivity and specificity of the history and physical examination for coronary artery disease. Ann Intern Med 118:81–90; 120:344–345, 1993.
30. Wasserman K: Dyspnea on exertion: Is it the heart or the lungs? JAMA 248:2039–2043, 1982.
31. Work Practices Guides for Manual Lifting. NIOSH Publication No. PB82–178948.
32. U.S. DHHS Social Security Administration: Disability Evaluation Under Social Security. Washington, DC, Dept of Health and Human Services, 1990.
33. Cocchiarella L, Andersson GBJ (eds): Guides to the Evaluation of Permanent Impairment, 5th ed. Chicago, American Medical Association, 2001.

CHAPTER

27

Peripheral Vascular Impairment

DENNIS J. WRIGHT, MD ■ STEPHEN L. DEMETER, MD, MPH

The evaluation of the patient with peripheral vascular disease (PVD) may be addressed by location (central versus peripheral; upper versus lower extremity) or by the type of disease (arterial versus venous). The impairment evaluation of PVD encompasses a thorough history, a detailed physical examination, physiologic testing to assess the degree of impairment, anatomic evaluation to evaluate the extent of disease, and an evaluation of therapeutic options that could return the patient to a compensated state of health. This chapter covers diseases of the aorta, peripheral occlusive disease of the lower and upper extremities, venous diseases, and lymphedema.

DISEASES OF THE AORTA

History

In the vascular evaluation of a patient, the history plays a key role in the overall assessment. A sample worksheet for obtaining a vascular history is shown in Figure 27–1. A checklist such as this helps to assure the completeness of the history. A consideration of the family history (including prior generations) in the patient with a disease of the aorta is vital.

When considering diseases of the aorta, the two principal concerns are aortoiliac occlusive disease and aneurysmal disease. The discussion of both of these entities begins with coexistent cardiovascular conditions such as hypertension, angina, myocardial infarction, congestive heart failure, and cardiac arrhythmia. Careful questioning may be necessary to obtain a history of hypertension, as many patients believe that once they are taking antihypertensive medication, they no longer have hypertension. A detailed list of patient medications is very valuable. Diabetes (including "borderline" diabetes) and hyperlipidemia, both treated and untreated, should be identified. Tobacco use is perhaps the single most important comorbid factor for the development of both aneurysmal and occlusive disease. The duration and intensity of tobacco use should be identified. A search for other tobacco-related problems such as cardiac disease and pulmonary problems is also important. Other significant aspects of the history include a history of renal vascular disease, stroke, arthritis, collagen vascular disease, and back disease (both degenerative and post-traumatic). A complete and detailed history of prior vascular interventions such as angioplasties, stents, and operations is mandatory.

The most indicative symptom of aortoiliac occlusive disease is claudication,[7] which presents with symptoms primarily in the hips, thighs, and buttocks but can present in or extend into the calves if there is a component of femoral or popliteal disease. Symptoms such as cramping, tightness, "giving out," and aching that occur while ambulating are typical descriptions. These symptoms are usually relieved by rest and are reproducible with resumption of activity. The details of the patient's symptoms of claudication must be sought. Symptoms that occur without activity or those that cannot be relieved unless the patient sits or lies down must be explored as symptoms similar to claudication can be caused by diseases in other organ systems.

The two major concerns in the differential diagnosis of claudication are neurovascular conditions and arthritis. Neurovascular claudication due to spinal stenosis and other neurospinal compressions may mimic claudication but often has distinctive qualities. Lateral and/or anterior distribution of leg pain is unusual with vascular disease and is more often seen in neurologic conditions. A numbing quality to the discomfort, especially with paresthesias at rest, may disclose a neurologic etiology.

VASCULAR HISTORY/PHYSICAL INTAKE EXAMINATION

Name ______________________ Age _____ Sex _____

General History

Medications ____

____

Allergies ____

Diabetes _____ Hyperlipidemia _____

Tobacco _____ Duration ____________ Currently Smoking? _____

Cardiac History _____ MI _____ Angina _____ CHF _____ Arrhythmia _____

Hypertension ____________ Duration ____________

CVA _____ COPD _____ Renal Insufficiency _____

Arthritis ________ Collagen Vascular Disease ________

Back Injury/Surgery ____________

Other Injury ____

Previous Operations ____________________________________

Prior Vascular Operations ______________________________

Family History of Vascular Disease, Cardiac Disease, and Thrombotic Disease

Description of Symptoms

____

____

____

____

____

EXAMINATION

Height ________ Weight ________ Pulse ________ BP R ________ L _____

Upper Extremity

Swelling R _____ L _____ Bilateral _____ Measurements R _____ L _____

Ulceration R _____ L _____ Description ____________________

____

Pulses	Right	Left	Comments (Bruit/Aneurysm)
Carotid			
Subclavian			
Axillary			
Brachial			
Radial			
Ulnar			

Figure 27–1. Sample worksheet for obtaining vascular history.

Figure continued on following page

Lower Extremity

Swelling R _____ L _____ Bilateral _____ Measurements R _____ L _____

Ulceration R _____ L _____ Description ______________________________

Pulses	Right	Left	Comments (Bruit/Aneurysm)
Aortic			
Iliac			
Femoral			
Popliteal			
D. Pedal			
P. Tibial			

Figure 27–1. *Continued*

Symptoms may be unilateral or bilateral depending on the site or level of the disease. Arthritic conditions can also be confused with vascular claudication, especially when exacerbated by exercise. A careful history may give clues to the etiology. The reproducibility of arthritic pain is often variable with respect to the degree of exercise needed to reproduce the symptoms, with pain often not occurring until after the exercise is completed. Arthritic pain may also vary with time of day or changes in weather, whereas vascular claudication remains fairly consistent under these conditions. If pain does not subside with cessation of activity or if it worsens after a period of rest, an arthritic etiology should be considered.

Further questioning may reveal other signs and symptoms of vascular disease. Changes in skin temperature and skin color (blanching, bluish discoloration, dependent rubor) are associated with decreased perfusion. Constant numbness, especially in the nondiabetic, may be a symptom of ischemic neuropathy. Loss of muscle mass may be seen in longstanding ischemia. When significant aortoiliac disease is present, impotence may be associated with symptoms of hip, thigh, and/or buttock claudication (Leriche syndrome).[7] Ischemic pain at rest and tissue loss is rare with aortoiliac disease alone.

Aneurysmal disease of the aorta presents with few symptoms. The occasional patient will report abdominal fullness or a sense of feeling that his or her heart is beating in the abdomen but this is rare. Significant back pain, rarely caused by aortic aneurysms unless they are active or leaking, is most often caused by musculoskeletal conditions. It is this quiescent nature of aortic aneurysms that makes them so difficult by history. A family history will occasionally identify family members who have had aneurysms.

Physical Examination

A thorough physical examination is the starting place in the patient with PVD. A thorough examination of the vasculature and the heart should precede a more complete branched examination of the abdomen. Abdominal palpation may reveal a pulsatile mass but the lack of this finding does not rule out an aortic aneurysm. Auscultation may reveal abdominal bruits but these may be of no significance. Significant disease may be present without any bruit and bruits may be present due to mesenteric, renal, or aortoiliac stenosis. Thus, although they may point to atherosclerosis of the aorta, they are nonspecific.

Examination of the pulses is extremely important and must be performed carefully and completely. The absence of one or both femoral pulses is very common with aortoiliac disease. Femoral bruits are often present. The remainder of lower extremity pulses should be detailed. With severe aortoiliac occlusion these pulses may be absent but in rare instances, with excellent collateral circulation, distal pulses may be weakly palpable. Exact recording of popliteal, posterior tibial, and dorsal pedal pulses is a must. It should be remembered that 5% of the normal population lacks a dorsal pedal pulse. When pulses are not palpable, an effort should be made to document the presence or absence of the pulse with a hand-held Doppler instrument. All pulses should be documented by their character, not only by their presence.

Other indicators of vascular disease include hair loss, decreased skin temperature, and poor capillary refill. Muscles and joints should be inspected for signs of muscle atrophy and joint swelling. The skin color should be examined in both dependent and elevated positions to assess for dependent rubor or pallor on elevation, both signs of vascular insufficiency. Any ischemic ulcer or necrotic tissue must be thoroughly documented by its extent and location. A single digit, or several digits, affected by ischemic changes in the face of apparently normal pulses may denote proximal aortic disease causing embolic events.

The hand-held Doppler examination is a very important adjunct to the physical examination. It is an excellent confirmatory examination that can document the character and presence of the pulses on simple physical examination. The presence of flow by the Doppler examination, even when it is quite good, does not eliminate the presence of vascular disease nor does it take the place of more formal noninvasive testing. It will, however, help to document the presence of flow. Also, if the Doppler signal is absent, severe disease is present and a prompt vascular referral should be considered.

Noninvasive Testing

Further evaluation for vascular disease is accomplished by multiple noninvasive means.[20] Physiologic testing with segmental pressures and plethysmographic waveforms offer reliable indicators of the location and severity of disease. Treadmill testing reproduces the conditions that induce the symptoms of claudication and can provide positive or negative results. A recommended method for treadmill testing is the protocol used by the Social Security Administration.[16] The patient is exercised on a treadmill for 5 minutes at 2 mph with at least a 10% grade. The AMA Guides has a similar recommendation.[4(p73)] Careful preassessment for cardiac or pulmonary disease should take place before treadmill testing as it may be contraindicated in some patients. Resting pulse pressures and waveforms need to be obtained in all patients. Patients need to be prescreened for the presence of cardiac or pulmonary disease that may contraindicate the treadmill test or cause the patient to terminate the test prior to the onset of claudication symptoms.

The normal ankle/brachial index (ABI) (blood pressure measured in the ankle/blood pressure measured in the arm) is considered to be 0.9 and above. Claudication symptoms may occur at any level below this level. Disabling claudication usually occurs with ankle/ brachial indices of less than 0.5, when the ankle blood pressure falls to less than 50% of baseline levels, or when it takes more than 10 minutes for the ankle blood pressure to return to baseline levels.[3] A recent article summarized the results of ankle/brachial indices and suggested that values greater than 1.30 are indicative of noncompressible vessels, values between 0.90 and 1.30 are normal, and values between 0.40 and 0.90 are indicative of mild to moderate peripheral arterial disease, with values less than 0.40 being found in severe peripheral arterial disease.[9]

The exercise test report should include the treadmill settings, the duration of the exercise, a description of any symptoms that develop, the reasons for stopping the treadmill testing if the desired level of exercise is not obtained, the postexercise ankle blood pressures, and the amount of time required to return the ankle pressure to baseline (pre-exercise) levels. This type of test is extremely valuable in impairment evaluations because it recreates the physiologic conditions that cause a claimant's symptoms.

Treadmill testing creates peripheral vasodilation in distal muscle beds. In the face of fixed vascular obstruction, a patient cannot compensate for the increased demand for flow, resulting in a drop in the perfusing pressure in the lower extremities. Patients who have a normal ankle/brachial index at rest may develop significant symptoms and/or physiologic changes when exercised on the treadmill. Conversely, patients may experience significant symptoms without any change in ankle/brachial indices. This may be seen particularly in patients whose symptoms are caused by neurologic or musculoskeletal conditions.

Patients with extensive vascular calcification and noncompressibility of their vessels may have falsely elevated ankle/brachial ratios. This is not uncommon in the diabetic and elderly populations. Plethysmography will show normal waveform patterns in vessels with normal compressibility. However, calcified, noncompressible vessels will have significantly flattened waveforms, despite pressures exceeding 200 mm Hg. Other techniques may be necessary to assess the full extent of the patient's vascular disease in these circumstances. Duplex imaging of the arterial system is one of these techniques. By combining techniques of flow velocity assessment with ultrasonagraphic imaging, a noninvasive mapping of the lower extremity arterial system may be ascertained. Beginning with the aortoiliac segment and continuing down the entire leg, areas of stenosis as well as occlusion may be identified. It must be stressed that this primarily documents anatomic abnormalities rather than confirming the causation of sympomatology caused by these blockages. In some patients, however, it may be the only confirmatory test available, especially if treadmill testing is either contraindicated or is unable to be easily interpreted owing to compressibility issues.[3,21]

Computed tomographic angiography and magnetic resonance angiography provide similar anatomic data. Both require the injection of contrast agents but are considerably less invasive than routine arteriography. As with duplex imaging, they provide anatomic confirmation of areas of disease within the vascular tree, but fail to provide any significant physiologic data that are necessary for translating the anatomic abnormalities into data needed for an impairment or disability evaluation. Newer generations of magnetic resonance imaging scanners, combined with gadolinium contrast injections, approximate the diagnostic accuracy of standard arteriographic techniques.[2,3,13,15,29]

The best screening test for a suspected abdominal aortic aneurysm is the abdominal ultrasound because it is both minimally invasive and very accurate in this diagnosis. It provides information about the location as well as the size of the suspected aneurysm. Computed tomographic scanning provides similar information but is more expensive and not recommended for screening purposes. It does, however, give more reliable information about the size, location, and involvement of the aneurysm.[2,3,13,15,29]

Invasive Testing

Arteriography is the gold standard for the anatomic evaluation of arterial occlusion. Patients who are referred for arteriography should have symptoms that would warrant intervention if an occlusion is identified. These symptoms include lifestyle limiting claudication, ischemic rest pain, or tissue loss. If purely diagnostic information is desired (with consideration for surgical intervention) or if the test is being performed to confirm significant disease in a patient in whom treadmill testing is unable to be performed, one of the previously mentioned noninvasive tests is more appropriate.

This information does not replace the physiologic testing provided by treadmill testing. However, in some patients, such as those with noncompressible vessels, it may be one of the few diagnostic modalities to completely assess the vascular system. Arteriography is also one of the primary tools used to assess for a source of atheroemboli as a cause of distal ischemia. Finally, although not a primary diagnostic test for aneurysmal disease, it may serve as an important diagnostic adjunct, especially if consideration is being given to endovascular aneurysmal repair or stent placement.

There are risks inherent to contrast arteriography. Renal failure or insufficiency can occur due to contrast exposure in a small but significant number of patients. Other risks include anaphylaxis, embolization, and puncture site complications. Therefore, invasive testing should be reserved for those patients who have significant symptoms, are not candidates for other types of investigations, or are candidates for invasive intervention.

Intervention for Aortoiliac Disease

The aortoiliac segment has, perhaps, the best long-standing results for peripheral revascularization than any other area of vascular disease. Recanalization by thromblytics plus intervention with angioplasty and stenting are very effective in restoring circulation. Standard operative procedures are also quite successful and have similar good long-term results. More complex lesions may require surgical intervention but a wider range of lesions is being approached interventionally.[29] Combined techniques also can make more severe lesions into those that can be addressed with a less aggressive operative approach.

Aneurysmal disease has long been approached by open operative techniques. The biggest drawbacks have always been the operative risk, prolonged recoveries, and potential for failure to return to a completely normal postoperative state. Newer endovascular techniques for aneurysm repair decrease these risks and significantly decrease postoperative recovery times.[29]

Impairment Due to Proximal Arterial Insufficiency

Arterial insufficiency results in impairment when an individual is no longer able to perform activities of daily living (ADLs) owing to a loss of the ability to walk, ischemic pain, or loss of limbs due to ischemic disease.

TABLE 27–1

Criteria for Rating Permanent Impairment Due to the Diseases of the Aorta

Class 1: **0% to 9% Impairment of the Whole Person**	**Class 2:** **10% to 29% Impairment of the Whole Person**	**Class 3:** **30% to 49% Impairment of the Whole Person**	**Class 4:** **50% to 100% Impairment of the Whole Person**
Asymptomatic during ordinary activities; has evidence of mild aortic abnormality that is unlikely to progress	Asymptomatic during ordinary activities; has a known progressive aortic abnormality **or** recovered from aortic surgery, asymptomatic, and is not expected to be at risk for future aortic disease as a consequence of surgery	Mild to moderate symptoms from aortic abnormality despite medication **or** recovered from aortic surgery, continues mild to moderate symptoms, or at risk for recurrence of aortic abnormality	Moderate to severe symptoms due to aortic abnormality that persist despite medication and that interfere with activities of daily living (functional class 3 or 4) **or** recovered from aortic surgery but moderate to severe symptoms persist despite medication

From Cocchiarella L, Andersson GBJ (eds): Guides to the Evaluation of Permanent Impairment, 5th ed. Chicago, American Medical Association, 2001, p 70, with permission.

TABLE 27–2

Criteria for Rating Permanent Impairment Due to Valvular Heart Disease

Class 1: 0% to 9% Impairment of the Whole Person	**Class 2: 10% to 29% Impairment of the Whole Person**	**Class 3: 30% to 49% Impairment of the Whole Person**	**Class 4: 50% to 100% Impairment of the Whole Person**
Evidence by physical examination or laboratory studies of valvular heart disease **and** no symptoms in the performance of ordinary daily activities (functional class I; 5 METS; Table 3–2) or with moderately heavy exertion (7 to 10 METS) **and** does not require continuous treatment, except for intermittent prophylactic antibiotics for surgical or dental procedure to reduce risk of bacterial endocarditis **and** no evidence of CHF **and** no signs of ventricular dysfunction or dilation, and severity of stenosis or regurgitation estimated to be mild (METS >7; TMET [Bruce protocol] >6 min) **and** in the individual who has recovered from valvular heart surgery, all above criteria are met	Evidence by physical examination or laboratory studies of valvular heart disease, and no symptoms in performance of daily activities, but symptoms develop on moderately heavy physical exertion (functional class II) **or** requires moderate dietary adjustment or drugs to prevent symptoms or to remain free of signs of CHF or other consequences of valvular heart disease, such as syncope, chest pain, and emboli **or** signs or laboratory evidence of cardiac chamber dysfunction and/or dilation, severity of stenosis or regurgitation estimated to be moderate, and surgical correction not feasible or advisable; METS >5 but <7; TMET (Bruce protocol) >3 min **or** has recovered from valvular heart surgery and meets criteria for functional class II	Signs of valvular heart disease and slight to moderate symptomatic discomfort during performance of ordinary daily activities (functional class III) **and** dietary therapy or drugs do not completely control symptoms or prevent CHF **and** signs or laboratory evidence of cardiac chamber dysfunction or dilation, severity of stenosis or regurgitation estimated to be moderate or severe, and surgical correction not feasible; METS >2 but <5; TMET (Bruce protocol) >1 min but <3 min **or** has recovered from heart valve surgery but continues to meet criteria for functional class III	Signs by physical examination of valvular heart disease, and studies at rest or in performance of less than ordinary daily activities (functional class IV) **and** dietary therapy and drugs cannot control symptoms or prevent signs of CHF **and** signs or laboratory evidence of cardiac chamber dysfunction or dilation, severity of stenosis or regurgitation estimated to be moderate or severe, and surgical correction not feasible; METS <2; TMET (Bruce protocol) <1 min **or** recovered from valvular heart surgery but continues to meet criteria for functional class IV

CHF, congestive heart failure; METS, metabolic equivalents.
From Cocchiarella L, Andersson GBJ (eds): Guides to the Evaluation of Permanent Impairment, 5th ed. Chicago, American Medical Association, 2001, p 30, with permission.

This impairment may be partial or complete based on the amount of symptoms that a person has or the degree of physiologic impairment assessed by diagnostic tests. Some problems such as aneurysmal disease may require limitations on work stressors (i.e., disabling) while not causing true impairment in ADLs.

The impairment caused by diseases of the aorta is based on the symptoms created by the aneurysm or the presence of a surgical repair of an aneurysm. Table 27–1 is reprinted from the fifth edition of the AMA Guides.[4] The symptoms that are referred to, when separating aneurysmal disease into categories, appear to be those created by the presence of congestive heart failure, by the effects of distal embolization, or from interference in the peripheral circulation. (See Examples 4–9 through 4–16.[4[pp70–72]]) Thus, it is not entirely clear, to these authors, why impairment is provided for aneurysmal disease as opposed to simply rating the effects of the aneurysm on other structures. For example, in a patient with a dilated aortic root and aortic regurgitation due to the aneurysm, the impairment rating is based on the symptoms created by the aortic regurgitation because the aneurysm itself is asymptomatic. Table 27–2 (Table 3–5 of the Guides which provides impairment ratings for Valvular Heart Disease) is provided to contrast and compare the categorization of the impairment created by aneurysmal disease and that created by valvular disease.

LOWER EXTREMITY ARTERIAL DISEASE

History

The history in lower extremity occlusive disease is similar to that for aortoiliac disease. The distribution of symptoms may differ based on the level of the occlusion. Superficial femoral occlusions are most often associated with calf claudication. Foot claudication symptoms alone are rare but may be seen in entities that cause severe infrapopliteal occlusive disease, such as thomboangiitis obliterans or Buerger's disease. Symptoms may be unilateral or bilateral depending on the site of the occlusion.

One symptom more commonly seen with distal disease is ischemic rest pain. This is usually described as limited to the foot or toes and may be associated with early ulceration. The pain can be unrelenting especially with the foot elevated. The only relief may be when the foot is kept in a constantly dependent position, thus recruiting extra perfusion by means of gravity. However, the patient's complaints may focus on the redness and swelling in the foot caused by the continuous dependent positioning. This is an important condition to identify owing to its ability to cause ischemic tissue loss.

Physical Examination

Here, as in aortoiliac disease, the examination of the pulses is extremely important. The hallmark of femoral-popliteal occlusive disease is the presence of good groin pulses combined with the absence of distal pulses. Prominent or aneurysmal pulses of the femoral or popliteal arteries should be documented, as these could be a source for either embolic or thrombotic arterial occlusions. The distal pulses may only be able to be documented with the hand-held Doppler. If these are absent, it suggests severe disease. Variances in the pulses from leg to leg should also be identified and described.

Careful examination of the feet is very important with distal disease. Nowhere is this more evident than in the diabetic patient. Diabetic patients may have a neuropathy that limits some of the pain of ischemic ulceration and diabetic retinopathy can impair their ability to see their feet well enough to identify early disease. Ulcers can occur between the toes and should be rigorously looked for, as should ischemic cracks of the heels and pressure point ulcers.

Noninvasive and Invasive Testing

Noninvasive testing for distal arterial occlusive disease is similar to that for aortoiliac disease. Initial steps are physiologic testing with segmental pressures, plethysmographic waveforms, and treadmill testing. If small vessel occlusive disease is in question (vasospastic or occlusive), individual toe pressures may be obtained and cold stress testing can be performed.[3]

The waveform analysis may be even more important than in more proximal disease, especially in patients with noncompressible vessels. Normal waveforms show a sharp upstroke, prompt downstroke, and the presence of a dichrotic notch. Progressive blunting of this waveform occurs as the occlusion worsens. Both the amplitude and the normal waveform appearance are diminished, with the most severe degrees of disease being represented by a flattened waveform (Figs. 27–2 and 27–3). Further anatomic testing is appropriate in patients with normal or supernormal ankle/brachial indices in the presence of abnormal waveforms.

Invasive testing is limited to those patients in whom intervention would be considered. In addition to rest pain and tissue loss, lifestyle limiting claudication is one such indication. This may be defined as claudication that prevents the patient from performing normal ADLs or his or her job. Arteriography may be done for its diagnostic benefits and as a means of interventional therapy.

Medical and Interventional Therapy for Peripheral Lower Extremity Occlusive Disease

Medical therapy may be the first step in attempting to alleviate claudication symptoms. The improvement in symptoms in clinical trials is measured by two indices: the pain-free walking distance (PFWD; also known as the initial claudication distance) and the maximal walking distance (MWD; also known as the absolute claudication distance). There are two current medications approved for the treatment of intermittent claudication. Pentoxifylline and cilostazol work by different means to improve flow to affected extremities. In recent years, pentoxifylline (a phosphodiesterase inhibitor) has fallen out of favor, with only modest treatment results being seen.[6,17] Cilostazol, a phosphodiesterase III inhibitor (which produces vasodilation and inhibition of platelet aggregation), has shown more consistent results in increasing the PFWD and MWD.[1,6] The goal of medical therapy is to diminish symptoms and allow for longer distances of walking prior to the onset of claudication. In some patients, the combination of a walking program and medication will provide sufficient relief to allow a return to normal activities. Other patients require more aggressive means of treatment.[7,13,1]

The various types of interventional therapies discussed for proximal disease are applicable for the patient with distal disease. However, the long-term

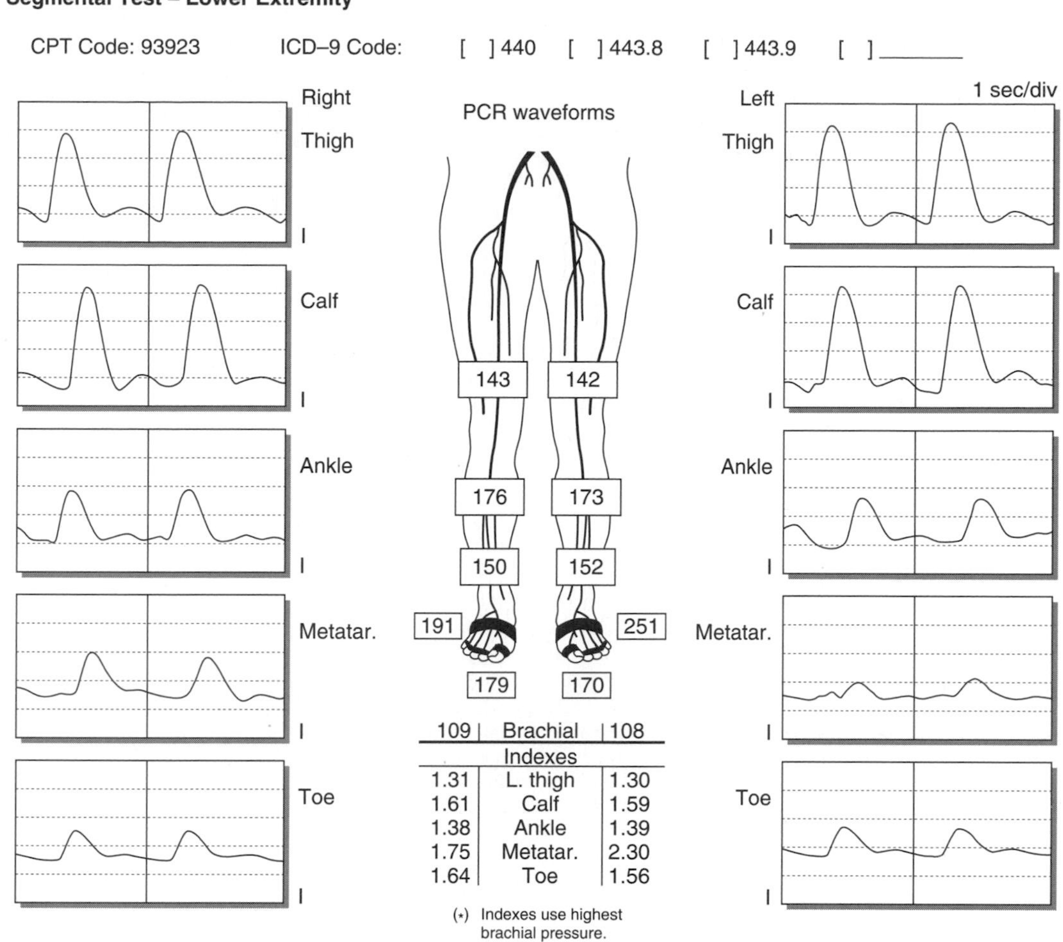

Figure 27–2. Normal Doppler examination of the lower extremities.

results and successes tend to be lower the more distal the level of the occlusion. Angioplasty and stenting are more successful in the femoral-popliteal system and less effective in the infrapopliteal vessels, where bypass surgery may be the only good alternative. In most instances, intervention is reserved for patients who fail medical therapy or for patients with more severe disease and symptoms.

Impairment Assessment in Lower Extremity Arterial Disease

Persons with lower extremity vascular disease will usually present for evaluation owing to severe claudication and rest pain. The impairment evaluation is dependent on the findings of a thorough history, physical examination, and diagnostic testing. If an individual has convincing symptoms but lacks consistent physical findings, other causations including musculoskeletal and neurologic etiologies should be considered.

The evaluation of lower extremity peripheral vascular impairment, using the AMA Guides, is found in two sections of the Guides.[4] Chapters 4 ("The Cardiovascular System: Systemic and Pulmonary Arteries") and 17 ("The Lower Extremities") both provide tables on the classification of lower extremity impairment due to peripheral vascular diseases. The two tables, reprinted as Tables 27–3 and 27–4, are similar but not identical. Impairment created by venous disease of the lower extremities is included in each of these tables. If the examinee has had an amputation, the impairment value for the amputation needs to be combined with the impairment value from the vascular disorder.[4(pp73,553)] The impairment values are given in lower extremity units in both sections and tables, not in whole person values.

As can be seen and as noted, the two tables appear to be identical, yet there are some differences. In Class 2, Chapter 4 of the Guides states that intermittent claudication is to be present "on severe usage of the lower extremity"; Chapter 17 states that it is to be present "on walking at least 100 yards at an average pace." The dis-

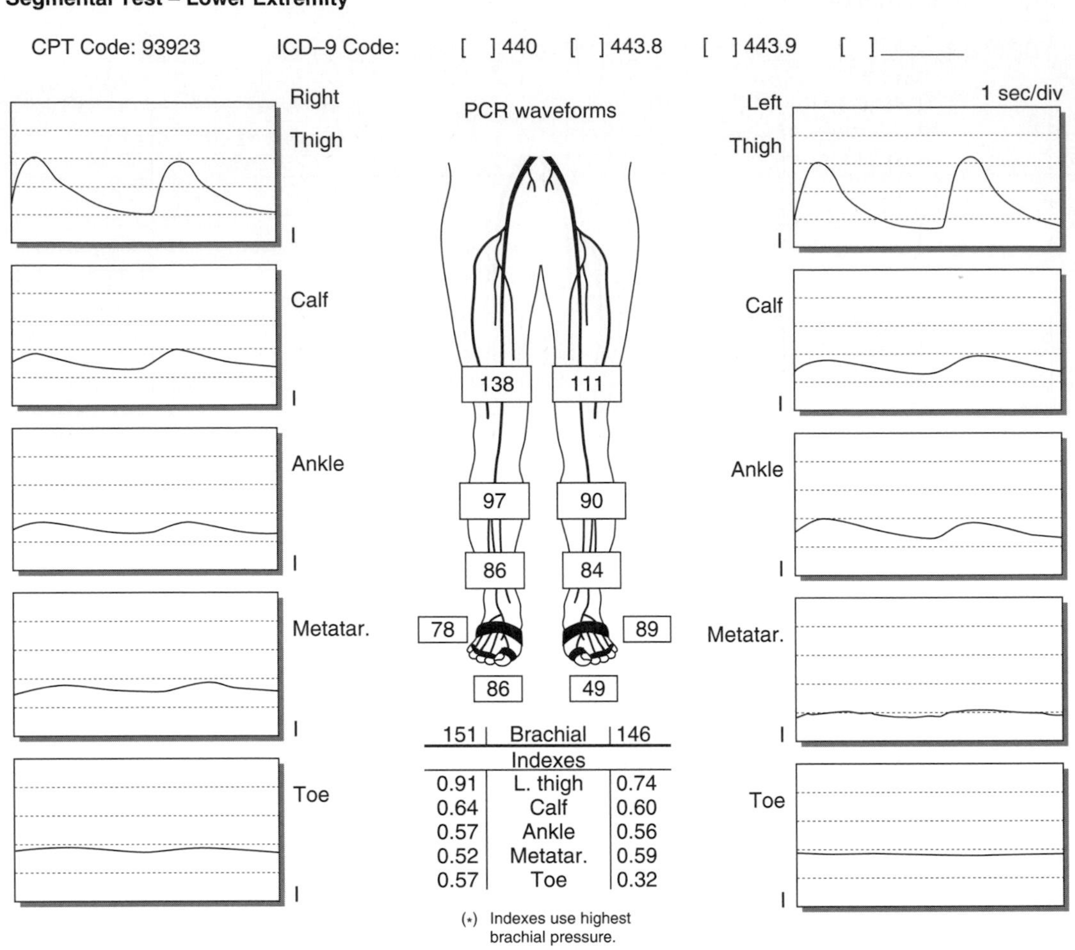

Figure 27–3. Abnormal Doppler examination of the lower extremities.

tinction of walking 25 to 100 yards for a Class 3 rating is the same in both tables. The concept "severe usage" is unclear and the evaluator is advised to use the 100-yard distance as a more reliable and easier method of analysis. The onset and presence of claudication pain is the same for Classes 4 and 5 in both tables.[4]

The concept of edema is similar in both tables except, again, in Class 2. Chapter 4 of the Guides states that the edema is "of a moderate degree controlled by elastic supports"; Chapter 17 states that the edema is only incompletely controlled by the elastic supports.[4]

In the section covering vascular damage, Chapter 4 of the Guides states that there should be "evidence of persistent, widespread, or deep ulceration involving two or more extremities." Chapter 17 states that there should be "evidence of persistent *vascular disease or of persistent*, widespread, or deep ulceration involving two or more extremities." The italicized words from Chapter 17 are missing from Chapter 4.[4]

Finally, the examples used in both sections cover venous disease and chronic edematous states in a similar fashion. There are no examples of arterial disease impairment rating in Chapter 17 of the Guides.[4] However, and importantly, Chapter 17 states in the introductory comments to this section (pp 553– 554), "when amputation due to peripheral vascular disease is involved, the impairment due to amputation should be evaluated according to the criteria in section 17.2i, and the impairment percent should be combined … with an appropriate percent based on Table 17–38 for the remaining vascular disease." A similar remark in seen in the introduction to section 4.3.[4(p73)] Unfortunately, Examples 4–23 and 4–24 both describe impairment of the lower extremity due to arterial disease and involving an amputation. Neither example combines the rating for the vascular disorder with a rating for the amputation.

TABLE 27-3

Criteria for Rating Permanent Impairment of the Lower Extremity Due to Peripheral Vascular Disease

Class 1: 0% to 9% Impairment of the Lower Extremity	Class 2: 10% to 39% Impairment of the Lower Extremity	Class 3: 40% to 69% Impairment of the Lower Extremity	Class 4: 70% to 89% Impairment of the Lower Extremity	Class 5: 90% to 100% Impairment of the Lower Extremity
Neither intermittent claudication nor pain at rest **or** only transient edema **and** on physical examination, not more than the following findings are present: loss of pulses; minimal loss of subcutaneous tissue; calcification of arteries as detected by radiographic examination; asymptomatic dilation of arteries or of veins, not requiring surgery and not resulting in curtailment of activity	Intermittent claudication on severe usage of the lower extremity **or** persistent edema of a moderate degree, controlled by elastic supports **or** vascular damage evidenced by a sign such as a healed, painless stump of an amputated digit showing evidence of persistent vascular disease, or a healed ulcer	Intermittent claudication on walking as few as 25 yards and no more than 100 yards at average pace **or** marked edema that is only partially controlled by elastic supports **and** vascular damage evidenced by a sign such as healed amputation of two or more digits of one extremity, with evidence of persisting vascular disease or superficial ulceration	Intermittent claudication on walking less than 25 yards, or intermittent pain at rest **or** marked edema that cannot be controlled by elastic supports **or** vascular damage as evidenced by signs such as an amputation at or above an ankle, or amputation of two or more digits of two extremities with evidence of persistent vascular disease; or persistent widespread or deep ulceration involving one extremity	Severe and constant pain at rest **or** vascular damage evidenced by signs such as amputation at or above the ankles of two extremities, or amputation of all digits of two or more extremities with evidence of persistent, widespread, or deep ulceration involving two or more extremities

From Cocchiarella L, Andersson GBJ (eds): Guides to the Evaluation of Permanent Impairment, 5th ed. Chicago, American Medical Association, 2001, p 76, with permission.

TABLE 27-4

Lower Extremity Impairment Due to Peripheral Vascular Disease

Class 1: 0% to 9% Impairment	Class 2: 10% to 39% Impairment	Class 3: 40% to 69% Impairment	Class 4: 70% to 89% Impairment	Class 5: 90% to 100% Impairment
Neither claudication nor pain at rest **and** only transient edema **and** on physical examination, not more than the following findings are present: loss of pulses; minimal loss of subcutaneous tissue; calcification of arteries as detected by x-ray examination; asymptomatic dilation of arteries or of veins, not requiring surgery and not resulting in curtailment of activity	Intermittent claudication on walking at least 100 yards at an average pace **or** persistent edema of a moderate degree, incompletely controlled by elastic supports **or** vascular damage as evidenced by a sign such as a healed, painless stump of an amputated digit showing evidence of persistent vascular disease or healed ulcer	Intermittent claudication on walking as few as 25 yards and no more than 100 yards at average pace **or** marked edema that is only partially controlled by elastic supports **or** vascular damage as evidenced by a sign such as healed amputation of two or more digits of one extremity, with evidence of persisting vascular disease or superficial ulceration	Intermittent claudication on walking less than 25 yards or intermittent pain at rest **or** marked edema that cannot be controlled by elastic supports **or** vascular damage as evidenced by signs such as an amputation at or above an ankle, or amputation of two more digits of two extremities with evidence of persistent vascular disease, or persistent widespread or deep ulceration involving one extremity	Severe and constant pain at rest **or** vascular damage as evidenced by such signs as amputations at or above the ankles of two extremities, or amputation of all digits of two or more extremities, with evidence of persistent vascular disease or of persistent, widespread, or deep ulceration involving two or more extremities

From Cocchiarella L, Andersson GBJ (eds): Guides to the Evaluation of Permanent Impairment, 5th ed. Chicago, American Medical Association, 2001, p 554, with permission.

Social Security

In the evaluation of the person applying for Social Security disability, the Social Security Administration requires one of four conditions to be present: amputation at or above the tarsal level; a resting ankle/brachial index of less than 0.5; a drop in the ankle pressure to less than 50% of resting levels after exercise or, in a person with an ankle/brachial index of greater than 0.5, if it takes the pressure 10 minutes to return to baseline; or failure to identify the common or deep femoral vessels on arteriography in a person with severe claudication or rest pain.[16]

Re-evaluation Timing

Most medical therapies for lower extremity arterial disease take as long as 3 months to become effective. If these treatments are not sufficient in providing symptom relief, invasive intervention will often be necessary. Most endovascular interventions allow a return to activities within days of their performance. Assessment of these procedures should be done with noninvasive physiologic arterial testing to provide a new postintervention baseline and to document the effectiveness of the procedure. Return to normal activities following revascularization surgery varies with the location and extent of the procedure, but in general requires about 4 to 6 weeks. Guidelines for postoperative testing are similar to those with interventional therapy.[7,15]

Correlation With Quality of Life Indices

White et al[18] described a number of quality of life (QOL) indices used in the evaluation of vascular surgical interventions in a chapter reviewing a variety of studies that integrated the results of vascular interventions (both operative and nonoperative) and patient expectations and outcomes. In that chapter, the authors provided clinical outcome categories that were similar to those found in Tables 4–4, 4–5, 16–17, and 17–38 of the Guides (Tables 27–3 through 27–6 of this chapter). A variety of QOL parameters were also provided with references to other indices. Unfortunately, whereas clinical measures such as ABI, vascular patency, and limb salvage all "effectively assess the physiological impact of vascular intervention," they "do not adequately describe overall patient benefit or adverse effect."[18(p33)] The chapter also specifically looked at four parameters: functional status, perceived health, psychological well-being, and role function. "Functional status" covered items similar to the types of parameters found in the concept of ADL as used by the AMA Guides.[4(pp4–5)] Their results indicated that the "relationship between various objective clinical parameters, such as ABI, and walking distance, and patient-reported outcomes of lower extremity ischemia do not show a high degree of correlation."[18(p34)] Thus, although outcome measures can address objective measurements of vascular disease and the results of interventions that can also be measured objectively, there does not necessarily appear to be as good of a correlation between the objective measurements of vascular disease (treated or untreated) and effects on ADLs, which is the principal goal of the AMA Guides.

UPPER EXTREMITY ARTERIAL DISEASE

History

Causes of upper extremity arterial occlusion are more varied than in the lower extremities. Complex disorders such as vasculitidies, collagen vascular diseases, thoracic outlet problems, and vasospastic disorders may all cause upper extremity occlusive disease. Although atherosclerosis may also cause upper extremity disease, it does so in a distinct minority of patients and tends to be a problem only of the elderly. A thorough general history is the starting point in discerning the etiology.[13,15]

The patient's presenting complaints are used to direct the initial questioning. A history of painful digits with associated color changes that occur in response to temperature change is often a sign of vasospastic disease. The classical color changes are a pattern of white, blue, and finally red that can be brought on by change in temperature or strong emotional stimuli. This history of Raynaud's phenomena should be followed by a careful interrogation to elicit a history compatible with any of the various types of collagen vascular diseases. Inquiries should be made about arthralgias, rashes, telangiectasias, dysphagia, sclerodactyly, and mouth ulcers. If any of these symptoms or signs is present, an evaluation for connective tissue disorders should be considered as part of the evaluation of upper extremity arterial disease. In addition to connective tissue disorders, there are a variety of other disorders associated with Raynaud's phenomenon including abnormal circulating globulins, myeloproliferative disorders, certain medications, and occupational causes. Approximately one third of cases will be idiopathic, another one third will be associated with connective tissue diseases, and the last third will include all other causes.[14(p1178)] These should be considered because the approach, treatment, and ultimate impairment will differ based on the etiologic causation of this condition.[14(pp1177–1179)] Unilateral Raynaud's phenomenon should be considered as caused by arterial emboli until excluded. However, it should be noted that a patient's Raynaud's phenomenon may be different in intensity from side to side and that this disparity, even when profound, should not be equated with unilateral Raynaud's.[10(p1121)]

Arterial insufficiency is relatively unusual in thoracic outlet syndromes. Patients may complain of either digital ischemia or upper extremity pain with exertion. These symptoms are commonly exacerbated during overhead work or with the arms adducted. The distribution of these symptoms may also help to distinguish thoracic outlet problems that are related to nerve compression from those caused by arterial insufficiency. When pain involves the entire arm and is of a fatiguing quality, it is usually associated with vascular problems, as opposed to pain that is in a brachial plexus distribution. Embolic phenomena must be considered if digital ischemia is present. Digital ischemia can also be seen in individuals with a history of repetitive trauma. Hypothenar hammer syndrome and other types of repetitive damage to the small vessels may cause digital arterial occlusions. A complete work history may discover conditions that predispose to the above conditions (see Chapter 61). The use of vibrating tools such as jackhammers may also be associated with upper extremity occlusive disease. Other causes of isolated digital ischemia include ergot intoxification, heavy metal poisoning, intra-arterial drug injection, and central sources for emboli.[7,15]

Arteritis is a significant cause of upper extremity occlusive disease. Takyasu's arteritis, giant cell arteritis, and Buerger's disease have all been associated with exertional pain and digital ischemia. Involvement of the great vessels with symptoms of cerebrovascular events or vertebrobasilar insufficiency, especially in a patient who fits the typical epidemiologic pattern for Takyasu's arteritis (female, 20 to 30 years of age), should prompt further evaluation. Giant cell arteritis affects an older population and is an unusual cause of upper extremity ischemia. However, this diagnosis should be considered in patients who have jaw pain with chewing, dysphagia, headaches, and/or visual disturbances associated with the upper extremity symptoms. Buerger's disease should be considered in the young male smoker with digital ischemia, especially when associated with superficial phlebitis.[7,13,15]

Atherosclerotic disease causes occlusion of the upper extremities in as few as 10% of patients with this condition. Typical symptoms include fatigue of the arms with repetitive activities such as hair combing. Digital ischemia is unusual except in advanced and severe cases of atherosclerotic disease and its presence should suggest a different etiology for the ischemic changes. Fibromuscular disease of upper extremity vessels may present with both fatigue symptoms and digital ischemia.

Physical Examination

The upper extremity examination should start with bilateral blood pressure measurements with special attention to any difference greater than 20 mm Hg. The examination of the subclavian, axillary, brachial, radial, and ulnar arteries should include an evaluation of the pulses, the Doppler flow, and the presence or absence of bruits. The fingers should be examined for current or remote ulcers and for the presence of nonhealing traumatic lesions. Muscle wasting in the hand should be identified and characterized as it can occur with both thoracic outlet syndromes and carpal tunnel syndrome. The Doppler flow to the palmar arch and digital arteries should be documented when digital ischemia is evident. Any significant abnormalities in the physical examination should prompt further investigation in the noninvasive laboratory.

Noninvasive and Invasive Testing

As in the lower extremity, testing for upper extremity occlusive disease should begin with physiologic testing. Segmental Doppler pressures and plethysmographic waveforms are performed and pressures are compared from arm to arm as well as from the upper arm to the lower arm. Digital pressures and waveforms can be assessed in both the resting and cold stressed states to evaluate for vasospastic disease. Exercise testing and testing with the arms in various positions may elucidate either physiologic or anatomic abnormalities.[3]

Arteriography is a more important diagnostic tool in the upper extremities than in the lower extremities. In the assessment of digital arterial occlusions, arteriography can delineate the extent of digital occlusion, assess for a proximal source for emboli, give a means for delivery of intra-arterial diagnostic medications, and identify associated stenoses. Arteriography may also offer a minimally invasive means for intervention with angioplasty and stenting. Operative strategies are developed from the information provided by arteriography.

Impairment Assessment in Upper Extremity Arterial Disease

Upper extremity arterial vascular occlusions cause impairment in one of three ways: symptoms of claudication, signs of vascular damage, and symptoms caused by Raynaud's phenomenon.

Exertional fatigue or rest pain may limit a person's ability to perform ADLs. This type of impairment should be evaluated aggressively by upper extremity Doppler examination, with activity challenge if needed, owing to the implication that symptoms suggest severe underlying disease. This impairment should be reassessed if medical or surgical intervention is successful in restoring at least part of the circulation.

Raynaud's phenomena, although limited in the extent of underlying permanent vascular damage, may significantly limit a person's ADLs. For example, simple tasks in the home may be impossible if the same activity is performed outside the home in colder weather. Medications may be of some value in reducing the vasospastic response to cold. Physical barriers are usually all that most persons need for symptom control, especially with mild disease. Sympathectomy, once considered a possible treatment for this disorder, has been abandoned owing to the lack of good long-term responses. The AMA Guides points out that the diagnosis of Raynaud's phenomenon must be secure. "Pain on exposure to cold or generalized paleness of the fingers on exposure to cold do not in themselves indicate Raynaud's."[4(p73)]

Vascular occlusive diseases, embolic events, and vasculitidies can all result in tissue loss in the upper extremity. In these disorders, the functional status of remaining digits as well as the degree of pain in the amputated digits may determine the impairment of the evaluee. Healed ulcers may not affect a person's ability to perform ADLs. However, the ulcers may give rise to sufficient pain that there may be functional impairment and inability to perform many ADLs. Revascularization surgery is limited in its role in improving a person's functional status.

Tables 4–4 (Table 27–5) and 16–7 (Table 27–6) are reprinted from the AMA Guides. As in the lower extremity, there are marked similarities in the two tables. However, there are some dissimilarities, and these are discussed in the following. Additionally, as in the lower extremity, amputations are to be combined with the appropriate impairment created by the vascular disease. All impairments in these two tables are for impairment of the upper extremity, not the whole person.[4]

Table 16–17 (Table 27–6) is separated into six categories of symptoms. These are really factors or indicators of disease as not all are symptoms. It tends to make this table easier to use than Table 4–4 (Table 27–5). There are several typographical errors in Table 16–17 (Table 27–6). The words "vascular disease" are missing after the word persistent ("...with evidence of persistent ... widespread, or deep...") in Classes 4 and 5. Of more importance is the concept of edema being controlled by elastic supports. This concept is found in the edema section of Table 4–4 (Table 27–5) but is absent in Table 16–17 (Table 27–6). Similarly, the concepts of pain at rest and medication control are missing from Table 4–4 (Table 27–5). The term "one extremity" is missing from the vascular damage section of Class 4 in Table 4–4 (Table 27–5) when referring to amputation at or above the wrist, although this should be clear from looking at Class 5 in the same table. The only major typographical error, is in Table 4–4 (Table 27–5) in the claudication section, where the word mild is used instead of moderate.[4]

VENOUS AND LYMPHATIC DISEASES

Venous insufficiency and lymphatic disease of both the upper and lower extremities have common features. They are manifest with swelling, discomfort, and, in the worst cases, ulceration. As with arterial disease, the history and physical examination are pivotal when establishing the appropriate diagnostic testing sequence.

History

A thorough general medical history should be performed. Patients should be questioned about cardiac and pulmonary problems. Problems that relate to swelling and pain in the extremity should be sought. Signs of chronic venous disease such as varicosities, dermatitis, and ulceration (both current and healed) must be looked for. The duration and pattern of each of these problems should be established.

Pain may present and its pattern gives clues to the etiology of the venous or lymphatic disease. Pain associated with venous ulceration is often quite remarkable and is fairly well localized to the area of the ulceration. Generalized aching pain that occurs after periods of standing is more insidious in nature than with arterial disease, but is often relieved once the extremity is elevated. Pain with exertion that feels like a bursting sensation in the muscles can also be felt and, when seen in the legs, is termed venous claudication. This is usually associated with advanced cases of venous insufficiency. Painless swelling (often described as an uncomfortable tightness) suggests lymphedema if not associated with other symptoms of venous disease.

A history of deep venous thrombosis must be rigorously questioned for. Essential information includes the dates, causes, treatments, sites, and complications of those episodes. Trauma in the home or workplace or of an iatrogenic nature (e.g., central venous lines) should be explored. A history of hypercoaguability (either in the patient or in the family) should be sought. A history of superficial phlebitis is also important. Prior use of stocking therapy including compliance and response to this form of treatment should be documented. Postphlebitic syndromes of pain, swelling, and ulceration are seen in up to 29% to 79% of patients who have experienced deep vein thromboses, with approximately 5% of the U.S. population having post-thrombotic changes (an estimated 6 to 7 million people with stasis changes and 0.4 to 0.5 million with leg ulcers).[11(p1931)] This history is especially important where impairment issues are concerned.

Physical Examination

Superficial varicosities were once thought to be a limited disease with no physiologic consequences. The fundamental pathophysiologic cause of chronic venous insufficiency is due to valvular incompetence (>90%). The remainder of patients have chronic venous obstruction as the underlying etiology. The valvular incompetency can be isolated to the superficial veins, the deep veins, the perforating veins, or may be a combination of any of these. In more than one third of patients with chronic venous insufficiency and skin ulceration, valvular incompetence is in the superficial veins, the perforating veins, or both, with half of these patients having disease isolated to the superficial veins.[5(p174)]

Swelling is the primary physical finding on examination. It may or may not be of a pitting variety. The swelling may be associated with brawny induration, a brownish-purple discoloration of the skin that does not blanch. Varicosities may be present or absent, and evidence of venous "spiders" or varicosity ruptures may be present. Venous eczema presents with dry, cracked, and

TABLE 27-5

Criteria for Rating Permanent Impairment of the Upper Extremity Due to Peripheral Vascular Disease

Class 1: 0% to 9% Impairment of the Upper Extremity	**Class 2: 10% to 39% Impairment of the Upper Extremity**	**Class 3: 40% to 69% Impairment of the Upper Extremity**	**Class 4: 70% to 89% Impairment of the Upper Extremity**	**Class 5: 90% to 10 Impairment of the Upper Extremity**
Neither intermittent claudication nor pain at rest **or** only transient edema **and** on physical examination, not more than the following findings are present: loss of pulses; minimal loss of subcutaneous tissue of fingertips; calcification of arteries as detected by radiographic examination; asymptomatic dilation of arteries or of veins, not requiring surgery and not resulting in curtailment of activity **or** Raynaud's symptoms with or without obstructive physiology (as documented by finger brachial indices of <0.8 or low digital temperatures with decreased laser Doppler signals that do not normalize with warming of affected digits) that completely responds to lifestyle changes and/or medical therapy	Intermittent claudication on severe upper extremity usage **or** persistent edema of a moderate degree, controlled by elastic supports **or** vascular damage evidenced by a sign such as a healed, painless stump of an amputated digit showing evidence of persistent vascular disease, or a healed ulcer **or** Raynaud's phenomena with obstructive physiology (as documented by finger/brachial indices of <0.8 or low digital temperatures with decreased laser Doppler signals that do not normalize with warming of affected digits) that incompletely responds to lifestyle changes and/or medical therapy	Intermittent claudication on mild upper extremity usage **or** marked edema that is only partially controlled by elastic supports **and** vascular damage evidenced by a healed amputation of two or more digits of one extremity, with evidence of persisting vascular disease or superficial ulceration	Intermittent claudication on mild upper extremity usage **or** marked edema that cannot be controlled by elastic supports **or** vascular damage as evidenced by signs such as an amputation at or above a wrist, or amputation of two or more digits of both extremities with evidence of persistent vascular disease; or persistent widespread or deep ulceration involving one extremity	Severe and constant pain at rest **or** vascular damage evidenced by signs such as amputation at or above the wrists of both extremities, or amputation of all digits of both extremities with evidence of persistent, widespread, or deep ulceration involving both upper extremities

From Cocchiarella L, Andersson GBJ (eds): Guides to the Evaluation of Permanent Impairment, 5th ed. Chicago, American Medical Association, 2001, p 74, with permission.

TABLE 27-6

Impairment of the Upper Extremity Due to Peripheral Vascular Disease

	Upper Extremity Impairment %				
Symptoms	**Class 1 (0% to 9%)**	**Class 2 (10% to 39%)**	**Class 3 (40% to 69%)**	**Class 4 (70% to 89%)**	**Class 5 (90% to 100%)**
Claudication	None	Intermittent with severe use	Intermittent with moderate use	Intermittent with mild use	Persistent
Pain at rest	None	None	None	Intermittent	Severe and constant
Edema	Transient	Persistent and moderate	Marked	Marked	Marked
Signs of vascular damage	Loss of pulses; minimal loss of subcutaneous tissue of fingertips; arterial calcifications on x-ray; asymptomatic dilation of veins or arteries not requiring surgery; no decreased activity	Healed painless amputation stump of one digit with persistent vascular disease or healed ulcer	Healed amputation stump of two or more digits with persistent vascular disease or superficial ulceration	Amputation of two or more digits of each extremity, or amputation at or above wrist of one extremity with persistent widespread or deep ulceration of one extremity	Amputation of all digits or amputation at or above the wrist of each extremity, with persistent vascular disease or widespread or deep ulcerations of both extremities
Raynaud's phenomenon	Raynaud's symptoms with or without obstructive physiology (as documented by finger brachial indices of <0.8 or low digital temperatures with decreased laser Doppler signals that do not normalize with warming of affected digits) that completely responds to lifestyle changes and/or medical therapy	Raynaud's phenomena with obstructive physiology (as documented by finger/brachial indices of <0.8 or low digital temperatures with decreased laser Doppler signals that do not normalize with warming of affected digits) that incompletely responds to lifestyle changes and/or medical therapy			
Medication control	Good	Good	Partial	Partial	Poor

From Cocchiarella L, Andersson GBJ (eds): Guides to the Evaluation of Permanent Impairment, 5th ed. Chicago, American Medical Association, 2001, p 498, with permission.

poorly nourished skin. It correlates with the severity and, especially, the longevity of the disease process.

Venous ulcers occur in the "gaiter distribution" of the lower third of the leg (midcalf to below the malleoli). Similar ulcers can also appear in the lower portion of the arm. These ulcers tend to have ill-defined margins, lacking sharply demarcated edges. They are often prone to large amounts of fluid exudation and/or transudation through the surface of the wound. There may be multiple areas of ulceration and they usually show evidence of good granulation tissue in their bases. Distal ulcers with sharply demarcated edges suggest an arterial cause. The presence of concomitant arterial and venous disease is not a infrequent occurrence and should be considered when appropriate associated risk factors are present.

Noninvasive Testing

Just as in the arterial system, there are a variety of tests available for testing the adequacy of the venous system. Noninvasive tests such as Doppler ultrasonography, plethysmography, thermography, radionuclide tests, and certain blood tests are of value for the diagnosis of venous thromboses, either acute or chronic. Measuring and physiologically quantitating chronic venous insufficiency is more difficult. Ambulatory venous pressures can be measured and have a good correlation with the presence of skin ulceration. In general, however, the diagnosis of chronic venous insufficiency, for the purpose of an impairment evaluation, will be clinical as opposed to physiological.

Treatment

Venous diseases are perhaps the most difficult problem faced by vascular specialists. There are few, if any, good, longstanding, surgical cures for venous disease. Ulcers are best treated by consistent wound care and compression. All other forms of venous disease are treated with compression garments. The lack of good interventional and surgical treatments, as well as lack of patient compliance with the more conservative measures, leads to chronic problems that often result in disability.[8,12]

IMPAIRMENT EVALUATION FOR VENOUS DISEASE AND LYMPHEDEMA

Lower Extremity Disease

Many levels of temporary and permanent impairment are evidenced in lower extremity venous disease. Superficial venous diseases such as varicose veins and superficial reflux disease (greater and lesser saphenous reflux) can result in significant pain. Many of these problems can be treated with compression stockings, which may significantly reduce symptoms. Occasionally, a patient may require direct treatment to alleviate symptoms. Examples of direct treatment include ligation, stripping, and sclerotherapy.

As noted previously, it has been traditionally held that most cases of superficial venous disease cause little impairment and interfere with the ADLs only in a very limited fashion. However, superficial disease may give rise to chronic venous insufficiency. When superficial disease presents without complicating features, it produces only a Class 1 lower extremity impairment, as seen in Tables 4–5 and 17–38 (Tables 27–3 and 27–4).[4] For more advanced disease, it should be rated using the schema used for the deep venous system.

More complex problems occur with disease of the deep venous system. Swelling can be a considerable problem even in situations where tissue loss is not a concern. Moderate, persistent edema may be present that is responsive to compression stocking therapy. This type of venous insufficiency causes little permanent impairment. The degree of impairment increases if the edema fails to respond to compression therapy. Tables 4–5 and 17–38 (Tables 27–3 and 27–4) allow for an impairment level as high as 89% of the lower extremity depending on the degree of edema, the response to treatment, and (although not directly stated) the degree of interference with ADLs. The examples in Chapters 4 and 17 of the Guides provide some insight into these high impairment ratings for venous diseases.[4(pp76–78,554)] Because of pronounced stasis, venous diseases can make a person prone to stasis ulceration. As noted previously, this is often recalcitrant to treatment. The skin can become prone to injury with even minor trauma producing lesions that eventually ulcerate. Even without ulceration, there are often prolonged recovery times. The stasis also increases the likelihood for developing thromboses in the affected areas that either compound the original problem or lead to embolic phenomena. If conservative treatment with elastic stockings fails to control the problem and if medications are inadequate or create unacceptable side effects or complications, the only treatment option is prolonged elevation of the legs. This creates marked interference with performing any of the activities of daily life.

When ulceration occurs, the level of impairment increases, even when the swelling can be controlled. Venous ulceration is one of the leading causes of lost work time in the United States. Recidivism is a prime cause of ongoing disability. Many people place a lower priority on venous ulcer care than they do on other medical or nonmedical concerns. In many cases, no thorough care plan is given to the individual, and the follow-up is erratic. Today, many excellent centers are available for wound care and the multidisciplinary approach offered in these centers is frequently able to achieve healing in a significantly reduced time. This type of consistent care reduces rates of recidivism and increases the rate of wound healing.

The ulcer itself may be a significant cause of pain and, in some severe uncontrolled instances, may even lead to tissue loss and amputation. Although these extreme instances are rare, less severe cases of venous ulceration may still impair a person's ability to perform normal activities. Many therapeutic regimens require the individual to limit the number of hours that they spend on his or her feet. In addition, many dressings are bulky and limit the footwear a person can wear. Specialty clinics that specifically deal with lower extremity venous disease may be used; however, they often require frequent visits and/or frequent therapeutic interventions to which the person must adhere for best results.[7,15]

Lymphedema is an unusual cause of significant impairment, more owing to its infrequent occurrence than to the nature of the disease. Swelling and infection are the major causes of impairment in this group of people. Similar to venous disease, if swelling becomes uncontrolled, use of the affected extremity can be severely limited. Significant surgical intervention has been disappointing in chronic lymphedema and it can be quite disfiguring. If conservative measures are ineffective, the impairment caused by lymphedema is assessed in a fashion similar to venous diseases.

Upper Extremity Disease

Venous disease and lymphedema of the upper extremity both create impairment by their inability to be controlled. The incidence of this problem may be increasing for venous disease and decreasing for lymphatic disease owing to increasing numbers of central venous lines and decreasing numbers of radical breast surgeries. Ulceration is a rare complication of upper extremity venous disease and is even more rare in lymphatic disease. Infection can occur in both situations but is more frequent in lymphedema. Recurring infections may further impair the lymphatic drainage of the upper extremity and lead to increased swelling. Compression garments are the mainstays of therapy for both of these diseases.[7]

The method of impairment assessment for venous disease and lymphedema of the upper extremities is found in Tables 4–4 and 16–17 (Tables 27–5 and 27–6). The amount of impairment is based on the degree of control over the edema and the presence of ulceration.[4]

References

1. Beebe HG, Dawson DL, Cutler BS, et al: A new pharmacological treatment for intermittent claudication: Results of a randomized, multicenter trial. Arch Intern Med 159:2041–2050, 1999.
2. Bernstein EF: Recent Advances in Noninvasive Diagnostic Techniques in Vascular Disease. St. Louis, Mosby, 2000.
3. Bernstein EF: Vascular Diagnosis, 4th ed. St. Louis, Mosby, 1993.
4. Cocchiarella L, Andersson GBJ (eds): Guides to the Evaluation of Permanent Impairment, 5th ed. Chicago, American Medical Association, 2001.
5. Criado E, Passman MA: Physiologic assessment of the venous system. In Rutherford RB (ed): Vascular Surgery, 5th ed. Philadelphia, WB Saunders, 2000, pp 165–191.
6. Dawson DL, Cutler BS, Meissner MH, Strandness DE Jr: Cilastazol has beneficial effects in treatment of intermittent claudication: Results from a multicenter, randomized, prospective, double-blind trial. Circulation 98:678–686, 1998.
7. Ernst CB, Stanley JC: Current Therapy in Vascular Surgery, 4th ed. St. Louis, Mosby, 2001.
8. Gloviczki P, Cho JS: Surgical treatment of chonic deep venous obstruction. In Rutherford RB (ed): Vascular Surgery, 5th ed. Philadelphia, WB Saunders, 2000, pp 2049–2066.
9. Hiatt WR: Medical treatment of peripheral arterial disease and claudication. N Engl J Med 344:1608–1621, 2001.
10. Johnston KW: Upper extremity ischemia: Overview. In Rutherford RB (ed): Vascular Surgery, 5th ed. Philadelphia, WB Saunders, 2000, pp 1111–1116.
11. Meissner MH, Strandness DE: Pathophysiology and natural history of acute deep venous thrombosis. In Rutherford RB (ed): Vascular Surgery, 5th ed. Philadelphia, WB Saunders, 2000, pp 1920–1937.
12. Moneta GL, Porter JM: Nonoperative treatment of chronic venous insufficiency. In Rutherford RB (ed): Vascular Surgery, 5th ed. Philadelphia, WB Saunders, 2000, pp 1999–2007.
13. Moore WS: Vascular Surgery: A Comprehensive Review, 5th ed. Philadelphia, WB Saunders, 1998.
14. Porter JM, Edwards JM: Occlusive and vasospastic diseases involving distal upper extremity arteries—Raynaud's syndrome. In Rutherford RB (ed): Vascular Surgery, 5th ed. Philadelphia, WB Saunders, 2000, pp 1170–1183.
15. Rutherford RB: Vascular Surgery, 5th ed. Philadelphia, WB Saunders, 2001.
16. Social Security Administration, U.S. Department of Health and Human Services: Disability Evaluation Under Social Security. Social Security Administration publication #64-039/ICN #468600. Washington, DC, Social Security Administration, U.S. Department of Health and Human Services, 1998.
17. Weitz JI, Byrne J, Clagett GP, et al: Diagnosis and treatment of chronic arterial insufficiency of the lower extremities: A critical review. Circulation 94:3026–3049, 1996.
18. White JV, Jones DN, Rutherford RB: Integrated assessment of results: Standardized reporting of outcomes and the computerized vascular registry. In Rutherford RB (ed): Vascular Surgery, 5th ed. Philadelphia, WB Saunders, 2000, pp 20–37.
19. Yao JST, Pearce WH: Progress in Vascular Surgery. Stamford, CT, Appleton and Lange, 1997.
20. Zierler RE, Sumner DS: Physiological assessment of peripheral arterial occlusive disease. In Rutherford RB (ed): Vascular Surgery, 5th ed. Philadelphia, WB Saunders, 2000, pp 140–165.
21. Zwiebel WJ: Introduction to Vascular Ultrasonography. Philadelphia, WB Saunders, 1992.

CHAPTER

28

Dermatological Impairment

JAMES S. TAYLOR, MD

PREVALENCE: DISABILITY AND SKIN CONDITIONS

In the United States, an estimated 35 to 43 million persons have a disability, costing the nation an estimated $176.7 billion annually.* According to U.S. Census data from 1990, an estimated 12.8 million persons aged 16 to 64 years had a work disability of 6 months or longer.[21,22] Many applications for federal disability benefits are are submitted with 6.3 million Americans drawing checks in 1993 in contrast to 4.6 million in 1988.[20] In 1993, the Centers for Disease Control and Prevention published data on the prevalence of selected chronic conditions in the United States for the period 1986 through 1988 based on the National Health Interview Surveys. Rates per thousand persons for 10 skin conditions and the percentage of each causing limitation of activity, one or more hospitalizations, and one or more physician visits are listed. Dermatitis leads the list with a rate of 38.1 per 1000 persons, of which 1.2% caused limitations of activity. In contrast, chronic ulceration of the skin had the lowest rate, affecting 0.9 per 1000 persons, but had the highest percentage (24.1%) causing limitation of activity.[1]

An updated report was published in 1996, based on 1992 data, listing the prevalence of chronic conditions from all causes associated with activity limitations. There were 362,000 cases of diseases of the skin and subcutaneous tissue (ICD-9-CM Codes 680–709) in these categories: contact dermatitis and other eczema—90,000; psoriasis and similar disorders—58,000; chronic ulcer of the skin—58,000; and other disorders—156,000.[12] According to State Workers' Compensation data reported to the Bureau of Labor Statistics through the Supplementary Data System, based on 1985–1986 data, but not published by Leigh and Miller until 1998, dermatitis was the third most common cause of compensable temporary total and partial disability and the sixth most common cause of permanent partial disability in the United States.[14]

DISABILITY PROGRAMS

Impairment caused by skin disorders, as with other organ systems, is rated using an accurate diagnosis; documentation of its effects on a person's occupation, activities of daily living (ADL), occupational risks and demands, response to treatment(s), and avoidance of precipitating factors; an estimation of the prognosis based on these factors; and a careful review of the information contained in the body of medical knowledge concerning the specific disorder.[2,15]

Disability caused by skin disorders, as with other organ systems, is decided using the rating system specific to each patient's case and is usually based on the referring source or the conditions of employment and exposure associated with the development of the skin disorder. Many of the rating systems and referring sources have peculiarities inherent to the style, format, or purpose of the source, and are discussed in this chapter.

Workers' Compensation

Occupational skin disease cases under workers' compensation account for most of the impairment evaluations performed by dermatologists. According to figures from the U.S. Bureau of Labor Statistics, work-related skin disorders were the second most common cause of occupational disease in the United States in 1999.[28] In 1984, when federal statistics were last available on time lost from work, approximately 25% of workers with occupational skin disease lost time from work, averaging 10 to 12 days each.[26]

Most claims based on occupational skin disease involve temporary total or permanent partial disability. Temporary total occupational disability occurs when an occupational disorder *prevents an individual from performing his or her job.*

Some states allow third party liability suits arising out of workers' compensation cases. For example, a machinist who has received workers' compensation for patch test–proven allergic contact dermatitis to a coolant germicide also can sue the manufacturer of the germicide for damages from the injury.

The U.S. Chamber of Commerce publishes an annual analysis of each state's workers' compensation laws. A much more detailed version published by the American Insurance Institute is also available through the U.S. Chamber of Commerce.[27]

Social Security Disability

The Disability Evaluation Under Social Security Handbook states:[24] "Skin lesions may result in a marked, long-lasting impairment if they involve extensive body areas or critical areas such as the hands or feet and become resistant to treatment. These lesions must be shown to have persisted for a sufficient period of time despite therapy for a reasonable presumption to be made that a marked impairment will last for a continuous period of at least 12 months."[(pp58–59)] Only five specific categories of skin impairments are listed, but medically equivalent impairments will also be considered. Skin impairments are also considered in the determination of residual functional capacity, which what a worker can still do despite his or her limitations (written communication, Ronal D. Fisher, Social Security Administration, Baltimore, May 10, 1994; confirmed by Dale Cox, Social Security Administration, Baltimore, (MD,) February 14, 2001).

Department of Veterans Affairs

The Department of Veterans Affairs' Physician's Guide for Disability Evaluation Examinations[29] has been formatted into the Automated Medical Information Exchange (AMIE) system. This system covers 11 types of benefit categories, ranging from VA disability, compensation, and pensions to former prisoners of war, Persian Gulf veterans, and a number of miscellaneous categories, including some VA employees and veterans exposed to environmental hazards. Results of the VA Compensation and Pension Examination are then rated by a Rating Board at a VA regional office in accordance with the Veterans Benefits Administration Schedule for Rating Disabilities, which is included in Title 38, Code of Federal Regulations.

Claims are filed with the Veterans Benefits Administration and the Veterans Health Administration schedules examinations. Physicians in the Department of Veterans Affairs access the AMIE examination worksheets from the Internet (personal communication, Clay Johnson, Department of Veterans Affairs, Washington, D.C., April 2001).

Specific skin conditions are listed by the VA, especially scars, eczema, various infections, psoriasis, and tumors. Other skin conditions can be considered (written communication, Teresa R. Oster, Department of Veterans Affairs, Atlanta, May 6, 1994). Specific Department of Veterans Affairs regulations relate to Agent Orange. Recently, porphyria cutanea tarda and Hodgkin's disease have been added to chloracne, non-Hodgkin's lymphoma, and soft tissue sarcoma as diseases with presumptive service connection, based on exposure to Agent Orange and other herbicides in Vietnam veterans.[30]

Military Services and Department of Defense

The military services have standards for induction and retention into the armed services (written communication, William D. James, MD, Walter Reed Army Medical Center, June 2, 1994). These standards include medical conditions. Those involving the skin include severe acne and eczema as well as a number of other inflammatory and malignant conditions such as psoriasis, collagen vascular diseases, chronic urticaria, and lymphomas. Also included are "any other chronic skin disorder of a degree or nature that requires frequent outpatient treatment or hospitalization or interferes with the satisfactory performance of duty."[6] The Department of Defense also has specific disability separation guidelines that will often tie in with specific VA benefits.[5]

Federal Employees' Compensation Act

The Federal Employees' Compensation Act (FECA) and program is administered by the Office of Workers' Compensation Programs (OWCP) in the U.S. Department of Labor. For employment-related disabling skin conditions FECA provides disability compensation for wage loss during the period of disability. Skin conditions are not covered under the scheduled permanent partial disability provisions of FECA. Occupational skin conditions may be covered under the disfigurement provision. "For serious disfigurement of the face, head, or neck of a character likely to handicap an individual in securing or maintaining employment, proper and equitable compensation not to exceed $3,500 shall be awarded in addition to any other compensation payable under this schedule." Please see the discussion and notes under FECA in Chapter 4 of this volume for useful information on benefits (written communication, John D. McLellan, Jr., JD, Alexandria, VA, February 13, 2001).

Longshore and Harbor Workers[2] Act

The Longshore and Harbor Workers' Compensation Act (LSA) is also administered by the OWCP in the U.S. Department of Labor. For employment-related disabling skin conditions, the LSA provides disability compensation for wage loss during the period of disability. Skin conditions are not covered under the scheduled permanent partial disability provisions of the LSA. Occupational skin conditions may be covered under the disfigurements provision: "proper and equitable compensation not to exceed $7,000 shall be awarded for serious disfigurement of the face, head, or neck or of other normally exposed areas likely to handicap the employee in securing or maintaining employment." This latter benefit would be paid after and in addition to the initial wage loss compensation. Please see the discussion and notes covering the LSA Compensation Program in Chapter 4 of this volume for more complete information (written communication, John D. McLellan Jr., JD, Alexandria, VA, February 13, 2001).

Fewer claims are now made for skin conditions because of the more frequent use of container ships. Some examples of skin-related conditions are dermatitis from cocoa and hemp (personal communication, John McLellan, Jr., JD, June 1994).

Americans with Disabilities Act (ADA)[2,18,19]

Nethercott[18] has recently reviewed fitness to work under the ADA. Only a few skin conditions make a potential employee excludable under specific job requirements as regulated by the ADA. An example is an individual with chronic hand dermatitis that may affect grip strength. Topical therapy for the hand dermatitis may also interfere with job function, such as driving heavy machinery. Other conditions that may exclude a worker under certain circumstances include infectious disease of the skin, skin diseases affecting thermoregulation, and physical agent intolerance. Work-aggravated skin diseases such as psoriasis and lichen planus, vitiligo, and eczema may require workplace accommodation for the worker under the ADA.

Dermatologic Disability Proposals

General guides to the evaluation of cutaneous impairment have been proposed by Sauer, Canizares, Kanof, and Robinson between 1962 and 1968.[23] However, it was not until 1971, with the publication of the first edition of the AMA Guides that a set of guidelines was proposed for all body systems, including the skin.[2] The basic definitions and concepts of permanent impairment and disability proposed by the members of the AMA Committee on Cutaneous Impairment still stand.

OCCUPATIONAL DERMATOSES

Direct causes of occupational skin disorders include exposure to chemical, physical, mechanical, and biological agents. Injuries (lacerations, cuts, abrasions, burns) cause the overwhelming majority of cases. Chemicals cause 90% of occupational skin diseases. Of these, 70% to 80% are irritant contact dermatitis. Twenty to thirty percent are allergic contact dermatitis. The hands are involved in 90% of patients with contact dermatitis. The remaining 10% of occupational skin disease cases include folliculitis and acne (e.g., oil acne, chloracne), pigmentary disorders (e.g., postinflammatory hyper- or hypopigmentation, contact leukoderma), granulomas (e.g., foreign body, infectious), ulceration (e.g., chrome holes), neoplasms (butchers warts, arsenic-induced squamous cell carcinoma), and miscellaneous disease of the hair and nails.[26]

Studies of the prognosis for occupational skin disease indicate that persistent disease ranges from 32% to 75% of cases. Improvement in the persistent cases has been seen in some reports. Frequent factors causing these conditions to persist include the presence of atopic dermatitis, allergy to chromate, and cases of chronic irritant contact dermatitis. Other reasons for persistence of dermatitis include misdiagnosis, secondary or iatrogenic allergic contact dermatitis, insufficient advice to workers, nondermatologic factors, and endogenous and multifactorial hand dermatitis. Other statistics, outcomes, factors that affect outcome, and social consequences of occupational disability have been discussed by Nethercott,[17] Cooley,[3] and Hogan.[10]

IMPAIRMENT EVALUATION OF PUTATIVE OCCUPATIONAL DERMATOSES

Dilemmas for the Physician[13]

Medical determinations in workers' compensation involve a number of issues for the examining and treating physician:

1. Patient assertions and demands concerning work-relatedness of their disease, job changes, and job modifications.
2. Social gatekeeping concerning time off from work, date for return to work ("why can't it be on Friday?"), and determination of work-relatedness of disease.

3. Lack of adequate workplace data, such as detailed job descriptions, lists of work contacts and exposures, including material safety data sheets, and in some cases samples of workplace chemicals. This is probably the major deficiency facing the physician. A plant visit is ideal but not often practical.
4. Clinical judgment versus technology (e.g., determining whether a machinist with hand eczema and negative patch tests has an occupational irritant contact dermatitis or endogenous hand eczema).
5. Conceptual differences in medical versus legal concepts of causation. Absolute proof fulfilling Koch's postulates is not required in workers' compensation cases. Determination by the physician that a cause-and-effect relation exists between a disease and a job "within a reasonable medical certainty or probability" is usually adequate. Statement of a "possible" relationship is not adequate.[13]

Medical Evaluation

The patient's history is an integral part of the evaluation. Published history forms may be used by physicians or their assistants or adapted for self-administration by patients.[8,9] An initial examination of the area of chief complaint often helps to direct the questioning. The history of the present illness should focus on the following:

1. Patient's description of the chief complaint(s).
2. Chronology, including previous treatments and frequency of occurrence.
3. Location of the lesions at onset.
4. Spread of the lesions, if any.
5. Morphology of the lesions.
6. Time away from work, including weekends, vacations, sick leave, and disability.
7. Unintended overexposure versus usual exposure to the precipitating chemical(s) or agent(s).

Determination of the timing of the reaction also is important. Onset of symptoms within minutes or 1 to 2 hours points more to contact urticaria or irritation. Onset after one or two days or as long as 1 week suggests contact allergy, especially in first-time cases of dermatitis or in recurrent, intermittent acute dermatitis. This distinction is blurred in chronic cases. It is also important to remember that irritation, contact urticaria, and contact allergy may coexist. The interval between initial exposure and onset of occupational acne or pigmentary disturbance is usually several weeks; for tumors, several years.[11]

The usual clinical course of occupational contact dermatitis is improvement away from work for a few days and exacerbation on re-exposure, unless there is a common contact both at home and at work. Exceptions to this rule clearly exist. Outcome studies in workers with industrial dermatitis, as reviewed by Nethercott[17] and Cooley and Nethercott,[3] show persistent dermatitis in one third or more of cases; reasons for this were previously discussed. A list of drugs and other medications should be included. Contact dermatitis is possible from the systemic administration of a number of drugs to which an individual is sensitive or cross-sensitive. The frequency and effect of systemic corticosteroids should be determined, especially for reports of improvement away from the job.

Work history should include:

1. A description of job and job title(s)
2. List of work contacts
3. Review of material safety data sheets
4. Dates of employment, hours worked per week, shift, and dates and effects of any job or task changes
5. Similar complaints of other workers, if any
6. Methods and frequency of cleaning the skin, including use of waterless hand cleaners and workplace solvents
7. Protective creams and protective clothing, especially gloves

Direct questions about specific causes of flares and improvements may be helpful[8]

Past history should include:

1. List of previous compensation claims and skin conditions
2. Allergies such as childhood eczema, asthma, and hay fever
3. Overt reactions to the major contact allergens, including metals, medicaments, cosmetics, dyes, and preservatives
4. Past medical history
5. Review of systems
6. Family and social history
7. Hobbies and second jobs[8]

In some instances a review of old medical and hospitalization records is important.[2]

The physical examination should include the location, description, and distribution of the eruption as well as a listing of other important cutaneous findings. A complete skin examination is often indicated. In contact allergy the area of most intense dermatitis usually corresponds to the site of the most intense contact with the allergen. Exceptions to this rule exist, as when allergens are transferred to distant sites. Volatile airborne chemicals may cause dermatitis on exposed body areas. Contact dermatitis may be symmetrical or asymmetrical, uniform or confluent, or may involve discrete patchy areas.

Results of diagnostic tests should be recorded, especially scrapings for microorganisms (a potassium hydroxide preparation for cutaneous fungal infections is the most common such procedure performed by dermatologists), cultures, laboratory tests, biopsies, and patch tests. Specific comments about their relevance should be included.[2]

Of the thousands of chemicals in commercial use today, only about 200 are commonly recognized as allergic contact sensitizers, hereas several thousand other potential contact allergens exist.[4] Valid positive patch tests are generally accepted as the gold standard for the diagnosis of allergic contact dermatitis. Thus patch testing plays a crucial role in the evaluation of patents with occupational hand dermatitis. Be aware that patch testing may yield false-positive and false-negative results. Selecting the proper concentration of the suspected allergen, vehicle, site of application, and type of patch is critical for procedure validity. Making such selections and determining test result relevance require considerable skill and experience. Interpret a positive or negative patch test result in conjunction with the clinical history and a detailed knowledge of testing procedures. Although appropriate test concentrations and vehicles have been established for many sensitizers, there are no established vehicle and concentration standards for the vast number of chemicals in use. Thus, a positive or negative patch test result should not be accepted at face value until the details of the testing procedures have been evaluated, and the direct clinical relevance of the test results to the workplace is accurately determined.[2]

Diagnosis and Treatment

The diagnosis should be listed along with other significant cutaneous findings. Associated diagnoses, such as asthma or significant systemic illness, should also be recorded. Other major symptoms purported by the patient to be occupationally related should be included, and recommendations made for appropriate evaluation by an occupational physician or other specialist. An assessment of the current medical status and statement of further medical plans and treatment also should be provided.[2]

CAUSATION

Determination of the precise cause-and-effect relation between a skin disorder and an occupation is not always easy. Key[11] lists five criteria to consider for the diagnosis of occupational skin diseases:

1. Appearance of the lesions
2. Site of the eruption
3. History
4. Course of the disease
5. Diagnostic tests

Mathias[16] has adapted these criteria for establishing occupational causation and aggravation in contact dermatitis. He proposes that a positive answer to four of the following seven questions would generally be adequate to establish probable cause:

1. Is the clinical appearance compatible with contact dermatitis?
2. Are there workplace exposures to potential irritants or allergens?
3. Is the anatomic distribution of the eruption compatible with job exposure?
4. Is the temporal relationship between exposure and onset consistent with contact dermatitis?
5. Have nonoccupational exposures been excluded as causes?
6. Does the dermatitis improve away from work exposure to the suspected irritant or allergen?
7. Do patch or provocation tests identify a probable cause?

Work Aggravation of Skin Diseases[25]

Although terminology may vary, some states make a legal distinction between work-connected and work-aggravated conditions. Pre-existing skin conditions will often be disqualified for workers' compensation. Clear-cut exceptions should be accepted as work related or aggravated. An example would be work-aggravation of a health-care worker with a history of remote or current atopic eczema who develops allergic contact dermatitis to a chemical in the workplace, such as glutaraldehyde or latex allergy from contact with rubber gloves.

EVALUATION OF TEMPORARY TOTAL IMPAIRMENT

As a prelude to impairment evaluation, the physician must determine the impact of the medical condition on life activities and whether the condition is stable and unlikely to change. If the worker has a new or recent condition that significantly precludes working on the current job, then temporary total impairment may exist, and an appropriate amount of time away from work may be warranted under most Workers' Compensation laws.

USE OF THE AMA GUIDES[2]

The AMA Guides to the Evaluation of Permanent Impairment may be used to evaluate permanent impairment of any body system, from both occupational and nonoccupational causes: they are not designed for use in evaluating temporary impairment. The Guides are a set of guidelines, not absolute recommendations, and are designed to bring objectivity to an area of great subjectivity by providing clinically sound and reproducible criteria useful to physicians, attorneys, and adjudicators. They espouse the philosophy that all physical and mental impairment affects the whole person. "A 95% to 100% whole-person impairment is considered to represent almost total impairment, a state that is approaching death." Before using the Guides for evaluating cutaneous impairment, the physician should read the two introductory chapters, the glossary, and then Chapter 8, on the skin. Chapter 2, "Practical application of the Guides," lists a suggested outline for a medical evaluation report:

1. Medical history
2. Clinical evaluation
3. Diagnoses
4. Stability of the medical condition
5. Impact of the medical condition on specific activities of daily living, including occupation
6. Explanation for concluding that the individual is or is not likely to suffer further impairment by engaging in usual activities
7. Explanation for concluding that accommodations or restrictions related to impairment are or are not warranted
8. A listing of specific impairment percentages

The Guides chapter on skin lists five classes of impairment, ranging from 0% to 95%. The impact of the disorder on activities of daily living (ADL) should be the major consideration in determining the class of impairment. The frequency and intensity of signs and symptoms and the frequency and complexity of medical treatment should guide the selection of an appropriate impairment percentage and estimate within any class.

ADLs include self-care and personal hygiene, communication, physical activity, sensory function, hand functions (grasping, holding, pinching, percussive movements, and sensory discrimination), travel, sexual function, sleep, and social and recreational activities. Because most occupational skin disorders involve the hands, chronic hand dermatitis may have a significant impact on ADLs. Other examples of specific ADLs are listed in the glossary of the Guides.

The examples within each class are very important guides for the first-time user. The AMA Guides divide skin impairment into five classes. Diagnoses of the following examples, by class, include:

- *Class 1 (0% to 9%):* allergic contact dermatitis (three examples); chronic urticaria; thermal burn scars
- *Class 2 (10% to 24%):* chronic hand eczema; hypertrophic burn scar; atopic dermatitis; chemical burn; chemically induced nail dystrophy; latex allergy
- *Class 3 (25% to 54%):* persistent occupational contact dermatitis; follicular occlusive triad with scarring; pemphigus vulgaris
- *Class 4 (55% to 84%):* stasis dermatitis and ulceration; scleroderma, pustular psoriasis, thermal burn scars; mycosis fungoides; basal cell nevus syndrome
- *Class 5 (85% to 95%):* xeroderma pigmentosum, epidermolysis bullosa dystrophica

The fifth edition of the Guides contains new examples of impairment from latex allergy and skin cancer as well as refinement of some of the previous examples. Most are not Workers' Compensation cases but are clearly applicable to such cases. It is critically important to remember that impairment is not determined by diagnosis alone but by the effect of the disease on ADL along with the frequency and intensity of the disease and the frequency and complexity of therapy; thus there are examples of the same disease in several different classes. Most cutaneous impairment falls within the first three classes ranging from 0% to 54%.

Certain therapies, such as PUVA (bath or systemic) for psoriasis or hand eczema and calcipotriol ointment for psoriasis, may have such a significant impact on disease outcome that the author believes they should be employed before making a final determination of permanent impairment.

Unique to the skin chapter are the discussions of pruritus, disfigurement, and scars and skin grafts. The evaluation of pruritus is based on its interference with ADLs and the extent to which the description of pruritus is supported by objective findings, such as lichenification, excoriation, or hyperpigmentation. Disfigurement usually involves no loss of body function and little or no effect on ADLs. Disfigurement may well impair self-image, cause lifestyle alteration, and result in social rejection. These changes are best evaluated in accordance with the criteria in the chapter on mental and behavioral conditions. Evaluation of scars and skin grafts is made according to the impact on ADLs. When impairment is based on peripheral nerve dysfunction, based on loss of range of motion, or caused by scarring, it should be evaluated in accordance with the criteria in the chapters on the nervous system and musculoskeletal system.

CONCLUSIONS AND RECOMMENDATIONS

All diagnoses should be listed and summarized. A summary statement regarding causation is then made; for example, "Within a reasonable degree of medical certainty, the disease is (or is not) related to work." A physician is not required to have such an opinion and in some cases may not be able to make a determination of probable cause. The diagnosis should include a description of specific clinical findings related to the impairment, and how they relate to and compare with the criteria in the Guides. The impairment value should also be explained. Specific recommendations for therapy should be included along with a brief explanation of the treatment. Recommendations for prevention including work restrictions are made next: this includes suggestions for environmental modification (exhaust ventilation, splash guards) and personal protective equipment. The effect of future exposures to chemical, physical, and biologic agents should be addressed, along with any need for rehabilitation.[2] Some states and insurance carriers provide rehabilitation services, several of which may be applicable to individuals with skin diseases; vocational evaluation, occupational therapy, and retraining programs may be helpful to motivated workers. Finally, the basis for the conclusions should be discussed, such as personal observations of the treating physician(s) with specified dates, a one-time independent medical evaluation, and findings from history, old records, physical examination, and patch tests, alone or in combination. Inconsistencies and other disclaimers should be listed.[2]

References

1. Centers for Disease Control and Prevention: Prevalence of Selected Chronic Conditions: United States (1968–88)—Vital and Health Statistics (Series 10, No. 182). Atlantan, National Center for Health Statistics, Centers for Disease Control and Prevention, 1993.
2. Cocchiarella L, Anderson GBJ (eds): Guides to the Evaluation of Permanent Impairment, 5th ed. Chicago, American Medical Association, 2001.
3. Cooley JE, Nethercott JR: Prognosis of occupational skin diseases. Occup Med 9:19–24, 1994.
4. Davidson CL: Occupational contact dermatitis of the upper extremity. Occup Med 9:56–74, 1994.
5. Department of Defense: Disability Separation. Washington, DC, American Forces Information Service, Department of Defense, 1988.
6. Department of Defense: Physical Standards of Enlistment, Appointment, and Induction Section 2–36, Skin and cellular tissues, p 14 (AR 40–501, Update Issue 1). Washington, DC, Department of Defense, Undated (received June 2, 1994).
7. Fisher TF: New developments in workers' compensation law. Ann NY Acad Sci 572:256–260, 1989.
8. Freeman S: Diagnosis and Differential diagnosis. In Adams RM (ed): Occupational Skin Disease, 3rd ed. Phildelphia, WB Saunders, 1999, pp 189–207.
9. Goldstein A: Writing report letters for patients with skin disease resulting from on-the-job exposures. Derm Clin 2:631–641, 1984.
10. Hogan DJ: The prognosis of occupational contact dermatitis. Occup Med 9:53–58, 1994.
11. Key M: Confusing compensation cases. Cutis 3:965–996, 1967.
12. LaPlante MP, Carlson D: Disability in the United States: Prevalence and Causes, 1992. Washington, DC, Office of Special Education and Rehabilitative Services, U.S. Department of Education, 1996.
13. Leavitt SS: Defining and Implementing Medical Standards for Workers' Compensation (Syllabus: Course on Workers' Compensation). Washington, DC, American Society for Law and Medicine, 1975.
14. Leigh JP, Miller TR: Job-related diseases and occupations within a large workers' compensation data set. Am J Indust Med 33:197–211, 1998.
15. Martin RA: Occupational Disability. Springfield, Thomas, 1975.
16. Mathias CGT: Contact dermatitis and workers' compensation: Criteria for establishing occupational causation and aggravation. J Am Acad Dermatol 20:842–848, 1989.
17. Nethercott JR: Disability due to occupational contact dermatitis. Occup Med 1:199–203, 1986.
18. Nethercott JR: Fitness to work with skin disease and the Americans with Disability Act of 1990. Occup Med 9:11–18, 1994.
19. Nethercott JR: The Americans with Disabilities Act. Am J Contact Derm 4:185–186, 1993.
20. Panetta warns of disability disaster. The Plain Dealer, November 11, 1993.
21. Prevalence of mobility and self-care disability—United States, 1990. MMWR Morb Mortal Wkly Rep 42:760–761, 767–769, 1993.
22. Prevalence of work disability—United States, 1990; MMWR Morb Mortal Wkly Rep 42:757–759, 1993.
23. Sauer GC: A guide to the evaluation of permanent impairment of the skin. Arch Dermatol 97:566–569, 1968; 98:202–204, 1968.
24. Social Security Administration: Disability Evaluation Under Social Security (SSA Pub. No. 64–039). Washington, DC, Social Security Administration, U.S. Department of Health and Human Services, 1994:58–59.
25. Specialized skills of clinical practice, Appendix 2. In Rosenstock, LR, Cullen MR (eds): Clinical Occupational Medicine. Philadelphia, WB Saunders, 1986, p 273.
26. Taylor J: Occupational dermatoses. In Alderman MH, Hanley MJ: Clinical Medicine for the Occupational Physician. New York, M. Dekker, 1982, pp 299–304.
27. U.S. Chamber of Commerce: Analysis of Workers' Compensation Laws. Washington, DC, U.S. Chamber of Commerce, 2000.
28. US Department of Labor: Non-fatal occupational illnesses by category of illness, private sector, 1995–1999. Washington, DC, Bureau of Labor Statistics, U.S. Department of Labor, 2000.
29. Veterans Administration: Physicians's Guide for Disability Evaluation Examinations. Washington, DC, Department of Medicine and Surgery, Veterans Administration, 1985.
30. VA adds benefits for Agent Orange. US Med, April 1994.

CHAPTER

29

Endocrinological Impairment

STEPHEN L. DEMETER, MD, MPH

The tenth chapter of the fifth edition of the AMA Guides[1] is a well-written chapter that stands on its own and does not need a lot of explanation. The material provided is excellent. It describes the clinical conditions and tests needed for diagnoses of various diseases and separates the classes of impairment in a rational fashion. The multiple examples are excellent and provide guidance for the evaluator when rating impairment owing to an endocrinologic condition.

There are, however, areas of concern that warrant explanation. First, many of the endocrine abnormalities are, by their nature, ongoing and progressive. They are never static and well stabilized and are therefore never at maximum medical improvement. This creates some problems when assessing impairment due to these disorders. Diabetes and its complications is probably the best example of this issue (see following discussion).

A second issue, of equal importance, is the concept of treatment for disease. On page 212, the fifth edition of the Guides states: "When an endocrine disorder results in decreased secretion of a hormone, it is usually possible to replace the hormone by either the oral or the parenteral route, resulting in virtual normalization of body physiology except, of course, for the inability to secrete the hormone. Apart from the need to take the medication on an ongoing basis, decreased secretion alone does not warrant an impairment rating."[1] Later on the same page is the following comment: "Disorders resulting in increased secretion of a hormone often can be effectively treated. In some cases, a treatment may leave the individual with a reduced ability to secrete the hormone. If so, the severity of the resulting condition and the effect on the ability to perform activities of daily living are evaluated to determine the impairment rating."[1] Yet on page 20, the Guides state: "A patient may decline surgical, phamacologic, or therapeutic treatment of an impairment. If a patient declines therapy for a permanent impairment, that decision neither decreases nor increases the estimated percentage of the individual's impairment."[1]

Every table found within Chapter 10 of the Guides rates impairment based on the effectiveness of treatment. For example, the first table (Table 29–1) states that a Class 1 impairment is based on the following criterion: "disease controlled effectively with continuous treatment ..."; Class 2 is for "related symptoms and signs from disease inadequately controlled by treatment ..."; and Class 3 is for "severe symptoms and signs of disease

TABLE 29–1

Criteria for Rating Permanent Impairment Due to Hypothalamic-Pituitary Axis Disorders

Class 1: 0% to 15% Impairment of the Whole Person	**Class 2: 16% to 25% Impairment of the Whole Person**	**Class 3: 26% to 50% Impairment of the Whole Person**
Disease controlled effectively with continuous treatment, with minimal impact on ability to perform activities of daily living	Related symptoms and signs from disease inadequately controlled by treatment and impact ability to perform activities of daily living	Severe symptoms and signs of disease persist despite treatment and significantly impact ability to perform activities of daily living

From Cocchiarella L, Andersson GBJ (eds): Guides to the Evaluation of Permanent Impairment, 5th ed. Chicago, American Medical Association, 2001, p 215, with permission.

[that] persist despite treatment ..."1(p215) Thus, this table (and a review of all the tables in this section) classifies individuals based on the effectiveness of treatment.

It is more logical to assess impairment based on the effect of treatment rather than on the untreated state because the concept of maximum medical improvement implies that a person is on treatment, that the treatment is effective, that the patient is compliant with the treatment program, and that the medically or surgically prescribed regimen is one that will achieve optimum health. Otherwise, the patient cannot be at a maximal improvement level.

The chapter also states: "as stated in chapter 2, even with appropriate medication, it is debatable whether the individual has regained the previous state of good health. Thus, the examiner may increase the impairment rating by a small percentage (1–3%) to account for an incomplete return to a condition of normal health."[1(p212)] However, many of the sections in Chapter 10 award higher amounts of whole person impairment (WPI) simply based on the need for and appropriate use of medications.

These issues are best exemplified in example 10–16.[1(p224)] A 32-year-old woman with a 10-year history of autoimmune thyroiditis is presented. Her symptoms, present for 1 year, include progressive fatigue, weakness, periodic nausea, weight loss, occasional postural dizziness, and craving for salt. She has a diagnosis of hypoadrenalism. She has a 10% impairment of the whole person. The stated reason for the 10% WPI is that "hypoadrenalism will be permanent, with the individual requiring lifelong treatment with an adrenal glucocorticoid and mineralocorticoid in order to perform usual activities of daily living."[1(p224)] In this individual, replacement therapy should cause her symptoms to disappear and allow her to lead a normal lifestyle. Yet if she were to decline treatment, she would likely have a Class 3 impairment (30% to 90% WPI) based on the severity and frequency of her symptoms. Furthermore, the 10% WPI is more than the 1% to 3% suggested in the introduction to both the Guides (p 20) and the Endocrine chapter (p 212).

One of the more important concepts discussed in Chapter 10 concerns WPI created by the effects of medications (as opposed to the WPI caused by the need to take medications). The most notable example is the use of corticosteroids. The importance of this issue is created by the frequency of usage of this class of medications as well as the frequency and severity of their side effects. Impairing side effects of corticosteroids include obesity and disfigurement, osteoporosis, bony fractures, skin disorders, psychological abnormalities, recurrent infections, fatigue, peripheral edema, cardiovascular problems, and ocular disease, to name a few. The difficulty with awarding WPI owing to the side effects of the corticosteroids revolves around the amount of WPI attributable to the hyperadrenal state alone, without the effects on other organ systems that are independently rated. In other words, looking at the long list of side effects, which are used for determining WPI due to this condition and which are not? The solution is found in a footnote to Table 10–6 (Table 29–2) that suggests that WPI caused by iatrogenic conditions be reserved for "impairments due to the general effects of adrenal steroids, such as myopathy, easy bruising, and obesity. The estimated percentages should be combined with those related to specific impairments, such as diabetes or fractures due to osteoporosis, by means of the Combined Values Chart ..." (1, p 226). In other words, this table is used for all those effects or complications that are not assessed using other chapters. These are the problems that fall through the cracks when a careful inventory of side effects is ascertained and assessed. For example, in a person with severe and unsightly bruising or excessive photosensitivity, one could use Chapter 8 (Dermatology) or Chapter 14 (Psychiatry) to rate the impairment. However, whichever chapter or table is used, only one impairment rating should be given. The evaluator should assess the impairment based on the chapter that best covers the interferences in activities of daily living. For some individuals, the principal disturbances caused by the bruising and photosensitivity will be psychological. For others, especially in more severe cases, they will be dermatologic. If they are neither, then the general effects of the disturbances in activities of daily living created by these complications should be assessed using Table 10–6, which is comprehensive. Thus

TABLE 29–2

Impairments Related to Hyperadrenocorticism*

Severity	% Impairment of the Whole Person
Minimal, as with hyperadrenocorticism that is surgically corrected by removal of a pituitary or adrenal adenoma or due to moderate pharmacologic doses of glucocorticoids	0%–14%
Moderate, as with bilateral hyperplasia that is treated with medical therapy or adrenalectomy or due to large pharmacologic doses of glucocorticoids	15%–39%
Severe, as with aggressively metastasizing adrenal carcinoma	Variable†

*This table should be used to evaluate impairments due to the general effects of adrenal steroids, such as myopathy, easy bruising and obesity. The estimated percentages should be combined with those related to specific impairments, such as diabetes or fractures due to osteoporosis, by means of the Combined Values Chart (p. 604) of the Guides.

†The degree of estimated impairment will depend on the effects of the tumor on other organ systems; appropriate Guides chapters should be consulted.

From Cocchiarella L, Andersson GBJ (eds): Guides to the Evaluation of Permanent Impairment, 5th ed. Chicago, American Medical Association, 2001, p 226, with permission.

if the disturbances in activities of daily living are created by multiple side effects (e.g., the dermatologic issues noted or obesity or fatigue), the evaluator should globally assess them rather than assigning particular numbers to them individually and adding or combining these numbers.

One last but major issue found in the endocrine chapter deals with the concept of impairment created by future considerations, with a confused WPI recommendation based upon anticipated worsening of a condition, or more commonly, the complication of a condition as based upon the risk of a deterioration or complication without a valid statistical base upon which to determine the frequency of such deteriorations.

Throughout the remainder of the book, and in accordance with the philosophy noted in Chapters 1 and 2, individuals are rated based on the concept of maximum medical improvement. This states that "an impairment should not be considered permanent until the clinical findings indicate that the medical condition is static and well stabilized, often termed the date of maximum medical improvement. It is understood that an individual's condition is dynamic. Maximum medical improvement refers to a condition or state that is well stabilized and unikely to change substantially in the next year with or without medical treatment."[1(p601)]

When assessing WPI created by an endocrine disease, it is important to remember that some problems are, by their nature, progressive and produce clinical deterioration as time passes. Diabetes mellitus creates problems in many organ systems, especially vascular and neurologic, which are ongoing and progressive. This disease will probably never reach a maximum medical improvement level because, by the nature of its complications, it is never static or well stabilized. This is reflected in Table 10–8 (Table 29–3), which assesses WPI in the patient with diabetes based on the disease's complications.

The evaluator can resolve this problem by making a subtle psychological shift if he or she takes the approach of "maximum medical worsening" as opposed to maximum medical improvement (which as defined on page 2[1] applies to a condition that is "unlikely to change substantially in the next year with or without medical treatment"). Many sections in the fifth edition (as well as previous editions) actually make a subtle philosophical substitution of maximum medical worsening as opposed to maximum medical improvement for assessment purposes. The interested reader can read this edition with this concept in mind and note multiple examples.

For example, diabetes mellitus will always be at maximum medical improvement if a patient has his or her blood sugars under control. Deterioration, sometimes rapid, due to vascular damage is one of the hallmarks of severe or uncontrolled diabetes of long duration. Therefore, these individuals will always be at maximum medical improvement but may require frequent changes in their WPI based on the effects in other organ systems. Therefore, in these individuals, WPI ratings may change significantly, even every 6 months, from the time of the initial rating because they are not at their maximum medically worsened state.

Another peculiarity of Chapter 10 is that WPI can be assigned based on risk of a future event. An instance is

TABLE 29–3

Criteria for Rating Permanent Impairment Due to Diabetes Mellitus

Class 1: 0% to 5% Impairment of the Whole Person	**Class 2: 6% to 10% Impairment of the Whole Person**	**Class 3: 11% to 20% Impairment of the Whole Person**	**Class 4: 21% to 40% Impairment of the Whole Person**
Type 2 diabetes mellitus that can be controlled by diet **and** may or may not have evidence of diabetic microangiopathy, as indicated by presence of retinopathy or albuminuria greater than 30 mg/dL	Type 2 diabetes mellitus **and** satisfactory control of plasma glucose level requires both a restricted diet and hypoglycemic medication (either an oral agent or insulin) **and** evidence of microangiopathy, as indicated by retinopathy or by albuminuria of greater than 30 mg/dL, may or may not be present; if retinopathy has led to visual impairment, evaluate as described in Chapter 12, The Visual System	Type 1 diabetes mellitus, with or without evidence of microangiopathy	Type 1 diabetes mellitus **and** hyperglycemia or hypoglycemia occurs frequently despite conscientious efforts of both individual and physician

From Cocchiarella L, Andersson GBJ (eds): Guides to the Evaluation of Permanent Impairment, 5th ed. Chicago, American Medical Association, 2001, p 231, with permission.

seen in example 10–8, which states that a person has a 10% impairment of the whole person because of "continued risk of the renal calculus."[1(p220)] Thus some parts of the chapter define impairment based on risk and possibilities as opposed to known abnormalities whereas other chapters do not.

Metabolic bone disease also deserves mention. Example 10–47 states that a person has a "15% impairment due to metabolic bone disease; combined with the estimated rating for musculoskeletal system impairment ..."[1(p241)] This section covers the issue of pain created by osteoporosis *without* "fracture, spinal collapse, or other complications of metabolic bone disease." However, pain in the osteoporotic patient is caused by bone fractures (as opposed to the patient with hyperparathyroidism, where bone pain is a common accompanying feature). This section also presumably covers the adjustments that a person makes in activities of daily living created by factors used to prevent a fracture (such as the prophylactic use of canes or walkers). However, both issues are unclear in this section and this section places itself at odds with the philosophy of the Guides wherein pain is usually included as part of a WPI for a given condition (especially orthopedic).

SUMMARY

The chapter on endocrine disorders in the AMA Guides was difficult for the chapter authors to prepare and is also difficult to critique. The WPI percentages are arbitrary. However, they represent consensus statements by physicians in this field. One can argue that the impairment percentages either over- or underestimate impairment in the evaluee. The authors of the Guides have recognized this problem and concern and note that this area of clinical medicine is an art and not a science and that "the Guides suggest that physicians use clinical judgment."[1(p11)]

Reference

1. Cocchiarella L, Andersson GBJ (eds): Guides to the Evaluation of Permanent Impairment, 5th ed. Chicago, American Medical Association, 2001.

CHAPTER

30

Gastrointestinal Impairment

JAMES R. McPHERSON, MD, MSc, FACP

Gastrointestinal symptoms are common in patients seeking medical consultation. Although a substantial number do not have diseased or injured organs, it is essential to investigate them in a comprehensive manner. Objective evidence is crucial to establish a definite diagnosis and attempt to achieve maximal medical improvement. The Impairment Evaluation Summary on pages 138 through 141 of the AMA Guides, fifth edition, provides a listing of diagnoses, symptoms, investigations, and statements regarding end organ damage. However, the most critical and helpful tests are not identified specifically for each diagnosis.

This chapter briefly describes some aspects of normal physiology and anatomy of the various gastrointestinal organ systems followed by descriptions of alterations produced by disease, genetic abnormalities, trauma, or surgical therapy, and also the development and progression of complications inherent to the diseases, all of which may lead to permanent impairment. Descriptions of disability are presented in Chapter 64.

The degrees of impairment listed in the Guides are consensus based and may be subject to increase or decrease as the natural history of the particular disease evolves and new therapies are developed.

The Oropharynx

Although this area is not specifically mentioned in the AMA Guides, its role in normal swallowing is important. When excessive dryness in the buccal mucosa occurs secondary to radiation or Sjögren syndrome, movement of particles toward the esophagus is greatly hampered. Groups of pharyngeal muscles must act in a coordinated way to move particles further and the larynx must close to prevent aspiration. Dysfunction secondary to neural damage can cause significant dysphagia. Separation between the muscle groups may provoke a pharyngeal–esophageal diverticulum (Zenker diverticulum) to develop and produce dysphagia by filling with food particles. Symptoms in this region are difficult to evaluate by simple studies and may require cineradiography during swallowing and motility studies.

Esophagus

After successful transit through the mouth and pharynx, food particles enter the proximal esophagus where a timed peristaltic wave is initiated and propagated down to the gastroesophageal sphincter. Relaxation of this muscle, which at rest is contracted to prevent reflux, must occur before particles enter the stomach.

Diffuse esophageal spasm is characterized by high pressure incoordinated contractions of the esophageal musculature resulting in pain and failure of propulsion of esophageal contents.[7] Stenosis in the lower esophagus from recurring reflux of erosive stomach acids or tumor may result in dilatation of the proximal esophagus causing deterioration of peristalsis.[6] Scleroderma involving the esophagus adversely affects normal peristalsis causing reflux and dysphagia. Achalasia—a failure of the sphincter to relax with the swallowing reflex—is ideally treated by muscle splitting pneumatic dilatations in early stages to prevent irreversible dilatation of the proximal esophagus.[8] Barium and motility studies or endoscopy provide objective evidence for specific diagnoses and assists in the evaluation of impairment.

Stomach

Food particles entering the stomach undergo mixing and grinding to make them of ideal size and shape to be pushed into the duodenum. The gastric antrum plays an important grinding role—likened to a grist mill—as well as producing the hormone gastrin, which is necessary for both acid production by the parietal cells and stimulation of gastric motility. The role of the vagus nerve is also significant and when patients have a surgical vagotomy, an emptying procedure such as gastroenterostomy may be required.

Distal gastrectomy for peptic ulcer disease is rare with current powerful antisecretory drugs to control acid production. However, patients who have undergone partial gastrectomy, and in some cases total gastrectomy, for severe hypersecretion have a distinct impairment of digestion and may have a mild degree of malabsorption secondary to the altered pathway and delayed mixing with pancreatic enzymes. Proximal gastrectomy or distal esophagectomy for malignant disease with anastomosis in continuity also results in significant impairment.

Diabetic gastroparesis may cause significant impairment due to nausea, vomiting, and dilatation of the stomach filled with retained food. Gastric emptying measurements, intraluminal pressure measurements, and scintigraphy with radioisotopes are needed for evaluation. The use of prokinetic drugs may help, but a feeding jejunostomy may be needed for survival. Total gastrectomy results in greater impairment as patients are usually unable to regain normal weight.

Duodenum

The duodenum is the source of important hormones influencing gut motility. Additionally, pancreatic secretions enter the intestinal system through the duodenum as does the bile. Intense mixing of pancreatic enzymes and bile with digested food particles of carbohydrate, fat, and protein occurs here in preparation for their absorption through the mucosal cells of the jejunum and ileum.

A gastrojejunostomy results in delayed and less efficient mixing of food particles now entering the jejunum instead of the duodenum. There is usually only a mild degree of malabsorption.

Small Intestine

The jejunum and ileum are vitally important, as they are the site of most of the absorption of nutrients and minerals for the body.

Investigation of disease in the small bowel is somewhat limited to x-rays and blood studies, although endoscopy is becoming more feasible.

A hereditary absence of lactase in the mucosa may produce diarrhea through the inability to absorb lactose. The remedy is relatively simple with the use of exogenous lactase and thus symptoms may be prevented.

Celiac-sprue can produce a severe type of malabsorption due to diffuse abnormalities of the mucosal cells. Early diagnosis by testing for antigliadin antibodies and a jejunal mucosal biopsy is crucial to prevent severe malnutrition. Most patients respond to removal of gluten from the diet but occasionally the disease is refractory and may require steroid use. Lymphoma may be a sequela of longstanding disease. Meticulous attention to the diet is essential. The offending gluten is found in many foods including wheat, rye, and barley. The ingestion of even minute amounts has been known to cause acute diarrhea and a shock-like state.

Crohn's disease may involve any part or all of the small intestine. This disease is a common cause of intestinal failure. More commonly it involves the distal ileum, producing intestinal obstruction and possibly abscesses and fistulae owing to its transmural characteristics. Surgery is reserved for complications. If necessary, resection of 100 cm or less is well tolerated. Following surgery, if there is no recurrence, only modest dietary adjustments are needed along with vitamin B_{12} injections on a regular basis.

Intestinal failure can occur with diffuse Crohn's disease, radiation enteritis, without massive resection, ischemic bowel disease, and diffuse motility disorders. Total parenteral nutrition is necessary and can rehabilitate slightly more than 50% of patients.[8] Long-term management necessitates a home parenteral nutrition program, which is discussed in Chapter 64.

Colon

Inflammatory bowel disease—specifically, ulcerative colitis and Crohn's disease of the colon—produces major impairment in many or most patients with the disease. Ulcerative colitis, a mucosal disease causing diarrhea, bleeding, and debility, may also cause joint, liver, and skin disease. Total colectomy is curative for most of these associated conditions with the exception of sclerosing cholangitis.[3] The formation of a Brooke ileostomy or ileal pouch–anal anastomosis is tolerated well but is considered a permanent impairment.[5] Disability caused by various stomas and anastomoses are discussed in Chapter 64.

Pancreas

Relapsing acute pancreatitis, whether idiopathic or related to alcohol abuse, creates significant impairment. Pancreatitis associated with biliary tract calculi is usually cured by removal of the gall bladder and ductal stones. Objective evidence of the severity of damage from the relapsing attacks includes calcification in the pancreas or stones in the ductal system, pseudocysts, the development of diabetes mellitus and malabsorption often with marked steatorrhea. The pancreas normally produces enzymes well in excess of the body's needs. When steatorrhea occurs, more than 90% of the capability of enzyme production has been destroyed. Replacement therapy is usually helpful.

The major impairment caused by pancreatic disease often comes from intractable pain, often leading to narcotic addition. Nerve blocks may be helpful but occasionally total pancreatectomy is considered as a last resort.[2]

Cystic fibrosis with pancreatic insufficiency requires dietary adjustment and enzyme replacement.

Liver and Biliary Tract

Chronic liver disease produces major impairment. The great variety of symptoms and signs are listed in the Impairment Evaluation Summary in the AMA Guides. A specific diagnosis of cause is crucial, thus differential studies should include hepatitis serologic markers, serum transferrin and ferritin levels, ceruloplasmin, and a liver biopsy, if feasible.

Alcoholic cirrhosis usually follows a minimum of 10 years of alcohol abuse. Alcohol abuse can cause recurring acute alcoholic hepatitis episodes which are characterized by jaundice, enzyme elevations, and, often, abdominal pain. Once the fatty degeneration caused by the alcoholic hepatitis has been replaced by dense scarring, cirrhosis exerts all its potential for overwhelming symptoms.

Primary biliary cirrhosis is a disease of uncertain etiology. It is characterized by damage to the epithelial cells of the small intrahepatic bile ducts followed by interlobular duct destruction. It is more likely an autoimmune disease.[4] The presentation may be with pruritus or an elevated alkaline phosphatase level in the blood and is corroborated by an elevated antimitochondrial antibody test. Over time, increasing cholestasis and liver failure occurs. Impairment is minimal at onset but ultimately liver transplant is the only effective therapy. Drug toxicity, causing prolonged cholestasis, must be included in the differential diagnosis.

Hemochromatosis deserves special mention because early diagnosis and therapy can prevent or reverse the development of cirrhosis.[4] The hereditary variety is associated with increased intestinal absorption of iron with deposition of excessive amounts in the liver and pancreas. Increased awareness of the possible diagnosis and inclusion of routine iron studies has resulted in earlier diagnoses prior to the development of cirrhosis and diabetes mellitus. Early symptoms include fatigue, joint aching, and impotence. Elevated transferrin saturations above 50% and elevated ferritin levels are corroborative. Weekly phlebotomy of 500 mL of blood until the transferrin saturation is below normal and the serum ferritin level is below 50 μgm/L is necessary. Most patients will then require four to eight phlebotomies per year on an indefinite basis. Secondary causes of hemochromatosis are usually related to iron overload as may occur in people with multiple transfusions, excessive iron ingestion, and some types of chronic hepatis. These do not have the progressive nature of the hereditary form if iron sources are eliminated.

Wilson's disease, although rare, deserves mention as it is treatable.[1] A genetic defect causes a low ceruloplasmin level with excessive accumulation of copper in body tissues such as the liver, nervous system, and eye, which produces harmful effects. Treatment with penicillamine to lower copper stores is effective. Dietary adjustments are not major. The prognosis in Wilson's disease with treatment is excellent except for patients presenting with fulminant liver failure.

Primary sclerosing cholangitis causes diffuse extra- and intrahepatic bile duct inflammation. It is diagnosed by a retrograde cholangiogram. The cause is unknown, but it may be associated with ulcerative colitis. Treatment is similar to that for primary biliary cirrhosis.

Impacted ductal stones and strictures in the biliary tree are usually amenable to treatment. Thus permanent impairment is less likely to develop currently than it was in the past.

Anorectal Disease

Anal incontinence can cause significant impairment. Careful and complete studies are important to provide an etiologic diagnosis. These tests include anorectal manometry, electromyographic studies, and a defecating proctogram. A diverting sigmoid colostomy may be required for permanent benefit.

References

1. Balan V, Scolapio JS, Harrison J, et al: Survival in Wilson's disease. Gastroenterology 106:A863, 1994.
2. Brandhagen D, Fairbanks V, Batts K: Update on hereditary hemochromatosis. Mayo Clin Proc 74:917–921,1999.
3. Cooper MJ, Williamson RCN, Benjamin IS, et al: Total pancreatectomy for chronic pancreatitis. Br J Surg 74:912–915, 1987.
4. Desmet VJ: Current problems in diagnosis of biliary disease and cholestases. Semin Liver Dis 6:233–245, 1986.
5. Kohler LW, Pemberton JH, Zinsmeister AR, et al: A comparison of Brooke ileostomy, Koch pouch and ileal pouch–anal anastomosis. Gastroenterology 101:679–684, 1991.
6. McCord GS, Staiano A, Clouse RE, et al: Achalasia, diffuse spasm and nonspecific disorders. Baillieres Clin Gastroenterol 5:307–335, 1991.
7. Pope CE II: Acid reflux disorders. N Engl J Med 331:656–660, 1994.
8. Scolapio JS, Fleming CR, Kelly DG, et al: Survival of home parenteral nutrition– treated patients: 20 years experience at the Mayo Clinic. Mayo Clin Proc 74:217–222, 1999.

CHAPTER

31

Genitourinary Impairment

INDER PERKASH, MD, FRCS (Edin), FACS

The urinary system consists of the upper urinary tract (the kidneys and the ureters), the bladder, and the urethra. The urethra is a common conduit for both urine and seminal ejaculation in men but only serves the sole purpose of urinary elimination in women. The kidneys are important homeostatic regulatory organs. The degree to which kidney and conduit abnormalities affect the whole person ranges from anemia to generalized manifestations of deterioration of the renal function leading to a degree of uremia with raised blood urea nitrogen, serum creatinine, and systemic acidosis.

Urinary and reproductive system impairment can also result from disorders in other systems; e.g., hematologic, endocrine, or neurologic disease that may produce significant urinary or reproductive system impairments. The primary source of the end-organ impairment of the genito-urinary system will influence the whole person impairment rating. Central nervous system (CNS) disorders with intracranial and spinal cord lesions will produce bladder dysfunction. Intracranial pathologies will produce detrusor hyperreflexia. Lesions below the pons will also be associated with bladder sphincter dyssynergia. Detrusor hyperreflexia leads to increased frequency of micturition and dysfunctional voiding, high pressure incomplete reflex voiding, and neurogenic incontinence. Patients with detrusor-sphincter dyssynergia do not empty their bladder well. High pressure voiding could result in vesico-ureteral reflux with repeated urinary tract infections, hydronephrosis, and possibly pyelonephritis. Impairment evaluations for CNS or spinal cord lesions may require inclusion of bladder function for a complete evaluation.

IMPAIRMENT EVALUATION

Urinary tract function impairments are manifested in both urinary and general (nonspecific) signs and symptoms including difficulty in voiding, frequency of micturition, dysuria, and hematuria. General signs and symptoms include loss of appetite, decreased sense of well being, weight loss, chills and fever, abdominal (renal angle) pain, suprapubic mass, hypertension, anemia, and uremia. Renal disease with renal functional impairment will also lead to changes in blood urea nitrogen, creatinine, and creatinine clearance.

EVALUATION OF KIDNEY FUNCTION

Glomerular Filtration Rate

The kidney performs a wide range of complex functions; therefore, the assessment of renal function requires measurement of different processes occurring in various portions of the kidney unit—the nephron. It is not practical to measure each one; therefore, selected functions are determined. The glomerular filtration rate (GFR) is one of the key functions of the nephron used to assess the normality of renal blood flow and glomerular integrity. Its measurement is based on the concept of clearance of a substance that is freely filtered at the glomerulus and one that is not metabolized, secreted, or reabsorbed by the tubule. Inulin clearance, using a constant intravenous infusion, would seem ideal. A normal GFR using inulin clearance for young adults is 130 mL/min for males and 120 mL/min for females per 1.73 in^2 of body surface area. Exercise lowers GFR; pregnancy may increase it by as much as 50%. Extreme overhydration or dehydration may also affect the filtration rate. Creatinine clearance is the most widely used clinical method for determining GFR. Its advantage over inulin is that it is endogenously produced by body muscles at a reasonably constant rate and, therefore, does not need infusion.

Creatinine Clearance and Radioisotope Studies for Effective Renal Plasma Flow

Serum creatinine and renal clearance of endogenous creatinine seem to be the best markers for a quantitative evaluation of renal function. The serum creatinine level reflects overall renal function. Under normal hydration conditions, serum creatinine levels are less than 1.5 mg/dL (133 μmol/L). The normal creatinine clearance ranges from 130 to 200 L/24 hours (90 to 139 mL/min) for men and 115 to 180 L/24 hours (80 to 125 mL/min) for women. The endogenous creatinine clearance gives a quantitative estimate of total functioning kidney units (nephrons) and the GFR. Although there are some difficulties with creatinine clearance, it serves as a useful clinical tool as long as its shortcomings are kept in mind. For example, muscle wasting may reduce the production of creatinine and thereby alter its constant production. Other causes of spurious serum creatinine values are seen in patients with diabetic ketoacidosis;[3] cirrhosis;[1] and following the administration of cephalosporin, trimethoprim and sulfamethoxazole, cimetidine, or proporanal.[2] Creatinine clearance is particularly useful when assessing changes in renal function over the long term. The normal individual excretes between 0.5 and 1.5 mg creatinine/hr/kg of body weight (roughly 1500 mg/24 hr). The clearance is performed by obtaining a 24-hour urine collection, recording the volume and creatinine content, and obtaining a serum creatinine concentration. If the urine collection does not have a total of about 1500 mg of creatinine it may indicate an incomplete urine collection in a male (height, 170 cm). Levels are lower in females.

Renal function impairment can also be measured by using radioisotopes. The GFR can be measured by using technetium-99m labeled albumin (^{99m}Tc-DTPA) or mercaptoacetyltriglycine (MAG3), the later being currently used in most institutions because it has better imaging properties. Both tubular secretion and filtration (effective renal plasma flow) can be measured by using ^{131}I-orthoiodohippurate (^{131}I-OIH).

Serious renal functional impairments are also reflected in changes in serum electrolytes. Parenchymal losses due to repeated infections or trauma will be seen on radiographic studies such as computed axial tomography scans with dye injection. To further determine renal impairment, metabolic studies such as tests of concentration and dilution, serum and urine electrolytes, urine osmolality, urine proteins, and urine cultures, and radiologic studies including renal computerized tomography may provide useful information.

BLADDER FUNCTION AND DISORDERS

The urinary bladder has a triple innervation. The parasympathetic innervation is from sacral nerves S2, S3, and S4. The sympathetic innervation is from T12 to L1. The bladder outlet, passing through the external urethral sphincter, is supplied by the pudendal nerve (also from S2, S3, and S4 segments). The bladder muscle is predominantly supplied by the S3 segment and the external urethral sphincter by the S2 segment. Autonomic innervation helps the bladder in storage and voluntary voiding, which is achieved by relaxation of the external urethral sphincter through pudendal innervation.

The bladder wall (detrusor muscle) is supplied by the autonomic nerves and is thus well suited for storage (filling) and expulsion (micturition) of urine. During filling a normal bladder accommodates 400 to 700 cc of urine and the intravesical pressure does not rise (stable and compliant) over 15 to 20 cm water. Micturition is under voluntary control. A neurogenic bladder is an unstable bladder causing involuntary contractions of the bladder muscle, releasing small volumes and resulting in urinary incontinence.

Bladder Disorders

Bladder dysfunction may be due to problems within or outside the urinary system. Intracranial lesions involving the brain and spinal cord, trauma, or other nervous system disorders can produce impairments in voiding. Bladder tumors, stone diseases, and inflammatory lesions may also produce urinary system impairment. Urethral lesions such as enlarged prostate, urethral stricture, or tumors lead to difficulty in voiding, dysuria, retention of urine, or overflow incontinence. Pelvic trauma can produce disruption of the urethra with subsequent stricture formation. Surgically created urinary diversions, by definition, also lead to urinary system impairment. Signs and symptoms reflecting bladder and sphincter dysfunction are manifest by irritative and obstructive symptomatology.

Functional Evaluation of the Bladder

On physical examination, a distended bladder can be palpated above the pubic symphysis. An abnormal neurologic examination of the saddle region can suggest problems with bladder innervation. Lack of buttock sensation is indicative of neurologic pathology. Rectal examination testing anal sphincter tone and voluntary contraction may indicate the degree of perineal striated muscle integrity, intact sacral spinal and supraconal segments, and intact neuroaxis. The presence of the bulbocavernosus reflex demonstrates that the sacral reflex is intact (although this reflex may be absent in normal individuals or with full rectum). In determining the presence of the bulbocavernosus reflex, the glans penis or clitoris is squeezed and the external anal sphincter is felt to contract on the previously inserted examining finger.

Diagnostic Procedures

Diagnostic procedures used to assess bladder function include urinalysis, intravenous pyelogram, spiral computed tomography with contrast, voiding cystourethrogram, and cystoscopy. Urodynamic studies serve to quantify the two major bladder functions of storage and expulsion of urine. Data are collected by various techniques describing what occurs as the bladder is filling (storage) and emptying (micturition). The bladder outlet (vesical neck) is studied by modalities including voiding cystourethrography, cystoscopy, and transrectal sonography. Emptying is also studied by uroflowmetry (urine flow rate). Thus urodynamic studies enable one to study bladder and sphincter activity as well as measure the activity of voiding. The results of cystometry, uroflowmetry, and the urethral pressure profile can suggest an underlying lesion, especially when studies are performed by well-qualified personnel, although results are sometimes subjective even in the best of hands. Simultaneous cystometry and electromyography of the urethral sphincter can assist in evaluating the status of the spinal cord. Normally, bladder contraction is associated with a relaxed sphincter, but patients with spinal cord lesions can show nonrelaxation of the sphincter (dyssynergia).

CLASSIFICATION OF IMPAIRMENT AND DISABILITY

Renal Function Impairment: Criteria for Rating Permanent Impairment Due to Renal Disease

Renal function impairment is well described in the chapter entitled "The Urinary and Reproductive Systems" in the AMA Guides.

Class 1: 0% to 14% Whole Person Impairment

Diminution of upper urinary tract function, as evidenced by creatinine clearance of 75 to 90 L/24 h (52 to 62.5 mL/min) or intermittent symptoms and signs of upper urinary tract dysfunction that do not require continuous treatment or surveillance or only one kidney is functioning.

Class 2: 15% to 34% Whole Person Impairment

Diminution of upper urinary tract function as evidenced by creatinine clearance of 60 to 75 L/24 h (42 to 52 mL/min) or symptoms and signs of upper urinary tract disease or dysfunction necessitating continuous surveillance and frequent treatment, although creatinine clearance is greater than 75 L/24 h (52 mL/min) or successful renal transplantation results in marked renal function improvement.

Class 3: 35% to 59% Whole Person Impairment

Diminution of upper urinary tract function as evidenced by creatinine clearance of 40 to 60 L/24 h (28 to 42 mL/min) or symptoms and signs of upper urinary tract disease or dysfunction are incompletely controlled by surgical or continuous medical treatment, although creatinine clearance is 60 to 75 L/24 h (42 to 52 mL/min).

Class 4: 60% to 95% Whole Person Impairment

Diminution of upper urinary tract function as evidenced by creatinine clearance below 40 L/24 h (28 mL/min) or symptoms and signs of upper urinary tract disease or dysfunction persist despite surgical or continuous medical treatment, although creatinine clearance is 40 to 60 L/24 h (28 to 42 mL/min) or renal function deterioration requires either peritoneal dialysis or hemodialysis.

Bladder: Criteria for Rating Permanent Impairment Due to Bladder Disease

Signs and symptoms resulting from bladder impairment vary with the nature of the injury or illness, its anatomic location, and its response to treatment. The AMA Guides have classified bladder impairment into four broad functional categories. The following is a rating system (adapted from the AMA Guides) using disorders seen by an examiner as a reference point, as well as the resultant scope of complications caused by disease or injury. Impairment ratings are assigned to each category, ranging from 0% to 15% whole person impairment for Class I impairments that result in intermittent symptoms without incontinence to 40% to 60% for Class IV impairments where the patient is totally incontinent.

Class 1: 0% to 15% Whole Person Impairment

Symptoms and signs of bladder disorder requiring intermittent treatment and normal function between episodes of malfunctioning.

Class 2: 16% to 40% Whole Person Impairment

Symptoms and signs of bladder disorder, e.g., urinary frequency (urinating more than every 2 hours) or severe nocturia (urinating more than three times a night), requiring continuous treatment.

Class 3: 41% to 70% Whole Person Impairment

Poor reflex activity (e.g., intermittent urine dribbling, loss of control, urinary urgency) or no voluntary control on micturition or reflex or areflexic bladder on urodynamics.

References

1. Burney TL, Senapati M, Desai S, et al.: Acute cerebrovascular accident and lower urinary tract dysfunction: a prospective correlation of the site of the brain injury with urodynamic findings. J Urol 156:1748–1750, 1996.
2. Kahn Z, Hertanu J, Yang WC, et al.: Predictive correlation of urodynamic dysfunction and brain injury after cerebrovascular accident. J Urol 126:86–88, 1981.
3. Perkash I: Detrusor-sphincter dyssynergia and dyssynergic responses: recognition and rationale for early modified transurethral sphincterotomy in complete spinal cord injury lesions. J Urol 120:469–474, 1978.
4. Walsh PC (ed): Campbell's Urology, 7th ed. Philadelphia, WB Saunders, 1998.
5. Cocchiarella L, Andersson GBJ (eds): Guides to the Evaluation of Permanent Impairment, 5th ed. Chicago, American Medical Association, 2001.
6. Baker JP, et al: Nutritional assessment: A comparison of clinical judgment and objective measurements. N Engl J Med 306:969, 1982.
7. Fine EJ, Blaufox MD, Rosseleigh MA: Urological applications of radionuclides. Clinical Urology, 2nd ed. Philadelphia, WB Saunders, 2000, pp 621–660.

CHAPTER

32

Hematologic and Oncologic Impairment

BARRY S. LEVINSON, MD ■ EUGENE P. FRENKEL, MD

In the evaluation of hematologic and oncologic disorders, specific tests may be a guide to the degree of impairment. Because the capability of a person to adapt to the degree of laboratory abnormalities varies from one individual to the next, the evaluation of laboratory changes needs to be related to the level of dysfunction. Guidelines are helpful, but each case must be determined individually; in addition, rapid and dynamic changes may be seen, particularly with hematologic disorders, making it critical to evaluate the individual during a stable period. However, these tests do not directly measure organ function, as do pulmonary function tests for lung disease or exercise tests for heart disease.

The function of blood is ubiquitous in the body but can be divided into several main categories. The red blood cells' primary function is to carry oxygen to the tissues and remove carbon dioxide. If this function is impaired, symptoms of anemia will result; if severe and prolonged dysfunction occurs, there may be diminished end organ function caused by inadequate tissue delivery of oxygen. In contradistinction, the presence of an excessive number of red blood cells, termed polycythemia, may be associated with increased viscosity and subsequent decreased blood flow and oxygen delivery, causing an increased predisposition for clotting (thrombosis) or bleeding (hemorrhage).

White blood cells function as an essential part of the immune system. The main components are neutrophils, lymphocytes, and monocytes, as well as eosinophils and basophils. Plasma cells, also an important component of the immune system, are responsible for the production of soluble immune proteins and immunoglobulins. Alterations in the number or function of these cells can contribute to immunologic abnormalities and impairment, and result in increased risk, frequency, and severity of infections.

Platelets are an essential component of clotting or coagulation. Abnormalities in either number or function can lead to a hemorrhagic or thrombotic state. Alterations in other components of the coagulation cascade such as clotting factors or anticlotting factors also may result in either hemorrhage or thrombosis.

ANEMIA

Anemia, defined as diminished red blood cell numbers or decreased hemoglobin (Hb) and hematocrit (Hct), causes impairment by reducing oxygen-carrying capacity, resulting in a variety of symptoms (see Table 32–1). Hb is the molecule within the red blood cells that actually binds oxygen. Therefore, if the amount of hemoglobin as measured by red blood cell count (RBC), Hb, or Hct is diminished in amount or in functional ability, there will be an impairment of oxygen delivery to the tissues with consequent symptoms of anemia.

The measurement of Hb, Hct, or RBC is essential in the evaluation of hematologic impairment and disability, but

TABLE 32–1
Signs and Symptoms of Anemia

Symptoms	Signs
Dyspnea on exertion	Skin pallor
Dizziness	Tachycardia
Throbbing headaches	Systolic ejection murmur
Palpitations	(Possible) peripheral edema
Easy fatigability	
Increased symptoms of pre-existent vascular disease	
Angina pectoris	
Claudication	
CNS	

the overall determination is more complex in cases of mild to moderate anemia where the rate of fall of the red cells and the duration of the condition are important parameters in a person's functional level. Additionally, the underlying state of cardiovascular health, pulmonary health, and age all contribute to a person's tolerance to different levels of anemia and his or her ability to endure or undertake exertional activities. Thus, the comorbid status of the individual needs to be correlated with the specific level of hemoglobin (or red cell number). For instance, mild anemia (Hb 1 g/dL; Class I impairment) would pose no significant impairment in a young, otherwise healthy man; by contrast, in a patient with organic heart disease or a pulmonary disorder (e.g., chronic obstructive pulmonary disease), such a modest decrease in oxygen carrying capacity could result in enough impairment to define true disability.

The causes of anemia are numerous. However, the degree of impairment more clearly relates to the rate of development and to the severity of the anemia than to the etiology. For instance, an acute decrease in Hb (or Hct), which may occur with hemorrhage, autoimmune hemolytic anemia, or acute leukemia, is often associated with rapid development of symptoms and significant concurrent impairment, even when the Hg is only 9 to 10 g/dL. Parenthetically, it is generally thought that chronic Hg levels of 9 g/dL or greater create no impairment and that a worker should be capable of normal job duties. A correlate parameter is that when the Hg falls to 7 g/dL or less, there is a reduction in work capacity. However, when anemia develops slowly (such as in megaloblastic anemia, chronic lymphocytic leukemia, or myelofibrosis), the individual may present to the physician with Hg levels in the 3 to 5 g/dL range and virtually no symptoms. Parameters used to define levels of impairment are defined in Table 32–2.

A suggested classification for activities of daily living (ADL) for hematologic disorders is available in the AMA Guides, fifth edition, which is reproduced as Table 32–3.

Such criteria must be carefully related to the rapidity of the development of the anemia because, as discussed, the absolute RBC count, Hb, and Hct are only one factor in the disability determination. The best definition of impairment for any individual can be achieved when the parameters that define permanent impairment (Table 32–2) are integrated into the data for functional classification (Table 32–3) to derive a final determination.

Anemia may be acquired or congenital. Congenital anemias such as hemoglobinopathies (most commonly sickle cell anemia or the thalassemias) are due to abnormal Hb. Red cell membrane disorders and enzyme disorders may also be causes of congenital anemias. The degree of anemia in congenital anemias is usually greater than in acquired forms. The longstanding history and lifestyle of these patients often allow tolerance and lesser impairment than similar levels in patients with acquired anemias. Anemia may also be due to a deficiency of erythropoietin, such as anemia of chronic disease or iron reutilization defects. Anemia may be secondary to nutritional deficiencies such as iron, B_{12}, or folate deficiency. These may result from an associated underlying mechanism (for example, gastrointestinal malignancy in iron deficiency or folate deficiency secondary to severe alcohol abuse). These acquired disorders may be readily reversible with appropriate supplementation and thus provide only transient impairment.

Primary bone marrow disorders such as myelodysplastic syndromes or refractory anemias may be manifested by a chronic low-grade anemia that does not impair function. However, with time, there is frequently a progression of the changes with worsening anemia causing associated symptoms and even the need for chronic red blood cell transfusion. These bone marrow disorders may also be associated with leukopenia (low white blood cell counts) and thrombocytopenia (low platelets). In determining impairment secondary to anemia one must consider the functional impairment in addition to the degree of

TABLE 32–2

Criteria for Rating Permanent Impairment Due to Anemia

Class 1: 0% to 10% Impairment of the Whole Person	**Class 2: 11% to 30% Impairment of the Whole Person**	**Class 3: 31% to 70% Impairment of the Whole Person**	**Class 4: 71% to 100% Impairment of the Whole Person**
No symptoms	Minimal symptoms	Moderate to marked symptoms	Moderate to marked symptoms
and	**and**	**and**	**and**
hemoglobin 10–12 g/dL	hemoglobin 8–10 g/dL	hemoglobin 5–8 g/dL*	hemoglobin 5–8 g/dL*
and	**and**	**and**	**and**
no transfusion required	no transfusion required	transfusions of 2–3 U required every 4–6 weeks†	transfusions of 2–3 U required every 2 weeks†

* Level before transfusion.

† Implies hemolysis of transfused blood.

From Cocchiarella L, Andersson GBJ (eds): Guides to the Evaluation of Permanent Impairment, 5th ed. Chicago, American Medical Association, 2001, p 193, with permission.

TABLE 32–3

Functional Classification of Hematologic System Disease

Class	Description
I (none)	No signs or symptoms of disease despite laboratory abnormalities; individual performs the usual activities of daily living
II (minimal)	Some signs or symptoms of disease; individual performs the usual activities of daily living with some difficulty
III (moderate)	Signs and symptoms of disease; individual requires varying amounts of assistance from others to perform the usual activities of daily living
IV (marked)	Signs and symptoms of disease; individual requires assistance to perform most or all activities of daily living

From Cocchiarella L, Andersson GBJ (eds): Guides to the Evaluation of Permanent Impairment, 5th ed. Chicago, American Medical Association, 2001, p 192, with permission.

anemia as determined by laboratory test. Also the prognosis will vary depending on whether the condition is reversible or readily treatable with chronic therapy (such as megaloblastic anemia secondary to B_{12} or folate deficiency) or irreversible (as in myelodysplastic states and leukemia).

The functional classification (Table 32–3) is actually a description of the ADL. In taking an individual's history, the examiner determines the level that the person was capable of prior to the illness and compares it to the activities tolerated at the time of evaluation with the reduced Hb to estimate the percentage of work or ADL capabilities lost.

■ A construction worker who regularly did heavy work, including lifting of 100 pounds or more, developed chronic myelocytic leukemia (CML). The disease process was controlled with therapy and his Hg levels were stable between 8 and 9 g/dL. He was unable to tolerate his previous heavy work but was able to tolerate light work. He was transferred successfully to the position of inspector and spent 8 hours per day walking, standing, or sitting with minimal demands for physical activity. One could estimate therefore that he lost approximately 50% of his preinjury capacity to work as a result of this hematologic disease. This correlates to 11% to 30% whole person impairment.

A similar worker with CML and more advanced disease maintained an Hg of only 7 g/dL and had chronic fatigue. He was only capable of working in a modified position in an office setting. A disability recommendation would restrict him to sedentary work only. The claimant is in a relatively stable state and has achieved maximal medical improvement. This correlates with 31% to 70% whole person impairment. ■

TABLE 32–4

Karnofsky Performance Status Scale

Functional Capability	Level of Activity
Able to carry on normal activity; no special care needed	100%—Normal; no complaints, no evidence of disease 90%—Able to carry on normal activity; minor signs or symptoms of disease 80%—Normal activity with effort; some signs or symptoms of disease
Unable to work; able to live at home; cares for most personal needs; needs varying amount of assistance	70%—Cares for self; unable to carry on normal activity or to do active work 60%—Requires occasional assistance but is able to care for most of own needs 50%—Requires considerable assistance and frequent medical care
Unable to care for self; requires equivalent of institutional or hospital care	40%—Disabled; requires special medical care and assistance 30%—Severely disabled; hospitalization indicated, although death not imminent 20%—Very sick; hospitalization necessary; active supportive treatment necessary 10%—Moribund; fatal 0%—Dead

An excellent way to estimate impairment in these clinical circumstances is to employ performance status scales that have been developed for patients with cancer (see Tables 32–4 and 32–5); these are discussed in the section on oncologic impairment.

TABLE 32–5

Eastern Cooperative Oncology Group Performance Status Scale

Grade	Level of Activity
0	Fully active; able to carry on all predisease performance without restriction (Karnofsky 90% to 100%)
1	Restricted in physically strenuous activity but ambulatory and able to carry out work of a light or sedentary nature; e.g., light housework, office work (Karnofsky 70% to 80%)
2	Ambulatory and capable of all self-care but unable to carry out any work activities; up and about more than 50% of waking hours (Karnofsky 50% to 60%)
3	Capable of only limited self-care, confined to bed or chair more than 50% of waking hours (Karnofsky 30% to 40%)
4	Completely disabled; cannot carry on any self-care; totally confined to bed or chair (Karnofsky 10% to 20%)

PLATELET DISORDERS

Platelets are fragments of cells derived from megakaryocytes in the bone marrow that are important in the clotting mechanism and may be associated with impairment and disability if inadequate numbers or function of the platelets exists, resulting in a hemorrhagic predisposition. The production defect may result from an infiltrative process within the marrow as seen with leukemia, lymphoma, granulomas, or carcinomas. There may be premature destruction, as seen in immune-mediated thrombocytopenia, or a consumption coagulopathy, such as disseminated intravascular coagulation or thrombotic thrombocytopenic purpura. These conditions may be chronic in nature, in which case the propensity to bleed is related to the absolute number of platelets. The chronicity of the condition has a bearing on the adaptability of the body to the predisposition to bleed. Some conditions, such as immune thrombocytopenic purpura (ITP), may be very responsive to therapy with steroids or splenectomy. Excessive numbers of platelets (thrombocythemia or thrombocytosis) may be a primary process under the category of myeloproliferative disorders and may be associated with hemorrhage or, more commonly, a thrombotic predisposition.

Generally, platelet counts above 50,000/μL do not cause bleeding unless there is an associated platelet dysfunction and therefore are not a cause for work or ADL restrictions. Between 10,000 and 50,000/μL, bleeding can occur with surgery or trauma but spontaneous bleeding is not likely to occur. At platelet counts below 10,000/μL, even minor trauma can cause bleeding and spontaneous bleeding may be seen. At platelet counts below 5,000/μL, there is high risk for spontaneous bleeding, including intracranial hemorrhage. Therapy with platelet transfusions, steroids, and/or splenectomy (if appropriate) is needed, as well as specific treatment for the disease process causing this disorder. At platelet counts below 5,000/μL, impairment may not be evident if bleeding has not occurred, but because of the high likelihood of spontaneous bleeding, the evaluator must consider the actual platelet count and estimate the risk of spontaneous, atraumatic bleeding. Impairment ratings reflect prophylactic restrictions of the ADL.

■ A clumsy housewife frequently cuts herself while preparing meals. She has ITP. Her platelet counts, after therapy, are approximately 20,000/μL or below. Her whole person impairment is 31% to 55% owing to the restrictions in her ADL. ■

COAGULATION DISORDERS

Coagulation disorders are associated with abnormalities in either the protein factors associated with the coagulation cascade, with the platelets, or due to an interaction of these two components. They predispose to bleeding because the complicated process that ultimately leads to clot formation is impaired.

Hemophilia is an abnormality of one of several clotting factors. The most common is a varying degree of deficiency in factor VIII. Although this can be an acquired defect, most cases are congenital. The degree of severity (the most severe cases have <1% factor activity) determines the likelihood of spontaneous hemorrhage, which can be disabling or life-threatening. The use of exogenous replacement factor can correct clotting to normal and help stop bleeding and the possible long-term complications from hemorrhage (such as severe arthropathies). Recognition, diagnosis, and treatment in early childhood has markedly reduced the degree of impairment, and many people with hemophilia now commonly function normally in the workplace. Other coagulation defects include factor IX deficiency or hemophilia B (which clinically resembles factor VIII deficiency). Von Willebrand disease is the result of a congenital deficiency of a complex protein that serves as a carrier for factor VIII. Although it is sometimes an acquired abnormality in conjunction with other diseases, it is the most common hereditary coagulopathy. In most individuals the abnormality is mild and significant bleeding only occurs after surgery or trauma. Indeed this may first be recognized in adulthood at the time of the first surgical incursion. Impairment is uncommon, except when transiently associated with trauma.

The disorders of coagulation that are associated with impairment largely focus on congenital lesions. Recognized impairment is the cumulative result of bleeding over a lifetime. Impairment relates not to the bleeding, but to the chronic tissue injury secondary to the repeated bleeds, which often results in joint scarring and dysfunction, pulmonary fibrosis, or renal failure; therefore, the evaluation of impairment is determined and rated by the end organ dysfunction. Most acquired coagulation disorders are transient and reversible, and do not lead to hematologic impairment. However, as with platelet disorders, an impairment rating is justified based upon prophylactic restrictions in the ADL using Table 9–4[1(p203)] as a guide.

THROMBOTIC CONDITIONS

Some vascular thrombotic events are the result of congenital or acquired deficiencies of clotting factors that primarily function to keep the blood fluid (antithrombin, protein C, or protein S) or congenital mutations (factor V Leiden, prothrombin 20210A). The result of these changes is a predisposition to clot formation in either the venous or arterial vasculature. The result can be the development of a myocardial infarction, a cerebrovascular accident, pulmonary emboli, or deep vein thromboses. In each of these clinical circumstances, the impairment is determined by the nature of the end organ damage rather than the hematologic abnormality, per se. Patients with recurrent thrombosis (i.e., a second episode) commonly require prolonged or even lifetime anticoagulation as a prophylactic measure. For that group, the definition of impairment requires an evaluation of the risks and limitations of performance due to the possibility of bleeding from their prophylactic medication. Such a numerical definition requires consideration of patient age, the nature of comorbid diseases, and the type of anticoagulant to be utilized.

Some uncommon clotting alterations can be associated with thrombosis and more rarely hemorrhage. The development of antiphospholipid antibodies and a related lesion, lupus anticoagulant, can be associated with fetal wastage and microvascular occlusions of the retina or in the brain. The clear biologic relevance of these laboratory findings is complicated by such findings in individuals with no apparent disease. Therefore, impairment is again determined by the specific end organ complications present in the individual.

LEUKEMIA

An abnormal proliferation of white blood cells (leukocytes) results in a leukemia. This may be associated with anemia and thrombocytopenia as well as the lack of normal white blood cells, which results in a diminished ability for the patient to properly handle infections. Such infections may be life threatening.

Leukemias are divided into acute and chronic types and by myeloid, lymphoid, or monocytoid cell lines. They vary based on the period of time one can have the disease before life-threatening complications occur. Acute leukemias require aggressive chemotherapy interventions and intensive antibiotic and blood product support. Such a course of treatment renders patients impaired for variable periods of time. Fortunately, more than 50% of patients with acute leukemia of virtually every type undergo remission and many are cured. In such patients a complete hematologic recovery after the conclusion of therapy may allow them to return to their previous activities and work environment. However, patients with acute leukemia should be considered 100% impaired until a durable (stable) remission is achieved.

Chronic leukemias vary greatly regarding the degree of disability encountered by the individual. Some patients, whose only manifestation of leukemia is an elevated white blood cell count (particularly those with chronic lymphocytic leukemia), may not require any intervention for a prolonged period of time (years and even decades). This is often true for early stage chronic lymphocytic leukemia (CLL). In the case of CML, new molecular based therapies (such as imatinib mesylate [Gleevec]) appear effective in prolonging the chronic phase of the disease or even achieving a complete and durable remission, making this a disease of prolonged duration without disability. Thus, impairment in the chronic leukemias is largely limited to periods when intensive treatment is needed, or in late stages, where terminal transition is common. Some parameters to help rate impairment are provided in Table 32–6.

Other conditions associated with leukopenia, especially neutropenia, may vary in their potential risk of infection and exposure to potential infectious pathogens may constitute an excessive risk. In this circumstance, the occurrence, nature, and severity of the infection determines the degree of impairment.

TABLE 32–6

Criteria for Rating Impairment Due to White Blood Cell Disease

Class 1: 0% to 15% Impairment of the Whole Person	Class 2: 16% to 30% Impairment of the Whole Person	Class 3: 31% to 55% Impairment of the Whole Person	Class 4: 56% to 100% Impairment of the Whole Person
Symptoms or signs of leukocyte abnormality	Symptoms and signs of leukocyte abnormality	Requires continuous treatment	Symptoms and signs of leukocyte abnormality
and	**and**	**and**	**and**
needs no or infrequent treatment	performs most daily activities, although requires continuous treatment	interference with the ability to perform daily activities, requires occasional assistance from others	requires continuous treatment
and			**and**
performs all or most daily activities			experiences difficulty in performing activities of daily living; requires continuous care from others

From Cocchiarella L, Andersson GBJ (eds): Guides to the Evaluation of Permanent Impairment, 5th ed. Chicago, American Medical Association, 2001, p 200, with permission.

MYELOPROLIFERATIVE DISORDERS

Excess production of one or more cell lines in the bone marrow such as polycythemia vera (red blood cells) or essential thrombocythemia (platelets) may be associated with excessive hemorrhage or thrombotic predisposition. When these conditions are successfully treated, the risk is markedly reduced and patients may be able to function normally. These conditions may ultimately progress to a condition of fibrosis in the marrow, which leads to low blood counts, possible transfusion dependence, and even leukemia.

Myelofibrosis, as a primary process, is usually initially associated with an elevated white blood cell count but may progress to anemia, which can be very severe. The chronicity of this disease may be associated with a reasonable functional state despite very low Hb and Hct levels. Eventually, however, such patients become symptomatic and impairment ensues. Parameters for estimation of whole person impairment are the same as those provided in Table 32–6, because clinical correlates are the same. In addition, Tables 32–4 and 32–5, used to define impairment in cancer patients, directly apply here as well.

SPLENIC DISORDERS

The spleen is the largest lymphoid organ in the body and serves a function as a filter of senescent red blood cells and a site of processing infections, especially of encapsulated organisms such as *S pneumococcus* and *Haemophilus.* Post-splenectomy, there may be a persistent elevation of the white blood cell and platelet counts. This is not a pathologic disorder, although patients may be predisposed to pneumococcal and *Haemophilus* infections. No specific impairment results from removal of the spleen in adults.

Patients may have splenomegaly secondary to a myeloproliferative or lymphoproliferative disorder, such as CLL, lymphoma, or portal hypertension. Depending on the size of the spleen, patients may have pain or decreased ability to eat secondary to compression of the stomach. There may also be relative thrombocytopenia, leukopenia, and even anemia, which are often asymptomatic. Impairment correlates best with the degree of anemia and the previously mentioned parameters therefore apply.

ACQUIRED IMMUNODEFICIENCY SYNDROME

Acquired immunodeficiency syndrome (AIDS) is a disorder that causes impairment because of immune disregulation. The likelihood of dysfunction is estimated by the CD4 count and the viral load. With progressive disease there is a greater risk of infectious complications, specifically opportunistic infections. The overall impairment is determined by assessing impairment of the organ systems involved with such infections, such as the gastrointestinal tract, skin, lungs, central nervous system, or blood.

An acute retroviral syndrome may develop early in human immunodeficiency virus (HIV) infection; symptoms include fever, fatigue, pharyngitis, rash, myalgia, and arthralgia. Quantitative HIV RNA measurements also indicate the extent of HIV infection. Early stages are characterized by a CD4 count greater than $0.50 \times 10^9/L$ (500 cells/mm^3); these individuals are often asymptomatic but may have lymphadenopathy, leukopenia, thrombocytopenia, and dermatologic conditions. Intermediate stages involve CD4 counts of $0.20 \times 10^9/L$ to $0.50 \times 10^9/L$ (200 to 500 cells/mm^3); antiretroviral therapy is often initiated to prolong this stage of disease. Individuals may have few or no symptoms or may develop constitutional symptoms, diarrhea, herpes simplex infections, oral or vaginal candidiasis, upper respiratory tract infections, sinusitis, or common bacterial infections. Advanced stages, often defined by CD4 counts less than $0.20 \times 10^9/L$ (200 cells/mm^3), are associated with an increased incidence of opportunistic infections and meet the Centers for Disease Control and Prevention definition for AIDS. At low CD4 levels, there is an increased incidence of complications, including infections such as *Pneumocystis carinii* pneumonia, *Toxoplasma gondii* encephalitis, tuberculosis, cryptosporidiosis, salmonellosis, and esophageal candidiasis; neoplasms including Kaposi sarcoma, lymphoma, and cervical cancer; and neurologic dysfunction, such as mononeuritis multiplex, peripheral neuropathies, cranial nerve palsies, and myelitis. At CD4 levels below $0.10 \times 10^9/L$ (100 cells/ mm^3), the following are more common: HIV-associated dementia, wasting syndromes, progressive multifocal leukoencephalopathy, cytomegalovirus retinitis, disseminated *Mycobacterium avium* complex, cryptococcal meningitis, disseminated coccidiomycosis, histoplasmosis, and invasive aspergillosis.

Patients with AIDS can develop malignancies such as squamous cell Hodgkin's carcinoma of the cervix, Kaposi sarcoma, and non-Hodgkin's lymphoma. Lymphomas are usually very aggressive and often involve extranodal sites such as the central nervous system or gastrointestinal tract or body cavities such as the pleura and peritoneum. These diseases may be associated with profound disability but sometimes may respond reasonably well to therapy.

The frequency and extent of the immunologic complications will determine the extent of the individual's impairment and disability.

Impairment can be assessed in several ways. It may be assessed by its effects on various organ systems; e.g., dermatologic or pulmonary. A global assessment, based on the estimated interference in activities of daily living, is also appropriate.

ONCOLOGIC DISORDERS AND IMPAIRMENT

There are many reasons for impairment in oncologic or malignant disorders. Impairment may arise from the primary cancer, from metastatic disease, or from the toxic effects of therapy—surgery, radiation, chemotherapy, or immunotherapy.

There are also systemic symptoms that can be secondary to a malignancy such as pain, anorexia, weight loss, or fatigue. Some malignancies, depending on the specific cell type and the stage of the disease at presentation, are amenable to therapy, with good outcomes. In such cases, patients may have initial symptoms followed by side effects of therapy, which ultimately leads to a restoration of function. Other patients, with more advanced disease, may become disabled but encounter some improvement of function with therapy. With progressive disease there is an inexorable decline of performance status and permanent impairment. Initial symptoms are commonly attributable to the primary site of disease.

Patients may also be initially debilitated by the presence of metastatic disease or may develop metastatic disease in the course of their illness. Symptoms can result from bone pain or fractures when disease has spread to bone, neurologic abnormalities when disease involves the brain, respiratory problems when the lungs are involved, or liver failure, which can cause anorexia, nausea, vomiting, fatigue, and fevers.

Even when patients respond well to therapy there may be prolonged sequelae of chemotherapy agents, which can cause impairment. Neuropathy can be secondary to vincristine, cisplatin, or taxanes; cardiotoxicity can result from anthracycline therapy; ototoxicity and nephrotoxicity can be associated with cisplatin; and pulmonary fibrosis may be secondary to bleomycin. Bone marrow toxicity may be related to alkylating agent exposure (e.g., cyclophosphamide).

Radiation therapy may be associated with fatigue, skin changes, fibrosis of underlying tissues, and bone marrow suppression. Many of these effects are temporary, but in some patients the residual effects are prolonged. Therefore, patients with cancer may have temporary, partial, or permanent impairment depending on a multiplicity of factors: primary site of disease, stage or extent of disease, toxicity secondary to therapy, and overall response to treatment.

Psychological factors may also lead to significant impairment in patients with cancer. Depression is common and may resolve when treated directly or when the patient recovers from therapy with a good prognosis. There is recent evidence that cognitive impairment occurs with chemotherapy and cranial radiation and that such changes may last for the rest of the individual's life, complicating the interpretation and definition of the role and degree that these need to be integrated into the post-therapy evaluation of impairment.

Medicines used to control symptoms such as narcotics for pain or phenothiazines for nausea may also have debilitating side effects, such as drowsiness or altered mental status, which can be disabling. Many patients with cancer try to conduct their lives as normally as possible during the course of their illness and wish for return to their normal life as quickly as possible. It is important in evaluating impairments in these patients to look at the overall prognosis and have realistic expectations for treatment and outcome.

Two commonly used scales of functional performance status are the Karnofsky scale (Table 32–4) and the Eastern Cooperative Oncology Group (ECOG) scale (Table 32–5). These refer to the level of activity of which a patient is capable. Parameters are related to the anatomic extent or histopathology of the cancer.

In the Karnofsky scale, a patient with performance status (PS) of 90% to 100% (or ECOG scale 0) should be able to continue to work at almost any occupation. A patient with Karnofsky PS 80% or ECOG 1 may be able to function in sedentary or office work. By definition, a patient with a PS of 70% or less or ECOG of 2 or higher is unable to work.

Reference

1. Cocchiarella L, Andersson GBJ (eds): Guides to the Evaluation of Permanent Impairment, 5th ed. Chicago, American Medical Association, 2001.

SECTION

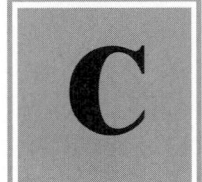

Neurological Impairment Assessment

CHAPTER

33

Neurological Diagnostic Techniques

SCOTT HALDEMAN, DC, MD, PhD, FRCP(C) ■ RAND S. SWENSON, DC, MD, PhD

The nervous system is the most complex system in the body. It influences the function of virtually every organ system and has primary control over movement, sensory function, higher cognitive function, and the interaction of the organism with the environment. A wide variety of disabling disorders affect the nervous system and many of the symptoms described by individuals seeking disability can be the result of nervous system damage. Although most of these symptoms can be adequately assessed by the clinical examination, in some cases the examination may not be able to adequately evaluate or quantitate the problem. This is particularly true as many complaints, particularly abnormal sensations, are subjective in nature.

The evaluation of the impaired patient begins with a proper diagnosis. However, when evaluating dysfunction resulting from neurologic disorders, it is problematic that the same condition can produce widely differing degrees of impairment. Patients with such diverse neurologic conditions such as multiple sclerosis, carpal tunnel syndrome, and spinal stenosis can have symptoms that range in severity from minimal to crippling. Because damage to neural structures can cause different degrees of dysfunction, it is essential that quantitative methods be developed to assess the levels of neurologic impairment.

Many of the systems of impairment rating, including those in the AMA Guides to the Evaluation of Permanent Impairment[5] and California guidelines, list the major neurologic functions and then attempt to organize them by defining specific whole person impairment percentages. The Social Security Administration,[138] on the other hand, lists specific diagnoses and symptom patterns. It is left to the clinician to reach conclusions on the ability of a patient to perform certain activities or control bodily functions.

Specialized diagnostic testing, especially of an objective nature, has been acknowledged as providing important information in the assessment of potential disability. The Social Security Administration requires the listing of laboratory results justifying a diagnosis. For example, the Social Security handbook specifically mentions the electroencephalogram (EEG) as one method of diagnosing epilepsy.[138] Another is the AMA Guides. Therefore, this chapter has been designed to explore the utility of many of the tests employed in patients with neurologic complaints, particularly with regard to their potential contribution to an impairment rating and the assessment of disability.

RATIONALE FOR TESTING

There are several roles for specialized testing in the evaluation of the individual with a potential neurologic impairment. A test is most helpful when it is selected appropriately for a particular clinical diagnosis and with knowledge of the strengths and weaknesses of the test relative to the diagnosis. Specialized tests should be driven by the clinical history and physical examination and are particularly useful when applied to filling gaps and answering questions remaining after careful consideration of the individual's history and examination. Careful clinical consideration allows for proper framing of remaining questions, permitting the selection of specialized tests that are most likely to provide satisfactory answers. Although an understanding of the sensitivity and specificity of these tests is important, the predictive value of diagnostic testing is greatly enhanced by applying a test selectively to a patient population with a high likelihood of having the condition. "Shotgun" screening of individuals with low probability of having the condition will produce many false positive results, even when the test itself has an acceptably high level of specificity. Therefore, the utility of a test is dependent on the population in whom it is used, and the clinical examination and history is critical for defining this population.

There are several potential roles for neurodiagnostic testing in the evaluation of individuals with impairment. The most important use is facilitating proper diagnosis. However, testing has also been employed in other ways, such as in an attempt to document loss of function, to confirm subjective complaints, and to rule out other intercurrent problems.

The tests included in this chapter that illustrate these points are listed in Table 33–1.

Determination of Diagnosis

The formulation of an accurate diagnosis is a necessary, if incomplete step, in the determination of impairment. However, a diagnosis alone is insufficient, because even individuals with the same diagnosis can have widely differing degrees of impairment. A diagnosis provides information on the nature of impairments that might be expected, the anticipated clinical course, the overall prognosis, and the availability of treatments or cures. All of these elements are necessary pieces of the puzzle when determining impairment and disability. Neurodiagnostic testing is often essential as an adjunct to the clinical examination in order to determine the diagnosis on which the impairment is based. For example, electro-

TABLE 33–1

The Utilization of Neurodiagnostic Testing in an Impairment Evaluation

Determination of the Diagnosis	Documentation of Loss of Function	Documentation of Subjective Complaints
1. Brain disorders a) Imaging (MRI, CT, etc.) b) Cognitive testing c) EEG d) Evoked potentials (VEP, BAEP) e) Spinal tap 2. Spinal cord disorders a) Imaging (CT, MRI) b) Evoked potentials c) Spinal tap 3. Radiculopathy a) Imaging b) EMG c) Reflex studies d) Evoked potentials 4. Peripheral neuropathies a) NCVs (motor, sensory) b) Reflex studies c) EMG 5. Bowel, bladder, and sexual disorders a) Cystometry b) Evoked potentials c) Anal EMG d) Penile tumescence 6. Muscle disorders a) Blood analysis b) EMG c) Repetitive stimulation d) Biopsy	1. Cognitive deficits a) Psychological test b) Event related potentials c) SPECT, PET 2. Motor deficits a) EMG b) Motor NCV c) Cortical motor evoked potentials 3. Sensory deficits a) Sensory NCV b) SEP 4. Coordination deficits a) Electronystagmography 5. Bowel and bladder deficits a) Cystometry b) Evoked potentials c) Penile tumescence	1. Pain None 2. Paresthesias ? Sensory NCVs 3. Muscle spasms ? Surface EMG ? Muscle evoked potentials 4. False positive testing on EMG/NCV/SEP EEG Imaging

MRI, magnetic resonance imaging; CT, computed tomography; VEP, visual evoked potential; BAEP, brainstem auditory evoked potentials; EMG, electromyography; NCV, nerve conduction velocity; SPECT, single photon emission computed tomography; PET, positron emission tomography; SEP, somatosensory evoked potential; EEG, electroencephalography.

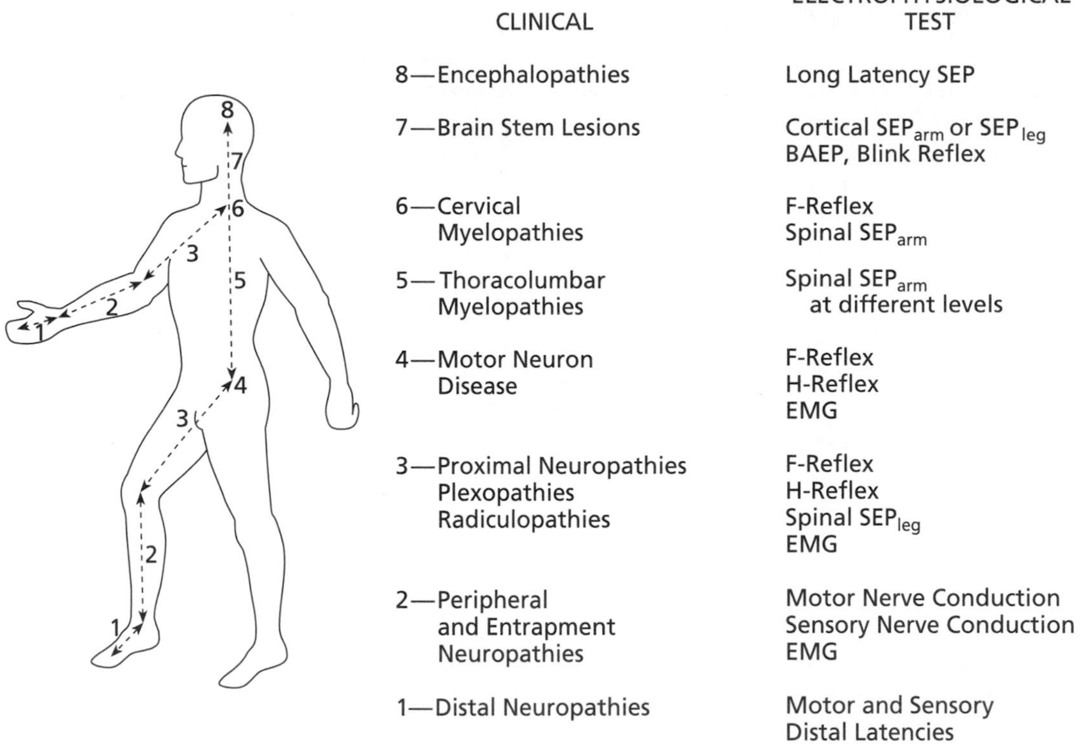

CLINICAL
ELECTROPHYSIOLOGICAL TEST
8—Encephalopathies
Long Latency SEP
7—Brain Stem Lesions
Cortical SEParm or SEPleg
BAEP, Blink Reflex
6—Cervical Myelopathies
F-Reflex
Spinal SEParm
5—Thoracolumbar Myelopathies
Spinal SEParm at different levels
4—Motor Neuron Disease
F-Reflex
H-Reflex
EMG
3—Proximal Neuropathies Plexopathies Radiculopathies
F-Reflex
H-Reflex
Spinal SEPleg
EMG
2—Peripheral and Entrapment Neuropathies
Motor Nerve Conduction
Sensory Nerve Conduction
EMG
1—Distal Neuropathies
Motor and Sensory Distal Latencies
8
7
6
5
4
3
2
1

Figure 33–1. Example of electrodiagnostic tests used for localizing a neurologic deficit in the extremities. SEP, somatosensory evoked potential.

diagnostic tests may be necessary to localize neurologic lesions affecting peripheral nerves (Fig. 33–1). The diagnosis is key to understanding prognosis, the nature of anticipated impairments, and available treatments.

Documentation of Loss of Function

A single disease can cause loss of neurologic function that ranges from mild to severe. Multiple sclerosis (MS), for example, may cause dysfunction ranging from a reversible, minor symptom of numbness or blurred vision to a combination of incapacitating deficits of cognitive, motor, and sensory function. A spinal radiculopathy can result in deficits ranging from isolated loss of myotonic reflexes to a devastating cauda equina syndrome. Therefore, the simple determination of a diagnosis is not sufficient to assess the level of impairment or disability. Testing, however, may be helpful and even necessary in some cases in order to document the degree of neurologic deficit caused by a specific diagnosis.

Confirmation of Subjective Complaints

Many individuals have neurologic symptoms that are subjective in nature or that cannot be objectively documented by clinical observation alone. Symptoms such as pain, muscle tenderness, vague feelings of weakness, fatigue, paresthesias, dizziness, and changes in memory are often difficult or impossible to confirm through the clinical examination. Because most impairment evaluation systems require some degree of objective verification of clinical symptoms, individuals with predominantly subjective complaints represent a particular challenge. In some circumstances, neurodiagnostic testing can provide objective verification of nervous system dysfunction, contributing to the accurate attribution of these subjective complaints.

Ruling Out Intercurrent Problems

In some cases a person may have several conditions that contribute to his or her overall presentation of neurologic impairment. An example of this would be the person with neck and limb pain as well as hand paresthesias. It is possible that this may represent a radicular syndrome, although the hand paresthesias may be due to a different pathology (such as carpal tunnel syndrome) than the neck pain. In such a case, electrodiagnostic tests might be helpful in evaluating the possibility of radiculopathy, but may be equally important in determining whether he or she has a carpal tunnel syndrome accounting for some of the complaints.

UTILITY OF NEURODIAGNOSTIC TESTING

There are several issues that must be addressed when considering the utility of any diagnostic test. First, it is important to know the range of conditions that can be evaluated by the test. Second, it is helpful to know the sensitivity and specificity of the test as well as the positive and negative predictive values of that test for the condition that is being assessed. (See also Appendix A for a better understanding of these statistical issues.)

Most neurodiagnostic tests are applied to several, if not many, conditions. Even tests that investigate a limited pathophysiology (such as nerve conduction studies) can be applied to many conditions, including polyneuropathy, peripheral entrapment neuropathy, plexopathy, or radiculopathy. Therefore, it is meaningless to discuss the utility of the diagnostic test without directly addressing each of the conditions to which it can be applied.

The issues of sensitivity, specificity, and predictive value are particularly thorny when discussing neurodiagnostic tests because the values for sensitivity and specificity (which are, themselves, intermediate steps in the determination of predictive values) have not been determined for many conditions. There are two main reasons for this. First, most neurodiagnostic tests are applied to at least several different disorders. Some of these disorders are common and some are rare. There are even subtypes of most of these conditions, for which the values of sensitivity and specificity would be expected to differ. Therefore, whereas it may be possible to give reasonably accurate values for sensitivity and specificity of tests for some common conditions, it is not possible for many others because they have not been adequately studied. Another problem is that a critical step in ascertaining sensitivity and specificity of any testing procedure is to know who does and does not have the condition. Therefore, it is considered necessary to have a "gold standard" for diagnostic comparison in order to accurately evaluate sensitivity and specificity. Unfortunately, most of the conditions that require neurodiagnostic testing do not have such a gold standard. In fact, for some problems, such as carpal tunnel syndrome, the neurodiagnostic tests (particularly electrodiagnostic tests) have been considered the gold standard despite the fact that these tests are recognized as having some limitations.

Because sensitivity and specificity are such important considerations in the evaluation of diagnostic testing, investigators have used several methods to get around the problem of lack of a gold standard. The classic neurologic gold standard has been the clinical examination. However, only recently has intraobserver and interobserver reliability of the neurologic examination been studied, and in many cases it has been shown not to be particularly reliable.[23,56] In place of a gold standard, the sensitivity of a test can be estimated by assessing the diagnostic value of the test in a population of patients with very clear-cut evidence of having the clinical syndrome in question. This approach is likely to overestimate the sensitivity of the test because these patient groups mostly include those with severe or advanced disease. Another approach has been to test the value of the diagnostic test against a flawed gold standard. Of course, when the diagnostic value of the comparison test is unknown, this can produce flawed findings. An example of this is the comparison of neurodiagnostic testing with radiographic imaging such as computed tomography (CT), magnetic resonance imaging (MRI), or myelography.[94,123] This comparison suffers from the wide variation in imaging findings in most diagnoses as well as from the fact that many abnormalities on imaging can exist in asymptomatic individuals and without producing any neurologic deficit.[22,24,29,32,79] Although comparison with imaging may be appropriate in some conditions for which imaging has a high diagnostic value (such as multiple sclerosis), it is problematic in other conditions where imaging is not definitive (such as radiculopathy). Finally, some studies have used the clinical response to specific therapy, such as surgery, as a gold standard against which to compare neurodiagnostic testing. Again, this approach is probably inadequate as a surgical population is highly selected. Additionally, there are important questions as to whether improvement after treatment (such as surgery) necessarily indicates the accuracy of the initial diagnosis and whether the nonblinded intraoperative observations of a surgeon can be used as a valid gold standard. When considering any report of specificity or sensitivity of a test, all of these issues must be recognized.

The evaluation of specificity presents additional concerns beyond those enumerated in the consideration of problems with sensitivity. For example, in order to determine the specificity of a test, it is necessary to know the distribution of normal in the general population. Whereas most neurodiagnostic tests (such as nerve conduction studies, evoked potentials, and spinal fluid analyses) have been done on large enough sample populations to establish a mean and standard deviations in the normal population, there is no consensus on whether to use 2, 2.5, or 3 standard deviations from the mean to determine the cutoff for normality. Clearly, the specificity of the test increases as one progresses from 2 to 3 standard deviations, where the percentage of normal subjects who would test as abnormal decreases from around 5% to less than 1%. However, the sensitivity of the test for identifying abnormal patients would significantly decrease by this change in cutoff. This issue may be less of a problem with some neurodiagnostic results, such as findings of acute denervation on needle electromyography, which are considered pathologic whenever encountered.

It would be ideal to know the positive and negative predictive values of each particular test. In fact, this is considered to be essential if a test is being employed for screening purposes. However, in order to determine the predictive value of a test one must not only know the sensitivity and specificity of the test but also the prevalence of the condition in the population that is being studied. This presents a problem, particularly if a diagnostic test is being applied to a highly selected patient population (such as those seeking disability). Because of the general lack of such data for neurodiagnostic tests, these tests should not and, indeed, cannot be utilized as a screening mechanism.

Although some research has been done to determine the specificity and sensitivity of testing for specific disease entities, substantially less is known about how various tests correlate with degree of impairment. An example of this is brain MRI, which is known to have a high degree of sensitivity for the diagnosis of multiple sclerosis but not for the degree of impairment.[24,58,87] This lack of correlation with impairment has been a particular problem in assessing spinal abnormalities, where degenerative changes, spondylolisthesis, disc herniation, and stenosis have been identified in large percentages of asymptomatic patients.[28,29,32,108,142] Imaging and laboratory tests (biopsy, blood tests, cerebrospinal fluid) may present relatively accurate anatomic or pathophysiologic diagnoses for many conditions but may not give information as to the symptoms, functional status, or degree of impairment of the nervous system.

Some neurodiagnostic tests have a slightly different problem; that is, they may be quite good at defining pathology, but not the etiology. For example, nerve conduction and evoked responses measure the function of a peripheral nerve or central pathway but are nonspecific as to the nature of the disease process causing the disruption in the pathway. Somatosensory evoked potentials can be abnormal in any disease affecting the spinal cord including demyelination, neoplasms, degenerative disorders, or central disc herniations. Nerve conduction studies only show the speed of conduction and amplitude of signal. These measures can be affected by several pathologic processes including focal neuropathies as well as more generalized polyneuropathies.

Unfortunately, there have been few, if any, well-constructed studies that have specifically addressed the relationship of neurodiagnostic tests to impairment and to the loss of functional capacity. This is a natural extension of the fact that most neurodiagnostic tests are poorly correlated with a person's day-to-day functions. A possible exception to this is neuropsychological testing, where functional tests of cognition are utilized. Even this may not help very much in accurately determining the degree of disability if the testing does not closely model tasks that a person is called upon to perform in daily life.

When reading this chapter and other papers on the use of neurodiagnostic testing in the evaluation of impairment, it is important to determine whether the test is being used for a pathologic diagnosis, the determination of loss of neurologic function, or the quantitation of degree of impairment. It is necessary to recognize that these factors are not interchangeable and that even though testing may be critical to the diagnosis, the contribution of most neurodiagnostic tests in the evaluation of impairment and disability is quite limited. Beyond their diagnostic utility, they may make some secondary contribution to evaluation of degree of severity of the condition and potentially permit objective follow-up evaluation of the progress of the condition. They are of limited (if any) use in screening or in the direct quantitation of degree of impairment.

DETERMINATION OF DIAGNOSIS

Confirmation of the presence or absence of specific pathology or loss of organ function is a necessary step in diagnosis. Neurodiagnostic testing is an integral part of this process. The choice of testing procedures must be focused by the history and clinical examination and is dependent upon several factors. These factors include the part of the nervous system that is presumed to be affected, the type of process that is thought to cause the symptoms, and the specific disease entities that are under consideration. It is not possible in this chapter to describe all of the vast array of diagnostic tests used by neurologists. The following section of this chapter is a simple outline of certain testing procedures that may be used to document neurologic diseases when impairment is an issue. Details of the methods for performance of these tests their accuracy, and idiosyncrasies are left to textbooks of neurology. Wherever possible, we consider the application of these tests to certain clinical conditions that commonly occur in the setting of impairment evaluations.

Most neurologic diseases are classified according to the region of the nervous system that is affected. Anatomic subdivisions commonly include the forebrain, brainstem, spinal cord, nerve roots, peripheral nerves, visceral nervous system, and muscles. Disorders of each of these subdivisions of the nervous system have specific tests that may be applied to the investigation.

Brain Disorders: Forebrain and Brainstem

The number of diseases that can affect the brain fills multiple textbooks on neurology. It is not appropriate or possible to discuss specific diseases in this chapter except as examples. Each brain disorder is diagnosed by a combination of clinical findings and diagnostic tests. Each test has different degrees of sensitivity and specificity depending on the nature of the disease entity and the severity of involvement. The tests that are used to confirm the presence of pathology, however, can be divided into several categories, discussed in the following.

Imaging Studies

Diseases of the brain that produce structural lesions can often be visualized by means of imaging studies. MRI, CT, angiography, and a variety of radiographic procedures fall under this heading. The accuracy of these studies is often enhanced by the infusion of intravenous contrast media and, more recently, by magnetic resonance spectroscopy and functional MRI.

Historically, imaging studies have been used to document anatomic and pathoanatomic structural changes in tissue that can cause nervous system dysfunction. The location and nature of these structural changes are predictive of the kind of abnormalities that might be anticipated. For example, a lesion affecting the dominant motor strip and Broca area would be expected to produce marked deficits in speech and contralateral motor function. On the other hand, infarction in the cerebellum would probably result in ipsilateral impairments in coordination and balance. Imaging is also important in documenting multiple sclerosis plaques, the presence and size of neoplastic lesions, and abscesses and infections.

Certain imaging findings, however, are of questionable importance in the determination of neurologic impairment. For example, there can be multiple, nonspecific punctate white-matter lesions reflecting asymptomatic vascular changes in the normal older population.[35,36] These white-matter lesions have been noted in over 50% of elderly volunteers free of neuropsychiatric or general disease.[116] The finding of one or more of these in a younger individual can raise questions of MS, stroke, vasculitis, or head injury, even though they may be an incidental finding.[21] Imaging, therefore, is generally a diagnostic tool that must be placed in clinical context. It is not a mechanism for determining the degree of impairment in neurologic disorders.

Cognitive Neuropsychological Tests

Significant psychological, cognitive, and psychiatric disorders can exist with an otherwise normal neurologic examination and in the absence of any imaging abnormality. In some cases, findings commonly seen in asymptomatic patients such as white matter hyperintensities may be associated with subtle cognitive changes on neuropsychological testing.[116] On the other hand, depending on the particular brain regions that are involved, large brain lesions my produce no obvious loss of cognitive or intellectual abilities. Psychological and cognitive disorders, however, may provide the principal explanation for impairment in disorders such as traumatic brain injury. It has been reported that even relatively minor head injuries may cause disturbances in performance on neuropsychological testing in patients with an otherwise benign examination.[20,60]

There is considerable overlap between psychiatric disorders and cognitive functions. Furthermore, cognitive test scores can be influenced by mood, alertness, concentration, and the nature of the test.[62] These factors often result in confusing differences in medical opinions when determining cognitive impairment and even more discrepancy when determining: the cause of impairment, the possibility that the impairment existed prior to injury, and how it is effecting recovery. Neuropsychological and cognitive tests are attempts to measure and document higher brain functions. The use of specific cognitive testing and is psychiatric evaluation is described in Chapter 38.

Electroencephalography

The EEG is one of the more established neurologic tests of brain function. EEG abnormalities can be differentiated into nonspecific (slowing) and specific (epileptiform and disease-specific) patterns that may be focal or generalized. The sensitivity and specificity of the test varies with each disease entity.

In the evaluation of episodic neurologic disorders such as epilepsy, the primary diagnostic tool is the clinical examination, with the EEG often utilized as a confirmatory test. Epilepsy carries very specific disability connotations and legal responsibilities for patients and physicians (e.g., driving, working at heights). The documentation of spikes and sharp waves from specific parts of the brain may confirm the diagnosis of seizures although not all individuals with spikes and sharp waves have epilepsy. The finding of epileptiform activity is reasonably specific as only around 4% of normal subjects will show such activity. However, there are a number of patterns that may be misinterpreted as abnormal or that have questionable clinical significance. These patterns may lead to the erroneous conclusion that the EEG supports a diagnosis of epilepsy.[30] The sensitivity of a single EEG in detecting epileptiform activity in patients with documented seizure disorders is not particularly high, being around 50%. Additionally, only about a third of patients with epilepsy will have abnormal findings on every EEG.[30] Therefore, normal EEGs do not rule out epilepsy.

There is a growing recognition that nonepileptic seizures (often referred to as pseudoseizures) account for about 20% of all cases of intractable epilepsy.[89] In some cases, the only way to effectively differentiate the two phenomena is to do simultaneous EEG recording and video monitoring. This may require hospitalization and observation during one or several epileptic events.

The EEG may also be of value in confirming a diagnosis of a generalized, toxic, or metabolic encephalopathy or coma.[37] Depressed brain function following trauma, metabolic disturbances, and many degenerative brain diseases may cause a generalized slowing of background activity. Certain causes of encephalopathy or encephalitis such as Creutzfeldt-Jakob disease, herpes simplex encephalitis, or hepatic failure can produce specific EEG patterns that may be important in the diagnosis. The EEG may also aid in differentiating between organic coma and catatonia in comatose patients.

In recent years, computer analysis of the EEG has become increasingly popular. This has largely paralleled the rise in use of digital EEG technology and in signals processing capability. The capacity to perform so-called brain mapping and computer assisted EEG can be found in many neurophysiologic laboratories. The use of computer-assisted EEGs to enhance the sensitivity of the test is gaining acceptance particularly in long-term monitoring settings. The use of quantitative measures (such as so-called brain mapping) to assist in the analysis of these signals was evaluated in 1997 by a committee of the American Academy of Neurology and the American Clinical Neurophysiology Society.[100] They concluded that these procedures were investigational for many of the conditions to which they have been applied, such as post-concussion syndrome, mild to moderate head injury, learning disability, attention disorders, and various behavioral disorders. Although this conclusion has been challenged,[73] there are significant concerns relative to the frequency of minor abnormalities with computer-generated EEG analysis and the interpretation of their significance. Such data have at times been assigned greater significance than ongoing research warrants. Brain mapping procedures remain controversial and there are questions relative to differentiation among artifacts, normal variants, and true abnormalities.

The EEG and, particularly, brain mapping must be interpreted with care in the person with potential impairment claim. However, well-defined, localized abnormalities and specific generalized activity changes can sometimes be the deciding factor in the diagnosis of cerebral disorders.

Evoked Potentials

With the development of computerized analysis of cerebral potentials, the past two decades have seen a marked increase in the use of evoked potentials to evaluate central nervous system sensory pathways. These tests may provide unique information as no other neurodiagnostic procedure gives objective data relative to central sensory systems.

Visual evoked potentials (VEPs) are most useful in documenting demyelinating or compressing lesions of the optic nerve or optic tracts. Nath et al[95] noted delayed conduction in 45% of patients with macular pathology. On the other hand, although the electroretinogram has been used to test the overall function of the retina, VEPs may be normal or near normal in macular disease. Therefore, a combination of a pattern-shift VEP together with the electroretinogram has been recommended to differentiate optic nerve from retinal disease.[77] VEPs have been used to differentiate hysterical blindness from true organic blindness although this should only be done in conjunction with a more complete examination. Furthermore, VEPs are nonspecific, because they are likely to be abnormal no matter what the cause of damage to optic pathways. For example, they are often delayed in such diverse conditions as Friedreich ataxia, vitamin B_{12} deficiency, MS, and diabetes. Although delayed VEPs are considered a hallmark of optic nerve demyelination, they do not correlate well with impairment. Chiappa[41] noted that when these potentials are normal, the examination is always normal, but in patients with MS, the test is commonly abnormal despite clinically normal vision. Therefore, VEPs have been reported to be useful in identifying subclinical damage to the optic system in conditions such as MS. However, there is a wide variation in the reported sensitivity of VEPs for demyelinating disease, with published values ranging between 47% and 96%.[42]

Brainstem auditory evoked potentials (BAEPs), also known as auditory evoked responses, can be an important adjunct to the testing and localization of problems related to hearing or to brainstem damage. Together with cochlear potentials, BAEPs may help distinguish cochlear from auditory nerve pathology. This test measures potentials from the cochlea through the auditory nerve and the brainstem as a series of well-defined peaks that are thought to be generated in different structures through this neural pathway. Lesions at different locations in the auditory pathway show different patterns of abnormality. The sensitivity and specificity are, again, disease specific. For example, there is a reported false-negative rate of 5% in the diagnosis of acoustic neuromas and cerebellopontine angle tumors.[51] In brainstem demyelinating lesions, a positive test is reported in only 32% to 64% of patients.[41] This test has been reported to be abnormal in head injury, even of a relatively minor nature. However, the reported sensitivity ranges widely, from 27% to 46%.[57]

Spinal Tap and Blood Analysis

The analysis of cerebrospinal fluid (CSF) and blood is an essential part of the diagnosis of certain central nervous system disorders, particularly of an inflammatory or infectious nature. For example, determination of the organism responsible for most nervous system infections is dependent upon blood and spinal fluid analysis. Testing CSF for immunoglobin (Ig) abnormalities and specifically determining oligoclonal bands and IgG synthesis rate has become an integral part in making the diagnosis of MS. However, it must be remembered that MS is only the most common of several disorders that result in abnormal immune globulins in the CSF. Many inherited metabolic disorders may similarly be confirmed by isolating specific abnormal proteins or polysaccharides. The tests are mentioned here simply for completeness. The sensitivity and specificity of these tests are, again, disease specific.

Tests of Vestibular and Cerebellar Function

Problems with balance, coordination, and eye movement can present particular challenges in evaluation as there are several systems involved in controlling these functions. For example, balance can be affected by conditions that affect sensory systems, including involvement of peripheral nerves in the feet or conduction pathways through the spinal cord (see following). It can also be adversely affected by weakness or by extrapyramidal motor problems (such as Parkinson's disease). Of course, balance is commonly affected by damage to the inner ear, vestibular nerves, and brainstem, which need to be tested independently. The general neurologic examination often provides some clues to disorders of these systems, potentially showing spontaneous nystagmus or signs of damage to neighboring structures, such as hearing, cerebellar function, or other brainstem functions. However, outside of the performance of positional testing, direct evaluation of the vestibular system may be quite difficult during the bedside examination. Electronystagmography (ENG) provides important information that cannot be obtained by any other method. This test is properly considered in the evaluation of individuals with vertigo, dizziness, or dysequilibrium who are suspected of having some level of damage to the vestibular apparatus of the inner ear or of the brainstem.[16]

Of course, vestibular disorders are only one of many problems potentially affecting balance. Posturography is a procedure that is used to assess the body's reactions to rapid motion of a platform on which a person is standing. Other parts of the test examine balance when individuals are presented with several different sensory challenges, including a moving visual surround and an unstable platform.[4] A committee of the American Academy of Neurology evaluated the literature in 1993 and concluded that dynamic posturography was promising but that the literature supporting the clinical utility of the procedure was sparse at that time.[17] The last decade has seen a substantial increase in the available literature[4] and most has supported the utility of posturography in the evaluation and monitoring of patients with gait instability that cannot be adequately characterized by more conventional means. Posturography probably has a sensitivity of between 50% and 77% and a specificity of between 50% and 71% for various vestibular disorders.[48,137] It may be particularly helpful in the assessment of vertigo of central nervous system origin. However, the issue of diagnostic utility of this procedure for many specific disorders remains open.

Spinal Cord Disorders

Injury or damage to the spinal cord (myelopathy) can cause substantial disability and impairment. Symptoms typically include motor and sensory dysfunction as well as problems with gait and coordination. Furthermore, there may be loss of control of bowel, bladder, and sexual function. The causes of spinal cord dysfunction include such diverse entities as spinal trauma, central disc herniation, spinal stenosis, severe spondylosis, neoplasm, congenital malformation, infection, vascular lesions, or demyelinating disease. The clinical examination usually gives a strong indication of myelopathy by the identification of a motor or sensory level, reflex changes, spinal percussive tenderness, Lhermitte sign, associated radiculopathy, or appropriate bladder and bowel changes. The clinical examination often is able to localize the approximate level of the lesion. However, individuals with myelopathy almost always require other testing to determine the type of lesion causing the impairment. Whereas this task has been simplified by the advent of advanced imaging, definitive answers relative to the nature and severity of myelopathy may require additional testing.

Imaging Studies

MRI scans, CT scans (with and without contrast), and myelography are the most common tests used for documenting spinal cord lesions. As in the case of brain disorders, there can be a significant discrepancy between lesions visualized on imaging studies and the symptoms and disability experienced by a person. Advanced degenerative changes, disc herniations, and even central stenosis may be found in individuals who are asymptomatic and who have normal functioning.[29,32,33,141,142]

Evoked Potentials

Somatosensory evoked potentials (SEPs) are commonly used in the evaluation of spinal cord lesions.[7] These potentials are generated by the stimulation of major nerves in the upper and lower extremities (Fig. 33–2). The impulses that produce the SEP signal travel through the posterior column system of the spinal cord and then through the lemniscal system of the brainstem to the thalamus and cerebral cortex. The usefulness of the test, therefore, is limited to lesions in these pathways. Patients with isolated damage to pathways mediating pain and temperature sensation, for example, usually have normal SEPs,[19,98] and SEPs are also quite insensitive to lesions of the cerebral cortex. Up to 90% of patients with definite MS and about half of MS patients without any sensory symptoms have abnormal SEPs.[43,101] Combining tests such as evoked potentials with an MRI may increase the sensitivity in the diagnosis of MS when compared with MRI alone.[24] Although lower limb SEPs are more sensitive for myelopathy, some patients only have abnormality in upper limb SEPs. Therefore, both should be done in the investigation of suspected spinal cord damage or disease. SEPs may also be abnormal in other forms of myelopathy including trauma, cervical spondylosis, and spinal cord tumors.[7] Restuccia et al have described abnormal SEPs in patients with confirmed lesions of the lumbosacral[110] and cervical[111] spinal cord. In contrast, SEPs have been found to be normal in 22 of 23 patients with asymptomatic compression of the cervical spinal cord by spondylosis and, therefore, may be of use in distinguishing individuals with clinically insignificant cervical stenosis from those with myelopathy.[132] Additionally, patients may have abnormal SEPs with limited findings on imaging studies.[148] Therefore, SEPs provide information that complements that from imaging studies and may contribute to the investigation of patients with suspected or questionable myelopathy.[55]

Motor Evoked Potentials

Motor evoked potentials are responses that are recorded from various muscle groups following magnetic stimulation of the motor cortex. If the latencies of cortically evoked motor responses are compared to those from magnetic stimulation of the spinal nerve roots, the central conduction time can be determined. This represents the amount of time for the motor signal to pass from the cerebral cortex through the brainstem and spinal cord. It has been proposed that this central conduction time may be utilized as a test of spinal cord lateral column function,[54] supplementing SEP testing which evaluates posterior column sensory functions. Nogues et al[99] found that the use of motor evoked potentials increased the sensitivity of SEPs alone in the evaluation of patients with syringomyelia. This test has been applied to many other causes of myelopathy, including cervical spondylotic myelopathy, where Tavy et al[131] found abnormalities in 27 of 28 patients. These investigators also reported that motor evoked potentials were normal in 22 of 25 patients with asymptomatic cervical spinal cord compression.[132]

Spinal Tap and Blood Analysis

The indications for spinal tap and specific blood tests in the diagnosis of spinal cord disease are similar to those for brain diseases. These tests may be of particular importance in the diagnosis of infectious diseases and inflammatory diseases (such as MS). There are numerous tests of CSF and blood, each with its unique diagnostic criteria, sensitivity, and specificity. Most of these tests, outside of the specific microbiologic tests, are nonspecific and have ranges of normal established in a manner similar to other clinical laboratory tests; i.e., as

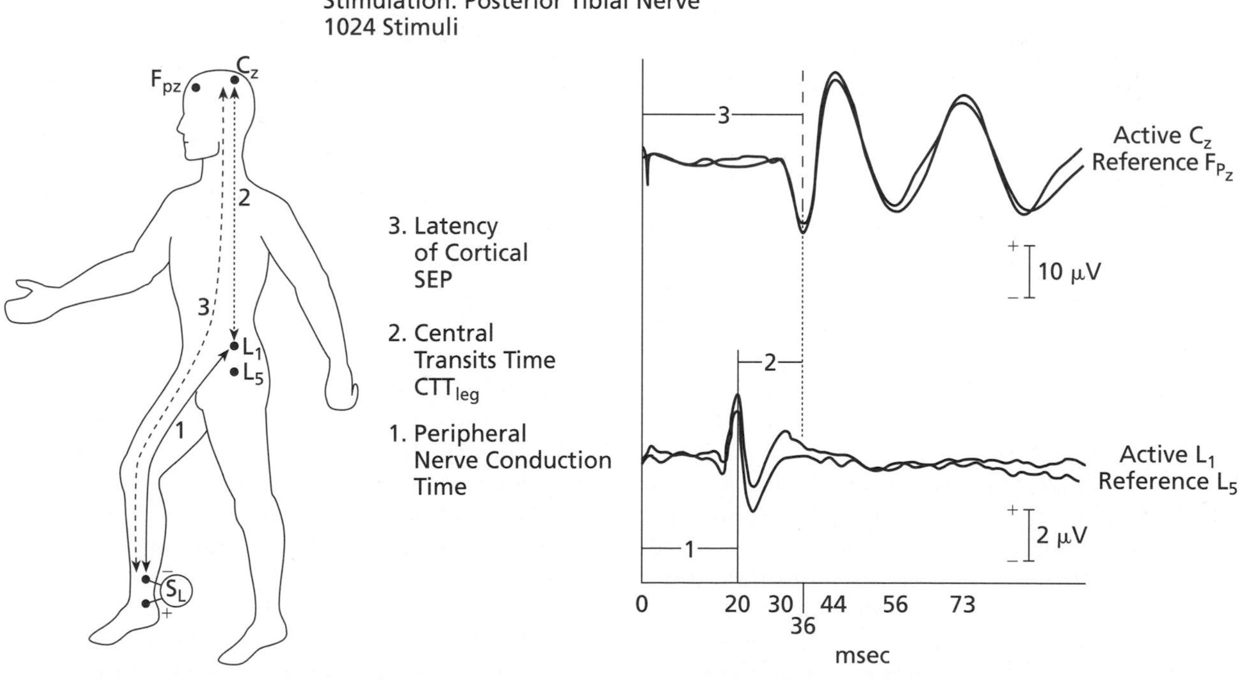

Figure 33–2. Pathways and form of somatosensory evoked potentials (SEP) from the lower extremities. (From Haldeman S: Spine 9:42, 1984.)

a mean and 2 standard deviations. Therefore, if the spectrum of normal is uniformly distributed, 5% of normal individuals will test as abnormal with 2.5% being high and 2.5% being low. Therefore, an abnormality that is further from the normal cutoff would more likely represent a real problem than would a value that is marginally outside of normal. An additional concern with diagnostic testing of blood and spinal fluid is that some tests can be abnormal in several disorders, some of which may not be related to the presenting complaint. For example, CSF protein can be slightly elevated by incidental disk disease or by clinically insignificant spinal stenosis. Diabetes mellitus may elevate CSF protein levels even when there is no involvement of the nervous system. It is not possible to address these tests in a short chapter and they are only included for completeness.

Radiculopathy

Many patients with radiculopathy have easily documented motor, sensory, and reflex abnormalities and a clinical pattern that does not require confirmation by specialized testing. However, other patients have a confusing clinical pattern of diffuse numbness or weakness and additional testing may be necessary to differentiate the presence or absence of radiculopathy. Electrodiagnostic studies and cystometry are perceived as important differentiators when assessing categories of impairment under the AMA Guides.[5] This is another area where research has been hampered by the lack of a gold standard with which to compare the diagnostic value of tests (see previous). This accounts for some of the variability between studies attempting to estimate the diagnostic value of these tests.

Imaging Studies

The imaging of lesions that impinge on the nerve root is covered primarily in Chapter 14. An important point to be reiterated is that the presence of compressive lesions seen on imaging studies does not necessarily document the presence or absence of radiculopathy, because such lesions can exist in the asymptomatic population.[32,72,142] Estimates of specificity of MRI for radiculopathy suggest that the value is about 50%, largely due to a high number of false-positives.[113] In addition, radiculopathy may be present without any anatomic abnormality. These observations have increased the importance of electrodiagnostic testing in an attempt to correlate pathophysiology with the anatomic pathology detected by imaging.[126,127] Increasingly, a combination of imaging and electrodiagnostic studies is being advocated to determine the nature and clinical importance of a suspected lesion.[32,65,113]

Needle Electromyography

Needle electromyography (EMG) remains a mainstay in the electrodiagnostic evaluation of radiculopathy.[10] Signs of acute denervation including positive sharp waves and fibrillation potentials are sought in muscles innervated by the nerve root in question. It is important to realize that needle EMG only becomes abnormal after 2 to 4 weeks of denervation as it can take that long for signs of irritability to develop in muscle fibers. Gradually these findings of acute denervation give way to reinnervation over a 9- to 12-month period, after which time giant polyphasic potentials may be evident. Because giant polyphasic potentials only develop when there has been substantial denervation and reinnervation, the needle study is less sensitive for remote radiculopathies than it is for acute ones or for chronic radiculopathies that have some ongoing damage. In addition, it must be remembered that the needle study can only examine the integrity of motor nerve fibers and that it is completely insensitive to damage of sensory nerve root fibers.

Several studies have investigated the sensitivity of needle EMG in the detection of radiculopathy. Typically, these reports have compared the needle study to a diagnosis by other means such as clinical tests with or without imaging correlation. Taken as a whole, these studies indicate a sensitivity that ranges between 95% and 100% on the high side[2,3,130] and 30% on the low side.[81] The majority of studies report sensitivities between 50% and 71%,[25,74,90,94,104,124,140,143,146] which appears to be the best estimate of the overall sensitivity of needle EMG for radiculopathy. Not surprisingly, the frequency of positive findings on EMG increases as one investigates persons with clinically definite radiculopathy as compared to possible radiculopathy.[94] Localization of the level of radiculopathy by needle EMG, however, is only as accurate as the understanding of the innervation of the muscles that are tested. Most muscles in the limbs are innervated by at least two nerve root levels and it is therefore necessary to sample multiple muscles in order to determine the specific nerve root or roots involved. For example, Young et al[147] found that needle EMG correctly predicted the level of radiculopathy in 84% of patients with clinical findings of radiculopathy. The needle study was negative in all patients without root pathology but failed to identify the correct level in 16% of cases. EMG is much less likely to produce a false-positive finding than imaging, such as with MRI.[94] Estimates of the specificity of needle EMG in radiculopathy are around 85%[113] and the needle study provides information that is complementary to that provided by imaging; i.e., information on the physiology of the nerve roots.

Reflex Studies

Conventional nerve conduction studies are poor predictors of radiculopathy as they do not test conduction across the level of the injury (see following). Electrophysiologic reflex studies, on the other hand, have the advantage of sending an impulse back to the spinal cord that, in the process of returning to the limb, crosses the level of the potentially injured nerve root on two occasions. An added benefit of reflex studies is that they become abnormal immediately after the onset of the radiculopathy. H-reflexes (Fig. 33–3) and bulbocavernosus reflexes (Fig. 33–4) measure both motor and sensory components of the nerve roots in question, whereas F-responses (Fig. 33–5) measure only the motor root function. The most commonly utilized reflex study is the H-reflex from the soleus-gastrocnemius muscle, which has been shown to have a very high correlation with S1 radiculopathy.[50] Both Braddom and Joynson[34] and Aiello et al[3] noted a 90% to 100% true positive rate and a 0% false negative rate in S1 radiculopathy.

The bulbocavernosus reflex response has been correlated with lower sacral nerve lesions at the S2–S3 level, and it is useful in documenting cauda equina syndrome and pudendal nerve injuries, although its sensitivity is not known.[65,67]

F-responses measure only the function of motor pathways as the electrical signal travels back to the spinal cord along the motor nerve fiber and then traverses the same axon back to the muscle from which the response is recorded. One limitation of this test is that the stimulated nerves and the muscles from which recordings are made all have innervation from multiple roots. Even if

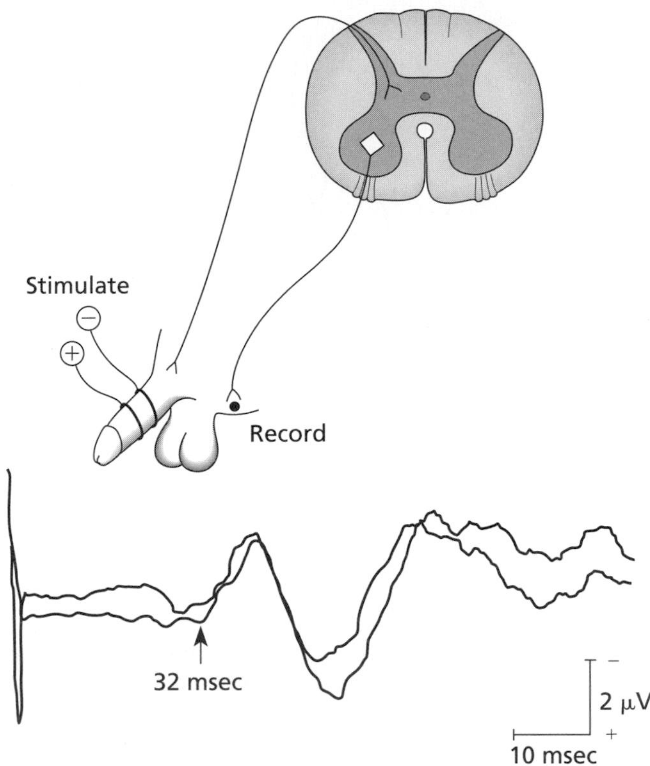

Figure 33–4. Pathways and form of a bulbocavernosus reflex. (From Haldeman S: Spine 9:42, 1984.)

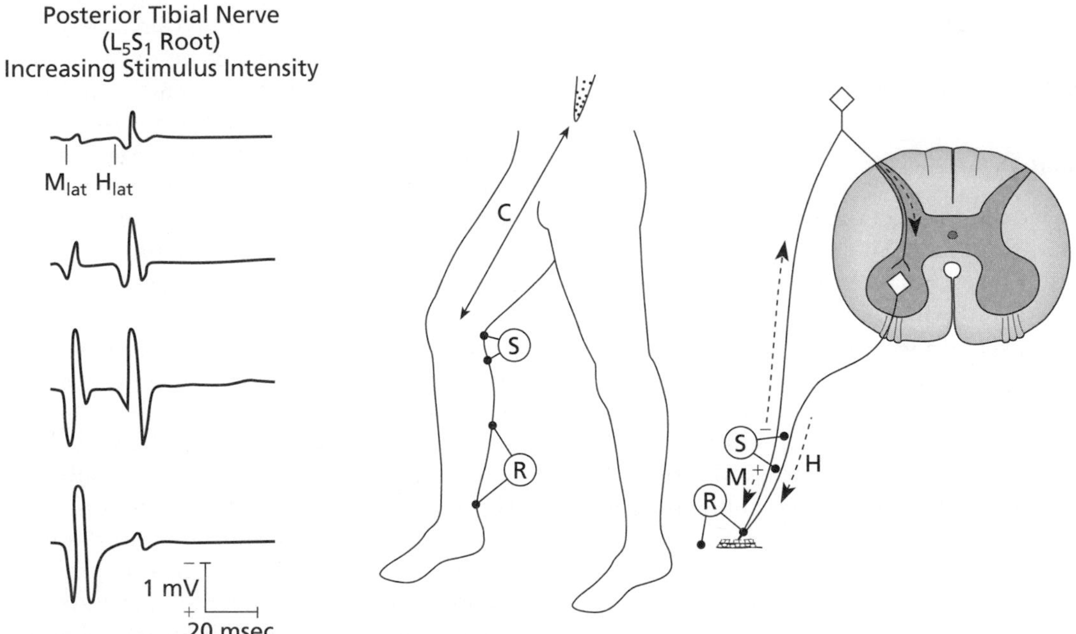

Figure 33–3. Pathways and form of an H-reflex providing the electrical equivalent of a stretch reflex. S, stimulus electrode; R, recording electrode; M, direct motor response; H, H-reflex. (From Haldeman S: Spine 9:42, 1984.)

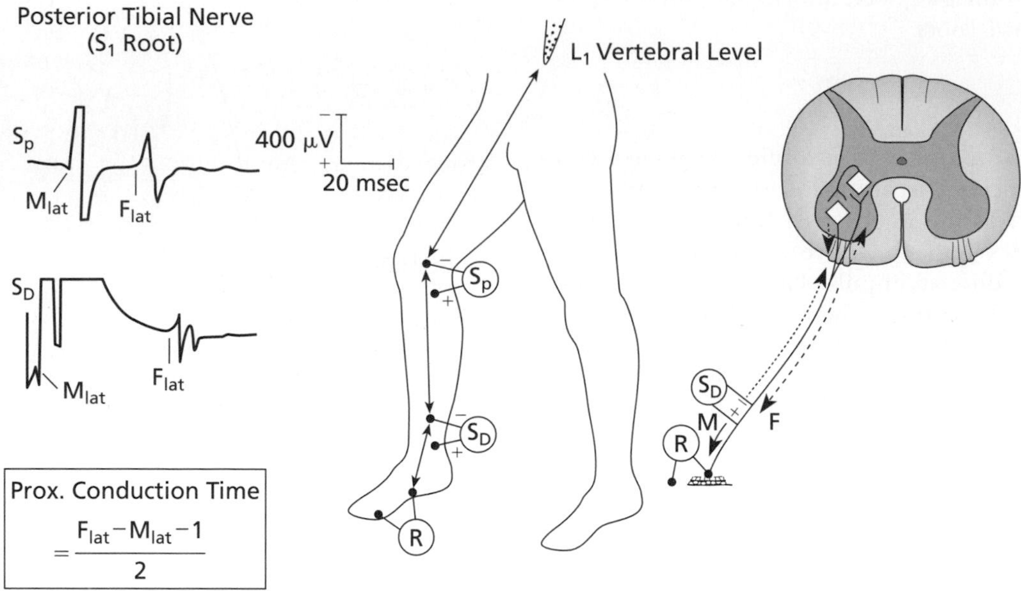

Figure 33–5. Pathways and form of an F-response, measuring conduction in the proximal portions of a motor nerve and the ventral root of the spinal cord. SD, distal stimulus; SP, proximal stimulus; R, recording electrode. (From Haldeman S: Spine 9:42, 1984.)

one nerve root contributing to the generation of the response is severely damaged, the overall response may be completely normal. This limits the sensitivity of the F-wave response for radiculopathy although it has been reported to be abnormally prolonged in 14% to 47% of patients with this condition. Additionally, it may be the only electrophysiologic abnormality in the first week following nerve root injury.[52,53,61] Nonetheless, the lack of sensitivity and the lack of specificity for radiculopathy in general, and specifically for particular root levels, limits the use of F-responses in the investigation of the patient with suspected radiculopathy.[143]

Nerve Conduction Tests

Conventional nerve conduction studies are normal in people with radiculopathy. There has been some enthusiasm for nerve root stimulation procedures in the diagnosis of radiculopathy with some reports of almost 80% sensitivity. However, these studies have not achieved widespread acceptance as of this time.[25,135] Magnetic stimulation of motor pathways has been reported to be abnormal in radiculopathic patients with weakness.[31] However, additional data on the clinical utility of the procedure would be needed prior to recommending it for the investigation of radiculopathy.

Evoked Potentials

The major limitation of needle EMG in the investigation of radiculopathy is its complete insensitivity to damage of sensory nerve roots. Attempts have been made to complement EMG with SEPs. SEPs elicited by stimulation of large, mixed nerves are mediated through multiple nerve roots. These do not appear to be of any value in documenting monoradiculopathy. The past 15 years has seen some enthusiasm for evoked potentials elicited by stimulation of a single dermatome in the evaluation of radiculopathy. There are several technical considerations including the fact that these potentials are small and can only reliably be identified at the level of the cerebral cortex. Therefore, a small lesion at the level of the nerve root would not be expected to substantially slow the arrival of the overall signal to the cerebral cortex. A recent review of the electrodiagnosis of radiculopathy concluded that nerve stimulation is diagnostically unhelpful in the investigation of radiculopathy, whereas cutaneous and dermatomal evoked potentials are insensitive.[143] Evoked potentials are rarely abnormal when the needle electromyogram is negative, and the reverse is frequently true.[146] The conclusion of the Committee on Technology Assessment of the American Academy of Neurology is that the use of dermatomal SEPs is investigational.[12]

In contrast to the relative lack of utility of evoked potentials for investigating monoradiculopathy, there is promise for SEPs in the assessment of lumbar spinal stenosis. Stolov and Slimp[129] found abnormal SEPs in 17 of 18 patients with surgically demonstrated spinal stenosis. Snowden et al,[123] using independent evaluation of dermatomal SEPs in spinal stenosis, demonstrated a sensitivity of 78% for multiple root disease and 93% for multiple plus single root disease. There were 3 false positive cases out of the 58 patients studied. Therefore, SEPs may provide supportive physiologic data in cases with imaging findings of questionable significance.

Other Tests

Several other procedures have been employed in an effort to document radiculopathy. Thermography has been shown to be abnormal in some patients with radiculopathy. However, the Committee on Technology Assessment of the American Academy of Neurology, after reviewing the literature, concluded that infrared thermography was of "limited value in the characterization of neurologic dysfunction or deficit."[13] Furthermore, they state that it has "not been shown to provide sufficient reliable characterizing information" for it to be useful in the evaluation of clinical problems including back, neck, or radicular disorders. A review of spinal ultrasound for back pain and radicular disorders found that there was no credible literature supporting the utility of this procedure.[14]

Peripheral Neuropathy

The variety of conditions that can affect peripheral nerves is truly staggering. They range from metabolic conditions such as diabetes mellitus and hypothyroidism to toxic exposures such as prolonged alcohol use and exposure to heavy metals or other industrial chemicals. Furthermore, deficiency syndromes (such as B vitamins like vitamin B_{12}), various medications, and infections (such as HIV and Lyme disease) must be considered. In the industrialized nations, there has been a rapid growth in recognition of repetitive traumatic injuries to nerves as they pass through narrow canals. Carpal tunnel syndrome, tardive ulnar palsy, and tarsal tunnel syndrome are among the most common of these entrapment neuropathies. Furthermore, peripheral nerves can be subjected to direct injury by a blow, penetrating wound, or direct compression. Radial and peroneal neuropathies are among the most common of this type of peripheral nerve injury. In addition, hereditary peripheral polyneuropathies as well as postinfectious polyneuropathies like the Guillain-Barré syndrome and brachial and sciatic plexopathies must be considered. All of these disorders can result in functional impairment and disability.

In many cases of neuropathy, the clinical examination and history are sufficient to make a diagnosis. However, testing is often necessary in individuals having primarily subjective feelings of numbness and/or pain in the extremities, especially if such symptoms are progressive and not well-delineated on the clinical examination. The following are the more commonly utilized neurodiagnostic tests for peripheral neuropathies.

Nerve Conduction

Nerve conduction studies are of two basic types: sensory and motor. These studies rely on the fact that damage to a peripheral nerve will either slow its conduction (by damaging the fast conducting, myelinated nerve fibers) or will cause the amplitude of the signal to decrease (by destroying axons or blocking their conduction). Entrapment neuropathies, for example, typically injure myelin and preferentially damage the largest diameter nerve fibers. Therefore, slowing of conduction is the chief finding in these conditions. The portion of the nerve that is injured will be the segment over which conduction will be most abnormal. In fact, the remainder of the nerve may conduct normally. Therefore, the shorter the segment of nerve around the damaged area that can be evaluated by the test, the more likely it is that an abnormality will be detected. One corollary of this is that some conditions are more amenable to evaluation by nerve conduction studies than others. These studies are particularly sensitive to problems in areas where nerves are accessible to stimulation all along its course so that short, diseased segments can be detected. Median neuropathies at the wrist,[8] ulnar neuropathies at the elbow,[9] and peroneal neuropathies at the knee fall into this category.

Motor nerve conduction studies have the advantage of recording a large voltage response (from muscle) when a motor nerve is stimulated at various sites along its course (Fig. 33–6). For example, it is possible to record a response from the thenar muscle in the hand upon stimulation of the median nerve at the wrist, above the elbow, in the axilla, and at the Erb point (the base of the neck). The localization of a lesion is made considerably easier by this kind of segmental approach.

Sensory nerve conduction studies are somewhat more difficult from a technical perspective as recordings must be made directly from the nerve and are therefore much smaller in amplitude. One limitation of these studies is that they only evaluate the fastest-conducting sensory nerve fibers. The loss of slowly conducting sensory nerve fibers (mediating pain and temperature) will not alter sensory conduction studies.

Generalized peripheral sensory neuropathies (polyneuropathies) are commonly studied by means of recording sensory and motor nerve conduction velocities and amplitudes in both the upper and lower extremities. These tests are quite sensitive for many types of polyneuropathy, particularly those that produce demyelination.[102]

Changes in sensory nerve conduction occur across many focal areas of entrapment. For some diagnoses, nerve conduction studies represent the most sensitive objective measure of abnormality, even though they are by no means perfect measures. In carpal tunnel syndrome, the best estimates of sensitivity of nerve conduction tests range from 49% to 84%.[39,46,78,84,115,121] These

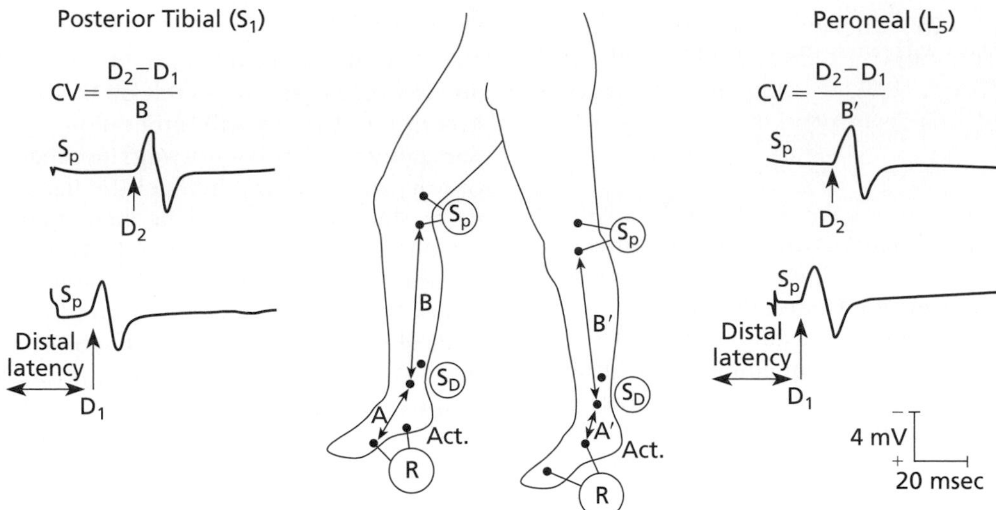

Figure 33–6. Pathways and form of standard motor nerve conduction studies in the posterior tibial and peroneal nerves. (From Haldeman S: Spine 9:42, 1984.)

figures would be higher in cases of severe carpal tunnel syndrome, and certain nerve conduction procedures appear to have greater sensitivity than others.[8] Specificity for carpal tunnel syndrome is high, ranging from 95% to 100%.[39,46,78,84,115] In the case of focal ulnar neuropathy at the elbow, the sensitivity of electrodiagnostic studies has been estimated to be between 37% and 84%.[27,70,86,88,105,107,109] Again, the specificity of the tests has been reported to be high (generally between 94% and 100%).[27,88,107,109] Not surprisingly, the study with the highest sensitivity (84%) reported a significantly lower specificity (50%), probably due to selection of criteria for abnormality.[70]

Reflex Studies

There are fewer studies of H- and F-responses in the investigation of a peripheral neuropathy. F-responses, however, are often the easiest and best tests for proximal neuropathies such as Guillain-Barré syndrome.[103] Olney and Aminoff found abnormalities in 31 of 44 nerves tested in 15 patients with Guillain-Barré syndrome. Disorders of the proximal portions of the peripheral nervous system, such as plexopathy and radiculopathy, may also show abnormalities of these responses. However, the sensitivity and specificity of F-responses for plexopathy has not been investigated and for radiculopathy is probably quit low.[143] On the other hand, H-reflexes are sensitive for certain radiculopathies, particularly S1 radiculopathy, but is only relevant to the study of a limited number of nerve roots.[143] F-responses have been reported to be useful in the investigation of generalized polyneuropathy, such as diabetes. One recent study describes the sensitivity of F-responses in detecting diabetic neuropathy as being between 61% and 85%.[133] F-responses may be the most sensitive electrodiagnostic finding in these patients.[6] However, the ability to generalize to other causes of polyneuropathy is limited because of the differences in pathophysiology between the various causes of neuropathy.

Needle Electromyography

The detection of denervation may be important in documenting traumatic damage to peripheral motor nerve fibers (see the previous discussion of EMG under the heading "radiculopathy"). Localization of an injury by means of the particular denervated muscles can be most helpful. In addition, the distribution of unaffected muscles is important in localizing the lesion. Motor neuron diseases, such as amyotrophic lateral sclerosis, enter into the differential of patients with progressive weakness. Needle EMG can be critical to diagnosis by demonstrating the diffuse nature of the denervation and fasciculations. It is also of value to know whether a nerve injury is complete or partial by looking for recruitment of units and recording muscle responses upon stimulation of the nerve proximal to an area of injury.

Other Tests

Several other tests have been proposed to evaluate and follow patients with a neuropathy. One of the more popular and documented among these tests is the current perception threshold test (CPT). This test evaluates the threshold for perception of several frequencies of electrical current and is somewhat limited by the subjective nature of the results. The American Association of Electrodiagnostic Medicine concluded that additional research is necessary to set normal values and to demonstrate sensitivity and specificity. They go on to state that the literature is "insufficient to make conclusions about the usefulness of this form of sensory testing at the present time."[15]

Bowel, Bladder, and Sexual Disorders

Often the most significant and distressing symptoms in certain cerebral disorders, partial myelopathies, and cauda equina syndrome are the associated disturbances in bowel, bladder, and sexual function. Because complaints of bowel or bladder urgency, sexual impotency, and anorgasmia are difficult to confirm in the clinical examination, testing is often important in order to make the diagnosis.[11,66]

Cystometry and Urodynamics

The utilization of cystometrogram and urodynamic studies to investigate bladder function has become increasingly sophisticated. Figure 33–7 demonstrates the testing that may be of value in isolating neurologic lesions affecting bowel, bladder, or sexual functioning. The cystometrogram has the capacity to differentiate peripheral from central nervous system disorders affecting the bladder. Peripheral neuropathies and injuries to the cauda equina are more likely to cause an areflexic cystometrogram, often with symptoms of urinary retention and overflow incontinence. Lesions affecting the central nervous system, and particularly the spinal cord, are more likely to cause hyperreflexia with symptoms of urinary urgency and frequency. Urodynamic studies can assist in determining the presence of dyssynergia of the urethral sphincter, which can result in urinary retention. Although 24-hour monitoring of bladder and urethral pressure has been reported, this remains an experimental procedure.[26]

Electrodiagnostic Studies

Somatosensory evoked potentials of the pudendal nerve (pSEP) evaluate the sensory pathways that traverse the S2–S4 nerve roots, the cauda equina, and the spinal cord. This nerve follows pathways similar to the pelvic nerves to the bladder and bowel. Abnormalities anywhere along the pudendal somatosensory neuraxis can result in an inability to record a cortical response or a delay in the response. These tests have been noted to be abnormal in patients with bowel, bladder, or sexual dysfunction due to diabetes, MS, or spinal cord injuries.[66–68]

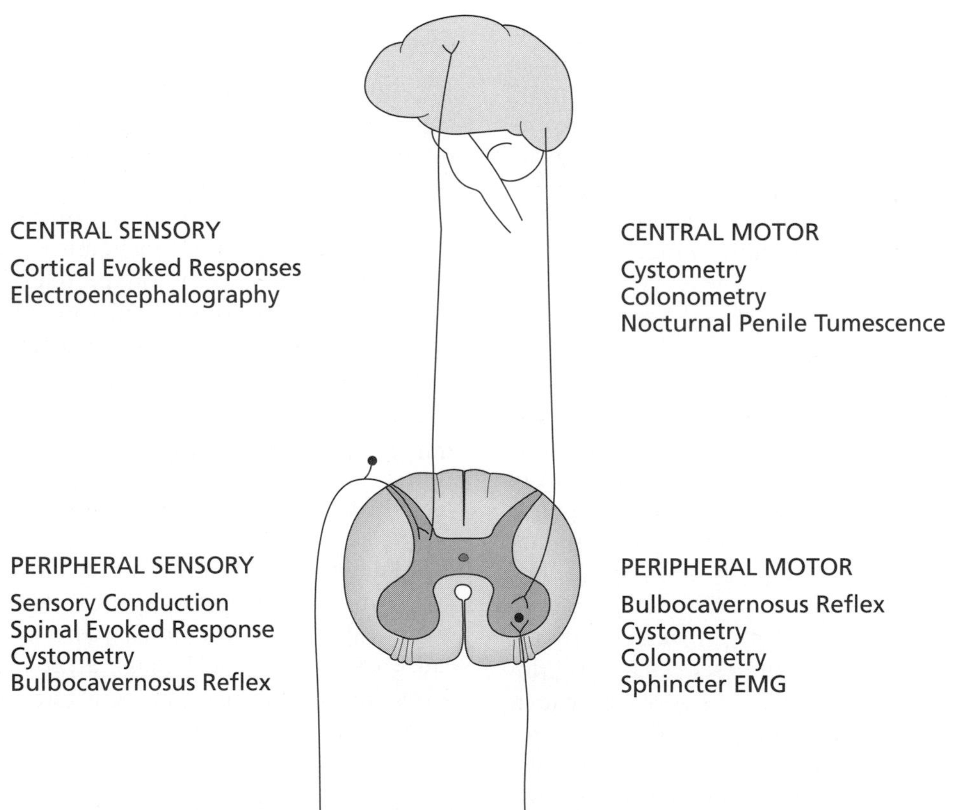

Figure 33–7. Tests used to evaluate neurologic lesions affecting bowel, bladder, or sexual dysfunction. (From Haldeman S, Bradley WE, Bhatia NN: Bull Clin Neurosci formerly Bull LA Neurol Soc 47:76, 1983, with permission.)

The test, however, does not differentiate between peripheral and central neurogenic pathways in most patients, because a spinal response is difficult to obtain. In a study of patients with MS, pSEPs were reported to be abnormal in all patients with bladder symptoms and in 8 out of 10 patients who did not have any bladder symptoms.[114] This procedure has been reported to be about 60% sensitive in detecting neurogenic impotence.[47]

The bulbocavernosus reflex response (BCR) records a reflex loop through the sacral spinal cord and the cauda equina. It is found to be abnormal in disorders affecting these structures including diabetes mellitus and tethered cord syndrome. This reflex has been estimated to be 70% sensitive in detecting patients with neurogenic causes of impotence.[47] The BCR may be complementary to pudendal evoked potential testing as some patients have abnormalities on only one of these two tests. Evaluation of the BCR aids in the differentiation between central and peripheral lesions particularly when combined with somatosensory pudendal evoked potentials, which traverse both the peripheral and central sensory pathways.

Anal EMG and Colonometry

The testing of neurologic dysfunction of the bowel is in its infancy. Needle EMG of the anal sphincter allows for the detection of denervation potentials when the pudendal nerve or sacral nerve roots are injured. Colonometry has been utilized in the same manner as cystometry for the bladder. In this situation, bowel pressure is recorded upon filling of the bowel. Hyperreflexia has been noted in spinal cord injuries and MS, whereas areflexic colonometry has been noted in diabetes mellitus.[63] These tests, however, have not been widely utilized and their sensitivity is not known.

Penile Tumescence and Rigidity

It is difficult, on clinical grounds, to differentiate organic from nonorganic causes of impotence. The differentiation commonly requires the measurement of penile erectile function by means of nocturnal penile tumescence testing over a period of one to three nights. Standard methods, using strain gages, are 85% to 90% sensitive in measuring erectile capacity, but there is a 15% to 20% false positive rate.[96,144] More recently the Rigi scan, which measures both tumescence and rigidity of the penis in the home setting, has replaced classic nocturnal penile tumescence testing in most routine settings. This test has the advantage of ease of use and also of being performed in the patient's normal home environment. One study using this method reported that of 11 patients with psychogenic impotence diagnosed by conventional methods, 3 (27.3%) showed abnormal nocturnal rigidity (false positives), whereas 8 of 94 (8.5%) with organic impotence showed normal nocturnal rigidity (false negatives).[82]

Muscle Disorders

Several common disorders associated with muscle pain, such as fibromyalgia and polymyalgia rheumatica, do not actually damage muscle fibers. On the other hand, there are some relatively uncommon disorders that can result in progressive damage to muscle fibers. These can be divided into the muscular dystrophies, metabolic myopathies (often with deficits in certain muscle enzymes), endocrinopathies (such as steroid-induced or due to hypothyroidism), toxic (occurring with several drugs or toxins), infectious (such as with trichinosis), or inflammatory (polymyositis, dermatomyositis, inclusion body myositis, or sarcoidosis). These disorders, with the possible exception of steroid myopathy, result in the breakdown of muscle tissue and a decrease in muscle strength. Inflammatory or infectious myopathies may also result in generalized pain or tenderness within the muscles. Myasthenia gravis (MG) and similar disorders have their primary effect on the neuromuscular junction with a resulting pattern of weakness that is mostly seen as fatigability.

Blood Analysis

The inflammatory and infectious myopathies are most commonly diagnosed by blood evaluation. The measurement of sedimentation rate, creatine phosphokinase, and aldolase may suggest breakdown of muscle tissue although these tests are quite nonspecific as to precise etiology. More specific biochemical tests of blood and urine may be necessary for the diagnosis of metabolic and rheumatologic muscle diseases. Immunologic tests may be necessary to detect parasitic and other infections affecting muscles.

Needle Electromyography

Needle EMG in generalized muscle diseases may be diagnostic. The finding of small, polyphasic motor units is indicative of myopathy, but the finding is not particularly sensitive, detecting about 46% of patients with myopathy.[97] It is also nonspecific in determining the cause of the muscle damage although the finding of myotonic discharges may help narrow the diagnostic focus.

Repetitive Stimulation

MG is a unique neuromuscular junction disease causing a high level of impairment, especially in its advanced stages. One of the most important diagnostic tools for MG is the response to repetitive stimulation of the muscle.[85] This has been reported to be abnormal in around 78% of patients with MG although the sensitivity of the test is directly proportional to the severity of the condition and its distribution in the body (generalized versus ocular, for example).[125] This test is usually combined with the tension test and immunologic studies to form the basis for the diagnosis.[75] Single fiber electromyography for the measurement of jitter has been reported to be more sensitive than repetitive stimulation for the diagnosis of neuromuscular junction disorders.[117,128] Electromyographic jitter is an assessment of neuromuscular transmission by recording the variation in latency between the potentials generated in two muscle fibers within the same motor unit. Stalberg et al[128] has gone so far as to state that if jitter is normal, one can rule out myasthenia.

Antibodies

MG is commonly associated with antibodies to the acetylcholine receptor (anti-AChR). The overall diagnostic sensitivity of anti-AChR antibodies has been reported to be 88%, the frequency of positive findings being related to the clinical subtype of the MG (ocular MG of early onset, 71%; ocular MG of late onset, 88%; severe generalized MG of early onset, 89%; severe generalized MG of late onset, 98%).[125] Additionally, the finding of anti-AChR antibodies is highly specific for MG (>99.9%).

Biopsy

The primary hereditary myopathies often require biopsy of a clinically affected muscle for diagnosis. The biopsy findings include the analysis of the staining characteristics as well as the morphology of the muscles. Muscle biopsy may also be important in the diagnosis of certain neurogenic problems such as amyotrophic lateral sclerosis.

DOCUMENTATION OF LOSS OF FUNCTION

The documentation of the loss of neurologic function is best determined by the clinical examination and can occasionally be extrapolated from the results of testing used in making the diagnosis. The diagnosis is of paramount importance in determining prognosis (i.e., is the condition reversible, stable, or progressive?). In some cases, even when the diagnosis is well established, it may not be clear whether a specific neurologic function has been affected or impairment has been caused by the disease. Neurodiagnostic testing may contribute to the analysis of these specific functions.

The ability to use neurodiagnostic testing to document impairment would require a quantitative component to the test as well as an ability to correlate the test findings to the degree of disability and impairment. Attempts at quantification of clinical neurodiagnostic testing have often led to very vague and descriptive 4- or 6-point scales of abnormality. These scales commonly describe normal, mild or minimal, slight or moderate, severe, and profound abnormalities or complete loss of the ability to record a test or perform a particular function. Similarly, there are disease-specific scales for such disorders as Parkinson disease, stroke,[45,49] and MS.[118,139] There are varying degrees of interobserver reliability for these scales, which typically rely on a combination of objective and subjective measures.

Because clinical scales often do not adequately capture the degree of impairment even for these single disorders, it is attractive to consider that neurodiagnostic tests might translate into a degree of impairment for the neurologic system being tested. This is particularly true as most of these tests are quantitative and objective in nature. However, although it may be possible to make some broad and general statements about severity, it is difficult to transfer the concept of neurodiagnostic testing directly into an impairment rating. For example, although myotatic reflexes may have a high interobserver correlation,[91] and notwithstanding the undoubted importance of this observation for a diagnosis, it has a poor correlation with the degree of impairment. Most of the neurodiagnostic tests described in the preceding section have poor correlation with the degree of loss of function. Nonetheless, the AMA Guides and other rating systems often require that sensory and motor loss and other abnormal neurologic function be quantified in rough terms. To a large extent this is dependent on the clinical evaluation and subjective considerations of the examinee and physician. This dependence on subjective elements has the potential to under- or overestimate the degree of impairment. In addition, there are no clinical measures that can reliably detect individuals who are malingering.[59] Neurodiagnostic testing may assist by documenting injury and, in selected cases, by contributing in general terms to determining the extent of loss of function. However, such correlations must be made with caution and in full recognition of the limitations of the testing procedures.

Cognitive Deficits

Cognitive and intellectual deficits following an injury or illness can vary over a wide range from normal to comatose. In addition, there is strong overlap between psychiatric illness and organic cognitive deficits with the two often coexisting. Although broad estimates of cognitive ability are relatively easy to make, it may be difficult in a basic clinical examination in a physician's office to define minor or specific degrees of loss of cognitive function. This is particularly important when deciding what problems a person might encounter in a work or home setting, and what limitations they may face. The neurologist is often dependent on cognitive testing by a neuropsychologist to determine which specific higher functions are affected and to what degree.[18] These concepts are discussed in Chapters 34 and 38.

Attempts to correlate objective neurodiagnostic testing with cognitive deficits have met with mixed results. The so-called event related potentials are based on the premise that it is possible to measure disturbances in the neuronal processes accompanying cognition.[64,71,93] These correlations, although statistically significant, have not proven to be sufficiently strong for diagnostic purposes.

The use of single photon emission CT (SPECT) and positron emission tomography scanning as a diagnostic tool for Alzheimer disease has shown a statistical relationship between dementia and metabolic changes in the brain as measured by these procedures.[38,44,106] The sensitivity noted by Claus et al[44] was 42% in mild, 56% in moderate, and 79% in severe Alzheimer disease; Hanyu et al report a sensitivity of 82% and specificity of 89%.[69] Some authors suggest that the use of SPECT be limited to cases of mild Alzheimer disease where there is considerable diagnostic doubt on clinical grounds.

Motor Deficits

The documentation and quantitation of weakness is primarily dependent on the clinical examination and on functional capacity assessments (outlined in Chapter 55). Neurodiagnostic testing is of limited assistance in this regard.

A crude estimation of the degree of denervation can be made by evaluating the interference pattern on the needle EMG examination. However, this is not easily transferred to the amount of weakness or impairment. Motor nerve conduction abnormalities are typically described as being mild, moderate, or severe, but these values do not accurately assess the degree of weakness. Testing is of value in the relatively uncommon case of complete neurogenic loss of motor function. The absence of motor response to motor nerve stimulation and the absence of active motor unit potentials during attempts to contract muscles would confirm this type of severe involvement.

The use of transcortical magnetic stimulation of the motor strip with recording from peripheral musculature may document interference with this pathway. However, there is no accepted method for correlating the evoked response to the degree of motor impairment.

Sensory Deficits

Sensory deficits can cause significant disability to people. The AMA Guides specifically rate pain with sensory loss as representing a greater impairment than pain without sensory loss. However, sensory loss is difficult to assess during a functional capacity evaluation and it is largely assessed by subjective means. There are quantitative tests of sensory function that are commonly available in neurophysiology laboratories.[145] It must be kept in mind that these tests rely on subjective reporting on the part of the claimant and therefore must be considered in light of psychophysical parameters. Objective signs of damage to sensory pathways, provided by nerve conduction studies and SEPs, can provide useful correlations for these more quantitative procedures. This is important given the high frequency of sensory complaints among people presenting for evaluation of impairment and disability and the importance of the sensory system in the determination of overall level of disability. Objective assessment can play a key role in the overall evaluation, especially because the subjective evaluation is only as good as the reporting ability of the claimant.

Sensory nerve conduction in peripheral nerve injuries and peripheral neuropathies can be of value in documenting whether such injuries exist and whether a clinical finding of sensory loss can be verified. As described, these sensory conduction studies can be very useful in conditions such as carpal tunnel syndrome and polyneuropathy, where the tests are quite sensitive. These tests are also of immense help in localizing the deficit and thereby determining the diagnosis. However, they have several limitations, including an inability to assess the function of slowly conducting (small pain and temperature) nerve fibers and a low sensitivity for many of the conditions to which they can be applied. Overall, they are crude methods of determining the severity or the degree of loss of sensory function. The sensory responses can be described as normal, slightly abnormal, moderately abnormal, severely abnormal, or unobtainable. The relationship of these terms to impairment, and especially an impairment rating, is not known.

SEPs have the ability to document a lesion within both the peripheral and the central somatosensory system. They are notably abnormal in peripheral neuropathies and in spinal cord lesions. However, the nature of evoked potentials does not permit extrapolation of a degree of impairment from the test abnormality. For example, they may be abnormal in a person with no sensory symptoms or impairments. In addition, as in the case of sensory nerve conduction studies, damage to the slowly conducting pathways for pain and temperature sensation will not affect the SEP.[19,98]

Coordination Deficits

Coordination deficits may reflect damage to many levels of the nervous system. Motor or sensory deficits can impact coordination whether the damage results from injury to the spinal cord, brain, or peripheral nerve. Disturbances of equilibrium and balance, including vertigo, may reflect diseases of the vestibular apparatus, brainstem, or cerebellum.

The primary test for impairment due to incoordination is the clinical examination. Clinical tests of gait and coordination are described in other chapters. Assessment of auditory, visual, and proprioceptive function may be aided by tests described earlier in this chapter. Inner ear function may be assessed by ENG, which can also help determine whether there is peripheral or central disturbance in vestibular function. The quantitation and evaluation of disorders of posture and stance may be aided by dynamic posturography (see previous). A tremorgram on EMG may help document and differentiate certain types of tremor but is rarely necessary.

VERIFICATION OF SUBJECTIVE COMPLAINTS

There is a strong emphasis within most disability rating systems on objective findings rather than subjective complaints. Social Security Administration guidelines specifically state that subjective complaints of impairment must manifest themselves in signs or laboratory tests confirming anatomic, physiologic, or psychological abnormalities.[138] However, many subjective complaints such as pain, muscle spasm, dysesthesia, minor cognitive problems, some psychological disturbances, vague weakness, or fatigue can present with a completely normal clinical examination. This has resulted in a proliferation of testing procedures in an attempt to confirm subjective complaints. The evaluation of minor cognitive and psychological symptoms is addressed in Chapter 38.

Pain

Despite being the most common cause of perceived impairment among examinees, pain cannot be measured or quantified by means of any neurologic testing. Therefore, it remains a subjective complaint on the part of the individual and can be influenced by psychological and emotional responses and is tied to concepts such as suffering.[40]

Because the AMA Guides rate pain associated with sensory deficits higher than pain with normal sensation, the importance of sensory nerve conduction and somatosensory evoked response testing has been raised beyond their purely diagnostic value. However, it is important to remember that these tests do not relate in any direct way to the sensation of pain. Testing to assess pain is discussed in Chapter 39.

There have been several reports relating thermographic abnormalities in various pain syndromes. However, with the possible exception of reflex sympathetic dystrophy and causalgia, most independent agencies, on review of the literature, have concluded that the test does not add sufficient diagnostic information to be useful.[13]

Paresthesias

Altered perception of sensory stimuli is a common complaint in the person being evaluated for impairment and disability. Often, this is not a reflection of damage to sensory systems. As described previously, a person with loss of sensation is treated differently in most disability rating systems. Therefore, a concerted effort should be made in the person with paresthesias to define any sensory loss and to determine whether this relates to any known physiologic pattern of sensory disturbance due to nervous system damage. It is only by doing so that appropriate neurodiagnostic tests can be selected, especially if one is to avoid the common problem of overutilization of testing. Indiscriminate use of tests may identify minor abnormalities that have no correlation with the clinical symptom patterns, potentially leading to inaccurate diagnosis.

Weakness

Similar to the evaluation of paresthesias, subjective statements of weakness in the absence of documentable pathology on imaging and other studies may lead the clinician on a long search for an explanation. The EMG may be helpful in distinguishing neurogenic weakness, particularly of the peripheral nervous system from weakness due to decreased effort or pain. However, the EMG has a significant subjective interpretive component that is dependent on the skill and experience of the electromyographer. The test results are rarely transferred to hard copy and the experience of clinicians in differentiating potentials can vary greatly. The AMA Guides[5] recommend that technicians be certified by the American Board of Electrodiagnostic Medicine and that testing should be done in a laboratory meeting the guidelines of the American Association of Electrodiagnostic Medicine. Minor EMG changes such as slight increase in insertional potentials and mild polyphasia may be falsely reported as abnormal and motor end plate potentials may be interpreted as fibrillations. The EMG should be considered an extension of the neurologic examination and should not stand alone as a documentation of organic weakness.

Muscle Spasm

Many individuals seeking disability describe muscle spasms and muscle tenderness. The AMA Guides recognize the presence of muscle guarding and nonuniform range of motion as being abnormal but consider this only in the category of minor impairment. Attempts to objectively evaluate muscle spasm have been disappointing. For example, needle EMG has shown areas of muscle tenderness to be electrically silent.[80] Certain experimental techniques such as the direct recording of muscle spindle activity[76] and the recording of cortical evoked responses on magnetic stimulation have shown some promise in looking at this issue.[149] However, these procedures have not been widely validated or accepted.

Surface EMG has been proposed as a method of recording muscle guarding and unequal muscle contraction leading to nonuniform balance. There are conflicting data relative to the presence or absence of static or resting abnormalities in surface EMGs of patients with low back pain. In contrast, several investigators have described differences in activation patterns of lumbar muscles during movement in patients with low back pain.[119,134] For example, Ahern et al[1] noted changes in surface EMG during dynamic flexion and extension in 89% of patients with low back pain. Despite this interesting finding, 13% of asymptomatic individuals in their study showed similar abnormality, indicating a lack of specificity that limits the use of the procedure in the disability setting. Sihvonen et al[120] similarly found abnormalities in chronic back pain but also in a significant number of control subjects. It is possible that further research will demonstrate the clinical utility of this procedure, but for now its utility in disability evaluation is limited.

FALSE-POSITIVE TESTING

The interpretation of normality on a test is dependent on a proper determination of the range of normal values. Even for individual diagnostic tests, there is some variation in the accepted range of normal. Technical performance factors such as stimulus strength, age-related factors, and temperature[83,92,122] play a role in this variability. Inaccurate calibration or measurement can introduce significant error. Ideally, each clinical laboratory should establish its own normative values including ranges based on age, sex, and skin temperature. This, however, is not always practical and most electrodiagnosticians use normative values published from an academic laboratory. Unfortunately, slight differences in technique and equipment can leave doubt as to the cutoff points for abnormality. Therefore, values at the borderline between normal and abnormal must be treated with caution in order to avoid overinterpretation of physiologic variations as pathologic. Comparisons between a symptomatic and an asymptomatic limb may provide important confirmatory data, although there can be fairly high variations within normal subjects.

Reflex and evoked responses are not identical on the two sides of the body and these responses vary greatly from individual to individual based on patient height. Therefore, normative data should be modified, particularly in individuals significantly outside the normal range of height or limb length. The interpretation of amplitude data on evoked potential and reflex studies is problematic due to a large degree of normal variability. For example, anything less than a 50% reduction in side-to-side amplitude of H-reflexes should be considered within normal limits. Additionally, the amplitude of SEPs can vary widely even when reproduced in the same individual on stimulation of the same nerve, rendering this value of limited (if any) clinical significance.

Many technical factors can influence evoked potentials, even in the most stable of these tests, such as BAEPs.[112] There are significant variations in interpeak latencies in the same patient when comparing one ear with the other or reproducing the test in the same ear after a 2-year interval.[136] Minor side-to-side differences should not be considered significant unless there are very tight controls on technique. Oken and Chiappa[101] reiterate the fact that when a normal value is taken as the mean plus 2 standard deviations, then 5% of normal patients may be considered to have abnormal test results. Furthermore, because evoked potential tests customarily measure the latency of several peaks and also several interpeak latencies, if 2 standard deviations are accepted as the range of normal for each value, there is a high chance of mischaracterization of a normal person as having disease. It is therefore recommended that mean plus 3 standard deviations be considered the basis of measuring normal values in evoked potentials.

Electroencephalographic findings may also be overinterpreted. There are several normal variant patterns that have characteristics suggestive of disease. Phantom spike, wave, and mu patterns, as well as movement artifact, may be misinterpreted as abnormalities by the unsophisticated electroencephalographer. Asynchronous, intermittent, focal, temporal slow delta transient potentials can be found in 30% to 60% of normal controls, yet have the appearance of being abnormalities. There are various procedures used by electroencephalographers to aid in discrimination of these normal variants and artifacts, but the overall value of the interpretation is highly dependent on the skill and experience of the examiner.

As described previously and in the chapter on imaging, the correlation of imaging studies with neurologic disability and impairment can be problematic. Numerous small white matter lesions can be seen in the brain of normal individuals and often do not correlate with clinical symptoms or impairment. Similarly, extensive degenerative changes and disc herniations in the cervical, thoracic, and lumbar spine are often present in the absence of symptomatology or disability.

CONCLUSION

Neurologic disorders are common causes of disability and impairment. In addition, there are many people who complain of symptoms that could potentially be caused by neurologic disorders. Neurodiagnostic testing is important, and at times critical to the evaluation of patients with neurologic diseases producing disability and impairment. Testing can be used to aid in the diagnosis of conditions, to provide objective verification of symptoms, or to quantitate disability. Of these three goals, neurodiagnostic tests have their greatest validity as part of the diagnostic process in concert with the history and clinical examination. At all times the choice of testing and the interpretation of test results is dependent on the suspected diagnosis. Neurodiagnostic tests can be of some utility in validating certain subjective complaints, although the tests are of limited (if any) use in excluding a physiologic basis for subjective complaints.

Neurodiagnostic testing is only of slight value in the documentation of loss of neurologic function and the quantification of such losses. The correlation between test results and the degree of impairment in most diseases and injuries has not been adequately studied. However, when closely correlated with an individual's clinical examination, the degree of abnormality of a test may help the clinician reach a conclusion as to the presence of a lesion and the amount of loss of function.

Neurodiagnostic testing cannot confirm the presence of pain, dysesthesias, or subjective muscle weakness in the absence of a well-defined disease entity. It is important to resist the temptation to overuse these tests on poorly focused clinical questions in order to rule out disease. In addition, extreme care must be taken in the evaluation of minor abnormalities in consideration of potential false-positive results, a problem that is magnified when multiple test procedures are employed. A full understanding of the factors causing variability in test results and the normal variations between laboratories and between patients is essential before giving credence to a test in the claimant without other corresponding clinical findings.

References

1. Ahern DK, Follick MJ, Council JR, et al: Comparison of lumbar paravertebral EMG patterns in chronic low back pain patients and non-patient controls. Pain 34:153–160, 1988.
2. Aiello I, Serra G, Migliore A, et al: Diagnostic use of H-reflex from vastus medialis muscle. Electromyogr Clin Neurophysiol 23:159–166, 1983.
3. Aiello I, Serra G, Tugnoli V, et al: Electrophysiological findings in patients with lumbar disc prolapse. Electromyogr Clin Neurophysiol 24:313–320, 1984.
4. Allum JH, Shepard NT: An overview of the clinical use of dynamic posturography in the differential diagnosis of balance disorders. Journal of Vestibular Research 9:223–252, 1999.
5. Cocchiarella L, Andersson GBJ (eds): Guides to the Evaluation of Permanent Impairment, 5th ed. Chicago, American Medical Association, 2001.
6. Andersen H, Stalberg E, Falck B: F-wave latency, the most sensitive nerve conduction parameter in patients with diabetes mellitus. Muscle Nerve 20:1296–1302, 1997.
7. Anonymous: Somatosensory evoked potentials: Clinical uses. Muscle Nerve 22(S8):S111–S118, 1999.
8. Anonymous: Literature review of the usefulness of nerve conduction studies and needle electromyography for the evaluation of patients with carpal tunnel syndrome. Muscle Nerve 22(S8):S145–S167, 1999.
9. Anonymous: The electrodiagnostic evaluation of patients with ulnar neuropathy: Literature review of the usefulness of nerve conduction studies and needle electromyography. Muscle Nerve 22(S8):S175–S205, 1999.
10. Anonymous: The electrodiagnostic evaluation of patients with suspected cervical radiculopathy: Literature review on the usefulness of needle electromyography. Muscle Nerve 22(S8): S213–S221, 1999.
11. Anonymous: Assessment: Neurological evaluation of male sexual dysfunction. Report of the Therapeutics and Technology Assessment Subcommittee of the American Academy of Neurology. Neurology 45: 2287–2292, 1995.
12. Anonymous: Assessment: Dermatomal somatosensory evoked potentials. Report of the Therapeutics and Technology Assessment Subcommittee of the American Academy of Neurology. Neurology 49:1127–1130, 1997.
13. Anonymous: Assessment: Thermography in neurologic practice. Report of the Therapeutics and Technology Assessment Subcommittee American Academy of Neurology. Neurology 40:523–525, 1990.
14. Anonymous: Review of the literature on spinal ultrasound for the evaluation of back pain and radicular disorders. Report of the Therapeutics and Technology Assessment Subcommittee of the American Academy of Neurology. Neurology 51:343–344, 1998.
15. Anonymous: Technology review: The Neurometer Current Perception Threshold (CPT). Muscle Nerve 22(S8):S247–S259, 1999.
16. Anonymous: Assessment: Electronystagmography. Report of the Therapeutics and Technology Assessment Subcommittee of the American Academy of Neurology: Neurology 46:1763–1766, 1996.
17. Anonymous: Assessment: Posturography. Report of the Therapeutics and Technology Assessment Subcommittee of the American Academy of Neurology. Neurology 43:1261–1264, 1993.
18. Anonymous: Assessment: Neuropsychological testing of adults. Considerations for neurologists. Report of the Therapeutics and Technology Assessment Subcommittee of the American Academy of Neurology. Neurology 47:592–599, 1996.
19. Anziska B, Cracco RQ: Short latency somatosensory evoked potentials. Studies in patients with focal neurological disease. Electroencephalogr Clin Neurophysiol 49:227–239, 1980.
20. Arcia E, Gualtieri CT: Association between patient report of symptoms after mild head injury and neurobehavioural performance. Brain Injury 7:481–489, 1993.
21. Autti T, Raininko R, Vanhanen SL, et al: MRI of the normal brain from early childhood to middle age. I. Appearances on T2- and proton density-weighted images and occurrence of incidental high-signal foci. Neuroradiology 36:644–648, 1994.

22. Awad IA, Spetzler RF, Hodak JA, et al: Incidental subcortical lesions identified on magnetic resonance imaging in the elderly: I—Correlations with age and cerebrovascular risk factors. Stroke 17:1084–1089, 1986.
23. Baldereschi M, Amato MP, Nencini P, et al: Cross-national interrater agreement on the clinical diagnostic criteria for dementia. Neurology 44:239–242, 1994.
24. Baumhefner RW, Tourtellotte WW, Syndulko K, et al: Quantitative MS plaque assessment with MRI. Its correlation with clinical parameters, EPs, and intra blood-brain barrier. Arch Neurol 47:19–26, 1990.
25. Berger AR, Busis NA, Logigian EL, et al: Cervical root stimulation in the diagnosis of radiculopathy. Neurology 37:329–332, 1987.
26. Bhatia NN, Bradley WE, Haldeman S, et al: Continuous monitoring of bladder and urethral pressure, a new technique. Urology 18:207–210, 1981.
27. Bielawski M, Hallett M: Position of the elbow in determination of abnormal motor conduction of the ulnar nerve across the elbow. Muscle Nerve 12:803–809, 1989.
28. Biering-Sorenson F, Hansen FR, Schroll M, et al: The relation of spinal x-ray to low back pain and physical activity among 60-year-old men and women. Spine 10:445–451, 1985.
29. Bigos SJ, Hansson T, Castillo RN, et al: The value of pre-employment roentgenographs for predicting acute back injury claims and chronic back pain disability. Clin Orthop 283:124–129, 1992.
30. Binnie CD, Stefan H: Modern electroencephalography: Its role in epilepsy management. Clin Neurophysiol 110:1671–1697, 1999.
31. Bischoff C, Meyer BU, Machetanz J, et al: The value of magnetic stimulation in the diagnosis of radiculopathies. Muscle Nerve 16:154–161, 1993.
32. Boden SD, Davis DO, Dina TS, et al: Abnormal magnetic resonance scans of the lumbar spine in asymptomatic subjects. J Bone Joint Surg [Am] 72:403–408, 1990.
33. Boden SD, McCowin PR, Davis DO, et al: Abnormal magnetic-resonance scans of the cervical spine in asymptomatic subjects. A prospective investigation. J Bone Joint Surg [Am] 72: 1178–1184, 1990.
34. Braddom RI, Joynson EW: Standardization of H reflex and diagnostic use in S1 radiculopathy. Arch Phys Med Rehabil 55:161–166, 1974.
35. Bradley WG Jr, Waluch V, Brant-Zawadzki M, et al: Patchy, periventricular white matter lesions in the elderly: A common observation during NMR imaging. Noninvasive Med Imag 1:35–41, 1984.
36. Brant-Zawadzki M, Fein G, et al: MR imaging of the aging brain: Patchy white matter lesions and dementia. AJNR Am J Neuroradiol 6:675–682, 1985.
37. Brenner RP: Utility of EEG in delirium: Past views and current practice. Int Psychogeriatr 3:211–292, 1991.
38. Burns A, Philpot MP, Costa AC, et al: The investigation of Alzheimer's disease with single photon emission tomography. J Neurol Neurosurg Psychiatry 52:248–253, 1989.
39. Caroll G: Comparison of median and radial nerve sensory latencies in the electrophysiological diagnosis of carpal tunnel syndrome. Electroencephalogr Clin Neurophysiol 68:101–106, 1987.
40. Chapman CR, Gavrin J: Suffering: The contributions of persistent pain. Lancet 353:2233–2237, 1999.
41. Chiappa KH: Evoked Potentials in Clinical Medicine. New York, Raven Press, 1989.
42. Chiappa KH, Jayakar P: Evoked potentials in clinical medicine. In Joynt RJ (ed): Clinical Neurology I. Philadelphia, J.B. Lippincott, 1992.
43. Chiappa KH: Short latency somatosensory evoked potentials: Interpretation. In Chiappa KH (ed): Evoked Potentials in Clinical Medicine. New York, Raven Press, 1990, pp 400–407.
44. Claus JJ, van Harskamp F, Breteler MMB, et al: The diagnostic value of SPECT with Tc-99m HMPAO in Alzheimer's disease: A population-based study. Neurology 44:454–461, 1994.
45. Cote R, Battista RN, Wolfson C, et al: The Canadian Neurological Scale: Validation and reliability assessment. Neurology 39:638–643, 1989.
46. DeLean J: Transcarpal median sensory conduction: Detection of latent abnormalities in mild carpal tunnel syndrome. Can J Neurol Sci 15:388–393, 1988.
47. Dettmers C, van Ahlen H, Faust H, et al: Evaluation of erectile dysfunction with the sympathetic skin response in comparison to bulbocavernosus reflex and somatosensory evoked potentials of the pudendal nerve. Electromyogr Clin Neurophysiol 34:437–444, 1994.
48. Di Fabio RP: Meta-analysis of the sensitivity and specificity of platform posturography. Arch Otolaryngol. Head Neck Surg 122:150–156, 1996.
49. D'Olhaberriague L, Litvan I, Mitsias P, Mansbach HH: A reappraisal of reliability and validity studies in stroke. Stroke 27:2331–2336, 1996.
50. Dvorak J: Neurophysiologic tests in diagnosis of nerve root compression caused by disc herniation. Spine 21 (Suppl. 24):39S–44S, 1996.
51. Eggermont JJ, Don M, Brackmann DE: Electrocochleography and auditory brain stem electric responses in patients with pontine angle tumors. Ann Otol Rhinol Laryngol 89(Suppl.):75, 1980.
52. Eisen A, Schomer D, Melmed C: The application of F-wave measurements in the differentiation of proximal and distal upper limb entrapments. Neurology 27:662–688, 1977.
53. Eisen A, Schomer D, Melmed C: An electrophysiological method for examining lumbosacral root compression. Can J Neurol Sci 4:117–123, 1977.
54. Eisen A, Shtybel W: Experience with transcranial magnetic stimulation. Muscle Nerve 13:995–1011, 1990.
55. El Negamy E, Sedgwick EM: Delayed cervical somatosensory potentials in cervical spondylosis. J Neurol Neurosurg Psychiatry 42:238–241, 1979.
56. Farrer LA, Cupples LA, Blackburn S, et al: Interrater agreement for diagnosis of Alzheimer's disease: The MIRAGE study. Neurology 44:652–656, 1994.
57. Fenton GW: The postconcussional syndrome reappraised. Clin Electroencephalogr 27:174–182, 1996.
58. Filippi M, Horsefield MA, Morrissey SP, et al: Quantitative brain MRI lesion load predicts the course of clinically isolated syndromes suggestive of multiple sclerosis. Neurology 44:635–641, 1994.
59. Fishbain DA, Cutler R, Rosomoff HL, Rosomoff RS: Chronic pain disability exaggeration/malingering and submaximal effort research. Clin J Pain 15:244–274, 1999.
60. Fisher JM, Williams AD: Neuropsychologic investigation of mild head injury: Ensuring diagnostic accuracy in the assessment process. Semin Neurol 14:53–59, 1994.
61. Fisher MA, Shivde AJ, Teixera C, et al: Clinical and electrophysiological appraisal of the significance of radicular injury in back pain. J Neurol Neurosurg Psychiatry 41:303–306, 1978.
62. Galasko D, Abramson I, Corey-Bloom J, Thal LJ: Repeated exposure to the Mini-Mental State Examination and the Information-Memory-Concentration Test results in a practice effect in Alzheimer's disease. Neurology 43:1559–1563, 1993.
63. Glick ME, Meshkinpour H, Haldeman S, et al: Colonic dysfunction in patients with thoracic spinal cord injury. Gastroenterology 86:287–294, 1984.
64. Goodin DS, Squires KC, Starr A: Long latency event-related components of the auditory evoked potential in dementia. Brain 101:635–648, 1978.

65. Haldeman S: The neurodiagnostic evaluation of spinal stenosis. In Andersson GBJ, McNeil TW (eds): Lumbar Spinal Stenosis. St. Louis, Mosby-Year Book, 1992.
66. Haldeman S, Bradley WE, Bhatia NN, et al: Neurologic evaluation of bladder, bowel and sexual disturbances in diabetic men. In Goto Y, Horiuchi A, Kogure K (eds): Diabetic Neuropathy. Proceedings of the International Symposium on Diabetic Neuropathy and Its Treatment, Tokyo, September 1981. Amsterdam, Excerpta Medica, 1982.
67. Haldeman S, Bradley WE, Bhatia NN, et al: Pudendal evoked responses in neurologic disease. Neurology 32:A67, 1982.
68. Haldeman S, Bradley WE, Bhatia NN, et al: Pudendal evoked responses. Arch Neurol 39:280–283, 1982.
69. Hanyu H, Abe S, Arai H, et al: Diagnostic accuracy of single photon emission computed tomography in Alzheimer's disease. Gerontology 39:260–266, 1993.
70. Hawley J, Capobianco J: Localizing ulnar nerve lesions by motor nerve conduction study. Electromyogr Clin Neurophysiol 27:385–392, 1987.
71. Hillyard SA, Kutas M: Electrophysiology of cognitive processing. Annu Rev Psychol 34:33–61, 1983.
72. Hitselberger WE, Witten RM: Abnormal myelograms in asymptomatic patients. J Neurosurg 28:204–208, 1968.
73. Hoffman DA, Lubar JF, Thatcher RW, et al: Limitations of the American Academy of Neurology and American Clinical Neurophysiology Society paper on QEEG. J Neuropsychiatry Clin Neurosci 11:401–407, 1999.
74. Hong CZ, Less S, Lum P: Cervical radiculopathy. Clinical, radiographic and EMG findings. Orthop Rev 15:433–439, 1986.
75. Howard JF Jr, Sanders DB, Massey JM: The electrodiagnosis of myasthenia gravis and the Lambert-Eaton myasthenic syndrome. Neurol Clin 12:305–330, 1994.
76. Hubbard DR: Sympathetic Spindle Spasm. Presented at the annual meeting of the California Medical Association, Anaheim, Calif, 1992.
77. Ikeda H, Tremain E, Sanders MD: Neurophysiological investigation in optic nerve disease: Combined assessment of the visual evoked response and electroretinogram. Br J Ophthalmol 62:227–239, 1978.
78. Jackson D, Clifford JC: Electrodiagnosis of mild carpal tunnel syndrome. Arch Phys Med Rehabil 70:199–204, 1989.
79. Jensen MC, Brant-Zawadzki MN, Obuchowski N, et al: Magnetic resonance imaging of the lumbar spine in people without back pain. N Engl J Med 331:69–73, 1994.
80. Johnson EW: The myth of skeletal muscle spasm. Am J Phys Med Rehabil 68:1, 1989.
81. Kahn MRH, McInnes A, Hughes SPF: Electrophysiological studies in cervical spondylosis. J Spinal Dis 2:163–169, 1989.
82. Kaneko S, Bradley WE: Evaluation of erectile dysfunction with continuous monitoring of penile rigidity. J Urol 136:1026–1029, 1986.
83. Kaplan PE: Sensory and motor residual latency measurements in healthy patients and patients with neuropathy: Part I. J Neurol Neurosurg Psychiatry 39:338, 1976.
84. Kimura J: The carpal tunnel syndrome: Localization of conduction abnormalities within the distal segment of the median nerve. Brain 102:619–635, 1979.
85. Kimura J: Electrodiagnosis in diseases of nerve and muscle: Principles and practice. Philadelphia, FA Davis, 1983.
86. Kimura J, Ayyar DR, Lippmann SM: Early electrodiagnosis of the ulnar entrapment neuropathy at the elbow. Tohoku J Exp Med 142:165–172, 1984.
87. Koopmans RA, Li DKB, Grochowski E, et al: Benign versus chronic progressive multiple sclerosis: Magnetic resonance imaging features. Ann Neurol 25:74–81, 1989.
88. Kothari MJ, Preston DC: Comparison of the flexed and extended elbow positions in localizing ulnar neuropathy at the elbow. Muscle Nerve 18:336–340, 1995.
89. Krumholz A: Nonepileptic seizures: Diagnosis and management. Neurology 53(Suppl. 2):S76–S83, 1999.
90. Leblhuber F, Reisecker R, Boehm-Jurkovic H, et al: Diagnostic value of different electrophysiological tests in cervical disk prolapse. Neurology 38:1879–1881, 1988.
91. Litvan I, Mangone CA, Werden W, et al: Reliability of the NINDS Myotatic Reflex Scale. Neurology 47:969–972, 1996.
92. Mayer RF: Nerve conduction studies in man. Neurology 13:1021, 1963.
93. Michalewski HJ, Rosenberg C, Starr A: Event-related potentials in dementia. In Cracco RQ, Bodis-Wollner I (eds): Evoked Potentials. New York, Alan R. Liss, 1986.
94. Nardin RA, Patel MR, Gudas TF, et al: Electromyography and magnetic resonance imaging in the evaluation of radiculopathy. Muscle Nerve 22:151–155, 1999.
95. Nath S, Sherman J, Bass S: VEP delays in macular disease (ARVO Suppl.). Invest Ophthalmol Vis Sci 22:60, 1982.
96. Nelson RP: Male sexual dysfunction: Evaluation and treatment. South Med J 80:69–74, 1987.
97. Nirkko AC, Rosler KM, Hess CW: Sensitivity and specificity of needle electromyography: A prospective study comparing automated interference pattern analysis with single motor unit potential analysis. Electroencephalogr Clin Neurophysiol 97:1–10, 1995.
98. Noel P, Desmedt JE: Somatosensory cerebral evoked potentials after vascular lesions of the brain-stem and diencephalon. Brain 98:113–128, 1975.
99. Nogues MA, Pardal AM, Merello M, Miguel MA: SEPs and CNS magnetic stimulation in syringomyelia. Muscle Nerve 15: 993–1001, 1992.
100. Nuwer M: Assessment of digital EEG, quantitative EEG, and EEG brain mapping: Report of the American Academy of Neurology and the American Clinical Neurophysiology Society. Neurology 49:277–292, 1997.
101. Oken BS, Chiappa KH: Somatosensory evoked potentials in neurologic diagnosis. In Cracco RQ, Bodis-Wollner I (eds): Evoked Potentials. New York, Alan R Liss, 1986.
102. Olney RK: Clinical trials for polyneuropathy: The role of nerve conduction studies, quantitative sensory testing, and autonomic function testing. J Clin Neurophysiol 15:129–137, 1998.
103. Olney RK, Aminoff MJ: Electrodiagnostic features of the Guillain-Barre syndrome: The relative sensitivity of different techniques. Neurology 40:471–475, 1990.
104. Partanen J, Partanen K, Oikarinen H, et al: Preoperative electroneuromyography and myelography in cervical root compression. Electromyogr Clin Neurophysiol 31:21–26, 1991.
105. Payan J: Electrophysiological localization of ulnar nerve lesions. J Neurol Neurosurg Psychiatry 32:208–220, 1969.
106. Perani D, De Piero V, Vallar G, et al: Technetium-99m HMPAO SPECT study of regional cerebral perfusion in early Alzheimer's disease. J Nucl Med 19:1507–1514, 1988.
107. Pickett JB, Coleman LL: Localizing ulnar nerve lesions to the elbow by motor conduction studies. Electromyogr Clin Neurophysiol 24:343–360, 1984.
108. Powell MC, Wilson M, Szypryt P, et al: Prevalence of lumbar disc degeneration observed by magnetic resonance in symptomless women. Lancet 13:1366–1367, 1986.
109. Raynor EM, Shefner JM, Preston DC, Logigian EL: Sensory and mixed nerve conduction studies in the evaluation of ulnar neuropathy at the elbow. Muscle Nerve 17:785–792, 1994.
110. Restuccia D, Di Lazzaro V, Valeriana M, et al: N24 spinal response to tibial nerve stimulation and magnetic resonance imaging in lesions of the lumbosacral spinal cord. Neurology 43:2269–2275, 1993.
111. Restuccia D, Di Lazzaro V, Valeriana M, et al: The role of upper limb somatosensory evoked potentials in the management of

cervical spondylotic myelopathy: Preliminary data. Electroencephalogr Clin Neurophysiol 92:502–509, 1994.

112. Robinson K, Rudge P: The stability of the auditory evoked potentials in normal man and patients with multiple sclerosis. J Neurol Sci 35:147–156, 1978.

113. Robinson LR: Electromyography, magnetic resonance imaging and radiculopathy: It's time to focus on specificity. Muscle Nerve 22:149–150, 1999.

114. Sau GF, Aiello I, Siracusano S, et al: Pudendal nerve somatosensory evoked potentials in probable multiple sclerosis. Ital J Neurol Sci 18:289–291, 1997.

115. Scelsa SN, Herskovitz S, Bieri P, Berger AR: Median mixed and sensory nerve conduction studies in carpal tunnel syndrome. Electroencephalogr Clin Neurophysiol 109:268–273, 1998.

116. Schmidt R, Fazekas F, Offenbacher H, et al: Neuropsychologic correlates of MRI white matter hyperintensities: A study of 150 normal volunteers. Neurology 43:2490–2494, 1993.

117. Schwartz MS, Stalberg E: Myasthenia gravis with features of the myasthenic syndrome: An investigation with electrophysiologic methods including single-fiber electromyography. Neurology 25:80, 1975.

118. Sharrack B, Hughes RA: Clinical scales for multiple sclerosis. J Neurol Sci 135:1–9, 1996.

119. Shirado O, Ito T, Kaneda K, Strax TE: Flexion-relaxation phenomenon in the back muscles. A comparative study between healthy subjects and patients with chronic low back pain. Am J Phys Med Rehabil 74:139–144, 1995.

120. Sihvonen T, Partanen J, Hanninen O, et al: Electric behavior of low back muscles during lumbar pelvic rhythm in low back pain patients and healthy controls. Arch Phys Med Rehabil 72:1080–1087, 1991.

121. Simovic D, Weinberg DH: The median nerve terminal latency index in carpal tunnel syndrome: A clinical case selection study. Muscle Nerve 22:573–577, 1999.

122. Simpson JA: Fact and fallacy in measurement of conduction velocity in motor nerves. J Neurol Neurosurg Psychiatry 27:381, 1964.

123. Snowden ML, Haselkorn JK, Kraft GH, et al: Dermatomal somatosensory evoked potentials in the diagnosis of lumbosacral spinal stenosis: Comparison with imaging studies. Muscle Nerve 15:1036–1044, 1992.

124. So YT, Olney RK, Aminoff MJ: A comparison of thermography and electromyography in the diagnosis of cervical radiculopathy. Muscle Nerve 13:1032–1036, 1990.

125. Somnier FE: Myasthenia gravis. Danish Medical Bulletin 43:1–10, 1996.

126. Spengler DM, Freeman CW: Patient selection for lumbar discectomy: An objective approach. Spine 4:129–134, 1979.

127. Spengler DM, Ouellette EA, Battie M, et al: Elective discectomy for herniation of a lumbar disc: Additional experience with an objective method. J Bone Joint Surg [Am] 72:230–237, 1990.

128. Stalberg E, Trantelj JV, Schwartz MS: Single-muscle-fiber recording of the jitter phenomenon in patients with myasthenia gravis and in members of their families. Ann NY Acad Sci 274:189, 1976.

129. Stolov WC, Slimp JC: Dermatomal somatosensory evoked potentials in lumbar spinal stenosis. In Proceedings, American Association of Electromyography and Electrodiagnosis/American Electroencephalography Society Joint Symposium, 1988, pp 17–22.

130. Tackmann W, Radu EW: Observations on the application of electrophysiological methods in the diagnosis of cervical root compressions. Eur Neurol 22:397–404, 1983.

131. Tavy DLJ, Wagner GL, Keunen RWM, et al: Transcranial magnetic stimulation in patients with cervical spondylotic myelopathy: Clinical and radiological correlations. Muscle Nerve 17:235–241, 1994.

132. Tavy DL, Franssen H, Keunen RW, et al: Motor and somatosensory evoked potentials in asymptomatic spondylotic cord compression. Muscle Nerve 22:628–634, 1999.

133. Toyokura: F-wave-duration in diabetic polyneuropathy. Muscle Nerve 21:246–249, 1998.

134. Triano JJ, Schultz AB: Correlation of objective measure of trunk motion and muscle function with low-back disability ratings. Spine 12:561–565, 1987.

135. Tsai CP, Huang CI, Wang V, et al: Evaluation of cervical radiculopathy by cervical root stimulation. Electromyogr Clin Neurophysiol 34:363–366, 1994.

136. Tusa RJ, Stewart WF, Shechter AL, et al: Longitudinal study of brainstem auditory evoked responses in 87 normal human subjects. Neurology 44:528–532, 1994.

137. Uimonen S, Laitakari K, Kiukaanniemi H, Sorri M: Does posturography differentiate malingerers from vertiginous patients? J Vestibular Res 5:117–124, 1995.

138. United States Department of Health, Education and Welfare: Disability Evaluation Under Social Security: A Handbook for Physicians. Washington DC: HEW Publication No. (SSA) 79–10089, 1979.

139. Verdier-Taillefer MH, Zuber M, Lyon-Caen O, et al: Observer disagreement in rating neurologic impairment in multiple sclerosis: Facts and consequences. Eur Neurol 31:117–119, 1991.

140. Waylonis GW: Electromyographic findings in chronic cervical radicular syndromes. Arch Phys Med Rehabil 49:407–412, 1968.

141. Weinreb JC, Wolbarsht LB, Cohen JM, et al: Prevalence of lumbosacral intervertebral disk abnormalities on MR images in pregnant and asymptomatic nonpregnant women. Radiology 170(Part 1):125–128, 1989.

142. Wiesel SW, Tsourmas N, Feffer HL, et al: A study of computer assisted tomography. I—The incidence of positive CAT scans in an asymptomatic group of patients. Spine 9:549–551, 1984.

143. Wilbourn AJ, Aminoff MJ: AAEM minimonograph 32: The electrodiagnostic examination in patients with radiculopathies. Muscle Nerve 21:1612–1631, 1998.

144. Wincze JP, Bansal S, Malhotra C, et al: A comparison of nocturnal penile tumescence and penile response to erotic stimulation during awake state in comprehensively diagnosed groups of males experiencing erectile difficulties. Arch Sex Behav 17:333–348, 1988.

145. Yarnitsky D: Quantitative sensory testing. Muscle Nerve 20:198–204, 1997.

146. Yinannikas C, Shahani BT, Young RR: Short-latency somatosensory evoked potentials from radial, median ulnar and peroneal nerve stimulation in the assessment of cervical spondylosis. Comparison with conventional electromyography. Arch Neurol 43:1264–1271, 1986.

147. Young A, Getty J, Jackson A, et al: Variations in the pattern of muscle innervation by the L5 and S1 nerve roots. Spine 8:616–624, 1983.

148. Yu YL, Jones SJ: Somatosensory evoked potentials in cervical spondylosis correlation of median, ulnar and posterior tibial nerve responses with clinical and radiological findings. Brain 108:273–300, 1985.

149. Zhu Y, Haldeman S, Starr A, et al: Paraspinal muscle evoked cerebral potentials in patients with unilateral low back pain. Spine 18:1096–1110, 1993.

CHAPTER

34

Central Nervous System Impairment

EDWIN H. KLIMEK, MD

WHAT ARE THE AMA GUIDES?

The American Medical Association's Committee on Rating of Mental and Physical Impairment first published the *Guides to the Evaluation of Permanent Impairment* in 1971 as a compendium of monographs.[37] The monographs dealing with different areas of impairment had been serialized from 1958 onward by *Journal of the American Medical Association.* The monographs were intended to correct confusion in the use of the terms "impairment" and "disability" as well as provide a series of practical guides to the evaluation of various types of permanent impairment. The preface to "Guides to the evaluation of permanent impairment: The central nervous system"[5] stated that permanent impairment was a permanent medical condition that can be measured with a reasonable degree of accuracy and uniformity on the basis of impaired function as evidenced by loss of structural integrity, pathology, or pain substantiated by clinical findings. Subsequent editions, including the fourth published in 1993[38] and the fifth published in 2001,[39] responded to political and administrative needs, internal shortcomings, and inconsistencies.

The process undertaken by the Committee on Rating of Mental and Physical Impairment was stated to include a careful study of the literature and the views of recognized authorities to establish recommended percentages related to provided criteria. A numerical value for rating impairment was preferred by the Committee because of difficulties in the application and variability of the terms in common use such as slight, marked, and moderate. The Guides were believed to be a uniform, detailed method requiring minimum computation. It was recommended that all final values of impairment be expressed in terms of the nearest 5%.

It is clear that the information and approach in the original monographs was achieved by consensus. There are no members of the original committee to elaborate on the consensus building required in the production of the original monographs. There is no recorded scientific basis for the ratings or approaches adopted and promulgated by the AMA in the Guides. In later revisions, the technical and legal staff of the AMA provided direction to the contributors and the editors. Over the decades the AMA has demonstrated an awareness of the importance of the Guides in litigation and mandated use by state and provincial bodies as an impairment schedule. The Guides have become a common starting point in estimating impairment and contributors were encouraged to work within established schedules and a conventional anatomic approach.

An impairment rating may be required by statute to serve as a surrogate for a loss of wage-earning capacity. By definition, impairment is "a loss, loss of use, or derangement of any body part, organ system, or organ function,"[39(p2)] or a condition that interferes with an individual's activities of daily living. The Guides clearly state, however, that impairment ratings are not intended for use as an indicator of work incapacity or loss of wage-earning capacity.[39(pp5,9)] The Guides direct that after WPI is estimated and an occupational activity is defined, one may assume an administrative responsibility and determine disability. In so doing, one must recognize that an impaired individual who is able to accomplish a specific task, with or without accommodation, is neither handicapped nor disabled with regard to that task. Thorough knowledge of the task requirements must be available, either by reference to an accepted database such as the *Dictionary of Occupation Titles* or in mutually agreed-upon detailed job requirements. Self-reported job requirements often correspond poorly with actual demands.

Disability determinations following CNS injury are challenging because manifestations may not only be transient and occult to the layperson, they can be contaminated by somatization. Somatization may result in stress-related symptoms and unnecessary exposure to dangerous, costly, and frustrating diagnostic procedures and treatments that may reinforce the perception of disability. Although the relative burden of different health conditions, in terms of disability, is fairly similar across the world, there are systematic and, in some cases, pronounced differences between cultures and informant groups.[35] The lives of individuals with disability around the world are usually far more limited by prevailing social, cultural, and economic constraints than by specific physical, sensory, psychological, or intellectual impairments.[15] Thus, disability determination depends on understanding the injury mechanism, neuropathology, and medical complications and requires the individual be evaluated in full light of his or her personal attributes. The respondent's tendency to provide personally desirable responses and distort responses to meet the examiner's expectations must also be carefully considered.

WHOLE PERSON IMPAIRMENT

The Guides follow the whole person concept in which evaluation of the whole person, not just the affected body part, is considered. Table 34–1 illustrates examples of WPI drawn from the Guides, fourth edition.[38] The Guides, fourth edition, establish a ceiling of 100% WPI, where "95% to 100% whole person impairment is … a state that is approaching death."[38(p8)] The fifth edition notes that a "90%–100% WPI indicates a very severe organ or body system impairment … approaching death."[39(p5)]

The Guides are for the evaluation of permanent impairment. Based upon the fourth edition, permanent means the impairment is unlikely to change substantially or by more than 3% in the next year with or without medical treatment and is not likely to remit despite medical treatment.[38(p315)] The Guides deals with CNS dysfunction for recognized categories, summarized in Table 34–2. Categories for evaluating CNS impairment were established in the first edition in terms of restrictions or limitations placed on a person's ability to perform the activities of daily living, not in terms of a neurologic diagnosis.[37] The Guides provides direction for evaluating a person with clinical findings in more than one impairment category and may permit the values to be combined. Within each recognized category, aid was provided in scaling cases of submaximal severity. It is an inherently difficult task to allocate functional subcategories into ordinal or linear representations of nondimensional phenomena. The Guides ranks subcategories of impairment severity at a point in time presumed to be permanent. However, the original monograph suggests that CNS impairment is not static and "all findings should be subject to review and the patient's condition revaluated at appropriate intervals for possible deterioration or improvement".[5]

The Guides avoids consideration of clinical or laboratory manifestations of disease deemed purely of diagnostic value. Unlike some organ systems, such as the respiratory system, in which laboratory testing of organ function is routine, the Guides precludes CNS impairment awards based solely on diagnosis or testing. It is not possible in this review of the Guides to fully address the validity of ancillary testing in CNS injury. However, the degree of confidence one places on test results must be understood to be defensible. For example, neuroimaging studies may corroborate the presence of an injury, but they are not the basis of a defensible impairment or disability determination in light of similar findings in asymptomatic individuals.[20] Likewise, psychological testing generates inferences about the people who achieve scores on a test.[26] Neuropsychological abnormalities indicating cognitive dysfunction should be consistent with the dose-response relationship seen in the spectrum of CNS injury and not arise from expectations in the individual. Abnormalities on neuropsychologic testing may support a diagnosis of CNS injury; but they do not make the diagnosis. Neuropsychologic testing that demonstrates dysfunction in a particular diagnosis is not pathognomonic. When patients demonstrate deficits disproportionate to impairment, further study of the confounding effects of age, pain, depression, and environmental demands are indicated.[33]

The diversity of manifestations in CNS disease is an argument for the use of disease-specific scales in forming an impairment rating because disease-specific scales include all manifestations of the disease of interest. For example, the Expanded Disability Status Scale (EDSS)[25] is composed of eight functional systems intended to be independent of each other and to reflect all manifestations of neurologic impairment in multiple sclerosis. The significance of each manifestation in terms of functional impairment is not clearly defined, although some hold that disability is irreversible beyond a score of 4.[7] A hierarchical progression such as in the EDSS suggests rankings are discrete, nonoverlapping, and reasonable in order, responsive to change and of proven reliability and validity.

Drawbacks to outcome scales are found in their applications and origins. During an application of a scale, an inadvertent aura of mathematical certitude and authority is implied. One tends to assume that differences in WPI among individuals are differences in disability severity. There is no scientific basis for these notions. Likewise, although the subcategories in the Guides are based on a measurable or estimable function, the range within each subcategory is not intuitively obvious,

TABLE 34-1

Comparative Whole Person Impairments

% WP	Condition	AMA Guides 4th edition	%WPI	AMA Guides 5th edition
100	Any state approaching death	Chapter 2.2, p 8	90–100	Chapter 1.2, p 5
85	Blindness	Chapter 8, Table 6, p 218	85	Chapter 12.4, pp 296–300
84	Paraplegia with loss of use of one arm	Chapter 3, Table 73, p 110	75% (Non-dominant arm), 82% (Dominant arm)	Chapter 13.5 and 13.6, pp 336–340
80	Loss of use of both arms	Chapter 4, Table 15, p 148	80+	Table 13–17, p 340
75	Paraplegia at lumbar level	Chapter 3, Table 72, p 110	94% when paraplegia is combined with the bladder, anorectal, and sexual impairments	Chapter 15.7, pp 395–398
70	Refractory seizures, total limitation of daily activity	Chapter 4, Table 5, p 143	70	Table 13–3, p 312
60	Amputation of one arm at shoulder	Chapter 3, Figure 2, p 18	60	Figure 16–2, p 441
40	Amputation of one leg at hip	Chapter 3.2 h, Table 63, p 83	40	Table 17–32, p 545
35	Deafness	Chapter 9, Table 3, p 228	35	Chapter 11.2, pp 240–251
33	Severe median nerve entrapment at elbow	Chapter 3, Table 16, p 57	40	Tables 16–15, p 492 and 16–3, p 439
29	C8 nerve root avulsion	Chapter 3, Table 13, p 51	29	Chapter 15.12, pp 423–426
24	Blindness in one eye	Chapter 8, Table 6, p 218	16	Chapter 12.4, pp 296–300
22	Loss of one thumb of either hand	Chapter 3, Tables 1–3, pp 18–20	22	Table 16–4, p 440
19	Paralysis of one side of face	Chapter 9, Table 4, p 230	19	Table 13–12, p 332
19	Peroneal nerve avulsion	Chapter 3, Table 68, p 89	18	Chapter 17.2l, pp 550–552
6	Loss of hearing in one ear	Chapter 9.1a, p 224	6	Chapter 11.2, pp 246–251
3	Loss of sense of smell	Chapter 9.3c, p 231	3	Chapter 13.4a, p 327
0	Uncomplicated incisional hernia	Chapter 10.9, Table 7, p 247	0	Table 6–9, p 136

From Doege T, Houston TP (eds): Guides to the Evaluation of Permanent Impairment, 4th ed. Chicago, American Medical Association, 1993; and Cocchiarella L, Andersson GBJ (eds): Guides to the Evaluation of Permanent Impairment, 5th ed. Chicago, American Medical Association, 2001, with permission.

scientifically validated, or precise. The origins of disease-specific scales to serve the needs of clinicians and the pharmaceutical industry to determine if an intervention may modulate the manifestations of a disorder prevents one from presuming that the change in a score truly reflects a change in a disease activity as influenced by the intervention in question. The importance of the change in disease activity in terms of activities of daily living is not always known and extrapolation to disability should be undertaken cautiously, if at all.

The Committee stated the following common impairments resulting from brain disorders were to be considered: sensory and motor disturbances, communication disturbances, complex integrated cerebral function disturbances, emotional disturbances, consciousness disturbances, and episodic disturbances. In the early editions of the Guides all but the sensory and motor disturbance categories were deemed to be maximal at 95% WPI. Estimates of impairment for sensory and motor disturbance and spinal cord injury were to be indirectly derived from the ability to stand, walk, use upper extremities, control bladder and bowel, breathe, and speak.[37]

The Guides' fourth edition includes the following nine functionally defined categories: consciousness and awareness, aphasia and communication, mental status/integrative functioning, emotional and behavioral disturbances, preoccupation or obsession, major motor or sensory abnormalities, movement disorders, episodic disorders, and sleep and arousal disorders. The fourth edition reduced the maximal WPI for all categories and directed that only the most severe of the first five forebrain impairments were to be considered. Any one of the subsequent four may then be combined with the previous selection from the first five.[38]

The fifth edition directs the evaluator to identify and use only the most severe of the following four CNS categories: 1) state of consciousness and level of awareness, whether permanent or episodic or due to sleep and arousal; 2) mental status; 3) use and understanding of language; and 4) influence of behavior and mood disorder. The broadening of state of consciousness and level of awareness incorporates the episodic disorders and sleep and arousal disorders found in the fourth edition. The broadening of behavior and mood incorporates the emotional and behavioral and the preoccupation and obsession found in the fourth edition.[39] This approach returns to the format of previous editions in which one forebrain impairment is combined with other categories of dysfunction. However, unlike some previous editions, the impairment maxima are less than 95%.

The forebrain categories of major motor or sensory disorders and movement disorders found in the fourth

TABLE 34-2

Central Nervous System Impairment in AMA Guides (4th and 5th editions)

Disorder Category	Maximum % WPI	Edition, Descriptor; Reference
Consciousness and awareness	90	4th, Table 4, p 142
	90	5th, irreversible coma; Table 13–2, p 309
Episodic disorders		
Syncope	70	4th, risk of bodily injury; Table 22, p 152
Convulsive	70	4th, total limitation; Table 5, p 143
Episodic loss of consciousness	70	5th, Table 13–3, p 312
Sleep and arousal	60	4th, unable to self care; Table 6, p 143
	90	5th, Table 13–4, p 317
Aphasia	60	4th, no communication; Table 1, p 141
	60	5th, no communication; Table 13–7, p 323
Mental status/integrative functioning	70	4th, no care for self; Table 2, p 142
	70	5th, no care for self; Table 13–6, p 320
Emotional and behavioral disturbance	70	4th, total dependence; Table 3, p 142
	90	5th, total dependence; Table 13–8, p 325
Preoccupation or obsession		4th, refer to Chapter 14
		5th, see emotional and behavioral
Major motor or sensory		See following
Station and gait	60	4th, Table 13, p 148
	60	5th; Table 13.5, p 336
One impaired upper extremity	45–60	4th; Table 14, p 148
	45–60	5th; Table 13–16, p 338
Two impaired upper extremities	80+	4th; Table 15, p 148
	80+	5th; Table 13–17, p 340
Movement disorder		4th; no specific guide
		5th; use major motor
Respiration	90+	4th; Table 16, p 149
		5th; Table 13–18, p 341
Bladder	60	4th; Table 17, p 149
		5th; Table 13–19, p 341
Anorectal	50	4th; Table 18, p 149
		5th; Table 13–20, p 342
Sexual	20	4th; Table 19, p 149
		5th; Table 13–21, p 342

From Doege T, Houston TP (eds): Guides to the Evaluation of Permanent Impairment, 4th ed. Chicago, American Medical Association, 1993; and Cocchiarella L, Andersson GBJ (eds): Guides to the Evaluation of Permanent Impairment, 5th ed. Chicago, American Medical Association, 2001, with permission.

edition remain in the fifth edition as station, gait, and movement disorders. According to the fifth edition, cranial nerve; station, gait, and movement disorders; extremity disorders related to central impairment; spinal cord; chronic pain; and peripheral nerve impairment are evaluated once the four categories of cerebral impairment are determined.[39] Movement disorder impairments remain estimates based on dysfunction of the upper extremities and station and gait. Thus estimates of CNS WPI will vary among editions of the Guides, despite the direction to contributors of the Guides to avoid changing WPI estimates. Disorders have been reassigned categories, subcategories have been adjusted, and permissible combinations have been reconsidered. For example, when considering disorders of impairment of consciousness and awareness, subcategories differ between the fourth and fifth editions. A persistent vegetative state or irreversible coma requiring total medical support is estimated at 50 to 90% WPI (fourth edition)[38] and 70 to 90% WPI (fifth edition).[39] The fifth edition no longer permits impairments derived from epileptic events to be combined with other CNS disorders such as mental status and integrative dysfunction.[39] In reviewing the comparison of the fourth and fifth editions' CNS WPI categories, one must be mindful that combinations are slightly more restrictive in the fifth edition (Table 34–2).

SPECIAL CONSIDERATIONS: AGE, HANDEDNESS

The WPI estimates generated by the AMA Guides are not adjusted by age. The Committee recommended that an age-related enhancement could be permitted for sexual capability and awareness of such function from a spinal disorder. Alternative impairment schedules for workers' compensation have permitted "enhancements" for age and handedness recognizing the socioeconomic influence of these personal attributes. For example, the report presented by Dr. D.E. Bell to the Association of Workmen's' Compensation Boards of Canada in 1960 included an impairment rating schedule. The numeric impairment derived from the schedule included consideration of personal attributes including age and handedness to "represent the loss of earning capacity" and fulfill the spirit of workmen's' compensation.[24]

In the 1964 monograph "Guides to the evaluation of permanent impairment: The peripheral spinal nerves,"[6] the Committee suggested that the basic tasks of daily living are more dependent on the preferred upper extremity when considering spinal cord injury. Dysfunction or loss of the preferred upper extremity results in greater impairment than the nonpreferred upper extremity. The Committee stated that all values are in terms of the preferred extremity and should be reduced for the nonpreferred extremity by 5% for impairment rating less than 50% and by 10% for upper extremity impairments greater than 50% before calculation of the WPI. The evaluation of the impairment of the preferred upper extremity should be subject to periodic review, as the unimpaired nonpreferred extremity sometimes becomes as accomplished as the previously preferred extremity. The Guides continued the use of the "preferred extremity" concept until the fifth edition, which refers to dominant extremity.[39]

Depending on which edition of the Guides an evaluator is using, the peripheral nervous system may be included in the chapter for the CNS. Peripheral nerve impairments are to be graded in terms of sensory (fourth edition Table 20,[38[p151]] fifth edition Table 13–23[39[pp346–347]]) and motor (fourth edition Table 21,[38[p151]] fifth edition Table 13–24[39[pp348–349]]) components. Multiple nerve impairments are to be combined within the affected limb and multiple extremity impairments may be combined after conversion to WPI.

LEVEL OF CONSCIOUSNESS AND AWARENESS

The criteria for evaluating disturbances of permanent responsiveness do not include sleep, seizures, or syncope, which are considered separately as episodic disorders. Similarly, the Guides, fifth edition, recognize that the disorders to be evaluated must be permanent, episodic, or due to sleep and arousal disorders (Tables 13–2, 13–3, and 13–4, respectively[39[pp309,312,317]]). An example in the Guides' fifth edition is symptomatic orthostatic hypotension of parkinsonian origin which is evaluated using Table 13–2.[39(p309)]

The relevant table from the Guides' fourth edition (Table 4, p 142; reprinted here as Table 34–3) or fifth edition (Table 13–2, p 309; reprinted here as Table 34–4) provides direction. To use the tables effectively one combines a WPI derived from the table with other CNS impairments as permitted by the specific edition. For the fourth edition, this includes major motor or sensory abnormalities, movement disorders, episodic disorders, or sleep or arousal disorders.[38] For the fifth edition, this includes station, gait, and movement; extremity disorders related to central impairments; spinal cord impairments; chronic pain; and peripheral nerve motor and sensory impairments. If one is unable to identify other impairments, relatively low values result compared to previous editions. Editions prior to the fourth assigned values as high as 95% WPI for the same categories (see Tables 34–3 and 34–4[39[pp312,317]]).

COMMUNICATION IMPAIRMENTS

Aphasia is the verbal manifestation of communication disturbance including expression, repetition, comprehension, dyslexia, dysgraphia, spelling, and pantomime. It is not a disturbance of phonation or articulation. The example of a left hemisphere stroke given in the Guides' fourth edition results in a 91% WPI after combining impairment for aphasia (45%), right upper limb impairment (55%), and gait impairment (65%).[38(p141)] Similarly, the Guides, fifth edition permits deficits from other dysfunctions to be combined (see Tables 34–5 and 34–6).[39]

TABLE 34-3

Impairment of Consciousness and Awareness

Impairment Description	% Impairment of the Whole Person
Brief repetitive or persisting alteration of state of consciousness, limiting ability to perform usual activities	0–14
Prolonged alteration of state of consciousness diminishing capabilities in personal care and other activities of daily living	15–29
State of semicoma with complete dependency and subsistence by artificial medical means	30–49
Persistent vegetative state, or irreversible coma requiring total medical support	50–90

From Doege T, Houston TP (eds): Guides to the Evaluation of Permanent Impairment, 4th ed. Chicago, American Medical Association, 1993, p 142.

TABLE 34–4

Criteria for Rating Impairment of Consciousness and Awareness

Class 1: 0% to 14% Impairment of the Whole Person	Class 2: 15% to 39% Impairment of the Whole Person	Class 3: 40% to 69% Impairment of the Whole Person	Class 4: 70% to 90% Impairment of the Whole Person
Brief repetitive or persistent alteration of state of consciousness **and** minimal limitation in performance of ADL	Brief repetitive or persistent alteration of state of consciousness **and** moderate limitation in performance of ADL	Prolonged alteration of state of consciousness, which diminishes capabilities in personal care and ADL	State of semicoma with complete dependency and subsistence on nursing care and artificial medical means of support **or** irreversible coma requiring total medical support

ADL, activities of daily living.

From Cocchiarella L, Andersson GBJ (eds): Guides to the Evaluation of Permanent Impairment, 5th ed. Chicago, American Medical Association, 2001, p 309.

MENTAL STATUS AND INTEGRATIVE FUNCTIONING

Functional deficits in this area commonly arise as a result of survival with moderate or severe impairments after a head injury.[34] The AMA Guides, fourth edition, recommends dysfunction in activities of daily living and the need for supervision to subcategorize severity.[38] The fifth edition continues this approach but introduces the Clinical Dementia Rating Scale (CDRS) in conjunction with one of the standardized mental status tests—the short Blessed, Neurobehavioral Cognitive Status Examination (NCSE), or Mini-Mental State Examination (MMSE)—to subcategorize cognitive dysfunction.[39]

These supplementary instruments are used to identify cognitive impairment. They correlate highly with each other but normative measurements of cognitive function in Alzheimer's disease (AD) in minority groups need to be validated.[31] The introduction of these instruments may introduce difficulties in distinguishing cognitive symptom severity from inherent measurement bias and intercurrent depression.[17] The differences in the onset and course characteristics and the specific differences among the various dementias call for careful diagnostic separation and consideration of caregiver burdens.[36] Thirty-two percent of adults with musculoskeletal pain seen in a physical medicine and rehabilitation (PM&R) outpatient clinic screened using the NCSE had impaired performance in at least one cognitive domain.[22] It remains to be seen whether the application of these instruments in estimating CNS impairment will be generally accepted and scientifically validated in disorders other than dementia of the Alzheimer type (DAT) (see Tables 34–7 and 34–8).

The CDRS is a global staging measure for DAT to assess the influence of cognitive losses on a person's ability to conduct everyday activities. It was developed to allow for a clinical diagnosis of DAT and to allow the clinician to judge its severity. The protocol uses semistructured interviews with the individual and an informant to rate the subject's cognitive performance and functional abilities. Criterion validity for both the global CDR and scores on individual domains have been demonstrated. The CDRS has been validated neuropathologically for the presence or absence of dementia and is widely accepted in the clinical setting as a reliable and valid global assessment measure for DAT.[28]

Extrapolation of the CDRS to the functionally derived subcategories found in Table 13–6 of the fifth edition[39(pp320–321)] requires testing of orientation, memory, attention, and abstraction, and judgment of the confounding effects of aphasia and personal deficiencies. Many capacities remain intact in patients with mild to moderate DAT, including the performance

TABLE 34–5

Impairments Related to Aphasia or Dysphasia

Description	% Impairment of the whole person
Minimal disturbance in comprehension and production of language symbols of daily living	0–9
Moderate impairment in comprehension production of language symbols of and daily living	10–24
Inability to comprehend language symbols; production of unintelligible or inappropriate language for daily activities	25–39
Complete inability to communicate or comprehend language symbols	40–60

From Doege T, Houston TP (eds): Guides to the Evaluation of Permanent Impairment, 4th ed. Chicago, American Medical Association, 1993, p 141.

TABLE 34–6

Criteria for Rating Impairment Due to Aphasia of Dysphasia

Class 1: 0% to 9% Impairment of the Whole Person	Class 2: 10% to 24% Impairment of the Whole Person	Class 3: 25% to 39% Impairment of the Whole Person	Class 4: 40% to 60% Impairment of the Whole Person
Minimal disturbance in comprehension and production of language symbols of daily living	Moderate impairment in comprehension and production of language symbols of daily living	Able to comprehend nonverbal communication; production of unintelligible or inappropriate language for daily activities	Complete inability to communicate or comprehend language symbols

From Cocchiarella L, Andersson GBJ (eds): Guides to the Evaluation of Permanent Impairment, 5th ed. Chicago, American Medical Association, 2001, p 323.

of self-care activities of daily living, such as eating, bathing, and grooming.[32] Because the Class I subcategory of Table 13–6 presumes normal performance of activities of daily living, a floor effect limits its application in mild traumatic brain injury (see Table 13–5 of the fifth edition of the Guides[39[pp320–321]]).

The fifth edition[39] also recommends conjoint use of the MMSE.[8] The MMSE has widespread popularity, ease of use, and a large body of research demonstrating its sensitivity in common neuropsychiatric disorders.[27] The MMSE has an expanded window suitable for only a narrow segment of the spectrum of impairment. Using a score of 23 as a cutoff, the sensitivity and specificity for the MMSE is 87% and 82%, respectively, for detecting delirium in hospitalized patients. The MMSE score does not provide a specific diagnosis; patients with dementia, delirium, retardation, schizophrenia, or depression have low scores. The MMSE score is age and educational dependent in the normal population, suggesting that the threshold to be considered abnormal must be adjusted for the individual.[14] The median MMSE score is 29 for individuals with at least 9 years of schooling, 26 for those with 5 to 8 years of schooling, and 22 for those with 0 to 4 years of schooling. The MMSE score fluctuates and is of limited value in individual patients with DAT for periods less than 3 years because of measurement error.[4]

The Guides' fifth edition[39] recommends the conjoint use of the Blessed Dementia Scale (BDS). The short version of the BDS may have equally good sensitivity, reliability, and neuropathologic validity.[11,18] The BDS has two parts. Part 1 (see Table 34–10) measures performance of everyday activities, changes in habits, changes in personality or interests, and drive. Information is obtained as much as possible from relatives or from those with close and continual contact. Part 2 is the "information–memory–concentration" test. It measures orientation for time, place, and person, the capacity to remember

TABLE 34–7

Mental Status Impairments

Impairment Description	% Impairment of the Whole Person
Impairment exists, but ability remains to perform satisfactorily most activities of daily living	1–14
Impairment requires direction and supervision of daily living activities	15–29
Impairment requires directed care under continued supervision and confinement in home or other facility	30–49
Individual is unable without supervision to care for self and be safe in any situation	50–70

From Doege T, Houston TP (eds): Guides to the Evaluation of Permanent Impairment, 4th ed. Chicago, American Medical Association, 1993, p 142.

TABLE 34–8

Criteria for Rating Impairment Related to Mental Status

Class 1: 1% to 14% Impairment of the Whole Person	Class 2: 15% to 29% Impairment of the Whole Person	Class 3: 30% to 49% Impairment of the Whole Person	Class 4: 50% to 70% Impairment of the Whole Person
Paroxysmal disorder with preimpairment exists, but is able to perform activities of daily living	Impairment requires direction of some activities of daily living	Impairment requires assistance and supervision for most activities of daily living	Unable to care for self and be safe in any situation without supervision
CDR = 0.5	CDR = 1.0	CDR = 2.0	CDR = 3.0

From Cocchiarella L, Andersson GBJ (eds): Guides to the Evaluation of Permanent Impairment, 5th ed. Chicago, American Medical Association, 2000, p 320.

TABLE 34-9

Clinical Dementia Rating (CDR)

Category	None: 0	Questionable: 0.5	Mild: 1	Moderate: 2	Severe: 3
Memory	No memory loss or slight inconsistent forgetfulness	Consistent slight forgetfulness; partial recollection of events; "benign" forgetfulness	Moderate memory loss; more marked for recent events; defect interfeces with everyday activities	Severe memory loss; only highly learned material retained; new material rapidly lost	Severe memory loss; only fragments remain
Orientation	Fully oriented	Fully oriented except for slight difficulty with time relationships	Moderate difficulty with time relationships; oriented for place at examination; may have geographic disorientation elsewhere	Severe difficulty with time relationships; usually disoriented to time, often to place	Oriented to person only
Judgment and Problem Solving	Solves everyday problems & handles business & financial affairs well; judgment good in relation to past performance	Slight impairment in solving problems, similarities, and differences	Moderate difficulty in handling problems, similarities, and differences; social judgment usually maintained	Severely impaired in handling problems, similarities, and differences; social judgment usually impaired	Unable to make judgments or solve problems
Community Affairs	Independent function at usual level in job, shopping, volunteer and social groups	Slight impairment in these activities	Unable to function independently at these activities although may still be engaged in some; appears normal to casual inspection	No pretense of independent function outside home Appears well enough to taken to functions outside a family home	No pretense of independent function outside home Appears too ill to be taken to functions outside a family home
Home and Hobbies	Life at home, hobbies, and intellectual interests well maintained	Life at home, hobbies, and intellectual interests slightly impaired	Mild but definite impairment of function at home; more difficult chores abandoned; more complicated hobbies and interests abandoned	Only simple chores preserved; very restricted interests, poorly maintained	No significant function in home
Personal Care	Fully capable of self-care		Needs prompting	Requires assistance in dressing, hygiene, keeping of personal effects	Requires much help with personal care; frequent incontinence

personal and recent autobiographical events and knowledge, and concentration or mental control.

The fifth edition recommends the conjoint use of the NCSE, which was developed for use in organic brain dysfunction and CNS lesions.[3] The NCSE is a screening examination that evaluates function within five major cognitive ability areas: language, constructions, memory, calculations, and reasoning. The examination separately assesses the levels of consciousness, orientation, and attention.[23] In patients with brain lesions, the MMSE has a false negative rate of 43% and the NCSE, 7%. The sensitivity of the NCSE is derived from two features of its design: the use of independent tests to assess skills within the five major areas of cognitive functioning and the use of graded tasks within each of these cognitive domains.[30] Some authorities recommend that the NCSE be used in persons with considerable cognitive impairment.[12]

TABLE 34–10

Blessed Dementia Scale Part 1

Changes in Performance of Everyday Activities	Points
1. Inability to perform household tasks	1 ½ 0
2. Inability to cope with small sums of money	1 ½ 0
3. Inability to remember short list of items; e.g. shopping list	1 ½ 0
4. Inability to find way about indoors	1 ½ 0
5. Inability to find way about familiar streets	1 ½ 0
6. Inability to interpret surroundings (e.g., to recognize whether in hospital or at home, to discriminate between patients, doctors and nurses, relatives and hospital staff)	1 ½ 0 1 ½ 0 1 ½ 0
7. Inability to recall recent events (e.g., recent outings, visits of relatives or friends)	1 ½ 0
8. Tendency to dwell in the past	1 ½ 0
9. Eating	
Cleanly with proper utensils	0
Messily with spoon only	2
Simple solids; e.g., biscuits	2
Has to be fed	3
10. Dressing	
Unaided	0
Occasionally misplaced buttons, etc	1
Wrong sequence, commonly forgetting items	2
Unable to dress	3
11. Continence	
Complete sphincter control	0
Occasionally wets bed	1
Frequently wets bed	2
Doubly incontinent	3
Change in personality, interests, drive	
No change	0
12. Increased rigidity	1
13. Increased egocentricity	1
14. Impairment in feelings for others	1
15. Coarsening of affect	1
16. Impairment of emotional control; e.g., increased petulance and irritability	1
17. Hilarity in inappropriate situations	1
18. Diminished emotional responsiveness	1
19. Sexual misdemeanor (appearing de novo in old age)	1
Interest retained	0
20. Hobbies relinquished	1
21. Diminished initiative or growing apathy	1
22. Purposeless hyperactivity	1

Scoring—0 = competent, 1/2 = partial competence, 1 = total incompetence in the particular activity.

EMOTIONAL OR BEHAVIORAL IMPAIRMENT

The AMA Guides recognizes the close relationship between neurologic and psychiatric illnesses. Both the fourth[38] and fifth[39] editions of the Guides permit use of the mental and behavioral disorders chapter (Chapter 14) for rating emotional or behavioral illness. The chapter is recommended if documented neurologic impairment is absent. In the Guides, fourth edition, Chapter 14 in turn recommends the use of the Diagnostic and Statistical Manual of Mental Disorders to establish a medically determinable diagnosis in a multiaxial evaluation.[38] The fifth edition, in Table 13–8 (reprinted here as Table 34–12), provides estimates ranging to a high of 90% WPI for people who are totally dependent on a caregiver.[39] The Guides also permits an assessment with the Neuropsychiatric Inventory (NPI).[10] The NPI is a validated clinical instrument for evaluating a wide range of psychopathology in previously diagnosed patients with dementia. It evaluates 12 neuropsychiatric disturbances common in dementia: delusions, hallucinations, agitation, dysphoria, anxiety, apathy, irritability, euphoria, disinhibition, aberrant motor behavior, nighttime behavior disturbances, and appetite and eating abnormalities.[9] A shortened version is under investigation.[21]

TABLE 34–11

Emotional or Behavioral Impairments

Impairment Description	% Impairment of the Whole Person
Mild limitation of daily social and interpersonal functioning	0–14
Moderate limitation of *some* but not all social and interpersonal daily living functions	15–29
Severe limitation impeding useful action in almost all social and interpersonal daily functions	30–49
Severe limitation of all daily functions requiring total dependence on another person	50–70

From Doege T, Houston TP (eds): Guides to the Evaluation of Permanent Impairment, 4th ed. Chicago, American Medical Association, 1993, p 142.

The severity of illness should be measured by alterations in the activities of daily living, social functioning, concentration, persistence, or pace, or deterioration or decompensation in work or work-like settings. The contribution of intercurrent depression is not always recognized in patients with left frontal lobe infarctions (see Tables 34–11 and 34–12).[29]

PREOCCUPATION OR OBSESSION

The Guides, fourth edition,[38] gives little practical assistance and does not specifically address this impairment; they refer the reader to Chapter 14 (p 297). Chapter 14 states, "a diagnosis alone can not be the basis for determining the presence of a disability"[38(p297)]; rather, "the basis is the severity of the individual's functional limita-

TABLE 34–12

Criteria for Rating Impairment Due to Emotional or Behavioral Disorders

Class 1: 0% to 14% Impairment of the Whole Person	Class 2: 15% to 29% Impairment of the Whole Person	Class 3: 30% to 69% Impairment of the Whole Person	Class 4: 70% to 90% Impairment of the Whole Person
Mild limitation of activities of daily living and daily social and interpersonal functioning	Moderate limitation of some activities of daily living and some daily social and interpersonal functioning	Severe limitation in performing most activities of daily living, impeding useful action in most daily social and interpersonal functioning	Severe limitation of all daily activities, requiring total dependence on another person

From Cocchiarella L, Andersson GBJ (eds): Guides to the Evaluation of Permanent Impairment, 5th ed. Chicago, American Medical Association, 2001, p 325.

TABLE 34–13

Classification of Impairments Due to Mental and Behavioral Disorders

Area or Aspect of Functioning	Class 1: No Impairment	Class 2: Mild Impairment	Class 3: Moderate Impairment	Class 4: Marked Impairment	Class 5: Extreme Impairment
Activities of daily living Social functioning Concentration Adaptation	No impairment is noted	Impairment levels are compatible with most useful functioning	Impairment levels are compatible with some, but not all, useful functioning	Impairment levels significantly impede useful functioning	Impairment levels preclude useful functioning

From Doege T, Houston TP (eds): Guides to the Evaluation of Permanent Impairment, 4th ed. Chicago, American Medical Association, 1993, p 301.

TABLE 34–14

Criteria for Rating Impairment of One Upper Extremity

Class 1: Dominant Extremity 1% to 9% Impairment of the Whole Person	Nondominant Extremity 1% to 4% Impairment of the Whole Person	Class 2: Dominant Extremity 10% to 24% Impairment of the Whole Person	Nondominant Extremity 5% to 14% Impairment of the Whole Person	Class 3: Dominant Extremity 25% to 39% Impairment of the Whole Person	Nondominant Extremity 15% to 29% Impairment of the Whole Person	Class 4: Dominant Extremity 40% to 60% Impairment of the Whole Person	Nondominant Extremity 30% to 45% Impairment of the Whole Person
Individual can use the involved extremity for self-care, daily activities, and holding, but has difficulty with digital dexterity		Individual can use the involved extremity for self-care, can grasp and hold objects with difficulty, but has no digital dexterity		Individual can use the involved extremity but has difficulty with self-care activities		Individual cannot use the involved extremity for self-care or daily activities	

From Cocchiarella L, Andersson GBJ (eds): Guides to the Evaluation of Permanent Impairment, 5th ed. Chicago, American Medical Association, 2001, p 338.

tions."[38(p297)] Given this direction, the evaluator is cautioned on p 301 that "…there are no precise measures of impairment in mental disorders." The Guides' fifth edition provides the evaluator with Table 13–8[39(p325)] (Table 34–12), which permits a maximum of 90% WPI for the individual requiring total dependence on another (see Tables 34–12 and 34–13).

MAJOR MOTOR OR SENSORY ABNORMALITIES

The AMA Guides recommends evaluation of other organ systems if relevant, or evaluation of ability to perform daily activities. The fifth edition's Table 13–16[39] (reprinted here as Table 34–14) is the only

TABLE 34–15

Criteria for One Impaired Upper Extremity

Impairment Description	% Impairment of the Whole Person: Preferred Extremity	Nonpreferred Extremity
Patient can use the involved extremity for self-care, daily activities, and holding, but has difficulty with digital dexterity	1–9	1–4
Patient can use the involved extremity for self-care, can grasp and hold objects with difficulty, but has no digital dexterity	10–24	5–14
Patient can use the involved extremity but has difficulty with self-care activities	25–39	15–29
Patient cannot use the involved extremity for self-care and daily activities	40–60	30–45

From Doege T, Houston TP (eds): Guides to the Evaluation of Permanent Impairment, 4th ed. Chicago, American Medical Association, 1993, p 148.

TABLE 34–16

Station and Gait Impairment Criteria

Impairment Description	% Impairment of the Whole Person
Patient can rise to a standing position and can walk but has difficulty with elevations, grades, stairs, deep chairs, and walking long distances	1–9
Patient can rise to a standing position and can walk some distance with difficulty and without assistance but is limited to level surfaces	10–19
Patient can rise to a standing position and can maintain it with difficulty but cannot walk without assistance	20–39
Patient cannot stand without help of others, mechanical support, and a prosthesis	40–60

From Doege T, Houston TP (eds): Guides to the Evaluation of Permanent Impairment, 4th ed. Chicago, American Medical Association, 1993, p 148.

place where handedness is recognized. It changes the nomenclature of "preferred extremity" seen in the fourth edition with "dominant" versus "nondominant" upper extremity.[38(p148)] The WPI estimates are unaltered. Because the use of the term "preferred extremity" was, in practice, synonymous with "handedness" or hemispheric speech dominance, in only a small number of cases will this change impairment. It would be a rare circumstance when a task-specific upper extremity preference for the nondominant upper extremity might occur. Adequate accommodation would likely be an overriding consideration (see Tables 34–14 and 34–15).

Impairment of station and gait caused by a CNS or peripheral neurologic disorder is determined according to the effect on ambulation. The ratings were unchanged from the fourth to the fifth editions (see Tables 34–16 and 34–17).

The evaluation of bibrachial injuries also remained unchanged between the fourth and fifth editions (see Tables 34–18 and 34–19).

MOVEMENT DISORDERS

Movement disorders can be broadly separated into disorders of excessive or decreased movement. Tremor is the most common involuntary movement disorder.[16] It is an involuntary, rhythmic, periodic, mechanical oscillation of a body part distinct from other involuntary movement disorders, such as chorea, athetosis, ballismus, tics, and myoclonus. Other intrusive movement disorders are either infrequent or are rarely as disruptive to limb dysfunction. CNS disorders manifesting poverty of movement, such as parkinsonian syndromes, more commonly demon-

TABLE 34–17

Criteria for Rating Impairments Due to Station and Gait Disorders

Class 1: 1% to 9% Impairment of the Whole Person	Class 2: 10% to 19% Impairment of the Whole Person	Class 3: 20% to 39% Impairment of the Whole Person	Class 4: 40% to 60% Impairment of the Whole Person
Rises to standing position; walks, but has difficulty with elevations, grades, stairs, deep chairs, and long distances	Rises to standing position; walks some distance with difficulty and without assistance, but is limited to level surfaces	Rises and maintains standing position with difficulty; cannot walk without assistance	Cannot stand without help, mechanical support, and/or an assistive device

From Cocchiarella L, Andersson GBJ (eds): Guides to the Evaluation of Permanent Impairment, 5th ed. Chicago, American Medical Association, 2001, p 336.

TABLE 34–19

Criteria for Rating Impairments of Two Upper Extremities

Class 1: 1% to 19% Impairment of the Whole Person	Class 2: 20% to 39% Impairment of the Whole Person	Class 3: 40% to 79% Impairment of the Whole Person	Class 4: 80% + Impairment of the Whole Person
Individual can use both upper extremities for self-care, grasping, and holding, but has difficulty with digital dexterity	Individual can use both upper extremities for self-care, can grasp and hold objects with difficulty, but has no digital dexterity	Individual can use both upper extremities but has difficulty with self-care activities	Individual cannot use upper extremities

From Cocchiarella L, Andersson GBJ (eds): Guides to the Evaluation of Permanent Impairment, 5th ed. Chicago, American Medical Association, 2001, p 340.

TABLE 34–18

Criteria for Two Impaired Upper Extremities

Impairment Description	% Impairment of the Whole Person
Patient can use both upper extremities for self-care, grasping, and holding, but has difficulty with digital dexterity	1–19
Patient can use both upper extremities for self-care, can grasp and hold objects with difficulty, but has no digital dexterity	20–39
Patient can use both upper extremities but has difficulty with self-care activities	40–79
Patient cannot use upper extremities	80+

From Doege T, Houston TP (eds): Guides to the Evaluation of Permanent Impairment, 4th ed. Chicago, American Medical Association, 1993, p 148.

TABLE 34–20

Impairments Related to Syncope or Transient Loss of Awareness

Level	Description	% Impairment of the Whole Person
1	Mild loss of awareness with drop in blood pressure of 15 mm Hg/ 10 mm Hg without compensatory increase in pulse rate, lasting more than 2 minutes after precipitating event	1–9
2	Moderate loss of blood pressure of 25 mm Hg/15 mm Hg, with loss of awareness or consciousness lasting 1–2 minutes	10–29
3	Levels 1 and 2 are present with repeated severe losses of blood pressure of 30 mm Hg/20 mm Hg, and additional neurologic symptoms or signs of focal or generalized nature also are present	30–49
4	Level 3 is present with uncontrolled loss of consciousness and muscle control without recognized cause and with risk of body injury	50–70

This table is applicable to patients receiving treatment.
From Doege T, Houston TP (eds): Guides to the Evaluation of Permanent Impairment, 4th ed. Chicago, American Medical Association, 1993, p 152.

strate incoordination or ataxia and are more readily rated with the Guides.

There is no specific table in the Guides for movement disorders. The Committee recommended the use of functional activity derangement to derive impairment. The fourth and fifth editions direct the evaluator to use tables relevant to the dysfunction resulting from the movement disorder for assistance. In effect, the evaluator is to assess the resulting motor dysfunction of the limbs or by station and gait.

EPISODIC NEUROLOGIC IMPAIRMENTS

The Guides, fourth edition,[38] consider episodic disorders that are intermittent but persistent. These include syncope, convulsions, and narcolepsy. Reflex forms of syncope (vasovagal syncope and carotid sinus syncope) seem to carry little risk of death but are associated with a high incidence of injury, particularly in elderly people. Sleep apnea, which is considered in the fourth edition's Chapter 5, is excluded.[38(p163)] A common error in evaluating epilepsy is to use this table to estimate impairment of persistent cognitive impairment instead of the appropriate mental status and integrative functioning sections (Chapter 4, Table 2[38[p142]]) (see Tables 34–20, 34–21, and 34–22).

The Guides, fifth edition,[39] requires episodic neurologic impairments to be persistent and permanent. These include syncope, convulsive disorders, and arousal and sleep disorders. The criteria for episodic loss of consciousness are given in Table 13–3 (reprinted as Table 34–23) and permit the physical examination findings to substitute for the limitation of activities.

TABLE 34–21

Impairments Related to Epilepsy, Seizures, and Convulsive Disorders

Impairment Description	% Impairment of the Whole Person
Paroxysmal disorder with predictable characteristics and unpredictable occurrence that does not limit usual activities but is a risk to the patient or limits performance of daily activities	0–14
Paroxysmal disorder that interferes with some activities of daily living	15–29
Severe paroxysmal disorder of such frequency that it limits activities to those that are supervised, protected, or restricted	30–49
Uncontrolled paroxysmal disorder of such severity and constancy that it totally limits the individual's daily activities	50–70

From Doege T, Houston TP (eds): Guides to the Evaluation of Permanent Impairment, 4th ed. Chicago, American Medical Association, 1993, p 143.

TABLE 34–22

Impairment Criteria for Sleep and Arousal Disorders

Description	% Impairment of the Whole Person
Reduced daytime alertness with sleep pattern such that patient can carry out most daily activities	1–9
Reduced daytime altertness requiring some supervision in carrying out daytime activities	10–19
Reduced daytime alertness that significantlylimits daily activities and requires supervision by caretakers	20–39
Severe reduction of daytime alertness that causes the patient to be unable to care for self in any situation or manner	40–60

From Doege T, Houston TP (eds): Guides to the Evaluation of Permanent Impairment, 4th ed. Chicago, American Medical Association, 1993, p 143.

Table 13–4[39(p317)] is specific for sleep and arousal disorders. An Epworth Sleepiness Scale (ESS)[19] score of 10/24 is defined as a Class 3 (30 to 69%) WPI. Despite the directions provided by the fifth edition, by some authorities reservations have been expressed that the score of the ESS "correlates with the multiple sleep latency test (MSLT), which supports pathologic sleep in narcolepsy and idiopathic hypersomnia."[39(p317)] No statistically or clinically significant association has been found between Epworth scores and mean sleep latency.[2]

A common issue generating antagonism in patients with epilepsy concerns the privilege to drive. The Epilepsy Foundation of America states: "While the Epilepsy Foundation of America opposes mandatory

TABLE 34–23

Criteria for Rating Impairment Due to Episodic Loss of Consciousness or Awareness

Class 1: 0% to 14% Impairment of the Whole Person	Class 2: 15% to 29% Impairment of the Whole Person	Class 3: 30% to 49% Impairment of the Whole Person	Class 4: 50% to 70% Impairment of the Whole Person
Paroxysmal disorder with predictable characteristics and unpredictable occurrence that does not limit usual activities but is a *risk* to the individual or limits daily activities **or** blood pressure drop of 15/10 mm Hg without compensatory increase in pulse rate and lasting more than 2 minutes after precipitating event, with mild awareness loss that limits daily activities	Paroxysmal disorder that interferes with *some* daily activities **or** moderate blood pressure drop of 25/15 mm Hg, with loss of awareness or consciousness lasting 1 to 2 minutes and that interferes with *some* daily activities	Severe paroxysmal disorder of such frequency that it limits activities to those that are supervised, protected, or restricted **or** repeated severe blood pressure losses of 30/20 mm Hg, with loss of awareness or consciousness lasting 1 to 2 minutes **and** additional neurologic symptoms or signs of focal or generalized nature	Uncontrolled paroxysmal disorder of such severity and consistancy that it severely limits individual's daily activities **or** repeated severe blood pressure losses of 30/20 mm Hg, with uncontrolled loss of consciousness and muscle control without recognized cause and with risk of body injury

This table is applicable to individuals receiving treatment.
From Cocchiarella L, Andersson GBJ (eds): Guides to the Evaluation of Permanent Impairment, 5th ed. Chicago, American Medical Association, 2001, p 312.

physician reporting laws, it does support state laws which give physicians 'good faith' immunity for participating in the driver licensing process, and for voluntarily reporting those patients who pose an imminent threat to public safety because they are driving against medical advice. 'Good faith' should be defined as acting in accordance with a reasonable standard of care."[13] Each jurisdiction may also have mandatory reporting requirements.

A second problem involving a first time witnessed seizure ensues after the evaluation is completed. Typically an employee will require a return to work clearance before resumption of employment. This decision requires careful consideration by the physician. It is uncommon that the occupation is overtly hazardous (scuba divers, steeple jacks). The possibility of self-injury or injury to office and factory coworkers and property may require temporary work restrictions until a firm prognosis is established. The employee may find that these restrictions jeopardize advancement in the workplace. The employer is often reluctant to allow these individuals to continue at the workplace, fearing workplace disruption or the repercussions of a workplace injury. Objections from employers or other partisan advocates become adversarial if reasonable accommodations cannot be agreed upon. The evaluator must note the working demands as they affect seizure threshold and comment on the potential of anticonvulsant side effects to cause impaired attention. The "reasonableness" of the accommodation is not a medical issue and should be left to administrative parties.

In refractory epilepsy the evaluation becomes focused on the impairment estimates because disability is generally accepted. One may use a seizure severity scale to bolster the subcategorization into several levels and document thorough consideration of all manifestations. Severity scales evolved because pharmaceutical instruments in which clinically significant changes in seizure frequency, type, and severity are measurements of interest in clinical trials. As a result, validated patient-based seizure severity scales[1] were developed to reflect interventional effects.

CRANIAL NERVES

The Guides considers dysfunction of a cranial nerve as it corresponds to its defined function. There is usually more than one section of the text to estimate impairment of a specific cranial nerve. The options are summarized in Table 34–24. Select issues and changes from the fourth to the fifth edition are reviewed in that table.

Speech is addressed separately in the Guides' fourth edition in Chapter 9 (ear, nose, throat, and related structures) and directions are given to estimate dysfunction (Tables 7, 8, and 9[38[pp232–234]]). A 35% maximal WPI is permitted for speech that meets no demands of everyday function. The Guides' fifth edition follows the same format, noting that there is no single acceptable proven test that will measure objectively impairment of the voice.[39]

Impaired binocular vision was determined in the Guides' fourth edition by the use of Figure 3.[38(p217)] It recognized diplopia in central fixation as a greater impairment than in peripheral fields. The fifth edition recommends considering best-corrected binocular visual acuity to estimate impairment.[39]

SPINAL CORD INJURY

The Guides' fourth edition offers two methods for evaluating spine injury. It directs the usage of the DRE method in the presence of trauma and the range of motion method if the injury is nontraumatic or not well represented by the DRE method. Spinal cord injury or paraplegia can be evaluated with the spine section in Chapter 3 or the CNS section in Chapter 4. After selecting the appropriate DRE of lumbosacral, cervicothoracic, or thoracolumbar spine impairment using Tables 72, 73, or 74 (respectively),[38(pp110–111)] one determines if the individual meets criteria for Category VI, VII, or VIII. This is combined with the highest impairment found in the lesser categories (I through V). An estimate of impairment limited to 84% WPI in the event of quadriplegia ensues. The alternative of using the CNS (Chapter 4) method permits combining impairments for all dysfunctions from Tables 13 through 19.[38(pp148–149)] The ensuing WPI readily exceeds 90% in typical cases of cervical cord injury resulting in quadriplegia.

The Guides' fifth edition eliminates this discrepant approach. The spine section of Chapter 15 directs the use of Tables 15–3 (lumbar spine injury), 15–4 (thoracic spine injury), and 15–5 (cervical disorders),[39(pp384,389,392)] but has eliminated Categories VI, VII, and VIII. It directs that all spinal cord (long tract) injury be evaluated using the CNS chapter exclusively. The relevant dysfunctions resulting from spinal cord injuries or other adverse conditions are identified in Tables 13–5 through 13–21[39(pp320–342)] and combined. These include impairments rated by dysfunction of station and gait, use of upper extremities, urinary bladder, anorectal and sexual dysfunction, and pain. Adjustment for age is considered for sexual system dysfunction according to Chapter 7 (urinary and reproductive systems).[39]

TABLE 34-24

Cranial Nerves Overview

Cranial Nerve	Max WPI	Descriptor	AMA Guides Edition, Reference
I Olfactory	5%	Anosmia	4th, Chapter 4.1, p 144 5th, Chapter 13.4a, p 327 5th, Chapter 11.4c, p 262
	3%	Anosmia	4th, Chapter 9.3, p 231
II Optic	85%	Blind	4th, Chapter 4.1, Tables 7 and 8, p 144 5th, Table 13–9, Table 13–10, p 328 also 5th edition, Chapter 12
	85%	Blind	4th, Chapter 8.4, Table 6, p 218
III Oculomotor IV Trochlear V Abducens	24%	Due to diplopia Determined by visual acuity	4th, Chapter 8.3, Figure 3, p 217 5th, Chapter 12
VI Trigeminal	35%	Debilitating pain	4th, Chapter 4, Table 9, p 145 5th, Table 13–11, p 331
VII Facial	45%	Bilateral palsy	4th, Chapter 4, Table 10, p 146 5th, Table 13–12, p 332 4th, Chapter 9, Table 4, p 230
	50%	Bilateral palsy	5th, Table 11–5, p 256
VIII Vestibular	95%	Confinement needed	4th, Chapter 9.1c, p 228 5th, Table 11–4, p 253
	70%	Confinement needed	4th, Chapter 4, Table 11, p 146 5th, Table 13–13, p 334
Cochlear	35%	Deaf	4th, Chapter 9, Table 3, p 228 5th, Table 11–3, p 250
	6%	Monaural hearing loss	4th, Chapter 9, Tables 2 and 3, pp 226, 228 5th, Tables 11–2 and 11–3, pp 248–250
IX Glossopharyngeal	60%	Neuralgia Neuralgia	4th, Chapter 4.2c, Table 12, p 147 5th, Table 13–14, p 334
X Vagus	60%	Speech/swallowing	4th, Chapter 4.2c, Table 12, p 147 5th, Table 13–14, p 334 4th, Chapter 9, Table 6, p 231 5th, Table 13–14, p 334
XI Accessory	60%	Swallowing/speech	4th, Chapter 9, Table 6, p 231 4th, Chapter 9, Tables 7 and 9, pp 233–234; also Chapter 3, cervical ROM
		Refers to deglutition	4th, Chapter 11.4b 5th, Table 11–7, p 262 also Chapter 11.4a, airway 5th, Table 11–6, p 260
XII Hypoglossal	60%	Choking	4th, Chapter 4.2c, Table 12, p 147 5th, Table 13–14, p 334

ROM, range of motion.

References

1. Baker G, Smith D, Dewey M, et al: The development of seizure severity scale as an outcome measure in epilepsy. Epilepsy Res 8:245–251, 1991.
2. Benbadis SR, Mascha E, Perry MC, et al: Association between the Epworth Sleepiness Scale and the Multiple Sleep Latency Test in a clinical population. Ann Intern Med 130:289–292, 1999.
3. Blostein PA, Jones SJ, Buechler CM, Vandongen S: Cognitive screening in mild traumatic brain injuries: Analysis of the Neurobehavioral Cognitive Status Examination when utilized during initial trauma hospitalization. J Neurotrauma 14:171–177, 1997.
4. Clark CM, Sheppard L, Fillenbaum GG, et al: Variability in annual Mini-Mental State Examination score in patients with probable Alzheimer disease. A clinical perspective of data from the Consortium to Establish a Registry for Alzheimer's Disease. Arch Neurol 56:857–862,1999.
5. Committee on Rating of Mental and Physical Impairment: Guides to the evaluation of permanent impairment: The central nervous system. JAMA 1–16, 1963.
6. Committee on Rating of Mental and Physical Impairment: Guides to the evaluation of permanent impairment: The peripheral spinal nerves. JAMA 189:128–142, 1964.

7. Confacreux C, Vukusic S, Moreau T, Adeline P: Relapses and progression of disability in multiple sclerosis. N Engl J Med 343:1430–1438, 2000.
8. Crum RM, Anthony JC, Bassett SS, Folstein MF: Population-based norms for the Mini-Mental State Examination by age and educational level. JAMA 269:2386–2391, 1993.
9. Cummings JL: The Neuropsychiatric Inventory: Assessing psychopathology in dementia patients. Neurology 48(Suppl. 6):S10–16, 1997.
10. Cummings JL, Mega M, Gray K, et al: The Neuropsychiatric Inventory: Comprehensive assessment of psychopathology in dementia. Neurology 44:2308–2314, 1994.
11. Davis PB, Morris JC, Grant E: Brief screening tests versus clinical staging in senile dementia of the Alzheimer type. J Am Geriatr Soc 38:129–135, 1990.
12. Doninger NA, Bode RK, Heinemann AW, Ambrose C: Rating scale analysis of the Neurobehavioral Cognitive Status Examination. J Head Trauma Rehabil 15:683–695, 2000.
13. Epilepsy Foundation of America Position Statement: http://www.efa.org/advocacy/efaposition.html. May 27, 2002.
14. Grigoletto F, Zappala G, Anderson DW, Lebowitz BD: Norms for the Mini-Mental State Examination in a healthy population. Neurology 53:315–320, 1999.
15. Groce NE: Disability in cross-cultural perspective: Rethinking disability. Lancet 354:756–757, 1999.
16. Habib-ur-Rehman: Diagnosis and management of tremor. Arch Intern Med 160:2438–2444, 2000.
17. Hargrave R, Reed B, Mungas D: Depressive syndromes and functional disability in dementia. J Geriatr Psychiatry Neurol 13:72–77, 2000.
18. Heun R, Papassotiropoulos A, Jennssen F: The validity of psychometric instruments for detection of dementia in the elderly general population. Int J Geriatr Psychiatry 13:368–380, 1998.
19. Johns MW: A new method for measuring daytime sleepiness: The Epworth Sleepiness Scale. Sleep 14:540–545, 1991.
20. Katzman GL, Dagher AP, Patronas AP: Incidental findings on brain magnetic resonance imaging from 1000 asymptomatic volunteers. JAMA 282:36–39, 1999.
21. Kaufer DI, Cummings JL, Ketchel P, et al: Validation of the NPI-Q, a brief clinical form of the Neuropsychiatric Inventory. J Neuropsychiatry Clin Neurosci 12:233–239, 2000.
22. Kewman DG, Vaishampayan N, Zald D, Han B: Cognitive impairment in musculoskeletal pain patients. Int J Psychiatry Med 21:253–262, 1991.
23. Kiernan RJ, Mueller J, Langston JW, Van Dyke C: The Neurobehavioral Cognitive Status Examination: A brief but quantitative approach to cognitive assessment. Ann Intern Med 107:481–485, 1987.
24. Klimek E: Disability and impairment schedules in Canadian workers' compensation systems compared to the AMA Guides. Disability 8:1–9, 1999.
25. Kurtzke JF: Rating neurologic impairment in multiple sclerosis: An Expanded Disability Status Scale (EDSS). Neurology 33:144–152, 1983.
26. Landy FJ: Stamp collecting versus science. Am Psychol 41:1183–1192, 1986.
27. Malloy PF, Cummings JL, Coffey CE, et al: Cognitive screening instruments in neuropsychiatry: A report of the Committee on Research of the American Neuropsychiatric Association. J Neuropsychiatry Clin Neurosci 9:189–197, 1997.
28. Morris JC: Clinical dementia rating: A reliable and valid diagnostic and staging measure for dementia of the Alzheimer type. Int Psychogeriatr 9(Suppl. 1):173–176, 1997.
29. Robinson AG, Price TR: Post-stroke depressive disorders: A follow-up study of 103 patients. Stroke 13:635–641, 1982.
30. Schwamm LH, Van Dyke C, Kiernan RJ, Merrin EL, Mueller J: The Neurobehavioral Cognitive Status Examination: Comparison with the Cognitive Capacity Screening Examination and the Mini-Mental State Examination in a neurosurgical population. Ann Intern Med 107:486–491, 1987.
31. Shadlen MF, Larson EB, Gibbons L, McCormick WC, Teri L: Alzheimer's disease symptom severity in blacks and whites. J Am Geriatr Soc 47:482–486, 1999.
32. Small GW, Rabins PV, Barry PP, et al: Diagnosis and treatment of Alzheimer disease and related disorders. Consensus statement of the American Association for Geriatric Psychiatry, the Alzheimer's Association, and the American Geriatrics Society. JAMA 278:1363–1371, 1997.
33. Stuss DT: A sensible approach to mild traumatic brain injury (editorial). Neurology 45:1251–1252, 1995.
34. Thornhill S, Teasdale GM, Murray GD, et al: Disability in young people and adults one year after head injury: Prospective cohort study. BMJ 320:1631–1635, 2000.
35. Üstün TB, Rehm J, Chatterji S, et al: Multiple-informant ranking of the disabling effects of different health conditions in 14 countries. Lancet 354:111–115, 1999.
36. Vetter PH, Krauss S, Steiner O, et al: Vascular dementia versus dementia of Alzheimer's type: Do they have differential effects on caregivers' burden? J Gerontol B Psychol Sci Soc Sci 54:S93–98, 1999.
37. American Medical Association: Guides to the Evaluation of Permanent Impairment. Chicago, American Medical Association, 1971.
38. Doege T, Houston TP (eds): Guides to the Evaluation of Permanent Impairment, 4th ed. Chicago, American Medical Association, 1993.
39. Cocchiarella L, Andersson GBJ (eds): Guides to the Evaluation of Permanent Impairment, 5th ed. Chicago, American Medical Association, 2001.

CHAPTER

35

Peripheral Nervous System Impairment

MARC T. TAYLOR, MD

The peripheralnervous system (PNS) is composed of neural structures that connect the brainstem and spinal cord with other tissues of the body. The PNS includes the spinal nerves as they exit and enter the spinal cord, the various plexuses, the major peripheral nerves, and all of the associated peripheral neural structures, excluding the cranial nerves. These special neural structures transmit neural impulses between the spinal cord and other tissues of the body. The spinal nerves contain nerve fibers that carry motor impulses, as well as sensory impulses, back and forth between the central nervous system and the specialized nerve tissues in the skin, muscles, tendons, ligaments, bones, and joints. The spinal nerves also contain the sympathetic and parasympathetic nerve fibers that make up the autonomic nervous system, which innervates blood vessels, viscera, and sweat glands.

Because of the complex nature of the PNS, pathologic conditions can impair the function of the system at many different points in the various neural pathways. A degenerative motor neuron disease can affect the proximal cell bodies in the spinal cord, whereas a pathologic process or condition, such as Guillain–Barré syndrome, diabetes mellitus, or chronic alcohol abuse, can create significant neuromuscular dysfunction in the more peripheral nerve structures. When evaluating peripheral nerve injuries, it is important to recognize the possible role that a pre-existing or underlying systemic pathologic process might have in any neuromuscular dysfunction.

This chapter presents methods for evaluation upper and lower extremity neuromuscular dysfunction as related to the spinal nerves, the brachial plexus, and the major peripheral nerves of the upper and lower extremities. It addresses specific conditions, such as entrapment neuropathies, and discusses some of the differences in the approach to peripheral nerve disorders in relationship to the different editions of the AMA Guides to the Evaluation of Permanent Impairment. Over the years there have been various papers and books published that have guidelines for the maximum percentage of loss of function of the whole person due to an injury to the PNS. Because of the common use and acceptance of the AMA Guides, the discussion and the description of methods of calculating a whole person impairment in this chapter use the principles and approach in that book.

This chapter does not deal with sensory deficits in the digits of the hand that are due to lesions in the digital nerves. Because an injury to the PNS structures has a different healing process than the healing of a laceration of a digital nerve of the finger, the impairment rating is calculated using different sections of the AMA Guides. Impairment due to digital nerve injuries is calculated according to the various tables and graphs under the specific sections related to the hand in the AMA Guides, which is section 16.3 in the fifth edition. Central nervous system and spinal cord injuries, mental and behavioral disorders, and pain disorders are addressed in other chapters of this book. Complaints of pain that are not consistent with the pathophysiology of injury or a disease process in a peripheral nerve structure cannot be given an impairment rating using this section.

THE EVALUATION PROCESS

When evaluating injuries of the PNS, a detailed history, with a review of all pertinent available medical records, and a thorough physical examination need to be performed in order to establish the diagnosis as accurately as possible. Although the final impairment rating is not dependent on the diagnosis or the etiology of the impairment, establishing the diagnosis can provide important information in terms of possible future progression or regression of any disease process and the possible need for future medical care. In certain clinical situations the evaluation process might require or include appropriate diagnostic studies, such as special imaging studies or a needle electromyographic evaluation done by appropriately trained and certified physicians. The evaluating physician should be able to determine if any abnormality found on any diagnostic testing is playing a role or has any clinical significance in terms of the overall clinical picture in a particular individual, as well as to recognize the possible role that a preexisting or underlying systemic pathologic process might have in any neuromuscular dysfunction. For example, the diagnostic accuracy of needle electromyographic tests can be greatly affected by such factors as age, sex, hand temperature, and anthropometric factors (see Chapter 33).

A detailed history and physical examination, as well as review of all pertinent medical records, are important to help determine whether an individual has reached maximum medical improvement (MMI). In the fifth edition of the AMA Guides, MMI is defined as "a condition or state that is well stabilized and unlikely to change substantially in the next year, with or without medical treatment. Over time, there may be some change; however, further recovery or deterioration is not anticipated."[(p601)]

Although this wording of the definition of MMI is somewhat different from previous editions of the Guides, the concepts that the medical condition is stable and not amenable to further treatment and that the employability and the impairment in an individual will not change significantly in the future are the same in all editions of the AMA Guides. When trying to determine whether an individual has reached MMI or should receive an impairment rating, it is also important for the evaluating physician to be aware of any regional, state, or jurisdictional differences in this basic concept of MMI. Once MMI has been reached, permanent impairment as a result of an injury to the PNS can be determined.

It should be noted that the tables of the peripheral nerve section of the AMA Guides cannot be used to give an impairment rating for complaints of generalized loss of strength, sensibility loss, or pain in the upper or lower extremities in an area where a nerve was not injured. In order to give an impairment rating, objective, reproducible physical findings or objective abnormalities on needle electrodiagnostic testing have to be present. Complaints of pain, loss of sensation, or loss of strength in the defined pathway of a nerve without objective evidence of an injury to the PNS do not receive any impairment.

As noted here, as well as in other chapters of the AMA Guides, the impairment has to be permanent and the result of an injury to the PNS in order to receive a rating using the tables of the peripheral nerve section of the AMA Guides. The temporary loss of function and complaints of pain seen with soft tissue inflammation associated with repetitive activities using the extremities, which resolve with conservative medical treatment or rest, cannot be rated through the peripheral nerve sections. In some situations these individuals may have a recurrent clinical picture of the development of musculoskeletal pain in an area from exertional myalgias and musculoskeletal inflammation after performing certain types of repetitive activities. These temporary musculoskeletal inflammatory clinical conditions may be work related and may respond to medical evaluation and treatment, but they are not permanent and, therefore, cannot receive a permanent impairment rating.

These clinical situations can be difficult to address with a claimant or patient when this recurrent clinical picture is associated with repetitive activities that are a part of the required essentials of a position within the workplace. At times it means that a person cannot physically perform on a regular basis the essentials of the workplace position, and a new position in the workplace should be found. If the musculoskeletal inflammation has resolved and all examinations and diagnostic studies are normal, then there is not an ongoing, underlying disease process or active medical condition for which the person can receive an impairment rating. Frequently in this situation, the inability to perform the essentials of a position in the workplace without developing a temporary inflammatory condition or the complaint of pain is a workplace issue. There is no permanent injury to the PNS; hence there is no impairment rating.

The evaluating physician must separate out the workplace issues from any underlying pathologic process involving the PNS that would benefit from active medical care or surgery. The results of tests, such as appropriate needle electrodiagnostic testing, the two-point discrimination test, the Semmes-Weinstein touch pressure threshold monofilament test, and imaging studies, can provide additional objective data. These test results can be used in combination with the findings of the physical examination to help the physician determine the permanent injury to the PNS for which the individual can receive an impairment rating.

DEFINING SENSORY AND STRENGTH LOSSES IN THE PNS

The permanent impairment rating as a result of a PNS disorder is based on the determination of losses of sensory and motor function that are the result of a PNS abnormality.

Because of the subjective nature of sensibility testing, documentation by clinical evaluation the degree of loss of sensation and the effects of any pain in a region as a result of a peripheral nerve injury can be challenging. In order to receive a permanent impairment, the complaints of pain and loss of sensation have to be consistent, reproducible, and in the defined anatomic pathway of the spinal nerve, brachial plexus, or major peripheral nerve that is diseased or was injured. The pathology that affects the PNS produces signs and symptoms in the extremities that are specific to the level or area of injury. Section 16.3 of Chapter 16 in the fifth edition of the AMA Guides discusses some important points concerning the clinical sensory evaluation of injured nerves. This section is excellent in explaining and clarifying many issues involved in the sensory examination, and it is a great improvement to the previous editions of the AMA Guides.

As pointed out in section 16.3, "The important difference between 'sensation' and 'sensibility' was clearly defined by George Omer in 1974. "Sensation is the acceptance and activation of impulses in the afferent nerve fibers of the nervous system ... "Sensibility is the conscious appreciation and interpretation of the stimulus that produced sensation." The clinical nature of the loss of the sensory function and the pattern of recovery after an injury to the PNS are different from that seen following a laceration to a digital nerve in the hand. Peripheral nerve injuries can alter the sensibility, or "conscious appreciation and interpretation of the stimulus that produced sensation," in the area of involvement. The static two-point discrimination test is most useful when evaluating injuries to the digital nerves of the hand. Although the static two-point discrimination test can be a useful part of the clinical examination when evaluating peripheral nerve injuries, frequently, it is necessary to use several different types of clinical tests to define the nature of the loss of sensibility. The Semmes-Weinstein monofilament pressure test, the pinprick test, and the moving two-point discrimination test are examples of clinical tests that can be used in addition to the standard static two-point discrimination test. Providing an appropriate, quiet testing environment to administer these tests is an important part of the examination process performed by the physician when trying to determine the loss of sensibility in a peripheral nerve injury.

It is important to realize that the calculation of the impairment rating for a loss of sensory function is based on the process and specific definitions that are given within the specific tables in the PNS sections of the AMA Guides. In previous editions of the AMA Guides, these were Table 10 or Table 11 of Chapter 3. In the fifth edition of the AMA Guides, Table 16–10 in Chapter 16 is used to determine the impairment as a result of a sensory deficit and pain from a peripheral nerve disorder (reprinted here as Table 35–3). The top half, or Section A, of Table 16–10, provides a clinical description for six different grades that can be used to place the nerve injury in a clinical category; these grades are based on the findings of the clinical examination. The bottom half, or Section B of Table 16–10, outlines the steps that should be followed to calculate the impairment. There are six different grades, ranging from Grade 5 to Grade 0. For each clinical grade in Section A, a range of minimum and maximum percentage relative values is given in the "% Sensory Deficit" column of the table. Based on the findings of the clinical examination, the examining physician must use his or her clinical judgment to place the nerve injury in the appropriate grade. Once the clinical grade category is determined, the physician must then estimate an appropriate percentage within the range of sensory deficit percentage values shown for that grade for the loss of function of the damaged nerve. The maximum percentage value in a grade should not be given automatically.

The first grade of Table 16–10 (Table 35–3) is Grade 5. Grade 5 is described as "No loss of sensibility, abnormal sensation, or pain." The percent sensory deficit relative value for Grade 5 is 0%. Grade 4 is described as "Distorted superficial tactile sensibility (diminished light touch), with or without minimal abnormal sensations or pain, that is forgotten during activity." The relative value given in this grade ranges from 1% to 25%. Grades 3, 2, and 1 have their own specific clinical descriptions and their own grade-specific range of deficit percentages. Grade 0 is described as "Absent sensibility, abnormal sensation, or severe pain that prevents all activity," and this grade is given a relative value of 100%. It is important to note that in order to receive any percentage at all, a sensory or sensibility deficit must be present on the clinical examination. Without this reproducible, objective finding, the effect of pain on activities cannot be rated.

Injuries to the PNS can create paralysis or an alteration in the motor power in the extremities by affecting the muscles or groups of muscles innervated by the involved nerves. Similar to the sensory examination, the clinical examination of motor strength in a particular muscle or muscle group relies on the cooperation of the examinee and has a subjective component to it. In order to receive a permanent impairment, the results of the examination has to be consistent, reproducible, and in the defined anatomic pathway of the spinal nerve, brachial plexus, or major peripheral nerve that is diseased or was injured. Documentation of any muscle atrophy and the results of needle electromyographic examinations can be helpful in providing objective signs of a nerve pathology resulting in loss of muscle function.

The calculation of the impairment rating for the loss of motor nerve function or power is based on the process and specific definitions that are given within the

TABLE 35–1

Determining Impairment of the Upper Extremity Due to Sensory Deficits or Pain Resulting From Peripheral Nerve Disorders

A. Classification

Grade	Description of Sensory Deficit or Pain	% Sensory Deficit
5	No loss of sensibility, abnormal sensation, or pain	0
4	Distorted superficial tactile sensibility (diminished light touch), with or without minimal abnormal sensations or pain, that is forgotten during activity	1–25
3	Distorted superficial tactile sensibility (diminished light touch and two-point discrimination), with some abnormal sensations or slight pain, that interferes with some activities	26–60
2	Decreased superficial cutaneous pain and tactile sensibility (decreased protective sensibility), with abnormal sensations or moderate pain, that may prevent some activities	61–80
1	Deep cutaneous pain sensibility present; absent superficial pain and tactile sensibility (absent protective sensibility), with abnormal sensations or severe pain, that prevents most activity	81–99
0	Absent sensibility, abnormal sensations, or severe pain that prevents all activity	100

B. Procedure

1	Identify the area of involvement using the cutaneous innervation chart (Figure 16–48) or the dermatome chart (Figure 16–49).
2	Identify the nerve structure(s) that innervate the area(s) (Table 16–12 and Figures 16–48, 16–49, and 16–50).
3	Grade the severity of the sensory deficit or pain according to the classification given above (a). Use clinical judgment to select the appropriate percentage from the range of values shown for each severity grade.
4	Find the maximum upper extremity impairment value due to sensory deficit or pain for each nerve structure involved: spinal nerves (Table 16–13), brachial plexus (Table 16–14), and major peripheral nerves (Table 16–15).
5	*Multiply* the severity of the sensory deficit by the maximum upper extremity impairment value to obtain the upper extremity impairment for each nerve structure involved.

From Cocchiarella L, Andersson GBJ (eds): Guides to the Evaluation of Permanent Impairment, 5th ed. Chicago, American Medical Association, 2001, p 482, with permission.

specific tables in the PNS sections of the AMA Guides. In previous editions of the AMA Guides these were Table 11 or Table 12 of Chapter 3. In the fifth edition of the AMA Guides, it is Table 16–11 of Chapter 16 (reprinted here as Table 35–2). Just as in Table 16–10 used for the sensory losses, the top half, or Section A, of Table 16–11 provides a clinical description for six different grades. These grades have specific definitions of muscle function that can be used to place the neural abnormality in a clinical category based on the findings of the clinical examination. The bottom half, or Section B, of Table 16–11, outlines the steps of the procedure that should be followed to calculate the impairment.

This clinical grading system uses the concept of manual muscle testing to determine the degree of loss of motor power in an extremity. The descriptions and standards for manual muscle testing are based on the standards that were set by the National Foundation of Infantile Paralysis. Through manual muscle testing, the examining physician uses clinical judgment to estimate the appropriate percentage of any motor deficit or loss of power in a muscle or muscle group from the dysfunctioning nerve. A normal muscle will contract and be capable of moving an extremity through its full range of motion with full resistance. When examining an individual and reviewing medical records, it should be remembered that there can be significant differences in the grading of muscle strength loss or power loss from one examiner to the next.

Each grade of Section A in Table 16–11 has a range of percent motor deficit, which is the range for the percentage given within each grade of the table that deals with motor and loss of power deficits. In this clinical grading system the grades are related to the results of manual muscle testing, and there are no additional objective, functional strength measurements, such as a Jamar hand dynamometer, a pinch gauge, or isometric or isokinetic testing, used for this process. Medical studies have shown that manual muscle testing grading results from one examination to the next in the same person are the most consistent when done by an experienced physician. One fault in the manual muscle testing system brought out in these studies is that the grade that the experienced physician selects in a particular person may be the same and consistent from one examination to the next, but the grade and percentages might have significant variation from one physician to another in the same person. Although objective testing that is performed using the Jamar, pinch gauge, isometric equipment, or isokinetic equipment has some advantages, these devices have limitations in terms of their ability to test specific nerves, muscles, or muscle groups.

Just like the sensory loss process used in Table 16–10, the examining physician must use clinical judgment to place the nerve injury in the appropriate grade. To determine the appropriate grade the physician uses the manual muscle testing system. After the clinical grade category is determined, the physician must then estimate the appropriate percentage within the range of motor deficit percentage values shown for that grade for the loss of function of the damaged nerve. The maximum percentage value in a grade should not be given automatically.

One should carefully review the design and definitions of the grades in Table 16–11. Based on the clinical descriptions and classifications of each grade that are found in Table 16–11, most patients will fall into a Grade 4 classification, because Grade 4 is defined as "Complete active range of motion against gravity with some resistance." The percentage range that can be given for a Grade 4 is 1% to 25%. If the physician finds on clinical

TABLE 35–2

Determining Impairment of the Upper Extremity Due to Motor and Loss-of-Power Deficits Resulting From Peripheral Nerve Disorders Based on Individual Muscle Rating

A. Classification

Grade	Description of Muscle Function	% Motor Deficit
5	Complete active range of motion against gravity with full resistance	0
4	Complete active range of motion against gravity with some resistance	1–25
3	Complete active range of motion against gravity only, without resistance	26–50
2	Complete active range of motion with gravity eliminated	51–75
1	Evidence of slight contractility; no joint movement	76–99
0	No evidence of contractility	100

B. Procedure

1	Identify the motion involved, such as flexion, extension, etc.
2	Identify the muscle(s) performing the motion and the motor nerve(s) involved.
3	Grade the severity of motor deficit of individual muscles according to the classification given above.
4	Find the maximum impairment of the upper extremity due to motor deficit for each nerve structure involved: spinal nerves (Table 16–13), brachial plexus (Table 16–14), and major peripheral nerves (Table 16–15).
5	Multiply the severity of the motor deficit by the maximum impairment value to obtain the upper extremity impairment for each structure involved.

From Cocchiarella L, Andersson GBJ (eds): Guides to the Evaluation of Permanent Impairment, 5th ed. Chicago, American Medical Association, 2001, p 484, with permission.

evaluation that the examinee is capable of providing complete active range of motion against resistance, the maximum relative value for Grade 4 that is used to determine the final percent for the nerve loss would be 25%. The clinical decision that the physician has to make is what percentage to use out of the range of 1% to 25%.

Grade 3 from Table 16–11 is defined as "Complete active range of motion against gravity only, without resistance." The range of values for the percent motor deficit is 26% to 50%. Grade 2 is defined as "Complete active range of motion with gravity eliminated," and the range is 51% to 75%. Grade 1 is defined as "Evidence of slight contractility; no joint movement," and a range of 76% to 99% is used. Grade 0 is defined as "No evidence of contractility," with a 100% deficit value. Based on these clinical descriptions, a final maximal percent motor deficit value greater than 25% from Section A of Table 16–11 is used only when the examinee falls into clinical Grade 3 or worse.

For instance, if on the physical examination the person can provide range of motion against gravity with some resistance, but there appears to be a 60% loss of strength or power in the specific muscle being tested, then the maximum value used for that clinical grade from Section A of Table 16–11 would be 15% (25% × 60%) and not 60%. A 60% value from Section A of Table 16–11 would be used to represent a higher grade of nerve damage in Table 16–11, which is Grade 2, defined as "Complete active range of motion with gravity eliminated." Using the 60% value as the final percent motor deficit value for a Grade 4 patient gives an excessively high impairment value to the individual with a Grade 4 muscle function, whereas on a comparative basis it diminishes the impairment in an individual with the more severe Grade 2 loss of muscle function.

CALCULATING THE IMPAIRMENT

Whether dealing with a spinal nerve root injury, a plexus injury, or a major peripheral nerve injury to the upper or lower extremity, the method of using the various tables in the PNS sections of the AMA Guides to determine the final impairment rating is the same. As discussed, the bottom half, or Section B, of Tables 16–10 and 16–11 outlines the steps of the procedure that should be followed to calculate the impairment due to the sensory and motor losses. Whether one is determining impairment from a sensory loss or motor loss, the basic approach is the same in the use of both tables. As discussed, the area of involvement of the sensory loss or the motor deficit is identified through clinical examination and using the appropriate cutaneous innervation charts, dermatome charts, and motor innervation charts provided in the Guides reprinted here as Figures 35–1 through 35–4 and Tables 35–1 and 35–2. The severity of the sensory deficits or motor deficits is then graded and given a percentage, based on the rating classification that is present in Section A of Table 16–10 and Table 16–11.

Each spinal nerve root, plexus, and major peripheral nerve structure has a "maximum % impairment" value assigned to it for its maximum functional contribution to the upper or lower extremity. Tables 16–13, 16–14, 16–15, and 17–37 give the maximum relative value percentages for the importance in the sensory and motor functions of the extremities of each nerve root, plexus, or major peripheral nerve structure (Tables 35–5, 35–6, and 35–7). Once the clinical percentage of loss of function from Section A has been determined, this percentage has to be multiplied times whatever the maximum value percentage is for that particular nerve structure in order to obtain the final impairment percentage. It should be noted that these final impairment percentages are in upper and lower extremity impairments, and they should be converted to a final whole person impairment.

Table 16–13 (Table 35–5) is used to obtain the maximum upper extremity impairment values due to a sensory deficit or pain or motor deficit due to an injury to individual spinal nerves. This table gives relative values for the spinal nerves C5–T1. Table 16–14 (Table 35–6) gives the maximum upper extremity impairment values due to a unilateral sensory or motor deficit in the brachial plexus. Table 16–15 (Table 35–7) is used to obtain the maximum values due to a unilateral sensory or motor deficit in the major peripheral nerves of the upper extremities. Table 17–37 is used to obtain the relative values for injuries to the major peripheral nerves in the lower extremities.

■ A 25-year-old man sustained a deep laceration to the radial side of the distal left forearm, which required surgical exploration. The soft tissues and a median nerve laceration were repaired. Two years later, he has healed well and returned to work. He complains of some strength loss with certain grasping and pinching type activities using the left hand. He also states that the sensation in the left thumb, index, and middle fingers on the palmar aspects is "not quite the same as the right." He denies problems in performing activities owing to the sensory loss and does not have any other complaints.

On examination he complains of minimal but consistent decreased sensation to light touch and pinprick in the left thumb, index, and middle fingers compared to the left ring and little fingers. Semmes-Weinstein monofilament testing has a similar abnormal pattern. There is decreased opposition strength on physical examination, slight wasting of the thenar muscles, and abnormal electromyographic testing of the thenar muscles in the left hand. There are no other physical abnormalities in the left upper extremity. ■

The procedure described in Section B of Table 16–10 is followed to determine the sensory impairment. Based on the history and the clinical findings of minimal problems due to the sensory loss, the claimant is placed in a

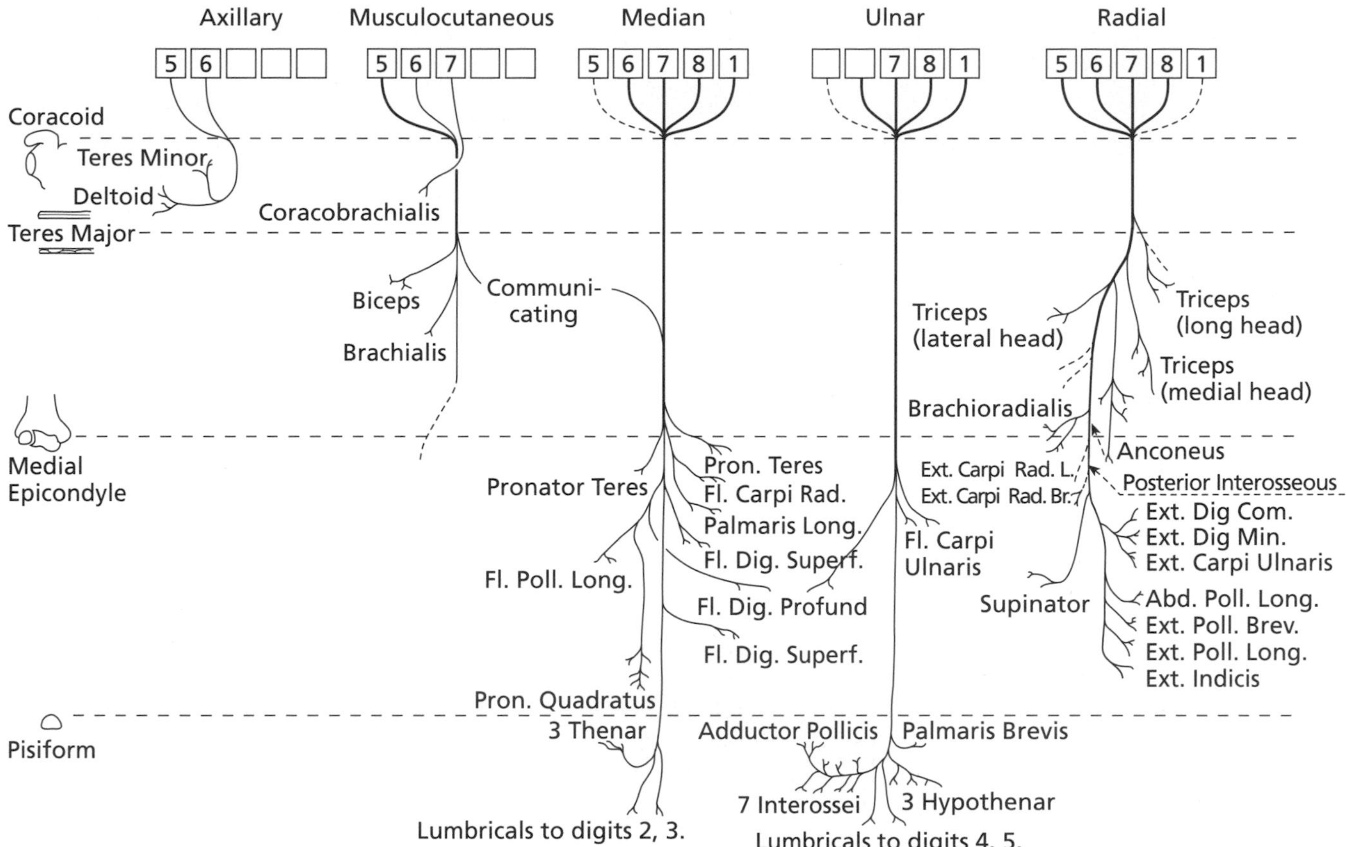

Figure 35–1. Motor innervation of the upper extremity. (From Swanson AB, de Groot Swanson G: Evaluation of permanent impairment in the hand and upper extremity. In Cocchiarella L, Andersson GBJ [eds]: Guides to the Evaluation of Permanent Impairment, 5th ed. Chicago, American Medical Association, 2001, p 487, with permission.)

Grade 4 classification in Section A of Table 16–10. Grade 4 has a 1% to 25% range allowed in the column for the percent sensory deficit. The examining physician has latitude in the percentage that can be chosen within this range. In this case a grade of 5% is chosen.

Returning to the procedure described in Section B of Table 16–10, the physician examines the middle section of Table 16–15 to find the nerve and region involved. In this case the section “Median nerve below midforearm” is used because of the level of the original laceration injury. From this section the physician obtains the maximum percent upper extremity impairment from the “Sensory deficit or pain” column of Table 16–15. In this case the value is 39%. This value is based on the concept that the “median nerve below midforearm” is considered to have 39% of the upper extremity sensory function.

The 5% for the value from Section A of Table 16–10 is multiplied by the 39% from Table 16–15 for a 2% upper extremity impairment due to the sensory loss and pain.

Similar to the sensory calculation, the procedure described in Section B of Table 16–11 is followed to determine the strength or power impairment. Based on the patient’s history and the clinical findings, he is placed in a Grade 4 classification in Section A of Table 16–11. Grade 4 has a 1% to 25% range allowed in the column for the percent motor deficit. As is true in the sensory impairment, the examining physician has latitude in the percentage that can be chosen within this range of 1% to 25%. In this case a grade of 10% is chosen, because of the significant clinical findings of thenar muscle wasting and electromyographic abnormalities.

Returning to the procedure described in Section B of Table 16–11, the physician again consults the middle section of Table 16–15 and the section “Median nerve below midforearm” because of the level of the original laceration injury. From this section the physician obtains the maximum percent upper extremity impairment from the “Motor deficit” column of Table 16–15. In this case the value is 10%. This 10% is given for the maximum value that the “Median nerve below midforearm” has in terms of the upper extremity motor function.

The 10% for the value from Section A of Table 16–11 is multiplied by the 10% from Table 16–15 for a 1% upper extremity impairment due to the motor loss.

The 2% upper extremity impairment due to the sensory loss and pain is combined with the 1% upper

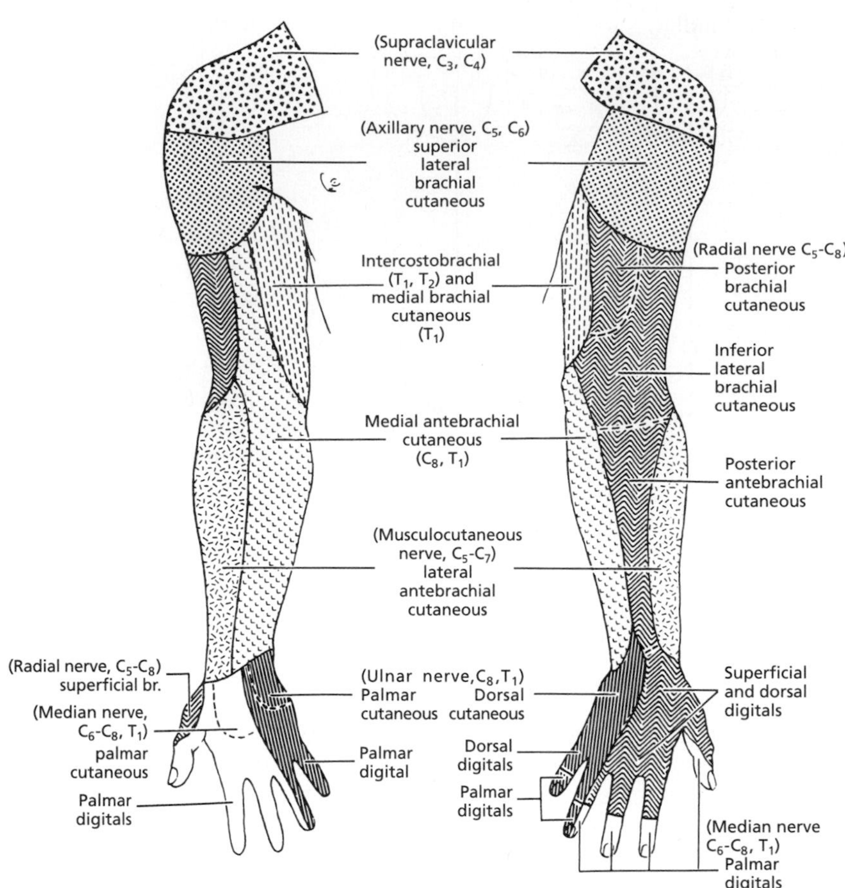

Figure 35–2. Cutaneous innervation of the upper extremity and related peripheral nerves and roots. (From Cocchiarella L, Andersson GBJ [eds]: Guides to the Evaluation of Permanent Impairment, 5th ed. Chicago, American Medical Association, 2001, p 488, with permission.)

extremity impairment due to the strength loss to give a total of a 3% upper extremity impairment. This converts to a 2% whole person impairment using Table 16–3 from Chapter 16 in the Guides.

SPECIAL POINTS TO CONSIDER

The tables in the peripheral nerve section of the AMA Guides use the concept of an alteration of sensibility. When evaluating the impairment from peripheral nerve dysfunction, it is not appropriate to give an impairment rating of 0% just because the individual has a normal static two-point discrimination test. Even though the alteration of sensibility as a result of a peripheral nerve dysfunction may result in a final whole person impairment rating value that is only one or two percentage points, this does not mean that the impairment is insignificant or should not be given. The sensory exam of the physical exam is very subjective in

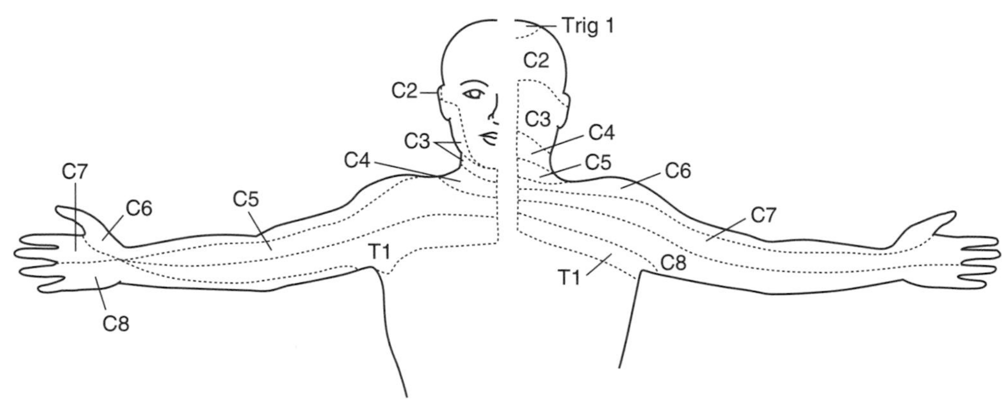

Figure 35–3. Dermatomes of the upper limb. (From Cocchiarella L, Andersson GBJ [eds]: Guides to the Evaluation of Permanent Impairment, 5th ed. Chicago, American Medical Association, 2001, p 490, with permission.)

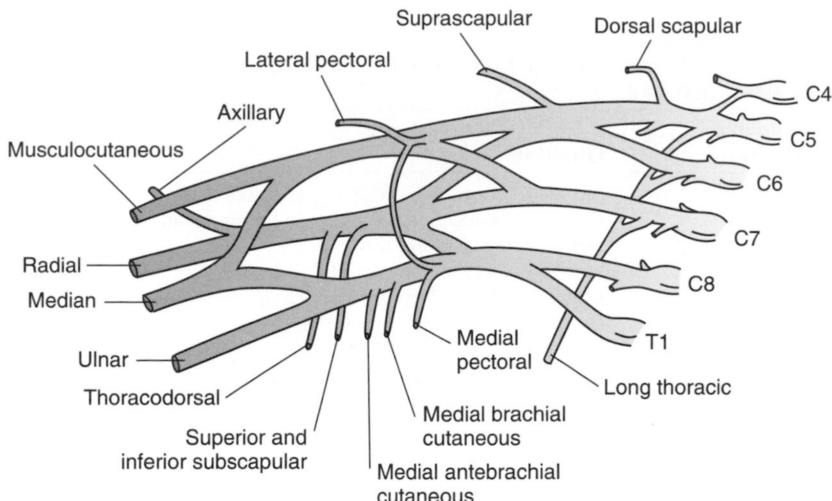

Figure 35–4. The brachial plexus. (From Cocchiarella L, Andersson GBJ [eds]: Guides to the Evaluation of Permanent Impairment, 5th ed. Chicago, American Medical Association, 2001, p 490, with permission.)

nature, and even some of the sensory testing parts of the electrodiagnostic testing performed with the needle and surface electromyographic tests are subjective in nature. If the other areas of the electrodiagnostic testing demonstrate additional objective evidence of compression or damage of a peripheral nerve, such as nerve conduction velocity testing demonstrating significant delay in the median nerve through the carpal tunnel, these objective findings can be correlated with the results of the physical exam. Even though there might be a normal static two-point discrimination test on physical examination, a sensibility loss in a defined anatomic pathway of the altered peripheral nerve that can be documented on a consistent, objective basis should be given an impairment rating using the appropriate peripheral nerve tables.

Although an individual may have a diagnosis of carpal tunnel syndrome, there are many clinical presentations of compression of the median nerve in the volar aspect of the wrist. When there are positive clinical findings of nerve dysfunction and abnormalities on nerve conduction study, the impairment is calculated as in the example using Tables 16–10, 16–11, and 16–15. If after surgery the clinical examination has normal sensibility and opposition strength testing findings, but there are abnormal motor latencies or electromyographic testing of the involved thenar muscles, a maximum 5% upper extremity impairment rating may be given. If the physical examination, sensibility studies, and nerve studies are normal, then impairment rating will be 0%.

Significant diseases of or injuries to the major peripheral nerves can create loss of strength and loss of motion of the joints of the extremities. The evaluating physician must be cautious not to give multiple impairment values for the same injury, which would result in an excessive final impairment rating. For instance, damage to the median nerve in the distal forearm can not only alter the sensory function of the digits of the hand, but also can affect the range of motion of the thumb and the strength measurements of the involved hand. In this instance of a median nerve injury, the final impairment rating should only be based on the value calculated using the tables and graphs of the peripheral nerve sections of the AMA Guides. The impairment values in these tables for damage to a peripheral nerve take into account the associated impairments, such as range of motion loss, strength loss, and pain. The impairment values from the other sections of the AMA Guides that are used specifically for loss of strength or loss of range of motion in the upper or lower extremities should not be used or combined when the injury is to the PNS. If an impairment value is given from all the different sections, an excessive impairment rating will result for the same disease or injury to the peripheral nerve structure.

An exception to this principle is when the extremity has a loss of range of motion in the joints that is due to a separate injury or medical condition. In this clinical situation it is appropriate to combine the impairment from the range of motion loss or strength loss with the impairment that has resulted from the peripheral nerve damage.

COMPLEX REGIONAL PAIN SYNDROME

Individuals with documented complex regional pain syndrome (CRPS)/reflex sympathetic dystrophy (RSD) are given an impairment rating using Section 13.8, Section 16.5e, and Section 17.2m of the fifth edition of the AMA Guides (Tables 35–8 through 35–10). These sections are new and were not present in prior editions of the AMA Guides. Unfortunately, these sections are not consistent

TABLE 35–3

Origins and Functions of the Peripheral Nerves of the Upper Extremity Emanating From the Brachial Plexus

Nerves of Plexus	Primary Branches	Secondary Branches	Function
Muscular branches	Unnamed		Motor to longus colli, scalenes, and subclavius
Dorsal scapular (C5)			Motor to rhomboideus major and minor, levator scapulae
Long thoracic (C5, 6, 7)			Motor to serratus anterior
Suprascapular (C5, 6)			Motor to supraspinatus and infraspinatus
Lateral pectoral (C5, 6, 7)			Motor to pectoralis major and minor
Medial pectoral (C8, T1)			Motor to pectoralis major and minor
Upper subscapular (C5, 6)			Motor to subscapularis
Lower subscapular (C5, 6)			Motor to teres major and subscapularis
Thoracodorsal (± C6, C7, 8)			Motor to latissimus dorsi
Medial brachial cutaneous (T1)			Sensory to anteromedial surface of arm (with intercostobrachial)
Intercostobrachial (T2)			Sensory to posteromedial surface of arm (with medial brachial cutaneous)
Medial antebrachial cutaneous (C8, T1)			Sensory to anterocentral surface of arm, anteromedial half of forearm, and posteromedial third of elbow, forearm, and wrist
Musculocutaneous (C5, 6, 7)	Unnamed		Motor to coracobrachialis, biceps brachil, brachialis
	Lateral antebrachial cutaneous		Sensory to anterolateral half and posterolateral third of forearm
Axillary (C5, C6)	Teres minor branch		Motor to teres minor
	Anterior		Motor to deltoid (middle and anterior thirds)
	Posterior	Muscular branches	Motor to deltoid (posterior third)
		Upper lateral brachial cutaneous	Sensory over lower half of deltoid
Radial (C5, 6, 7, 8 ± T1)	Unnamed		Motor to triceps brachii, brachialis (lateral part), brachioradialis, extensor carpi radialis longus, anconeus
	Ulnar collateral		Motor to triceps brachii (medial head)
	Posterior brachial cutaneous		Sensory to distal posterocentral surface of arm as far as olecranon
	Inferior lateral brachial cutaneous		Sensory to distal posterolateral surface of arm and elbow
	Posterior antebrachial cutaneous		Sensory to posterocentral surface of forearm
	Superficial terminal	Dorsal branches	Sensory to posterolateral half of wrist and hand
		Dorsal digitals (5 branches)	Sensory to dorsum of thumb, index, middle, and ring (radial half) fingers up to middle phalanx
	Deep terminal (posterior interosseous)	Unnamed	Motor to extensor carpi radialis brevis, and supinator
		Superficial branch	Motor to extensor digitorum communis, extensor digiti minimi, extensor carpi ulnaris
		Deep branch	Motor to extensor pollicis longus, extensor pollicis brevis, abductor pollicis longus, extensor indicis proprius Sensory to wrist joint capsule

From Cocchiarella L, Andersson GBJ (eds): Guides to the Evaluation of Permanent Impairment, 5th ed. Chicago, American Medical Association, 2001, p 485, with permission.

TABLE 35–4

Origins and Functions of the Peripheral Nerves of the Upper Extremity Emanating From the Brachial Plexus

Nerves of Plexus	Primary Branches	Secondary Branches	Function
Median (± C5, C6, 7, 8, T1)	Unnamed	Cubital fossa and forearm branches	Motor to pronator teres, flexor carpi radialis, palmaris longus, flexor digitorum superficialis
	Anterior interosseous		Motor to radial half of flexor digitorum profundus (index and middle fingers), flexor policis longus, pronator quadratus
	Palmar cutaneous		Sensory to central proximal surface of palm
	Thenar muscular		Motor to abductor pollicis brevis, flexor pollicis brevis (superficial head), opponens pollicis
	Common palmar radial digital	1st lumbrical branch	Motor to 1st lumbrical
		Proper palmar digitals (3 branches)	Sensory to 1st web space (palmar), palmar, and distal dorsal surfaces of thumb (both sides) and index (radial side)
	Common palmar central digital	2nd lumbrical branch	Motor to 2nd lumbrical
		Proper palmar digitals (2 branches)	Sensory to 2nd web space (palmar), palmar, and distal dorsal surfaces of contiguous sides of index and middle fingers
	Common palmar ulnar digital	Proper palmar digitals (2 branches)	Sensory to 3rd web space (palmar), palmar, and distal dorsal surfaces of contiguous sides of middle and ring fingers
Ulnar (± C7, C8, T1)	Unnamed	Forearm branches	Motor to flexor carpi ulnaris, ulnar half of flexor digitorum profundus (ring and little fingers)
	Palmar cutaneous		Sensory to ulnar surface of palm and wrist
	Dorsal cutaneous	Dorsal branches	Sensory to ulnar dorsum of wrist and hand
		Dorsal digitals (3 branches)	Sensory to dorsum of ring finger (ulnar proximal half), little finger (up to nail root), and 4th web space
	Superficial palmar	Palmaris brevis br	Motor to palmaris brevis
		Proper palmar digitals (3 branches)	Sensory to palmar and distal dorsal surface of ring (ulnar half), and little finger (both sides)
	Deep palmar		Motor to adductor pollicis, flexor pollicis brevis (deep head), abductor digiti minimi, flexor digiti minimi brevis, opponens digiti minimi, 3rd and 4th lumbricals, all interossei

From Cocchiarella L, Andersson GBJ (eds): Guides to the Evaluation of Permanent Impairment, 5th ed. Chicago, American Medical Association, 2001, p 486, with permission.

in their discussions of the pathology, the methods of clinically defining the disease process, or the way the impairment rating is calculated in individuals with complaints of pain in the upper and lower extremities.

Table 16–16 (Table 35–8), found in Section 16.5e, outlines objective criteria for the diagnosis of CRPS. In order to make a diagnosis of CRPS, at least eight of these objective physical or diagnostic findings must be present concurrently. This table can be very useful to the examining physician who needs a standardized, reproducible method for documenting the presence or absence of CRPS in a particular individual.

Section 16.5e outlines steps used to determine upper extremity impairment when CRPS is present. Section 13.8 has Table 13–22 (Table 35–9) to rate the upper extremity, but this table is used to rate chronic pain in one extremity. Activities of daily living (ADLs) are used as a basis for the impairment using Table 13–22, and the complaints and limitations of ADLs are self-reported by the individual with chronic pain. In Section 13.8, the statement is made that Table 13–15 (Table 35–10) should be used for a lower extremity impairment for "causalgia, posttraumatic neuralgia, or RSD." Table 13–15 has "Criteria for rating impairments due to station and gait disorders." The examining physician calculates the impairment using the self-reported complaints and limitations in ADLs by the individual with chronic pain.

It is unfortunate that these differences in the various chapters of the AMA Guides exist in the method of rating the claimant with complaints of pain. Section 16.5e and Table 16–16 are excellent additions to the AMA Guides, providing standards and guidelines that can be modified by the examining physician are used to give an impairment in the upper and lower extremity in an individual with CRPS and complaints of pain.

TABLE 35–5

Maximum Upper Extremity Impairment Due to Unilateral Sensory or Motor Deficits of Individual Spinal Nerves or to Combined 100% Deficits

Spinal Nerve	Maximum % Upper Extremity Impairment Due to: Sensory Deficit or Pain*	Motor Deficit†	*Combined* Motor/Sensory Deficits
C5	5	30	34
C6	8	35	40
C7	5	35	38
C8	5	45	48
T1	5	20	24

* See Table 16–10a to grade sensory deficit or pain.
† See Table 16–11a to grade motor deficit.
From Cocchiarella L, Andersson GBJ (eds): Guides to the Evaluation of Permanent Impairment, 5th ed. Chicago, American Medical Association, 2001, p 489, with permission.

TABLE 35–6

Maximum Upper Extremity Impairments Due to Unilateral Sensory or Motor Deficits of Brachial Plexus or to Combined 100% Deficits

Brachial Plexus and Trunks	Maximum % Upper Extremity Impairment Due to: Sensory Deficit or Pain*	Motor Deficit†	Combined Motor/ Sensory Deficits
Brachial plexus (C5 through C8, T1)	100	100	100
Upper trunk (C5, C6, Erb-Duchenne)	25	75	81
Middle trunk (C7)	5	35	38
Lower trunk (C8, T1, Déjerine-Klumpke)	20	70	76

* See Table 16–10a to grade sensory deficit or pain.
† See Table 16–11a to grade motor deficit.
From Cocchiarella L, Andersson GBJ (eds): Guides to the Evaluation of Permanent Impairment, 5th ed. Chicago, American Medical Association, 2001, p 490, with permission.

TABLE 35–7

Maximum Upper Extremity Impairment Due to Unilateral Sensory or Motor Deficits or to Combined 100% Deficits of the Major Peripheral Nerves

Nerve	**Maximum % Upper Extremity Impairment Due to: Sensory Deficit or Pain**	**Motor Deficit†**	**Combined Motor and Sensory Deficits**
Pectorals (medial and lateral)	0	5	5
Axillary	5	35	38
Dorsal scapular	0	5	5
Long thoracic	0	15	15
Medial antebrachial cutaneous	5	0	5
Medial brachial cutaneous	5	0	5
Median (above midforearm)	39	44	66
Median (anterior interosseous branch)	0	15	15
Median (below midforearm)	39	10	45
Radial palmar digital of thumb	7	0	7
Ulnar palmar digital of thumb	11	0	11
Radial palmar digital of index finger	5	0	5
Ulnar palmar digital of index finger	4	0	4
Radial palmar digital of middle finger	5	0	5
Ulnar palmar digital of middle finger	4	0	4
Radial palmar digital of ring finger	3	0	3
Musculocutaneous	5	25	29
Radial (upper arm with loss of triceps)	5	42	45
Radial (elbow with sparing of triceps)	5	35	38
Subscapulars (upper and lower)	0	5	5
Suprascapular	5	16	20
Thoracodorsal	0	10	10
Ulnar (above midforearm)	7	46	50
Ulnar (below midforearm)	7	35	40
Ulnar palmar digital of ring finger	2	0	2
Radial palmar digital of little finger	2	0	2
Ulnar palmar digital of little finger	3	0	3

* See Table 16–10a to grade sensory deficits or pain.
† See Table 16–11a to grade motor deficits.
From Cocchiarella L, Andersson GBJ (eds): Guides to the Evaluation of Permanent Impairment, 5th ed. Chicago, American Medical Association, 2001, p 492, with permission.

TABLE 35-8

Objective Diagnostic Criteria for CRPS (RSD and causalgia)

Local clinical signs

Vasomotor changes
- Skin color: mottled or cyanotic
- Skin temperature: cool
- Edema

Sudomotor changes
- Skin dry or overly moist

Trophic changes
- Skin texture: smooth, nonelastic
- Soft tissue atrophy: especially in fingertips
- Joint stiffness and decreased passive motion
- Nail changes: blemished, curved, talonlike
- Hair growth changes: fall out, longer, finer

Radiographic Signs

- Radiographs: trophic bone changes, osteoporosis
- Bone scan: findings consistent with CRPS

Interpretation

≥8 Probable CRPS
<8 No CRPS

From Cocchiarella L, Andersson GBJ (eds): Guides to the Evaluation of Permanent Impairment, 5th ed. Chicago, American Medical Associaiton, 2001, p 496, with permission.

TABLE 35-9

Criteria for Rating Impairment Related to Chronic Pain in One Upper Extremity

Class 1		Class 2		Class 3		Class 4	
Dominant Extremity 1% to 9% Impairment of the Whole Person	**Nondominant Extremity 1% to 4% Impairment of the Whole Person**	**Dominant Extremity 10% to 24% Impairment of the Whole Person**	**Nondominant Extremity 5% to 14% Impairment of the Whole Person**	**Dominant Extremity 25% to 39% Impairment of the Whole Person**	**Nondominant Extremity 15% to 29% Impairment of the Whole Person**	**Dominant Extremity 40% to 60% Impairment of the Whole Person**	**Nondominant Extremity 30% to 45% Impairment of the Whole Person**
Individual can use the involved extremity for self-care, daily activities, and holding, but is limited in digital dexterity		Individual can use the involved extremity for self-care and can grasp and hold objects with difficulty,but has no digital dexterity		Individual can use the involved extremity but has difficulty with self-care activities		Individual cannot use the involved extremity for self-care or daily activities	

From Cocchiarella L, Andersson GBJ (eds): Guides to the Evaluation of Permanent Impairment, 5th ed. Chicago, American Medical Association, 2001, p 343, with permission.

TABLE 35-10

Criteria for Rating Impairments Due to Station and Gait Disorders

Class 1: 1% to 9% Impairment of the Whole Person	Class 2: 10% to 19% Impairment of the Whole Person	Class 3: 20% to 39% Impairment of the Whole Person	Class 4: 40% to 60% Impairment of the Whole Person
Rises to standing position; walks, but has difficulty with elevations, grades, stairs, deep chairs, and long distances	Rises to standing position; walks some distance with difficulty and without assistance, but is limited to level surfaces	Rises and maintains standing position with difficulty; cannot walk without assistance	Cannot stand without help, mechanical support, and/or an assistive device

From Cocchiarella L, Andersson GBJ (eds): Guides to the Evaluation of Permanent Impairment, 5th ed. Chicago, American Medical Association, 2001, p 336, with permission.

Bibliography

American Academy of Neurology: Clinical Utility of Surface EMG. St. Paul, MN, American Academy of Neurology, 2000.

Bell JA: Sensibility evaluation. In Hunter J, Schneider L, Macklin E (eds): Rehabilitation of the Hand. Philadelphia, Mosby, 1978, pp 278–279.

Callahan AD: Sensibility assessment: Prerequisites and techniques for nerve lesions in continuity and nerve lacerations. In Hunter J, Macklin E, Callahan AD (eds): Rehabilitation of the Hand, 5th ed. Philadelphia, Mosby, 1995, pp 129–152.

Cocchiarella L, Andersson GBJ (eds): Guides to the Evaluation of Permanent Impairment, 5th ed. Chicago, American Medical Association, 2001.

Doege TC, Houston TP (eds): Guides to the Evaluation of Permanent Impairment, 4th ed. Chicago, American Medical Association, 1993.

Engelberg AL (ed): Guides to the Evaluation of Permanent Impairment, 3rd ed. Chicago, American Medical Association, 1988.

Kendall H, McCreary EK, Provance P: Muscles: Testing and Function, 4th ed. Baltimore, Williams & Wilkins, 1993.

Moberg E: Sensibility in reconstructive limb surgery. In Fredericks S, Brody GS (eds): Symposium on the Neurologic Aspects of Plastic Surgery. St. Louis, Mosby, 1978, pp 30–35.

Nathan PA, Keniston RC, Myers LD, et al: Natural history of median nerve sensory conduction in industry: Relationship to symptoms and carpal tunnel syndrome in 588 hands over 11 years. Muscle Nerve 21:711–721, 1998.

Omer GE Jr: Sensation and sensibility in the upper extremity. Clin Orthop 104:30–36, 1974.

Redmond DM, Rivner MH: False positive electrodiagnostic tests in carpal tunnel syndrome. Muscle Nerve 11:511–517, 1988.

Salerno DF, Franzblau A, Werner RA, et al: Median and ulnar nerve conduction studies among workers: Normative values. Muscle Nerve 21:999–1005, 1998.

Stokes HM: The seriously injured hand: Weakness of grip. J Occup Med 25:683–684, 1983.

Tubiana R, Valentin P: Opposition of the thumb. Surg Clin North Am 48:967–977, 1968.

C H A P T E R

36

Visual Impairment

AUGUST COLENBRANDER, MD

Ophthalmology has experienced many firsts in the practice of medicine, especially in the area of impairment evaluation. After the invention of the ophthalmoscope in 1851, ophthalmology became the first organ-based specialty. Impairment evaluation received early attention. In the 1890s, Magnus, in Germany, developed detailed scales.[1] In 1925, the AMA Committee for the Compensation of Eye Injuries[2] adopted a new set of compensation scales for vision loss that were based on an employability study by Snell[3] and a mathematical formula developed by Snell and Sterling.[4] Through its fourth edition, the Vision chapter in the AMA Guides[5] has been based on Snell's Visual Efficiency scale. From 1925 to 2000, however, insights into disability have changed while numerous revisions have led to internal inconsistencies. The Vision chapter in the fifth edition has undergone radical changes. A detailed listing of the steps and procedures is provided in Chapter 12 (the Visual System) of the AMA Guides[19] and is not repeated in this chapter. The purpose of this chapter is to explain the underlying philosophy and the consequences of the changes that were made. The discussion assumes that the Vision chapter of the AMA Guides is available for reference.

ASPECTS OF VISION LOSS

As has been described in the introductory chapters, ability loss can be approached from various points of view. Just as all aspects of a complex sculpture cannot be captured in a single snapshot, so must the description of vision loss, with all its consequences, take into account multiple aspects.

The most commonly used set of aspects[6] is the one promoted by the World Health Organization (WHO)'s International Classification of Impairments, Disabilities and Handicaps (ICIDH).[7] This publication, intended as a companion to WHO's International Classification of Diseases (ICD-9[8] and ICD-9-CM[9]), was prepared in the 1970s and published in 1980. Its successor is the International Classification of Functioning (ICF[10]), published in 2001. The aspects and ranges are also the subject of a recent (2002) standard of the International Council of Opthalmology (ICO).[10a] It is interesting to note, however, that the terminology of impairment, disability, and handicap had already been used in a report on Rehabilitation Codes[11] prepared in 1968 for the predecessor of the National Eye Institute. This appears to be another instance in which developments in ophthalmology were ahead of those in other specialties.

The four most important aspects of vision loss are summarized in Table 36–1. Although these aspects can be applied to any functional loss, this chapter mainly discusses their application to vision loss. The first two aspects refer to the organ system. The first aspect is that of anatomic and structural changes (diseases, injuries, anomalies, etc.). The second aspect is that of functional changes at the organ level, such as visual acuity loss and visual field loss. These aspects are the traditional domain of clinical ophthalmology. The third and fourth aspects describe how these changes affect the individual. The third aspect describes the skills and abilities of the individual. This would include such items as reading skills, mobility skills, and daily living skills (ADL; activities of daily living; also termed impairments). The last aspect points to the social and economic consequences of a loss of abilities. This might include effects such as the loss of a driver's license, loss of earning capacity, or loss of social contacts (or disabilities; see Chapter 1 for definitions).

TABLE 36–1
Aspects of Vision Loss

Variable	The Organ		The Person	
Aspects	Structural change Anatomic change	Functional change at the organ level	Skills, abilities of the individual	Social, economic consequences
Negative terms		Impairment	Disability	Handicap
Neutral terms	Health condition	Organ function	Activities	Participation
Application to Vision	Eye diseases Disorders, injuries	"Visual functions" measured quantitatively	"Functional vision" described qualitatively	Vision-related Quality of life
Examples	Corneal scar Cataract Retinal degeneration Optic atrophy	Visual acuity Visual field Color vision Dark adaptation	Reading skills Mobility skills Daily living skills	Social isolation Job loss Loss of earnings

Vision loss can be approached from different points of view (see text). The different aspects are sometimes described by different names.

Anatomic and Structural Changes

The first aspect describes the underlying disorders or diseases at the organ level. Describing only the deviations from normal is a negative approach. The term "health conditions" is a more neutral term that could include the normal condition. Ophthalmoscopy and slit-lamp biomicroscopy have given ophthalmology tools to describe anatomic changes in more detail than is possible for many other organ systems. Yet these descriptors give relatively poor clues to the severity of their functional consequences.

This aspect is extensively coded in ICD-9 and ICD-9-CM. Because these are classifications of diseases, normal conditions are referred to in an appendix. ICIDH used the term disorders to describe this aspect. ICF prefers the term structural change. This book uses the term impairment.

Visual Functions

The second aspect describes functional changes at the organ level. Visual functions are not limited to visual acuity and visual field, but also include functions such as contrast sensitivity, color vision, dark adaptation, and binocularity. The term impairment is commonly used to describe this aspect; like the term disease or disorder, it describes loss. In contrast, the general term organ function and the vision-specific term visual function are neutral terms. The distinction between negative and neutral terms has consequences for the use of scales. A scale of organ function (on which a higher value refers to better function) can easily include acuity levels that are better than standard vision (better than 20/20). An impairment scale (on which a higher value refers to lesser function) would require negative numbers to recognize such acuity levels. Here again, ophthalmology has developed unique tools that can measure organ functions, such as visual acuity and visual field, objectively and in great detail.

To describe this aspect, ICIDH used the term impairment. ICF uses the term functional change as well as the term impairment. The AMA Guides[19] also use the term impairment as does this book.

It is important to recognize that measurements of visual functions can be used for two purposes: to assist in diagnosing the underlying disorder or to estimate the functional consequences (see Fig. 36–1). This distinction has consequences for the choice of tests used; for example, tests such as electroretinography and visual evoked potentials are helpful in diagnosing the underlying condition, but are poor predictors of the functional consequences. Because visual acuity loss can have many different causes, visual acuity testing adds little to the differential diagnosis, but can help in estimating the impact on activities of daily living (ADL). The Ishihara color test is good at diagnosing even minor red-green deficiencies for genetic studies, but overestimates the functional consequences. The D15 color test, on the other hand, was designed to be insensitive to minor deficiencies and to detect only those that might have functional consequences. The discussion in this chapter is oriented toward the functional consequences.

Functional Vision

The third aspect reaches beyond the description of organ function by describing the skills and abilities of the individual. It describes how well the individual is able to perform certain activities. In the field of vision,

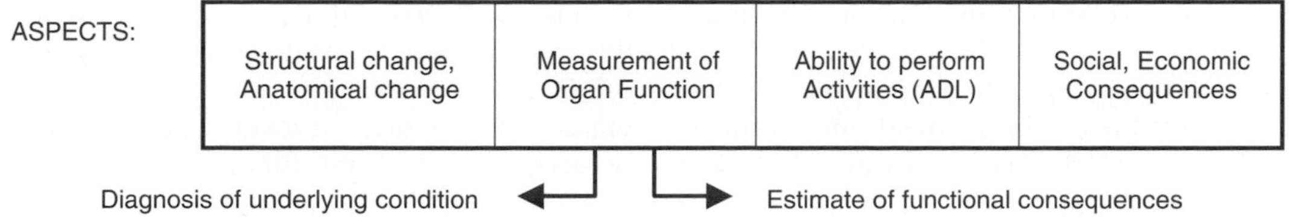

Figure 36–1. Use of visual function measurements. Different tests serve different purposes (see text).

the term functional vision is used to distinguish this aspect from the previous one (visual functions). Each descriptor for this aspect must have two parts: one specifying the activity and the other specifying the ability to perform it. In ICIDH, ability loss was described as disability. Its successor, ICF, discourages the use of negative terms and changed the heading for this aspect to the "Activities" aspect. In the AMA Guides,[19] the term *impairment* refers to organ function, whereas the term *impairment rating* refers to the functional vision aspect; i.e., an estimate of the ability to perform generic ADLs. Note that the concept of ability describes how well an individual can perform a certain activity. This is distinct from whether the individual actually does perform the activity.

Societal and Economic Consequences

The fourth and last aspect describes the societal and economic consequences for the individual caused by an impairment or by a loss of ability. This aspect is also referred to as quality of life. Whether one's quality of life is considered satisfactory or not depends in part on personal and societal expectations and demands. In ICIDH, this aspect was described as handicap and measured in terms of loss of independence; in ICF, it is described under the heading of participation which lists a variety of higher-order social functions. These terms describe two sides of the same coin: handicap refers to the barriers that need to be overcome, participation to the success in overcoming them. Here, again, it is important to differentiate between how well an individual can participate and how well the individual does participate. The story of Helen Keller is one example of how some people can achieve full participation in spite of extraordinary handicaps. Yet it is clearly not realistic to expect such performance from all individuals with a similar impairment.

The AMA scales aim at providing generalizable scales based on the estimated ability to perform generic daily living skills.[19] They do not extend to quality of life issues and to the environmental adaptations that can be made to improve the quality of life (including employability) of an individual. This does not mean, however, that such factors should not be mentioned in an evaluator's report.

INTERVENTIONS FOR REHABILITATION

The four aspects of vision loss are not independent. There is a chain of cause and effect, running from the left to the right, but the links are not rigid. The fact that rehabilitation is at all possible is a direct result of this flexibility. The art of rehabilitation is manipulating each of these links so that a given disorder results in the least possible handicap or the greatest possible participation. Different professionals must

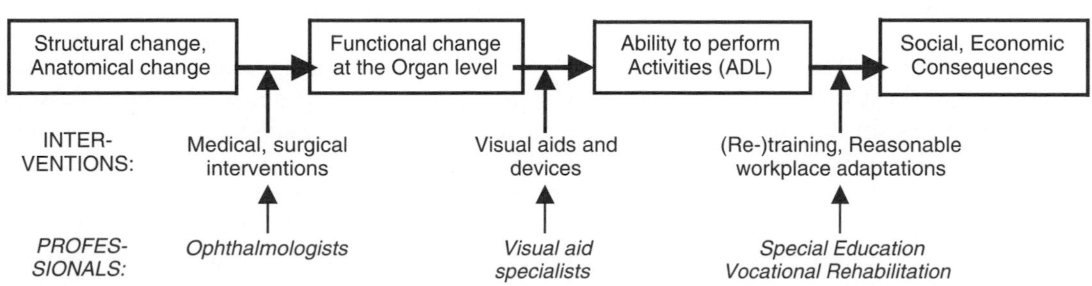

Figure 36–2. Various interventions. The links between the various aspects are flexible and can be influenced by various external interventions (see text).

contribute their expertise at various steps, as shown in Figure 36–2.

The first link, from anatomic changes to their functional effects, can be changed by medical and surgical interventions. For vision, this is the domain of the ophthalmologist. The AMA Guides discuss mainly permanent impairment; i.e., residual impairment after maximal medical improvement. The scales, however, could be used to characterize transient impairment as well.[19]

The next link, from visual functions to functional vision, can be influenced by the use of various vision enhancement and vision substitution devices. The most obvious form of vision enhancement is the use of magnification to restore reading ability. What constitutes effective vision enhancement may not be the same for all persons: some patients benefit from higher illumination levels; others, with glare sensitivity, do better with reduced light levels. For more severe vision loss, vision substitution skills may be needed, such as the use of Braille and talking books or the use of a long cane for mobility. This is the domain of visual aid specialists.

The last link, from the skills and abilities of the individual to their social and economic consequences, can be influenced by modifying the physical environment. Examples include curb cuts for wheelchair users, better lighting and contrast for individuals with vision loss, and reasonable workplace adaptations as required by the Americans with Disabilities Act (ADA). Another option is education aimed at changing the individual's capabilities and/or societal expectations; this may include retraining of the individual and/or job adaptations. This is the domain of special educators, counselors, and vocational specialists.

Recognizing the flexibility of the links shown in Figure 36–2 is crucial for an understanding of disability and rehabilitation. Not only is it this flexibility that makes rehabilitation possible, but the variable effect of rehabilitative interventions also makes it impossible to simply predict one aspect from the other in any individual case. Two patients with similar impairments (acuity, field) will have different abilities with regard to ADLs if one has access to visual aids and the other does not. Two patients with equal ability losses will achieve different levels of participation if one has access to a workplace where reasonable accommodations (as required by the ADA) have been made and the other does not. The best that can be done when producing tables like those in the AMA Guides[19] is to make statistical estimates. Magnus realized this a century ago when he called his work "rules for estimation."[1]

The wide array of possible interventions makes it mandatory that rehabilitation involves a team of different professionals. Figure 36–2 also makes it clear that the effects of their interventions must be measured with different yardsticks. Measurement of visual acuity and other visual functions can be used as an outcome measure for medical and surgical interventions. For the prescription of visual aids and other vision enhancement techniques, visual acuity and visual field are the starting point; the effect of these interventions must be measured by recording improved performance of ADL. Unfortunately, scales have not yet been developed to do this, although various efforts are underway. Retraining and job modifications may result in greater participation. Changes in this area (except earning potential) are even harder to measure objectively.

DISABILITY EVALUATION

The different points of view that can be used in disability evaluation affect the relative emphasis that is placed on the evaluation of different aspects.

The Social Security Act (SSA) defines disability as the inability to engage in any substantial gainful activities by reason of any medically determinable physical or mental impairment(s) which can be expected to result in death or which has lasted or can be expected to last for a continuous period of not less than 12 months.[20] This definition clearly addresses the economic consequences by evaluating the earning potential (aspect 4). It is a reasonable definition for the purpose of the law. Yet one should realize that the use of different terminologies may give rise to seemingly contradictory statements. For example, Helen Keller certainly had profound impairments (in the sense of ICIDH), yet she achieved full participation (in the sense of ICF) and would not have been considered disabled (for the purpose of the SSA, excepting, of course, the automatic qualifier of blindness).

Rehabilitation specialists and educators who prepare an individual rehabilitation plan are most interested in evaluating the various skills of the individual (aspect 3) so that rehabilitation efforts can be concentrated on those skills in which the individual is deficient. For this purpose, creating a visual ability profile is more useful than collapsing all information into a single number. This approach stresses the differences between individuals and takes into account the adjustments they have already made. On the other hand, an administrator who needs to assign a disability compensation package for vision loss may not be so interested in the adjustments different individuals have made. For benefit purposes it may be more desirable to give individuals, with the same loss, the same compensation so that individuals who have made good adjustments do not get penalized with lesser benefits. This approach is best served by calculating a single number that estimates the average impact on daily living skills (aspect 3) based on the measurement of visual acuity and visual field (aspect 2). The advantage of this approach is that the measurement of visual acuity and visual field can be much more objective than the direct assessment of vision-related daily living skills.

The difference in the two approaches is summarized in Figure 36–3. The AMA Guides[19] were constructed to support the last approach. As discussed, the fact that individual skills and skill differences are ignored means that the approach of the AMA Guides cannot be used for the determination of individual rehabilitation needs.

The AMA approach[19] makes the assignment of benefits a two-step procedure. The first step is the medical measurement of the impairment. This is the responsibility of the physician. The second step is the assignment of benefits. This is the responsibility of the plan administrator. This two-step procedure is different from Snell's visual efficiency scale, which tried to establish a direct link from visual acuity to employability in 1925.

Because two or more parties will be involved, it is of the utmost importance that they understand each other's responsibilities and the differences involved in the various approaches. Although the physician's primary responsibility is to accurately measure the impairment and to apply the formulas provided in the AMA Guides,[19] the physician may also be asked about rehabilitation and employment options, and should therefore have a basic familiarity with those issues as well (see Chapter on communication).

Administrative decisions for the same impairment may or may not be the same for different plans. A plan aimed at compensation for work-related injuries may pay a disability compensation, even if the individual is still gainfully employed. A plan aimed at providing compensation for loss of earnings would deny the claim of the same individual, because he or she is still gainfully employed.

TERMINOLOGY

To help various professionals to have an understanding of each other's roles and the use of shared terminology, this section lists various terms and the way in which they are used in various contexts (see also Chapter 1 for definitions).

Impairment—In this chapter, the term *impairment* is used to refer to functional changes at the organ level (visual functions); e.g., a cataract is an anatomic change—the resulting visual acuity loss is the impairment. Other texts, however, may also extend the term impairment to anatomic changes. *Impairment rating* is used in the AMA Guides[19] to indicate the impact of the

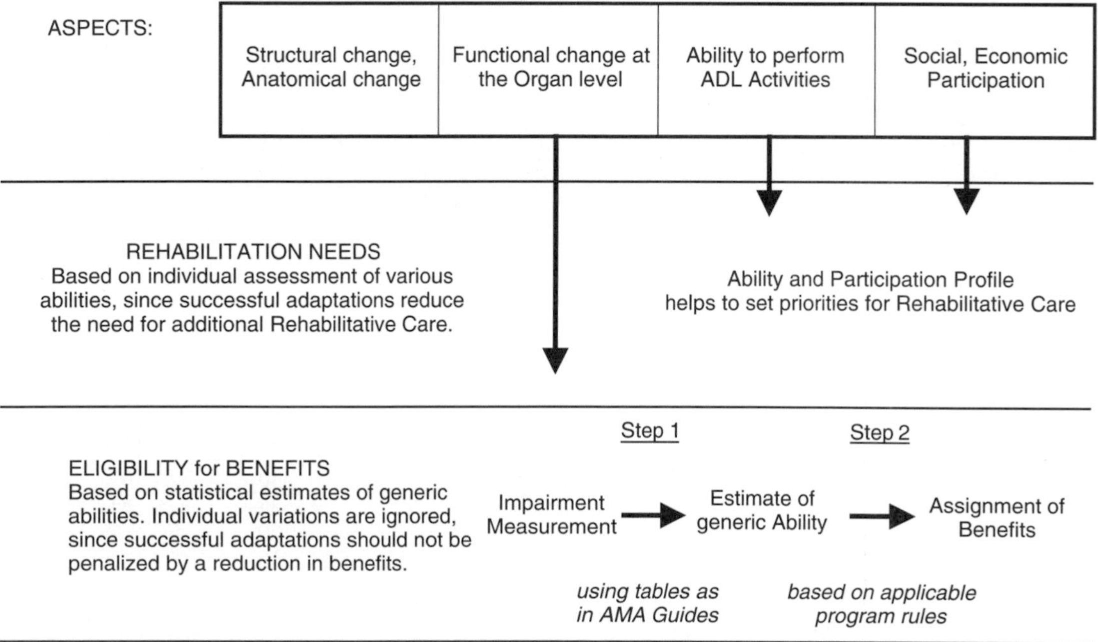

Figure 36–3. Rehabilitation needs versus eligibility for benefits. Disability and impairment evaluations are for different purposes and may choose to look at different aspects (see text).

impairment on the ability to perform daily living skills (functional vision). In the vision chapter, the estimated impact is primarily derived from the impairment measurement (visual acuity, visual field).

Disability—Use of this term is avoided in ICF, partly because it is a negative term and partly because it is used with many different meanings. *Having a disability* may be used as a synonym for having an impairment (aspect 2). *Being disabled* may refer to the fact that the individual is unable to perform certain ADLs (aspect 3). *Being on disability* may indicate that the individual receives benefits, one of the possible social consequences of an ability loss (aspect 4). Disablement is a term used in ICF to avoid the term disability. Curiously, its counterpart, enablement, which is the basis of rehabilitation, is never used in ICF. Visual efficiency was the name given to Snell's scale, which was used up to the fourth edition of the AMA Guides.[5] It aimed at providing a direct translation of visual acuity values to employability in 1925. Use of this scale is discontinued in the current, fifth edition.

Visual acuity score, visual field score—In the fifth edition,[20] these scores are used to translate the (nonlinear) results of visual acuity and visual field measurement to linear scores that can be used in calculations. They refer to the measurements made for each eye separately.

Functional acuity score, functional field score—These scores refer to the functional vision of the individual rather than the eye. They are calculated from the visual acuity score and visual field score. They estimate the impact of vision loss on daily living skills; i.e., on reading skills for the functional acuity score and on orientation and mobility skills for the functional field score. Because normal vision is binocular vision, calculation of the functional scores is weighted heavily in favor of binocular visual acuity and the binocular

TABLE 36-2

Functional Vision Scores versus Visual Efficiency Scores

		Visual Acuity			Visual Field			
ICD-9-CM Ranges		**Visual Acuity Score**	**Visual Efficiency Distance**	**Visual Efficiency Near**	**Average Radius (if Loss is Concentric)**	**Visual Field Score**	**Visual Efficiency (AMA)**	**Visual Efficiency (Esterman)**
Range of Normal Vision	20/125	110				110		
	20/16	105				105		
	20/20	100	100%	100%	60°	100	96%	89%
	20/25	95	95%	100%	55°	95	88%	83%
Near-normal Vision (mild loss)	20/32	90	90%	95%	50°	90	80%	77%
	20/40	85	85%	90%	45°	85	72%	69%
	20/50	80	75%	50%	40°	80	64%	61%
	20/63	75	65%	40%	35°	75	56%	53%
Moderate Low Vision	20/80	70	55%	20%	30°	70	48%	46%
	20/100	65	50%	15%	25°	65	40%	35%
	20/125	60	40%	10%	20°	60	32%	24%
	20/160	55	30%	5%	15°	55	24%	15%
Severe Low Vision	20/200	50	20%	2%	10°	50	16%	6%
	20/250	45			9°	45	14%	
	20/320	40	15%		8°	40	13%	
	20/400	35	10%		7°	35	11%	
Profound Low Vision	20/500	30			6°	30	10%	
	20/630	25			5°	25	8%	0%
	20/800	20	5%		4°	20	6%	
	20/1000	15			3°	15	4%	
Near-Blindness	20/1250	10			2°	10	2%	
	20/1600	5			1°	5		
	20/2000	0						
Total Blindness	NLP				0°	0	0%	

Adapted from Cocchiarella L, Andersson GBJ (eds): Guides to the Evaluation of Permanent Impairment, 5th ed. Chicago, American Medical Association, 2001, p 284, with permission.

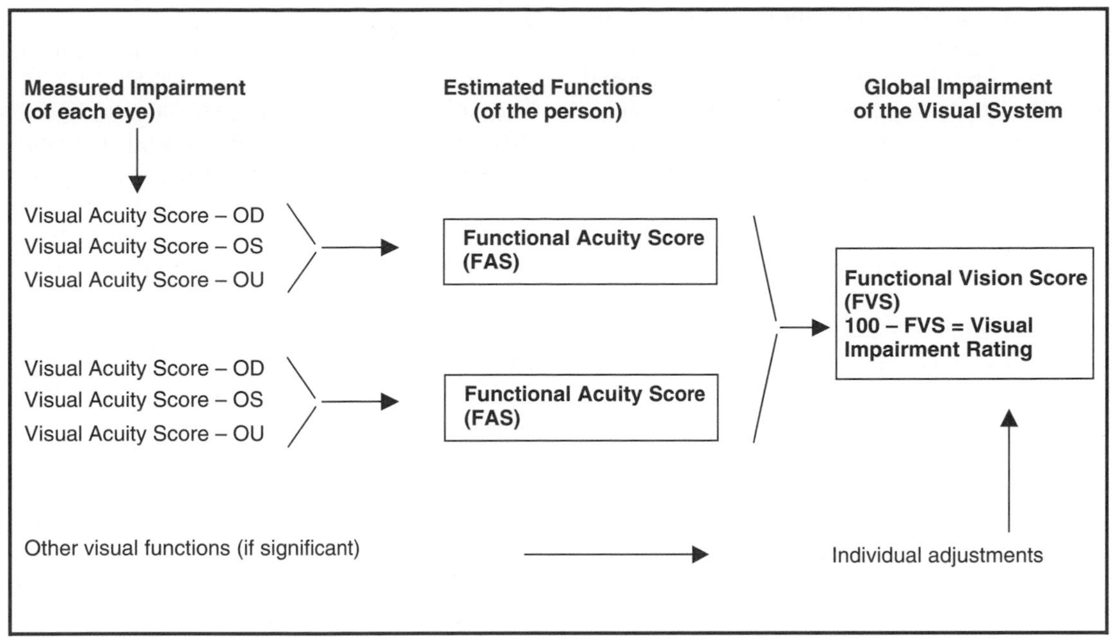

Figure 36–4. From impairment measurement to ability estimate (Adapted from Cocchiarella L, Andersson GBJ [eds]: Guides to the Evaluation of Permanent Impairment, 5th ed. Chicago, American Medical Association, 2001, p 279, with permission.)

field. The calculation of these estimates is distinct from the direct assessment of various visual abilities. Direct assessment would result in a visual ability profile as would be needed for individual rehabilitation plans (see Fig. 36–3). Efforts are underway in various quarters to construct scales for the latter purpose, but there is no consensus yet on their validity and applicability.

Functional vision score—This score is a theoretical construct and provides a composite of the acuity and field score for those situations where it is desirable to collapse the multifaceted reality of vision into a single number.[12] A conversion table between the old visual efficiency scale and the functional vision score is offered in Table 36–2. Figure 36–4 summarizes the relationship between these scores.

The scores mentioned are ability scores; i.e., higher numbers represent better function. The impairment scales and impairment rating scales used in the AMA Guides[19] indicate loss; i.e., higher numbers represent poorer function. The AMA scales are obtained by subtracting the various scores from 100.

UNIFORM MEASUREMENT SCALES

Different organ functions are measured in different units. Visual acuity is measured in terms of visual angle, hearing loss is measured in dB, lung function is measured in volume/minute. Such disparate measurements obviously cannot be compared directly. However, one of the reasons for measuring organ function is to predict the performance of daily living skills. Regardless of the specific skill

TABLE 36–3
General Ability Ranges

	Type of Aids for Rehabilitation	Range descriptors	Ability	Point Score	Impairment
		Above normal	Exceptional ability	>110	—
	No aids required	Normal	Has reserves	100 ± 10	0
Normal or near-	↓	Mild loss	Losing reserves	80 ± 10	0
normal performance	Enhancement aids	Moderate loss	Needs some aids	60 ±10	40
	Enhancement aids	Severe loss	Restricted with aids	40 ± 10	60
Restricted	↓	Profound loss	Marginal with aids	20 ± 10	80
performance	Substitution aids	(Near-) total loss	(Near-) impossible	0–10	100

involved, the ability to perform most skills can be expressed on a uniform scale, as shown in Table 36–3.

This scale has six main ranges (seven if exceptional ability is added). In the top three, performance is normal or near-normal, in the lower three it is restricted. The ranges can easily be fitted with a 10- or 100-point score and can be applied to any ability, as is demonstrated in the following discussion with examples from the mobility and locomotion domain.

Exceptional performance—Some individuals have exceptional abilities; e.g., the person is an Olympic runner. (Note that this range could not be covered by an impairment scale, where normal = 0.)

Range of normal performance—Most human functions have a reserve capacity; e.g., the person can run and walk.

Mild ability loss—In this range the reserve is lost, but everyday performance is not yet significantly compromised; e.g., the person can walk, but not run.

Moderate ability loss—In this range the disabling effect can be overcome with appropriate performance enhancing aids; e.g., the person can walk with the support of a cane.

Severe ability loss—In this range performance starts to fall below normal and endurance is limited, even with assistive devices; e.g., the person can move around with a walker.

Profound ability loss—In this range, the options for enhancement are limited. Performance must rely equally on substitution skills; e.g., the person can move around in a wheelchair, substituting arm power for leg power.

Near-total or total inability—In this range, the original skills, if any, have become unreliable and may at most serve as an adjunct; e.g., the person must be wheeled around passively.

Note that this scoring system is expressed in points, rather than in any specific measurement unit or in percentages of a measurement unit. The impairment (and the impairment rating in the AMA Guides) can then be expressed in percentages of this point scale.

The ranges discussed above will be used in various tables in this chapter. It should be understood that these ranges are part of a smooth, continuous scale of abilities and do not indicate any stepwise increases in ability. The visual acuity values may be compared to mileposts along a road. They provide useful reference points, but the landscape does not suddenly change when a marker is passed; rather the landscape changes gradually in the interval between the markers.

VISUAL ACUITY SCALES

How can these principles be applied to visual acuity measurement? Traditional visual acuity charts often had an irregular progression of letter sizes, uneven spacing, and a different number of letters on different lines. Newer, standardized charts have a geometric progression of letter sizes, proportional spacing, and five letters on each line.[13–15] These charts, often referred to as ETDRS-type charts (because they were first used in the Treatment Diabetic Retinopathy Study), allow for more consistent accuracy at all levels of visual acuity.

Table 36–4 offers the opportunity for various comparisons.

The left side of the table shows the ranges of visual acuity defined in ICD-9-CM, the official U.S. Health Care classification. Each range covers four lines on a standard, ETDRS-type chart.

The center section of the table indicates the visual acuity score (VAS) for each visual acuity level. The AMA Impairment rating is obtained by subtracting the VAS from 100.[19] Note that the VAS is an ability scale and extends beyond 100, as normal acuity is better than the 20/20 standard. The impairment scale is truncated at 20/20.

The right side of the table presents ranges of reading ability. It assumes that the examinee is literate and that reading is only limited by the visual impairment.

This layout allows several comparisons. Comparing the VAS scale to the ICD-9-CM ranges, it is seen that each line correctly read counts for five points. Because each line on a standard chart has five characters, the VAS can simply be interpreted as a count of the total number of letters read correctly, with the 20/2000 line counting as 0. The 20/2000 level is a convenient and appropriate baseline, as this level of acuity normally exists far into the periphery.

Comparing the VAS scale to the reading ability ranges, it is seen that the VAS scale also fits the general ability ranges in Table 36–3.

Finally, the reading ability ranges need to be compared to the acuity ranges. For this purpose, the visual acuity values on the left side of the Table are expressed in three ways. The first column shows the standard U.S. notation for 20 feet, the preferred testing distance for normal and near-normal vision (see AMA Guides, section 12.2b.1[19[p281]]). The next column shows the notation for 1-meter testing, which is the preferred testing distance for the low vision range (see AMA Guides, section 12.2b.2[19]). The third visual acuity column indicates the distance at which 1 M print (average newsprint) would be recognizable. This distance is important because it indicates the focal length of glasses or magnifiers needed at each acuity

TABLE 36–4
Visual Acuity Ranges

Impairment Ranges (ICD-9-CM)	Visual Acuity US Notation	1 m Notation	1 M Print Read at	Visual Acuity Score	Impairment Rating	Estimated Reading Ability
Range of Normal Vision	20/12.5	1/0.63	160 cm	110	—	Normal reading speed
	20/16	1/0.8	125 cm	105	—	Normal reading distance
	20/20	1/1	100 cm	100	0%	Reserve capacity for small print
	20/25	1/1.25	80 cm	95	5%	
Near-normal Vision (mild loss)	20/32	1/1.6	63 cm	90	10%	Normal reading speed,
	20/40	1/2	50 cm	85	15%	reduced reading distance,
	20/50	1/2.5	40 cm	80	20%	no reserve for small print
	20/63	1/3.2	32 cm	75	25%	
Moderate Low Vision	20/80	1/4	25 cm	70	30%	Near-normal with reading
	20/100	1/5	20 cm	65	35%	aids, uses low power magnifier
	20/125	1/6.3	16 cm	60	40%	or large print books
	20/160	1/8	12.5 cm	55	45%	
Severe Low Vision	20/200	1/10	10 cm	50	50%	Slower than normal with
	20/250	1/12.5	8 cm	45	55%	reading aids, uses high-power
	20/320	1/16	6.3 cm	40	60%	magnifiers
	20/400	1/20	5 cm	35	65%	
Profound Low Vision	20/500	1/25	4 cm	30	70%	Marginal with reading aids,
	20/630	1/32	3.2 cm	25	75%	may use magnifiers for spot
	20/800	1/40	2.5 cm	20	80%	reading, but may prefer talking
	20/1000	1/50	2 cm	15	85%	books
Near-Blindness	20/1250	1/63	1.6 cm	10	90%	No visual reading,
	20/1600	1/80	1.25 cm	5	95%	uses nonvisual sources,
	20/2000	1/100	1 cm	0	100%	talking books, Braille
Total Blindness	No light perception					

See sections 12.1 and 12.2 of the AMA Guides for more detailed instructions on visual acuity measurement.
Adapted from Cocchiarella L, Andersson GBJ (eds): Guides to the Evaluation of Permanent Impairment, 5th ed. Chicago, American Medical Association, 2001, p 284, with permission.

level. (Note: The listed distance indicates the minimum power for high plus reading glasses or for magnifiers held close to the eye. Magnifiers held at a distance from the eye are somewhat less effective and need to be somewhat stronger. Also, letter chart acuity refers to threshold acuity, whereas comfortable reading may require some additional magnification [stronger lenses].)

As long as the viewing distance for 1 M print is 30 cm or more (i.e., in the normal or near-normal range), no significant difficulty in reading newsprint should be encountered. In the moderate low vision range, the viewing distance becomes 25 cm or less. (Note that 25 cm is the distance to which the magnification of magnifiers is referenced.) In the severe low vision range (20/200 or less), the viewing distance becomes 10 cm or less, a distance at which binocular vision, even with prisms, is no longer possible. In the profound low vision range, the viewing distance for newsprint becomes less than 5 cm (less than 2 inches). With this magnification requirement, visual reading becomes marginal.

Because each of these comparisons shows a good fit, the VAS can be used as a reasonable estimate of the reading ability loss caused by loss of visual acuity.

CHANGING PERCEPTIONS AND "LEGAL" BLINDNESS

Table 36–4 shows that the ICD-9-CM category for severe vision loss corresponds to what, in various U.S. statutes, is described as legal blindness. The term legal blindness is a regrettable misnomer, as 90% of the people who are so labeled are not blind, but have residual vision. The continued use of the term legal blindness supports the popular misconception of a black-and-white dichotomy between those who are legally sighted and those who are legally blind. The reality is that there is a gradual transition with a large gray area of individuals with low vision. The word *low* indicates that these individuals have less than normal vision; the word *vision* indicates that they are not blind. Describing a person with a severe vision loss as legally blind is as preposterous as describing a person with a severe heart ailment as legally dead.

The term legal blindness dates from the depression years, when it replaced the earlier, more descriptive term of industrial or economic blindness. At that time, little attention was given to the use of residual vision. Children with vision loss were placed in schools for the blind, where they were blindfolded and taught blind skills. Indeed, the concept of sight-saving classes treated vision like money in the bank that was best preserved by not using it. It was not until the early 1950s that the first low vision rehabilitation services were opened at the Industrial Home for the Blind and at the Lighthouse in New York.

Snell's visual efficiency scale dates from this early era. It gave 20/200 acuity an efficiency value of "20." His scale left little room for differentiation among those with less than 20/200 acuity. Today it is realized that those with 20/200 vision may have lost 80% of their employability in 1925, but certainly not 80% of their vision. In accordance with the general ability scale in Table 36–3, the new scale places 20/200 at "50," thus preserving as much room for differentiation above as below this level. See Table 36–2 for a more detailed comparison.

Attention should also be paid to the psychological effect of the term legal blindness. When we tell a person that he or she is "blind," we have categorized that person with the unspoken implication that nothing more can be done (about the underlying disorder). When we tell a person that he or she has low vision, the implication is that he or she has a problem. The next question, then, is what can be done about the problem. The answer is that many things can still be done to preserve and enhance that person's quality of life.

VISUAL FIELD SCALES

Table 36–5 provides scales for visual field loss. Its layout is similar to that of Table 36–4. The traditional assump-

TABLE 36–5
Visual Field Ranges

Impairment Ranges (ICD-9-CM)	Special Conditions	Average Radius (Concentric)	Visual Field Score	Impairment Rating	Estimated Ability for Visual Orientation and Mobility (O + M)
Range of Normal			110	—	Normal visual orientation
Vision		65°	105	—	Normal mobility skills
		60°	100	0%	
		55°	95	5%	
Near-normal		50°	90	10%	Normal O + M performance, needs
Vision		45°	85	15%	more scanning, occasionally surprised
(mild loss)	Loss of	40°	80	20%	by events on the side
	one eye	35°	75	25%	
Moderate		30°	70	30%	Near-normal performance, requires
Low Vision		25°	65	35%	scanning for obstacles
	Lost upper	20°	60	40%	
	field	15°	55	45%	
Severe	Hemianopia	10°	50	50%	Visual mobility is slower than normal,
Low Vision		9°	45	55%	requires continuous scanning, may
	Lost lower	8°	40	60%	use cane as adjunct
	field	7°	35	65%	
Profound		6°	30	70%	Must use long cane for detection of
Low Vision		5°	25	75%	obstacles, may use vision as adjunct
		4°	20	80%	for identification
		3°	15	85%	
Near-Blindness		2°	10	90%	Visual orientation unreliable; must
		1°	5	95%	rely on long cane, sound, guide dog,
Total Blindness	No visual field		0	100%	and other blind mobility skills

See section 12.3 of the AMA Guides for more detailed instructions on visual field measurement.
Adapted from Cocchiarella L, Andersson GBJ (eds): Guides to the Evaluation of Permanent Impairment, 5th ed. Chicago, American Medical Association, 2001, p 289, with permission.

tion that a visual field loss to a 10° radius (20° diameter) is equally disabling as a visual acuity loss to 20/200 is maintained. Both receive a score of 50. Also maintained are the ICD-9-CM definitions for profound and near-total visual field loss (10° and 5° diameter). ICD-9 and ICD-9-CM had no definitions for lesser losses.

The fourth edition of the AMA Guides[5] offered several methods of visual field assessment that were incompatible with each other and with the common definition of legal blindness. The AMA formula gave the same value to central field loss as to peripheral field loss and to the upper and lower half fields; it gave a score of "20" to field loss to a 12.5° radius. Esterman introduced the use of preprinted overlay grids. His grids gave different weights to different areas and gave the lower half field twice the weight of the upper half field. The monocular version of his grid gave a score of "20" to a 15° radius; the binocular version gave that same score to a 20° radius (twice the legal definition).

The new formula can be implemented manually or with an overlay grid. The use of preprinted grids is possible, but not needed, because the layout is so simple that the grids can be constructed by hand. The new layout gives 50% of the weight to the central 10°, which is consistent with the fact that this area corresponds to 50% of the visual cortex. The new layout gives 50% extra weight to the lower half field, which is a reasonable compromise between the AMA and the Esterman approach. The new layout scores a left or right hemianopia as a 50-point loss (equivalent to tunnel vision to a 10° radius); loss of the upper half field is a 40-point loss and loss of the lower half field is a 60-point loss. This is more appropriate than the old scale, where only a loss of more than three quadrants would qualify as legal blindness.

Implementation

The new layout is implemented by drawing 10 meridians: two in each of the upper quadrants and three in each of the lower quadrants. Along each meridian one point is counted for every 2° up to a 10° radius and one point per 10° beyond the 10° radius. Thus, a 60° radius scores 10 points. The upper and nasal meridians will not reach 60°, but the lower and temporal meridians will extend further; thus, a normal field will score 100 points. This is summarized in Figure 36–5.

ESTIMATING FUNCTIONAL VISION

Having measured the visual functions (visual acuity, visual field), an estimate of the overall functional vision of the person needs to be calculated. This process is summarized in Figure 36–4.

Because normal vision is binocular vision, the formula for converting the visual acuity/field scores for each eye to functional acuity/field scores for the person is heavily weighted in favor of the binocular function in the fifth edition of the Guides. The formula is as follows: (OD + OS + 3 × OU)/5. This is different from the formula used in prior editions of the Guides. That formula did not consider binocular function; it first combined visual acuity and visual field for each eye separately and then combined the two eyes as if they were independent organs.

Binocular visual acuity is routinely measured. The binocular field, however, is not easily measured. Existing visual field equipment has no means of monitoring fixation when the head is centered and no means of ensuring that the two eyes converge the appropriate amount for the short viewing distance in the field-testing bowl. Therefore, it is recommended that monocular visual fields be obtained in the usual way and that the binocular field be constructed from an overlay of the two monocular fields.

INTERPRETATION OF THE FUNCTIONAL SCORES

At this point it is appropriate to repeat what the functional scores (functional acuity score, functional field score, functional vision score) do and do not provide.

They are called scores because they are directly derived from a scoring system for visual acuity and visual field (number of letters seen on a standard chart, number of dots seen on a standard field plot). No individual judgments enter into this calculation. The term rating, on the other hand, leaves room for some individualized judgment. In the AMA Guides (section 12.4 and Table 12–10[19[p298]]), this adjustment room is provided in converting the functional vision score to an impairment rating (see Table 36–6).

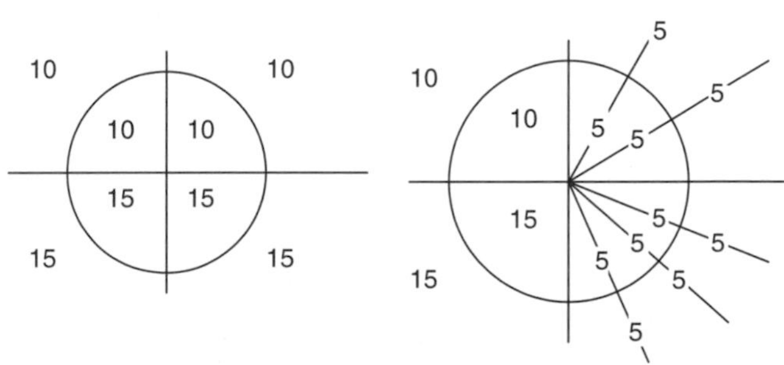

Figure 36–5. Arrangement of the measurement points for visual field scoring. Note that the arrangement of the meridians within the quadrants avoids the need for special rules for hemianopias. (From Cocchiarella L, Andersson GBJ [eds]: Guides to the Evaluation of Permanent Impairment, 5th ed. Chicago, American Medical Association, 2001, p 288, with permission.)

Because functional score calculations are based on visual acuity and visual field measurements, they are more reproducible than a direct assessment of vision-related skills and abilities would be. The visual system is fortunate in that visual functions can be measured accurately and that the results show a good correlation with functional vision (see Table 36–4 and Fig. 36–4). For other organ systems the correlation between measured organ function and estimated abilities may not be as obvious or as precise. For those organ systems some direct assessment of ADL abilities may be required.

The scores do not take into account that some individuals will have made better adaptations to vision loss than others. This has advantages for the assignment of benefits, as the judgment calls of the evaluator are reduced and individuals who have made good adaptations are not penalized by a reduction of benefits. On the other hand, reducing the complex and multifaceted reality of vision to a single number requires an enormous amount of oversimplification and thus may throw out significant information.

Whereas the functional acuity score is related to visual reading skills and the functional field score is related to visual orientation and mobility skills, the functional vision score, which combines the two, is a more abstract concept, no longer related to any particular real-life skill. When visual impairment ratings have to be combined with impairment ratings for other organ systems, the resulting value becomes even more abstract.

The relationship between letter chart acuity and reading ability, as expressed in Table 36–4, assumes the availability of glasses and some basic magnifiers. It also assumes literacy. If these conditions are not met, visual performance may be worse than expected.

Use of Braille, talking books, and voice output devices can compensate significantly for a loss of visual reading skills. Use of a long cane or a dog guide can compensate significantly for a loss of visual mobility skills. Because the objective of a scoring system is to assess the effects of vision loss, the scores do not take into account how these nonvisual skills can enhance actual performance.

The relationships in Tables 36–4 and 36–5 are based on some general assumptions about the abilities needed for generic ADL (aspect 3). They specifically exclude additional job-related or environment-related demands (see AMA Guides, Chapters 1 and 2[19]). The vision requirements for navigating a mountain trail may be higher than those for navigating a sidewalk. The scores do not reflect such unusual demands. An extreme example may clarify this: a hobbyist working with an unprotected power tool lost some digits from his little finger. Even if this were his dominant right hand, his loss of ADL abilities (aspect 3) would not be significant; if it were his left hand, the loss would be even less. If he is a professional violinist, he could still hold the bow with his damaged right hand, but even a partial loss of his left-hand function might signal the end of his career (aspect 4). Workmen's compensation insurance would not pay, because the loss was not work-related. However, professional disability insurance might pay a significant amount.

COMMENTS ON SOME OF THE PROCEDURAL STEPS

The following section provides some comments and clarifications on selected procedural steps. They are referenced to the Vision chapter (Chapter 12) in the AMA Guides.[19]

Section 12.2—Impairment of Visual Acuity

Because the vast majority of cases of vision loss involve visual acuity loss, determination of best-corrected visual acuity is never skipped. See section 12.3 regarding possible skipping of visual field tests.

Section 12.2b.1—Testing in the Normal Range

ETDRS-type charts (geometric progression, proportional spacing, five letters per line) are preferred. If such charts are not available, traditional charts may be used. If the visual acuity is around 20/200, the criterion "20/200 or less" should be interpreted as "less than 20/160" or as "less than 10/80" on a traditional chart moved to 10 feet. Otherwise, on traditional charts, the criterion "20/200 or less" effectively becomes "less than 20/100."

Section 12.2b.2—Testing in the Low Vision Range

In this range, testing at 1 meter is recommended over the use of vague estimates such as "count fingers" or "hand movements." Charts for use at this distance are available commercially.[16]

Section 12.2b.2—Monocular versus Binocular Acuity

The new rules specify testing of binocular acuity, rather than assuming that the binocular acuity equals the acuity of the better eye. For most practitioners, testing of the binocular acuity already is a part of the routine eye examination.

Section 12.2c—Steps for Assigning a Visual Acuity-based Impairment Rating

These steps have been discussed previously (see Table 36–4 and Fig. 36–4). Determination of reading acuity has been made optional because most reading measurements are notoriously inaccurate. Most practitioners record only the print size read, without the exact distance. Furthermore, the commonly used Jaeger numbers have no numeric basis, whereas point sizes may differ with the type style (e.g., 8-point Arial = 9-point Times Roman). The progression of the reading efficiency scale in the old rules was very irregular. If reading acuity is to be considered, accurate measurement guidelines are provided in section 12.5.

Section 12.3—Impairment of the Visual Field

Impairment of the visual field is much less frequent than impairment of visual acuity. If there are no complaints that might point to visual field loss, and if the history and screening tests (such as a tangent screen test or confrontation test, or a central-30 automated field test) provide no suspicion of visual field loss, visual field testing might be skipped. In that case, the functional field score is assumed to be 100 (no impairment) and the functional vision score equals the functional acuity score. The examiner should, of course, be prepared to defend this decision, if challenged.

Section 12.3a.4—Automated Perimetry

Although the Social Security Administration still prefers Goldmann-type testing,[20] such tests are increasingly difficult to obtain. There is a theoretical concern that static and kinetic testing might not always give the same results (static-kinetic dissociation). Such discrepancies, however, are probably exceedingly rare. As in previous editions, the AMA Guides allow the construction of a pseudo-isopter from an automated field plot (see Example 12–9 and Figs. 12–8 and 12–9 in the Guides[19]). Most automated plots are therefore limited to the central 30° (radius), because this area is the most informative for diagnostic purposes. For orientation and mobility, the far periphery is more important. Any visual field test for an impairment evaluation should therefore test to 60° or beyond. A normal central 30° test may at best be used as supportive evidence in skipping field testing. Although a commercially automated test sequence is not yet available, the feasibility of such a program has been demonstrated[17] and future development is expected.

Section 12.3a.5—Binocular Fields

As pointed out earlier, there is no equipment that allows reliable binocular field testing. Existing equipment does not allow fixation monitoring when the head, rather than the eye, is centered, and there is no way to ascertain that the examinee maintains the proper amount of convergence for the short viewing distance in the test bowl. It is recommended, therefore, that the binocular field be constructed by superimposing the monocular field plots (see Figs. 12–10 and 12–11 in the Guides for Examples 12–10 and 12–11[19[pp294–295]]).

Section 12.3b.1—Testing Grid

The construction of the testing grid is simple enough to be remembered and constructed by hand. Alternatively, preprinted grids can be obtained.

Section 12.3c—Assigning a Field-based Impairment Rating

The Impairment Rating can be calculated or counted on an overlay grid as the number of dots within the criterion isopter. Use of the overlay grid is recommended especially when scotomata are present,.

Section 12.4—Impairment of the Visual System

The new system (i.e., fifth edition of the Guides[19]) combines the VAS for the right eye, left eye, and both eyes to a functional acuity score and then combines that score with a similarly determined functional field score. This is different from the old system (i.e., editions one to four[5]), which first combined acuity and field values for the better eye and then combined them with a similar value for the lesser eye, as if the two eyes were independent organs. The new system accounts better for the fact that good visual acuity in one eye can compensate for poor acuity in the other eye. A good field in one eye can compensate for field loss in the other eye. However, visual acuity cannot compensate for field loss or vice versa.

Section 12.4a.1—Basic Rule

The formula to combine the visual acuity/field scores to a functional acuity/field score uses a weighted average. This formula produces the same result, whether applied to the scores or to the impairment ratings (100 – score). By contrast, the formula used to combine the functional acuity score with the functional field score is a multiplication and will produce very different results when applied to the scores or to the impairment ratings. The formula should be applied to the scores, which are positive ability scales, rather than to the negative impairment scales. The difference in result is graphically illustrated in Figure 36–6.

Section 12.4a.2—Additional Rules

The new system (i.e., fifth edition of the Guides[19]) treats visual acuity and visual field as independent variables, which they usually are. However, additional rules are needed to prevent the same loss from being counted twice, when the visual acuity loss and the visual field loss are not independent.

Section 12.4a.3—Rule for Central Scotomata

A central scotoma (a scotoma covering the point of fixation) causes both a visual acuity loss and a visual field loss. The Esterman grids solved this problem by ignoring any paracentral field losses. This is not appropriate because a pericentral ("doughnut") scotoma can be extremely debilitating, even if the central acuity for single letters is still reasonable. The new system solves this dilemma by disregarding the central field loss when visual acuity loss is present. The greater the visual acuity loss, the greater the area of central field loss that is ignored (see Table 12–9 and Examples 12–13, 12–14, and 12–15 in the Guides[19[pp297,299,300]]). The central field loss is ignored only for the calculation of the functional vision score. Peripheral field loss is never ignored.

Section 12.4b—Individual Adjustments

Although visual acuity loss and visual field loss account for most cases of visual impairment, other visual functions may also be impaired. In this case the functional vision score may be adjusted downward and the impairment rating upward. The same rule as for central scotomata applies: the additional impairment is counted only to the extent that its effects exceed the effects of the concurrent visual acuity and/or visual field loss. The size of the adjustment is limited to 15 points. The need for such an adjustment must be well documented. Contrast sensitivity is included in this group because its measurement is not yet well standardized and because it most often (but not always) is accompanied by visual acuity loss.

Section 12.4c—Impairment of the Whole Person

Total blindness should be rated as a 100% impairment of the visual system. Yet even totally blind persons can lead productive lives. Therefore, total impairment of the visual system does not equal total impairment of the whole person. The difference lies in the use of vision substitution skills. In the previous edition of the AMA Guides,[5] 100% visual impairment was equated with 85% whole person impairment. This equivalence is maintained in the fifth edition.[19] The 15-point difference is the same as allowed for additional impairments. Because the use of substitution skills hardly plays a role if the ability score is >50 (see Table 36–3), the adjustment has been made only for the range of 50 to 0 ability (50% to 100% impairment). Table 36–6 compares the adjusted scales.

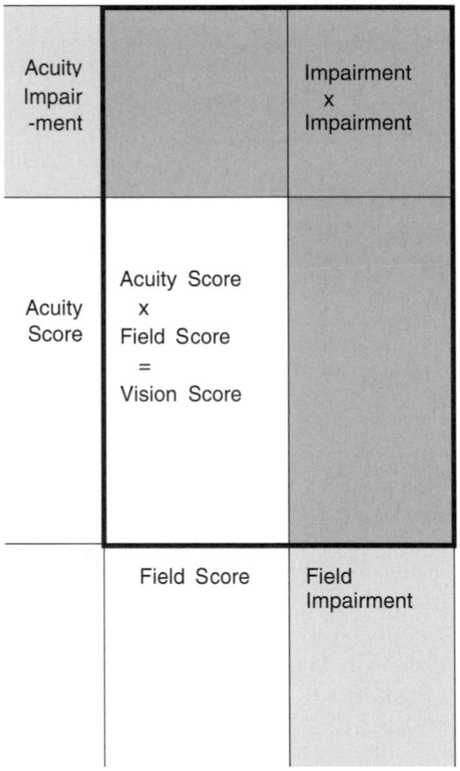

Acuity Impair -ment		Impairment x Impairment
Acuity Score	Acuity Score x Field Score = Vision Score	
	Field Score	Field Impairment

Figure 36–6. Multiplying ability scores versus multiplying impairment ratings. The acuity score (white) and the acuity impairment rating (gray) add up to 100. So do the field score and the field impairment rating. Note that the effect of multiplying the scores is entirely different from multiplying the impairment ratings. The functional vision score is represented by the white rectangle; the impairment rating of the visual system (100 – functional vision score) is represented by the sum of the other three rectangles (gray), rather than by the impairment x impairment rectangle only.

Section 12.5—Reading Acuity

As stated earlier, consideration of reading acuity is optional. If done in the context of a functional assessment it should be done with continuous text reading segments, rather than with a miniature letter chart. Reading cards with a geometric progression and uniform, proportionally spaced reading segments are preferred, because they allow the assessment of reading rates. Such cards are available commercially in various languages.[16] Letter sizes should be given in M-units, because this is the only unit that allows comparison to letter charts and distance acuity values.

Section 12.5d—Modified Snellen Formula

Use of a modified Snellen formula is recommended where the viewing distance is expressed in diopters (1/distance in m rather than in cm). This converts the Snellen formula from a fraction to a multiplication and the viewing distance from a fraction-within-a-fraction to a whole number. This results in much easier calculations. It also provides a direct reference to the dioptric power of the reading add.

TABLE 36–6

Converting Visual System Impairment in Whole Person Impairment

	Visual Acuity Score	**Visual Impairment Rating**	**Whole Person Impairment Rating**	
Impairment Ranges (ICD-9-CM)	Estimated Visual Ability	Estimated Loss of Visual Ability	Estimated Loss of Overall Ability	Estimated Ability to Perform Activities of Daily Living
Range of Normal Vision	110	—		Normal performance with reserve capacity
	105	—		
	100	0%		
	95	5%		
Near-normal Vision (mild loss)	90	10%		Normal performance, losing reserve capacity
	85	15%		
	80	20%		
	75	25%		
Moderate Low Vision	70	30%		Near-normal performance, need for some vision enhancement aids
	65	35%		
	60	40%		
	55	45%		
Severe Low Vision	50	50%	50%	Visual performance slower than normal, even with vision enhancement aids
	45	55%		
	40	60%	57%	
	35	65%		
Profound Low Vision	30	70%	64%	Visual performance becomes marginal, uses vision substitution for some tasks
	25	75%		
	20	80%	71%	
	15	85%		
Near-Blindness	10	90%	78%	Visual performance impossible, needs vision substitution skills for all tasks
	5	95%		
Total Blindness	0	100%	85%	

Modified from Cocchiarella L, Andersson GBJ (eds): Guides to the Evaluation of Permanent Impairment, 5th ed. Chicago, American Medical Association, 2001, p 298, with permission.

APPENDIX 1

Comparison of the Fourth and Fifth Editions

Changes from the fourth to the fifth edition are based on the scales and classifications of ICD-9-CM (1978) and ICIDH (1980). They were elaborated in the Guide for the Evaluation of Visual Impairment (1999), prepared by an international working group for the International Society for Low Vision Research and Rehabilitation.[18]

Several changes were discussed earlier. Changes in the calculation procedure were indicated in Figure 36–4.

The extra scale for diplopia was removed because diplopia measurement is not standardized. Whether its presence is disturbing may depend on factors in the visual environment. If diplopia is disturbing and interferes with daily living skills, the functional vision score and the visual system impairment rating may be adjusted, as they can be for other factors, indicated in section 12.4b.[19(p297)]

The considerable extra impairment rating for monocular aphakia was removed. The extra rating was based on the fact that monocular aphakia with spectacle lens correction caused disturbing differences in image size between the eyes in the past. This problem was eliminated by the introduction of implant lenses, which are now the standard treatment. The extension to monocular pseudophakia was a mistake, introduced when lens implantation was still considered an experimental procedure.

The most obvious difference is the change of scales, where 20/200 acuity and a field of 10° radius were moved from "20" to "50" on the ability scale (from 80% to 50% on the impairment scale). A comparison with other chapters of the fifth edition shows that the new scale fits better with the scales used for other organ systems. The new scales also allow for more differentiation in the lower ranges, an area that was considered unimportant in 1925 and is now the domain of low vision rehabilitation programs. The new scales also give more appropriate representation to hemianopias.

Use of the new scales does not change any eligibility rules, except that SSA regulations that state that legal blindness is equivalent to an 80% loss on Snell's visual efficiency scale[20(p28)] should now be read as equivalent to a 50% loss on the functional vision scale.

Table 36–2 offers a more detailed comparison between the old visual efficiency scale and the new functional vision score. This can be used to convert old ratings to the new score.

Table 36–2 shows the inconsistencies that had crept in over various revisions. The visual efficiency scale for distance vision had little room for differentiation in the lower ranges. The visual efficiency scale for near vision stopped even sooner and showed values that did not correspond to the distance scale. Inexplicably, the near vision rating dropped from 90% to 50% for a one-line difference from 20/40 (newsprint at 50 cm) to 20/50 (newsprint at 40 cm).

The visual field scores show similar discrepancies between the AMA formula and the Esterman monocular grid. Neither conformed to the common legal blindness definition, which states that field loss to a 10° radius is equivalent to an acuity loss to 20/200 (20 points on the visual efficiency scale).

References

1. Magnus H, Wuerdeman HV: Visual Economics, With Rules for Estimation of the Earning Ability After Injuries to the Eyes. Milwaukee, Porth, 1902. Earlier publications in German.
2. Report of the Committee on Compensation for Eye Injuries. JAMA 85:113–115, 1925.
3. Snell AC: Visual efficiency of various degrees of subnormal visual acuity. Its effect on earning ability. JAMA 85:1367–1373, 1925.
4. Snell AC, Sterling S: The percentage evaluation of macular vision. Arch Ophthalmol 54:443–461, 1925.
5. American Medical Association: Guides to the Evaluation of Permanent Impairment. Chicago, American Medical Association; 1st ed, 1971; 2nd ed, 1984; 3rd ed, 1988; 3rd ed, rev, 1990; 4th ed, 1993.
6. Colenbrander A: Dimensions of visual performance: Low Vision Symposium, American Academy of Ophthalmology. Trans AAOO 83:332–337, 1977.
7. International Classification of Impairments, Disabilities and Handicaps (ICIDH). Geneva, World Health Organization, 1980.
8. International Classification of Diseases, 9th Revision (ICD-9). Geneva, World Health Organization, 1977. Its successor for international reporting is ICD-10, 1995.
9. International Classification of Diseases, 9th Revision: Clinical Modification (ICD-9-CM). First edition: Ann Arbor, Mich,

Commission on Professional and Hospital Activities, 1978. Later editions in the public domain. ICD-9-CM, the official US Health Care Classification is based on ICD-9 but contains additional detail. The impairment ranges used in the AMA Guides are based on ICD-9-CM.

10. International Classification of Functioning, Disability and Health (ICF), Geneva, World Health Organization, 2001. ICF is a companion classification to the ICD. The ICD classifies diseases and disorders; ICF classifies their functional consequences.

10a. International Council of Ophthalmology: Visual Standards, Aspects and Ranges of Vision Loss with Emphasis on Population Surveys. San Francisco, Pacific Vision Foundation. To order: fax 415-346-6562 ($5 per copy).

11. [M. Riviere, 1970] Rehabilitation Codes. Classification of Impairment of Visual Function. Final Report 1968, [U.S. National Institute of Neurological Diseases and Blindness].

12. Colenbrander A: The functional vision score. A coordinated scoring system for visual impairments, disabilities and handicaps. In Kooijman AC, Looijestijn PL, Welling JA, van der Wildt GJ (eds): Low Vision—Research and New Developments in Rehabilitation. Studies in Health Technology and Informatics. Amsterdam, IOS Press, 1994, pp 552–561.

13. Bailey IL, Lovie JE: New design principles for visual acuity letter charts. Am J Optom Physiol Ophthalmol 53:740–745, 1976. Bailey and Lovie introduced the proportionally spaced layout with five letters/line that is now the standard.

14. Ferris FL, Kassov A, Bresnick GH, Bailey I: New visual acuity charts for clinical research. Am J Ophthalmol 94:91–96, 1982.

15. National Eye Institute: Measurement Guidelines for Collaborative Studies. Bethesda, Md, National Eye Institute, 1982. The NEI (ETDRS) guidelines popularized the standardized layout. The NEI rules specify a rating system similar to the Visual Acuity Score.

16. Low Vision Test Chart. One side: letter chart from 50 M to 1 M (acuity: 1/50, 20/1000 to 1/1, 20/20), 1 m cord attached. Other side: reading segments from 10 M to 0.6 M, diopter ruler included, standardized segments for reading rate measurements. Available in English, Spanish, Portuguese, German, Dutch, Finnish, and Swedish. Folds to fit a briefcase. The reading segments are also available separately on $8\frac{1}{2} \times 11$-inch cards. Precision Vision, 944 First Street, LaSalle, IL 61301; fax: 815-223-2224.

17. Colenbrander A, Lieberman MF, Schainholz DC: Preliminary implementation of the functional vision score on the Humphrey field analyzer. Proceedings of the International Perimetric Society, Kyoto, 1992. In Perimetry Update 1992/1993. New York, Kugler Publications, 1993, pp 487–496.

18. International Society for Low Vision Research and Rehabilitation: Guide for the Evaluation of Visual Impairment. San Francisco, Pacific Vision Foundation, 1999.

19. Cocchiarella L, Andersson GBJ (eds): Guides to the Evaluation of Permanent Impairment, 5th ed. Chicago, American Medical Association, 2001.

20. Social Security Administration, US Department of Health and Human Services: Disability Evaluation Under Social Security (Social Security Administration publication #64-039/ICN # 468600). Washington, DC, Social Security Administration, 1998.

CHAPTER

37

Otolaryngological (ENT) Impairment

ROBERT T. SATALOFF, MD, DMA

This chapter reviews impairment and disability resulting from dysfunction of selected structures in the head and neck. The head and neck are rich in sensory and motor structures that are important for communication, cosmesis, deglutition, olfaction, and other functions important to an individual's quality of life and ability to function in the workplace. This chapter does not discuss all aspects of otolaryngologic impairment and disability, but rather is limited to a few topics selected for their high incidence, important individual consequences, and complexity.

There are numerous methods of evaluating otolaryngologic impairment and disability. Self-reporting methods take two forms: questionnaires and personal interviews. Self-reporting methods are subject to many variables. For example, the results can be influenced by the objectives of the questioner and/or the interviewer. Unless the material used by the interviewer is standardized, intertest results will not be comparable. Furthermore, unsupervised, self-completed questionnaires will be influenced by the attitude and education of the subject who is completing the questionnaire. For example, young and old subjects will respond differently. Older subjects tend to be more forgiving of their impairments or loss of function. When the impairments are equal, older subjects describe themselves as being less affected than younger subjects.[24]

When specific measurements are used to rate impairment, the results are influenced by the measurement materials.[10] The limitations of assessment techniques have not been overcome for otolaryngologic impairments. Many of the practices described in this chapter have shortcomings, but they represent the best and most standardized approaches currently available. Research is constantly in progress exploring more precise assessment methodologies.

HEARING IMPAIRMENT

Hearing loss may be sensorineural, conductive, mixed, and central. Sensorineural hearing impairment is caused by pathologic processes taking place in the cochlea, the acoustic nerve, or the brainstem. There are many causes of sensorineural hearing impairment including excessive noise exposure, ototoxic medications, childhood diseases, meningitis, tumors, and head injuries.[25,45] Conductive hearing impairment is due to pathology in the external or middle ear, including but not limited to otosclerosis, otitis media, congenital deformities, otitis externa, and impacted cerumen. Mixed hearing impairment occurs when there is combined sensorineural and conductive pathology. Examples include advanced otosclerosis and chronic otitis media. Central hearing loss involves the inability to process auditory signals; it may be seen and associated with multiple sclerosis, head trauma, brain tumors, and other conditions.

The need for some way of calculating or deriving impairment for patients with hearing loss became evident in the early 1940s. One of the first useful formulas was suggested by E.P. Fowler, Sr., in 1942. It included hearing measured at 500 Hz (hertz or cycles per second), 1,000 Hz, 2,000 Hz, and 4,000 Hz and weighted the losses in these frequencies.[9] Subsequently, in 1959, the American Medical Association introduced a formula that was similar but that had different weightings and included only 500 Hz, 1,000 Hz, and 2,000 Hz. Various combinations of frequencies have been suggested since then (Table 37–1). These formulas were used to determine impairments in hearing and understanding speech under everyday conditions. All the original formulas were based on tests performed with the subject listening

TABLE 37–1

Hearing Loss Formulas Proposed for Evaluating Impairment

Source	Frequencies (kHz)	Formula	Low Fence (dB re ISO 1960)
Fowler (1942)	0.5, 1, 2, 4 0.4, 0.15	Weighted 0.15, 0.3	10
AMA (1947)	0.5, 1, 2, 4	Variable weights (depending on HTLs)	20
AAOO (1959)	0.5, 1, 2	Unweighted average	25
ISO (1971, 1975)	0.5, 1, 2	Unweighted average	25
NIOSH (1972)	0.5, 1, 2	Unweighted average	25
Macrae (1975–6)	0.5, 1, 1.5, 2, 3, 4	Weighted 0.2, 0.25 0.2, 0.15, 0.1	<3 kHz: 20 4 kHz: 25
CHABA (1975)	1, 2, 3	Unweighted	35
B5 5330 (1976)	1, 2, 3	Unweighted average	30
Berney (Ginnold, 1979)	0.5, 1, 2, 4	Unweighted average	25
Oregon (Ginnold, 1979)	0.5, 1, 2, 4, 6	Unweighted average	25
ISO (1972a)	—	None standardized	—
AAO (1979)	0.5, 1, 2, 3	Unweighted average	25
British Association of Otolaryngologists (1983)	1, 2, 4	Unweighted average	20

kHz, kilohertz; dB, Decibels; ISO, International Standards Organization; AMA, American Medical Association; HTL, hearing threshold level; AAOO, American Academy of Ophthalmology and Otolaryngology; NIOSH, National Institute of Occupational Safety and Health; CHABA, Committee on Hearing and Bioacoustics of the American Standards Institute; BS, Bureau of Standards; AAO, American Academy of Otolaryngology.

in a quiet environment. The original American Academy of Ophthalmology and Otolaryngology formula (1959) was modified in 1979 when 3,000 Hz was added because it was considered to better represent speech perception and the ability to hear in noisy environments.

Why were all the formulas and assessment methods based on pure tones of various frequencies? Not because this provides the best representation of a person's ability to hear, but rather because pure tone audiometry is the best practical test available. It is standardized, valid, and reliable for determining the ability to detect soft sounds in a quiet environment in most cases. This provides a fairly useful guide to a person's ability to hear speech.[5–7] Other common tests, such as the speech reception threshold test, which uses bisyllabic spondaic words (e.g., "baseball," "flytrap," "backstop"), and the speech discrimination score, which uses single-syllable phonetically balanced word lists, provide additional information, but have important practical limitations that preclude their routine use in compensation formulas. Attempts to formulate useful and acceptable representative sentence lists and word lists for use in medical-legal settings have been unsuccessful.

The human ear has a frequency range from about 20 to 20,000 Hz. It is also extremely sensitive in detecting sounds of low intensity. Pure tone measurements are made with an instrument called an audiometer. Earphones are placed over the ears and tones are controlled for intensity and frequency to determine the hearing threshold, which is the lowest sound pressure level that can be heard by the individual. Routine audiometry requires a voluntary response such as raising a finger or hand or pushing a button. Hearing is usually measured with pure tone signals at 250, 500, 1,000, 2,000, 3,000, 4,000, 6,000, and 8,000 Hz.

Standard zero hearing level for each frequency tested by the audiometer is based on the hearing of a group of individuals whose age varied between 18 and 24 years and who had no history of previous ear problems. Pure tone tests may be done by air conduction or bone conduction. Air conduction tests measure the status of the external, middle, and inner ear, including the cochlea, acoustic nerve, brainstem, and cortex. Bone conduction tests measure sensorineural function more directly, bypassing the external and middle ear. Speech is tested by using spondee and phonetically balanced words as described previously.

There are more sophisticated and specialized tests, such as brainstem evoked response audiometry, also called auditory brainstem response or auditory evoked potential; electrocochleography; otoacoustic emission tests; and middle ear impedance measurement. These tests, along with other medical evaluations, are used by otologists to help determine the nature and specific cause of hearing impairment in selected individuals. They are often useful in differentiating noise-induced hearing impairment from other causes.

Specific criteria have been established that are also helpful in distinguishing noise-induced hearing loss from hearing loss resulting from other causes. The criteria state that occupational, noise-induced hearing loss characteristics are as follows:

1. It is always sensorineural, affecting the hair cells in the inner ear.
2. It is always bilateral. Audiometric patterns are usually similar bilaterally.
3. It almost never produces a profound hearing loss. Usually, low-frequency limits are about 40 dB (decibels) and high-frequency limits are about 75 dB.
4. Once the exposure to noise is discontinued, there is no substantial further progression of hearing loss as a result of the noise exposure.
5. Previous noise-induced hearing loss does not make the ear more sensitive to future noise exposure. As the hearing threshold increases, the rate of loss decreases.
6. The earliest damage to the inner ears reflects a loss at 3,000, 4,000, and 6,000 Hz. There is always far more loss at 3,000, 4,000, and 6,000 Hz than at 500, 1,000, and 2,000 Hz. The greatest loss usually occurs at 4,000 Hz. The higher and lower frequencies take longer to be affected than the 3,000 to 6,000 Hz range.
7. Given stable exposure conditions, losses at 3,000, 4,000, and 6,000 Hz will usually reach a maximal level in about 10 to 15 years.
8. Continuous noise exposure over the years is more damaging than interrupted exposure to noise, which permits the ear to have a rest period.[44]

HEARING DISABILITY

Hearing disability is defined as auditory difficulties caused by hearing impairment. Examples include problems with communicating by speech in work, social, or other settings; difficulties hearing warning signals; problems listening to music; and inability to localize sound sources or recognize different sounds. Communication by speech is considered to be generally the most important function of the auditory system. Therefore, communication difficulty is undoubtedly the most serious hearing disability.

Individuals with severe hearing loss may feel isolated and become introverted, refusing to go to parties, movies, religious services, and family gatherings. Participation in discussions may be limited. However, other individuals with similar hearing impairments may feel and function essentially normally, especially if they use amplification (hearing aids) effectively. Age adds a deleterious effect. The same dysfunction in older individuals causes more difficulty than it does in the younger person, although this does not necessarily correlate with the individual's tolerance of the problems.[24]

In general, the effects of hearing impairment on individuals vary as a function of their psychological makeup and daily activities. The effects are modified by the use of compensatory measures such as hearing aids, assistive devices, and speech reading (lip reading), as well as an individual's self-confidence and willingness to request assistance from others.

HANDICAP

A handicap caused by a hearing impairment is a disadvantage that prevents or limits an individual from completing a task that is normal or useful for that individual. Handicaps are nonauditory problems that arise because of a hearing impairment or disability. According to the World Health Organization, hearing handicaps can be classified into the following categories[20]:

1. Orientation handicaps—situational disorientation due to hearing loss, such as the inability to follow conversations
2. Physical independence handicaps—inability to maintain a strictly independent existence
3. Occupational handicaps—restriction of job or career choice
4. Economic self-sufficiency handicaps
5. Social integration handicaps—these cause numerous difficulties in carrying out ordinary daily activities, such as responding to warning signals and verbal messages
6. Inability to cope with occupational requirements—loss of earning capacity

EVALUATION

Pure tone thresholds are used to quantify impairment and determine compensation. Formulas average pure tone thresholds from selected frequencies. Although this methodology is less than perfect, it is the current standard. A good example is the formula used by the American Academy of Otolaryngology and the American Medical Association. This formula is based on the average of the thresholds at 500, 1,000, 2,000, and 3,000 Hz. This formula determines the average threshold at these four frequencies in one ear; subtracts 25 dB (the point above which handicap is said to begin [low fence] [Fig. 37–1]); and multiplies the difference by 1.5 to determine percentage of impairment in that ear. The average threshold in the remaining ear is treated the same way. This yields a percent impairment in each ear. However, because one's possible handicap is based on binaural hearing, the percent impairment in each ear is combined by weighting the better ear as 5 and the poorer ear as 1, then obtaining the average percentage of the two ears. This provides the percent of binaural handicap. An average of 25 dB equals 0% impairment and an average of 92 dB equals 100% impairment. An example is seen in Figure 37–2. The concept of using 25 dB as the cutoff point for hearing impairment (Fig. 37–3) is based on a study of hearing losses in over 1,000 patients who were tested and stratified by self-selection.[13] The patients answered the following question: "Do you think your hearing is good, fair, or poor?" They were then tested for hearing losses. All patients who stated that their hearing was "good" had intact 25 dB hearing. No patient with greater than 25 dB hearing threshold responded by saying his or her hearing was "good."

This formula has been widely adopted in the United States and in various other countries since it was proposed by the American Academy of Otolaryngology and approved by the American Medical Association in 1979. However, there has been controversy because the standard does not include frequencies above 3,000 Hz. More recent studies have suggested that it may not truly represent speech intelligibility.[33] Research is currently directed toward improving the presently accepted AMA method. However, considerable additional research and experience will be needed before any change in the currently accepted, standardized methodology can be justified (Table 37–2). Table 37–3 presents an example of how the formula is used.

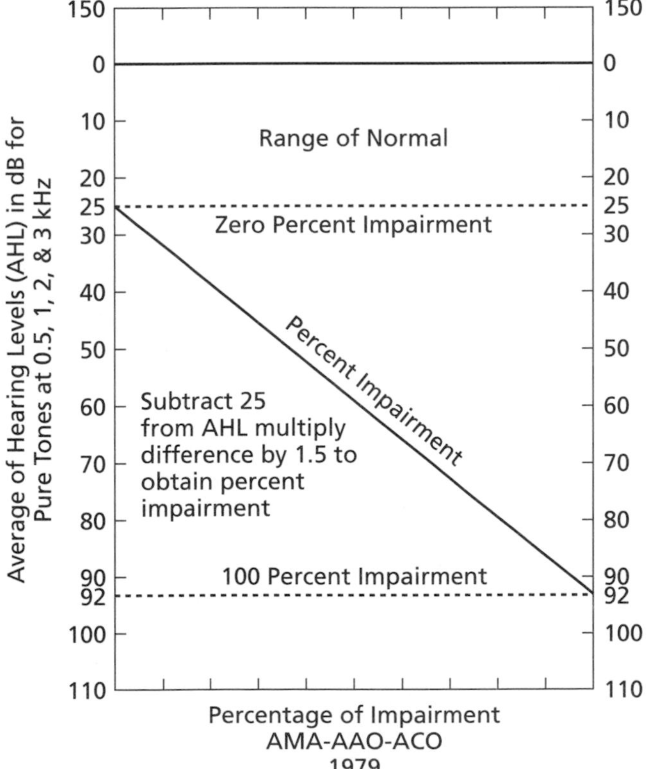

Figure 37–1. The present American Medical Association (AMA) formula for hearing impairment in graphic form. AAO = American Academy of Otolaryngology; ACO = American College of Occupational Medicine (now ACOEM, American College of Occupational and Environmental Medicine).

OTHER CONSIDERATIONS

In assessing any individual's disability from hearing loss, it is important to remember that there are millions of people in the United States with hearing loss from various causes unrelated to noise, injury, or other occupational cause. For medical and legal reasons, it is important to establish an accurate diagnosis in any individual with hearing loss or related dysfunction, such as tinnitus or vertigo.

It is also important to recognize that much can be done to ameliorate hearing disabilities and thereby mitigate the handicaps. Rehabilitative techniques include the use of hearing aids, including in-the-ear, behind-the-ear, body aids, programmable aids, magnetic middle ear implants, and cochlear and brainstem implants; and assistive listening devices, including telephone amplifiers, infrared, microwave, and FM systems. With the proper amplification, counseling, and auditory training, most people with hearing impairments function extremely well, and many function normally.

■ A 50-year-old police officer complained of having difficulty hearing everyday communication, especially in noisy environments. He also complained of tinnitus in both ears, which he described as a constant, high-pitched tone. The tinnitus appeared to be worse in a quiet environment and bothered him when he was trying to go to sleep.

Physical examination of his ears, nose, and throat was unremarkable except for a moderate bilateral high-frequency, sensorineural hearing loss demonstrated by pure tone audiometry. His occupational history revealed that he had been a police officer for 25 years. His duties required him to practice with his 9 mm handgun on a monthly basis and each time he would fire from 50 to 60 rounds of ammunition. He did not use ear protection for the first 15 years, but used it regularly for the remaining 10 years.

When impairment is calculated according to the present AMA Guides formula, the patient shows an 8.8% binaural handicap. His audiogram shows a pure tone hearing loss as follows:

Hz	500	1,000	2,000	3,000	4,000	6,000
Right ear	15	15	30	60	70	60
Left ear	10	15	40	70	80	60 ■

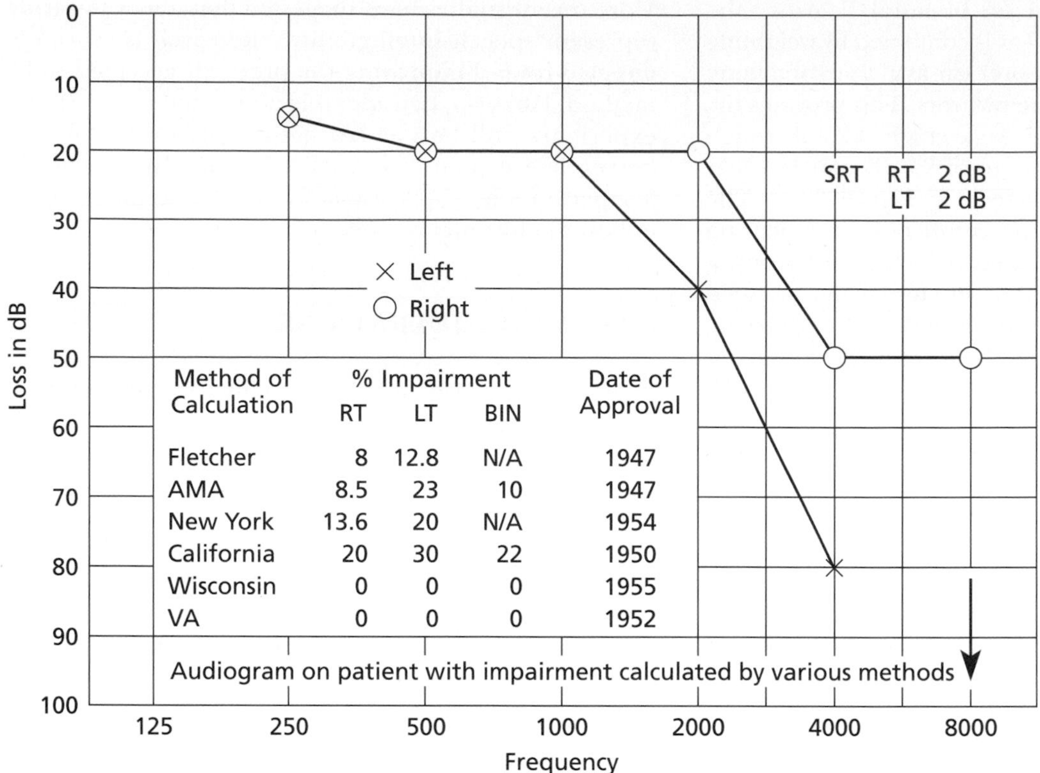

Method of Calculation	% Impairment RT	LT	BIN	Date of Approval
Fletcher	8	12.8	N/A	1947
AMA	8.5	23	10	1947
New York	13.6	20	N/A	1954
California	20	30	22	1950
Wisconsin	0	0	0	1955
VA	0	0	0	1952

Figure 37–2. Audiogram of sample patient. The inset table shows impairment of that patient by various rating systems. AMA = American Medical Association; VA = Veteran's Administration; SRT = Speech Reception Threshold Test; RT = Right ear; LT = Left ear; dB = Decibels; BIN = Binaural; ↓ at 8000 = Arrow showing hearing level at 8 kHz is beyond limits of audiometer. (Data compiled from Fletcher H: A method of calculating hearing loss for speech from the audiogram. Acta Otolaryngol 90[Suppl.]: 26–37; American Medical Association, 1947; New York Workman's Compensation Board, 1954 [amended 1958]; California Industrial Accident Commission, 1950 and 1962; Wisconsin Industrial Commission, 1955; Chief Medical Director, Veterans' Administration, Washington, DC, 1952.)

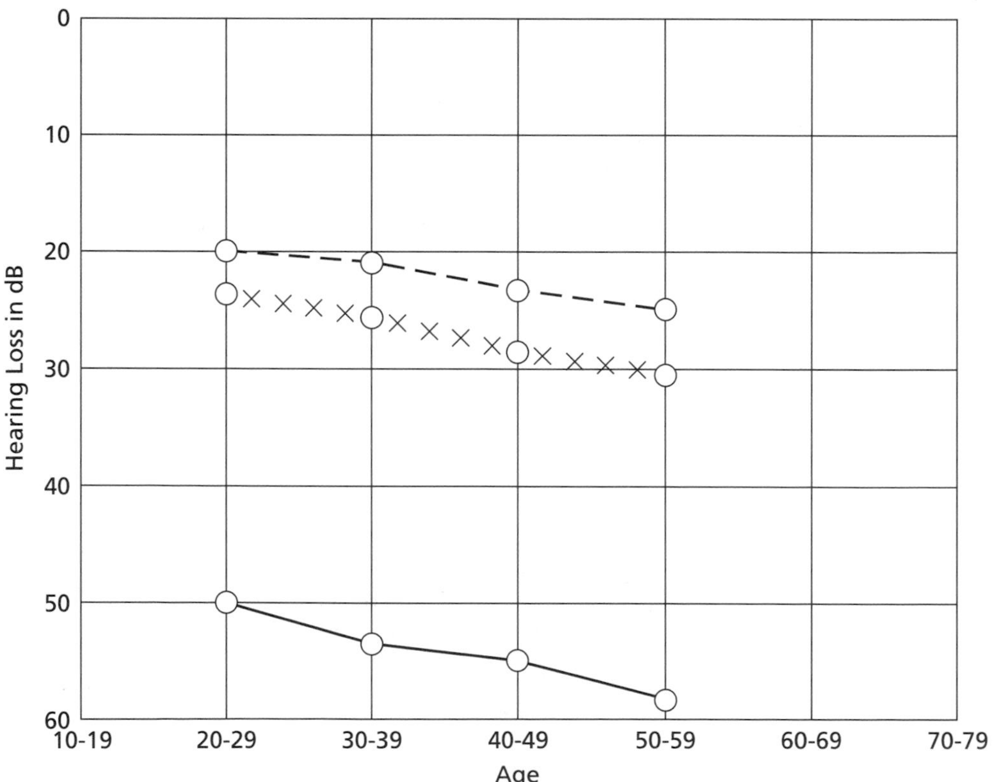

Figure 37–3. Rationale for choosing 25 db as cutoff point for hearing impairment.

TABLE 37–2

Formulas Used by Various States: Occupational Hearing Loss Statutes

State	OHL Compensable	Time Limit to File	Separation From Noise Before Filing	Minimum Exposure in Last Employment	Hearing Loss Formula	Presbycusis Deduction for Aging	Deduction for Pre-Existing Loss	Benefits (Scheduled Injury) One Ear	Both	Choice of Physician	Aural Rehabilitation Provided?	Waiting Period	Award for Tinnitus (Ringing Noise)
AL	Y	1 y–q	NIS	NIS	ME	N	Y	$11,6600	$35,860	Carrier	P	N	(1)
AK	Y	D–2 y	NIS	NIS	ME	N	N	[2]	[2]	Employee	P	N	Y
AZ	Y	1 y	NIS	NIS	59 AAOO	N	Y	$28,110	$84,006	Employee	Y	N	N
AR	Y	2 y	NIS	NIS	ME	N	N	$11,802	$44,398	Carrier	Y	N	P
CA	Y	D–1 y	NIS	NIS	79 AAOO	N	Y	[2]	[2]	Employee	P	N	Y
CO	Y	3–5 y	NIS	NIS	ME	N	Y	$9,991	$39,681	Carrier	Y	N	N
CT	Y	D–1 y	NIS	NIS	59 AAOO	N	N	$32,656	$97,968	Employee	N	N	P
DE	Y	D–y	NIS	NIS	ME	N	Y	$30,833	$71,944	Employee	Y	N	P
DC	Y	1 y	6 m	NIS	47 AMA	P	Y	$43,410	$166,964	Employee	Y	N	P
FL	Y	D–2 y	NIS	NIS	ME	N	Y	[3]	[3]	Carrier	Y	N	Y
GA	Y	1 y	6 m	90 d	59 AAOO	N	Y	$24,375	$48,750	Carrier	Y	6 m	N
HI	Y	D–1–2 y	NIS	NIS	59 AAOO	N	N	$26,998	$103,800	Employee	P	N	Y
ID	Y	1 y	NIS	NIS	ME	N	Y	[4]	$43,890	Carrier	Y	N	NIS
IL	Y	3 y	NIS	90 d	ME	N	Y	$43,140	$172,560	Employee	N	N	NIS
IN	Y[5]	2–3 y	NIS	NIS	ME	N	Y	$12,500	$39,500	Carrier	Y	N	N
IA	Y	2 y	6 m	90 d	ME	Y	Y	$43,600	$152,600	Carrier	Y	N	Y
KS	Y	1 y	NIS	NIS	47 AMA	N	N	$10,980	$40,260	Carrier	Y	N	N
KY	Y	1–3	6 m	90 d	59 AAO	N	Y	[4]	[4]	Employee	N	N	P
LA	Y	D–4 m	NIS	NIS	ME	Y	N	[6]	[6]	Carrier	Y	N	NIS
ME	Y	2 y	30 d	90 d	59 AAOO	Y	Y	$33,050	$88,200	Employee	Y	30 d	Y
MD	Y	2 y	6 m	90 d	59 AAOO	Y	Y	$56,500	$150,516	Employee	Y	6 m	NIS
MA	Y	D–1 y	NIS	NIS	ME	N	N	$20,297	$53,892	Employee	P	N	P
MI	N	D–4 m	NIS	NIS	ME	N	Y	[7]	[7]	Carrier	Y	N	N
MN	Y	D–3 y	NIS	NIS	ME	N	N	[3]	[3]	Employee	Y	N	P
MS	Y	D–2 y	NIS	NIS	ME	N	Y	$11,714	$43,929	Carrier	Y	N	P
MO	Y	D–1 y	6 m	90 d	59 AAOO	Y	Y	$14,442	$53,051	Carrier	N	6 m	N
MT	Y	D–30 d	6 m	90 d	59 AAOO	Y	Y	[2]	[2]	Employee	Y	6 m	N
NE	Y	D–6 m	NIS	NIS	59 AAOO	N	Y	$23,400	[8]	Employee	N	N	Y
NV	Y	D–90 d	NIS	NIS	79 AAOO	N	Y	[2]	[2]	Employee	P	N	Y
NH	Y	2 y	NIS	NIS	59 AAOO	P	N	$25,200	$103,320	Carrier	Y	N	Y
NJ	Y	D–1/2 y	4 weeks	1 y 3 d 40 weeks	47 AMA (Plus 3,000 Hz)	P	N	$8,640	$50,400	Carrier	N	N	N
NM	Y	1 y	NIS	NIS	ME	NIS	Y	$15,682	$58,808	Carrier	NIS	N	N
NY	Y	90 d–2 y	3 m	90 d	59 AAOO	N	Y	$24,000	$60,000	Panel	P	6 m	Y
NC	Y	D–2 y	6 m	90 d	59 AAOO	N	Y	$39,200	$84,000	Carrier	Y	6 m	N
ND	Y	1 y	NIS	NIS	AMA	N	N	$20,850	$83,400	Employee	Y	5 d	N
OH	Y	6 m	NIS	NIS	ME	N	Y	$14,175	$70,875	Employee	Y	N	Y
OK	Y	D–3–18 m	NIS	NIS	AMA	N	N	$21,300	$63,900	Carrier	Y	N	Y
OR	Y	D–180 d To 5 y	NIS	NIS	500-6K	Y	Y	$27,240	$87,168	Employee	Y	N	Y
PA	Y	3 y	NIS	NIS	AMA(9)	N	Y	$35,280	$152,880	Carrier	N	N	N
RI	Y	D–2 y	6 m	NIS	59 AAOO	P	Y	$5,400	$18,000	Employee	Y	6 ms	N
SC	Y	D–2 y	NIS	NIS	ME	P	Y	$38,678	$79,773	Carrier	Y	N	Y
SD	Y	2 y	6 ms	90 d	AMA	Y	Y	[10]	$61,200	Carrier	Y	N	N
TN	Y	1–3 y	NIS	NIS	ME	N	N	[10]	$77,250	Panel	N	N	P
TX	Y	6 m	6 m	NIS	59 AAOO	N	Y	[10]	$54,9000	Carrier	Y	N	Y
UT	Y	1 y	6 m	NIS	ME	Y	Y	[10]	$32,5000	Carrier	N	6 m	N
VT	Y	1 y	NIS	NIS	ME	N	Y	$37,804	$130,860	Employee	Y	N	Y
VA	Y	D–2 y	NIS	NIS	59 AAOO	N	Y	$26,700	$53,400	Panel	Y	N	Y
WA	Y	D–1 y	NIS	NIS	59 AAOO	N	Y	[11]	[11]	Employee	NIS	N	P
WW	Y	D–3 y	NIS	NIS	59 AAOO	N	N[2]	[2]	[2]	Employee	Y	N	P
WI	Y	NONE	14 d	90 d	CHABA	Y	Y	$6,624	$39,744	Employee	Y	2 m	N
WY	Y	D–1–3 y	NIS	NIS	ME	P	N	$12,400	$24,800	Employee	Y	N	N

[1] Alabama: Courts have the authority for establishing criteria to be used in determining the degree of hearing loss.
[2] Alaska, California, Montana, Nevada, and West Virginia: Ratings for compensation purposes are determined as a percentage of permanent total disability.
[3] Florida and Minnesota: Benefits paid according to degree of impairment and loss of earnings.
[4] Idaho and Kentucky: Weekly benefit amount is 55% of the state average weekly wage (SAWW).
[5] Indiana: Yes. If traumatic injury.
[6] Louisiana: No hearing loss schedule.
[7] Michigan: Hearing loss compensation based on wage loss.
[8] Nebraska: Loss of hearing in both ears constitutes permanent total disability.
[9] Pennsylvania: No award for under 10%.
[10] South Dakota, Tennessee, Texas, and Utah: Monaural loss is determined as a percentage of binaural loss.
[11] Washington: Benefits based on percentage of disability, or combination thereof, at the time of injury.

OHL, occupational hearing loss; P, possible; D, discovery rule; N, no; Y, yes; AMA, American Medical Association; AAOO, American Academy of Ophthalmology and Otolaryngology; NIS, not in statute; CHABA, Committee on Hearing, Bioacoustics and Biomechanics (working group of the National Academy of Sciences); ANSI, American National Standards Institute.

Modified from Herman AM, Anderson BE, Kerr TM (eds): State Workers' Compensation Laws. Washington, DC, U.S. Department of Labor, 1999, pp 160–163.

TABLE 37-3
How the Formula is used

	500 Hz	1,000 Hz	2,000 Hz	3,000 Hz
Right ear	15	25	45	55
Left ear	20	30	50	60

Example: mild hearing loss.

1. Right ear $\frac{15 + 25 + 45 + 55}{4} = \frac{140}{4}$ = 35-dB average
2. Left ear $\frac{20 + 30 + 50 + 60}{4} = \frac{160}{4}$ = 40-dB average

Monaural impairment

3. Right ear 35–25 = 10 dB × 1.5% = 15%
4. Left ear 40–25 = 15 dB × 1.5% = 22.5%
5. Better ear 15 × 5 = 75
6. Poorer ear 22.5% × 1 = 25.5
7. Total 97.5 ÷ 6 = 16.25

TINNITUS

The problems caused by tinnitus, its quantification, and its effect on human performance have been subjects of discussion and study for many years. Review of past and recent literature indicates that physicians have learned little of significance about tinnitus over the past century. Serious attempts are being made to develop animal models, measurement techniques, and self-scaling methods that should lead to a better understanding of the sources and mechanisms of the phenomenon. Such knowledge will undoubtedly also lead to better methods of management and treatment.

Tinnitus is not a disease. Rather, it is a symptom that may be the result of a disease or injury. However, tinnitus is so common that establishing causation is frequently difficult. The principal reason for the increasing interest in tinnitus within the context of a discussion of impairment and disability is its effect on the daily activities of those individuals who have it. The major problem with tinnitus is that it is primarily a subjective phenomenon. Consequently, it is frequently difficult to verify even the presence of tinnitus, let alone its consequences.

Definition and Prevalence

Tinnitus, or noise in the head or ear, is one of the most challenging symptoms in otology. It has been speculated that tinnitus may be the result of a continuous stream of discharges along the auditory nerve to the brain caused by abnormal irritation in the sensorineural pathway. Although no sound is reaching the ear, the spontaneous nerve discharge may cause the patient to experience a false sensation of sound. Although this theory sounds logical, there is no scientific proof of its validity.

Tinnitus is a term used to describe perceived sounds that originate within a person, rather than in the outside world. Although nearly everyone has mild tinnitus momentarily and intermittently, continuous tinnitus is abnormal. The National Center for Health Statistics reports that about 32% of all adults in the United States acknowledge having had tinnitus at some time.[28] Approximately 6.4% of affected individuals characterize their tinnitus as debilitating or severe. The prevalence of tinnitus increases with age up until approximately 70 years and declines thereafter.[37] This symptom is more common in people with otologic problems, although tinnitus also can occur in otologically normal patients. Nodar reported that approximately 13% of school children with normal audiograms report having tinnitus at least occasionally.[34] Sataloff et al studied 267 normal elderly patients with no history of noise exposure or otologic disease and found that 24% had tinnitus.[46] As expected, the incidence is higher among patients who consult an otologist for any reason. Fowler questioned 2,000 consecutive patients and 85% of them reported tinnitus.[8] Heller and Bergman found that 75% of patients complaining of hearing loss reported tinnitus, and Graham found that approximately 50% of deaf children also complained of tinnitus.[16,17] According to Glasgold and Altmann, nearly 80% of patients with otosclerosis have tinnitus,[12] and House and Brackmann reported that 83% of 500 consecutive patients with acoustic neuromas had tinnitus.[19]

One of the surprising features about tinnitus is that not everybody has it. Consider that the cochlea is exquisitely sensitive to sounds, and relatively loud sounds are being produced inside each human's head, such as the rushing of blood through the cranial arteries as well as the noises made by muscles in the head during chewing. That an individual rarely hears these internal body noises may be explained partially by the way that the temporal bone is situated in the skull and by the depth at which the cochlea is embedded in the temporal bone. The architecture and the acoustics of the head ordinarily prevent the transmission of these noises through the bones of the skull to the cochlea and thus to consciousness; yet the cochlea is built and situated in such a way that normally it can respond to very weak sounds carried by the air from outside the head. Only when there are certain changes in the vascular walls—perhaps caused by arteriosclerosis—or in the temporal bone structure does the ear pick up these internal noises. Patients may say that they hear their own pulse as a result of a vascular disorder, and it may seem to be louder when the room is quiet, or at night when they are trying to go to sleep. Pressing on various blood vessels in the neck rarely stops this type of tinnitus, which is not associated with hearing loss.

In addition to being troublesome, tinnitus may also serve as an early warning of auditory injury. For example, a high-pitched ringing or hissing may be the first indication of impending cochlear damage from ototoxic drugs—a clear signal that the drug should be stopped or its dosage reduced whenever possible. Generally, the tinnitus disappears and no measurable hearing loss results, although in some instances the tinnitus may persist for months or even years.

Among the common drugs capable of producing tinnitus are aspirin and quinine in large doses, and many antibiotics.[44] These drugs should be used with extreme caution, especially when kidney function is deficient.

Among the common misconceptions about tinnitus is that it is idiopathic and incurable. Neither of these assumptions is always correct. Awareness of conditions that cause tinnitus, however, has not been as helpful to tinnitus research as might be expected. Recognizing a causal relationship has not shed much light on the actual mechanisms by which internal sounds are created.

Tinnitus usually poses a difficult problem for the physician and patient. Tinnitus may be either subjective (audible only to the patient) or objective (audible to the examiner as well). Objective tinnitus is comparatively easy to detect and localize because it can be heard by the examiner using a stethoscope or other listening device. It may be caused by glomus tumors, arteriovenous malformations, palatal myoclonus, and other conditions. Subjective tinnitus is much more common; however, it cannot be confirmed by current objective tests. Consequently, it is usually difficult to document its presence and quantify its severity, although a few tests are currently available to help. Although the character of tinnitus is rarely diagnostic, certain qualities are suggestive of specific problems. Seashell-like tinnitus is often associated with endolymphatic hydrops, swelling of the inner ear membranes associated with Meniere syndrome, syphilitic labyrinthitis, trauma, and other conditions. Unilateral ringing tinnitus may be caused by trauma, but it is also suggestive of an acoustic neuroma. Pulsatile tinnitus may be caused by arteriovenous malformations or glomus jugulare tumors, although more benign problems are more common.

Evaluation and Rating

Tinnitus is found in large numbers of people, but it is not a frequent unsolicited complaint or a significant handicap. Nevertheless, workers' compensation boards in many states require a statement regarding tinnitus-related impairment. How does one rate or scale "annoyance" or "debilitating" subjective reactions to tinnitus? There is no way to do this scientifically from the information presently available. Consequently, because physicians are often required to rate tinnitus, a variety of individually devised systems that seem reasonable based on available data is used. However, these are not standardized or generally accepted by any official medical organization, such as the American Academy of Otolaryngology–Head and Neck Surgery or the American Medical Association. As an example, tinnitus may be scaled as slight, mild, mild–moderate, moderate, or severe.[36] These ratings, used in California, are based on judgments, or perhaps more correctly, educated guesses, derived from the patient's reported complaints. These are derived through answers to a set of questions designed to determine whether tinnitus is present, and if so, how much of a problem it poses. The questionnaire is not sufficiently extensive to permit a diagnosis. In the following questionnaire, numerical values, indicated in parentheses, are used for rating quantification:

A. Do you have ringing or noises in your ears or head?
   Yes ( )   No ( )
   (If yes, continue to B)
B. Is the noise constant or intermittent?
   Constant ( ) (3)   Intermittent ( )
   If intermittent, is it:
     On more than off ( ) (2)
     Off more than on ( ) (1)
C. Does it prevent you from going to sleep?
   Yes ( ) (2)   No ( ) (0)
D. Is it worse in quiet?
   Yes ( ) (1)   No ( ) (2)
E. Is it worse when you are not busy doing something?
   Yes ( ) (1)   No ( ) (2)
F. What does it sound like?
   High-pitched tone ( ) (2)
   Low-pitched tone ( ) (1)
   Rushing air ( ) (1)
   Static ( ) (2)
   Any other pitch problems (e.g., buzzing or humming) ( ) (1)
G. How much does it bother you?
   Mildly ( ) (1)
   Moderately ( ) (2)
   Severely ( ) (3)

When this is adapted to the California scale, the results are:

5	=	Slight
6–7	=	Mild
8–9	=	Mild-to-moderate
10–11	=	Moderate
12	=	Severe

These ratings are based strictly on the patient's answers. If a physician has any reason to believe that the answers are not truthful and correct, supporting evidence must be presented.

Various other questionnaires and methods for tinnitus evaluation have been proposed. Most prominently, these include techniques for tinnitus matching. Although these are well described and widely used, and are in fact used by the author, they have significant shortcomings.

Recently, instruments have been developed to measure tinnitus handicap. One of the best divides the 25-question assessment into functional, emotional, and catastrophic response categories.[29,32] This tinnitus handicap inventory is well designed and psychometrically validated,[30] but it still depends entirely on voluntary, subjective responses. Objective criteria for detecting exaggerated responses or malingering have not been developed. Similar handicap indices have also been proposed for dizziness[21] and hearing loss.[31,52] Extensive additional research will be required before a fair and reasonable rating system for tinnitus can be developed on a scientific basis. Such a system would be a substantial improvement over current arbitrary practices such as the 5% added impairment for the presence of tinnitus according to the AMA Guides.[1]

Verification

Verification of the presence of tinnitus is an exceedingly difficult task, except in the uncommon cases of objective tinnitus. Measurements of tinnitus loudness and pitch can be made in some patients by matching techniques. It is argued that if the tinnitus can be matched to known signals, it must be present. However, numerous other studies have shown that measurements using these techniques are often unreliable for loudness and pitch, especially for pitch. In individual cases, this may be due to test artifact or fluctuation of the tinnitus. Such measurements are fraught with pitfalls, and in the hands of many, the results can be questionable. Nevertheless, in some cases, these studies are helpful. The author often uses tinnitus masking and matching studies on the same individual, repeated at subsequent evaluations over a period of months. If the individual consistently reports tinnitus at the same frequency and intensity, this is considered reasonably good supporting evidence that the tinnitus is present. All studies agree that subjective complaints of tinnitus do not correlate with measurement findings in most patients.

Experience suggests a direct correlation between compensation amounts and severity of tinnitus complaints. Consequently, it appears particularly important to devise criteria that will help sort out the merits of various claims. A set of criteria developed by a colleague working with tinnitus claims in the Veterans Administration provides interesting guidelines. Before such a tinnitus claim may be considered meritorious, the following conditions have to be met:

1. The complaint (or claim) that tinnitus was present and disabling must have been unsolicited. If the complaint was not present in the medical records before the claim, it seems reasonable to assume that it arose as a consequence of the interview and medical history process.
2. The tinnitus must accompany a compensable level of hearing loss.
3. The treatment history must include one or more attempts to alleviate the perceived disturbance by medication, prosthetic management, or psychiatric interview.
4. There must be evidence to support the idea of personality change or sleep disorders.
5. There must be no contributory history of substance abuse.
6. The complaint of tinnitus must be supported by statements from family members, a spouse, or others close to the patient.[23]

Although these criteria may seem somewhat severe, the difficulties of objective verification and the potential for abuse of the compensation system necessitate such rigor. Awards for tinnitus at jury trials have varied from $15,000 to $1,500,000. When compared, these cases show little, if any, difference in their descriptions of patients' hearing or tinnitus complaints, and some patients have had no compensable hearing loss. With this monetary potential, claimants alleging tinnitus are often familiar with the subject and are aware that its presence cannot be definitively confirmed or refuted in most cases. The listed criteria are designed to elicit some objective corroborating evidence that tinnitus is present. A medical record of tinnitus complaints and evaluations that substantially predate considerations of compensation litigation may be some such evidence. However, issues of causation remain challenging even under these circumstances. At present, one must recognize the hazards of providing compensation for a totally subjective alleged complaint, the presence of which cannot usually be verified, and the personal consequences of which are also extremely difficult to measure. Compensation for tinnitus should be considered appropriate only in a very small percentage of alleged cases.

DIZZINESS

Dizziness, like deafness and tinnitus, is a subjective experience and is a symptom, not a disease. Its cause must be sought carefully in each case. The term "dizziness" is used by patients to describe a variety of sensations, many of which are not related to the vestibular system. It is convenient to think of the balance system as a complex conglomerate of senses that send information to the brain about one's position in space. Components of the balance system include the vestibular labyrinth, the eyes, neck muscles, proprioceptive nerve endings, and cerebellum. If all components of the balance system are providing accurate information, one has no equilibrium problem. However, if most of the components indicate to the brain that the body is standing still, for example, but one component indicates that the body is turning left, the brain becomes confused and a person will experience dizziness. It is the physician's responsibility to analyze systematically each component of the balance system to determine which component or components are providing incorrect information, or whether correct information is being provided and analyzed in an aberrant fashion by the brain.

Typically, labyrinthine dysfunction is associated with a sense of motion. It may be true spinning, a sensation of being on a ship or of falling, or simply a vague sense of imbalance when moving. In many cases, it is episodic. Fainting, body weakness, spots before the eyes, general lightheadedness, tightness in the head, and loss of consciousness are generally not of vestibular origin. Such descriptions are of only limited diagnostic help. Even some severe peripheral (vestibular or eighth nerve) lesions may produce only mild unsteadiness or no dizziness at all, as with many patients having acoustic neuromas. Similarly, lesions outside the vestibular system may produce true rotary vertigo, as seen with trauma or microvascular occlusion in the brainstem and with cervical vertigo.

Dizziness is a relatively uncommon problem in healthy individuals. In contrast to a 24% prevalence of tinnitus, Sataloff et al found only a 5% prevalence of dizziness in their study of 267 normal senior citizens.[46] However, most of the population is not as healthy as the highly selected sample in this study. From 5% to 10% of initial physician visits involve a complaint of dizziness or imbalance, accounting for over 11 million physician visits annually.[54] Dizziness is one of the most common reasons for a visit to a physician in patients older than 65 years. Approximately one-third to one-half of people age 65 years and older fall each year, and the consequences can be serious.[22] Falls result in approximately 200,000 hip fractures per year, and this injury carries a 10% mortality rate. Falls are the leading cause of death by injury in people 75 years and older.[22] Dizziness is also a common consequence of head injury. Over 450,000 Americans suffer serious head injuries annually.[53] A majority of these people complain of dizziness for up to 5 years after the injury, and many are disabled by this symptom.[11] Dizziness may also persist for long periods of time after minor head injury.[25]

In addition to deafness and tinnitus, vertigo is an important symptom associated with disorders of the ear. The intimate relationship of the vestibular portion of the labyrinth to the cochlea makes it easy to understand why many diseases and lesions such as Meniere disease, head trauma, and vascular conditions affect both balance and hearing. Some diseases such as mumps classically affect only the cochlea. Certain toxins and viruses affect only the vestibular portion without affecting the hearing. Intense noise damages only the cochlea.

Causes of dizziness are almost as numerous as causes of hearing loss, and some are medically serious, such as multiple sclerosis, acoustic neuroma, diabetes, and cardiac arrhythmia. Consequently, any patient with an equilibrium complaint needs a thorough examination. For example, although dizziness may be caused by head trauma, the fact that it is reported for the first time after an injury is not sufficient to establish causation without investigating other possible causes.

It is important to carry out a systematic inquiry in all cases of disequilibrium, not only because the condition is caused by serious problems in some cases, but also because many patients with balance disorders can be helped. Many people believe incorrectly that sensorineural hearing loss, tinnitus, and dizziness are incurable, but many conditions that cause any or all of these may be treated successfully. It is especially important to separate "peripheral," or noncentral, causes, which are almost always treatable, from more central causes, such as brainstem contusion, in which the prognosis is often worse.[44]

Balance Testing

The balance system is extremely complicated, and ideal tests have not been developed. Research is currently underway to develop tests that will assess accurately the entire composite functioning of the balance system and test each component in isolation. At present, the most commonly performed tests are electronystagmography (ENG) and computerized dynamic posturography (CDP). Vestibular evoked potential testing is under investigation.

Electronystagmography

ENG is a technique for recording eye movements and detecting spontaneous and induced nystagmus. It allows measurement of eye movements with eyes open and closed, and permits quantification of the fast and slow phases, time of onset and duration, and other parameters. Although some centers use only horizontal leads, the use of both horizontal and vertical electrodes is preferable. ENG must be done under controlled conditions with proper preparation, which includes avoidance of drugs (especially those that affect the central nervous system). Even a small drug effect may cause alterations in the ENG tracing. The test is performed in several phases. These include calibration, which assesses cerebellar function; tests for gaze nystagmus, sinusoidal tracking, optokinetic nystagmus, and spontaneous nystagmus; Dix Hallpike (see Box 37–1) and positional testing; and caloric irrigations. The test may give useful information about peripheral and central abnormalities in the vestibular system. Interpretation is complex and difficult.[4,44] The performance of ENG is especially helpful when a unilateral reduced vestibular response is identified in conjunction with other signs of dysfunction in the same ear. In such cases, it provides strong support for a peripheral (eighth nerve or end organ) cause of balance dysfunction.

Computerized Dynamic Posturography

For more than 20 years, platforms have been used to try to assess more complex integrated functioning of the balance system. Until recently, most were static posture platforms with pressure sensors used to measure body sway while patients tried to maintain various challenging positions, such as the Romberg and Tandem Romberg maneuvers (see Box 37–1). Movement was measured with eyes closed and opened. The tests had many drawbacks, including an inability to separate proprioceptive function and eliminate visual distortion. In 1971, Nasher introduced a system of CDP which has been developed into a test system that is available commercially (Equitest) and is used widely.[14]

Dynamic posturography uses a computer-controlled moveable platform with a sway-referenced surrounding visual environment. In other words, both the platform and visual surround move, tracking the anterior-posterior sway of the patient. The visual surround and platform may operate together or independently. The system is capable of creating visual distortions or totally eliminating visual cues. The platform can perform a variety of complex motions, and the patient's body sway is detected through pressure-sensitive strain under the platform.[27]

The typical test protocol evaluates sensory organization through six test procedures and movement coordination through a variety of sudden platform movements. Balancing strategies and responses are assessed using both the sensory organization and movement coordination test batteries. Dynamic posturography provides a great deal of information about total balance function that cannot be obtained from tests such as the ENG alone. Dynamic posturography is also valuable in distinguishing organic from nonorganic disequilibrium, an asset that is particularly valuable in some cases of alleged disability.[23]

BOX 37–1 Clinical Balance Tests

Dix Hallpike Testing: A part of the electronystagmography (ENG) that is specific for paroxysmal spasmodic vertigo.

Romberg Testing: A cerebellar test. The individual with clumsiness of all movements of gait with the eyes closed only, usually indicates peripheral ataxia. No change with the eyes open or closed indicates a cerebellar origin.

Tandem Romberg Testing: Gait is tested by asking patient to walk using heel to toe movements.

Evoked Vestibular Response

Evoked vestibular response testing is analogous to brainstem auditory evoked testing. However, vestibular evoked potentials are not being used clinically.

Impairment and Disability

In many cases, it is possible to document an impairment in the balance system. In others, the subjective complaint of dizziness may be the only abnormality. When present, vertigo and other conditions of disequilibrium may be disabling, particularly for people working in hazardous job situations. Persons who lose their balance even momentarily may injure themselves or others severely when working around sharp surfaces, rotating equipment, driving a forklift, or working on ladders or scaffolding.

There are many other examples of occupations that are not possible for people with disequilibrium disorders. The problem is even worse in conditions that typically cause intermittent severe disequilibrium, such as Meniere disease. The inability to test the balance system thoroughly makes it impossible in some instances to disprove, objectively, workers' contentions that they have spells of dizziness. For example, if a worker is struck in the head while performing his job and claims that he has intermittent "dizzy spells" afterward, even if he has a normal ENG, his assertion may be true. Even if malingering is suspected, in the absence of objective proof, if a physician contests this claim and declares him fit to return to work without sufficient evidence, both the physician and the industry may incur substantial liability if the worker has a period of disequilibrium and seriously injures himself or other workers. Considerable research is needed to develop more sophisticated techniques of assessing equilibrium.

Criteria for classifying equilibrium have been proposed by Sataloff and Hart.[43] This classification is intended to be used following a comprehensive clinical evaluation, appropriate testing, and establishment of a valid estimate of the individual's balance capacity and causation when possible. The classification is intended for use with disturbances caused by organic dysfunction in any part of the spatial orientation system. It is important to recognize that such disorders are commonly dynamic. Hence, judgments regarding the permanency of impairment are most credible following attempts at treating the condition, and after enough time has passed to allow the condition to stabilize.

Classification

Dizziness and especially vertigo can be very disabling symptoms, and are often accompanied by nausea, vomiting, anxiety, headache, and other complaints. Symptoms may be constant, may occur in episodic "attacks," frequently without warning, or may be constant with exacerbations.

Some findings on clinical examination may be entirely objective, such as a third degree spontaneous nystagmus, whereas others may be entirely feigned, e.g., an alleged post-traumatic ataxia of gait. Many others fall between these extremes. Clinical and laboratory assessment are used to establish data that determine impairment and disability classification. Organizing the history and physical and laboratory findings helps to simplify and clarify this process.

Symptoms Elicited by History

1. No complaint of dizziness/unsteadiness
2. Mild dizziness—does not interfere substantially with daily activities
3. Mild to moderate dizziness—interferes with some activities but they can be resumed
4. Moderate dizziness—interferes with many activities, but important activities can usually be accomplished with effort and with lifestyle adjustments
5. Severe dizziness—interferes with most activities; unable to drive or ambulate without assistance
6. Profound dizziness—bedridden or wheelchair-dependent

Signs on Physical Examination

1. None
2. Mild unsteadiness with reduced visual or proprioceptive input
3. Paroxysmal positioning nystagmus or moderate unsteadiness with reduced visual or proprioceptive input
4. Staggering when walking with the eyes closed
5. Inability to stand or walk without the assistance of another individual, even with eyes open

Laboratory Test Results

Laboratory test results correlate well with, and indeed are the primary measure of, impairment of function, but they may not correlate well with disability. This is especially true if the brain and related structures are intact, and if the onset of the impairment occurred months or years prior to the evaluation. Nevertheless, laboratory test results are usually helpful in determining whether there is a physical basis for the individual's complaints.

In correlating symptoms with laboratory tests, it is useful to rate the overall results of the tests as follows:

1. Normal
2. Mildly impaired test results
3. Moderately impaired test results
4. Markedly impaired test results
5. Complete loss of function on testing
6. Consistency among history, physical examination, and test results that is in keeping with organic etiology
7. Inconsistency among history, physical examination, and test results that is not in keeping with organic etiology

The outcome of the symptoms evaluation, the physical signs, and the laboratory test results should be correlated, with emphasis on the validated symptoms—i.e., those confirmed by the history, physical findings, and results of laboratory tests—as best representing the subject's true state of disability.

Consistency

Findings should be fairly consistent across subsets of the evaluation process if otolaryngologic complaints are organic in etiology. Overall review should look for:

1. Consistency among history, symptoms, physical examination, and laboratory tests
2. Inconsistency among history, symptoms, physical examination, and laboratory tests

Impairment Criteria Resulting From Loss of Spatial Orientation and Equilibrium

(See also Table 11–4 of the fifth edition of the AMA Guides.[1[p253]])

Class 1: Impairment of the Whole Person (0%)

A designation of Class 1 is assigned when symptoms or signs of dysequilibrium are present without supporting clinical or objective evidence of organic disease and the dizziness has no effect on the usual activities of daily living.

Class 2: Impairment of the Whole Person (1% to 10%)

A designation of Class 2 is assigned when symptoms or signs of dysequilibrium are present with supporting clinical and/or objective findings, and dizziness may interrupt activities for a brief period of time, but activities can be resumed as soon as the dizziness resolves. Activities of daily living can be performed without assistance except for complex activities.

Class 3: Impairment of the Whole Person (11% to 30%)

A designation of Class 3 is assigned when symptoms or signs of dysequilibrium are present with supporting clinical and/or objective findings, and dizziness has required the patient to change plans and make allowances for dizziness. The person can continue to perform simple activities of daily living such as self-care and household duties, drive, engage in most recreational activities, and work, but is unable to perform complex activities.

Class 4: Impairment of the Whole Person (31% to 60%)

A designation of Class 4 is assigned when symptoms or signs of dysequilibrium are present with supporting clinical and/or objective findings, and the patient's dizziness requires constant adjustments in activities and budgeting of the patient's energies. Activities of daily living cannot be performed without assistance, except for self care.

Class 5: Impairment of the Whole Person (61% to 95%)

A designation of Class 5 is assigned when symptoms or signs of dysequilibrium are present with supporting clinical and/or objective findings, and dizziness prevents the patient from doing most of the activities that he or she could do prior to the onset of dizziness, including drive, work, and take care of a family in the usual fashion. Even essential activities must be limited. Higher values are used when symptoms of dysequilibrium are present with supporting clinical and/or objective findings and the usual activities of daily living cannot be performed without assistance, except for self-care not requiring ambulation, and confinement to the home or other residential facility is necessary under most circumstances.

Disability

Disability rating is beyond the scope of this discussion. However, it is an important and complex subject that requires knowledge of an individual's professional activities. The same impairment rating may produce substantial differences in disability. For example, a computer data entry clerk with Class 3 impairment may have little or no disability, whereas a skyscraper construction worker with the same impairment may be totally disabled for his usual occupation.

Treatment

Dizziness may be curable in some cases. A comprehensive discussion of treatment is beyond the scope of this chapter. However, medications, surgery, manipulation, physical therapy, and other modalities may be successful in some patients, especially when a specific etiology can be identified.[44]

VOICE AND SPEECH

For many years, "voice" and "speech" were treated as one subject under the heading "speech." Since the late 1970s, voice and voice science have evolved as subspecialties in the field of otolaryngology and speech-language pathology. Technology and standards of practice now permit appropriate consideration of both aspects of verbal communication. Voice refers to production of sound of a given quality, ordinarily using the true vocal folds. Speech refers to the shaping of sounds into intelligible words. The disability and handicap associated with severe impairment of speech are intuitively obvious: if a person cannot speak intelligibly, verbal communication in the home, workplace, and social settings is extremely difficult or impossible. However, voice disorders have been underappreciated for so long that their significance may not be as immediately apparent. Nevertheless, if a voice disorder results in hoarseness, breathiness, voice fatigue, decreased vocal volume, or other similar voice disturbances, the worker may be unable to be heard in the presence of even moderate background noise, to carry on telephone conversations for prolonged periods, or to perform work-related and many other kinds of functions. Communication with hard-of-hearing family members and friends may be particularly difficult and frustrating for everyone involved.

Numerous conditions can result in voice or speech disturbances; such information is readily available in the literature.[2,15,39] Briefly, voice and speech afflictions may be due to injury of or trauma to the brain, face, neck, or chest; exposure to toxins and pollution;[41,42] cerebrovascular events; voice misuse; cancer; psychogenic factors; and other causes. The following discussion concentrates on the consequences of voice and speech dysfunction.

Evaluation

For the purposes of this chapter, it should be assumed that the evaluation of voice and speech involves assessment of the ability to produce phonation and articulate speech and does not involve assessment of content, language, or structure. There is no single, generally accepted measure to quantify voice or speech function. Therefore, the standard of practice requires the use of a battery of tests.

Various tests and objective measures of voice have become clinically available since the late 1970s and are used in a growing number of centers. Tests such as strobovideolaryngoscopy, acoustic analysis, phonatory function assessment, and laryngeal electromyography are recognized as appropriate and useful in the evaluation of speech and voice disorders.[3,18,39,40] Evaluation of voice requires visualization of the larynx by a physician trained in laryngoscopy, usually an otolaryngologist, and the determination of a specific medical etiology for voice dysfunction. Assessment of the quality, frequency range, intensity range, endurance, pulmonary function, and function of the larynx as a valve or airflow regulator can be performed easily and inexpensively using readily available equipment. Normative values have been established.[38] More sophisticated techniques to quantify voice function, such as spectrography and inverse filtering, are even more helpful. Slow-motion assessment of vocal fold vibration using strobovideolaryngoscopy is an established procedure first described over 100 years ago and is necessary to establish a diagnosis.[47,48]

A battery of tests is required to determine the audibility, intelligibility, and functional efficiency of speech. Audibility permits the patient to be heard over background noise. Intelligibility is the ability to link recognizable phonetic units of speech in a manner that can be understood. Functional efficiency is the ability to sustain voice and speech for a period of time sufficient to permit useful communication.

There are many approaches available for speech assessment, most of which are described in standard speech-language pathology textbooks.[2] However, for the purposes of determining impairment and disability, the method recommended in the AMA Guides is used most commonly.[23] This assessment procedure uses "The Smith House" reading paragraph, which reads as follows:

> Larry and Ruth Smith have been married nearly fourteen years. They have a small place near Long Lake. Both of them think there's nothing like the country for health. Their two boys would rather live here than any other place. Larry likes to keep some saddle horses close to the house. These make it easy to keep his son amused. If they wish, the boys can go fishing along the shore. When it rains, they usually want to watch television. Ruth has a cherry tree on each side of the kitchen door. In June they enjoy the juice and jelly.

The patient is placed approximately 8 feet from the examiner in a quiet room. The patient is then instructed to read the paragraph so that the examiner can hear plainly and understand the patient, Patients who cannot read are asked to count to 100 (and should be able to do so in under 75 seconds). Patients are expected to be able to complete at least a 10-word sentence in one breath, sustain phonation for at least 10 seconds on one breath, speak loudly enough to be heard across the room, and maintain a speech rate of at least 75 to 100 words per minute.

The advantages of the system described in the AMA Guides are its simplicity and wide use. However, this approach does not take advantage of the many standardized speech evaluation tests available in the literature, of technology for better quantification, or of techniques available to help identify psychogenic and intentional voice and speech dysfunction. These advanced methods should be used when the results of simple confrontation testing as described in the AMA Guides are unconvincing.

More sophisticated criteria for rating voice and/or speech impairment and disability have been proposed by Sataloff.[39(pp795–800)] Disability related to voice disorders is common not only among voice professionals such as singers and actors, but also among broadcasters, teachers, clergy, sales personnel, politicians, attorneys, telephone receptionists, and shop foremen who must shout over noise, and many other professionals who depend on vocal quality and endurance. An appropriate determination of voice-related disability requires a comprehensive understanding of voice science and medicine and legal definitions and issues, and consideration of the vocal needs of each individual with voice impairment. For the purposes of classifying voice and/or speech impairment and disability, audibility, intelligibility, and functional efficiency must be taken into account. Audibility is based on the person's ability to speak at a level sufficient to be heard. It generally reflects the condition of the voice. Intelligibility is based on the ability to articulate and to link phonetic units of speech with accuracy sufficient to be understood. Functional efficiency is based on the ability to produce a satisfactorily rapid rate of speaking and to sustain this rate over a period of time sufficient to permit useful communication. Determination should be based on subjective and objective assessments of voice and speech, and reports pertaining to the individual's performance in every-

TABLE 37–4

Classification of Voice/Speech Impairment

	Class 1 0%–14% Voice/ Speech Impairment	**Class 2 15%–34% Voice/ Speech Impairment**	**Class 3 35%–59% Voice Speech Impairment**	**Class 4 60%–84% Voice Speech Impairment**	**Class 5 85%–100% Voice/ Speech Impairment**
Audibility	Can produce speech of an intensity sufficient for *most* needs of everyday speech, although this sometimes may require effort and occasionally may be beyond individual's capacity	Can produce speech of an intensity sufficient for *many* needs of everyday speech and is usually heard under average conditions; however, may have difficulty being heard in noisy places—such as cars, buses, trains, train stations, or restaurants	Can produce speech of an intensity sufficient for *some* needs of every-day speech such as close conversation; however; has considerable difficulty at a distance or in noisy places—such as cars, buses, trains, train stations, or restaurants—because the voice tires easily and tends to become inaudible after a few seconds	Can produce speech of an intensity sufficient for *a few* needs of everyday speech, but can barely be heard by a close listener or over the telephone and may be able to whisper per audibly but with no louder voice	Can produce speech of an intensity sufficient for *no* needs of everyday speech
Intelligibility	Can perform *most* articulatory acts nec-essary for everyday speech, but may occasionally be asked to repeat and find it difficult or impossible to produce some phonetic units	Can perform *many* articulatory acts nec-essary for everyday speech and be under-stood by a stranger, but may have numer-ous inaccuracies and sometimes appears to have difficulty articulating	Can perform *some* articulatory acts nec-essary for everyday speech and can usually converse with family and friends, but may be under-stood by strangers only with difficulty and often may be asked to repeat	Can perform a *few* articulatory acts necessary for every-day speech, can pro-duce some phonetic units, and may have approximations for a few words such as names of own family members, but is unintelligible out of context	Can perform *no* articulatory acts necessary for everyday speech
Functional Efficiency	Can meet *most* demands of articula-tion and phonation for everyday speech with adequate speed and ease, but occa-sionally may hesitate or speak slowly	Can meet *many* demands of articula-tion and phonation for everyday speech with adequate speed and ease, but some-times speaks with difficulty and speech may be discontinuous, interrupted, hesitant, or slow	Can meet *some* demands of articula-tion and phonation for everyday speech with adequate speed and ease, but can sustain consecutive speech only for brief periods and may give the impression of being easily fatigued	Can meet a *few* demands of articula-tion and phonation for everyday speech with adequate speed and ease (such as single words or short phrases), but cannot maintain uninterrupted speech flow; speech is labored and rate is impractically slow	Can meet *no* demands of articula-tion and phonation for everyday speech with adequate speed and ease

From Cocchiarella L, Andersson GBJ (eds): Guides to the Evaluation of Permanent Impairment, 5th ed. Chicago, American Medical Association, 2001, p 265, with permission.

day living and occupational situations. The reports or evidence should be supplied by reliable observers. The standard of evaluation is the normal speaker's performance in average situations for everyday living for the nonprofessional voice user. For the profes-sional voice user, the standard of evaluation is the expected performance in professional and everyday situations of comparable voice professionals. Table 37–4 summarizes voice and speech impairment crite-ria. In evaluating functioning efficiency, everyday speech communication shall be interpreted as includ-ing activities of daily living as well as routine voice and speech requirements of the person's profession. A judgment is made regarding his or her speech and voice capacity with regard to each of the three columns of the classification chart (Table 37–4). The degree of impairment of voice/speech is equivalent to the greatest percentage of impairment recorded in any one of the three columns of the classification chart. For example, if a person's speech impairment is judged as follows—audibility, 10% (Class 1); intelligi-bility, 50% (Class 3); and functional efficiency, 30%

TABLE 37–5

Speech Impairment Related to Impairment of the Whole Person

% Speech Impairment	% Impairment of the Whole Person Occupational Class 1	% Impairment of the Whole Person Occupational Class 2	% Impairment of the Whole Person Occupational Class 3
0	0	0	0
5	2	4	5
10	4	8	10
15	5	10	15
20	7	14	20
25	9	18	25
30	10	20	30
35	12	24	35
40	14	28	40
45	16	32	45
50	18	36	50
55	19	38	55
60	21	42	60
65	23	46	65
70	24	48	70
75	26	52	75
80	28	56	80
85	30	60	85
90	32	64	90
95	33	66	95
100	35	70	97

Intended as a guideline for converting percentage speech impairment to percentage impairment of the whole person. From Sataloff RT: Professional Voice: The Science and Art of Clinical Care, 2nd ed. San Diego, Singular Publishing Group, 1997, pp 798–799.

(Class 2)—then the voice/speech impairment is judged to be equivalent to the greatest impairment (50%).

Converting an impairment of voice and speech into impairment of the whole person requires knowledge of the individual's occupational voice and speech requirements. These may be divided into three classes, as follows:

Class 1: Voice/speech impairment should not result in significant change in ability to perform necessary occupational functions. Little or no voice/speech required for most daily occupational requirements. Examples: manuscript typist, data entry clerk, copyeditor.

Class 2: Voice/speech is a necessary component of daily occupational responsibilities, but not the principal focus of the individual's occupation. Impairment of voice or speech may make it difficult or impossible for the individual to perform his or her occupation at his or her preimpairment level. Examples: stockbroker, nontrial attorney, supervisor in noisy shop.

Class 3: Voice/speech is a primary occupational asset. Impairment seriously diminishes the individual's ability to perform his or her job, or makes it impossible to do so. Examples: classroom teacher, trial attorney, opera singer, broadcast announcer. Table 37–5 is intended as a guideline for converting percentage of speech impairment to percentage impairment of the whole person.

Patient Example

■ A 20-year-old woman, a singer and artist, has come for an impairment evaluation. She had experienced no voice difficulties until she was exposed to fumes during art classes. An investigation of the art classroom revealed that the room had no windows and poor ventilation. The students worked with acrylics, oil paints, and some materials that were heated in flames. Within the first week of classes she noticed a cough, shortness of breath, and headaches during class. Her requests for room ventilation went unanswered. By the end of the first semester, she could not sing or speak for prolonged periods without becoming hoarse. She also developed severe hoarseness and a headache within 30 minutes of exposure to acrylics and after exposure to other art supplies.

Four years later, her symptoms persisted. She became severely dysphonic and short of breath when exposed to acrylics, perfumes, and many other art supplies. Thus she is unable to continue her career as an artist. In addition, the pulmonary consequences of her exposure have left her with airway reactivity-induced asthma in singers (ARIAS syndrome) and multiple chemical sensitivities, making it impossible for her to pursue a career as a singer or public speaker. In addition to singing, exercise, cold air, and exposures to smoke, dust, and fumes also induce her asthmatic symptoms, which include shortness of breath, wheezing, and coughing. She also becomes hoarse and develops a stuffy nose at these times.

Treatment has included the use of antihistamines and decongestants, which she still takes twice a day. When she does not use these medications, she notices the gradual onset of increasing nasal congestion, sinus drainage, and headaches within 24 hours. To help her breathing difficulties, she takes three puffs of ipratropium bromide three times a day, three puffs of beclomethasone dipropionate three times a day, and two puffs of cromolyn sodium three times a day. She is intolerant of theophylline, even at low doses. In addition, she uses an albuterol inhaler on an as-needed basis. She generally needs an average of two puffs per day.

Despite these medications, she has occasional episodes of respiratory infections. She averages one sinus infection (characterized by pain, fever, and the production of yellow to green discharge) approximately once every 2 to 3 months. She develops lower respiratory infections (characterized by increasing episodes of shortness of breath, wheezing, cough, and the production of yellow to green sputum) approximately once every 4 months. On these occasions, she is treated with antibiotics and a 10-day course of oral steroids. In addition, she requires steroid injections two to three times a year for wheezing. ■

Physical Examination and Test Results

Rhinomanometric studies of the patient's nose reveal moderate resistance to airflow that is completely reversed with phenylephrine. Wheezes are heard in both lungs. A computed tomography scan of her sinuses shows concha bullosa in both maxillary sinuses with generalized sinus mucosal thickening. A screening spirometry test is obtained after she has been off her medications for 24 hours. Her forced expiratory volume at 1 second is 44% of predicted. This improves to 62% after an aerosolized bronchodilator is administered. A methacholine challenge test is also obtained and shows a PC_{20} mg/mL of 0.40.

Using the criteria currently advocated in the AMA Guides,[1] this patient would be classified as Class 1 for audibility, Class 3 for intelligibility, and Class 2 for functional efficiency. This would result in an overall Class 3 designation, with speech impairment rated at 50%. This corresponds to an impairment of the whole person of 18%. This value, of course, should be combined with the value assessed for her asthma (Class 3, 26%–50% whole person impairment; see Chapter 5 of the AMA Guides[1] or Chapter 25 of this book) and a value for her sinus condition (see Table 37–6). A representative value would be 18% combined with 40% combined with 3% or 52% whole person impairment.

NOSE, SINUSES, OLFACTION, AND TASTE

Rhinitis, rhinorrhea, allergic "sinus" conditions, and related maladies are so common that establishing a casual relationship between occupational exposures and these conditions is often difficult. Nevertheless, exposure to various pollutants and irritants, especially organic pesticides, can produce such symptoms, and it is possible for these symptoms to persist even after the worker has been removed from the causal environment. In most cases, mild nasal congestion and rhinorrhea are not serious health problems. However, exposure to some products, including sawdust and radium, may be associated with the development of cancers in the nose and sinuses. These may cause serious permanent impairment and even loss of life. No criteria have been established to measure impairment associated with rhinorrhea, and this condition is usually not a serious disability or handicap for most

TABLE 37–6

Permanent Impairment of the Whole Person Related to Abnormalities of the Nose and Sinuses, and Taste and Smell

Classification	Symptoms	Percentage Impairment of the Whole Person
Mild	Mild rhinorrhea; occasional partial nasal obstruction; no impairment of taste or smell	0% to 1%
Moderate	Chronic rhinorrhea, intermittently purulent; frequent partial nasal obstruction; intermittent sinusitis, resolves (asymptomatic) between episodes, intermittent impairment of taste and/or smell	1% to 2%
Severe	Chronic purulent rhinorrhea; frequent infectious sinusitis; need for sinus surgery; loss of taste and/or smell	3% to 5%

professionals. Nasal obstruction can be a disturbing symptom, and it may even impair work performance in a small number of professions such as those requiring maximal athletic effort and certain musical occupations including singing and the playing of double reed instruments (oboe and bassoon). Measurement of nasal airflow remains controversial. Rhinomanometry may provide an objective measure of nasal resistance at a specific point in time, but rhinomanometry has many limitations and cannot provide a diagnosis or establish causation.[26,35] When used, it must be interpreted expertly, with full understanding of the limitations and variably of the technique. When nasal abnormalities are also associated with loss of olfaction or taste, more important consequences may ensue. Table 37–6 suggests impairment criteria for rhinosinusitis and disorders of taste and smell.

Impairment of smell and taste may also be caused by exposure to inhaled pollutants or those absorbed into the body through points of entry other than the respiratory tract such as the gut or skin. Bilateral complete loss of either sense results in disturbing impairment and disability, especially when there is loss of olfaction, causing an inability to detect toxic fumes and other hazards. In the past, taste and smell assessment have depended entirely on subjective response. However, more sophisticated taste and smell testing is now available and capable of sorting out typical organic and nonorganic responses.[49,51] The AMA Guides suggests a value of 3% impairment of the whole person for patients in whom there is complete loss of olfaction and taste.[1] The 3% figure was not derived from scientific studies and must be considered a "best guess" assignment. Partial loss or distortion of taste and smell may be a more serious impairment or disability for persons in certain industries, such as those involving food and fragrance. Impairment and disability assessment must be individualized in such cases. Complete loss of olfaction in some cases has also led to serious psychiatric disorders and malnutrition.[50]

OTHER AREAS OF OTOLARYNGOLOGY

Impairment of the face, oral cavity, temporomandibular joint, neck, lungs, or the systems for mastication and deglutition may also occur in some people. The AMA Guides divide facial impairment and disfigurement into classes, citing percentage impairments of the whole person in each class.[1,23] These designations are also the result of subjective estimates and are not yet validated by quality-of-life studies or other scientific research (Tables 37–7 and 37–8).

The Guides also provides a classification for respiratory impairment (dyspnea). Neck abnormalities are not widely discussed in terms of impairment. However, neck injury or surgery that produces cranial nerve injury may produce substantial disability in some occupations. This is especially true of injury to the eleventh cranial nerve in anyone who requires upper arm strength and the ability to work with arms above shoulder level. The evaluation of mastication and deglutition has traditionally depended on subjective assessment, such as reports on a patient's dietary tolerance. However, recent advances in the science of deglutition have produced better assessment techniques, including swallowing assessment with flexible fiberoptic endoscopy, three-phase radiographic swallowing studies, and others. These techniques should be used to specify and quantify, when possible, the nature and severity of impairment of mastication and deglutition. There is little precedent and no agreement or standardization regarding quantification of impairment, disability, or compensation levels for most of these conditions. Consequently, until further research has been completed, disability judgments must be made taking into account the individual's impairment and response to this type of impairment; interference with daily activities; interference

TABLE 37–7

Facial Disfigurement and Impairment (Summary of Recommendations in AMA Guides)

Disfigurement	Percentage Impairment of the Whole Person
Mild scars or pigmentation	0% to 5%
Loss of supporting structure (depressed bone)	5% to 10%
Loss of a portion of anatomic part (such as nose)	10% to 15%
Unilateral facial paralysis	1% to 19%
Bilateral facial paralysis	5% to 45%
Loss or deformity of outer ear	0% to 5%
Nasal distortion	0% to 5%
Loss of entire nose	25% to 50%
Massive distortion of facial anatomy	16% to 50%

TABLE 37–8

Permanent Impairment of the Whole Person Related to Abnormalities of Mastication and Deglutition (Summary of Recommendations in AMA Guides)

Disfigurement	Percentage Impairment of the Whole Person
Soft foods only	5% to 19%
Liquid food only	20% to 39%
Dependent on gastrostomy or tube feeding	40% to 60%

with occupational, social, or recreational requirements; and other factors.

References

1. Cocchiarella L, Andersson GBJ (eds): Guides to the Evaluation of Permanent Impairment, 5th ed. Chicago, American Medical Association, 2001.
2. Aronson A: Clinical Voice Disorders, 3rd edition. New York, Thieme Medical Publishers, 1990, pp 117–145.
3. Baken RJ: Clinical Measurements of Speech and Voice. Boston, College Hill Press, Little Brown, 1987.
4. Barbarh O, Stockwell GW: Manual of Electronystagmography. St. Louis, CV Mosby, 1976.
5. Doerfler LG, Nett EM, Matthews J: The relationships between audiologic measures and handicap: Part I. JOHL I:103–152, 1998.
6. Doerfler LG, Nett EM, Matthews J: The relationships between audiologic measures and handicap: Part II. JOHL I:213–235, 1998.
7. Doerfler LG, Nett EM, Matthews J: The relationships between audiologic measures and handicap: Part III. JOHL I:243–264, 1998.
8. Fowler EF: Tinnitus aurium: Its significance in certain diseases of the ear. NY State J Med 12:702–704, 1912.
9. Fowler EP Sr: A simple method of measuring percentage of capacity for hearing speech. JASA 13:373, 1942.
10. Gatehouse S: The role of non-auditory factors in measured and self-reported disability. Acta Otolaryngol (Suppl. 476):249–256, 1991.
11. Gibson WPR: Vertigo associated with trauma. In Dix MR, Hood JD (eds): Vertigo. New York, John Wiley and Sons, 1984.
12. Glasgold A, Altmann R: The effect of stapes surgery on tinnitus in otosclerosis. Laryngoscope 76:1642–1652, 1966.
13. Glorig A: Personal communication, 1995.
14. Goebel JA, Sataloff RT, Hanson JM, et al: Posturographic evidence of non-organic sway pattern in normal subjects, patients and suspected malingers. Otolaryngol Head Neck Surg 117:293–302, 1997.
15. Gould WJ, Sataloff RT, Spiegel JR: Voice Surgery. St. Louis, CV Mosby, 1993.
16. Graham JM: Tinnitus in children with hearing loss, CIBA Foundation Symposium 85. Tinnitus 172–181, 1981.
17. Heller MR, Bergman M: Tinnitus aurium in normally hearing persons. Ann Otol Rhinol Laryngol 62:73–83, 1953.
18. Hirano M: Clinical Examination of the Voice. New York, Springer-Verlag, 1981, pp 1–98.
19. House JW, Brackmann DE: Tinnitus: Surgical Treatment, CIBA Foundation Symposium. Tinnitus 204–212, 1981.
20. International Classification of Impairments, Disabilities, and Handicaps. Geneva, World Health Organization, 1980.
21. Jacobson JP, Newman CW: The development of the dizziness handicap inventory. Arch Otolaryngol Head Neck Surg 116:424–427, 1990.
22. Jenkins HA, Furman JM, Gulya AJ, et al: Disequilibrium of aging. Otolaryngol Head Neck Surg 100:272–282, 1989.
23. Knox: Personal communication (to Glorig A), 1985; Glorig A, personal communication, 1995.
24. Lutman ME: Hearing disability in the elderly. Acta Otolaryngol (Suppl. 476):239–248, 1991.
25. Mandel S, Sataloff RT, Schapiro S: Minor Head Trauma: Assessment, Management and Rehabilitation. New York, Springer-Verlag, 1993.
26. McCaffrey TV, Kern ED: Clinical evaluation of nasal obstruction: A study of 1,000 patients. Arch Otolaryngol 105:542–545, 1979.
27. Nasher LN: A model describing vestibular detection of body sway motion. Acta Otolaryngol Scand 72:429–436, 1971.
28. National Chapter for Health Statistics: Hearing Status and Ear Examinations: Findings Among Adults. United States, 1960–1962. Vital and Health Statistics, Series 11, No. 32. Washington, DC, U.S. Department of HEW, 1968.
29. Newman CW, Jacobson JP, Spitzer JB: Development of the tinnitus handicap inventory. Arch Otolaryngol Head Neck Surg 122:143–148, 1996.
30. Newman CW, Sindrige SA, Jacobson JP: Psychometrically adequacy of the tinnitus handicap inventory (THI) for evaluating treatment outcome. J Am Acad Audiol 9:153–160, 1998.
31. Newman CW, Weinstein BE, Jacobson JP, Hug GA: The hearing handicap inventory for adults: Psychometric adequacy and audiometric correlates. Ear Hearing 11:176–180, 1990.
32. Newman CW, Wharton JA, Jacobson JP: Retest stability of the tinnitus handicap questionnaire. Ann Otol Rhinol Laryngol 104:718–723, 1995.
33. Nilsson M, Soli SD, Sullivan JA: Development of the hearing in noise test for the measurement of speech reception thresholds in quiet and in noise. JASA 95:1085–1099, 1994.
34. Nodar RH: Tinnitus aurium in school-age children: Survey. J Aud Res 12:133–135, 1972.
35. Pallanch JF, McCaffrey TV, Kern ED: Normal nasal resistance. Otolaryngol Head Neck Surg 93:778–785, 1985.
36. Physicians' Guide to Medical Practice in the California Workers' Compensation System. Industrial Medical Council, State of California, 1994, 3:37.
37. Reed GF: An audiometric study of two hundred cases of suspected tinnitus. Arch Otol 71:94–104, 1960.
38. Sataloff RT: Professional Voice: The Science and Art of Clinical Care. New York, Raven Press, 1991.
39. Sataloff RT: Professional Voice: The Science and Art of Clinical Care, 2nd ed. San Diego, Singular Publishing Group, 1997.
40. Sataloff RT: The human voice. Sci Am 267:108–115, 1992.
41. Sataloff RT: The impact of pollution on the voice. Otolaryngol Head Neck Surg 106:701–705, 1992.
42. Sataloff RT: Vocal tract response to toxic injury: Clinical issues. J Voice 8:63–64, 1994.
43. Sataloff RT, Hart CW: Assessing balance impairment. J Occup Hearing Loss 2:191–197, 1999.
44. Sataloff RT, Sataloff J: Occupational Hearing Loss, 2nd ed. New York, Marcel Dekker, 1993, pp 371–372.
45. Sataloff RT, Sataloff J: Occupational Hearing Loss, 3rd ed. New York, Marcel Dekker, 1998.
46. Sataloff J, Sataloff RT, Luenebury W: Tinnitus and vertigo in healthy senior citizens with a history of noise exposure. Am J Otol 8:87–89, 1987.
47. Sataloff RT, Spiegel JR, Carroll LM, et al: Strobovideolaryngoscopy in professional voice users: Results and clinical value. J Voice 1:359–364, 1988.
48. Sataloff RT, Speigel JR, Hawkshaw MJ: Strobovideolaryngoscopy and clinical value. Ann Otol Rhinol Laryngol 100:725–727, 1991.
49. Serby MJ, Chobor KL: Science of Olfaction. New York, Springer-Verlag, 1992, pp 279–584.
50. Spiegel JR, Frattali M: Olfactory consequences of minor head trauma. In Mandel S, Sataloff RT, Schapiro SR (eds): Minor Head Trauma: Assessment, Management and Rehabilitation. New York, Springer-Verlag, pp 225–234.
51. Spielman AI, Brand JG (eds): Experimental Cell Biology of Taste and Olfaction: Current Techniques and Protocol. Boca Raton, Fla, CRC Press, 1995, pp 15–430.
52. Ventry I, Weinstein BE: The hearing handicap inventory for the elderly: A new tool. Ear Hearing 3:128–134, 1982.
53. U.S. Department of Health and Human Services: Head Injury: Hope Through Research. National Institutes of Health Publication. U.S. Department of Health and Human Services, 1989, 84:2478.
54. U.S. Department of Health and Human Services: Public Health Services: National Center for Health Statistics (Series 13). U.S. Department of Health and Human Services, 1978, p 56.

SECTION

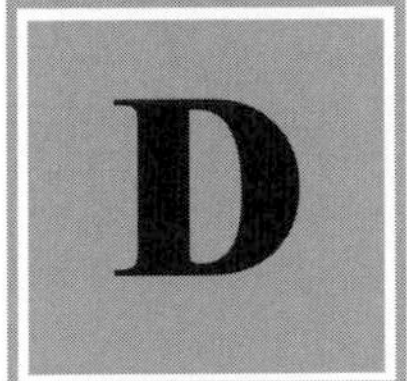

Psychiatric Impairment Assessment

C H A P T E R

38

Psychiatric Diagnostic Techniques

MOSHE S. TOREM, MD

It has been said that physicians determine impairment and lawyers determine disability. In many respects, this is a true statement. The physician's role in determining impairment, as seen in the previous chapters in this section, is one of arriving at diagnoses, describing the limitations that an individual has due to these diagnoses, and deriving an impairment rating based on the severity of the diseases and the patient's limitations. That formulation is used to determine the limitations that individuals have in their activities of daily living and, at times, how these translate into limitations in the workplace.

By the very nature of their specialty, psychiatrists and psychologists, in the usual course of practicing their specialty, must be aware of the circumstance of their patient's life and job. These activities of occupational and daily living are integral parts of a person's psychiatric illness, treatment, and placement. For these reasons, those involved in the psychiatric profession are better equipped to assess the impact of a person's psychiatric illness on occupational and daily living activities than are other members of the medical profession.

The third and fourth editions of the Guides, published in 1988 and 1994[1,2] departed from the traditional concept of impairment rating found in other sections of the book, as well as in previous editions of the Guides, by stating the following:

> Unlike the situations with some organ systems, there are no precise measures of impairment in mental disorders. The use of percentages implies a certainty that does not exist, and the percentages are likely to be used inflexibly by adjudicators, who then are less likely to take into account the many factors that influence mental and behavioral impairment. Moreover, because no data exist that show the reliability of the impairment percentages, it would be difficult for the *Guides* users to defend their use in administrative hearings. After considering this difficult matter, the Committee on Disability and Rehabilitation of the American Psychiatric Association advised *Guides'* contributors against the use of percentages in the chapter on mental and behavioral disorders of the fourth edition.[1(pp301–302)]

There are other reasons arguing against the use of impairment percentages in the psychiatric impairment section. The first is the lack of external verification. For an orthopedic impairment, for example, one starts with a diagnosis, measures a functional impairment by means of a variety of tests, and is then in a position of describing impairments by using these validating tests. When a patient presents with arthritic pain in a shoulder caused by a prior rotator cuff injury, there will be limitation in the range of motion and in some circumstances a muscle weakness caused by these two disorders. The diagnosis is thus "validated" by means of the restriction of motion and diminished muscular strength. These diagnostic and examination abnormalities are then assessed by testing many individuals with similar diagnoses and restrictions and then measuring the degree of impairment in activities of daily living or occupational functioning due to these conditions. Similar examples can be given for other organ systems. However, with psychiatric impairments, this middle step is missing. A diagnosis can be given and tests can be administered. Yet for all their reliability and validity, few of these tests have any objective method of validation. The disturbances in functional activities are driven by the diagnosis rather than by test results.

A more subtle argument can be made against the use of impairment percentages. When using the Guides, physicians measure impairment as opposed to disability. Disability is described more frequently by the psychiatric evaluator. In other words, impairment is translated into situational restrictions. As a result of a psychiatric/psychological evaluation, the evaluator may give a diagnosis and state that, because of the particular diagnosis, the strength of symptomatology, and the response to treatment, an individual is precluded from certain situational activities. Thus psychiatric evaluations more often result in a true disability evaluation than solely an impairment rating.

Both the Social Security Guidelines[32] and the AMA Guides[41] restrict impairment evaluation for psychiatric patients to permanent disorders. The Social Security department defines disability as "the inability to engage in any substantial gainful activity by reason of any medically determinable physical or mental impairment(s) which can be expected to result in death or which has lasted or can be expected to last for a continuous period of not less than 12 months."[32(p2)] The Guides state that "an impairment should not be considered 'permanent' until the clinical findings, determined during a period of months, indicate that the medical condition is static and well stabilized."[1(p9)] By applying such criteria, many of the acute, situational difficulties that arise because of behavioral or psychiatric disturbances will be eliminated. The evaluator of psychiatric impairment, from material previously developed on these individuals, not only will be aware of a patient's diagnosis and restrictions on both the activities of daily and occupational life, but also should be aware of the response to treatment. This information will then be incorporated into the impairment rating. As such, greater opportunity is afforded the psychiatric evaluator to assess disability, as opposed to strictly impairment.

DSM-IV

In 1994, the American Psychiatric Association published the fourth edition of the Diagnostic and Statistical Manual of Mental Disorders (DSM-IV).[4] This almost 900-page book is described as a "team effort. More than 1,000 people (and numerous professional organizations) have helped us in the preparation of this document."[4(pXIII)] The book lists and describes the criteria necessary to arrive at various psychiatric diagnoses. The World Health Organization has published a similar classification, entitled International Statistical Classification of Diseases and Related Health Problems (ICD-10),[34] and the authors of the DSM-IV state that the two systems are fully compatible.

In recent years, the number of people claiming disability due to psychiatric illness has been steadily increasing. This phenomenon may be due in part to an increased public awareness and knowledge of the nature of mental illness as a result of regular patient education campaigns by professional organizations, such as the American Psychiatric Association, and the increased popularity of self-help publications. In addition, DSM-III introduced a new diagnostic category making it easier to identify psychiatric illness as a result of trauma (post-traumatic stress disorder),[2] and a new diagnostic category was added in DSM-IV—acute stress disorder.[4]

DSM-III introduced a new system of diagnosing mental illness based on a multi-axial paradigm. This approach has been continued and refined in the following editions of DSM-III-R[3] and DSM-IV.[4] This multi-axial system requires that the mental health professional diagnose the patient's condition on five different axes or categories.

Axis I: Clinical Disorders and/or Other Conditions That May be a Focus of Clinical Attention

Axis I is used for reporting all the various mental disorders or conditions except for personality disorders and mental retardation (which are reported on Axis II). If more than one mental disorder is diagnosed, the first and principal diagnosis listed will be the one that is the major cause of the person's psychiatric illness.

Axis II: Personality Disorders and/or Mental Retardation

Axis II is used for reporting personality disorders and/or mental retardation. Here, the clinician is expected to assess a person's lifelong behavioral patterns that define his or her character and personality. Many individuals have a diagnosis on both Axis I and Axis II: however, some may only have a diagnosis on Axis I and none on Axis II.

Axis III: General Medical Conditions

Axis III refers to the person's general medical health, determined by a review of medical records and examinations, and should include all coexisting medical diagnoses. When an individual has more than one clinical diagnosis for Axis III, all diagnoses should be reported. Some individuals may have no diagnoses on Axis III, indicating that they are in good physical health.

Axis IV: Psychosocial and Environmental Problems

In this section, the examiner is expected to report any psychosocial and environmental problems that may impact on a person's condition, treatment, and prognosis. A psychosocial or environmental problem may be a stressful life event, an environmental difficulty or deficiency, a family or interpersonal stressor, an inadequacy of social support or personal resources, or any other problem relating to the context and setting in which the individual's difficulties have developed. Some people have so-called positive stressors, such as a job promotion, falling in love, getting married, having children, or getting a prestigious award. These should be listed only if they lead to a specific identified problem or contribute to the patient's maladaptive functioning.

In some cases, psychosocial problems may develop as a consequence of the psychopathology found on Axis I and/or II and/or a medical condition on Axis III. In some individuals, multiple psychosocial or environmental problems may be identified and in these cases, clinicians are required to list as many as are judged to be relevant. The general guideline, according to DSM-IV,[4] is that clinicians should note only those psychosocial and environmental problems that have been present during the year preceding the current evaluation. However, DSM-IV states, "the clinician may choose to note psychosocial and environmental problems occurring prior to the previous year if these clearly contribute to the mental disorder or have become a focus of treatment—for example, previous combat experiences leading to Posttraumatic Stress Disorder." For convenience, DSM-IV has grouped the problems into nine categories (Table 38–1).

Axis V: Global Assessment of Functioning

According to DSM-IV,[4] Axis V was created for reporting the individual's overall level of functioning. This information is useful not only in assessing the severity of the impairment, but also in planning treatment, measuring its impact, and predicting outcome. Assessing the overall level of functioning in Axis V is done by using the Global Assessment of Functioning (GAF) scale (found in the appendix of DSM-IV).[4] The GAF scale is to be used only with respect to psychological, social, and occupational functioning (disability). The instructions clearly specify: "Do not include impairment in functioning due to physical (or environmental) limitations."[4] In many cases, it is useful to rate the individual's global level of functioning at the time of the examination and, separately, the highest level of functioning for at least 3 months during the past year preceding the examination.

The rating of overall psychosocial functioning is done on a scale of 0 to 100 and was operationalized by Luborsky.[18] Endicot et al[9] developed a revision of Luborsky's Health-Sickness Rating Scale, which they called the Global Assessment Scale. The GAF is a modified version of the Global Assessment Scale.

Other than the GAF scale, Axis V also utilizes the Defensive Functioning Scale and the Social and Occupational Functioning Assessment Scale, which are also found in the appendices of DSM-IV.[4]

TABLE 38–1

DSM-IV—Axis IV: Psychosocial and Environmental Problems

1. Problems with primary support group
2. Problems related to the social environment
3. Educational problems
4. Occupational problems
5. Housing problems
6. Economic problems
7. Problems with access to health care services
8. Problems related to interaction with the legal system/crime
9. Other psychosocial and environmental problems

THE PSYCHIATRIC EXAMINATION

To determine psychiatric disability and impairment, a competent evaluation begins with a thorough psychiatric and medical history that includes the following items: the date that a person's symptoms began, the existing environment in which the symptoms took place, the level of stress or dissatisfaction in an individual's home life and work environment, what the person thought was going on at the time that the symptoms started, and to what he or she attributed the source of the symptoms (e.g., to being overworked, to a specific injury, to a harsh and critical boss, to the threat of losing one's job, to being required to do work without proper training, to family and marital conflicts, to a recent death in the family, or to being sinful and unfaithful). Such a history should also include the actions taken to relieve these symptoms, including visits to other medical practitioners including psychiatrists and other mental health professionals, such as psychologists, counselors, or ministers. This history should also include the response to such treatments as well as whether medications have been used, their positive effects in controlling symptoms, their side effects, and which medications created no significant changes. Moreover, the history should include past events prior to the beginning of the present illness symptoms or work impairment and should provide information regarding past treatment, hospitalizations, suicide attempts, or personal losses. In addition, the history should include data about the individual as a person, including such significant elements as a history of childhood abuse, trauma, school functioning and level of education, as well as personal habits, such as the use of caffeine, alcohol, or nonprescription drugs. A history of possible addiction, such as laxative abuse, cigarette smoking or use of other forms of tobacco, alcohol use, or illicit drug use should be noted. The current marital relationship (if applicable) and any possible forms of stress and family dysfunction should be detailed. It is also important to inquire into the health of the person's parents, grandparents, and siblings, as certain psychiatric conditions have a strong hereditary component, including bipolar mood disorders, obsessive-compulsive disorder, attention-deficit disorder, certain forms of mental retardation, communication disorders, anxiety disorders, alcoholism, depressive disorders, and personality disorders.

Before a claimant is seen, it is helpful to use a self-assessment questionnaire to elicit his or her own words in describing, in writing, the nature of the distress, what relieves it, what makes it worse, and his or her opinion about possible solutions, including the desire for disability and one's own assessment of the level of impairment. It is also important to include in such a self-assessment form a section that relates to the claimant's wishes about the future, as well as concrete plans regarding one's job and plans for a source of income.

The examination is based on a thorough mental status examination, which includes the following sections: general observations of the claimant's appearance, how well he or she is dressed and groomed, and how that is compatible with his or her socioeconomic and occupational status. General observations should also include the claiment's general demeanor, to what extent he or she was spontaneous in describing his or her perceived problems, and to what extent he or she was overtly negativistic, hostile, mistrustful, or suspicious, or pleasant and cooperative. Other important observations include items that are relevant to the claimant's general behavior and activity during the interview and psychiatric examination. Such observations may include any of the following: hyperactivity, hypoactivity, silliness, agitation grimaces, mannerisms, tics, compulsions, hypervigilence, boredom, tearfulness, sitting in a stooped fashion, pacing, or elation. It is often helpful to observe if the claimant's facial expressions and posture were appropriate to the interview. The overall comprehensive findings of the psychiatric examination should be recorded on a structured form. An example is provided in Figure 38–1 (which may be copied from this chapter by any person for the purposes of a psychiatric evaluation without permission from the publisher).

The psychiatric examination proceeds with examination of the person's mood; affect; thought processes; thought content; somatic functioning and concern; perception; sensorium; cognitive functions; judgment; insight; attitude towards one's illness; and potential for self injury, suicidal behavior, or violence.

The examination should also evaluate the claimant's attitude toward the examiner as well as possible barriers to communication, including deficiencies in speaking English, necessitating an interpreter; deafness, necessitating a sign language interpreter; poor quality of speech due to aphasia or severe stuttering; refusal to cooperate; or conscious falsification of information. These data determine the reliability and completeness of information, which should be assessed and reported by the examiner.

The examiner should rate the overall severity of illness and its impact on the person's life on a scale of mild, moderate, marked, severe, or extremely severe. Once these are completed, the examiner should provide a formulation of the data, including the person's strengths and assets. This formulation should lead to a consideration of possible diagnoses on Axis I according to DSM-IV.

EVALUATING PSYCHIATRIC IMPAIRMENTS

As mentioned previously, to meet the criteria for disability, a person must have an impairment that disrupts his or her level of adaptive functioning in activities of daily living at home or in the workplace. According to the U.S. Department of Health and Human Services' Disability Evaluation Under Social Security,[32] the assessment of the severity of mental impairments includes four different aspects: limitations in activities of daily living; social functioning; concentration, persistence, and pace; and deterioration or decompensation in work or work-like settings. These are discussed in detail in that source.[32]

PSYCHOLOGICAL TESTS

There are hundreds of psychological tests. Some of the tests that are especially helpful in performing a thorough psychiatric impairment or disability examination are listed below. Some are given to the claimant to be self-administered and later interpreted by the examining psychiatrist.

1. **Beck scales to assess anxiety and depression:** Each of these two widely used scales consists of a 21-item inventory of the individual's self-report on his or her emotions, feelings, and behaviors related to anxiety or depression. The Beck scales for anxiety or depression are easy to score and provide valuable information on the severity of anxiety and depression, rating them as minimal, mild, moderate, severe, or extreme.[5–7]
2. **Zung scales to assess anxiety and depression:** These two scales consist of 20 questions each with four possible answers on a Likert-type scale. The interpretation is simple and provides information on the claimant's level and severity of anxiety or depression.[35–40]
3. **Hamilton scales to assess anxiety and depression:** Hamilton[14–16] developed specific scales that assist in the assessment of anxiety and depression. However, they require active assessment by the examiner of the person's mental state. The patient is rated on a

THE CENTER FOR MIND-BODY MEDICINE

PSYCHIATRIC ASSESSMENT AND MENTAL STATUS EXAMINATION*

Basic Data:

Name: ______________________ DOB: __________ Age: ________

Social Security No.: ______________________

Claim Number: ______________ Injury Date: ______________

Employer's Name: ______________________

Policy Number: ______________________

Name of Examiner: ______________________

Place of Examination: ______________________

Date of Examination: ______________________

Primary Care Physician: ______________ Tel#: __________

Additional Current Physicians: ______________________

____

____

Referral Source and Reason for Assessment and Examination:

____

____

____

____

*** Developed by Moshe S. Torem, M.D., FAPA**
Medical Director, The Center for Mind-Body Medicine
4125 Medina Road, Akron, Ohio, 44333

Figure 38–1. Sample of a psychiatric assessment and mental status examination form. (Developed by Moshe S. Torem, MD, FAPA, Medical Director, The Center for Mind-body Medicine, 4125 Medina Road, Akron, OH 44333.)

Figure continued on following page

PSYCHIATRIC ASSESSMENT AND MENTAL STATUS EXAMINATION

Psychiatric Interview and Medical History:

Chief Complaint(s) and Current Symptoms:

Relevant Data from History of Present Illness:

Relevant Data from Past Psychiatric and Medical History:

Relevant Data from Personal History:

Relevant Data from Family History:

Figure 38–1. *Continued*

PSYCHIATRIC ASSESSMENT AND MENTAL STATUS EXAMINATION

Current Medical Conditions and Recent Surgeries:

Current Medications and Dosage:

Personality Style:

Adjustment to Illness and Coping Skills:

Future Plans:

Relevant Additional Information:

Figure 38–1. *Continued*

PSYCHIATRIC ASSESSMENT AND MENTAL STATUS EXAMINATION

MENTAL STATUS EXAMINATION: (Circle all items that apply)

Apparent Physical Health: poor fair good

Appearance:					
	clean clothes	neatly dressed	well groomed	disheveled	bispeckled
	unkempt	sloppy	dirty clothes	casual	

General Demeaner:				
	spontaneous	demanding	friendly	cordial
	preoccupied	manipulative	cold/aloof	agreeable
	regressed	negativistic	animated	irritable
	mistrustful	hostile	suspicious	ingraciating

Eye Contact:				
	avoids direct gaze	most of the time	often	occasionally
	stares into space	most of the time	often	occasionally
	glances furtively	most of the time	often	occasionally

Psychomotor Behavior:					
	stooped	relaxed	fidgeting	tremors	hyperactive
	tics	restless	overall slowing	hypervigilant	hypoactive

Facial expressions and body posture appropriate for setting and examination.

Mood:					
anxious	angry	sad	apathetic	helpless	loneliness
hopeless	futureless	tearful	euthymic	elated	anhedonia
constricted	diurnal variation	silly	giggling	ambivalence	

Affect:					
tearful	angry	sad	constricted	full range	anxious
flat	inappropriate for setting	helpless	labile	full supple	panicky
animated	appropriate for setting	hopeless		vivacious	euphoric

Comments on mood/affect:

____

____

____

____

Speech and Thought Process:				
	clear	slurred	incoherent	irrelevant
	loose associations	evasiveness	blocking	word play
	circumstanciality	flight of ideas	loud	monotonous
	whispering	comprehensible	perseverations	logical
	concrete thinking	neologisms	stuttering	articulate

Figure 38–1. *Continued*

PSYCHIATRIC ASSESSMENT AND MENTAL STATUS EXAMINATION

Rate of Speech: fast slow average

Comments on Speech and Thought Process:

____
____
____
____

Thought Content:

grandiosity	ideas of reference	delusions
suspiciousness	self derogatory	obsessions
ambivalence	persecutory	phobias
autistic thinking	religiosity	self harm
erotomania	suicidal	somatic
paranoid	resentful	death and dying
thought insertion	nihilistic	bizarre
shame	guilt	hypochondriacal worries

Major focus of thoughts:

____
____
____
____

Comments on Thought Content:

____
____
____
____

Somatic Functions and Concerns:
(in the past three months)

Appetite Changes:	none	decreased	increased		
Eating Issues:	none	binging, overeating	purging	self starvation	dieting
Weight Changes:	none	gained ____ lbs.	lost ____ lbs.	current weight ____ lbs. current height ____	BMI ____
Energy Changes:	none	low energy	excessive energy		
Libido Changes:	none	decreased from usual	increased from usual		

Figure 38-1. *Continued*

PSYCHIATRIC ASSESSMENT AND MENTAL STATUS EXAMINATION

Sleep Problems:

none	increased from usual	decreased from usual
problem falling asleep	sleeps ____ hours in 24 hour period	nightmares
frequent awakenings at night	sleep walking	sleep apnea
early morning awakening	heavy snoring	daytime sleepiness
nocturnal myoclonus	nocturnal incontinence	bruxism
feels tired in a.m.	feels refreshed and rested in a.m.	somniloquy

Somatic Preoccupation and Worries:

none	diarrhea	pain	shortness of breath	headaches
nausea	vomiting	tremor	palpitations	backaches
disuria	itching	sweating	blurred vision	constipation
hoarseness	vertigo	beltching	fatigue	edema

Other concerns: ______________________________

____

Perception: (circle all items that apply)

Hallucinations: ______________________________ Yes No

Illusions: ______________________________ Yes No

Depersonalization: ______________________________ Yes No

Derealization: ______________________________ Yes No

Misperceptions of role: ______________________________ Yes No

Misperception of meaning: ______________________________ Yes No

If "yes" to any of the above, please give details: ______________________________

____

____

____

Sensorium: (circle all items that apply)

Fully oriented in time, place and person: ______________________________ Yes No

Disorientation to time: ______________________________ Yes No

Disorientation to place: ______________________________ Yes No

Disorientation of person: ______________________________ Yes No

Disorientation of context: ______________________________ Yes No

Clouded consciousness: ______________________________ Yes No

Dissociation: ______________________________ Yes No

Figure 38–1. *Continued*

PSYCHIATRIC ASSESSMENT AND MENTAL STATUS EXAMINATION

Give details for any pathological findings: ______________________________

____

____

____

Cognitive Functions:

Memory Impairment:	immediate memory impairment ______________	Yes	No
	recent memory impairment ______________	Yes	No
	remote memory impairment ______________	Yes	No
Attention Deficit: ______________		Yes	No
Distractibility: ______________		Yes	No

If "yes" to any of above, give details: ______________________________

____

____

Abstraction capacity (test for Proverbs): preserved impaired

If impaired specify with examples: ______________________________

____

____

Intelligence: retarded borderline below average average above average

Judgment:

Family relations: ______________ Other social relations: ______________ Finances: ______

Employment: ______________ School: ______________ Future plans: ______________

Insight:

recognition of one's problem or illness ______________	Yes	No
awareness of one's contribution to problem or illness ______________	Yes	No
motivation to get well ______________	Yes	No

Additional comments on insight: ______________________________

____

____

____

Reliability of Information:	very good	good	fair	poor
Attitude Towards Examiner:	positive	neutral	ambivalent	negative
Cooperativeness in the examination:	guarded	only answers questions		fully cooperative

Figure 38–1. *Continued*

PSYCHIATRIC ASSESSMENT AND MENTAL STATUS EXAMINATION

Overall Severity of Illness: mild moderate marked severe

Assets and Strengths:

adaptable	ambitious	animated	articulate
assertive	astute	attentive	believable
brave and careful	broad-minded	charming	courteous
educated	efficient	flexible	future oriented
industrious	intelligent	motivated to get well	enduring
persevering	pragmatic	psychological-minded	energetic
reasonable	resourceful	stable and helpful	introspective
stable work history	confident	support system	thoughtful

Additional comments on Assets and Strengths: ______________________________

____

____

Psychological Scales and Tests Administered:

____

____

____

Discussion and Formulation:

____

____

____

____

Diagnoses:

Major Psychiatric Illness(es) (DSM-IV, Axis I): ______________________________

Personality Disorder(s) (DSM-IV, Axis II): ______________________________

Medical Illness(es) exacerbated by Psychiatric Condition (DSM-IV, Axis III): ______________________________

____

____

Figure 38–1. *Continued*

PSYCHIATRIC ASSESSMENT AND MENTAL STATUS EXAMINATION

Psychosocial and Environmental Problems (DSM-IV, Axis IV) (check all that apply)

_____ Problems with primary support group
_____ Problems with access to health care services
_____ Educational problems
_____ Problems related to the social environment
_____ Economic problems
_____ Housing problems
_____ Occupational problems

Elaborate on checked items: ____

____

____

____

Global Assessment of Functioning Score (GAF) (DSM-IV, Axis V) Current _______ Highest level in past year _____

Prognosis: Poor Fair Good Excellent Unknown

Medical Opinion and Recommendations:

____

____

____

____

____

____

____

____

____

____

____

Name of Examiner Examiner's Signature Date

Figure 38–1. *Continued*

specifically structured rating scale after a thorough psychiatric examination.

4. **Incomplete sentences Blank—adult form:** This is a projective test in which the patient projects his or her thoughts and feelings into words that are interpreted by the examining psychiatrist. This instrument, which has been found helpful by psychologists and psychiatrists, instructs the person to complete a list of 40 sentences that begin with one, two, or three words, allowing the examinee to indirectly reveal some of his or her inner feelings, ambivalence, thought content, thought processes, and richness of vocabulary by communicating in written form. The psychiatrist looks for the existence of any central themes as well as internal inconsistencies and contradictions within one sentence as well as in the full 40 sentences.
5. **Assessing the patient's strengths:** Here, a person is asked to complete a questionnaire focusing on his or her strengths and health rather than psychopathology, illness, and symptoms. This form includes information on such items as one's hobbies, health habits, strength of social support systems, favorite foods, favorite movies, use of leisure time, religious practices, ability for imaginary capacity and daydreaming, personal style of relating to the external world, ability to manage and handle finances, and ability to utilize available resources.
6. **Minnesota Multiphasic Personality Inventory (MMPI):** This particular test has been widely used in the United States and consists of over 500 declarative statements that may be answered "true," "false," or "I can't say." The results are scored by a computer and provide hypotheses for the psychologist to explore with more specific testing. A new updated version of this test has recently been introduced, called the MMPI-II.
7. **Tests of intellectual functioning:** These tests measure the person's apparent level of intellectual functioning as well as intellectual capacity. Commonly, they are known as IQ tests. The most reliable and best validated tests for intellectual functioning are the Wechsler tests. The one commonly used for adults is called the Wechsler Adult Intelligence Scale–Revised.
8. **The Pain Experience Scale:** This is a 19-item self-report instrument; items in the scale represent common experiences found in persons who experience pain. Individuals are requested to rank each statement on a scale of 0 to 6 in terms of how frequently they experience the sensation, feeling, or thought associated with pain.[31]
9. **Neuropsychological testing:** In the last decade, a growing awareness has developed of the not uncommon presence of impaired higher functioning originating from within the neocortex. Some authors[14] believe that about 20% of individuals previously diagnosed as having a psychogenic disorder actually have some type of organic brain syndrome. Neoropsychological tests are performed by psychologists with special training in the field and they are designed to measure a wide range of cortical functions influencing behavior. Some of these brain–behavior functions assessed by neuropsychological testing include the following:
   1. The capacity for learning new skills and ideas
   2. The ability for complex conceptual cognitive processing without being distracted
   3. The capacity to make fine sensory discriminations
   4. The capacity to perform fine motor coordination
   5. The adequacy of perceptual–motor functions
   6. The adequacy of perception and perceptual reasoning
   7. The adequacy of short-term memory
   8. The adequacy of constructional skills
   9. The capacity to persist in performing difficult tasks without being distracted in the face of environmental pressure
   10. The ability to flexibly shift one's expectations, focus, and efforts in the face of a change in conditions of the external environment
   11. The adequacy of language-related functions
   12. The ability to control one's impulses, especially during a stressful situation

   It is important to note that these neuropsychological tests are useful in detecting impairment in cortical brain functions, especially in patients in whom computed axial tomography scan, magnetic resonance imaging, or electroencephalography may be within the normal range and do not reveal a specific disorder. Filskov and Boll[11] provide an excellent resource for learning more about neuropsychological testing and its place in the assessment of functional impairments of the brain.
10. **Projective personality tests:** These tests systematically measure a person's psychological strengths and weaknesses by assessing how well he or she copes when emotionally aroused. The person taking the test is required to respond to ambiguous and vague stimuli, such as inkblots. The most commonly used tests are the Rorschach Inkblot[29] and the Thematic Appreception Test.[20]
11. **Global Assessment of Functioning:** Axis V requires the psychiatrist to assess the claimant on a GAF scale that provides a score on a scale of 0 to 100, with zero meaning inadequate information, 1 to 10 meaning "persistent danger of severely hurting self or others (e.g., recurrent violence) or persistent inability to maintain minimal personal hygiene or serious suicidal act with clear expectation of death," and 91 to 100 indicating "superior functioning in a wide range of activities, life's problems never seem to get out of

hand, is sought out by others because of his or her many positive qualities. No symptoms."[4]

Another scale that has been found helpful is the Jenkins Activity Survey (JAS),[17] a 52-item self-report that evaluates a measure of coping with stress because it focuses on the cognitive and perceptual characteristics of the individual that mediate responses to stress. The JAS has shown predicted validity in the population of patients with coronary heart disease.

The Social Adjustment Scale–Self Report, comprised of 42 questions rated on a five-point scale of severity, was developed by Weissman and Bothwell.[33] It covers such issues as emotional and instrumental qualities in role performance, social and leisure activities, relationships with the extended family, marital role, parental role, family unit, and economic independence. Norms are available for non-patient community samples, acute and recovered depressed patients, patients with schizophrenia, and patients with drug addiction.

PSYCHIATRIC RATING SYSTEMS

Because disability determination is basically a social decision with medical input, various jurisdictions have different rules and requirements. Social Security Disability Insurance determinations are binary; the patient/client is either qualified or not.[12,21,22,32] In the Veterans Administration and workers' compensation systems, disability may range from mild to partial to marked to total.[13,19,25] Obviously, disability measurements must consider the specific system requirements as well as the observable psychiatric impairments.

The New York State Department of Social Services, Office of Disability Determinations, requests semiquantitative ratings in the following "work-related mental activities"[21–23]:

1. Understanding and memory
2. Sustained concentration and persistence
3. Social interaction
4. Adaption (i.e., adaptation to environmental change and demand)

In California, the Industrial Accidents Medical and Chiropractic Advisory Committee, Subcommittee on Permanent Psychiatric Disability, devised a list of eight work functions with five degrees of impairment[10]:

1. The ability to comprehend and follow instructions
2. The ability to perform simple and repetitive tasks
3. The ability to maintain a work task appropriate to a given workload
4. The ability to perform complex and varied tasks
5. The ability to relate to other people beyond giving and receiving instructions
6. The ability to influence people
7. The ability to make generalizations, evaluations, or decisions without immediate supervision
8. The ability to accept and carry out responsibility for direction, control, and planning

The Social Security System[32] categorizes behavioral and psychiatric impairment into the following categories: organic mental disorders; schizophrenic, paranoid, and other psychotic disorders; affective disorders; mental retardation and autism; anxiety-related disorders; somatoform disorders; personality disorders; and substance addiction disorders. Additionally, a special section is devoted to mental disorders for children and young adults (under the age of 18). There are 11 diagnostic categories for these individuals, including organic mental disorders; schizophrenic, delusional (paranoid), schizoaffective, and other psychotic disorders; mood disorders; mental retardation; anxiety disorders; somatoform, eating, and tic disorders; personality disorders; psychoactive substance dependence disorders; autistic disorder and other pervasive developmental disorders; attention deficit hyperactivity disorder; and developmental and emotional disorders of newborn and younger infants.

Various criteria are used to establish inclusion in the categories used by the Social Security system and are found in references 4 and 32. Some of these categories are described in greater detail owing to their pervasive inclusion within rating systems.

The AMA Guides follow the Social Security listings very closely. However, there are special notations made about substance abuse, personality disorders, mental retardation, and pain. Pain is covered in a separate chapter. Table 38–2 reproduces the classification of impairments due to psychiatric abnormalities from the AMA Guides.

ORGANIC BRAIN DISEASES

Organic brain diseases are expressed clinically as either dementia or delirium. By definition, delirium is an acute brain disorder characterized by clouding of consciousness. Delirious patients are almost universally unable to function vocationally or socially. They require intensive medical treatment for the underlying medical condition; for example: delirium tremens due to alcohol withdrawal or delirium caused by septicemia.

Most disability decisions for organic brain disease involve dementias that are chronic disorders with impairment of cognitive and intellectual functioning. In the appraisal of disability related to dementia, accurate quantification of specific cognitive functions is essential.

TABLE 38–2

Classes of Impairment Due to Mental and Behavioral Disorders

Area of Aspect of Functioning	Class 1 No Impairment	Class 2 Mild Impairment	Class 3 Moderate Impairment	Class 4 Marked Impairment	Class 5 Extreme Impairment
Activities of daily living Social functioning Concentration Adaptation	No impairment is noted	Impairment levels are compatible with most useful functioning	Impairment levels are compatible with some, but not all, useful functioning	Impairment levels significantly impede useful functioning	Impairment levels preclude useful functioning

From Cocchiarella L, Andersson GBJ (eds): Guides to the Evaluation of Permanent Impairment, 5th ed. Chicago, American Medical Association, 2001, p 363, with permission.

In addition to the standard battery of psychological tests, including the Wechsler Adult Intelligence Scale, detailed neuropsychological tests may be indicated. These results should be integrated with workplace appraisals. If an employee cannot function in his or her usual assignment, other jobs may be considered before disability is considered. For example, W.C. was a bright, competent accountant prior to an automobile accident in which he sustained frontal and temporal lobe brain damage. Neuropsychological testing revealed substantial loss of short-term memory and appreciable interference with attention and concentration. These impairments were also obvious in a trial of work in his usual profession. As an accommodation, he was given an administrative assignment. He remained employed until the clerical/administrative work was taken over by a contractor. His employer, unable to find a suitable place for him, then determined that he was totally disabled. W.C.'s story illustrates the relationship between impairment and disability; he became vocationally disabled when the workplace no longer could provide work that he could perform with his chronic cognitive impairments.

SCHIZOPHRENIA

The diagnostic category of schizophrenia includes a diverse group of disorders, some with a formal subtype designation—e.g., catatonic or paranoid. Impairments range from moderate, with ability to function in carefully structured environments, to profound, with severe chronic impairment requiring institutionalization.[24] Although there is good inter-rater agreement about global function assessment, there is generally no accepted list of critical functions, let alone techniques for their quantitative measurement.[8,10,19,22,23,28] The principal impairments associated with schizophrenia that interfere with work capacity are cognitive functions and social skills. Cognitive/intellectual functioning can be assessed in the mental status examination and with psychometric tests, such as the Wechsler Adult Intelligence Scale. Social skills, however, often vary from one setting to another, and therefore are best measured in specific situations; e.g., a workplace or a sheltered workshop.[19,25,26] In occupational environments, managers usually offer the best appraisal of an employee's work capacity.[27]

In quantifying the degree of disability associated with schizophrenia, the claimant's job skills must be weighed and considered as thoroughly as the cognitive and social impairments. For example, D.S., a 50-year-old man with chronic schizophrenia, works as a computer programmer; he remains employed despite severe introversion and bizarre appearance because of his superior technical skills and a protective manager. Occasionally he needs counseling from the company's employee assistance program. His programming talent has enabled him to maintain a job despite marginal social capacity. An unusually empathic manager has buffered him from the many corporate environmental pressures. D.S. clearly has an impairment due to schizophrenia; however, he is not disabled.

AFFECTIVE DISORDERS

Affective disorders vary significantly in severity, chronicity, and periodicity. The range of impairment varies from mild, in chronic dysthymia, to severe, in rapid-cycling bipolar disorder or in refractory major depression. Many of these individuals have prolonged periods of well-being with normal social and vocational functioning. For those individuals with intermittent illness, disability is often measured by the amount of time lost from work. For example, C.E., an electrical engineer/programmer, remained employed despite several episodes of mania. His contributions to the department were considered acceptable by his manager. The Veterans Administration, however, comparing his position and pay with that expected of a person with his education and experience, awarded him a permanent partial disability (33%).

People with chronic, noncyclical affective disorders usually manifest impairments in cognition and volition.[26,27] A mental status examination and psychometric testing can provide measures of impairment in work-related skills and capacities. However, the measurement of disability is best served by an accurate and honest work appraisal; e.g., comparing the employee's contribution to that of his or her peers. Usually the degree of chronic depressive impairment is reflected in a reduction of productivity that can be quantified by management.[13,26,27]

ANXIETY DISORDERS

Current standard nomenclature—e.g., DSM-IV and ICD-10[4,34]—groups anxiety disorders together. The behavioral manifestations of these disorders range from internal preoccupation with no external signs, as in mild obsessions, to severe anxiety or panic attacks with secondary agoraphobia. A housebound, markedly phobic person may appear cognitively intact on formal examination and yet deserves a very high or total disability rating because he or she cannot maintain regular attendance in the workplace.[26,27] In each of the following anxiety disorders, specific impairments may compromise vocational and social functions:

- Generalized anxiety disorder—concentration, attention, and memory
- Panic disorder—episodic interruption of cognitive capacities
- Phobic disorders—avoidance, including inability to travel
- Obsessive-compulsive disorder—inability to make decisions
- Dissociative disorders—inconsistent cognitive performance and interpersonal behaviors with peers and managers

The quantitative measurement of impairment depends on the nature of the disorder as well as the requirements of his or her work and the interferences with other aspects of daily living. For example, E.M., a gifted research scientist with an obsessive-compulsive disorder, developed an original technique in computer science. He was unable to apply for a patent and to publish his work because of an obsessive inability to limit the literature citations in his paper. What began as a research disclosure grew into a review article, then a monograph, and finally a textbook. During this long delay, other scientists published similar work, thereby diminishing the value of E.M.'s efforts to the scientific community and to his company. Although he remained employed, he could have been awarded a disability in some jurisdictions proportionate to his reduced effectiveness. Here, again, the most salient measures derive from the workplace and not from the physician's office.

SOMATOFORM DISORDERS

Somatoform disorders encompass a wide variety of physical complaints for which little or no organic pathology can be found.[25] Many individuals with somatoform disorders present with pain or fatigue—two perceptions or experiences that cannot be accurately measured or externally validated. In other words, they have symptoms without signs. How, then, can impairment or disability be evaluated? The question is relevant because of the extensive absence from work or avoidance of life responsibilities associated with these conditions.

At present, there is no consensus in measuring impairment or disability related to somatization. The Social Security Administration, taking a functional approach, has awarded full disability benefits to some patients with chronic fatigue syndrome. Many private corporations have argued that they cannot award benefits to people with symptoms in the absence of physical, laboratory, or psychometric pathology. Other companies have been willing to consider disability awards after unsuccessful treatment, including integrated pain clinics. Some employees with chronic fatigue syndrome, multiple environmental allergies, multiple chemical sensitivities syndrome, or chronic benign intractable pain syndrome have sued corporations after the rejection of disability applications. They claim that their inability to perform activities of daily living, because of fatigue and/or pain, should be accepted despite the lack of corroborating evidence. In the absence of definitive legislation, an appellate level court decision must clarify this critical question (see also Chapter 42).

PERSONALITY DISORDERS

Personality disorders are characterized by aberrant behavior, usually in the absence of major affective or intellectual disturbances. The most important diagnostic information is derived from a person's history rather than the mental status examination or formal psychological tests.[19,25,27] Valuable data can be gathered from a patient's personal history, especially areas devoted to school, military service, employment, and criminal behavior, when applicable.

The question of impairment quantification and disability determination is as difficult for personality disorders as it is for substance abuse (see below). Many jurisdictions hold to a long-established position equating personality disorders with character traits; that is, they develop early, are relatively immutable, and do not represent a disease or illness. Therefore, personality disorders are processed through administrative channels and employees are separated from these organizations without disability benefits.[26,27]

Recent research and clinical interest in severe personality disorders—e.g., borderline and narcissistic personality disorders—have led to a reopening of the disability issue and have cast doubt on the exclusion of these disorders from other psychiatric diseases. Some companies will review personality disorders on a case-by-case basis, using functional rather than diagnostic criteria for disability determinations. If approved, most of these employees are awarded total disability, because their behavior is considered incompatible with the needs of the organization. For example, L.M. worked for several years as an administrative assistant. She had two advanced degrees and unusual creative gifts. Her behavior, however, was characterized by impulsiveness, grandiosity, suspiciousness, and somatization. Repeated mental status examinations uncovered significant distortions in reality testing with primitive coping skills. Treatment by several psychiatrists was unsuccessful. On the verge of her forced separation from the business for unsatisfactory performance and insubordination, she was reviewed for medical disability and adjudicated unable to function because of severe borderline personality pathology. Here, again, her behavior was the determining factor, not the diagnosis or her impairments measured by formal tests. Psychiatric tests were able to establish that her unacceptable behavior was derived from the effects of a severe character pathology.

SUBSTANCE ABUSE

Substance abuse and drug addiction are among the most controversial topics in the impairment and disability field. Should people with drug addiction, whose problems appear to be self-induced, derive benefits, especially if their economic support can be used to prolong their disease and disability? Why can these people not maintain sobriety? Should society reward a relapse by providing benefit programs?

Recovering substance abusers who are able to maintain sobriety with continued community support should be able to resume their customary activities of daily living, including work. In the absence of comorbid disorders, such as mental illness, substance abuse in remission is not a disabling condition.

What about alcohol or drug abusers who frequently relapse or who remain chronically drug dependent? Under mandate of federal regulations, business and government organizations must be drug free. Consequently, individuals who continue to use drugs cannot be employed.[27] Exceptions include sheltered workshops and medically supervised methadone maintenance programs.

Various organizations and entitlement programs differ dramatically in the determination of disability for substance abusers. Private industry usually separates employees after two or three rehabilitation efforts, in an administrative separation rather than medical disability. Conversely, the Social Security system considers substance abuse that is unresponsive to rehabilitation techniques a totally disabling condition.[32] There are no elements of partial disability or measures of degree of disability. Because of legal and social sanctions, chronic, relapsing substance abuse is not compatible with employment.

References

1. American Medical Association: Guides to the Evaluation of Permanent Impairment, 4th ed. Chicago, American Medical Association, 1993.
2. American Psychiatric Association: Diagnostic and Statistical Manual of Mental Disorders, 3rd ed. Washington, DC, American Psychiatric Association, 1982.
3. American Psychiatric Association: Diagnostic and Statistical Manual of Mental Disorders, 3rd ed, rev. Washington, DC, American Psychiatric Association.
4. American Psychiatric Association: Diagnostic and Statistical Manual of Mental Disorders, 4th ed. Washington, DC, American Psychiatric Association 1994.
5. Beck AT: The Beck Depression Inventory. San Antonio, TX, The Psychological Corporation/Harcourt Brace, 1987, 1993.
6. Beck AT: Beck Anxiety Inventory. San Antonio, TX, The Psychological Corporation/Harcourt Brace, 1990, 1993.
7. Beck AT, Ward CH, Mendelson M, et al: An inventory for measuring depression. Arch Gen Psychiatry 4:561–571, 1961.
8. Bonder BR: Disease and dysfunction: The value of Axis V. Hosp Commun Psychiatry 41:959–960, 1990.
9. Endicot J, Spitzer RL, Fleiss JL, Cohan J: The global assessment scale: A procedure for measuring overall severity of psychiatric disturbance. Arch Gen Psychiatry 33:766–771, 1976.
10. Enelow AJ: Assessing the effect of psychiatric disorders on work function. Occup Med 3:621–627, 1988.
11. Filskov SB, Boll TJ (ed): Handbook of Neuroclinical Psychology. New York, John Wiley & Sons, 1981.
12. Goldman HH, Runck B: NIMH Report. Social Security Administration revises mental disability rules. Hosp Commun Psychiatry 36:343–345, 1985.
13. Grant B, Robbins D: Disability, worker's compensation, and fitness for duty. In Kahn J (ed): Mental Health in the Workplace: A Practical Psychiatric Guide. New York, Van Nostrand Reinhold, 1993, pp 83–105.
14. Hamilton M: The assessment of anxiety states by rating. Br J Med Psychol 32:50–55, 1959.
15. Hamilton M: A rating scale for depression. J Neurol Neurosurg Psychiatry 23:56–61, 1960.
16. Hamilton M: Development of a rating scale for primary depressive illness. Br J Soc Clin Psycol 6:278–296, 1967.
17. Jenkins CD, Rossman RH, Friedman J: Development of a psychological test for the determination for the coronary-prone behavior pattern in employed men. J Chronic Dis 20:371–379, 1967.
18. Luborsky L: Clinicians' judgments of mental health. Arch Gen Psychiatry 7:407–417, 1962.
19. Massel HK, Liberman RP, Mintz J, et al: Evaluating the capacity to work of the mentally ill. Psychiatry 53:31–43, 1990.
20. Murray HA: Thematic Apperception Test Manual. Cambridge, MA, Harvard University Press, 1943.
21. New York State Department of Social Services, Office of Disability Determination: Reporting Requirements for Psychiatric Consultative Examinations. Albany, NY, New York State Department of Social Services, 1985.

22. Nussbaum K, Schneidmuhl AM, Shaffer JW: Psychiatric assessment in the Social Security program of disability insurance. Am J Psychiatry 126:897–799, 1969.
23. Pincus HA, Kennedy C, Simmens SJ, et al: Determining disability due to mental impairments: APA's evaluation of Social Security Administration guidelines. Am J Psychiatry 148:1037–1043, 1991.
24. Reich J: DSM-III diagnoses in Social Security disability applicants referred for psychiatric evaluation. J Clin Psychiatry 47:81–82, 1986.
25. Robbins D: Medical Disability Absence From Work. Valhalla, NY, New York Medical College, 1989.
26. Robbins D: Psychiatric conditions in worker fitness and risk evaluation. Occup Med 3:309–321, 1988.
27. Robbins D: The psychiatric patient at work. Occup Med 1:549–558, 1986.
28. Rosen A, Hadzi-Pavlovic D, Parker G: The life skills profile: A measure assessing function and disability in schizophrenia. Schizophr Bull 15:325–337, 1989.
29. Rorschach H: Psychodiagnostics. New York, Grune and Stratton, 1949.
30. Strub RL, Black FW: The Mental Status Examination in Neurology. Philadelphia, F.A. Davis, 1977.
31. Turk DC, Rudy TE: Pain experience: Assessing the cognitive component. Abstract from the Fifth Annual Meeting of the American Pain Society, Dallas, March 3–8, 1985.
32. U.S. Department of Health and Human Services: Disability Evaluation Under Social Security (SSA Publication No. 64–039) Washington, DC, U.S. Department of Health and Human Services, Social Security Administration, 1998.
33. Weissman MM, Bothwell S: Assessment of social adjustment by patient self report. Arch Gen Psychiatry 33:111–115, 1976.
34. World Health Organization: Manual of the International Statistical Classification of Diseases, Injuries, and Causes of Death: International Classification of Diseases (ICD). Geneva, World Health Organization, 1992.
35. Zung WWK: A self-rating depression scale. Arch Gen Psychiatry 13:63–70, 1965.
36. Zung WWK: Evaluating treatment methods for depressive disorders. Am J Psychiatry 124(Suppl.):40–48, 1968.
37. Zung WWK: A rating instrument for anxiety disorders. Psychosomatics 12:371–379, 1971.
38. Zung WWK: From art to science: The diagnosis and treatment of depression. Arch Gen Psychiatry 29:328–337, 1973.
39. Zung WWK: Prevalence of clinically significant anxiety in a family practice setting. Am J Psychiatry 143:1471–1472, 1986.
40. Zung WWK, Wonnacott TH: Treatment prediction in depression using a self-rating scale. Biol Psychiatry 2:321–329, 1970.
41. Cocchiarella L, Andersson GBJ (eds): Guides to the Evaluation of Permanent Impairment, 5th ed. Chicago, American Medical Association, 2001.

CHAPTER

39

Evaluating and Rating Impairment Caused by Pain

GERALD M. ARONOFF, MD, FAADEP, DABPM

PAIN: IMPAIRMENT AND DISABILITY ISSUES

Chronic pain is a major public health problem that inflicts not only tremendous personal suffering but also economic loss to individuals and society. Direct and indirect costs of chronic pain in the United States are estimated to be $125 billion.[54] If the pain remains intractable, the health care professional and the patient become increasingly uncertain as to the appropriate course of treatment and both develop a sense of impotence and helplessness. As each becomes frustrated and disappointed in the other, their interaction becomes more strained and less direct.[7,10]

As defined by the International Association for the Study of Pain, pain is "an unpleasant sensory and emotional experience with actual or potential tissue damage or described in terms of such damage."[50] The operational definition of pain that this author has found most useful is that of a complex personal, subjective, unpleasant experience involving sensations and perceptions that may or may not be related to physical injury, tissue damage, or nociception (the perception of pain based on organic pathology, transmitted from peripheral receptors to the central nervous system). Its expression may be influenced by psychosocial, ethnocultural, genetic, biochemical, religious, and other factors.[15] Some people will actually take the definition further and say chronic pain, per se, is what an individual says it is.[33] It is a subjective experience that cannot adequately be measured. Studies have found that there is no direct relationship between the extant tissue damage and the severity of pain.[17]

Loeser's paradigm[46] in conceptualizing chronic pain syndromes is useful. He suggests that the initial noxious stimulus leading to nociception seems to be less important in the management of chronic pain syndromes than the suffering, which is an emotional experience, and the pain behaviors that the patient exhibits. This is not meant to discount that nociception may have initiated the pain process. It does, however, suggest that in chronic pain syndromes, central more than peripheral factors may be prolonging the suffering and contributing to delayed recovery and disability. Nociception, if still present, may not be directly treatable by conventional techniques (such as analgesics, nerve blocks, or surgery).

Clinically, physicians cannot prove or disprove the existence of pain in a given individual. A person complaining of pain may or may not have nociception, suffering, pain behavior, impairment, or disability. Pain behaviors are any and all actions that communicate to an observer that an individual is in pain. Examples include grimacing, groaning, limping, using visible pain relieving or support devices, and requests for pain medications, among others. Pain behaviors are often conditioned, learned, and goal directed. As such they are amenable to behavioral interventions and psychotherapies and can be modified or replaced by wellness behaviors that are more adaptive.

CHRONIC PAIN AND PSYCHIATRIC ILLNESS

Pain is an extremely common complaint in patients with known emotional disorders and may be an associated symptom in virtually any psychiatric illness. There has been extensive clinical research indicating the tendency for affective and personality disorders to occur with intractable chronic pain.[19,20,43,59,69] The Diagnostic and Statistical Manual of Mental Disorders, third edition (DSM-III) listed the term psychogenic pain syndrome.[3] The revision, DSM-III-R, deleted the preceding term and substituted somatoform pain disorder.[4] The latest revision, DSM-IV, uses the term pain disorder.[5] These terms apply to only a relatively small percentage of the chronic pain population. Many of the remainder have underlying organic pathophysiology as well as an emotional disorder. Table 39–1 lists emotional disorders associated with chronic pain syndromes.

TABLE 39–1

Emotional Disorders Associated With Chronic Pain Syndrome[10]

I. Somatoform disorders
   A. Somatization disorder
   B. Conversion disorder
   C. Pain disorder
   D. Hypochondriasis
   E. Undifferentiated somatoform disorder

II. Affective disorders

III. Personality disorders

IV. Psychological factors affecting medical or "organic" conditions

V. Malingering

VI. Schizophrenia

VII. Substance use disorders

Frequency			
Intermittent	Occasional	Frequent	Constant
Minimal			
Slight			
Moderate			
Marked			
Intensity			

Somatoform Disorders

Somatoform disorders are those in which physical symptoms suggest a physical disorder for which there is evidence of underlying psychopathology but no demonstrable organic findings or known physiologic mechanisms. It should be emphasized that the creation of the physical symptom in a somatoform disorder is not intentional.

Somatization Disorder

Somatization disorder, formerly known as Briquet syndrome and often referred to as hysteria, is a chronic, polysymptomatic disorder generally with the onset early in life, before age 30. Chiefly affecting women, the condition's main feature is a repetitive or chronic concern with physical symptoms lacking objective findings to substantiate the subjective complaints. These individuals tend to consult many physicians in an attempt to validate their symptoms and frequently have surgical procedures with minimal pathologic findings. They often have prolonged phases of incapacity, are at high risk for iatrogenic complications, and should be managed conservatively unless there are clear signs of objective pathology warranting more aggressive treatment. Frequently individuals may experience somatization but do not meet diagnostic criteria for a somatization disorder.[6] Consideration should be given to the diagnosis of an atypical somatoform disorder.

Conversion Disorder

Individuals said to have underlying hysterical personality patterns are prone either to exaggerate the magnitude of their complaints or to present these complaints in a melodramatic fashion. It should be emphasized, however, that in no way do these statements imply that the patient's pain is not real or that it is not organically based. Working with these patients, one learns that their choice of words as descriptors for their pain usually involves emotionally laden and flamboyant language that often prejudices the clinician. Therefore, it should be emphasized that some symptoms initially felt to represent conversion may later be found to have a neurologic or musculoskeletal basis. Conversion symptoms are those that result from an emotional conflict, are not related to bodily disease directly, and are ultimately in accordance with the patient's concept of functional loss of a part rather than an actual anatomic or physiologic loss. If the symptoms affect the body, they are called conversion symptoms. Comparable symptoms not affecting the body, such as hysterical loss of memory, are known as dissociative symptoms. When pain is the only conversion symptom, the term pain disorder associated with psychological factors should be used. Several factors are noteworthy. Patients with conversion disorders truly believe that they have the deficits they claim. Their inability to move or appropriately use body parts often leads to secondary impairments through, for example, disuse atrophy or joint contractures. An ominous combination is found in individuals with conversion disorders and dependent personality traits (or dependent personality disorders) because they are at increased risk to develop a chronic sick role or chronic disability syndrome.

Pain Disorder

Pain disorders are not infrequent occurrences among patients going to pain centers. Clinically, the primary feature is the complaint of pain without adequate physical findings but associated with evidence of the etiologic role of psychological factors. It is not, however, a diagnosis of exclusion. Patients with nondiagnosed chronic pain or chronic pain of uncertain etiology should not be presumed to have psychogenic pain. To do so is incorrect and does the individual with pain a disservice. It should be established that no other mental (or physical) disorder is contributing to the disturbance. It has been the author's impression that the premorbid personalities of these individuals commonly reveal evidence of neurotic functioning and, less often, borderline personality organization preceding the trauma of an injury or painful medical illness. These patients often become quite incapacitated and are at risk to become invalids unnecessarily if the sick role is reinforced by health care providers or significant others.

Pain itself may become the focal aspect within a neurotic conflict. It is then called a pain neurosis and it may be linked with the possibility of financial compensation as with a compensation neurosis. Sometimes a core issue involves unmet dependency needs and both primary and secondary gain. The diagnosis of a pain disorder associated with psychological factors must be made cautiously and periodically re-examined to rule out the possibility that the pain may be explained on an organic basis.

If a specific treatment for a pain disorder is available and if the potential benefits to the patient outweigh the risks, that treatment should be suggested. If, however, invasive treatment offers no distinct advantage over conservative treatment, and carries an increased risk, conservative treatment should be suggested.

Hypochondriasis

Hypochondriasis implies a fascinated absorption and preoccupation with physical symptoms. It is not uncommon among pain patients. That is not to say that these individuals may not have underlying organic pathology and mechanical causes of pain, but rather that the degree of somatic preoccupation becomes an obsession. They fail to be reassured by clinical or laboratory evaluations and remain fixated in their belief that they need more diagnostic tests and evaluations. Arguing with these individuals and trying to dissuade them from their convictions is generally futile. The intensity of their concerns often causes significant psychosocial dysfunction and may impair occupational functioning, depending on the extent of psychopathology and the extent to which their lives revolve around the sick role. One must, of course, exclude true organic disease. However, it should be emphasized that the presence of true organic disease does not rule out the possibility of coexisting hypochondriasis. These patients are at increased risk for iatrogenic complications because of the excessive diagnostic procedures they undergo, as well as the multiple medication trials they attempt.

Undifferentiated Somatoform Disorder

Undifferentiated or atypical somatoform disorder is a category used to describe physical symptoms or complaints not explained by demonstrable organic findings or a known pathophysiologic mechanism and apparently linked to psychologic factors but without adequate symptoms to make a diagnosis of somatoform disorder.

Psychologic Factors Affecting Medical Conditions

According to DSM-IV, the category psychological factors affecting medical condition can be used to describe disorders that in the past have been referred to as either psychosomatic or psychophysiologic. A very common problem with pain patients is a tendency to suppress emotional expression and internalize feelings. The physiologic expression of these tendencies is manifested in autonomic hyperactivity and muscle tension, both of which directly contribute to the pain. Included in this category are tension and migraine headaches, angina pectoris, painful menstruation, sacroiliac pain, neurodermatitis, arthritis, peptic ulcers, and other conditions. The author would suggest that fibromyalgia be considered as an addition to the above list.

Malingering

Malingering implies a conscious and voluntary fabrication of a physical or psychological symptom for personal gain. This may involve financial compensation, drug seeking, personal manipulation, vocational disability, or other attempts to manipulate the individual's environment through the use of pain. To be classified as a malingerer, the person must be consciously feigning illness. These individuals are often difficult to treat because the obvious gain is so overwhelming. Frequently they perceive themselves as having more to gain by retaining the symptom than by relinquishing it. There is commonly a great deal of underlying psychopathology, and the primary treatment of malingering, if amenable to treatment at all, must be psychiatric. It is the author's belief that whereas malingering in the general medical population is not common, conscious symptom magnification or embellishment (for personal gain) is a significantly greater issue among workers' compensation or personal injury pain patient populations, both of which may involve active litigation. That is not to imply that all or even most of these individuals are malingerers. Experienced pain clinicians can generally distinguish the patient's underlying motivation. The clinician performing impairment evaluations must understand that many individuals presenting for this assessment do so involuntarily as part of an adversarial process. In this context, the incidence of symptom embellishment and submaximal effort is greater than in the general population.

Schizophrenia

Patients with schizophrenia attending a pain center with primary pain complaints are uncommon, but this can occur. Symptoms are often discussed as part of a bizarre somatic delusion. A British study[73] of 78 hospitalized schizophrenic patients found 29 to have pain complaints. Of these, 13 had an appropriate physical cause. The remainder were felt to have somatoform pain. The head, leg, and back were the most common sites of pain. Complaints were most often described in sensory terms. The report summary indicated that patients with schizophrenia may have less pain than those with anxiety or depression but may experience pain from both physical and psychological causes.

Substance Use Disorders

Patients with chronic pain are often very experienced in the use of medications. When evaluating psychoactive substance use disorders one must recognize varying patterns of medication usage. For some, the pattern is sporadic and intermittent with medications taken only by prescription from one primary physician. This is appropriate medication use. Some patients believe they are taking prescribed (or over the counter) medication appropriately, but later find out they were not. This is medication misuse. Some patients take medication for reasons other than that for which it was prescribed. This is substance abuse. For others there are multiple physicians writing many prescriptions, each unaware of the actions of the others. The patient is knowingly involved in a process of deception. They may receive medication from illicit sources outside the medical system. These are individuals whose illicit use of medications may have preceded the onset of their pain and who now hope to have this use legitimized by physicians. This is substance addiction and it should be considered as a psychological and behavioral process. Portenoy[57] describes three characteristics of the addiction process: 1) loss of control over drug use, 2) compulsive drug use, and 3) continued use despite harm. It is inappropriate to use the term addiction interchangeably with drug abuse or drug dependence (although there may be some common features).

Other persons who never would have considered illicit drugs are now faced with chronic pain and are unable to obtain what they feel is adequate medication. They develop a pattern often diagnosed as addiction when, more accurately, it should be considered as pseudoaddiction.[75] The problem is complex and often iatrogenic, related to inadequate pain treatment. The patient's behavior, although consistent with criteria for addiction, is motivated by obtaining adequate pain relief and not by "getting high." When pain relief occurs, addictive behaviors cease. Aronoff and Gallagher have suggested guidelines for maintenance opioid use in chronic pain[14] and has described the relatively low risk of addiction in appropriately selected chronic pain patients maintained on long-term opioids.[8] It has become established that there is a subpopulation of patients with chronic pain who, if appropriately maintained on analgesic medication, can remain functional and productive. If inadequately treated, they will become disabled. For many patients, the process of disability is preventable with the appropriate use of analgesics (often involving use of sustained action opioids) and adjuvant analgesics coupled with training in pain management techniques.

CHARACTERISTICS OF PATIENTS WITH CHRONIC PAIN SYNDROME

With chronic pain syndromes there are often complex interactions between physical and psychological factors. These patients share many of the characteristics listed in the following[9]:

Preoccupation with pain
Strong and ambivalent dependency needs
Feelings of isolation and loneliness
Characterological masochism (meeting others needs at their own expense)
Inability to take care of self needs
Passivity
Lack of insight into patterns of self-defeating behavior
Inability to deal appropriately with anger and hostility
Use of pain as a symbolic means of communication

The pain-prone individual, described initially by Engel[36,37] and later by Blumer and Heilbronn,[20,21] has a significant developmental history notable for unhappiness and trauma during childhood, often involving physical and sexual abuse, emotional neglect, high incidence of alcoholism in the family, and a personal and family history of illness, disability, and chronic pain. These individuals often had to assume early adult responsibilities and are described as having been hyperresponsible children. They may have had many early unmet dependency needs subsequently gratified through the pain experience. Later in life, following an injury or illness, pain may be their way of saying "Now it's my turn to be taken care of."

There is growing evidence that depression lowers pain tolerance, increases analgesic requirements, and adds to the debilitating effects of pain.[51] Studies of the relationship between chronic pain and depression in hospital patients in whom there was no organic lesion[47] found consistently that a greater percentage of patients seen in the hospital or pain clinic with what was called chronic indeterminate pain have clinical depression than in a comparative population who had chronic pain explained by underlying pathophysiology. A higher percentage of subjects with chronic indeterminate pain were found to have a family history of depression and depressive spectrum disease.

Currently, tricyclics are among the most common nonanalgesic medications used in the management of chronic pain syndromes. Their usage for the treatment of chronic pain has been summarized by Aronoff and Evans,[13] Aronoff and Gallagher,[14] Oxman and Denson,[55] Atkinson,[16] and Monks.[53] The newer class of serotonin reuptake inhibitors including fluoxetine, sertraline, and paroxetine are less well studied with the chronic pain population but should also be considered as they have been found to be useful in the management of depression and appear to have a favorable side effect profile. In patients with chronic pain, depression, and insomnia, the use of sertraline or citalopram in the morning combined with a sedating tricyclic in the evening often achieves excellent efficacy with a lower incidence of side effects than a higher dose of the sedating tricyclic alone.

Are there distinguishing personality characteristics in individuals prone to develop chronic pain syndrome or become disabled by pain? Although studies suggest that there may be, there are no clear findings indicating to what extent well-defined personality traits are associated with the development of a chronic pain syndrome as opposed to having the pain amplify traits that are then maintained by operant mechanisms. In addition to pain-prone personality characteristics, other common personality characteristics include being antisocial, passive-dependent, histrionic, and masochistic self-neglectful.[60] The latter refers to individuals who meet others' needs at their own expense and whose behaviors, therefore, can be considered self-defeating.

DISABILITY INTERVENTION

There is no linear relationship between the degree of medical or psychiatric impairment and the resulting disability rating. The findings of a multidisciplinary medical panel from the Boston University Medical Center emphasize this.[63] In this study, 111 consecutive patients with chronic low back pain referred by the Office of Workers Compensation Programs were assessed. The mean age of the cohort was 49.4 years with an average length of predetermined disability of 4.92 years. Of these, only 13 (11.7%) were found to have evidence of significant objective impairment that, by itself, warranted total disability. Of the 13, roughly half were physically impaired and half were psychiatrically impaired. One finding was that in none of the six patients granted psychiatric disability was the psychiatric impairment found to be work-related. In other words, in each of these cases (100%), the insurance carrier for the employer was paying for a claim that was not their responsibility. Among those found not to be totally disabled, only 5 of the 98 patients (5.1% or 4.5% of the total sample) had returned to work at least part time by the time of their evaluation. It was noted that of the 98 patients with a partial or full work capacity, 93 patients (94.9% or 83.8% of the total sample) had incorrectly overestimated their own impairments from a narrow and strict medical perspective and had not returned to work.

Strang[63] discusses the "chronic disability syndrome" in which individuals who are capable of working choose to remain disabled. They often lack the motivation to recover and return to productivity. The disability is often the result of a fairly minor injury but actually represents an inability to cope with other life problems. Unfortunately, physicians and other health care providers who overly estimate impairment and impose limitations and restrictions that make little sense and pose barriers to vocational re-entry reinforce the disability syndrome. In vulnerable individuals, this is a major factor leading to iatrogenic disability

Brena and Chapman[23] describe the "5 D's," a cluster of symptoms often seen in chronic pain patients: dramatization (of vague, diffuse, nonanatomic pain complaints); drug abuse (misuse of habit-forming pain medications); dysfunction (bodily impairments related to various physical and emotional factors); dependency (passivity, depression, and helplessness); and disability (pain contingent on financial compensation and pending litigation claims). The fourth edition of the AMA Guides adds three other "D's," including duration (longer than is considered normal for a given process); diagnostic dilemma (clinical impressions are often inconsistent, inaccurate, and vague despite extensive evaluations); and disuse (from prolonged inactivity). The Guides suggests the need for at least four of these eight characteristics to establish a presumptive diagnosis of chronic pain syndrome.[2]

Several authors have contributed to an understanding of why pain-related disability and litigation are such major problems. Brena and Chapman[22] reviewed several studies of the disability process, indicating that certain patient characteristics made the patients prone to be involved in a disabling injury. In one study, Weinstein[74] noted these factors: 1) low self esteem in a dependent person, 2) inability to deal competently with stress, 3) demanding job, and 4) tension at home. The injury was viewed as a socially acceptable way out of a stressful situation.

Ellard[35] enumerates some characteristics of patients who have significant psychological reactions to injury. 1) The patients lack the usual objective signs of suffering (a disparity between verbal pain complaints and untroubled manner). 2) Objective clinical findings do not correlate with the complaint (for example, no atrophy of the paralyzed limb). 3) Poor motivation is exhibited (patients remain passive sufferers, vehemently asserting a problem and a desire to get well, yet failing to effectively participate in the treatment). 4) The patients exhibit unusual treatment responses. Initially, these patients may not actively seek treatment; once treated, they fail to benefit from it, although they continue to pursue it. Ellard notes that, in many of these patients, there is no evidence of a stated psychopathologic condition preceding the injury episode. He summarizes the diagnostic and treatment dilemma these patients create, stating that the symptoms may represent a conscious or unconscious desire for the person to establish that he or she is sick, "not so much because of his personal pathological condition, but because of the social consequences of the sick role." He notes that, when financial gain is involved, the complaints are more often remedied by legal rather than by medical processes. Brena and Chapman[22] noted the demoralized behavior of many patients in chronic pain management programs when consistently confronted with situations in which they could not control the outcome. They demonstrated elements of depression, passivity, and lack of initiative in attempting to affect situation outcomes. They point to the common features between these behaviors and those previously noted in workers prone to chronic disability following a work-related injury.

Disability is more difficult to treat once it has continued for 6 months or longer. Thus early recognition of features predicting poor prognosis and prompt intervention are important. Seres and Newman note that 80% to 90% of workers with back injuries return to work within days or weeks of the injury. Of the remaining injured, 5% to 15% have prolonged or permanent disability.[61] This author's impression is that the latter group does not necessarily have more significant impairment than the former group that returned to work earlier.

McGill[48] noted in his study of industrial back problems that a lengthy period of disability predicted a low likelihood of ever returning to work. Those out of work longer than 6 months had a 50% probability of return, those out of work for over 1 year had a 25% chance of return, and those out of work longer than 2 years were extremely unlikely to return. These statistics are consistent with more recent data.[70]

Aronoff has described the "disability epidemic"[7,11] that is most prominent in the United States and other countries where entitlement programs are viewed as appealing alternatives to gainful employment. If this epidemic is to be reversed, the compensation and disability systems must be changed so that they encourage early intervention, prevention of chronicity with incentives toward rehabilitation, and early return to work.

Often the patient's attitude and motivation, coupled with the support system, are likely to determine whether the patient allows pain to be totally disabling. It is especially a reflection of the patient's underlying personality style and life goals. These factors are better predictors for a successful outcome than is the medical diagnosis.

Chronic pain research indicates that decreased function depends not only on pathophysiology but also on "illness behaviors" or "pain behaviors" (such as inactivity, drug misuse, and learned helplessness).[24] Patients with lengthy disabilities are special in several respects. Snook et al[62] found that patients receiving workers' compensation for back injuries were less likely to have objective findings or a definitive diagnosis than were those with back injuries who were not receiving compensation.

In discussing patients with chronic low back claims, Carron[28] indicated the three most striking factors were as follows: 1) 78.7% of the subjective complaints were not supported by objective findings; 2) 60% of patients were taking dependency-inducing drugs; and 3) 49.3% of patients had a previous back injury. In those injuries (occult) that were neither witnessed nor reliably documented, and with pain as the major manifestation of injury, he noted a high incidence of a previously compensable injury, drug dependency, obesity, low income, and nonsupervisory work. In one study by Leavitt et al,[45] 70% of workers receiving compensation for back injuries reported that a specific work activity or event triggered the pain or injury, but only 35% of workers not receiving compensation for low back pain reported a clearcut work-related event.

Catchlove and Cohen's[29] retrospective review of two groups of chronic pain patients receiving workers' compensation emphasizes the importance of return to work as a goal of pain management programs. When a directed return-to-work approach was incorporated into their treatment, 60% of patients returned to work, and 90% continued to work an average of 9.6 months later. They were also receiving fewer compensation benefits and less additional pain treatment than a group of patients similarly treated, but for whom a return-to-work directive was not included. Although the improvements may have been related both to selection factors (a treatment contract that patients had to affirm) and to treatment efficacy, the results were significant. Similar findings were noted by Hall et al,[38] who found that physicians' recommendations for restricted or light duty were associated with a worse prognosis for successful return to work. One should not underestimate the importance of physicians' authoritarian guidance, which can be offered as supportive paternalism. Patients will either live up to medical expectations that they need not be disabled or conversely become invalids unnecessarily through learned helplessness. Their physical, emotional, social, and spiritual well-being is more likely to be realized with the self-esteem that results from feeling useful because of gainful employment than with a disability award.[7]

Of back pain patients treated at pain programs, many have undergone multiple pain-related surgeries. In Waddell et al's study of failed lumbar disc surgery in workers' compensation patients following industrial injuries, 97% had some persistent pain complaints, 77% continued with impaired functioning, and of those who had third or fourth operations, outcomes were progressively worse, with increased psychological dysfunction.[71] These individuals typically claim to be no better following one or more surgical procedures, have limitations in functional activities of daily living (ADL), have behavioral sequelae consistent with the term chronic pain syndrome, and often have significant associated depression. Common denominators for many of these problems include a well-intentioned, but perhaps overzealous surgeon, who may feel guilty or responsible for the patient's persistent pain and suffering, a demanding and persistent patient who insists on being fixed or cured, a health care system that is procedure-driven, and the inefficiency of a disability system that often reinforces disability rather than rehabilitation. In general, it is recommended that the following patients should have a second opinion prior to elective surgery:

Two or more pain-related surgeries without beneficial results
One or more pain-related surgeries with negative findings
Attorney referred patients involved in pain-related litigation
Known or highly suspected major psychopathology
History of unjustified overuse of the health care system

Seres and Newman[61] indicate that low back injuries are the most frequently litigated claims and represent the most common type of "cumulative trauma" injury. Many studies[45,48,62] indicate that pain treatment is less successful for those receiving workers' compensation or with pending litigation than for those not receiving it.

Dworkin et al[34] found that in 454 chronic pain patients, only the employment status at initial evaluation predicted treatment response (employed patients had better outcomes than those not employed). Neither litigation nor compensation was a significant predictor of treatment outcome. Similarly, Peck et al[56] found no significant effects of either litigation or representation by an attorney on the pain behavior of patients with pending workers' compensation claims.

In evaluating workers' compensation or personal injury–related pain patients, the screening process is extremely important, especially when the issue of disability compensation is involved. If, on the basis of the initial evaluation, it is thought that the patient's motivation toward behavioral change is marginal or that he or she is content to collect compensation and to have others in attending roles, thus assuming a passive-dependent attitude, treatment at a pain program should generally be deferred. This must be clearly expressed to the patient in a nonjudgmental way. It should be the patient's right to continue with the pain and suffering if he or she so chooses. An interpretation and clarification should address the issues very candidly. The primary concern should not be with the patient's reaction, but rather with assisting the patient to recognize motivational and attitudinal deficits, psychological factors complicating the disability, and issues of primary, secondary, and tertiary gain.

One should attempt to clarify life stressors, traumatic life events, past patterns of disability in the patient or other family member, repetitive patterns of self-defeating behaviors, a family history of chronic pain, illness, or disability, unmet dependency needs, childhood deprivations, and substance abuse. Having information about all of these is important in understanding how the patient became the person who is now seeking treatment. This information is essential in formulating a treatment plan and understanding prognosis, as well as in making statements about vocational matters and disability.[12]

IMPAIRMENT ASSESSMENT OF PAIN

In performing an impairment evaluation, it is essential to take a detailed medical, developmental, behavioral, and psychosocial history to assess an individual's current and premorbid level of functioning. Only then can one try to understand the impact of an injury or illness with subsequent pain. In the assessment one should always comment on whether there appears to be significant suffering and demonstrable pain behaviors. In attempting to address issues of causality or to apportion all or a part of an impairment to a specific incident or injury, one must know how the individual was functioning prior to the incident in question. Turk and colleagues have suggested three essential questions useful in assessing chronic pain[67,68]:

1. What is the extent of the patient's disease or injury?
2. What is the magnitude of the illness? That is, to what extent is the patient suffering, disabled, and unable to enjoy usual activities?
3. Is the illness behavior appropriate to the disease or injury, or is there evidence of amplification of symptoms for psychological or social reasons?

In addition to the above, the following questions are useful in performing evaluations related to chronic pain and psychiatric illness:

1. Was your childhood happy, difficult, stressful, or traumatic? Unless it was happy, get details. Specifically, look for dysfunctional family issues, physical or sexual abuse, emotional neglect, and unmet needs.
2. Were there any traumas during childhood, adolescence, or later in adulthood? This can often add clarification to an understanding of post-

traumatic stress disorders, phobias, pain prone characteristics, and other psychopathology.

3. How did you do in school? Were there specific problems? If an individual dropped out of school at an early age or repeated grades, get details. If you get a sense that the individual was driven to excel to the point of its becoming pathologic, get details.
4. Is there any prior history of emotional problems or past treatment? If so, get details including use of medications, duration of drug trials, and dosages. Did treatment help? What precipitated prior problems? Specifically, attempt to evaluate the developmental, psychosocial, and family histories for pain-prone characteristics.
5. Have you been able to make friends easily in the past? Do you have close friends now? Other than the nuclear family, what type of support system has there been? Is there evidence of inadequacies in personality development?
6. If there were abnormalities in usual developmental transitions, inquire. For example, what led to your leaving home at 16? To never leaving home by 50? To your five divorces?
7. Do any family members have emotional problems now or have they had these in the past? Other than the details, obtain an understanding of the impact on the person you are evaluating. Does the person believe he or she is just like that relative and will develop the same problems? What was it like growing up in the home with the ill relative? Who did the care taking?
8. Is there a personal or family history of substance dependence or abuse? Medical illness or chronic pain can occasionally be used for secondary gain to perpetuate a pre-existing substance use problem. Also evaluate the possibility that substances may be diverted to other family members.
9. Is there a history of prior psychosomatic illness or unexplained physical symptoms? Evaluate the role of stressors. Is there any insight by the individual?
10. Have there been prior medical problems or injuries similar to the current ones? Specifically, get details regarding a prior history of similar complaints of pain. What was the location of symptoms? Types of treatment? Duration of treatment? Severity of symptoms? Response to treatment? Was there any pain prior to the present illness? Was the individual in treatment? With whom? When did he or she last see this individual prior to the present illness? Was the person taking any medication for pain prior to the present illness? If there was pain prior to the present illness, were there any limitations of restrictions? Did the pain interfere with normal ADLs?
11. Does the person believe that he or she has been adequately evaluated and that everything that can and should be done has been? This is extremely important because people are less likely to accept recommendations about getting on with their lives and returning to work if they believe they require more diagnostic testing and interventional treatments (e.g., nerve blocks, surgery, spinal cord stimulators). The physician should be prepared to comment, with a reasonable degree of medical certainty, whether the current injury or illness has exacerbated or aggravated a pre-existing condition. Aggravation indicates a permanent worsening of a pre-existing condition. Exacerbation indicates a temporary recurrence of the prior symptoms that can be expected to subside with the individual's returning to baseline premorbid functioning.
12. Has disability been an issue in the past? Has the person either been disabled or applied for disability? The evaluator should have a good understanding of the many issues that may have precipitated the request for disability status.
13. Is litigation pending related to the present illness or injury? Has there been prior litigation related to other health issues or injuries? The extent to which litigation can prolong physical and emotional symptoms and complicate disability is discussed in detail in other works.[7,25,44,45,61,67,68,72]

The above list is not all-inclusive but rather is meant to give the reader guidelines for some of the subjects that should be explored. In evaluating the responses to the above questions, the likelihood of psychosocial issues influencing disability is as follows:

0 to 2 positive responses: Not suggestive
3 to 5 positive responses: Suggestive
6+ positive responses: Highly suggestive/probable

Occasionally resistance has been encountered from the individual being evaluated who cannot or will not appreciate the relevance of the questions to the current evaluation. One should clarify the importance of understanding past events and behaviors to accurately assess current as well as future functioning.

MEASURING AND RATING PAIN

One of the more difficult questions asked of the evaluating physician will relate to the measurement or rating of pain. Because clinical pain is a subjective process there are no purely objective physiologic measures currently available to measure pain. The best methods use subjective reports by the individual with pain. Although there are inherent limitations in relying on self-report measures, these ratings are felt to be the most reliable tools available.[39] However, it must be recognized that some individuals may bias their reporting for personal gain.

One of the simplest single-dimension measures of pain intensity is the verbal scale in which an individual is asked to estimate pain on a continuum from no pain, mild, moderate, severe, to horrible or excruciating.

Perhaps the most commonly used pain rating scale is the linear visual analog scale (VAS), as follows:

NO PAIN ←——→ WORST PAIN IMAGINABLE

The individual places a mark on the line indicating the pain estimate between no pain and the worst imaginable pain. The rater can measure the distance from 0 to 10 and form a quantified measure. The advantage of the VAS is its simplicity; the disadvantage is its oversimplicity, treating pain as if it were unidimensional. Revill et al[58] found that patients produce estimates on the VAS that are reliable over time. It has also been shown that the scale can predict outcome 6 months later,[77] whereas others have found that the VAS only reflects a single point in time.

A similar method is used in the AMA Guides fourth edition relating pain intensity with pain frequency (Fig. 39–1).[2] Because pain is known to be multidimensional in nature, other self-report tools commonly used in pain management programs include pain drawings and pain diaries. Pain drawings are assessed in terms of being appropriate (corresponding to the pathophysiologic process), inappropriate (not corresponding to the pathophysiologic process), or, depending upon how bizarre the drawing, suggestive of various types of psychopathology. Pain diaries, which monitor pain intensity as well as daily activities, medication usage, sleep patterns, and pain behaviors, are helpful in assessing the frequency, intensity, and duration of pain and how it affects ADL.

The McGill Pain Questionnaire (MPQ)[49] was developed to measure clinical pain as a multidimensional experience. Specifically looking at sensory and affective components, intensity, and miscellaneous dimensions of the pain experience, the MPQ also includes a pain drawing. A review by Hinnant[40] indicates that although the MPQ shows reliability and validity, there is significant disagreement over the accuracy of the test and its ability to discriminate diagnostic groups of patients.

		Frequency			
		Intermittent	Occasional	Frequent	Constant
Intensity	Minimal				
	Slight				
	Moderate				
	Marked				

Figure 39–1. Pain intensity-frequency grid. (From Hall H, McIntosh G, Melles T, et al: Effect of discharge recommendations on outcome. Spine 19:2033–2037, 1994, with permission.)

The Dartmouth Pain Questionnaire (DPQ)[31] is used as an adjunct to the MPQ because its authors believe that the MPQ neglects measurements of somatic interventions, impaired function, remaining positive aspects of function, and changes in self-esteem since the onset of pain. Cronbach[32] notes that the DPQ can be used to differentiate between patients who have and have not benefited from pain treatment.

The Pain Disability Index (PDI)[67] is a self-reporting inventory that is useful in assessing the degree to which chronic pain interferes with daily activities. According to Tait et al, high scores on the PDI relate to "time spent in bed, psychosomatic symptoms, stopping activities because of pain, work status, pain duration, usual pain intensity, quality of life, pain extent, and education."[65] Hebben[39] notes that the measure appears to possess both test-retest reliability and validity with regard to pain-based disability.

The Vanderbilt Pain Management Inventory[26] evaluates patients' response to pain in terms of their use of active versus passive coping styles, noting that the more active copers had less pain, depression, helplessness, and impairment.

The West Haven–Yale Multidimensional Pain Inventory[41] focuses on the "impact of pain on the patient's life, the responses of others to the patient's communication of pain, and the extent to which patients participate in common daily activities."

The Pain Patient Profile (P-3)[66] test is a self-report, multiple choice assessment that helps screen for the presence of depression, anxiety, and somatization, factors frequently associated with chronic pain. The P-3 test can be used in multiple settings to identify psychological variables hindering a patient's recovery from an injury as well as evaluate the patient's emotional readiness for surgery. In addition, the P-3 test can be used to clarify psychological variables in medical-legal assessments and long-term disability issues.

Several psychological tests that are not specific to either pain or disability evaluation but have achieved popularity in clinical evaluation of both include the Minnesota Multiphasic Personality Inventory (MMPI)[64] and the updated revision the MMPI-2,[1] the Symptom Checklist 90-revised,[42] and the Millon Behavioral Health Inventory.[52] These are used to measure psychopathology in medical and psychiatric populations with attention to various personality characteristics that may influence treatment outcome and prognosis. None of these should be used as definitive tests of psychogenicity or organicity of a specific pain problem. In the well-known and often quoted Boeing study, Bigos et al[18] found the MMPI useful in predicting subjects most likely to report back injuries at work. For a detailed discussion of clinical pain measurement the reader is referred to chapters by Hebben,[39] White,[76] and Hinnant.[40] The Battery for Health Improvement (BHI)[27] test is a self-report, multiple choice assessment that helps provide objective information and practical treatment strategies to professionals who treat injured patients in a variety of settings. The BHI is often used as an adjunct in the assessment of occupational and other personal injuries and in long-term disabilities.

SOCIAL ISSUES

It can be anticipated that issues such as unemployment during an economic recession, job dissatisfaction, and financial or job insecurity may influence the worker's demands on the treating physician to recommend temporary or permanent disability as a way of coping with economic stressors. As difficult as it may be, physicians must, with understanding and compassion, objectively assess impairment, and not confuse their role as the patient's advocate with their responsibility for objectivity. Perhaps it is an independent physician rather than the treating physician who can most objectively, accurately, and unemotionally rate impairment, thus maintaining the uniqueness of the treating physician's relationship with his or her patient.

Physicians must realize that rehabilitation is preferable to disability, and that there is a need to improve the ability to reinstate people with pain so that they remain functional and productive. Invalidism is a process that can and must be addressed by the health care system. Individuals who must endure chronic pain suffer less when their lives have purpose and meaning. Gainful employment frequently can serve as a distraction from pain. Rehabilitation and occupational health personnel can help facilitate the process of returning the injured worker to employment by creatively devising employment opportunities geared toward the limitations of the individual.

IMPAIRMENT FROM CHRONIC PAIN

The fourth[2] and fifth[30] editions of the AMA Guides recognize that chronic pain involves altered perceptions and maladaptive behaviors; that pain per se cannot be validated objectively or quantitated; that the subjective complaints may be disproportionate to objective findings, which may be lacking; that "chronic pain is a self-sustaining, self-reinforcing, and self-regenerating process"[2(p307)]; and that there may be no ongoing nociception. The AMA Guides note, however, that chronic pain is a medical and not a psychiatric disorder.

On the issue of impairments, the AMA Guides take the position that "chronic pain and pain-related behaviors are not, per se, impairments, but they should trigger assessments with regard to ability to function and carry out daily activities."[2(p304)] The fourth and fifth Guides also state that other rating systems (Social Security, private insurance companies, Veterans Administration) take similar positions that pain, per se, is not a cause of impairment but that the underlying medical (both organic and psychiatric) conditions are.

The fifth edition of the Guides distinguishes between mechanical failure and pain as the basis for an impairment. Mechanical failure is viewed as the objective pathoanatomic or pathophysiologic process that causes a decrement in ADLs. This is the more traditional biomedical model which does not take into account the subjective experience of pain and is in keeping with the other chapters in the Guides that rate impairment based on organ system dysfunction. Examples used include impairment from amputations or spinal cord lesions producing objective deficits. The Guides acknowledge, however, the reality of subjective experience of pain as well as the challenge to the Guides system of impairment rating because of the subjectivity.[2,30] For the purposes of this chapter, the remarks that follow address impairment from the subjectivity of the pain experience because impairment from mechanical failure is addressed in the Guides conventional impairment ratings.[2,30]

The chapter on pain in the fifth edition[30] (pp 566–584) describes an alternative conceptual model for painful conditions and makes three assumptions: 1). Pain is influenced significantly by psychosocial factors. 2) There is often no direct correlation between pain and mechanical dysfunction. 3) Pain may significantly impact patients' ability to perform ADLs. (These factors were all emphasized in the fourth edition as well.[2]) Guidelines from the new chapter on pain are felt to be most appropriate for those conditions in which pain is not based in mechanical failure and when the conventional rating system is inadequate in assessing the actual ADL deficit the examinee experiences. Specific guidelines for using the pain chapter to evaluate pain-related impairment include the following situations: 1) when there is excess pain in the context of verifiable conditions that cause pain; 2) when there are well-established pain syndromes without significant, identifiable organ dysfunction to explain the pain—examples taken from the Guides include most headache, postherpetic neuralgia, tic douloureux, erythromyalgia, complex regional pain syndrome I (reflex sympathetic dystrophy), any injuries to the nervous system; and 3) when there are other associated pain syndromes—examples given include neuropathic pain states such as painful peripheral neuropathy, complex regional pain syndrome II (causalgia), thalamic pain syndrome, nerve entrapment syndromes, postparaplegic pain, syringomyelia pain, and brachial plexus avulsion pain.[30(p571)]

Guidelines for not using the pain chapter to rate pain-related impairment include 1) when conditions are adequately rated in other chapters of the Guides, 2) when rating individuals with low credibility, and 3) when there are ambiguous or controversial pain syndromes.[30(p571)] However, the pain chapter may be used to rate ambiguous or controversial pain syndromes if the person being evaluated meets all three of the following criteria: 1) the symptoms and/or physical findings match a known medical condition; 2) the individual's presentation is typical of the diagnosed condition; and 3) the diagnosed condition is widely accepted as having a well-defined pathophysiologic basis. If any of these criteria is not met, the pain condition is not ratable by the Guides.[30]

The authors of the pain chapter give significant weight to self-reports by individuals being evaluated (specifically concerning pain intensity, pain-related emotional distress, and ADL deficits, with the latter given the greatest weight).

The reader is referred to the pain chapter of the Guides[30(pp566–584)] for further discussion of detailed protocols for assessing pain-related impairments, which are divided into four general classes: mild, moderate, moderately severe, and severe. Although the chapter emphasizes that some pain may be real but unratable, it is this author's opinion that the new chapter will frequently be used to give this population a rating, which ultimately will be based on conditioned dysfunctional pain behavior, poor coping, and embellished self-reports by individuals having an impairment evaluation as part of an adversarial process, rather than on objective pathology. As emphasized earlier, pain behavior is modifiable, need not be permanent, and does not represent a stable or static condition. Therefore, to rate this as an impairment goes against the fundamental premise of the Guides.

The critical issues for there to be impairment are that the pain or pain-related condition has become stabilized and is unlikely to change substantially within the next year with or without medical treatment (defines MMI) and that there is significant diminished capacity to carry out ADLs (not merely that the daily activity is painful). Both of these issues appear to be problematic for physicians not accustomed to treating chronic pain patients, and there can be an overestimation of its contribution to impairment. As noted earlier, pain behavior is learned and goal-directed. As such it is modifiable. Because pain behavior often is the reason for diminished ADLs, physicians should not consider someone as having a permanent impairment solely on the basis of pain behavior. The author, therefore, had difficulty with the pain intensity-frequency grid (see Fig. 39–1) in the AMA Guides fourth edition, because, if used by the inexperienced rater, it allows for a pain rating based on modifiable pain behaviors.

Individuals with chronic pain should not be considered to have reached MMI unless they have 1) been evaluated by physicians knowledgeable about chronic pain, 2) had a multidisciplinary evaluation, and 3) had an adequate trial of adjuvant analgesics (for example, many patients with chronic pain and comorbid depression lose their symptoms when adequately treated with antidepressants, and similarly for some patients with neuropathic pain treated with anticonvulsants).

Brena and Turk[25] have noted that according to the World Health Organization's definition of impairment, chronic pain could be rightly viewed as a sensory impairment affecting at least two bodily systems: the musculoskeletal system through altered pattern of daily activity and the nervous system through altered central neuronal activity. Chronic pain also affects psychological functioning as pain-perceived emotional difficulties from pain. Impairments could be classified as primary, resulting from a demonstrable pathologic lesion affecting organ systems, and secondary, resulting from the consequences of the painful experience (such as from inactivity or substance dependence and abuse).

The AMA Guides allow for emotional factors resulting in alterations in mental health and it should be emphasized that psychogenic pain is not the same as chronic pain. Rather, it is a psychiatric disorder that should be treated by specialists in that field.

CONCLUSION

Pain perception may be distorted by psychiatric illness. It is very important to evaluate motivation, which the AMA Guides notes cannot be ignored as a connecting link between impairment and disability. Impairment may lead to an almost total or minimal disability depending on motivational factors. Attitude, motivation, and support systems are often more important prognosticators than any one physical finding.

There may be concurrent impairment related to the etiology of pain and to the psychiatric condition. Chronic pain may or may not affect daily activities, social functioning, concentration, or adaptation to stressful circumstances. It is important to defer the evaluation of impairment from chronic pain until it has been appropriately evaluated and managed, including by a physician specializing in pain medicine, if necessary. Multidisciplinary pain center treatment may reverse the effects of chronic pain syndromes by diminishing suffering, increasing functional daily activities, decreasing pain behaviors, improving coping skills, and decreasing or eliminating disability.

The AMA Guides notes that with chronic pain there may or may not be impairment, and variable amounts of disability, but there is almost certainly a handicap.

Physicians must rate impairment by objective criteria whenever possible. The fifth edition of the Guides[30] describes situations in which the patient's subjective pain experience can be used as the basis for an impairment rating. Chronic pain behaviors and psychopathology can contribute to and result from the suffering that coincides with the chronic pain syndrome. These can impede an individual's ability to function and carry out ADLs. However, the evaluation of these factors should be performed by those experienced and trained in pain medicine and impairment evaluation to prevent overestimation of impairment based on modifiable pain behaviors and unnecessary disability.

Acknowledgement: Supported by a research grant from Purdue Pharmaceuticals.

CLINICAL EXAMPLES

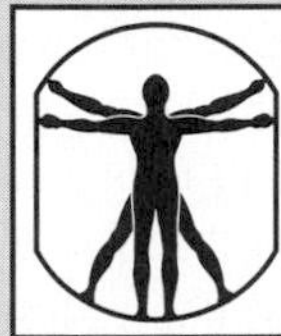

EXAMPLE

History

■ A 33-year-old divorced secretary has come to the Pain Therapy Center with complaints of chronic low back pain, cervical pain, and diffuse myalgias for approximately the past 2 years. Her symptoms developed insidiously, and, although no specific antecedent trauma was noted, the symptoms were concurrent with strenuous activity while moving furniture into her new home. When her symptoms persisted after several days of rest, she consulted her primary care physician who put her on a regimen of nonsteroidal anti-inflammatory agents, muscle relaxants, and several days off work. Pain continued and gradually increased despite medication and a trial of physical therapy, including TENS and massage. The initial diagnostic impression was acute cervical and lumbar strain. Over the next 3 to 6 months, she missed increasing numbers of work days. Currently her symptoms include generalized myalgias and arthralgias.

Her significant associated history includes her mother having had a cardiovascular accident 1 year before the patient's symptoms began. The examinee was involved in her mother's ongoing care until her death which occurred approximately 9 months before the onset of her symptoms. Also of note are significant marital stresses and work-related stresses with anxiety over possible layoffs.

The initial evaluation indicates that the examinee developed increased somatic preoccupation associated with depression and gradually progressive life disruption, including diminished efficiency at work, increased absenteeism, and increased pain with prolonged sitting, lifting, bending, or typing. She is already on medical leave and has applied for disability. She spends approximately half of her day recumbent using a heating pad for her various myalgias. She claims an inability to perform her usual household activities as a result of pain and debilitating fatigue and requires assistance for shopping. Associated with her complaints of neck and upper back pain are complaints of daily headaches of increasing severity. She feels that is unable to maintain herself vocationally and has considerable difficulties with other activities of daily living. She is also having increasing difficulties in her marital relationship. ■

Physical Examination

■ The musculoskeletal examination notes 14 of 18 fibrositic tender points. The neurologic examination is normal. The mental status evaluation reveals depression with matching affect and vegetative symptoms, including insomnia, complaints of fatigue, and diminished appetite and libido. ■

Test Results

■ The laboratory evaluation is essentially normal, including a normal sedimentation rate and rheumatoid factor levels. Cervical magnetic resonance imaging indicates a mild bulging disc without nerve root compression. ■

CLINICAL EXAMPLES *Continued*

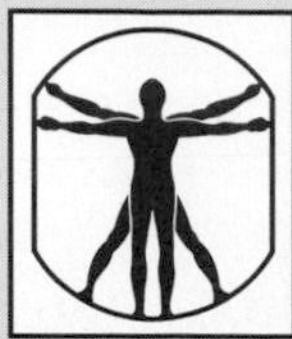

Assessment Process

■ This examinee is not rated because she has not yet reached maximum medical improvement (MMI). She is believed to have chronic pain and meets the diagnostic criteria for fibromyalgia, chronic tension type headaches, and major depression, single episode. Although she has not responded to conventional approaches with conservative treatment, her symptoms do not seem stable and are likely to change in the future with appropriate therapy. She is referred for an outpatient pain management approach through a pain center.

At the time of discharge from this pain center, her symptoms are considerably improved. Her pain is now occasional and the intensity is slight. Her headaches are significantly improved and respond to simple analgesics (acetominophen). She is increasingly aware of a psychophysiologic component to her symptoms, which increase during stressful times. She has become more aware of personality characteristics that often interfere with her getting her own needs met, as well as her tendency to become increasingly passive and dependent with greater reliance on the health care system. ■

Evaluation

■ The pain center evaluation indicates that, although she continues to complain of pain, there are no objectively validated limitations in daily activities. Based on the fifth edition of the Guides she would be considered unratable. That is, she does not meet criteria for having an impairment using the conventional rating system and has no ratable pain impairment. The pain chapter states "the pain of individuals with ambiguous or controversial pain syndromes is considered unratable." Although she meets two of the three criteria mentioned on p 572, she does not meet the third—that her condition be "widely accepted by physicians as having a well-defined pathophysiological basis."

It is also noted that, although she meets criteria for major depression, she is not found to have a psychiatric impairment. Therefore, at discharge she is felt to be at MMI and has no quantifiable or ratable impairment. ■

References

1. Ahles TA, Yunus MB, Gaulier B, et al: The use of contemporary MMPI norms in the study of chronic pain patients. Pain 24:159–163, 1986.
2. American Medical Association: Guides to the Evaluation of Permanent Impairment, 4th ed. Chicago, American Medical Association,1993.
3. American Psychiatric Association: Diagnostic and Statistical Manual of Mental Disorders, 3rd ed. Washington, DC, American Psychiatric Association, 1982.
4. American Psychiatric Association: Diagnostic and Statistical Manual of Mental Disorders, 3rd ed, rev. Washington, DC, American Psychiatric Association, 1987.
5. American Psychiatric Association: Diagnostic and Statistical Manual of Mental Disorders, 4th ed. Washington, DC, American Psychiatric Association, 1993.
6. Aronoff GM: Are pain disorder and somatization disorder valid diagnostic entities? Curr Rev Pain 4:309–312, 2000.
7. Aronoff GM: Chronic pain and the disability epidemic. Clin J Pain 7:330–338, 1991.
8. Aronoff GM: Opioids in chronic pain management: Is there a significant risk of addiction? Curr Rev Pain 4:112–121, 2000.
9. Aronoff GM: Psychodynamics and psychotherapy of the chronic pain syndrome. In Aronoff GM: Evaluation and Treatment of Chronic Pain, 3rd ed. Philadelphia, Lippincott Williams & Wilkins, 1999, pp 283–290.
10. Aronoff GM: Psychological aspects of nonmalignant chronic pain: A new nosology. In Aronoff GM: Evaluation and Treatment of Chronic Pain. Baltimore, Williams & Wilkins, 1992, pp 399–408.
11. Aronoff GM: The disability epidemic (Editorial). Clin J Pain 1:187–188, 1986.
12. Aronoff GM: The role of the pain center in the treatment of intractable suffering and disability from chronic pain. Semin Neurol 3:377–381, 1983.

13. Aronoff GM, Evans WO: Doxepin as an adjunct in the treatment of chronic pain. J Clin Psyciatry 43:42–45, 1982.
14. Aronoff GM, Gallagher RM: Pharmacological management of chronic pain: A review. In Aronoff GM: Evaluation and Treatment of Chronic Pain, 3rd ed. Philadelphia, Lippincott Williams & Wilkins, 1999.
15. Aronoff GM, McAlary PW: Pain centers: Treatment for intractable suffering and disability resulting from chronic pain. In Aronoff GM: Evaluation and Treatment of Chronic Pain, 2nd ed. Baltimore, Williams & Wilkins, 1992, p 416.
16. Atkinson JH: Psychopharmacologic agents in the treatment of pain syndrome. In Tollison CD (ed): Handbook of Chronic Pain Management. Baltimore, William & Wilkins, 1989, pp 69–99.
17. Beecher HK: Relationship of significance of wound to the pain experienced. JAMA 161:1609, 1956.
18. Bigos SJ, Battie MC, Spengler DM, et al: A prospective study of work perceptions and psychosocial factors affecting the report of back injury. Spine 16:1–6, 1991.
19. Blazer D: Narcissism and the development of chronic pain. Int J Psychiatry Med 10:69–77, 1980–1981.
20. Blumer D, Heilbronn M: Chronic pain as a variant of depressive disease: The pain-prone disorder. J Nerv Ment Dis 170:381–406, 1982.
21. Blumer D, Heilbronn M: The pain-prone disorder: A clinical and psychological profile. Psychosomatics 22:395–402, 1981.
22. Brena SF, Chapman SL: Pain and litigation. In Wall PD, Melzack R (eds): Textbook of Pain. New York, Churchill Livingstone, 1984, pp 832–839.
23. Brena SF, Chapman SL: The learned pain syndrome. Postgrad Med 69:53–62, 1981.
24. Brena SF, et al: Chronic pain states: Their relationship to impairment and disability. Arch Phys Med Rehabil 60:387–389, 1979.
25. Brena SF, Turk DC: Vocational disability: A challenge to pain rehabilitation programs. In Aronoff GM: Pain Centers: A Revolution in Health Care. New York, Raven Press, 1988.
26. Brown GK, Nicassio PM: Development of a questionnaire for the assessment of active and passive coping strategies in chronic pain patients. Pain 31:53–64, 1987.
27. Bruns D, Disorbio JM, Disorbio JC: BHI™ (Battery for Health Improvement™). Minneapolis, National Computer Systems, 1996.
28. Carron H: Compensation aspects of low back claims. In Carron H, McLaughlin RE (eds): Management of Low Back Pain. Boston, PSG, 1982.
29. Catchlove R, Cohen K: Effects of a directive return to work approach in the treatment of workers' compensation patients with chronic pain. Pain 14:181–191, 1982.
30. Cocchiarella L, Andersson GBJ (eds): Guides to the Evaluation of Permanent Impairment, 5th ed. Chicago, American Medical Association, 2001.
31. Corson JA, Schneider MJ: The Dartmouth Pain Questionnaire: An adjunct to the McGill Pain Questionnaire. Pain 19:59–69, 1984.
32. Cronbach LJ: Test validation. In Thorndike RL (ed): Educational Measurement. Washington, DC, American Council on Education, 1971, p 462.
33. Crue BL: Personal communication, 1985.
34. Dworkin RH, Handin DS, Richlin DM, et al: Unraveling the effects of compensation, litigation and employment on treatment response in chronic pain. Pain 23:49–59, 1985.
35. Ellard J: Psychological reactions to compensable injury. Med J Aust 349–355, 1970.
36. Engel G: Guilt, pain, and success. Psychosom Med 24:37–48, 1962.
37. Engel G: Psychogenic pain and the pain-prone patient. Am J Med 54:899–918, 1959.
38. Hall H, McIntosh G, Melles T, et al: Effect of discharge recommendations on outcome. Spine 19:2033–2037, 1994.
39. Hebben N: Toward the assessment of clinical pain in adults. In Aronoff GM (ed): Evaluation and Treatment of Chronic Pain. Baltimore, Williams & Wilkins, 1992, p 384–393.
40. Hinnant DW: Psychological evaluation and testing. In Tollison CD (ed): Handbook of Pain Management, 2nd ed. Baltimore, Williams & Wilkins, 1994, pp 18–35.
41. Kerns RD, Turk DC, Rudy TE: The West Haven–Yale Multidimensional Pain Inventory (WHYMPI). Pain 23:345–356, 1985.
42. Kinney R, Catchell RJ, et al: The SCL-90R: An alternative to the MMPI for psychological screening of chronic low back pain patients. Presented at the Annual Meeting of the International Society for the Study of the Lumbar Spine, Kyoto, Japan, May 1989.
43. Kramlinger KG, Swanson DW, Maruta T: Are patients with chronic pain depressed? Am J Psychiatry 140:747–749, 1983.
44. Krusen EM, Ford DE: Compensation factors in low back injuries. JAMA 166:1128–1133, 1958.
45. Leavitt SS, Beyer RD, Johnson TL: Monitoring the recovery process: Pilot results of a systematic approach to case management. Med Surg 41:25–30, 1972.
46. Loeser J: In Stanton-Hicks M, Boas R (eds): Chronic Low Back Pain. New York, Raven Press, 1982, pp 145–148.
47. Magni G, Arsie D, DeLeo D: Antidepressants in the treatment of cancer pain: A survey in Italy. Pain 29:347–353, 1987.
48. McGill CM: Industrial back problems: A control program. J Occup Med 10:174–178, 1968.
49. Melzack R: The McGill Pain Questionnaire. Pain 1:277–299, 1975.
50. Merskey H (ed): Classification of chronic pain: Description of chronic pain syndromes and definition of pain terms. Pain (Suppl. 3):S1, 1986.
51. Merskey H: The effect of chronic pain upon the response to noxious stimuli by psychiatric patients. J Psychosom Res 8:405–419.
52. Millon T, Green CJ, Meagher RB: Millon Behavioral Health Inventory, 3rd ed. Minneapolis, Interpretive Scoring System, 1982.
53. Monks R: Psychotropic drugs. In Bonica JJ (ed): The Management of Pain. Philadelphia, Lea & Febiger, 1990, p 1677.
54. Okifuji A, Turk DC, Kalauokalani D: Clinical outcome and economic evaluation of multidisciplinary pain centers. In Block A, Kremer E, Fernandez E (eds): Handbook of Pain Syndromes. Mahway, NJ, Lawrence Erlbaum, 1999, pp 77–98.
55. Oxman T, Denson DD: Antidepressants and adjunctive psychotrophic drugs. In Raj RP (ed): Practical Management of Pain. Chicago, Year Book Medical Publishers, 1988, pp 528–538.
56. Peck JC, Fordyce WE, Black R: The effect of pendency of claims for compensation upon behavior indicative of pain. Wash Law Rev 53:257–278, 1978.
57. Portenoy RK: Opioid therapy for chronic nonmalignant pain: A review of the critical issues. Special section on opioids for nonmalignant pain. Part 1. J Pain Symptom Manage 11:203–217, 1996.
58. Revill SI, Robinson JO, Rosen M, et al: The reliability of a linear analogue for evaluating pain. Anesthesia 31:1191–1198, 1976.
59. Romano JH, Turner JA: Chronic pain and depression: Does the evidence support a relationship? Psych Bull 97:18–34, 1985.
60. Rutrick D, Aronoff GM: Combined psychotherapy for chronic pain syndrome patients at a multidisciplinary pain center. In Aronoff GM (ed): Evaluation and Treatment of Chronic Pain. Baltimore, Urban & Schwarzenberg, 1985, pp 491–492.
61. Seres JS, Newman RI: Negative influences of the disability compensation system: Perspectives for the clinician. Semin Neurol 3:4, 1983.
62. Snook SH, et al: A. Study of three preventive approaches to low back injury. J Occup Med 20:478–481, 1978.
63. Strang JP: The chronic disability syndrome. In Aronoff GM (ed): The Evaluation and Treatment of Chronic Pain, 1st ed. Baltimore, Urban & Schwarzenberg, 1985.

64. Strassberg DS, Reimherr F, Ward M, et al: The MMPI and chronic pain. J Consult Clin Psychol 49:220–226, 1981.
65. Tait RC, Chibnall JT, Krause S: The Pain Disability Index: Psychometric properties. Pain 40:171–182, 1990.
66. Tollison DC, Langley JC: P3 (Pain Patient Profile). Minneapolis, National Computer Systems, 1992, 1995.
67. Turk DC: Evaluation of pain and disability. J Disability 2:24–43, 1991.
68. Turk DC, Rudy TE: Persistent pain and the injured worker: Integrating biomechanical, psychosocial, and behavioral factors in assessment. J Occup Rehab 1, 1991.
69. Turner JA, Roman JM: Review of prevalence of coexisting chronic pain and depression. In Benedetti C, Chapman CR, Moricca G (eds): Advances in Pain Research and Therapy, vol 7. New York, Raven Press, 1984.
70. Waddell G: Biopsychosocial analysis of low back pain. Baillieres Clin Rheumatol 6:523–527, 1992.
71. Waddell G, et al: Failed lumbar disc surgery following industrial injuries. J Bone Joint Surg 61:201–207, 1979.
72. Walsh NE, Dumitru D: Financial compensation and recovery from low back pain. Spine 2:109–121, 1987.
73. Watson GD, Chandarana PC, Mersky N: Relationships between pain and schizophrenia. Br J Psychol 138:33–36, 1981.
74. Weinstein MR: The concept of the disability process. Psychosomatics 19:94–97, 1978.
75. Weissman DE, Haddox JD: Opioid pseudoaddiction—an iatrogenic syndrome. Pain 36:363–366, 1989.
76. White P: Pain measurement. In Warfield CA (ed): Principles and Practice of Pain Management. New York, McGraw-Hill, 1993, pp 27–42.
77. Yang JC, Wagner JM, Clark WC: Psychological distress and mood in chronic pain and surgical patients: A decision theory analysis. In Bonica JJ (ed): Advances in Pain Research and Therapy. Florida, American Pain Society, 1983, pp 901–906.

CHAPTER

Evaluating and Rating Impairment Caused by Stress

BRIAN SCHULMAN, MD, CIME

The single most remarkable historical fact concerning the term stress is its persistent widespread usage in biology and medicine in spite of almost chaotic disagreement over its definition."[25]

PROBLEMS IN ASSESSING STRESS IN MEDICAL PRACTICE

Whereas it is widely accepted by physicians that excessive stress may be deleterious to a person's health, there is a lack of consensus on what constitutes stress or why some individuals are more vulnerable to stress than others. In the midst of this ambiguity, most physicians intuitively believe that stress plays a contributory role in the evolution of disability. The problem in assessment is creating a systematic process for the consideration of stress as a factor in disability. The complex causal nexus connecting life events, along with the variability of individual response and illness, lies at the core of impairment and disability assessments.

Several problems complicate the objective assessment of stress. Foremost, there is lack of agreement on the definition of stress. As Haan noted, "Stress is whatever stresses people, but its essential properties are not clear."[17] Stress has numerous meanings and descriptions; consequently, it is an elusive concept to understand and measure. It is difficult to examine stressful life events independently of other aggravating or modifying life events. Individuals may focus on a particular event or condition and ignore other seemingly more troublesome or distressing conditions.

Individuals respond differently when coping with similar events and conditions. The impact of stress is mollified or accelerated by individual variability, including coping style, personality functioning, temperament, and the absence or presence of comorbid mental disorders. It is difficult for a physician to integrate all the necessary information into a diagnostic formulation. With so many factors to consider, the only constant is variability of response.

Nonetheless, there is a body of empirical evidence linking stress with medical illness. Stressful life events have been shown to increase mortality in widows,[30] accelerate cardiovascular disease,[37] worsen Graves disease,[21] exacerbate psoriasis,[1] cause recurrent episodes of multiple sclerosis,[38] and increase susceptibility to common colds,[11,12] as well as contribute to the worsening of many other conditions.

The core problem in assessment is to understand each individual's particular sensitivity to stress, and to differentiate that stress vulnerability from other conditions that contribute to disability. In practice, the complaints of "being under stress" or feeling "unable to cope with stress" are findings that are heavily weighted in reaching conclusions about impairment and function. A physician may disproportionately focus on the severity of the stressor as a criterion of disability. Thus, an examiner may erroneously conclude that a very stressful event is more likely to lead to a severe impairment and may not consider personal vulnerability, comorbidity, or the effect of psychosocial factors as causes of disability.

The subjective experience of stress is not necessarily a sign of pathology. The stress response may be an adaptive mechanism, leading to a conservation of energy and a reassessment of goals. Stress may prompt one to yield in response to unresolvable conflict or to disengage from unobtainable goals as a protective mechanism.[27] Stress, as a transient state, may reflect a normative response, a measure of one's fitness and drive for survival.

A particular difficulty in stress assessment is predicting individual vulnerability in response to stressful circumstances. A person's projected response to a stressful circumstance is a criterion for rating the severity of a mental or behavioral impairment. The American Medical Association's Guides to the Evaluation of Permanent Impairment, fourth edition,[2] suggests that an examiner look for deterioration or decompensation in work or worklike settings as illustrative of repeated failure to adapt to stressful circumstances. An examiner is encouraged to adapt the legal standard of the "reasonable person" to make such a determination of the stressfulness of a circumstance or condition. The question of assessing what condition is sufficiently stressful to prompt an individual to withdraw from the situation or experience an exacerbation of signs and symptoms of a mental disorder, or aggravate or accelerate an existing disorder is critical to the impairment rating. However, this determination is largely speculative and regards stress vulnerability as a static condition. Predicting what circumstance will be stressful is problematic. Erroneous determinations can interfere with vocational restoration and contribute to invalidism. Similar statements are made in the fifth edition including adherence to the "reasonable man" standard.[40(p326)]

An examiner may draw conclusions about impairment without adequately assessing the motivation for improvement. For example, a bank teller who develops post-traumatic stress disorder (PTSD) and has persistent anxiety is likely to be advised not to return to work in a bank to avoid stressful circumstances that will likely trigger a recrudescence of symptoms. The subsequent loss of function in certain occupational settings will contribute to an impairment rating. However, a survivor of a vehicular accident who develops PTSD and persistent anxiety would likely be encouraged to start driving again as soon as possible after the accident. In most instances, the anxious driver would not be advised to stop driving or riding in motor vehicles. Consequently, the "recovered" survivor of a vehicular accident would have little functional loss and would less likely be rated with a permanent medical impairment.

In summary, the stressfulness of a traumatic event is but one element in assessment. The impact of such an event and the resultant impairment are influenced by many intangible factors, including coping, resilience, and motivation. Stress, personal response, and adaptation are inextricably entwined. Following a vehicular accident, the need to drive and resolve the fear of driving is an adaptive response that minimizes the severity of the consequent impairment. In assessment, the factors of attitude and motivation, as well as the response to treatment and social support, are critical determinants of residual impairment.

ASSESSMENT OF STRESS: THE IMPORTANCE OF INDIVIDUAL VARIABILITY

Hans Selye, considered by many to be the father of stress medicine, explained that stress is first and foremost a simple consequence of living,[34] and that essentially any event or condition that disrupts the state of homeostasis (termed a stressor) causes stress. If unresolved, the acute stress then leads to a physiologic state of chronic strain. His General Adaptation Theory regarded stress as a neutral, but inevitable, consequence of living. His frequently quoted advice to business executives cautions "It's not what happens to you that matters but how you take it." Stress was inescapable, and, for those who tried to find a stress-free environment, he advised, "the only condition where there is no stress is death."

In assessing stress, one should appreciate the adaptative value of stress as a nociceptive alerting response. The neurobiological stress response is a biological alerting system critical for defense and protection. Biological necessity, not pathologic response, underlies the stress response.

All too often, a physician, in the role of patient advocate, recommends that his or her patient be placed in a "stress-free environment" or be given a "low-stress job." It is never quite clear what the physician intends to have done in such cases. Are employers truly able to measure the "stressfulness" of a job or assignment? Is such an accommodation possible? Often, the exercise of finding a "less stressful" job produces dubious benefit. To a large measure, variability of response to stress determines the stressfulness of a job. Each person will respond differently to deadlines, overtime, or authority. Mikhail surveyed the literature and highlighted a consensus in the historical development of the stress concept.[26] To summarize, the following are considered important considerations in the assessment of stress:

1. Individuals show considerable variability in their reactivity to stress.
2. Stress is largely determined by an individual's perception of the stressful situation or the individual's anticipation of the inability to respond adequately to a given demand rather than the situation itself.
3. The extent of stress depends partly on the capability of an individual to cope.

Coping, which refers to adaptation under relatively difficult conditions, plays a critical function in "metabolizing" or resolving stress. Coping capabilities are the diverse skills that allow one to control the intensity and pace of external demands. Such skills confer the ability to maintain psychological and physiologic equilibrium under challenging conditions and when confronting difficult circumstances. By maintaining equilibrium, an individual can conserve resources and focus on the external situation.

Resilience refers to the speed, elasticity, and smoothness of restoration of equilibrium. Resilient systems (and people) respond quickly, with minimal expenditure of unnecessary effort. Resilient people are less likely to develop chronic emotional and physical strains. They possess the ability to muster additional energy (the ability to get a "second wind") and the capacity to respond to substitutes and access new opportunities, as well as the capacity for constructive use of anxiety and aggression. It is the dynamic interplay between a stressful condition and an individual's coping style, defense mechanisms, and inherent resilience that comprises the variability of response.

STRESS, PATIENTS, AND PHYSICIANS

Physicians and patients speak a colloquial language regarding stress. It is an informal, user-friendly language. The word stress has universal acceptance and frank appeal. Unlike "pyschogenic," "stress" is not stigmatizing. Rather, stress is an honorable designation that does not imply personal failing or moral weakness. Stress happens to everyone. It connotes drive, ambition, and determination. An individual rarely thinks about creating stress as a function of ineffective coping. It comes with the territory of ambition and confers a high status.

It has been said that the word "stress" is a doctor's best friend. It places closure on the consultation. The patient asks the physician, "Do you think it could be stress?" The doctor nods affirmatively. This assures the patient that the problem is not serious; at least the patient does not have cancer or a brain tumor. For a physician, the stress explanation circumvents having to pursue further, unnecessary tests. It provides some reasonable closure and reassurance, and suggests a solution.

The nonspecificity of stress enhances its therapeutic utility. It suggests a wide assortment of disturbances, but a singular response: change the deleterious aspects of your lifestyle. When patients speak of being under stress, they are advising their physician that the circumstances of their lives are not quite right. In a comparable way, when physicians speak of stress to their patients, they are cautioning their patients that factors related to lifestyle are affecting their state of health and contributing to their suffering.

The language of stress broadens the dialogue between physicians and patients, by including the psychosocial and environmental factors that affect health and disease. It is consistent with several models that propose to expand the physician's understanding of the biological context of health and disease. Engel's work expanded the understanding of illness and illness behavior by proposing a biopsychosocial model that depicts concentric and overlapping systems from the submolecular elements to the social and cultural system.[16] He emphasized the interaction of biological with environmental systems, where illness has a ripple effect disrupting all aspects of a person's life. Cassell emphasized the human elements of suffering and urged physicians to appreciate the multiple dimensions of "personhood."[9] For a physician to assist patients in the "transcendence" of suffering, medical therapeutics must encompass psychological, cultural, and even spiritual issues. Stress is a medium of expression that opens the door for a discussion of all of these important issues.

BIOLOGICAL CONCEPT OF STRESS

Human stress encompasses the study of environmental stimulus and biological response. The history of human stress research began with studies of physiologic response, but now includes psychological, psychosocial, and social studies.

Stress is a biological mediator of survival. All living organisms experience stress, especially Homo sapiens. Beginning with the Neanderthal, who was forced to find water and shelter from the cold, to the modern commodities trader shouting orders into two telephones simultaneously, stress has been linked to survival.

Threats to personal security or the anticipation of danger trigger neurochemical activation of the central nervous system resulting in hormonal secretion and alterations in behavior. The stress response allows one to fight or flee. Without a bolt of adrenaline to escape the predatory animals roaming the tundra, the evolution of Homo sapiens would have terminated on the Paleolithic food chain. Over millions of years, little has changed. Commodities traders still relish the "thrill of the pit," as they rely on the adrenal surge to barter a profit. Man is dependent upon, perhaps even addicted to, stress. This is a tense, potentially explosive, relationship. Stress is an essential adaptive mechanism, but also a force of destructive potential.

A biological understanding of the interaction of systems unfolded in the eighteenth century. The French physiologist Claude Bernard advanced the concept of living beings existing in a "harmonious whole," and emphasized that survival under difficult external conditions was dependent on the maintenance of a constant internal environment.[4]

The American physiologist Walter Cannon advanced the principles by which living systems survived in nature, noting that only when cells grow in masses and selectively differentiate into specialized functional units can they maintain the internal stability capable of separating them from disturbances due to shifts in the external environment.[7] The maintenance of internal stability in the face of changing external conditions is biological homeostasis. Any factor or condition that alters the state of homeostasis creates strain in the system.

Cannon correctly identified the critical role of sympathetic activation as a signal alerting the body to the physiologic dangers of cold, hemorrhage, lowered blood sugar, or toxins. Activation of the sympathetic system initiates a "fight versus flight" response with resultant activation of the hypothalamic-pituitary-adrenal (HPA) axis and biochemical reactions designed to restore homeostasis.

Cannon proposed that the biological homeostasis of living systems could be applied to social systems as well. He observed, "Only when human beings are grouped in large aggregations is there an opportunity of developing an internal organization which can offer mutual aid and the advantage, to many, of special ingenuity and skill." Stress could be generated by shifts in the social as well as the biological environment. Expanding the concept of biological homeostasis to include human stability in the social order served to integrate the biological with the psychological condition of stress.

In 1936, Selye published a seminal paper, "A syndrome produced by diverse noxious agents," in *Nature*, describing the general adaptation syndrome. He identified three physiologic stages for the stress response: alarm, resistance, and exhaustion. For Selye, stress was a nonspecific response to essentially the wear and tear of life: "the unconscious, wired in stress responses mediated by the neurohumoral system." The deleterious effect of stress was chronic activation of the HPA axis, resulting in biochemical and structural tissue changes and the clinical syndrome of "just being sick." Stress is a state of chronic activation of interdependent physiologic events initiated by virtually any toxic demand. Selye was less concerned with defining the first mediator of the alarm process than understanding the physiologic consequences of organ exhaustion. "Whatever the nature of the first mediator, however, its existence is assured by its effects, which has been observed and measured."

STRESS, IMMUNITY, AND DISEASE

Some of the most exciting developments in stress research have emerged from the field of psychoneuroimmunology, the study of the relationship between the brain and the immune system. Rabin has extensively reviewed the literature and described the multiple effects between psychological and physical stressors and alterations in humeral and cellular immune function.[32] As the brain responds to changes in an individual's environment, neurons throughout the brain activate the HPA, creating neurochemical activity that, among other actions, triggers immune activity. In turn, the immune system releases cytokine messengers to provide feedback to the brain, completing a feedback loop. The brain responds by releasing hormones that prevent excessive activation of the immune system.

To ensure homeostasis, the body's hormonal milieu is continuously being altered, primarily by the release of glucocorticoids and catecholamines. Stress influences the functional capabilities of the immune system. Stress also influences complex interactions of genetic, physiological, behavioral, and environmental factors that affect the body's ability to maintain health and resist disease. What several years ago was merely a fascinating area for speculation has become the subject of diverse biobehavioral research, which has produced extensive empirical data. The stress-immunity-disease literature provides the empirical nexus linking stress to the initiation or progression of arthritis, thyroid disease, infectious disease, cancer, human immunodeficiency virus disease, and cardiovascular disease.

Immune response is mediated by psychological variables. The ultimate outcome, essentially the ability to maintain health and resist disease, is not dependent on the severity of the stressor, but on the individual response. The evidence suggests that the quality of health can be ameliorated by adopting stress-buffering behaviors. As Rabin, who has extensively reviewed the stress-immunity literature, observed, "It is not the characteristics of the stressor that are of importance in determining hormonal alterations, but rather how the stressor is perceived by the brain and the availability of coping skills that will influence how the stress will alter the hormonal milieu in which the immune system resides."[32]

The finding that stress—whether associated with a single or repeated exposure to an experimentally designed stressor—increases neurochemical activity in the brain has important implications for understanding pathophysiology. Cognitive function and behavior have the capacity to alter the stress response. The empirical evidence suggests that social interactions, belief systems, humor, exercise, and intimacy can all influence immune function. There is also evidence that altering thoughts and behavior may create the distress-resistant brain.

STRESS AND PERSONALITY FUNCTION

Not unlike the way in which the immune system scans the molecular environment for pathogens, the personality metabolizes distress and protects the individual from the deleterious effects of stress. An individual with a functional personality neutralizes distressing cognitions and maintains emotional stability. An individual's ability to control aggression and hostility, prevent obsessive thoughts, or employ humor to maintain perspective are examples of the protective capabilities of the personality.

Healthy personality functioning is critical to the management of life stressors. Whereas it is beyond the scope of this chapter to discuss the complexities of personality, an awareness of how one's personality influences coping and adaptation is essential in assessing the impact of stress on medical impairment.

Briefly, personality encompasses a complex system of biological, mental, and behavioral factors that form an enduring pattern of response. Each person develops a unique personality style—a descriptive set of responses to stressors. Many factors contribute to the development of personality. In the biopsychosocial model, multiple etiologic factors are described; however, the model does not quantitate the relative contribution of each factor. In contrast, the diathesis-stress model is heavily biased to consider the biological predisposition of the individual, factors that comprise the inheritable predisposition.[29] In this model, a person's particular genetic and biological predisposition serve as the infrastructure of personality. Adult personality develops as a result of the particular experience of an individual. For example, studies of individuals with antisocial personality have demonstrated that traits such as impulsivity, as well as aggressive and irritable temperament, can be identified in childhood, well before the diagnosis of the personality disorder.[8]

GOODNESS OF FIT AND THE ADJUSTMENT TO DISABILITY

Chess and Thomas's Goodness of Fit model evolved from the New York Longitudinal Study of children and their families. They identified the importance of temperament and "goodness of fit" as ways of understanding the difficulties that children experience in their families.[10] Temperament is a biological factor derived from genetic influences and expressed in various patterns broadly categorized as difficult, easy, or slow to warm up. The "fit" between an individual's temperament and the demands of the environment was a critical variable interacting with other factors that influenced personality development. When there is a comfortable compatibility or fit between the capacities and characteristics of the individual and the demands and expectations of the environment, normal development and/or function is likely to occur. Conversely, when there is "poor fit" between temperament and the demands of the environment, impaired psychological functioning is probable.

TEMPERAMENT AND THE ASSESSMENT OF DISABILITY

Temperament and "goodness of fit" are valuable concepts for understanding an individual's response to convalescence following an injury or illness. Temperament influences an individual's response to disruption in normal routines. Changes in lifestyle and interpersonal dynamics occasioned by illness and injury affect the individual's fit. For example, the person with a high activity temperament who relishes being on the go and doing physical work will find convalescence from an injury and the sedentary lifestyle particularly disruptive and stressful. In such cases, symptoms of emotional distress, including unhappiness, sleep disturbance, or irritability, may occur and be erroneously attributed to clinical depression. For the most part, however, these are transient symptoms that are alleviated by a resumption of more temperamentally desirable activities, often including the restoration of a more active, structured lifestyle.

Individuals with difficult temperaments or those who are slow to warm up to new situations may resist change and therapeutic recommendations. These individuals adjust slowly to the sequelae of an injury or illness. Persistent symptomatology, rebellious behavior, and angry responses toward case managers, physicians, or family members are commonly encountered. An individual with a difficult temperament will demonstrate slow adaptability, intense reactions, and frequent negative moods. These temperamental characteristics blend into adult personality traits. The demands of these individuals may prompt unnecessary diagnostic procedures or excessive, redundant medical treatment. Frequently, this difficult, demanding behavior may be misdiagnosed as a mental or behavioral disorder.

An evaluator of disability should be aware of temperament and "goodness of fit" as variables in assessment. It is important to assess the difficulty an individual experiences adjusting to an altered lifestyle or the limitations imposed by an impairment. Whereas the adjustment difficulty should be therapeutically addressed, it should not be a primary factor in rating impairment. The assessment of impairment should include consideration of coping style, personality traits, and temperament as transient factors affecting a person's adjustment to changes in lifestyle and routines. An understanding of these variables will prevent misdiagnosis and potential errors in the rating of permanent mental and behavioral impairment.

STRESS AND PERSONALITY DISORDERS

Personality disorders may be diagnosed when the clinician identifies an enduring pattern of inner experience and behavior that is inflexible and pervasive. The inflexible pattern of cognition and behavior is manifest in a broad range of situations and leads to distress and impairment.[3] Personality disorder has an early onset and is unlikely to change over time, but may show a variable level of severity along a behavioral continuum. Nonetheless, personality disorder is a state disorder that is most obvious in stressful conditions.

Variations of normal personality functioning occur where a person is under stress. The normal personality may be strained, revealing vulnerabilities. It may appear that the individual, at least transiently, is not coping well. In the impairment evaluation, a physician may intuitively identify personality dysfunction, but may be uncertain if the condition is a transient response that will normalize following removal of the stressor or whether the behavior supports evidence of a state personality disorder. This is particularly problematic if the examiner is doing a single evaluation or does not have access to medical records. In practice, the distinction is circumvented by references to "functional overlay," "a psychogenic presentation," or "hysteroid reaction" to indicate that behavioral factors are protracting the disability.

The possibility that exposure to stress can induce a personality disorder is controversial. The Diagnostic and Statistic Manual of Mental Disorders, fourth edition (DSM-IV), does not allow for the possibility of a stress-induced personality disorder, whereas the International Classification of Diseases–10 allows for a personality disorder to be created by stress. Reich conducted an empirical study and found evidence suggesting that the state group of personality disorders could be distinguished from a "stress-induced personality disorder group" on the basis of clinical characteristics such as having a higher lifetime rate of suicide attempts, higher Hamilton Anxiety and Depression Scale scores, and a higher family incidence of other personality disorder clusters.[33] The hypothesis is that under stressful conditions certain individuals have personality vulnerabilities that are amplified, making them appear to have state personality disorders. The implication is that the stress-induced personality disorder is reversible with treatment. Certainly, being able to identify transient personality dysfunction is important in disability assessment, as it would, among other factors, bring the issue of permanency into question.

COPING AND DISABILITY

A complex and dynamic relationship exists between stress, coping, and disability. Coping has been used in a variety of contexts and ascribed a variety of meanings. It refers to the process of managing problems or troubles. In the context of adaptation and medicine, it is regarded as the problem-solving efforts made by an individual when the demands he or she faces are highly relevant to his or her welfare and when the demands tax his or her adaptive resources.[22] Experienced psychiatrists, familiar with performing impairment evaluations, can attest to the importance of coping as a factor in therapeutic outcome and rehabilitation. However, the influence of problem solving and mastery is not easily accounted for in impairment evaluation.

The DSM-IV addresses the issue of coping style in the section "Other conditions that may be a focus of clinical attention" as "Coping style and personality traits affecting ... a particular medical condition." The category is sufficiently broad to allow for inclusion of many different conditions where a deficient coping style aggravates an underlying medical condition.

For example, a patient with chronic pain who insists on a complete ablation of pain may "doctor shop" to find medical solutions. The development of iatrogenic complications may only intensify an individual's desire to find a medical solution. Meanwhile, functional restoration may be ignored and relationships strained. The individual may become increasingly hostile and noncooperative. This familiar course of events suggests a problematic coping style.

Personality traits also affect coping. For example, a police officer who is excitable may demonstrate excessive arousal in response to a variety of routine work events. If, in time, that officer develops coronary artery disease, his or her propensity to be excessively aroused (a personality trait) would render him or her vulnerable to aggravation or acceleration of the ischemic heart disease. In this circumstance, the medical disability might be considered diagnostically under the DSM-IV category "Stress-related physiological response affecting ischemic heart disease," which is listed under "Other conditions that may be a focus of clinical attention."

THE POSTTRAUMATIC STRESS SYNDROMES

The emotional impact of trauma may produce a posttraumatic stress disorder (PTSD). The first descriptions of this disorder involved victims of combat. Symptoms of palpitations, chest pain, headaches, and dimness of vision were observed among British troops in India and Crimea. During the Civil War, Dr. Jacob Mendes DaCosta studied a group of physically healthy soldiers with cardiac complaints and correctly theorized that the syndrome of "irritable heart" or "soldiers' heart" was attributed to excessive and persistent activation of the sympathetic nervous system. Similar observations were made in soldiers during World War I, World War II, and the Korean War, and the syndrome of a traumatically induced emotional disorder was variously called "shell shock," "traumatic war neurosis," and "battle fatigue." Following World War II, Kardiner and Spiegel identified the biological arousal of the disorder and called it a physioneurosis.[19] After the Vietnam War, investigators became aware of the delayed onset and chronicity of PTSD.

Post-traumatic stress syndromes have also been identified in survivors of noncombat events. Lindemann's classic study of the survivors of the Coconut Grove Fire was one of the first prospective studies of the effects of a noncombat disaster.[23] Investigators have studied survivors of serious events including, but not limited to, mass shootings,[28] building collapses,[39] and vehicular accidents.[20]

Assessment of PTSD

Exposure to severe trauma may precipitate PTSD. The disorder is characterized by recurrent and intrusive (upon consciousness) revivifications of the traumatic environmental event; persistent avoidance of stimuli associated with the trauma; and persistent symptoms of increased arousal. The criteria for PTSD also require that the symptoms persist for at least one month.[3]

PTSD has a variable course and is frequently confounded by comorbid psychiatric disorders. The psychophysiologic reactions to stressful stimuli may recur for decades after the event. The DSM-IV also recognizes Acute Stress Disorder (ASD) as a separate diagnostic entity. Symptoms develop within a month after exposure and, in addition to the characteristic symptoms of PTSD, an individual develops at least three dissociative symptoms, including numbing, detachment, reduced awareness of surroundings, derealization, depersonalization, or dissociative amnesia.

Three possible mechanisms are offered to explain the causation and tenacity of these symptoms.[36] Stress sensitization refers to a stressor-induced increase in physiologic and psychological response following exposure to stressors of the same or lesser magnitude. Presumably, the perceptual mechanisms mediating stressors are sensitized by exposure to the stressor. Fear conditioning is a second possible mechanism. This occurs when fear-inducing stimuli are associatively linked with neutral stimuli. For example, a Vietnam veteran and survivor of the Tet Offensive experiences a fear response conditioned by the distinctive chopper sound of a "Huey" helicopter. PTSD may be triggered, even decades later, by industrial sounds of a similar pitch and frequency. A third mechanism is the facilitation of memory by sympathetic arousal. In this mechanism, emotionally charged memories are believed to be more deeply embedded or "overconsolidated" in the memory centers of the brain.

One might question the evolutionary value of the posttraumatic response. Ideally, a "normal" fear reaction should be self-limiting. In PTSD, it is likely that fear extinction, which would normally occur over time, is inhibited, causing what is initially a protective mechanism to become a chronic alerting response leading to a clinical disorder. What originates as a normative response to danger may, under certain circumstances, become a pathologic condition.

Arguably, stress sensitization serves a protective function. Making the distinction between a protective reaction and a clinical disorder is critical in assessing a permanent impairment. For example, a steel worker who barely avoids a critical injury after falling several stories develops a phobia of heights. Is the phobia an adaptive response? Clearly, additional investigation is warranted to understand the adaptive value engendered by trauma and to differentiate the normal from the pathologic.

To assess the severity of PTSD, one should evaluate the medical impairment generated by the disorder. Recurrent symptomatology, marked restriction in the activities of daily living, and a severe, persistent disturbance in lifestyle are indications of psychopathology and impairment. Some attention should be given to the influences of psychosocial factors, particularly relational and occupational difficulties. Another concern is the influence of therapeutic interventions that encourage withdrawal and hamper desensitization.

THE ASSESSMENT OF LIFE EVENTS

Life events may be perceived as stressful. If the event is of sufficient severity, it may disrupt normal coping and, possibly, precipitate psychological or physical illness.

In recent years, there has been much interest in environmentally induced illness, particularly illness precipitated by events that impact life change. Virtually any life event can be included in this category, from the death of a spouse to a financial setback. In the life events model, events have psychological significance because they have a propensity to initiate social change and cause disruption of the adaptational balance. Surveys have been developed to quantify the relationship among life events, lifestyle impact, and distress. In 1967, Holmes and Rahe devised and published the Social Readjustment Rating Scale, which, in survey form, defined and listed life change events ranging from severe, such as the loss of a spouse, to more commonly experienced, such as job changes or financial difficulties.[18] Rater groups, serving as judges, assigned values to each event on the list, producing a hierarchy of stressful events. The result was a standardized rating of events that could be administered to assess the magnitude of social readjustment. It was widely quoted, but unfortunately of minimal clinical utility.

The life event–social readjustment scaling has questionable validity, as it valuates an event, any event, independent of other modifying or accelerating events and conditions. For example, the stressfulness of a divorce may be influenced by many environmental and constitutional factors. Timing, sequencing, and social circumstances play modifying roles. Moreover, personality factors, as well as the broadly defined abilities of coping defense, and mastery are critical determinants. Social support and cultural factors play a critical role in determining the response of an individual to a specific event.

To more fully assess the stressfulness of an event, investigators refined measuring systems for life events that encompass both the quantitative and the various qualitative aspects of the event. Dohrenwend et al devoted considerable effort to assessing the applicability of a life event scale to a particular population. They developed the Psychiatric Epidemiological Research Interview–Life Event Scale as part of a study in New York City to develop methodology to study life change and psychiatric illness in a particular community.[15] Paykel et al developed assessment instruments to correlate life events that occurred within 6 months of illness. In an effort to gain greater specificity, they categorized life events by activity (work, school, family), whether the event was socially desirable or undesirable, and whether the life change occasioned by the event represented an entrance or an exit from a person's social field.[31]

To account for variability of response, Dohrenwend and Dohrenwend designed their research to delineate group variability within event categories.[13] The authors felt that any scale designed to measure the stressfulness of events needed to take into consideration the relevant variables that would likely influence the respondent's reaction to the event. For example, when an individual "stopped working," it was important to know the sequence of events that led to the job loss. Did the person anticipate the event and was it desirable?

The impact of life events is variable across cultural, educational, and socioeconomic groups.[14,35] Consequently, the stressfulness of a particular event must be assessed within the context of a person's psychosocial environment. The "appearance" of an event does not indicate the degree of life change. For example, the birth of a child may be planned and anticipated or unplanned and unwanted. Moreover, the expectations for childrearing and the life change created by childbirth are variable experiences across cultural, ethnic, and sociocultural groups. The most elusive aspect to assess may be the "desirability" of the event. Events that are perceived as undesirable or events over which an individual has little control may have a disproportionately negative impact and create significant life change including protracted disability. The variability of response to a life event can best be assessed through a careful history.

In addition to life change events, usual and ordinary events, such as everyday problems,[6] the absence of uplifting events, and the occurrence of hassles,[5] have been considered as sources of stress. Burks and Martin[6] identified everyday problems, defined as ongoing and often chronic situations, which produced recurring unpleasantness and distress, and developed an inventory for assessment. Everyday problems, including financial problems, poor health, or unsatisfactory living conditions, are ubiquitous and can, like life change events, be stressful and cause psychological symptoms. The Hassles Scale was designed to assess the impact of ongoing life situations from both a quantitative and qualitative perspective. It consists of 117 items that are commonly experienced in the course of life and cover a full range of work, family, social, and practical considerations, such as time pressures, absence of opportunity, and losing things. The results are tabulated on the basis of frequency, intensity, and cumulative severity. Results from the application of the Hassles Scale support the finding that variance in reported psychological symptoms can be accounted for by hassles considered independently of major life change events. Early work with the Hassles Scale suggested that the broadly defined concept of life hassles might be more strongly associated with adaptational outcomes and presumably the development of illness rather than the life events themselves.

A final consideration in assessing the nexus between life events and life change is the independence of occurrence of events. Independence of events refers to a life event occurring independently of the predisposition of the individual. Events that occur as a function of a person's psychiatric illness or as a consequence of disordered personality functioning are dependent events. For example, if a person has a history of impulsive, angry, or disruptive behavior, and then has a serious automobile accident because of driving irresponsibly at an excessive speed or in an intoxicated state, the accident event would be rated dependent on, not independent of, the psychological state. A thorough history will provide useful information suggesting that many stressful events do not occur entirely independently of the underlying predisposition.

In summary, the assessment of recent life events, along with ongoing life hassles, provides important psychosocial information. In taking a history, an examiner should inquire about the context as well as the consequences of an event. An unexpected, negative event over which an individual has little control has a particularly pathogenic impact. Events that cause role transitions or interpersonal conflicts may result in protracted disability. This problem is frequently encountered in assessing industrial injuries where the blame for an accident is contested.

STRESS AND THE DSM-IV

The etiologic role of stress in the development of mental disorders is continuously being defined through a variety of empirical studies and is evident in the multiaxial diagnostic model.

Diagnostically, PTSD was officially delineated in 1980 as a clinical diagnosis within the Axis I category of anxiety disorders as a condition that develops as a result of exposure to one or more traumatic events. The essential feature of PTSD is the development of the characteristic features following exposure to an extreme traumatic stressor. The criteria allow for the delayed onset of symptoms, noting that clinical symptoms may not appear for up to 6 months following exposure to the stressor. The definition of extreme stressor is quite broad and encompasses virtually all serious negative events. The characteristic symptoms include re-experiencing of the event in any of four ways: intrusive distressing recollections, recurrent distressing dreams, acting or feeling as if the distressing event was recurring, and intense arousal in response to internal or external cues. Other primary symptoms include persistent avoidance of the stimuli associated with the trauma, numbing of general responsiveness, and persistent symptoms of arousal. The syndrome is considered acute if the duration of the symptoms is less than 3 months, or chronic if the symptoms are still present more than 6 months after the trauma.

After extensive review of the empirical literature, a second trauma-induced psychiatric disorder, ASD, was introduced into the DSM-IV.[3] The essential features of this disorder are the development of characteristic anxiety, dissociation, and other symptoms within 1 month after exposure to an extreme traumatic stressor. The diagnosis requires the presence of at least three dissociative symptoms (numbing, detachment, a reduction in awareness of surroundings, derealization, depersonalization, or dissociative amnesia), as well as re-experiencing of the trauma, marked avoidance of stimuli that arouse recollections of the trauma, marked symptoms of anxiety, and increased arousal. The disturbance lasts for at least 2 days and does not persist beyond 4 weeks after the traumatic event. However, prospective studies have not supported the current DSM-IV criteria for prominent dissociative symptoms and have brought into question the validity of ASD as a distinct disorder.[24]

In the DSM-IV, Adjustment Disorder is considered as a separate Axis I disorder—a syndrome characterized by the development of clinically significant emotional or behavioral symptoms in response to an identifiable psychosocial stressor or stressors. Criteria include evidence of significant impairment in occupational or social functioning. Adjustment disorder should be distinguished from a normative response to an unpropitious event or condition. The criteria require that an individual have either "marked distress that is in excess of what would be expected from exposure to the stressor" (criterion B-1) or "significant impairment in social or occupational (academic) functioning" (criterion B-2).[3(p626)] Adjustment disorder is manifest by emotional or behavioral symptoms occurring within 3 months of the onset of the stressor(s). The disorder is presumed to exist until the stressor is removed or, if the stressor persists, until an individual develops sufficient coping skills to adapt to its presence. A time limit of 6 months is placed on the duration of symptoms following resolution of the stressor.

Diagnostic uncertainty will impede the impairment evaluation. Particular attention should be given to the diagnosis (and misdiagnosis) of an adjustment disorder as a cause of permanent impairment. This is a transient disorder with specific criteria. For example, the criteria call for the disorder to be of limited duration. If symptoms persist beyond six months, it is prudent to examine for other comorbid conditions.

Additionally, the multiaxial dimension of the DSM-IV allows Axis IV reporting of psychosocial and environmental problems that may affect the diagnosis, treatment, and prognosis of mental disorders. Axis IV allows for the listing of a broad range of life problems that may be considered stressors, including problems with the primary support group, problems related to the social environment, educational problems, occupational problems, housing problems, economic problems, problems with access to health care, and problems related to interaction with the legal system.[3] This is an extremely useful inventory of life and living problems that should be thoroughly explored during assessment.

STRESS AND IMPAIRMENT

The response to stressful conditions is modified by many factors, including the severity, character, and context of stressors as well as the unique qualities of an individual. Variability of response is the rule, not the exception. Biological, psychological, and attitudinal factors influence the process of coping and adaptation and determine the extent of disability. Thus the assessment should explore individual variability and seek to identify the particular individual characteristics of the stress response.

The contribution of stress to medical impairment is most apparent when the stressful events and conditions occur just proximate to the onset of medical impairment and clinical improvement occurs spontaneously following removal of the noxious condition. Conversely, protraction of symptoms following removal of the stressor suggests an underlying problem with coping and/or personality function or the presence of comorbid illness. An examiner should explore a history of recent life events, individual vulnerability, and comorbidity and integrate these factors into a comprehensive mental and behavioral assessment of impairment.

It is important to bear in mind that stress is a ubiquitous condition of all living organisms and systems. It serves a protective and adaptive function. Severe stress may transiently hamper an individual's coping resources or reveal personality vulnerabilities. This is a normative response. In other individuals with either a significant state personality disorder or a comorbid mental illness, even a minor stress may result in serious impairment, suggesting that pre-existent vulnerability, not the stress response, is the causative problem.

In assessment, a detailed developmental history attentive to educational, military, and occupational performance is likely to provide evidence of recurring maladaptive patterns, suggesting a state personality disorder. Supportive medical documentation provides invaluable longitudinal information about response to treatment, attitude, and motivation. To best assess the mental and behavioral aspects of impairment, it is well to develop expertise in the psychiatric interview, with particular attention to observational skills, process awareness, and open-ended investigation.

The assessment of stress requires time and attention to detail. A balanced exploration of stressful psychosocial conditions, an examination of the personal responses to stressful conditions, and an evaluation of the psychosocial and occupational factors are minimal requirements for the assessment of function. Specifically, the assessment of stress should include the following items:

1. A thorough identification of the individual's age, sex, marital and familial status, current occupational status, and living condition.
2. A detailed history of his or her recent stressful conditions and life changes, along with an assessment of the impact of those changes on lifestyle.
3. A history of recent medical and psychiatric treatment, with particular attention to evidence of excessive treatment, lack of expected efficacy, and the individual's perception of benefit or harm. Treatment history should include a complete medication and prescription history, including current drug usage.
4. A substance and ethanol history. The Michigan Alcohol Screening Test (MAST) or a similar profile is recommended. An examiner should inquire about multiple prescribers of medication as an indication of potential impairment.
5. An educational and occupational history that includes all relevant training and acquired skills. Inquiry into the employment history, length of employment, reasons for changing employment, and assessment of occupational progression provides valuable information in response to external demands.
6. A relational and social history, with specific attention to the stability and quality of familial and social networks. Particular attention should be given to disruptions, separations, and contentious relationships.
7. A detailed analysis of the routine activities of daily living, including an assessment of the circadian pattern, quality and duration of sleep, nutrition, avocation, recreation, social interaction, and ability to perform such activities.
8. A mental status examination including an assessment of alertness, span of attention, mental acuity, affective stability, mood, level of depression or depressive equivalents, and anxiety. The Mini-Mental State Examination, the Hamilton Rating Scales for Depression and Anxiety, the Luria-Nebraska Brief Neuropsychological Screening, and the Beck Depression Inventory are useful adjunctive tools.
9. A clinical and, if possible, self-administered assessment of personality function. The clinical examination relies on the important developmental, social, school, and occupational history. One should also assess the relationship to significant caregivers, health providers, supervisors, and coworkers, as well as the examinee's response to the examiner and examining situation. The Minnesota Multiphasic Personality Inventory–II is the most widely utilized and reliable instrument to augment the clinical examination.
10. An assessment of phase of life, transcultural, and financial factors, including the issues of gain and protracted effect of current and potential litigation.

SUMMARY

Stress is a common complaint that brings patients to physicians. As a medium of communication, it conveys a multitude of meanings. It is an idiom of distress and a compact explanation for myriad symptoms. Stress plays a contributory role in the creation and protraction of serious disability. An extensive battery of empirical data is emerging to identify many of the mechanisms through which stress affects health and influences disease processes. Individual variability plays a very significant role in determining a person's response to stressful circumstances. An examiner's ability and willingness to assess individual variability and understand the psychosocial and environmental context of an individual's lifestyle are critical factors in assessing permanent disability.

EXAMPLES

Assessing Job Stress

Complaints of mental and physical symptoms attributable to job stress are commonly encountered in a psychological impairment evaluation. The problem usually involves either excessive workload or, far more commonly, interpersonal conflicts with coworkers or supervisors. Such complaints are often accompanied by accusations of harassment or discriminatory treatment.

The problem of work/resource imbalance is generally easier to assess than complaints attributed to interpersonal conflict. Guidelines established by the American College of Occupational and Environmental Medicine (ACOEM) define job stress as an imbalance between demand and resources. Elements of excessive demand include workload, time-sensitive deadlines, or the requirement to work excessively long hours. A deficiency of resources may result from a lack of technical or clerical support, insufficient supervision, or inadequate training and preparation. Stress results from a discrepancy between work demand and personal resources resulting in a failure of adjustment. Often, the person with job stress enjoys the content of his or her work, but is unable to keep up with responsibilities. In other circumstances, the work/resource imbalance is subtler, and stress is a function of a poor fit between a job and a particular worker.

Example 1: Excessive Workload

■ Mr. Simon was a 47-year-old married man who worked for a public agency as a computer maintenance specialist. As the agency gradually increased the number of computers, his workload increased. Although he genuinely enjoyed his work and got along well with his coworkers, he found it increasingly difficult to keep up with the expanding workload. An additional maintenance specialist was added, but the maintenance staff still was not able to meet the demands of the agency.

Mr. Simon felt personally responsible for getting the job done. To meet the expanded demand, he arrived earlier each morning and stayed later in the afternoon. Even working longer hours, he felt as if he could never catch up. He developed a "nervous stomach" and complained of throbbing, holocephalic headaches. After consulting with his private physician, no physical problem was found and no treatment was rendered. Nonetheless, the physician recommended that he take some time off. Mr. Simon refused to take time away from the job, claiming that he could not afford to get further behind. His work performance declined. He was easily angered and became quite irritable with even routine requests. After several discourteous confrontations, his supervisor referred him for psychiatric evaluation.

Discussion

The psychiatrist diagnosed major depression, recurrent. He opined that the depression was precipitated, at least in part, by the cumulative stress of the demand/resource imbalance. After a detailed assessment, the psychiatrist determined that Mr. Simon's self-esteem and self-worth were dependent on positive feedback from his occupational role. When he was unable to keep up with the demands of the job and get accolades from his coworkers, he suffered a significant loss. A treatment plan, which included a plan for return to work, allowed for a restoration of the positive feedback he needed from his work. This was done by limiting his overtime (which had been uncompensated) and working out a plan with the employer for quantitative work limits. Following his return to work, an assessment of medical impairment revealed mild deficits in endurance and mild limitations in his ability to adapt to highly pressured time deadlines. Job accommodations that addressed these problems greatly reduced the medical impairment.

Example 2: Poor Job/Person Fit

■ Mr. Jones, a 49-year-old systems analyst, was one of four analysts in a work group. Because he was the most technically knowledgeable, the vice president for information science made him the group leader, a job that required some supervision of the other three group members' work. Mr. Jones protested, claiming that he had neither management training nor experience. The vice president insisted that he take the job and assured him that there really was not much supervision involved.

From that time on, Mr. Jones manifested myriad psychosomatic and emotional problems. He missed time for a variety of doctor visits and for diagnostic assessments. He was placed on an out of work status, with the diagnosis of "job stress." Further, his physician provided a note stating that he was totally incapacitated.

Discussion

Two years after being promoted to the managerial position, Mr. Jones was granted Social Security Disability Income (SSDI). He expressed no interest in a return to work plan. Although the diagnosis of major depression had been accepted by SSDI as the basis for his impairment, the depression has been treated with fairly good response. Whereas he claimed to have loved his job as a systems analyst, he hated the "stress of managing others." He explained that he was always "thin-skinned" and very sensitive to criticism.

The supervisory job revealed Mr. Jones' personality vulnerabilities, problems that had not been previously evident in the workplace. Even more alarming, he was placed on disability status as a consequence of a stress-related job experience. The assessment of Mr. Jones' permanent medical impairment was based entirely on evidence of major depression without consideration for the poor job/person fit that preceded the depression and also precluded vocational restoration.

Job Stress and Interpersonal Conflict

Frequently, complaints of job stress emanate from interpersonal conflict. The job-stressed worker's emotional distress, which ranges in severity from irritability and nervousness to symptoms of major depression, is attributed to the adverse influence of a particular workplace relationship, usually with a supervisor. The worker's complaints usually stem from some unpleasant event or interaction. Getting a factual history may prove difficult. The worker may describe a series of confrontations or events, or may simply decline to discuss the problems, either on advice of counsel or to avoid "reliving a terrible experience." In either case, an examiner is offered only a partial and possibly biased description of the workplace experience.

Because the totality of the issues is not always made clear and an examiner rarely has access to both sides of the story, it is important to get additional information from the employer as well as from available records.

The medical records may provide important contributory information, but may also draw unsupported or inaccurate conclusions, particularly in regard to causality. For example, the worker may present documentation from a private physician, either a family physician or a mental health provider. Medical reports typically document a variety of somatic complaints such as headache, gastrointestinal problems, elevations in blood pressure, or chest pain. Although the medical information is inconclusive, the diagnostic assessment is "job stress," implying, but not objectively substantiating, a causal nexus between physical symptoms and alleged events in the workplace. The mental health report may describe anxiety, sleep disturbance, and/or depression with the assertion that these symptoms were generated by job stress. The typical recommendation is the prescription of a psychoactive medication and an off-work status.

When a return to work release is issued, the accommodation may request a change of venue or supervisor. There is rarely a medical rationale presented for such action. The implementations of such recommendations without adequate evaluation of the job-stressed worker is potentially disastrous. First, it validates the assessment of the worker's private physician, who is, by role, an advocate of his or her patient. Second, such diagnoses are heavily weighted by the worker's perception. Third, the treating physician has usually not provided a causal nexus relating the identified impairment to a particular event or condition. Consequently, an accommodation may be ineffective and, moreover, medically unnecessary.

Example 3: Confusing Personality Disorder With Job Stress

■ Ms. Edwards worked as an administrative clerk for a large company processing hundreds of routing forms each day. She developed symptoms of depressed mood, anxiety, sleep disturbance, and loss of appetite. She was very angry with her supervisor, who, she claimed, was harassing her. However, there were very few specific examples provided by either the worker or the employer to substantiate her allegations. Rather, Ms. Edwards claimed that she did not want to discuss the matter, or that discussions of the relationship made her ill—"It gives me a headache to talk about it."

Nonetheless, Ms. Edwards' psychiatrist concluded that she was suffering from job stress, and indicated that she was not fit for duty. No supportive medical documentation was provided to support his assessment. Ms. Edwards remained on a sick status for 18 months. She was then released to return to work by her psychiatrist if certain guidelines could be followed, including "reasonable isolation from her coworkers and the marked and inappropriate harassment," assignment to a new supervisor, and construction of a "private cubicle." Without seeking independent consultation regarding the medical necessity for such accommodation, the employer implemented those recommendations.

Six months later, Ms. Edwards was terminated for inappropriate and aggressive behavior. She filed a grievance and was reinstated. The arbitrator relied on the prior medical reports that indicated that Ms. Edwards has suffered job stress and considered that stress was a mitigating factor in recommending a reinstatement. There were no independent assessments done to question the diagnosis of job stress. However, prior to allowing a return to work, the medical director sent Ms. Edwards for an independent psychiatric assessment to determine if an accommodation of a private cubicle was still necessary.

Discussion

The independent medical examiner's assessment found limited evidence of a mental impairment and no indication that a "private cubicle," designed to shield Ms. Edwards from the presumed hostile and harassing behavior of her coworkers, was indicated. Rather, the assessment, which included a review of medical records, indicated that Ms. Edwards had a long history of aggressive and angry behavior, manifest in a wide variety of settings. On examination, she consistently demonstrated immature defenses of isolation of affect, displacement, and projection. Her behavior vacillated from childlike pleadings to discourteous and aggressive comments.

The private cubicle was not medically necessary as a job accommodation. It was deemed likely that Ms. Edwards' concern about the hostility of her coworkers was a perception heavily influenced by immature psychological defenses. The prior implementation of such an accommodation placed an excessive burden on her coworkers and supervisor to treat Ms. Edwards in a cautionary and dissimilar manner that was not medically warranted.

Assessing the Contribution of Stress to Impairment

Stress may herald the onset of anxiety, sleep disturbance, cognitive dysfunction, and affective instability. In most instances, those symptoms are transient, are of mild to moderate severity, and resolve with the restoration of homeostasis. This neural-mediated mechanism is operative in all living systems and plays a critical role in survival. Whereas stress may exacerbate (temporarily worsen) mental and behavioral symptoms, under most circumstances stress is unlikely to permanently worsen an impairment.

However, a permanent worsening of an underlying mental condition or the development of a stress-induced illness may occur if neurophysiologic mechanisms fail to restore homeostasis. The severity of the resultant impairment can be determined by an assessment of an individual's disturbance in function, consistent with the methodology described in Chapters 38 and 41 on the assessment of mental and behavioral disorders.[2]

In assessing impairment, ratings may be influenced by stress in the following ways:

1. When stress is determined to be a causative condition that precipitates an Axis I mental disorder, such as PTSD or Adjustment Disorder;
2. When stress is determined to have aggravated or accelerated a pre-existing mental disorder; for example, this might occur if an individual with panic disorder and agoraphobia is kidnapped and placed in a hostile situation. Such an intensely stressful experience may aggravate or accelerate a phobic disorder and result in a worsening of the preexistent impairment;
3. A stress-related condition may be induced when an individual is continuously or repeatedly exposed to extremely stressful states. The contribution of stress to a resultant impairment is most evident when the persistence of the stressful circumstance is determined by factors clearly outside the control of the affected individual; for example, as a prisoner or a hostage.

More commonly encountered cases involve workers subjected to continuous harassment, domestic partners coerced to remain in abusive relationships, or disabled workers restricted from any meaningful vocational restoration by a physical impairment. There is often a subjective predisposition that influences vulnerability. Consequently, the contribution of chronic stress must be distinguished from other comorbid states, including personality traits, coping style, and nonmedical issues. The use of stress differentiators—factors that help distinguish stress from other identified causes of mental or behavioral impairment—are helpful (a list of commonly encountered differentiators is included in the following section). A person's propensity to decompensate in response to specific identifiable stressful circumstances should be documented and considered in the assessment of impairment.

In commonly encountered examples, individuals may decompensate in response to job stress. However, implicating job stress as a casual factor may be made without unbiased assessment and reflect a subjective interpretation of either the worker or the worker's physician. Poorly documented and largely unsubstantiated allegations of job stress do not contribute medically reliable information about either the worker or the conditions of employment. Rather, the physician or evaluator should carefully assess a particular employment circumstance—for example, a demand-resource discrepancy, where the demands of a particular job exceed the resources of the worker. Other more difficult cases involve claims of harassment and discrimination. In assessing the contribution of stress generated from such circumstances, the examiner should be patient and detailed in his historytaking. The case method, wherein the details of a particular stress claim are systematically and chronologically examined, is time intensive, but necessary to arrive at meaningful conclusions about causation and impairment.

Example 4

■ John specialized in repairing computers. Following a reduction in force and a reorganization of the workplace, he was promoted to be in charge of the intelligence systems division. He was still required to fix computers, but now had to supervise six other people. He repeatedly advised his supervisor that he lacked the necessary skills to be head of the intelligence systems division. As time passed he was unable to keep up with the demands of his supervisory role and was missing time from work secondary to illness.

His physician wrote that John was experiencing a stress-related disorder manifest by chronic headaches, sleep disturbance, gastrointestinal hypermotility, and cognitive confusion. No specific medical diagnosis was made other than "stress at job, too much work, feels overwhelmed." Although his symptoms improved when he was on a sick status, they worsened when the doctor released him to return to work. The process was repeated several times, and his symptoms became chronic. After several recurrences, John was placed on a disability status. The stress emanating from the demand-resource discrepancy contributed to his impairment.

Stress Differentiators

To better understand the particular contribution of stress to medical impairment, the physician or examiner may consider certain stress differentiators or clinical findings based on case analysis. The presence of a differentiator may assist in identifying the cause of a particular symptom or finding, and help attribute it to a more specific causation.

Stress differentiators include the following:

1. An Axis I disorder
2. An Axis II disorder (personality disorder)

3. An Axis III disorder
4. An Axis IV disorder (psychosocial problem)
5. Coping style and personality traits
6. A history suggesting chronic dysfunction in school, the military, occupational settings, or other structured settings
7. Nonspecificity of the stressor—attribution of stress to the institution, supervisors, or the "attitude" of people/coworkers in general
8. Shifting or mutable stressors (the sense that if it is not one thing, it is another)
9. The absence of medical justification for the level of dysfunction
10. Malingering

Example 5

■ Megan, a 34-year-old woman, was terminated from her position as a stockbroker for repeatedly using poor judgment and acting rudely with clients and her supervisor. She filed a claim against the employer for sexual discrimination, citing a gender-hostile work environment. Following the termination, she claimed that her emotional distress prevented her from seeking other employment. She then sought coverage for psychiatric treatment for PTSD under the company's workers' compensation plan.

An examination and review of Megan's prior medical records revealed a 12-year history of intermittent psychiatric treatment for personality disorder, anxiety, and relational problems. The occupational history indicated that she had been previously terminated three times by investment firms for comparable reasons. Performance evaluations revealed that although she was "knowledgeable and industrious," she was "very defensive and argumentative with an explosive temper."

Discussion

The circumstances at her employment were not unusual or excessively demanding beyond the inherent requirements of the investment business. On examination, she did not meet criteria for PTSD. However, she did have evidence of Generalized Anxiety Disorder (mild severity) and Borderline Personality Disorder (moderate severity), as well as interpersonal problems that distracted her from her work (stress differentiators). Environmental or occupational stress did not significantly contribute to a worsening of her impairment.

Assigning a Severity Rating

A functional model should be employed to assess the contribution of stress to medical impairment. Criteria defined by the American Medical Association's Guides to the Evaluation of Permanent Impairment, fourth and fifth editions, require the assessment of four categories: activities of daily living; social functioning; concentration, persistence, and pace; and adaptation to stressful circumstances ("deterioration or decompensation in work or work-like settings").[2,40] In assessing the contribution of stress, the resultant change in function must be caused by the stress and be deemed to be permanent.

Example 6

■ A 28-year-old assistant manager of a bank was held at gunpoint during a robbery. The perpetrator was extremely nervous and threatening to shoot. The assistant manager was able to maintain her composure and assisted the perpetrator, believing that the quicker he got out of the bank, the less likely it would be that anyone would be injured. After she filled his sack, he raced to the door. Then, with no provocation, he turned and shot the security guard, who later died.

Subsequently, the assistant manager developed an acute stress disorder, which resolved within 30 days. Specifically, her flashbacks, avoidance, sleep disturbance, and heightened anxiety all improved. She was able to resume her usual socialization; run errands, including going to the bank for personal business; and maintain her concentration. However, when she returned to work, she developed the recurring thought that money was dirty. She felt compelled to wash her hands 20 or more times during the day. Consequently, her work performance declined.

Discussion

Her functional impairment was not due to persistent PTSD. Rather, the stress of the robbery aggravated a pre-existent obsessive compulsive personality trait and produced a hand-washing compulsion that affected the persistence and pace of her work performance. Stress had caused the aggravation and worsened a trait into a behavioral disorder. The stress impairment was mild, but required a medical accommodation; specifically, a change of occupational venue to a workplace where she did not handle cash.

Example 7

■ Joan was a high school graduate with 5 years of experience as an administrative assistant. She was hired as the executive assistant to the director of a large trade association. Although she had excellent recommendations and brought considerable energy and enthusiasm to the job, her resume did not meet the published job requirements. Additionally, Joan was the mother of two young children and her husband worked an evening shift, making it difficult for her to remain late at the office.

The executive director was extremely short tempered and frequently yelled at Joan, who was repeatedly intimidated by his behavior. Rather than seek clarification on certain work-related issues, she avoided the executive director whenever possible and tried to "figure out solutions" on her own. Because the resolution of many of the problems required considerable experience or technical knowledge, Joan's work was flawed with many errors. Subsequently, instead of addressing the deficiencies directly with Joan, the executive director criticized her performance to a secretary. On one occasion, Joan overheard the executive director refer to her as a "moron."

Although humiliated, she persisted in her job at the association. However, she felt isolated and unappreciated. Although she tried to complete her assignments, she found the work difficult and often beyond her expertise. She developed frequent stomach pains and headaches, requiring numerous physician visits, which further reduced the time she had to finish her assignments. She felt discouraged, lost confidence in her ability, and was easily upset by the smallest problem. She complained of feeling "stressed" to her primary care physician.

Joan met criteria for Adjustment Disorder. She was treated with psychotherapy and later improved. However, after resolution of the Adjustment Disorder, she had evidence of permanent impairment as demonstrated by functional loss. She complained that after her experience at the association, she "wasn't the same person." She no longer thought of herself as a smart person and was certain that people looked down on her because she had only a high school education. She reduced her social contacts and appeared less confident to her husband, who referred to his wife's experience at the association as the "worst experience of her life."

Discussion

Joan demonstrated a change in social function and a subtle loss of confidence, which were due to her exposure to the workplace conditions. Applying the stress differentiators did not suggest an alternative diagnosis or cause for the permanent behavioral changes. She was able to function at home and returned to work in an administrative position consistent with her education and experience. Although she did not decompensate in the workplace, she remained in a clerical position and complained that she lacked the confidence to seek a promotion.

The assessment of impairment demonstrates mild loss of function caused by prolonged exposure to particularly stressful workplace conditions, some of which were avoidable but some of which occurred outside of Joan's control.

References

1. Al'Abadie MS, Kent GG, Gawkrodger DI: The relationship between stress and the onset and exacerbation of psoriasis and other skin conditions. Br J Dermatol 130:199–203, 1994.
2. Cocchiarella L, Anderson GBJ (eds): Guides to the Evaluation of Permanent Impairment, 5th ed. Chicago, American Medical Association, 2001.
3. American Psychiatric Association: Diagnostic and Statistical Manual of Mental Disorders, 4th ed. Washington, DC, American Psychiatric Association, 1994.
4. Bernard C: Introduction to the study of experimental medicine. In Caplan AL, Engelhardt HT, McCartney JJ: Concepts of Health and Disease: Interdisciplinary Perspectives. Reading, Mass, Addison-Wesley, 1981.
5. Bonner AD, Coyne JC, Schaefer C, et al: Comparison of two modes of life stress measurement: Daily hassles and uplifts versus major life events. J Behav Med 4:1–39, 1981.
6. Burks N, Martin B: Everyday problems and life change events: Ongoing versus acute sources of stress. J Hum Stress 11:27–35, 1985.
7. Cannon WB: Relations of biological and social homeostasis. In Caplan AL, Engelhardt HT, McCartney JJ: Concepts of Health and Disease: Interdisciplinary Perspectives. Reading, Mass, Addison-Wesley, 1981.
8. Caspi A, Moffit TE, Newman DL, Silva PA: Behavioral observations at age three predict adult psychiatric disorders: Longitudinal evidence from a birth cohort. Arch Gen Psychiatry 53:1033–1039, 1996.
9. Cassell E: The Nature of Suffering. New York, Oxford University Press, 1991.
10. Chess S, Thomas A: Temperament in Clinical Practice. New York, Guilford, 1986.
11. Cohen S, Doyle WJ, Skones DP, et al: Social ties and susceptibility to the common cold. JAMA 277:1940–1944, 1997.
12. Cohen S, Tyrell DA, Smith AP: Psychological stress and susceptibility to the common cold. N Engl J Med 325:606–612, 1991.
13. Dohrenwend BP, Dohrenwend BS: Socioenvironmental factors, stress and psychopathology. Part I: Quasi-experimental evidence on social causation–social selection issue posed by class differences. Am J Community Psychol 9:129–146, 1981.
14. Dohrenwend BS, Dohrenwend BP: Some issues on research on life stress events. J Nerv Ment Dis 153:207–234, 1978.
15. Dorhenwend BS, Krasnoff L, Dohrenwend BP: Exemplification of a method for scaling life events. The PERI life events scale. J Health Soc Behav 19:205–229, 1978.
16. Engel G: The need for a new medical model: A challenge for biomedicine. In Caplan AL, Engelhardt HT, McCartney JJ (eds): Concepts of Health and Disease: Interdisciplinary Perspectives. Reading, Mass, Addison-Wesley, 1981.
17. Haan N: The assessment of coping, defense, and stress. In Goldberger L, Breznitz S (eds): Handbook of Stress: Theoretical and Clinical Aspects. New York, Free Press, 1993.
18. Holmes TH, Rahe RH: The Social Readjustment Rating Scale. J Psychosom Res 11:213–218, 1967.
19. Kardiner A, Spiegel H: The Traumatic Neurosis of War. New York, Hombre, 1947.
20. Kore D, Arnon I, Klein E: Acute stress response and posttraumatic stress disorder in traffic accident victims: A one year prospective follow-up study. Am J Psychiatry 156:367–373, 1999.
21. Kung AWC: Life events, daily stresses and coping in patients with Graves disease. Clin Endocrinol 42:303–308, 1995.
22. Lazarus RS, Averill JR, Opton EM: The psychology of coping: Issues of research and assessment. In Kohl G, Hamburg D, Adams J (eds): Coping and Adaptation. New York, Basic Books, 1974.
23. Lindemann E: Symptomatology and management of acute grief. Am J Psychiatry 101:141–148, 1944.
24. Marshall RD, Spitzer R, Liebowitz MR: Review and critique of the new DSM-IV diagnosis of acute stress disorder. Am J Psychiatry 156:1677–1685, 1999.
25. Mason J: Historical view of the stress field: Part I. J Hum Stress 1:6–12, 1975.
26. Mikhail A: Stress: A psychophysiological conception. In Monat A, Lazarus RS: Stress and Coping: An Anthology. New York, Columbia University Press, 1985.
27. Nesse RM: Is depression an adaptation? Arch Gen Psychiatry 57:14–20, 2000.

28. North CS, Smith EM, Spitznagel EL: Posttraumatic stress disorder in survivors of a mass shooting. Am J Psychiatry 151:82–88, 1994.
29. Paris J: A diathesis-stress model of personality disorders. Psychiatric Annals 9:692–697, 1999.
30. Parkes CM, Benjamin B, Fitzgerald RG: Broken heart: A statistical study of increased mortality among widowers. Br Med J 1:740–743, 1969.
31. Paykel ES, Prusoff BA, Uhbenhuth EH: Scaling of life events. Arch Gen Psychiatry 25:340–347, 1971.
32. Rabin BS: Stress, Immune Function and Health. New York, Wiley-Liss, 1999.
33. Reich J: An empirical examination of the concept of "stress-induced" personality disorders. Psychiatric Annals 29:701–706, 1999.
34. Selye H: History and present status of the stress concept. In Monat A, Lazarus RS: Stress and Coping: An Anthology. New York, Columbia University Press, 1985.
35. Skodol SE, Dohrenwend BP, Link BG, et al: The nature of stress: Problems of measurement. In Noshpitz JD, Coddington RD (eds): Stressors and the Adjustment Disorders. New York, John Wiley & Sons, 1994.
36. Southwick SM, Yehuda R, Wang S: Neuroendocrine alterations in posttraumatic stress disorder. Psychiatric Annals 28:436–442, 1998.
37. Steptoe A: Psychological Factors in Cardiovascular Disease. London, Academic Press, 1981.
38. Stip E, Truelle JG: Personality syndrome in multiple sclerosis and the effects of stressor recurrent attacks. Can J Psychiatry 39:27–33, 1994.
39. Wilkinson CB: Aftermath of a disaster: The collapse of the Hyatt Regency Hotel catwalks. Am J Psychiatry 140:1134–1139, 1983.
40. American Medical Association: Guides to the Evaluation of Permanent Impairment, 4th ed. Chicago, American Medical Association, 1994.

CHAPTER

41

Psychological Impairment

BYRON A. ELIASHOF, MD ■ JON STRELTZER, MD

The chapter on mental and behavioral disorders in the American Medical Association's Guides to the Evaluation of Permanent Impairment[2] (AMA Guides) indicates that the evaluation of mental and behavioral disorders consists of taking a history of mental or behavioral disorders, assessing current clinical status, and making a diagnosis. The psychiatric evaluation is then analyzed to determine the extent of impairment, utilizing impairment categories defined by the United States Social Security Administration.[19]

This chapter discusses this analysis. Psychiatric causes of impairment are delineated. Principles in making assessment ratings are described, and numerous examples are given. This chapter describes the assessment of mental impairment of varying severity levels, and will also discuss contributions to impairment by different psychiatric conditions that may coexist in a given individual. Frequently encountered special issues that make the assessment more complex are also discussed.

DETERMINING IMPAIRMENT ACCORDING TO THE AMA GUIDES

Criteria defined by the AMA Guides require the assessment of mental and behavioral impairment under four categories: activities of daily living; social functioning; concentration, persistence, and pace; and adaptation (also described as "deterioration or decompensation in work or work-like settings").[2]

Activities of daily living include such aspects of behavior as eating, sleeping, dressing, obtaining shelter, shopping, communicating, traveling, managing finances, and sexual and recreational functioning. A mental illness may cause impairment in these activities. For instance, a depressed individual may have anorexia, insomnia, and loss of libido. An individual with severe anxiety may be unable to leave home to travel, shop, or pursue recreational activities.

■ Case 1—impaired activities of daily living: A 46-year-old woman prided herself on her efficiency and neatness as a maid. After being sexually harassed at work, she developed a severe depressive illness. This caused her to lose her appetite, to have difficulty sleeping with frequent awakenings, and to be unable to enjoy sexual relations with her husband. She lost interest in housekeeping and her previously neat house was now untidy. ■

Social functioning includes behavior associated with interpersonal relationships and interaction with others. Specific areas one should consider when assessing impairment of social functioning include relationships with family members, friends, and associates. Also, one should consider the ability to interact with peers, coworkers, supervisors, and the general public. Such interactions should be assessed in the context of the individual's expected level of functioning and the specific circumstances of the situation. A mental illness may impair a manager of a company, for instance, such that he or she will be unlikely to be able to supervise or give instructions—abilities that might not be required of another worker.

■ Case 2—impaired social functioning: A 37-year-old jewelry sales representative developed an anxiety disorder after being in an airplane that made an emergency landing. He was physically unhurt, but subsequently this formerly genial man became irritable, snapped at people, and began losing accounts. His formerly happy relationship with his wife of 10 years also deteriorated, and they argued frequently. ■

Concentration, persistence, and pace refer to attention span, memory, and cognitive abilities in general. Issues for consideration in an impairment evaluation of this category include the ability to perform activities within a required schedule, to maintain proper focus on the required activities without unnecessary distractions, and to have an appropriate memory for such things as instructions, procedures, and locations. For instance, an assembly line worker with schizophrenia may be too distracted by hallucinations to work without making errors or creating safety hazards. A depressed individual may not be able to complete his or her work day without taking excessive rest periods owing to an overwhelming sense of fatigue.

■ Case 3—impaired concentration, persistence, and pace: A 32-year-old taxi driver was almost killed in a motor vehicle accident. Afterward, he developed a posttraumatic stress disorder that included severe anxiety when driving. He sometimes got lost trying to find streets in unfamiliar neighborhoods. He had to stop working because of his inability to pay attention to street directions and his inability to maintain concentration sufficiently to follow a map. ■

Adaptation refers to the ability to perform tasks, collaborating with others if necessary, when faced with the vicissitudes of workplace conditions, including the idiosyncrasies of coworkers. This might include the ability to make generalizations, evaluations, and independent decisions or judgments; the ability to negotiate with, instruct, be supervised by, or supervise others; the ability to respond appropriately to changes; and the ability to perform complex or varied tasks. For instance, a man with schizophrenia may function satisfactorily as a janitor if he has a fixed, daily routine with little direct contact with others, but he is vulnerable to psychotic decompensation if his routine is changed, or if he is criticized by a supervisor.

■ Case 4—impaired adaptation: A 46-year-old legal secretary worked for several bosses, each of whom would give her projects simultaneously. An irate client came to the office and threatened the staff with a knife. Although the secretary was unhurt, she developed an obsessive-compulsive anxiety disorder and could no longer tolerate frequent changes in assignments. She became overly meticulous and inefficient, and unable to adapt to previously manageable work stress. ■

Diagnosis and Psychiatric Symptoms

Psychiatric diagnoses are based on criteria that include clusters of symptoms and contain inclusionary and exclusionary elements.[3] A diagnosis is described on five axes, with specific mental disorders being listed on Axes I and II. Axis I consists mostly of clinical syndromes and Axis II consists mostly of personality disorders. Axis III designates general medical conditions relevant to the understanding or treatment of the mental disorder or disorders. This becomes particularly significant when there is a diagnostic issue between a mental disorder and a general medical condition, as is often the case in chronic pain. Axis IV consists of psychosocial and environmental problems that are not mental disorders themselves but may influence the understanding and management of the Axis I and II disorders. Axis V is a rating of psychosocial functioning. It correlates with mental impairment to a degree, but it is not the same, and it has limitations in validity (see also Chapter 38).[18]

Diagnosing psychopathology is not only important for assessing psychiatric impairment, but it can also influence the extent of disability caused by a physical impairment.[4,21] Psychological issues may also interfere with the accurate assessment of physiologic functioning, such as may occur in a functional capacity evaluation.[11]

Mental impairment is related to diagnosis, but not entirely, because disorders can range from mild to severe. Certain diagnoses tend to be associated with more severe impairment. For instance, schizophrenia and other psychotic disorders are more likely to be associated with problems in functioning at all levels. Adjustment disorders are more likely to be associated with minimal impairment, and when psychiatric disability is present, it tends to be transient.

Diagnoses are made up of constellations of signs and symptoms. These may be categorized into disturbances of consciousness, memory, emotion, thought, perception, speech, motor behavior, intelligence, insight, and judgment.[12] By definition, the symptoms must be of clinical significance in order to be considered part of a mental disorder. Nevertheless, they may occur within a great range of severity, and thus the degree of impairment within any particular diagnosis can vary substantially.

Following are two examples of patients with the same diagnosis, but in whom symptoms cause strikingly different functional sequelae.

■ Case 5: An adult man with chronic undifferentiated schizophrenia suffers from auditory hallucinations and has speech that tends to be illogical and difficult to understand. He has no friends, as he fears and avoids people. He lives in a halfway house where meals are provided. He is dependent on welfare for his subsistence. He spends his time alone, usually watching television and smoking cigarettes. Activities of daily living are markedly impaired in that he cannot independently provide for his own needs. He can dress himself but launders his clothes infrequently. He cannot travel alone beyond his immediate neighborhood without getting lost. He has severe limitations in his ability to socialize. The auditory hallucinations prevent him from concentrating on a task for any length of time. He requires constant structure and cannot adapt to changes in his routine. He is unable to work.

■ Case 6: In contrast to Case 5, another adult man with chronic undifferentiated schizophrenia has responded well to treatment. He has auditory hallucinations, but he recognizes that the voices are not real, and is able to ignore them much of the time. He has three friends. The relationships are superficial but provide companionship. He was a watch repairman prior to the onset of his illness, and he remains skillful at this, earning a good living. He is independent in all activities of daily living. Social functioning is impaired in that he has been unable to develop intimate relationships. He is able to concentrate satisfactorily when performing his skilled occupation. He has shown no difficulty adapting to busy times at the workplace. He takes medication daily and consults his psychiatrist monthly. ■

Levels of Severity of Impairment

As described in Chapter 38, the AMA Guides define five classes of mental impairment, ranging from none to mild (compatible with most useful function), moderate (compatible with some but not all useful functioning), marked (significantly impeding useful functioning), and extreme (precluding useful function).[2]

Cases 6 (previous) and 7, 12, and 13 (following) are examples of mild impairment. Functioning is generally satisfactory in all categories, although there are some areas of difficulty (see Table 41–1).

An example of moderate impairment would be an individual who performs somewhat marginally on the job owing to a chronic anxiety disorder with symptoms of excessive worry, apprehension, and panic attacks. He has difficulty adjusting to periodic increases in the volume of work, and uses excessive sick leave during those times. The fear of panic attacks causes him to decline most invitations to social events with family and friends. This would be considered an impairment compatible with some but not all useful function. Cases 9 and 11 following are further examples of moderate impairment.

An example of marked impairment might be an individual whose psychiatric illness interferes with rational thinking and whose delusions and hallucinations limit work ability to intermittent volunteer work sorting files, when not hospitalized. Case 5 (previous) and 10 (following) are examples of marked psychiatric impairment. The class of extreme impairment is limited to those cases in which there is essentially no ability to function independently. Cases 8 and 15 (following) represent extreme impairment.

For some disability evaluations, the examiner need only determine ability to work and limitations in that regard. For these purposes, the AMA Guides,[2] with its five impairment classes, is sufficient. Often, however, the examiner is asked to rate permanent impairment using percentages. The chapter on mental and behavioral disorders in the AMA Guides does not use specific percentages to estimate the extent of mental impairment, noting a lack of empirical evidence to justify such use. Frequently, third parties such as attorneys and administrative judges need to have percentages of impairment in order to make such decisions as monetary awards, eligibility for reimbursement by special funds, and other purposes. Although specific percentages represent, at best, an educated medical judgment, the clinician trained in the evaluation of impairment has the education and experience that are likely to make these estimates more valid and reliable than those of a layperson.

The only exception where the Guides fifth edition assigns percentages to individuals with emotional, mood or behavioral disturbances is in the chapter on the central and peripheral nervous system. Impairment ratings are given in 2 sections in this chapter, *only* when neurologic impairment is also present. In Tables 13–5 and 13–6 of the nervous system chapter, individuals with neurologic deficiencies such as organic brain syndrome, dementia and some specific, focal and neurologic deficiencies, along with psychological impairment,

TABLE 41–1

Classes of Impairment Due to Mental and Behavioral Disorders

Area or Aspect of Functioning	Class 1 No Impairment	Class 2 Mild Impairment	Class 3 Moderate Impairment	Class 4 Marked Impairment	Class 5 Extreme Impairment
Acitivities of daily living Social functioning Concentration Adaptation	No impairment noted	Impairment levels are compatible with most useful functioning	Impairment levels are compatible with some, but not all, useful functioning	Impairment levels significantly impede useful functioning	Impairment levels preclude useful functioning

From Cocchiarella L, Andersson GBJ (eds): Guides to the Evaluation of Permanent Impairment, 5th ed. Chicago, American Medical Association, 2001, p 363, with permission.

may be rated for their psychological impairment using the clinical dementia rating score (Tables 13–5 and 13–6).[1(p320)] Mild impairments are defined as the ability to satisfactorily perform most activities of daily living with only mild limitations of social and interpersonal functioning. This corresponds to 0% to 14% impairment. A mental impairment that may require an individual to have some direction and supervision of daily living activities or that causes moderate limitation of some but not all social and interpersonal interactions corresponds to 15% to 29% impairment. An impairment that requires one to have directed care under continued supervision and confinement in the home or another facility, or that causes severe limitations impeding useful action in almost all social and interpersonal daily functions, corresponds to 30% to 49% impairment. An impairment that renders an individual unable to care for self or unable to be safe without supervision, or that causes severe limitation of daily functions requiring total dependence on another person, corresponds to 50% to 70% impairment. Again, Table 13–6 is a useful paradigm for rating neurologic and psychiatric impairments and is illustrated in this chapter.

■ Case 7—low percent impairment: A 33-year-old man, employed as a groundskeeper, suffered a back injury at work. He developed substantial depressive symptoms that prevented him from returning to work, although his back had improved. Initial psychiatric evaluation determined that he was depressed and dependent on alcohol. These problems were treated, and 1 year later, he was maintaining sobriety and had no residual depressive symptoms. This man was rated as having no impairment in all categories except adaptation, in which he was considered to have very mild impairment. This was related to his need for ongoing antidepressant medication and his need for vigilance regarding relapse to alcoholism.

■ Case 8—high percent impairment: A 51-year-old woman performed satisfactorily as a semiskilled machine operator. She was considered "odd" because she often spoke of the supernatural and sometimes talked to herself. A careless coworker caused a malfunction that severely injured and almost killed her. She recovered physically, but feared for her life, and increasingly ruminated about the accident. Over the next year, her mental condition deteriorated, so that she was speaking in a bizarre and disorganized fashion, even with her family. She failed to improve over the next several years. Psychiatric impairment was determined to be marked to extreme in all categories. She needed help in almost all activities of daily living, although she could bathe and dress herself most of the time. She would eat only when food was given to her, but she had favorite foods. With regard to social functioning and concentration, she was unable to communicate coherently to others. She accompanied her daughter shopping, and could be directed to pay the cashier money, but she was unable to select items to buy. She could maintain attention at only the simplest tasks, such as chopping vegetables or pushing the cart in the store. With respect to adaptation, she had little ability to exercise independent judgment, even when attempting the daily chores necessary to maintain her home. Permanent psychiatric impairment was rated as marked class (Table 41–1).[1] ■

Assigning a percentage of impairment is an exercise in judgment based on the available data. These guidelines can be helpful in making an assessment of the degree of psychiatric impairment. It should be emphasized that records from employers, vocational counselors, and case managers, if available, often provide useful information regarding the individual's capabilities, attitudes, and motivation. The candor of the interviewee, the thoroughness of the diagnostic interview, the interpretation of psychological testing, and the availability of comprehensive past medical records for review will affect the assessment. The higher the quality of the information that is available, the greater the reliability and validity of impairment determinations.[15,16]

When performing an impairment rating, it is the individual's overall level of functioning that is to be considered. Thus an examine might be mildly impaired in one or more areas of functioning, but may still be moderately or markedly impaired overall. In order to gain perspective, it is often helpful to consider capacities that are intact, not just limitations. The following are more detailed examples of impairment ratings based on the AMA Guides.[1,2]

■ Case 9—moderate impairment: A 38-year-old motor patrol officer experienced minor bruises when she dove out of the way to avoid being intentionally run over by a drunken driver to whom she was attempting to give a citation. Afterward she was diagnosed with symptoms that met Diagnostic and Statistical Manual of Mental Disorders, fourth edition (DSM-IV) criteria for post-traumatic stress disorder.

After 3 years of treatment, her condition reached a plateau and was thought to be stable. When examined, she reported frequent episodes of tearfulness, diminished energy, distractibility, and occasional intrusive thoughts of the accident. She had less interest in her former recreational activities and no longer participated in many of them. She was irritable and became impatient with coworkers. She was easily angered in stores if she had to wait, and sometimes lashed out verbally if someone annoyed her. Although she formerly filled out paperwork in the police department after a day on the road, she now became distracted if others were speaking within earshot. She no longer trusted her judgment in an emergency. She was working part-time at a desk job that did not involve dealing with the public or require frequent interaction with coworkers. She was using excessive sick leave. She was irritable with her family, but generally continued to get along satisfactorily with them. She had little interest in being physically intimate with her husband.

Permanent partial impairment levels were rated as follows:

Activities of daily living: Class 2—mild impairment.

There was mild insomnia, reduced libido, and difficulty shopping for personal needs.

The examinee was able to do her housework and her laundry and care for herself. She could cook, shop, communicate, travel, use the telephone, manage her finances, and manage medication.

Social functioning: Class 3—moderate impairment.

There was friction in the relationship with her husband, family, friends, and coworkers owing to irritability. She refused to entertain. She no longer participated in social functions and attended family functions only at the extreme urging of her husband. She sometimes lost her temper when dealing with clerks and salespeople if she felt that they were inefficient or "stupid."

She was able, however, to relate adequately to coworkers and persons in authority. Her behavior at work was satisfactory, as were her work activities, as long as they involved minimal interactions with others.

Concentration: Class 2—mild impairment.

She was more easily distracted and had more difficulty completing tasks than before the development of her depressive disorder.

She was able to perform most activities within a schedule, maintain regular attendance, be punctual, and complete her limited work assignments. She could perform, for the most part, at a consistent pace.

Adaptation: Class 3—moderate impairment.

She had lost confidence in her ability to make decisions in novel situations and to respond appropriately. She had reduced tolerance for frustration. She could not satisfactorily perform tasks that required collaboration with others.

She was able, on the other hand, to make independent decisions and judgments in a restricted range of activities, accept realistic goals, and carry out limited responsibilities. She could adjust to changing directives to a degree.

Overall level of impairment: Class 3—moderate.

■ Case 10: Marked impairment: A 58-year-old gastroenterologist had a recurrence of diverticulitis. When the symptoms only partially responded to treatment, he began to worry about having cancer. He had difficulty sleeping, waking by 3 AM and lying in bed obsessively ruminating about his health. He had little appetite and had lost 22 pounds. He suffered intense fatigue. He would lie down throughout the day, attempting to rest, but would become too anxious, get up, and pace around the house, chain-smoking. He would attempt to read, but could not keep track of more than a sentence or two. He felt hopeless, was depressed, and had a furrowed brow. He developed a belief that other physicians had conspired to steal his patients. He was preoccupied with his abdominal symptoms. He then became preoccupied with episodes of tachycardia. He became irritable, socially withdrawn, and was concerned about having a grave and a marker for him and his family. He denied suicidal ideation. Although he agreed to take medication, he would take one or two doses, experience tachycardia, attribute it to the medication, and discontinue use. After two hospitalizations and extensive treatment with psychotherapy and various antidepressants, his condition showed minimal improvement. He refused electroconclusive therapy.

A physician who examined him 2 years later on behalf of his disability insurance carrier found him unable to practice medicine for the foreseeable future. The DSM-IV diagnosis was major depression, single episode, severe, with psychotic features.

Permanent partial impairment levels were rated as follows:

Activities of daily living: Class 4—marked impairment.

The examinee did not eat unless urged by someone. He had insomnia, had lack of libido, and no longer participated in recreational activities such as golf and watching movies. He could not shop, manage his finances, or read the newspaper.

He bathed occasionally, and dressed reasonably appropriately. He could communicate basic needs adequately.

Social functioning: Class 4—marked impairment.

He was unable to deal with clerks and the general public. He no longer sought out interpersonal contacts. He was unable to cooperate with others in simple tasks for more than about 15 minutes.

He had some limited ability to relate to family members and close friends, expressing interest in their activities.

Concentration: Class 3—moderate impairment.

The examinee had a severely reduced attention span, frequently being distracted by fears of cancer. He could not persist at a task for more than 10 or 15 minutes. With encouragement, he could perform serial subtraction of sevens and digit span testing satisfactorily. He could help prepare meals and clean up afterward, and do minor household and garden chores on his "good days."

Adaptation: Class 4—marked impairment.

He was unable to deal with even minor frustrations. He quickly became annoyed and angry. His speech sometimes became irrational when family members disagreed with his delusional beliefs.

He could converse reasonably on neutral topics not associated with health. He had some tolerance for delay such as waiting for meals or for a ride to take him on an outing. Decision-making activities were reduced to basic functions such as choosing what to wear and selecting programs to watch on television.

Overall level of impairment: Class 4—marked. ■

Temporary versus Permanent Impairment

Permanent impairment may be different from impairment that exists at any particular point in time. Ratings of permanent impairment need to filter out any portion of impairment that is current or temporary, including that which may be temporary because it has not yet been effectively treated. At times this may be difficult, because some mental disorders may improve very slowly over a long period of time. The examiner may be asked if the mental condition is now stable and stationary, or has reached maximum medical improvement.

The mental disorder may be considered stable when it is relatively unchanging. Stability may be present even when symptoms fluctuate, if periodic fluctuations are a part of the underlying condition, such as in bipolar disorder or borderline personality disorder. Symptoms may also vary from time to time in response to environmental events, but the basic mental illness, its severity, and its effect on functioning remain essentially the same. Maximum medical improvement can be considered to have been achieved when appropriate treatment has been rendered and there is relatively little likelihood of further improvement in the foreseeable future.

Frequently, permanent impairment is less severe than impairment present at the time of an examination. This is typical for psychiatric disorders. For example, a depressed individual may experience worsened symptoms due to a situational problem. However, time and/or further treatment may allow him or her to return to baseline.

There are situations in which an individual has a mental disorder causing impairment that is reduced by taking medication. An examinee with schizophrenia, for instance, may have symptoms sufficiently controlled so that he or she is able to work when taking antipsychotic medication. There may be residual symptoms, however, such as reduced socialization. The impairment assessment is based on the actual level of functioning when the patient is taking medication and should also take into account the effects of residual limitations. Medication side effects may be a concern if they affect an individual's level of functioning. New psychotropic medications are being introduced rapidly, however, and side effects can often be eliminated or minimized with careful psychopharmacologic management.

■ Case 11: A 34-year-old waitress was mugged in a hotel parking lot. She continued working, but was less efficient than previously because of a persistent insomnia that left her fatigued most days. Two months later she was criticized for slow work. She became depressed, ruminated constantly about the robbery, lost interest in her children, and developed guilt about her inability to work as efficiently as previously. She was diagnosed as having a major depressive disorder, severe, of a melancholic subtype. When evaluated, she was found to have stopped doing many household chores and was often irritable and socially withdrawn. A psychiatric impairment rating based on her level of functioning at that time would have placed her at a moderate level of impairment. She had, however, been minimally treated. Ordinarily, a melancholic depression has a good likelihood of response to treatment. Therefore, future treatment was recommended before permanent psychiatric impairment could be determined. ■

Occasionally, permanent psychiatric impairment is greater than appears to be the case at the time of examination. For example, an individual with bipolar disorder may be evaluated during a period in between episodes, while functioning perfectly normally. The bipolar condition, however, may be incompletely controlled with medication, subjecting him or her to periodic episodes of mania or depression. During those periods, the individual may demonstrate some impairment in social functioning and in adaptation to ordinary demands in the workplace. Because of these periodic episodes, and perhaps because of the need to plan for or adapt to them, such an individual might be evaluated as having a mild psychiatric impairment overall due to bipolar disorder, even though he or she is completely normal on the day of the psychiatric evaluation.

Etiology and Apportionment

Depending on the nature of the examination, the examiner may be asked not only to determine the presence of overall impairment, but also to assess the timing of the onset of impairment, the etiologic factors, and an apportionment of the percent of impairment due to the various causes under consideration. For instance, a claimant with pre-existing post-traumatic stress disorder may have subsequently developed additional anxieties due to a severe motor vehicle accident. There may be a need to divide the percent of permanent impairment into that which was pre-existing and that which was due to the accident.

■ Case 12: A 50-year-old factory worker slipped and fell 6 feet while trying to fix a problem with her machine. She complained of dizziness and pain in her left knee. Physical examination revealed a very frightened woman with multiple contusions, but no serious injury was found. She continued to work for the next 2 months, but increasingly complained of multiple aches and pains. Finally she stopped working because of these pains. At her impairment evaluation 3 years later, she complained of aching pain in her head, shoulders, ribs, and hips—in fact, she stated that her whole body hurt all day, every day. She also felt weak, making it difficult for her to walk or lift her right hand. She complained that her symptoms were exactly the same as immediately following her original injury. Because no objective physical findings had explained her symptoms, and because of nonphysiologic sensory changes and inconsistencies in strength and range of motion testing, she had been referred for psychiatric treatment 6 months after her injury.

She was found to have symptoms of depression at that time, which were successfully treated with medication and marital therapy. Her physical symptoms remained unchanged, however. Her daily activities consisted of spending time with her immediate and extended family. Her husband and children did most of the household chores, including shopping and cooking. Her psychiatrist was concerned that she was preoccupied with her insurance entitlements such that she would not improve until there was a settlement of her workers' compensation claim. This examinee was diagnosed to have a pain disorder associated with psychological factors.

Her permanent psychiatric impairment rating was as follows:

Activities of daily living: Class 2—mild impairment (sexual dysfunction, dependence on others).

Social functioning: Class 1–no impairment.

Concentration, persistence, and pace: Class 2—mild impairment (preoccupation with her pain).

Adaptation: Class 3—moderate impairment (focused on pain in response to demands for performance).

Overall level of impairment: Class 2—mild.

Apportionment: 4% permanent psychiatric impairment is apportioned to the specific injury, owing to residuals of depression as well as fear and anxiety about reinjuring herself. Eight percent is related to pre-existing tendencies to somatize in response to conflict and anxiety (consistent with the past history and documentation in medical records). ■

SPECIAL ISSUES

Stress

Psychiatric disability and impairment do not automatically occur in the presence of stress. Psychiatric impairment is related to a mental disorder. At times, a mental disorder may be precipitated by a stressful event or an ongoing stressful situation. In the workers' compensation setting, stress claims occur when a psychosocial cause leads to a claim for mental disorder. Stress claims have often been found to be precipitated by interpersonal conflicts on the job or to be associated with personality disorders in the claimants.[8] Cases 1 through 4, 9, and 18 through 20 are examples of mental conditions arising from psychosocial precipitants. Issues associated with the concept of stress are elaborated in Chapter 40.

Personality Disorders

Personality disorders are mental disorders that are enduring patterns of experience and behavior that are typically present throughout adult life.[10] The diagnosis is difficult when the patient is seen for a single evaluation, although reviewing medical records, personnel records, psychological tests, and perhaps collateral interviews may allow greater confidence in making such a diagnosis. Personality disorders typically cause mild, and occasionally moderate, psychiatric impairment. This is usually in the area of social functioning or adaptation. Personality disorders tend to cause difficulties with interpersonal relationships, and associated rigidities of character may interfere with adaptation. The impairments are often somewhat subtle, and adequate and even excellent functioning at work is often possible.

■ Case 13: A 55-year-old divorced man had been employed as a resident manager for a large apartment complex. He claimed disability from a back injury sustained while standing on a ladder changing a light bulb. He believed that a joint in his back was "loose." He reported that if he consciously tightened his muscles, making them rigid or tense, his condition was "controlled." It became "particularly bad," however, when he slept, because then he was "too relaxed." He drove a motorcycle, and he went ballroom dancing, sometimes competitively, four to five times per week, stating that these activities forced him to keep his muscles tight, thus minimizing dysfunction from his "loose joint." Although he was barely able to support himself financially and he had only one close relationship, he presented himself as a man of many talents.

He usually wore a suit and carried a briefcase. He claimed to have been a wealthy businessman in the past, frequently traveling overseas, but said that he was cheated out of his businesses by a jealous ex-wife. He also claimed to have been a professional musician and a professional artist in his younger days, although he could not provide meaningful details about the types of music and art with which he was involved. He earned money as a volunteer research subject in psychiatric drug studies. He was proud of his ability to ascertain what was needed for acceptance in a study, and to provide responses accordingly. The examinee's condition was chronic and characterologic, without acute symptoms. He fulfilled criteria for the diagnosis of narcissistic personality disorder. A permanent psychiatric impairment rating was as follows:

Activities of daily living: Class 1—no impairment.

Social functioning: Class 2—mild impairment (regularly boasting and exaggerating his achievements causing an inability to sustain more than superficial relationships).

Concentration, persistence, and pace: Class 1—no impairment.

Adaptation: Class 3—moderate impairment (major inability to empathize with others' needs or to recognize his own limitations).

Overall level of impairment: mild. ■

Substance Abuse

Substance abuse or dependence is commonly encountered in impairment evaluations. This complicates the evaluation because an individual may function very differently during periods of sobriety compared to periods of active use of alcohol or other drugs.

■ Case 14: A 50-year-old appliance repairman had been unable to return to work following an uncomplicated hernia repair operation. He complained of ongoing pain in his groin, but his greater problem was difficulty concentrating so that he had lost confidence in his ability to do the skilled tasks required at work. Psychiatric evaluation revealed a history of gradually increasing difficulties with alcohol dependence, binges and blackouts, and two arrests for driving under the influence. In recent years, he developed a pattern of drinking throughout the day, including on the job, and using excessive sick leave. When he was hospitalized for his surgical operation, he went through a period of alcohol withdrawal, becoming tremulous and diaphoretic and having vivid illusions. He did not report this to his doctor or nurses, but constantly asked for more pain medication. Subsequent to his hospitalization, he stopped drinking, but continued to take large amounts of a narcotic pain medication. His primary diagnosis was now opiate dependence, with a history of chronic alcohol dependence. He was judged currently unable to work because of cognitive impairment secondary to his high level of narcotic intake. With treatment of his substance dependence, however, it was thought that he would have no to minimal permanent impairment. In fact, if sober, he should be able to function better at work and at home than he had previously.

■ Case 15: A 55-year-old man with severe alcoholism lost his job 3 years prior to being evaluated for Social Security benefits. His family had given up on him and he was now homeless. Psychiatric evaluation revealed an unkempt, emaciated man with significant memory deficits and a lack of insight into his condition. Activities of daily living were substantially impaired as he could not provide for basic needs, including food, clothing, and shelter. Social functioning was similarly impaired. He had lost all his friends and alienated his family. Tests of memory and concentration revealed substantial impairment. He had lost the ability to function even in the highly structured setting of a sheltered workshop. Permanent psychiatric impairment was rated as extreme. ■

In Case 15, the patient's chronic alcoholism had resulted in a moderately severe dementia that interfered with all aspects of functioning. This contrasts with Case 14, in which the substance dependence was treatable and reversible.

Pain and Somatization

Somatic complaints are common in the general population, even when organic findings are absent.[13] Such complaints are often of particular concern in the context of an impairment evaluation.

■ Case 16: A 32-year-old construction worker slipped and fell on the job. He sprained his ankle and was off work for 3 weeks. His ankle recovered but he then complained of back and neck pain, which kept him off work for the next 9 months, despite repeated medical evaluations that revealed only minor degenerative changes in the spine. A psychiatric evaluation revealed that the man was unhappy with his job and that he needed to stay home to help his sickly parents. He was diagnosed as having a pain disorder that was primarily associated with psychological factors. There was no impairment in his activities of daily living, and he helped his parents with their daily needs. There was no impairment in social functioning; his relationship continued in their usual fashion. There was no deficit in his ability to concentrate and attend to whatever activities he desired. If psychiatric impairment were present it would be in the area of adaptation, a difficult area to evaluate in this case. Because of his pain complaints, he did not work at his job, which required heavy lifting. Medical evaluation indicated that, on a physiologic basis, he should be able to lift the objects required at his job. The fact that he was not working was solely due to psychological issues. ■

Does this case represent psychiatric impairment? From a psychological perspective, the claimant had the mental capability to do his job. In fact, it would probably be psychologically healthy for him to resume working. The availability of disability payments and compensation has been shown to correlate with prolonged disability and time away from work.[5,9] Thus rating the examinee as having a significant psychological impairment with regard to work would tend to reinforce and even create disability. This examinee was rated as having a mild impairment in the area of adaptation. This reflected the individual's difficulties in adapting to his discontent at work, and the development of somatic symptoms in response to his psychological conflicts about work and responsibilities at home. The permanent impairment rating was mild. None of this was attributed to work related factors. Instead, it was attributed to pre-existing personality issues that led to a somatic response to psychological conflict in association with unhappiness at work. In essence, his dissatisfaction with work is not considered a psychological impairment. His proclivity to somatize is a psychological impairment, but not one that was created by work-related conditions.

Among the somatizing disorders, pain disorders associated with psychological factors are probably the most common encountered with impairment evaluations. Chronic pain remains an enigma despite volumes having been written about it. Traditionally, pain has been thought to be a condition whereby neither a purely biological nor a purely psychological explanation suffices; it is a classic biopsychosocial condition. In impairment evaluations, however, pain disorders in which psychosocial factors clearly predominate are frequent,[20] as in the following case. (See Chapters 39 and 42 for additional discussion about pain and somatoform disorders.)

■ Case 17: A 47-year-old architect reported intractable pain in his neck after he was struck by a falling piece of lumber. Repeated physical examinations had demonstrated no objective abnormalities, and range of motion appeared normal when he was distracted but limited when he was directly examined. During the evaluation he stated that he could not sit or stand for more than half an hour at a time, which was not long enough to work at his drafting table. He, nonetheless, sat quietly through several hours of interviewing, was not observed to move about or shift in his chair, and there was no tension in his face. He smiled frequently, except when describing how the poor economy had devastated his previously successful practice. His voice became angry and he gesticulated broadly as he described problems with the opposing attorney during a deposition. ■

Motivation

Psychosocial problems may be present in the absence of a mental diagnosis or psychologically disabling symptoms. These may influence motivation to function according to one's abilities, especially at work. An individual may be angry with coworkers or supervisors. He or she may believe that he or she is being treated unfairly or even discriminated against, and may demand that a coworker be transferred or fired as a condition of returning to work. Such feelings and desires may or may not be justified. By themselves, however, such perceptions and feelings do not represent mental illness or mental impairment.

If no mental disorder is present, the evaluator may consider that the problem is the examinee's motivation to work under specific conditions. The examinee may be as capable of doing the job as before the confrontation. The worker chooses, however, not to continue working in association with a coworker or supervisor with whom there is conflict. In such a situation, it is generally the area of adaptation in which the impairment may be present. The question becomes, however, whether the difficulties in this area are due to a mental disorder or to personal preferences and desires. To examine this issue in another light, one might consider the category of social functioning. If one chooses not to associate with another individual, or a group of individuals, this does not necessarily reflect the presence of a mental disorder.

■ Case 18: A 60-year-old woman had been working in middle management for more than 20 years. She considered herself quite knowledgeable, and resisted her new boss's proposed changes. When she was given a less than satisfactory annual evaluation, she became enraged, complaining of unfair treatment and harassment, and refused to continue working under that boss. She continued to function well in all other areas, and sought transfer to another department, confident that she could do the work. She had conflict only with her supervisor, and was very angry in response to the conflict. An impairment evaluator found no mental disorder. ■

Likewise, a worker may report a symptom such as fatigue that prevents him or her from working. The problem, however, may be a monotonous or unpleasant job rather than a psychiatric illness.

■ Case 19: A 46-year-old single woman stated that she did not receive a promotion at work owing to sexual discrimination. She reported that she was so depressed that she lacked the energy and desire to do basic housework, much less return to her job as a department store cashier. Sometime later in the interview, when asked about her hobbies, she stated that she breeds Labrador retrievers, has eight of them, and that one is expecting a litter. When asked who feeds, cleans, and generally cares for the dogs, she responded, "I do." Such information raises a question as to whether the individual is too depressed to keep house and to work, or whether the issue is lack of desire to perform unpleasant tasks. ■

Desire for Compensation

Claimants seeking disability compensation frequently view the psychiatric impairment examination as a means to achieve their goal. This can influence the manner in which the claimant presents his or her story and it will consequently influence the manner in which the examination is performed and how the findings interpreted. Recent evidence confirms that in settings in which compensation is awarded, symptom presentations can be altered.[6,7,20] The compensation system may also influence whether an individual continues working or how rapidly he or she returns to work. In some settings this seems to be minor[17]; in others, the effects are striking.[5,9]

■ Case 20: A 54-year-old teacher felt that fellow teachers were ostracizing her and that the principal did not give her adequate support. She stayed home from work after being given an extra assignment by the principal. Two months later she had not returned to work. She then reported symptoms of severe depression and was receiving psychiatric treatment. She complained of insomnia because she could not stop thinking about the perceived mistreatment at work. She insisted that she deserved workers' compensation benefits because she had devoted the past 22 years of her life to her job, and complained that she had been underpaid and unappreciated for her dedication. When asked about her activities, she stated that she went dancing with friends and to karaoke bars several nights a week. At home she was busy painting her kitchen and sewing new curtains. Her activities were thought to be inconsistent with severe depression. A Minnesota Multiphasic Personality Inventory (MMPI) report noted exaggeration of symptoms, including a marked elevation of the F scale. After 1 1/2 years off work, with little change in her symptoms, she was evaluated for permanent impairment. She was judged to have no permanent psychiatric impairment because of many examples of intact functioning in each of the four impairment categories. ■

Symptom Magnification

Symptom magnification is a term (not a diagnosis) frequently used by medical evaluators when referring to a psychological phenomenon in which the examinee has reported symptoms greater than are consistent with the objective findings. It occurs in both psychiatric and nonpsychiatric medical conditions. There is often disagreement between examiners as to whether symptom magnification is present and concerning its significance. Symptom magnification can occur on a conscious or unconscious basis, and there may be a continuum from one to the other. It may represent a tendency to dramatize (reflecting a personality style), a cry for help (possibly reflecting intense suffering or the presence of a specific mental disorder), a tendency to somatize (such as in the presence of a somatoform disorder), or a desire for compensation or other secondary gain (which may or may not involve overt malingering).

Whether the component of symptom magnification is to be considered part of the permanent impairment will vary with the specific situation. In an individual with histrionic traits, the tendency to magnify symptoms stems from the pre-existing personality and may be permanent. If the symptom magnification stems from a desire for secondary gain, such as to avoid an unpleasant work situation, to be vindicated, or to obtain a financial reward, the magnified component may be expected to diminish or disappear after the litigation is over.

Symptom magnification, however, is usually not an element of permanent psychiatric impairment. In particular, a specific physical trauma or injury is sometimes followed by magnification of physical symptoms. Such symptom magnification is not likely to have been caused by the physical injury. Rather the cause is likely to be psychological.

The problem for the examiner is to determine to what degree the symptoms and altered function reported by the examinee are genuinely experienced, and to what degree the symptoms are generated in response to factors such as personal style or desire for benefits. There is no simple guideline, but, in general, the symptoms need to be evaluated in the context of the entire history and mental status examination. Psychological tests, although not a litmus standard, can often provide helpful information.

Malingering

Malingering is intentional, implying conscious production of false, distorted, or grossly exaggerated symptoms.[14] Although gross malingering is probably rare among disability claimants, the examining clinician frequently encounters distortions of pathology along a spectrum that extends from the unconscious to the partially conscious to the wholly conscious, and progresses from mild exaggeration of existing symptoms or dysfunctions to the total fabrication of symptoms and disability.

In addition to the magnification and fabrication of symptoms, another form of malingering is false attribution of an injury from an area that is not compensable to one that is. An example would be that of a chef who injures his back on his day off while moving furniture; however, he claims that he injured his back at work while carrying a heavy pot of soup and proceeds to file a workers' compensation claim. Sometimes the injury itself is intentionally staged, such as being struck by an automobile.

To conclude that malingering is present, one must carefully weigh all the data from all available sources, the examination, medical records, psychological testing, the history, and often statements by third parties. Because malingered complaints are most likely to involve subjective symptoms, such as depression, anxiety, pain, weakness, and poor concentration, they may be difficult or impossible to verify by an interview alone. Independent, third party verification (e.g., surveillance) may be the only means of providing this information. Such a recommendation to the referring source should be made extremely cautiously. In any event, this decision is one that belongs to the referring source, not to the examining/evaluating physician.

■ Case 21: A 37-year-old construction worker stated that because of his back injury he felt vulnerable to being attacked and had become afraid of leaving his home. A surveillance film showed him at a high-rider's meeting demonstrating his customized pickup truck and signing autographs as president of the club. He was deemed to have no psychiatric impairment due to anxiety associated with the back injury. ■

■ Case 22: The owner of a small company filed suit when a major customer canceled its contract. Among her claims were anxiety and depression due to resulting financial loss. Her alleged symptoms were incapacitating severe depression and anxiety that caused her to be unable to work. She denied any previous history of psychiatric illness or previous lawsuits. A comprehensive review of medical records showed that she had filed a suit for symptoms of post-traumatic stress disorder several years earlier when she was in a hotel that had a small fire that had caused no physical injury to her. The impairment examiner concluded that there was no permanent psychiatric impairment associated with the financial loss, but there was impairment associated with a long-standing personality disorder. ■

■ Case 23: A 31-year-old welder filed a claim for a shoulder injury while at work. After extensive physical therapy, he was deemed to have permanent impairment, and received an $18,000 settlement. Years later, he revealed that he never had any significant shoulder problem, but had feigned weakness and limitations of motion in order to receive compensation. The feigned symptoms were mild at first, but he became angry with the insurance company, which had initially denied benefits, and then he escalated the degree of supposed dysfunction, demanding more treatment. In his outrage, he actually came to believe that his shoulder was indeed injured. Only after he received his settlement did the awareness return that, in reality, there was nothing wrong with his shoulder. ■

SUMMARY AND CONCLUSIONS

Psychiatric impairment evaluations depend on an accurate assessment of the individual's psychiatric condition, including past history, symptoms, diagnoses, current activities and level of functioning, and motivation. Particular attention must be given to certain issues such as stress, personality disorders, substance abuse, pain and somatization, symptom magnification, and malingering, all of which add complexity to the evaluation. Furthermore, psychological issues may influence impairment attributed to nonpsychiatric medical conditions.

Although psychiatric impairment cannot be counted or measured, the AMA Guides provide principles on which to make impairment ratings. The emphasis is not on diagnosis, but rather on the effect of mental illness on functioning in four critical areas: activities of daily living; social functioning; concentration, persistence, and pace; and adaptation. The examiner needs to distinguish permanent from temporary impairment, and sometimes needs to apportion impairment among various causes. The level of severity is estimated sometimes with the use of specific percentages. It is likely that impairment determinations will be more specific and objective as knowledge is gained from scientific research. It is also likely that it will be difficult, if not impossible, to achieve complete objectivity, owing to philosophical and societal considerations that inevitably underlie judgments about mental impairment.

References

1. Cocchiarella L, Andersson GBJ (eds): Guides to the Evaluation of Permanent Impairment, 5th ed, chapter 13. Chicago, American Medical Association, 2001, pp 305–356.
2. Cocchiarella L, Andersson GBJ (eds): Guides to the Evaluation of Permanent Impairment, 5th ed, chapter 14. Chicago, American Medical Association, 2001, pp 357–372.
3. American Psychiatric Association: Diagnostic and Statistical Manual of Mental Disorders, 4th ed. Washington, DC, American Psychiatric Association, 1994.
4. Armenian HK, Pratt LA, Gallo J, Eaton WW: Psychopathology as a predictor of disability: A population-based follow-up study in Baltimore, Maryland. Am J Epidemol, 148:269–75, 1998.
5. Awerbuch MS: Whiplash in Australia: Illness or injury? Med J Aust 157:193–196, 1992.
6. Binder LM, Rohling ML: Money matters: A meta-analytic review of the effects of financial incentives on recovery after closed-head injury. Am J Psychiatry 153:7–10, 1996.
7. Ciccone DS, Just N, Bandilla EB: A comparison of economic and social reward in patients with chronic nonmaligant back pain. Psychosom Med 61:552–563, 1999.
8. Eliashof BA, Streltzer J: The role of "stress" in workers' compensation stress claims. J Occup Med 34:297–303, 1992.
9. Greenough CG: Recovery from low back pain. Acta Orthop Scand 64(Suppl. 254):1–34, 1993.
10. Gunderson JG, Phillips KA: Personality disorders. In Kaplan HI, Sadock BJ (eds): Comprehensive Textbook of Psychiatry/VI. Baltimore, Williams & Wilkins, 1995, pp 1425–1461.

11. Kaplan GM, Wurtele SK, Gillis D: Maximal effort during functional capacity evaluations: An examination of psychological factors. Arch Phys Med Rehabil 77:161–164, 1996.
12. Kaplan HI, Sadock BJ: Typical signs and symptoms of psychiatric illness. In Kaplan HI, Sadock BJ (eds): Comprehensive Textbook of Psychiatry/VI. Baltimore, Williams & Wilkins, 1995, pp 535–543.
13. Kroenke K, Spitzer RL, Williams JB, et al: Physical symptoms in primary care: Predictors of psychiatric disorders and impairment. Arch Fam Med 3:774–779, 1994.
14. Mills MJ, Lipian MS: Malingering. In Kaplan HI Sadock BJ (eds): Comprehensive Textbook of Psychiatry/VI. Baltimore, Williams & Wilkins, 1995, pp 1614–1622.
15. Okpaku SO, Sibulkin AE, Schenzler C: Disability determinations for adults with mental disorders: Social Security Administration vs independent judgments. Am J Public Health 84:1791–1795, 1994.
16. Pincus HA, Kennedy C, Simmens SJ, et al: Determining disability due to mental impairment: APA's evaluation of Social Security Administration guidelines. Am J Psychiatry 148:1037–1043, 1991.
17. Rosenheck R, Frisman L, Sindelar J: Disability compensation and work among veterans with psychiatric and nonpsychiatric impairments. Psychiatr Serv 46:359–365, 1995.
18. Roy-Byrne P, Dagadakis C, Unutzer J, Ries R: Evidence for limited validity of the revised global assessment of functioning scale. Psychiatr Serv 47:864–866, 1996.
19. Social Security Administration: Disability Evaluation Under Social Security. (Publication No. 64–039). Baltimore, Md, Social Security Administration, 1986.
20. Streltzer J, Eliashof BA, Kline AE, Goebert D: Chronic pain disorder following physical injury. Psychosomatics 44:227–234, 2000.
21. Von Korff M, Ormel J, Katon W, Lin EH: Disability and depression among high utilizers of health care. A longitudinal analysis. Arch Gen Psychiatry 49:91–100, 1992.

CHAPTER

42

Functional Somatic Syndromes

DANIEL J. CLAUW, MD

Virtually nothing regarding functional somatic syndromes (FSS) is agreed upon in the medical community. There is disagreement about the appropriate semantic terms that should be used to describe these conditions, whether these conditions have a primarily physiologic or psychological origin, and in particular, whether these are truly disabling conditions. In this review, fibromyalgia and chronic fatigue syndrome (CFS) are chosen as the prototypical FSS, and these particular conditions are discussed. However, the many other systemic and regional syndromes that fall within this spectrum are touched upon as well, and a contemporary view of the mechanisms regarding these illnesses, as well as an approach to both management and rehabilitation, is offered.

Although the terms currently used to describe chronic pain and fatigue syndromes are relatively new, these conditions are not. For centuries in the medical literature, there have been descriptions of symptom complexes nearly identical to those now labeled as fibromyalgia and CFS.[93] Many terms previously used to describe these conditions, such as myofibrositis, fibrositis, chronic Epstein-Barr Virus (EBV) syndrome, or chronic candidiasis, were attempts to link the symptom complex to an underlying pathophysiologic process. The more generic terms that are now used to describe these illnesses reflect the recognition that we know what does not cause these illnesses, but not what does. Thus we are fairly certain that there is no *-itis* (i.e., inflammation) of the muscles in fibromyalgia, and that CFS is not caused by chronic Candida or EBV infection.[136,159]

The existence of these conditions remains controversial. Some contend that these are "wastebasket" terms to describe patients who otherwise defy explanation, and others suggest that these are primary psychiatric conditions.[16,59,83,88] There are valid arguments refuting many of the current concepts on the definition and pathogenic mechanisms of these illnesses. However, refuting the existence of large numbers of individuals who suffer from multisymptom somatic syndromes is difficult.

DEFINITION AND CLINICAL FEATURES OF CHRONIC SYSTEMIC MULTISYMPTOM ILLNESSES

The most commonly recognized systemic conditions that fall within this spectrum include fibromyalgia, CFS, somatoform disorders, and multiple chemical sensitivity syndrome (MCSS). These entities and their characteristics are listed in Table 42–1. There are also a variety of less frequent conditions that share considerable homology with these illnesses. Some of these conditions are referred to as exposure syndromes because the illness is defined on the basis of an exposure suspected to cause the symptom complex (e.g., Persian Gulf syndrome, sick building syndrome). Other illnesses within this spectrum affect only one organ system or portion of the body, with the seminal features being pain and/or dysfunction in this region (e.g., migraine headaches, irritable bowel syndrome (IBS), temporomandibular joint dysfunction). A Venn diagram outlining this overlap is presented in Figure 42–1.

Fibromyalgia

Fibromyalgia is the second most common rheumatologic disorder after osteoarthritis.[156,157] In contrast to the three other disorders noted in Table 42–1, which are defined entirely on the basis of symptoms, the diagnostic criteria for this illness also require a

TABLE 42–1
Systemic Conditions Characterized by Chronic Pain and Fatigue

	Fibromyalgia	Chronic Fatigue Syndrome	Somatization Disorders	Multiple Chemical Sensitivity Syndrome
Definition	Diffuse, widespread pain, presence of "tender points" on examination	Severe fatigue, plus four of eight symptoms: myalgia, arthralgia, sore throat, tender neck, cognitive difficulty, headache, postexertional malaise, sleep disturbance	Variable numbers of medical symptoms not explained by known cause	Sensitivity to numerous environmental exposures, with resultant unexplained symptoms in multiple organ systems
Nondefining symptoms	Severe fatigue, headaches, irritable bowel symptoms, rash, cognitive symptoms, insomnia, chest pain, chemical sensitivity, psychiatric disturbances	Chemical sensitivity, psychiatric disturbances, rash, low grade fevers, dyspnea	Virtually any medical symptoms	Fatigue, myalgia, cognitive symptoms, HA, irritable bowel symptoms, psychiatric disturbances
Demographics	80% female	70% female	Females >males	Females >males
Epidemiology	2–4% of population	1% of population	Approximately 4%	?
Proposed triggers	Physical or emotional stressors, infections, immune activation	Infections, physical or emotional stressors, immune activation	Stress	Environmental exposure, stress

physical finding on examination: diffuse tenderness. To fulfill the criteria for fibromyalgia established in 1990, an individual must have both chronic widespread pain involving all four quadrants of the body (and the axial skeleton) and the presence of 11 of 18 tender points on examination (Box 42–1).[157]

The validity of the idea of tender points in fibromyalgia has been challenged.[34] A tender point is defined as an anatomic site where an individual complains of pain when approximately 4 kilograms of pressure is applied.

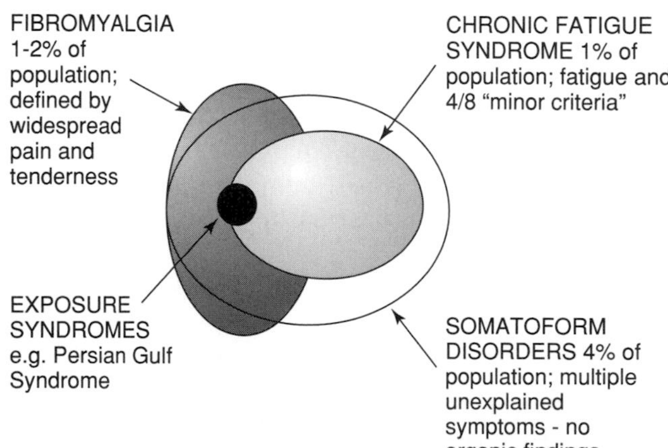

Figure 42–1. Overlap between systemic disorders characterized by chronic pain and fatigue.

Although early studies suggested that patients with fibromyalgia experienced tenderness only in these discrete regions, recent data show that individuals with fibromyalgia display increased sensitivity to pain throughout the body.[56,96,159] This recognition that the pain threshold of patients with fibromyalgia is globally diminished, even in regions such as the forehead or thumbnail, is important because it helped move the focus on the pathogenesis of fibromyalgia from the periphery to the central nervous system (CNS).

There are other potential problems with using tender points to substantiate the diagnosis of fibromyalgia. Many studies have demonstrated that this measure of tenderness is more susceptible to an individual's level of distress than are alternative measures of pain thresholds, such as a dolorimeter (a pressure gauge applied against the skin).[140,155] Also, tenderness is influenced by many factors, with female sex, increasing age, poor aerobic fitness, and mood disorders all tending to increase cutaneous pressure sensitivity.[55,125] Thus any criteria that require a certain number of tender points to establish the diagnosis of fibromyalgia will be biased toward identifying older women with poor aerobic fitness, a high level of distress, and concurrent mood disorders.

Although there may be problems with the current definition of fibromyalgia (particularly when it is used to diagnose an individual patient), this definition is the only one of those in Table 42–1 to undergo extensive testing for diagnostic sensitivity and specificity.[157]

Furthermore, these criteria have allowed a standardization of research in this area. One important type of study that has been performed using these criteria is population-based research to estimate the frequency of this illness in the general population. These studies have shown that in several different countries, the prevalence of fibromyalgia is fairly constant, ranging from 1% to 4% in the general population.[65,113,156] In all of these studies, the prevalence increases with age, and females are four to eight times more likely to be affected than males. The reason for this large sex difference in the prevalence of fibromyalgia is largely because women are more tender than men when tenderness is measured by sensitivity to cutaneous pressure. As an example, females in the population are about 10 times more likely than males to have 11 tender points.[155,156] However, there is not nearly as large a sex difference in the prevalence of chronic widespread pain, the symptom required for the diagnosis of fibromyalgia. About 10% of the population suffers from this symptom, but this symptom is only about 1.5 times more common in females than males.

Finally, these studies have shown that pain and tenderness occur as a continuum in the general population; thus, some individuals rarely experience pain, some experience continuous widespread pain, and others have occasional pain. There is no bimodal distribution, with a group of patients who are very tender. These same characteristics are seen when examining the frequency or severity of nearly any somatic symptom in the population, and create difficulty with defining this spectrum of illness. Furthermore, these aggregate in the population, with individuals with chronic pain much more likely to experience chronic fatigue, and vice versa. This illustrates the difficulty in using the severity of one or more of these subjective symptoms in an illness definition. Also, this suggests that common mechanisms may be responsible for the development of chronic pain, fatigue, and other somatic symptoms, and

BOX 42–1 The American College of Rheumatology 1990 Criteria for the Classification of Fibromyalgia

1. History of widespread pain

   Definition—Pain is considered widespread when all of the following are present: pain in the left side of the body, pain in the right side of the body, pain above the waist, and pain below the waist. In addition, axial skeletal pain (cervical spine or anterior chest or thoracic spine or low back) must be present. In this definition, shoulder and buttock pain is considered as pain for each involved side. "Low back" pain is considered lower segment pain.

2. Pain in 11 of 18 tender point sites on digital palpation

   Definition—Pain, on digital palpation, must be present in at least 11 of the following 18 tender pain sites:

   Occiput: bilateral, at the suboccipital muscle insertions
   Low cervical: bilateral, at the anterior aspects of the intertransverse spaces at C5–C7
   Trapezius: bilateral, at the midpoint of the upper border
   Supraspinatus: bilateral, at origins, above the scapula spine near the medial border
   Second rib: bilateral, at the second costochondral junctions, just lateral to the junctions on upper surfaces
   Lateral epicondyle: bilateral, 2 cm distal to the epicondyles
   Gluteal: bilateral, in upper outer quadrants of buttocks in anterior fold of muscle
   Greater trochanter: bilateral, posterior to the trochanteric prominence
   Knee: bilateral, at the medial fat pad proximal to the joint line

   Digital palpation should be performed with an approximate force of 4 kg. For a tender point to be considered "positive" the subject must state that the palpation was painful. "Tender" is not to be considered "painful."

* For classification purposes, patients will be said to have fibromyalgia if both criteria are satisfied. Widespread pain must have been present for at least 3 months. The presence of a second clinical disorder does not exclude the diagnosis of fibromyalgia.

From Wolfe F, Smythe HA, Yunus MB, et al: The American College of Rheumatology 1990 criteria for the classification of fibromyalgia. Arthritis Rheum 33:160–172, 1990.

perhaps even that these mechanisms may be variations on normal physiology responsible for these symptoms in the general population.

Although chronic widespread pain is the defining feature of fibromyalgia, a number of nonmusculoskeletal symptoms occur in increased frequency in patients with this disorder.[29,146,158] There is also considerable overlap between patients who fulfill criteria for fibromyalgia and those who fulfill criteria for other systemic disorders such as CFS, somatoform disorders, and exposure syndromes. This challenges the notion that any of these illnesses are discrete or unique diseases (Fig. 42–1).

Fibromyalgia is arguably the best studied of the illnesses in Table 42–1 regarding precipitating factors or triggers. There are many accepted triggers of fibromyalgia, all of which fall into the general category of stressors. Physical trauma such as motor vehicle accidents, emotional distress, and a variety of autoimmune and infectious illnesses seem capable of either initiating or exacerbating this illness.[57,62,121,147,157]

Chronic Fatigue Syndrome

CFS is another enigmatic disorder that has attracted increasing attention in recent years. Although the symptom of chronic fatigue affects 5% to 10% of the general population, CFS as currently defined is much less common.[24,47] The current definition for CFS requires that the affected individual display severe chronic fatigue without a defined cause as well as the presence of four of the following symptoms: myalgias, arthralgias, sore throat, tender nodes, cognitive difficulty, headache, postexertional malaise, or sleep disturbance (Box 42–2).[45] This definition was only recently adopted. The definition used before 1994 was more restrictive, and excluded individuals with concurrent psychological conditions (the new definition only excludes individuals with more severe forms of psychiatric disorders). There were several perceived reasons for a need for a new definition, including the fact that some objective findings required in previous criteria (e.g., pharyngitis, lymphadenopathy) were actually uncommonly noted in CFS. More frequently, the patient with CFS experiences a sore throat rather than inflammation of the pharynx, and tender nodes rather than enlargement of the lymph nodes. In the new CFS definition, it is of note that five of the eight minor criteria are pain-based, reinforcing the fact that diffuse pain (without accompanying abnormalities in the peripheral tissues) is also common in this condition. Besides the defining symptoms noted in the criteria, there are a variety of other symptoms seen with increased frequency in CFS. These are extremely similar to those noted for fibromyalgia.[29,76,93] The demographics of CFS are also similar to those of fibromyalgia, with a strong female predominance.[45]

BOX 42–2 Diagnostic Criteria for Chronic Fatigue Syndrome

1. Clinically evaluated, unexplained, persistent or relapsing chronic fatigue:
   A. Of new or definite onset (has not been lifelong)
   B. Is not the result of ongoing exertion
   C. Is not substantially alleviated by rest
   D. And results in substantial reduction in previous levels of occupational, educational, social, or personal activities
2. The concurrent occurrence of four or more of the following symptoms, all of which must have persisted or recurred during 6 or more consecutive months of illness and must not have predated the fatigue:
   A. Self-reported impairment in short-term memory or concentration severe enough to cause substantial reduction in previous levels of occupational, educational, social, or personal activities
   B. Sore throat
   C. Tender cervical or axillary lymph nodes
   D. Muscle pain
   E. Multi-joint pain without joint swelling or redness
   F. Headaches of a new type, pattern, or severity
   G. Unrefreshing sleep
   H. Postexertional malaise lasting more than 24 hours

From Fukuda K, Straus SE, Hickie I, et al: The chronic fatigue syndrome: A comprehensive approach to its definition and study. International Chronic Fatigue Syndrome Study Group. Ann Intern Med 121:953–959, 1994.

A brief review of the history of CFS is helpful to understand how we have arrived at our present understanding of this entity. Because the cardinal features of CFS resemble those of an infectious illness (e.g., myalgias, sore throat, fatigue), and because this illness has frequently been described as beginning in an epidemic, the study of this entity has been focused on identifying an infectious agent that causes the illness. None has been identified. Emerging evidence suggests that although CFS or fibromyalgia may be triggered by an infectious agent, in most individuals the chronic symptoms of these conditions are unlikely to be caused by an active infection.

One reason for this is that recent epidemiologic studies have cast doubt on the notion that CFS is an uncommon disorder that occurs in epidemics. Fukuda and colleagues at the Centers for Disease Control and Prevention (CDC) investigated an epidemic of CFS reported by a physician in a rural Michigan town.[47] The residents of two towns within the epidemic region were selected as the cases, and residents of two distant towns were selected as controls. There were two noteworthy results. First, there was no difference between the prevalence of prolonged fatigue (8%) or CFS (2%) between the two groups of residents. This calls into question the validity of many reports of apparent epidemics of CFS, as it shows that a pseudoepidemic can result when there is active surveillance for a disorder with a high background rate of undiagnosed individuals in the population. This study also found that the minimum prevalence of CFS in four rural Michigan towns was greater than 1% (this assumes that none of the nonresponders had CFS), which is much higher than previous estimates. One reason for this increased prevalence is that the new, less restrictive definition of CFS was used in this study. These prevalence figures are supported by another community-based study performed in the Chicago region that also used the new definition and arrived at a similar value.[67] Yet another recent population-based study estimated a lower point prevalence of CFS (0.1 to 0.2%), but was performed on a cohort of health maintenance organization patients, where individuals with a chronic illness might have been excluded from enrollment.[24]

Another reason that the viral/immune theory of CFS has come into question is the lack of specificity of the studies suggesting that these factors are causal. Early work demonstrated that many individuals with CFS had evidence of an enhanced antibody response to EBV.[136] In fact, for a brief period, the terms used to describe this condition suggested that the EBV virus was the sole cause of this entity. Subsequent reports showed that many patients with CFS lacked evidence of EBV reactivity, and that many others displayed elevated antibody titers to a number of other viruses, including human herpesvirus (HHV)-6, cytomegalovirus, and varicella, as well as various enteroviruses and retroviruses.[2] The finding of elevations of serum antibodies to numerous ubiquitous infectious agents in CFS obviously weakens the role for any single virus in the chronic phase of the disease. Moreover, there are substantial data demonstrating that a global increase in humoral immune responses is seen in a number of chronic stress states, and that neurohormonal changes account for these and other immune aberrations.[74,131] These phenomena are reviewed in greater detail in the following discussion on potential mechanisms.

Perhaps the most compelling evidence that CFS is unlikely to be caused by a persistent viral infection are the aggregate data contained in Table 42–1. Of note, viral infection and immune dysfunction are not postulated to play a role in any of the other illnesses that overlap with CFS, including fibromyalgia and somatoform disorders. Moreover, none of the organ-specific syndromes seen in high frequency in individuals with CFS are suspected to be due to an active viral infection.

Somatoform Disorders

Somatoform disorders are a group of classified psychiatric disorders defined by the presence of physical symptoms that are not fully explained by a known medical condition. These disorders include somatization disorder, hypochondriasis, conversion disorder, and pain disorder.[69] Somatization disorder, formerly called Briquet syndrome, is diagnosed when an individual has multiple somatic complaints that begin before age 30 for which medical attention has been sought but the complaints are not due to a known physical disorder. To meet criteria for this disorder the individual must have at least eight unexplained symptoms over a lifetime. As defined, this condition is uncommon (0.1 to 1.0% of the population). However, a less severe form of somatization is diagnosed when an individual displays one or more unexplained symptoms for greater than 6 months, and is much more common (affecting approximately 4% of the population). This illness has been variously termed subsyndromal somatization disorder and undifferentiated somatoform disorder (Diagnostic and Statistical Manual of Mental Disorders, fourth edition - [DSM-IV]).[6] Therefore, if the symptoms of fibromyalgia or CFS are considered unexplained, most individuals who meet criteria for one of these illnesses will also meet criteria for a somatoform disorder (see also Chapters 38 to 41).

Just as with fibromyalgia and CFS, there is considerable controversy regarding somatoform disorders. This controversy generally takes a different form than that surrounding fibromyalgia and CFS. For example, there has been little burden of proof placed on proponents of the concept of somatoform disorders, as by definition these conditions are acknowledged to have a psychiatric rather than physical basis. This is problematic, as there are multiple objective physiologic abnormalities noted in individuals with fibromyalgia and CFS that might explain symptomatology. Thus it becomes difficult to characterize these symptoms as physiologically unexplained.[11,111] Moreover, even undeniably psychiatric disorders, such as schizophrenia and major depression, are characterized by symptoms that are no longer considered biologically unexplained, as we learn that these illnesses are likely to be mediated in large part by central neurochemical imbalances. The failure of science to define the precise physiologic basis for the symptoms seen in these disorders is no excuse to label an individual with a psychiatric rather than medical diagnosis. In fact, this dualistic view should probably be abandoned for any disease.

However, just as with fibromyalgia and CFS, there have been research findings in the investigation of somatoform disorders that are of irrefutable value. Perhaps the most important are that somatic symptoms are very common, cluster in the population, and exert a tremendous cost in terms of both health care and related disability.[10] For example, it is estimated that about 25% of patients attending a primary care clinic will meet criteria for subsyndromal somatization disorder, and up to 50% of primary care visits are for somatic complaints within this spectrum.[75,80,81] Patients with somatization disorder (the most severe form of somatoform disorder) use 10 times the mean outpatient and inpatient medical services as those in the general population.[129] Given the high percentage of outpatient and inpatient visits that are due to symptoms within this spectrum, the economic costs of somatoform disorders—or any other semantic term that is clearly chosen—are substantial.

Other Miscellaneous Systemic Disorders

There are a number of other systemic conditions that fall within this spectrum. Some of these conditions are even more contentious than fibromyalgia and CFS. MCS is an example. Although there is no accepted definition of this entity, perhaps the best broad definition of MCS is that individuals display symptoms in several organ systems in response to multiple environmental stimuli. Thus an individual may experience nausea, paresthesia, and headaches in response to exposure to perfume, and myalgias, fatigue, and diarrhea in response to exposure to petrochemicals. Although there is disagreement regarding whether there is a physiologic link between these environmental exposures and the resultant symptoms, one cannot deny that there are patients who complain of symptoms of environmental sensitivity. Furthermore, the clinical overlap between this condition and CFS and fibromyalgia has been well established (see Box 42–3).[22]

Other symptom complexes are not defined on the basis of symptoms or signs, but instead by an environmental exposure that is alleged to cause the illness. Such environmental exposures that have been purported to cause illness are "sick buildings," deployment to the Persian Gulf War, and silicone breast implants, to name a few.[20,27,54,102] Usually, the clinical features and laboratory abnormalities described for these illnesses are difficult to distinguish from those of fibromyalgia, CFS, and somatoform disorders.

Regional or Organ-specific Syndromes Within the Same Spectrum

Although the defining features of fibromyalgia and CFS are pain and fatigue, respectively, most individuals with these illnesses also experience a high lifetime and

BOX 42–3 **Diagnostic Criteria for Multiple Chemical Sensitivity Syndrome**

1. Symptoms acquired in relation to some initial identifiable environmental exposure(s)
2. The symptoms involve more than one organ system
3. The symptoms recur and abate in response to predictable stimuli
4. The symptoms are elicited by exposures to chemicals of diverse structural classes and toxicologic modes of action
5. The exposures that elicit symptoms are very low; i.e., many standard deviations below the threshold limit values and at levels not known to cause adverse human responses
6. No single widely available test of organ system function can explain symptoms

From Cullen MR: The worker with multiple chemical sensitivities: An overview. In Cullen M (ed): Workers with Multiple Chemical Sensitivities. Philadelphia, Hanley & Belfus, 1987, pp 655–662; and Fiedler N, Kipen H: Neurobehavioral and psychosocial aspects of multiple chemical sensitivity. In National Research Council: Multiple Chemical Sensitivities. Addendum to Biologic Markers in Immunotoxicology. Washington, DC, National Academy Press, 1992, pp 109–116.

current prevalence of nondefining symptoms. Some investigators have used the term allied conditions to describe these closely related symptoms and syndromes; the number of such conditions has expanded, as seen in Figure 42–2.[29,62,159] It has become increasingly clear that there is a substantial overlap between these regional syndromes and the aforementioned systemic syndromes, in that individuals who have the systemic syndrome are much more likely to have these regional problems and vice versa. We devote a separate section to the overlap between psychiatric disorders and this spectrum of illness, because this inter-relationship is both complex and contentious.

Fibromyalgia has long been considered to be characterized by a high frequency of nonmusculoskeletal conditions, and the clinical features of this illness have been more completely characterized than those of the other systemic conditions within this spectrum.[29,62,76,93,159] Most patients with fibromyalgia and all patients with CFS complain of fatigue. Because early fibromyalgia research focused on the study of sleep, many fibromyalgia symptoms, including fatigue, had been considered primarily due to a disruption of deep (stage III/IV) sleep.[97] Sleep has also been extensively studied in CFS.[89] Current evidence does not support the notion that poor sleep is the primary cause of these illnesses. Many individuals with either of these illnesses have normal sleep studies, and sleep abnormalities such as alpha-delta sleep (which had previously been thought to be specific for these disorders) are seen in other conditions, as well as in normal individuals.[114] Furthermore, improvement in fibromyalgia symptoms with pharmacologic treatment does not correlate with improvement in sleep parameters.[5] Nonetheless, poor sleep is likely to contribute to some symptoms and physiologic abnormalities seen in these conditions, especially in disrupting the circadian secretion of hormones that are released during sleep (e.g., growth hormone). Poor sleep is also likely to participate in a vicious cycle of pain, disrupted sleep, and worsened fatigue and pain.

Other constitutional symptoms that may be seen in these individuals include large fluctuations in weight, heat and cold intolerance, and the subjective sensation of weakness. Individuals with this spectrum of illness also experience a variety of neurologic symptoms. Patients with both fibromyalgia and CFS have a higher than expected prevalence of both tension and migraine headaches.[157] Numbness or tingling, typically fleeting in nature and in a nondermatomal distribution, is also a common complaint.[126] Cognitive complaints, especially difficulty with attention and short-term memory, are seen frequently in patients with these entities, and in some may be the most debilitating aspect of their illness.[68,92] Objective abnormalities on neuropsychological testing have

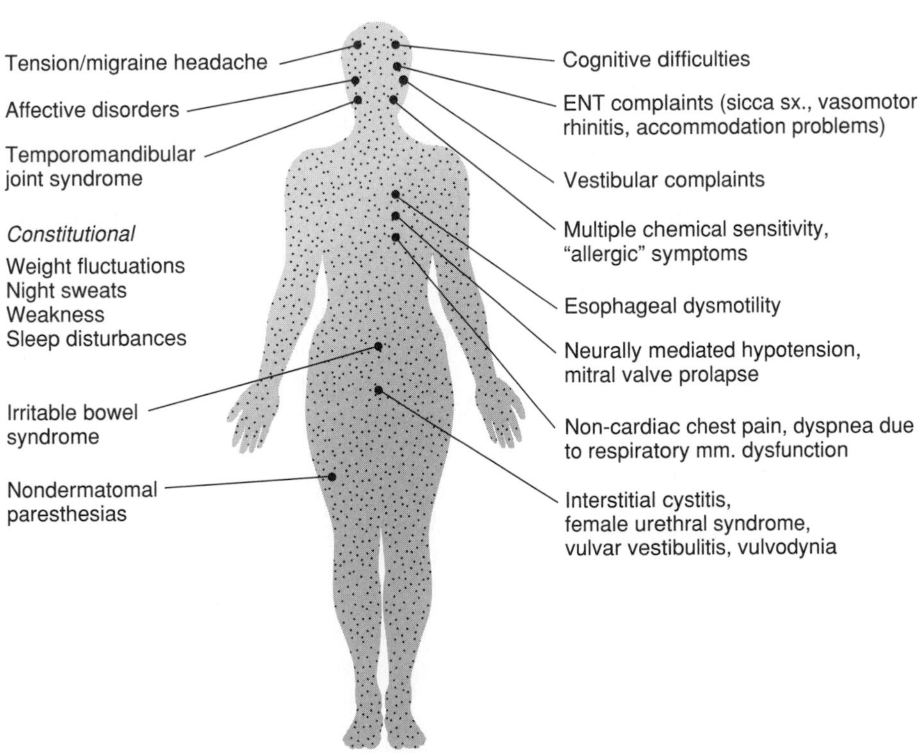

Figure 42–2. Localized or organ-specific syndromes.

also been noted, although these findings are not consistent.[32,35,68,92]

Patients with these illnesses also display a wide array of allergic symptoms, ranging from adverse reactions to drugs and environmental stimuli (as seen in MCSS), to higher than expected incidences of rhinitis, nasal congestion, and lower respiratory symptoms.[22,33] Although some of these individuals may truly be atopic, there are likely nonallergic mechanisms that contribute substantially to these symptoms.[31] Hearing, ocular, and vestibular abnormalities have also been noted, including a 70% incidence of a decreased painful sound threshold, 40% exaggerated nystagmus and ocular dysmotility, and 27% asymptomatic low frequency sensorineural hearing loss in fibromyalgia.[50,116] Other accompanying symptoms include sicca complex and temporomandibular joint dysfunction.[18,41]

Individuals with fibromyalgia likewise suffer from a number of symptoms of functional disorders of visceral organs, including a high incidence of recurrent noncardiac chest pain, heartburn, palpitations, and irritable bowel symptoms.[100,157] Prospective studies of randomly selected individuals with fibromyalgia have detected objective evidence of dysfunction of several visceral organs, including a 75% incidence of echocardiographic evidence of mitral valve prolapse, a 40% incidence of esophageal dysmotility, and diminished static inspiratory and expiratory pressures on pulmonary function testing.[61,86,105] Neurally mediated hypotension and syncope also appear to occur more frequently in individuals with both fibromyalgia and CFS.[118] Similar syndromes characterized by visceral pain and/or smooth muscle dysmotility are also seen in the pelvis. Well-established examples of such symptoms are the association with dysmenorrhea as well as with urinary frequency and urgency.[144] There may also be an association between fibromyalgia and other genitourinary conditions such as interstitial cystitis, endometriosis, and vulvar vestibulitis or vulvodynia (the latter of which are characterized by dyspareunia and sensitivity of the vulvar region).[44,79]

A discussion of the localized conditions within this spectrum must include the fact that it is common for any type of regional pain syndrome (e.g., temporomandibular joint dysfunction, vulvodynia, myofascial pain, or costochondritis) to eventually spread to become more systemic and involve the entire body; i.e., transform into fibromyalgia. Animal studies of allodynia and of phenomena such as central sensitization may provide clues about why this may occur.

Relationship With Psychiatric Disorders

As noted previously, the symptoms of chronic multisymptom illnesses and those of psychiatric disorders overlap significantly. Although some contend that all of these symptoms are supratentorial in origin, others counter that the rate of psychiatric comorbidities in these conditions is similar to that of any chronic disease.[4,88,160] A review of the accumulated data in these conditions supports a few consistent observations:

1. Approximately 20% to 40% of individuals with fibromyalgia or CFS seen in tertiary care centers have an identifiable current mood disorder such as depression or anxiety disorder.[4,17,88] Some studies have suggested that the frequency of psychiatric comorbidity is lower in individuals identified in primary care practices or in the general population, whereas other studies have found equally high percentages.[1,149] Regardless of the precise percentage of individuals with psychiatric comorbidities, at least 60% of individuals with fibromyalgia or CFS have no identifiable concurrent psychiatric condition. Thus there must be nonpsychiatric mechanisms capable of causing all of the symptoms seen in these disorders.
2. The lifetime history of mood disorders in individuals with fibromyalgia or CFS is high, averaging about 40% to 70% over several studies.[4,17,63] These data are among those used by Hudson and colleagues to posit that there is a spectrum of disorders including fibromyalgia, migraines, irritable bowel, and affective disorders that may share a common genetic predisposition and underlying pathogenic mechanisms. Again, some of these differences in the lifetime history of depression may be due to health care seeking behaviors, because lower lifetime incidences of affective disorders are typically noted in individuals with fibromyalgia who are identified in the general population.[1,155]
3. There are a myriad of complex psychosocial factors that play a significant role in some individuals with these illnesses, as with nearly any chronic medical illness. These include behavioral pathways, such as sick role behavior and maladaptive coping mechanisms, cognitive pathways, such as victimization and loss of control, and social pathways, such as interference with role functioning and deterioration of social or other support networks. Psychosocial factors are known to play a particularly prominent role in the transition from acute pain to chronic pain and disability. As pain progresses from the acute phase into chronicity, problems emerge for the individual such as job loss, financial constraints, and distancing of friends. If a patient's responses to these problems are maladaptive, such as avoidance of work, friends, financial responsibilities, and physical activity, the patient may become distressed and

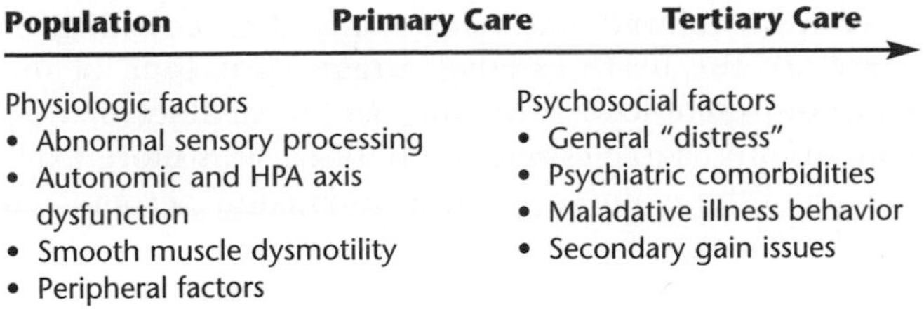

Population	Primary Care	Tertiary Care

Physiologic factors
- Abnormal sensory processing
- Autonomic and HPA axis dysfunction
- Smooth muscle dysmotility
- Peripheral factors

Psychosocial factors
- General "distress"
- Psychiatric comorbidities
- Maladative illness behavior
- Secondary gain issues

Figure 42–3. Relationship between physiologic and psychobehavioral factors in chronic multisymptom illnesses.

> overwhelmed by the pain and its negative impact on life. Increased stress, learned helplessness, depression, increased anxiety, anger, distrust, entitlement, and somatization can all emerge and worsen symptoms, probably by inter-related physiologic and psychological mechanisms. All of these factors can be important in dictating how individuals report symptoms, how and when they seek health care, and how they respond to therapy. This may also explain why cognitive-behavioral therapy, which addresses many of these issues, has generally been effective in the treatment of individuals with fibromyalgia, as well as nearly any other chronic medical condition.[101]

Figure 42–3 summarizes the relationship between physiologic factors and psychobehavioral factors in this spectrum of illness. At the far left of the graph, perhaps when individuals first develop symptoms, there may be primarily physiologic factors that are responsible. Such factors are discussed in more detail in the following. With chronicity of illness, some individuals may develop psychological and behavioral cofactors that exacerbate or perpetuate the illness. These factors, in combination with the physiologic factors, are likely to be the largest determinants of disability in this spectrum of illness. These latter factors are seen much more commonly in individuals who attend tertiary care clinics, and conversely, individuals who are found with these syndromes in the general population, or in primary care, are less likely to have such factors, and are likely to respond much better to purely physiologic (e.g., pharmacologic) interventions.

POTENTIAL MECHANISMS

There have been several objective abnormalities noted in individuals with fibromyalgia and CFS. There has been little study of underlying pathophysiologic mechanisms in the other conditions noted in Table 42–1, such as somatoform disorders and MCSS, so no comparable information is available. However, further insights into potential pathogenic mechanisms can be elucidated by examining the data collected on organ-specific disorders that commonly are associated with these conditions, such as migraine headaches and IBS. Table 42–2 summarizes the results of these areas of investigation.

Reproducible objective abnormalities that have been noted in these conditions are presented and placed within a theoretical construct that unites many findings that at first glance appear disparate. In the model of illness proposed, there are a group of individuals who are genetically predisposed to develop this entire spectrum of illness. Susceptible individuals commonly experience a number of organ-specific illnesses before finally progressing to develop the more debilitating systemic conditions later in life. These illnesses may develop indolently or abruptly, and in the latter instances typically follow exposure to a stressor or series of stressors. Once an individual develops this illness, there is evidence of blunting of the human stress response, which may be manifest as blunting of one or more hypothalamic-pituitary axes (HPA), globally increased peripheral

TABLE 42–2

Summary of Studies Examining Potential Pathogenic Mechanisms in Disorders of Chronic Pain and Fatigue

	Fibromyalgia	Chronic Fatigue Syndrome	Irritable Bowel Syndrome	Migraine Headaches
Familial aggregation	Yes	NS	NS	Yes
Increased peripheral nociception	Yes	Yes	NS	Yes
Increased visceral nociception	Yes	NS	Yes	NS
Neurotransmitter abnormalities	Yes	Yes	NS	Yes
HPA dysregulation	Yes, blunted	Yes, blunted	NS	NS
Autonomic dysfunction	Yes	Yes	Yes	Yes
Smooth muscle dysmotility	Yes	NS	Yes	Yes

NS, not studied.

and/or visceral nociception, or instability of the autonomic nervous system. These different axes of the stress response can either independently or concurrently function aberrantly, which may in part be responsible for the tremendous heterogeneity of symptoms. In this model, psychiatric illnesses can occur concurrently and significantly modulate disease activity and symptom expression, and vice versa. Finally, in this paradigm, changes in the immune system and in the peripheral tissues are de-emphasized, because there are data suggesting that these anomalies occur because of these central alterations in the stress system (see Chapter 40).

Genetic or Familial Predisposition

There is some evidence of familial aggregation for nearly all of the illnesses within this spectrum, although often these data are inferential rather than definitive. Several prospective studies have suggested that relatives of patients with fibromyalgia display higher than expected rates of fibromyalgia.[62,106,135] Family members of patients with fibromyalgia also display a high frequency of a number of conditions related to fibromyalgia, including IBS, migraine headaches, and mood disorders.[62] Many of these allied conditions, such as migraine headaches, have also independently been noted to have a familial predilection.[95]

Somatoform disorders and somatization have also long been considered to be familial, although until recently it had not been clear whether this tendency was due to genetics or to familial environmental effects (i.e., nature versus nurture). In arguably the best genetic study within this entire spectrum of illness, a large twin registry was used to examine what degree of variance in somatoform symptoms is predicted by genetics, and what percentage is predicted by environment. This study found that genetic factors accounted for 25% to 50% of the total variance in self-report of symptoms of somatization, whereas familial environmental effects accounted for virtually no variance.[73] Studies performed by this group have also expanded on the well-established familial nature of major depression, by demonstrating that subtypes of depression aggregate in families.[72] This observation may be particularly important when exploring the relationship between the biology of affective disorders and of illnesses such as fibromyalgia and CFS.

Triggering Events

Both the systemic and organ-specific syndromes within this spectrum can be triggered or exacerbated by a variety of physical, emotional, and immune stressors. Well-described examples include triggering or worsening of fibromyalgia by physical trauma such as motor vehicle accidents, of CFS by viral infections, and of all of these illnesses by emotional stressors.[37,38,53,60,147] Although these are the best described triggers for each of the symptom complexes, this may be an artifact of how patients are characterized and defined. It is more likely that all of these illnesses can be initiated or perpetuated by all of these types of stressors.

One recent study of CFS demonstrated this phenomenon.[122] A total of 134 consecutive patients who met CDC (Center for Disease Control) criteria for CFS were seen by an infectious disease specialist and had a comprehensive evaluation, including serologic studies for infectious agents postulated to cause this illness. These individuals also completed self-report questionnaires that examined the number and type of stressful events that occurred in the year before the diagnosis of CFS. Although 72% of these patients felt they had an infectious cause of illness, the evaluation revealed that 52% had no serologic evidence of infection, and only 20% had evidence of probable or definite infection. In contrast, 85% of the CFS patients reported at least one major stressful event in the year before the diagnosis of CFS (the average was 1.7 such events/patient), compared with only 6% of a control group (average of 0.1 events/control).

The epidemic of Gulf War–related illnesses that occurred in troops deployed to the Persian Gulf in 1990 and 1991 also affords an excellent example of how illnesses such as fibromyalgia and CFS may be triggered. To review, in 1990 and 1991 the United States deployed approximately 700,000 troops to the Persian Gulf to liberate Kuwait from Iraqi occupation. Fortunately, there were relatively few combat-related injuries and diseases during this conflict, but up to 45% of deployed veterans (as compared to 15% of nondeployed veterans) developed a constellation of symptoms and syndromes including muscle and joint pain, fatigue, memory problems, headaches, and gastrointestinal complaints.[46] This experience was not unique to U.S. troops, because veterans of this conflict from the United Kingdom experienced a similar increase in this spectrum of illness.[139]

Several expert panels have been convened to examine these illnesses. There is agreement that this is not a single illness, but rather a constellation of symptoms and syndromes similar to that seen in fibromyalgia and CFS. There is no single environmental exposure that is likely to have contributed to this illness. Instead, there are data from many sources that suggest that certain persons who are exposed to stressors, including infections or other types of immune stimulation, drugs or chemicals, physical trauma, or emotional stress, will develop a chronic multisystem illness.[30] Because of the recognized link with emotional stress, however, these illnesses have been characterized as psychosomatic illnesses. The problem with this categorization is similar to the problem with the concept of somatoform disorders: these constructs are based in large part on the now antiquated dualistic notion that illnesses are either functional or organic, and nearly all chronic illnesses can be influenced by a number of biological stressors.

Mechanisms Potentially Responsible for Continued Symptoms

Just as with other aspects of these disorders, there is legitimate disagreement regarding which of the objective abnormalities that have been identified are most likely to be most important. Many of the abnormalities are likely to represent secondary phenomena (epiphenomena) that are the result rather than the cause of the disorder. In this review, abnormalities that have been noted in the peripheral tissues as well as changes in immune function are considered to represent epiphenomena.

The Discarded Peripheral and Immune/Infection Hypotheses

Early studies examining the pathogenesis of fibromyalgia focused on the hypothesis that the principal abnormality was a histologic or metabolic abnormality in the areas of painful muscle. Biopsies of tender points have generally demonstrated histologically normal muscle, except for a higher incidence of ragged red fibers, a nonspecific finding.[13] Other investigators focusing on metabolic abnormalities demonstrated a decrease in muscle high energy phosphates and decreased muscle tissue oxygenation.[14] This constellation of findings led to the hypothesis that local tissue hypoxia was in part responsible for the pain and weakness seen in this condition, and that this hypoxia may occur because of sustained muscular contraction and the resultant decreased blood flow.

More recent findings, however, diminish the likelihood that fibromyalgia is a pathologic process localized to tender points or primarily affects muscle or peripheral tissues. As previously noted, all recent studies of fibromyalgia have indicated that the tenderness is not localized to tender points, or even to soft tissues. Moreover, the advent of phosphorus-31 magnetic resonance spectroscopy (MRS) has allowed the study of muscle metabolism in vivo. None of these studies has demonstrated any statistically significant difference in ratios of high-energy phosphate compounds between patients and controls.[39,66,127] Although there is not support for a primary role of peripheral tissue abnormalities in the pathogenesis of these conditions, it is plausible if not likely that there are secondary effects on these tissues that may contribute to symptomatology.

Another theory regarding the pathogenesis of these disorders is that these illnesses are caused by an active viral infection. This hypothesis has been primarily confined to CFS, and has not been proffered for any other systemic or organ-specific disorder in this spectrum. There have been a number of in vitro and in vivo immunologic abnormalities that have been described in CFS to support this thesis. Many of these data are difficult to interpret because these studies have lacked clinical and immunologic standardization, and have failed to realize the relevance of psychological profiles, duration of illness, methodologic differences, and rigorous controls.[82] Nonetheless, some generally reproducible results have emerged, and most abnormalities have been noted in both fibromyalgia and CFS.

A variety of cellular immune responses are diminished in these conditions.[9,26,98,103] The most consistent of these abnormalities has been low natural killer (NK) cell number and function. Other commonly noted changes are suppressed T cell proliferative responses to mitogens and antigens, changes in T lymphocyte subsets (increased activated CD8+ cells), and occasionally modest changes in cytokine concentrations.

In contrast, humoral immune responses are generally enhanced in these conditions. Although the number of circulating B lymphocytes is normal, increases in total serum immunoglobulins (Ig) and changes in IgG subsets have been noted.[9,112,124] In addition to these changes in overall Ig levels, there are also increases in the levels of a number of specific antibodies. Cohorts of patients with either CFS or fibromyalgia have been noted to have high titers of antibodies to a number of ubiquitous viruses, as previously noted.[2] There is also an increase in antinuclear antibodies in these conditions, although this issue has been debated.[124]

The immune changes seen in CFS and fibromyalgia are common to a number of chronic stressful conditions. Thus similar abnormalities in NK cell number and function, mitogen stimulation, and antibody levels have been noted in a number of chronic stressful situations: prisoners released from concentration camps, participants in desert survival training, students taking examinations, and recent widows or spouses of patients with Alzheimer disease, as well as in animal studies of chronic stress.[23,40,49,64,131] Interestingly, these animal studies have repeatedly demonstrated that immune changes are more prominent with exposure to inescapable or unavoidable stress, which may have interesting implications if this is also true in humans.

The Proposed CNS Dysregulation Hypothesis

The principal components of the human stress response are the corticotropin-releasing hormone (CRH) and locus ceruleus-norepinephrine/autonomic (sympathetic/LC-NE) nervous systems.[28,52] The CRH system is primarily centered in the hypothalamus and the sympathetic/LC-NE system in the brainstem. Activation of these systems by physical or emotional stimuli propagates a series of physiologic changes known as the stress response.

The model proposed posits that many of the symptoms and clinical features that occur in the spectrum of chronic pain and fatigue illnesses are due to dysregulation of the human stress response. There are many reasons why the stress response may be functioning abnormally in these conditions. These include an inherited abnormality in the activity of this system and/or an acquired abnormality in function, which might occur with repeated exposure to stressors. Regardless, most of the phenomena noted in this spectrum of illness may be explained by blunting of various axes of the human stress response. There is a substantial body of literature regarding this system, which cannot be reviewed in detail. There are several observations regarding the stress response, however, that must be emphasized because of the potential importance to the proposed hypothesis:

1. Several authors have noted that although this system is adaptive in animals and early human species, it may be maladaptive in the twentieth century. In everyday life this system is much more likely to be activated by daily events that have no threat to survival (e.g., sitting in traffic) than for the intended purposes of this system; e.g., to protect against predators or starvation.[94,115]
2. Different types of stress lead to markedly different biological responses, in both animals and humans. Stressors perceived as inescapable or unavoidable, or that are accompanied by lack of predictability or support, evoke the strongest adverse biological consequences.[28,52,115,143] This could conceivably explain why victims of trauma, such as motor vehicle accidents, appear to have a much higher rate of development of fibromyalgia and myofascial pain than those who are responsible for the accident.[57]
3. Early life stressors can have a permanent and profound impact on the subsequent biological response to stress in animals, because of the plasticity of the nervous system. Studies in rodents have demonstrated that exposure to endotoxin, trauma, or separation in the neonatal period all lead to permanent changes in the subsequent biological response to stress, extending throughout the life of the animal.[115,123,132,143] This plasticity may be due to changes in the number of neurons and number of circuits and/or increases or decreases in gene expression, leading to permanent changes in molecules that define the function of the system.[51,133] This permanent effect of early stressors could explain why individuals who develop fibromyalgia, CFS, somatoform disorders, IBS, and other disorders in this spectrum display a higher

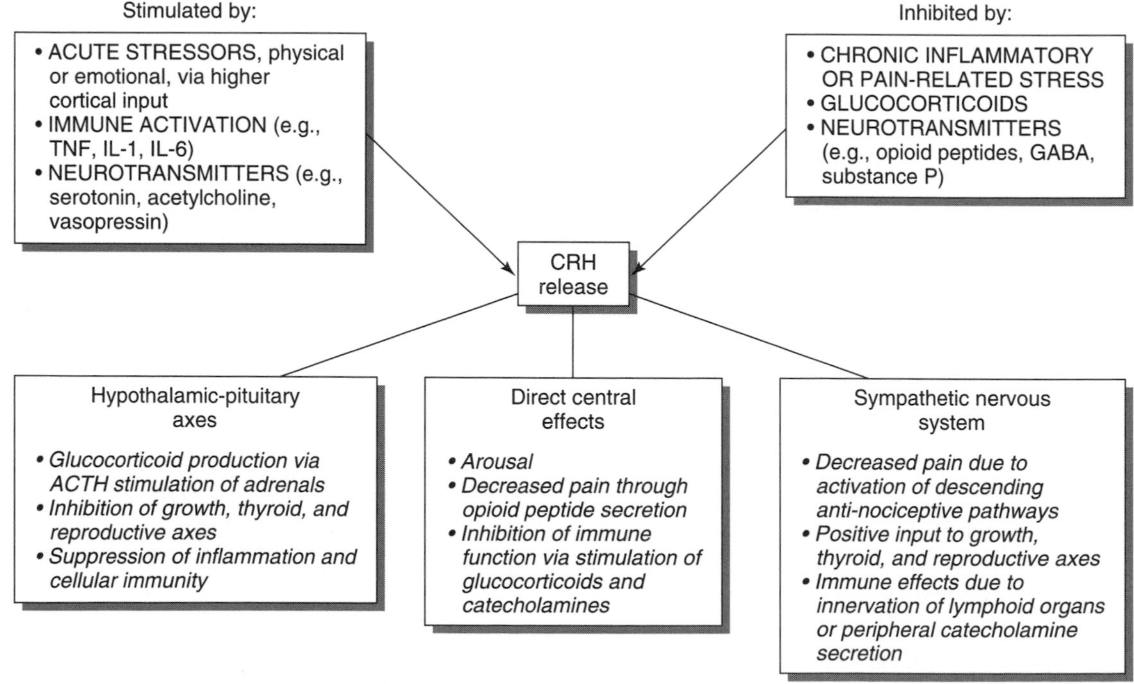

Figure 42–4. The human stress response. IL, interleukin; TNF, tumor necrosis factor; CRH, corticotropin releasing hormone; GABA, gamma-aminobutyric acid; ACTH, adrenocorticotropic hormone.

than expected incidence of childhood physical and sexual abuse.[12,130,145]

4. Within any species, there are genetic differences in the activity of the biological stress response.[94,134] It is possible that the genetic predisposition to develop this spectrum of disorders is actually due to inherited differences in the activity of the stress response.

Figure 42–4 outlines the principal features of the stress response. As noted, CRH is a principal modulator in this system. Although most CRH-containing neurons are in the paraventricular nucleus of the hypothalamus, these neurons and their projections are widely distributed throughout other portions of the CNS, and may be uniquely able to coordinate the overall stress response. The release of CRH is enhanced and inhibited by a number of factors that are noted, and then CRH exerts a number of direct and indirect effects on the various effector axes of the stress response. This system not only plays a well-recognized role in the control of hormonal and autonomic responses, but also directly mediates arousal as well as so-called stress-induced analgesia, via opioid-peptide secreting neurons in the arcuate nucleus of the hypothalamus that project to the brainstem and spinal cord.[21,28,137] In addition, the locus ceruleus is important in controlling other descending antinociceptive pathways, which under normal circumstances act to diminish the upward transmission of pain. Thus low CRH and/or sympathetic output is capable of causing diffusely increased nociception, because descending CRH or opioid peptidergic and sympathetic pathways act in the spinal cord to diminish pain.

The accumulated information suggests that the biological stress response is blunted in the chronic phase of fibromyalgia, CFS, and allied conditions. The expected biological consequences of this low CRH state are the opposite of those seen in acute stress, and are very similar to those noted in chronic pain and fatigue states: hypoarousal or fatigue, diffusely increased peripheral and visceral nociception, and dysautonomia conceivably leading to a number of consequences, including smooth muscle dysmotility and abnormalities in cardiovascular function.

Areas of CNS Dysfunction in this Spectrum of Illness

The areas of nervous system function that may be playing some role in the pathogenesis of fibromyalgia include sensory processing, autonomic and neuroendocrine, and psychobehavioral influences.

Abnormalities in Sensory Processing

Sensory processing, and pain transmission in general, has been best studied in fibromyalgia, because this condition is defined on the basis of pain and tenderness. Much of what has been demonstrated in fibromyalgia with respect to sensory transmission has been likewise found in other conditions in this spectrum, such as IBS, tension headache, and other conditions characterized by regional pain.

Several investigators have moved beyond determinations of tender point counts and dolorimeter values in fibromyalgia to more extensively examine the basis for widespread pain and tenderness in this condition. Such studies have demonstrated that patients with fibromyalgia cannot detect electrical, pressure, or thermal stimuli at lower levels than normal controls, but the point at which these stimuli cause pain or become unpleasant is lower.[8,85] Other studies have examined regional differences in pain sensitivity, and have demonstrated that although tender points are anatomic locations that are more sensitive to pressure, these regions are actually less responsive to both electrical and thermal stimuli than are "control points."[85] In studies examining the precise location of the hyperalgesia in fibromyalgia, it appears as though the largest difference in pain sensitivity is deep to the skin, but not exclusively in muscle.[77]

Other modulating influences have been examined to elucidate the precise mechanism(s) involved in pain transmission. One possible link between the systemic symptoms that these individuals experience and the diffuse pain seen in this condition is the sympathetic nervous system. There is emerging evidence that fibromyalgia may be characterized by a decrease in the activity of descending, antinociceptive pathways that begin in subcortical structures, including the locus ceruleus, and descend into the spinal cord. Under normal conditions, these pathways are tonically active, and inhibit the upward transmission of pain. Kosek and colleagues demonstrated that isometric contraction of muscle exerted the expected analgesic effect on pressure pain threshold in normal subjects, whereas fibromyalgia patients responded to this maneuver with a paradoxically lowered pain threshold.[78] Other investigators studied the effect of a tonic painful stimulus on pain threshold in fibromyalgia patients, and found that, in contrast to controls, there was no increase in pain threshold.[84] They suggested that this indicated a lack of descending noxious inhibitory control mechanisms in the fibromyalgia patients.

Other investigators have used functional brain imaging in persons with fibromyalgia to substantiate the notion that there may be a disturbance in pain processing in this condition. In both of these studies, persons with this condition were studied at baseline rather than with response to a painful (or other) stimulus. Mountz et al collected SPECT data on women with fibromyalgia and found evidence of regional differences in blood flow in areas involved in pain transmission, such as the caudate nucleus.[99] In contrast, Yunus performed baseline positron emission tomography scans on 10 subjects with fibromyalgia, and found these to be normal (personal communication).

Although nearly all of the research on sensory processing in fibromyalgia has focused on the processing of pain, there are some data suggesting a more generalized disturbance in sensory processing. For example, many persons with fibromyalgia experience sensitivity to loud noises, bright lights, odors, drugs, and chemicals. These symptoms of generalized sensitivity to multiple stimuli account for the significant number of persons with fibromyalgia who also could be classified with MCSS (an acknowledged misnomer for these symptoms).[128]

Other investigations have attempted to identify specific neurochemical abnormalities that may be associated with abnormal pain transmission. In arguably the most important biologic studies performed in this illness, several groups have demonstrated that patients with fibromyalgia have approximately threefold higher concentrations of substance P (SP) in cerebrospinal fluid (CSF) than normal controls.[19,119,141,148] SP is a pronociceptive peptide stored in the secretory granules of sensory nerves and released upon axonal stimulation. There is remarkable consistency between the findings of these groups of investigators, and in all cases there is very little overlap in SP levels between the fibromyalgia patients and normal controls.

The meaning of these elevated CSF SP levels is not entirely clear. The SP could theoretically be derived from overactive peripheral nociceptive fibers, or from central neurons. An elevated CSF SP is not specific for fibromyalgia, as this finding has also been noted in patients with osteoarthritis of the hip and chronic low back pain. It is likely that these findings are related to the presence of pain, as persons with CFS do not display this finding.[43] Russell et al have demonstrated that these SP levels in fibromyalgia are stable, or rise, over time, and do not change in response to acute painful stimuli. Also, the same magnitude of elevation of CSF SP is found in fibromyalgia patients with and without psychiatric comorbidities.[119] Animal models suggest that SP and excitatory amino acids (EAA) act synergistically at the level of the dorsal column of the spinal cord to contribute to the development of allodynia (a diffuse state of heightened sensitivity to normally nonpainful stimuli as seen in fibromyalgia). In these models, EAA act rapidly to acutely change the pain threshold, whereas SP acts more slowly and is likely more operative in chronic pain states.

There are several other substances known to have prominent effects on nociception that may be abnormal in fibromyalgia. For example, norepinephrine has an antinociceptive function centrally, and the level of its principal metabolite, 3-methoxy-4-hydroxyphenethylene (MHPG), is low in the CSF of fibromyalgia patients.[120] This finding again supports the possibility that descending antinociceptive influences from the autonomic nervous system could be a potential mechanism for the allodynia and hyperalgesia seen in fibromyalgia. It is also of note that some of the most effective drugs in treating central pain syndromes such as fibromyalgia act by augmenting central adrenergic activity.

Finally, there is some evidence to justify a role for low central levels of serotonin in several disorders within this spectrum. There are data suggesting a generalized defect in serotonin synthesis or metabolism in fibromyalgia, indicated by low levels of serotonin and its precursor, L-tryptophan, in the serum, as well as low levels of the principal metabolite, 5-HIAA, in the CSF (serotonin is undetectable in the CSF of humans).[120,161]

Although most evidence suggests that fibromyalgia is a disorder characterized by a dysregulation of the CNS, recent evidence from Rosner et al suggests that a subset of patients with this symptom complex may be suffering from unrecognized cervical spinal stenosis, or a Chiari malformation.[117] In this setting, compression of the cervical cord, or restriction of vertebral blood flow, could conceivably be responsible for diffuse pain, fatigue, and autonomic dysfunction. In several case series, patients with symptoms of fibromyalgia and CFS have markedly improved with decompressive surgery. Controlled studies that are underway should help delineate whether this is a common or rare cause of fibromyalgia symptoms.

Hypothalamic-Pituitary Dysfunction

There are substantial data indicating that the HPA function abnormally in subsets of persons with these disorders.[36] Each of these disorders differs somewhat with respect to the precise perturbations, and in all instances hypothalamic function is only abnormal in a small subset of subjects. In fibromyalgia, most studies have revealed low 24-hour free urinary cortisol, exaggerated ACTH release in response to CRH challenge, and abnormal diurnal rhythmicity of secretion of cortisol and other hormones. Adrenal insufficiency also occurs in response to exercise in fibromyalgia, as cortisol levels paradoxically fall rather than rise in response to physical exertion.[142] This postexercise adrenal insufficiency, as well as the decreased sympathetic response to exercise noted in the following, might in some way contribute to the severe postexertional pain and fatigue that both fibromyalgia and CFS patients experience. These changes in the HPA axis are opposite to those seen in melancholic depression, which is characterized by chronically increased stress system activity.[28]

Changes have also been noted in the growth hormone axis that suggest abnormal hypothalamic function. Insulin-like growth factor-1 (IGF-1) is produced in the liver, primarily in response to growth hormone (GH), and is responsible for many of the biological activities of GH. Bennett et al have demonstrated that IGF-1 is very low in about a quarter of fibromyalgia patients.[15] The defect in GH secretion that leads to the low IGF-1 appears to be hypothalamic in origin, because these individuals fail to secrete GH in response to a variety of types of stimulations.[15] Although administration of recombinant GH to this subset of fibromyalgia patients has been demonstrated to be of clinical benefit, the expense of this treatment and the likelihood that other less expensive treatments may be of similar efficacy has limited the use of this modality.

Autonomic Nervous System

There are also identifiable abnormalities in autonomic nervous system function in many of the disorders in this spectrum. Just as with studies of neuroendocrine function, only a subset of fibromyalgia patients will have abnormal autonomic function, depending on how this is defined. In summary, various studies have demonstrated that subsets of persons with fibromyalgia, as well as other similar disorders such as CFS, display low baseline sympathetic tone and an inability to respond to stressors.[42,110,142] The clinical manifestations that are related to autonomic dysfunction are not entirely clear, but may include orthostatic intolerance (e.g., as in neurally mediated hypotension), vasomotor instability, and visceral dysfunction.

Dysautonomia has likewise been documented in both IBS and migraine headaches, and is felt to play a central role in the genesis of both disorders.[25,87,90,108] In IBS, there have been several studies suggesting abnormalities in both central sympathetic and parasympathetic influences, and some studies have suggested that the abnormalities in the autonomic nervous system can predict certain types of symptoms (e.g., diarrhea or constipation-predominant).[3,48,91] Defects in autonomic function have also been delineated in migraine, with the aggregate data in these studies suggesting that there is baseline sympathetic hypofunction as well as instability of the sympathetic response.[104,108,109,162] Furthermore, studies in both IBS and migraine suggest that there is a dissociation between the symptoms of pain and autonomic dysfunction, which supports the hypotheses proposed regarding the independence of the axes of the stress response.[7,87,90,104,108,151]

Smooth Muscle Dysmotility

Smooth muscle dysmotility may be partially related to the dysautonomia in these conditions, and has been observed in numerous syndromes within this spectrum, including fibromyalgia, IBS, migraine headaches, and dysmenorrhea. The best studied of these entities in this regard has been IBS. Although the finding of smooth muscle dysmotility in IBS in the intestine is not surprising, these individuals have also been shown to display similar motility changes throughout the entire body, including the bladder, lung, and esophagus.[70,71,150,152,153] Similar changes in esophageal motor tone have been noted in fibromyalgia patients.[61]

DIAGNOSIS

Because of the breadth of this topic, it is impossible to cover the diagnostic approach to this spectrum of illness. Many of these conditions represent diagnoses of exclusion, and the appropriate testing paradigms for each of the illnesses within this spectrum are reviewed elsewhere. However, there are several points that bear mentioning because they apply to most or all of these syndromes.

Before making the diagnosis of a FSS, the practitioner should consider whether this label will help the patient. Hadler, in particular, has argued eloquently that the labeling of illnesses such as fibromyalgia may be harmful.[58] There is nothing unique about fibromyalgia in this regard, because labeling has been shown to be harmful in many medical conditions, such as hypertension. In contrast to hypertension, however, where labeling can be justified because of an increased risk of mortality in the absence of intervention, there is no evidence that treating fibromyalgia changes mortality. This places a burden on the treater of any condition that causes symptoms, but not damage, to ensure that a label is accompanied by a treatment plan that improves function.

Laboratory and other diagnostic testing should be used judiciously in the evaluation of the patient with clinical features consistent with this spectrum of illness. There are two primary reasons for this. First, excessive diagnostic testing can reinforce the notion that an individual is "sick" rather than just having a symptom that may occur commonly in the population and require no specific intervention (i.e., iatrogenically moving the patient from the left to the right side of Figure 42–3). This is particularly true if the symptoms within this spectrum have been present for a long period of time, wherein the patient may be coming in for an evaluation to be reassured that nothing serious is wrong.

The other reason to avoid unnecessary diagnostic testing in this spectrum of illness is that this can lead to inappropriate diagnoses and management. For example, because there is such a high rate of positive antinuclear antibodies and abnormal MRIs of the axial skeleton in the healthy, asymptomatic population, ordering these tests in individuals with nondiscriminative symptoms will lead to erroneous diagnoses in individuals with this spectrum of illness.

COMPLICATIONS AND PROGNOSIS

Frequent complications of FSS are loss of function, distress, maladaptive illness behaviors, psychiatric comorbidities, and disability or compensation claims. Most who study or treat this spectrum of illness believe that early diagnosis, appropriate education, and aggressive treatments in selected patients (e.g., using multidisciplinary therapy) will help prevent these complications, although there are few data to support this. There are compelling data to suggest that once a person develops these complications, and psychobehavioral issues predominate, then this spectrum of illness will be much less amenable to any type of therapy.

Good longitudinal studies examining the predictors or determinants of disability in this spectrum of illness are virtually nonexistent. Longitudinal studies examining this issue in nearly any other chronic medical illness, however, typically demonstrate that an individual's level of formal education, pattern of coping, level of distress, maladaptive beliefs about illness, level of social support, job satisfaction, and work environment are the most important predictors of who will become disabled from work.[107,138] Peripheral or objective factors such as the degree of damage or abnormality on radiograph or MRI, or any other objective laboratory or physical examination finding, are either poor predictors of who will become disabled or are not predictive at all. Those in clinical practice intuitively know this; they have "poster child" patients with crippling rheumatoid arthritis or severe neurodegenerative diseases who never miss a day of work despite severe peripheral disease. However, the disability process focuses on the documentation of these peripheral factors, helping to perpetuate the misconception that these are the most important factors that should be considered when assessing disability.

This focus on peripheral factors has led to some, almost comical attempts, to improve the disability process for persons with fibromyalgia and related conditions. Being asked to document the number of tender points displayed by an individual is one example. It is important to recognize that individuals with fibromyalgia are diffusely tender, and these points are merely regions of the body where everyone experiences increased tenderness. Although performing a tender-point examination certainly gives some measure of an individual's overall pain threshold, in population-based studies the number of tender points that individuals have is strongly correlated with their levels of distress. Counting tender points is an artifactual method for measuring pain threshold, as there are other methods of assessing tenderness that are not influenced by distress or other psychological factors. However, these techniques are cumbersome to use in clinical practice. Thus, a tender-point examination is a surrogate of how distressed an individual is, so much so that Wolfe has suggested that tender points are a "sedimentation rate for distress."[154]

Thus, even though it is likely that the same factors that predict disability in other chronic medical disorders (e.g., low back pain, rheumatoid arthritis, coronary artery disease) predict disability in these illnesses, this information presents a tremendous conundrum to the health care provider who is asked to make an impairment evaluation. If peripheral factors are of limited value in determining who will become disabled, then why do we not just ask our patients how distressed they are, why they are contemplating disability, and what barriers are preventing them from working? Actually, the answers to these questions can be tremendously enlightening. Frequently, the noted longitudinal data are correct. Patients are rarely contemplating disability because their knees will not fully extend, or because their rheumatoid factors are positive, but instead because of a multiplicity of biopsychosocial factors that have overwhelmed their abilities to continue to work in their current environments. The current disability systems sometimes do little to truly accommodate the worker, but instead are frequently adversarial and serve (as described by Dr. Hadler) as a "vortex" to pull down the worker.[58]

Thus, if a provider is making a disability determination on his or her own patient, when the patient initially raises the issue of disability, a prolonged visit should be scheduled to discuss the subject. During these encounters, it is useful to ask the patient in detail why he or she is contemplating applying for disability and what he or she expects to accomplish from it. In particular, patients should be warned that, although disability may look like the solution to their problems, it usually is not. If, despite this effort, the physician and patient cannot design a series of interventions that allows the patient to continue to work, then the examiner must decide whether to support the individual's disability claim. This is a difficult decision, and there are some basic principles that can be used as a guide. Again, the patient's "disease label" should not influence this decision. Although there is collective discomfort in the various FSS symptom complexes such as fibromyalgia, CFS, and Gulf War syndrome, reasonable judgments about the individual's abilities to continue to work must still be attempted.

References

1. Aaron LA, Bradley LA, Alarcon GS, et al: Psychiatric diagnoses in patients with fibromyalgia are related to health care–seeking behavior rather than to illness. Arthritis Rheum 39:436–445, 1996.
2. Ablashi DV: Viral studies of chronic fatigue syndrome. Clin Infect Dis 18(Suppl. 1):S130–S133, 1994.
3. Aggarwal A, Cutts TF, Abell TL, et al: Predominant symptoms in irritable bowel syndrome correlate with specific autonomic nervous system abnormalities [see comments]. Gastroenterology 106:945–950, 1994.
4. Ahles TA, Khan SA, Yunus MB, et al: Psychiatric status of patients with primary fibromyalgia, patients with rheumatoid arthritis, and subjects without pain: A blind comparison of DSM-III diagnoses. Am J Psychiatry 148:1721–1726, 1991.
5. Alvarez Lario B, Teran J, Alonso JL, et al: Lack of association between fibromyalgia and sleep apnoea syndrome. Ann Rheum Dis 51:108–111, 1992.
6. American Psychiatric Association: Diagnostic and Statistical Manual of Mental Disorders. Washington, DC, American Psychiatric Press, 1994.
7. Appel S, Kuritzky A, Zahavi I, et al: Evidence for instability of the autonomic nervous system in patients with migraine headache. Headache 32:10–17, 1992.

8. Arroyo JF, Cohen ML: Abnormal responses to electrocutaneous stimulation in fibromyalgia [see comments]. J Rheumatol 20:1925–1931, 1993.
9. Barker E, Fujimura SF, Fadem MB, et al: Immunologic abnormalities associated with chronic fatigue syndrome. Clin Infect Dis 18(Suppl. 1):S136–S141, 1994.
10. Barsky AJ, Borus JF: Somatization and medicalization in the era of managed care. JAMA 274:1931–1934, 1995.
11. Bell IR. Somatization disorder: Health care costs in the decade of the brain. Biol Psychiatry 35:81–83, 1994.
12. Bendixen M, Muus KM, Schei B: The impact of child sexual abuse—a study of a random sample of Norwegian students. Child Abuse Neglect 18:837–847, 1994.
13. Bengtsson A, Henrickson KG, Larsson J: Muscle biopsy in fibromyalgia. Scand J Rheumatol 15:1–6, 1986.
14. Bengtsson A, Henrickson KG, Larsson J: Reduced high energy phosphate levels in the painful muscles of patients with primary fibromyalgia. Arthritis Rheum 29:817–821, 1986.
15. Bennett RM, Cook DM, Clark SR, et al: Low somatomedin-C in fibromyalgia patients: An analysis of clinical specificity and pituitary/hepatic responses. Arthritis Rheum 36(9S):62, 1993.
16. Bohr T: Problems with myofascial pain syndrome and fibromyalgia syndrome [editorial]. Neurology 46:593–597, 1996.
17. Boissevain MD, McCain GA: Toward an integrated understanding of fibromyalgia syndrome. II. Psychological and phenomenological aspects. Pain 45:239–248, 1991.
18. Bonafede RP, Downey DC, Bennett RM: An association of fibromyalgia with primary Sjögren's syndrome: A prospective study of 72 patients. J Rheumatol 22:133–136, 1995.
19. Bradley LA, Alberts KR, Alarcon GS, et al: Abnormal brain regional cerebral blood flow and cerebrospinal fluid levels of substance P in patients and non-patients with fibromyalgia. Arthritis Rheum 39:1109, 1996.
20. Bridges AJ, Conley C, Wang G, et al: A clinical and immunologic evaluation of women with silicone breast implants and symptoms of rheumatic disease [see comments]. Ann Intern Med 118:929–936, 1993.
21. Brown MR, Fisher LA, Spiess J, et al: Corticotrophin-releasing factor: Actions on the sympathetic nervous system and metabolism. Endocrinology 111:928–931, 1982.
22. Buchwald D, Garrity D: Comparison of patients with chronic fatigue syndrome, fibromyalgia, and multiple chemical sensitivities. Arch Intern Med 154:2049–2053, 1994.
23. Buchwald D, Komaroff AL: Review of laboratory findings for patients with chronic fatigue syndrome. Rev Infect Dis 13(S1):S12–S18, 1991.
24. Buchwald D, Umali P, Umali J, et al: Chronic fatigue and the chronic fatigue syndrome: Prevalence in a Pacific Northwest health care system. Ann Intern Med 123:81–88, 1995.
25. Buzzi M, Bonamini M, Cerbo R: The anatomy and biochemistry of headache. Funct Neurol 8:395–402, 1993.
26. Caro XJ, Ojo-Amaize EA, Agopian MS, Peter JB: Natural killer cell function in primary fibrositis (fibromyalgia) syndrome. Arthritis Rheum 36:D114, 1993.
27. Chester AC, Levine PH: Concurrent sick building syndrome and chronic fatigue syndrome: Epidemic neuromyasthenia revisited. Clin Infect Dis 18(Suppl. 1):S43–S48, 1994.
28. Chrousos GP, Gold PW: The concepts of stress and stress system disorders. Overview of physical and behavioral homeostasis. JAMA 267:1244–1252, 1992.
29. Clauw DJ: Fibromyalgia: More than just a musculoskeletal disease. Am Fam Physician 52:843–0851, 1995.
30. Clauw DJ: The "Gulf War syndrome": Implications for rheumatologists. J Clin Rheum 4:173–174, 1998.
31. Clauw DJ, Gaumond E, Radulovic D, et al: The role of true IgE mediated allergic mechanisms in the allergic symptoms of fibromyalgia. Arthritis Rheum 39:R20, 1996.
32. Clauw DJ, Morris S, Starbuck V, et al: Impairment in cognitive function in individuals with fibromyalgia. Arthritis Rheum 37:R29, 1994.
33. Cleveland CH, Jr, Fisher RH, Brestel EP, et al: Chronic rhinitis: An underrecognized association with fibromyalgia. Allergy Proc 13:263–267, 1992.
34. Cohen ML, Quintner JL: Fibromyalgia syndrome, a problem of tautology. Lancet 342:906–909, 1993.
35. Cope H, Pernet A, Kendall B, David A: Cognitive functioning and magnetic resonance imaging in chronic fatigue. Br J Psychiatry 167:86–94, 1995.
36. Crofford LJ: Neuroendocrine abnormalities in fibromyalgia and related disorders. Am J Med Sci 315:359–366, 1998.
37. Culclasure TF, Enzenauer RJ, West SG: Post-traumatic stress disorder presenting as fibromyalgia. Am J Med 94:548–549, 1993.
38. Dailey PA, Bishop GD, Russell IJ, Fletcher EM: Psychological stress and the fibrositis/fibromyalgia syndrome. J Rheumatol 17:1380–1385, 1990.
39. de Blecourt AC, Wolf RF, van Rijswijk MH, et al: In vivo ^{31}P magnetic resonance spectroscopy (MRS) of tender points in patients with primary fibromyalgia syndrome. Rheumatol Int 11:51–54, 1991.
40. Dekaris D, Sabioncello A, Mazuran R, et al: Multiple changes of immunologic parameters in prisoners of war. JAMA 270:595–599, 1993.
41. Dworkin SF, Massoth DL: Temporomandibular disorders and chronic pain: Disease or illness? J Prosthet Dent 72:29–38, 1994.
42. Elam M, Johansson G, Wallin BG: Do patients with primary fibromyalgia have an altered muscle sympathetic nerve activity? Pain 48:371–375, 1992.
43. Evengard B, Nilsson CG, Lindh G, et al: Chronic fatigue syndrome differs from fibromyalgia. No evidence for elevated substance P levels in cerebrospinal fluid of patients with chronic fatigue syndrome. Pain 78:153–155, 1998.
44. Friedrich EG: Vulvar vestibulitis syndrome. J Reprod Med 32:110–114, 1987.
45. Fukuda K, Straus SE, Hickie I, et al: Chronic fatigue syndrome: A comprehensive approach to its definition and study. Ann Intern Med 121:953–959, 1994.
46. Fukuda K, Nisenbaum R, Stewart G, et al: Chronic multisymptom illness affecting air force veterans of the Gulf War. JAMA 280:981–988, 1999.
47. Fukuda K, Wilson L, Dobbins J: A community-based study of unexplained prolonged and chronic fatiguing illness in a rural area of Michigan. In AACFS 1994 Proceedings. New York, Haworth Medical Press, 1994.
48. Fukudo S, Suzuki J: Colonic motility, autonomic function, and gastrointestinal hormones under psychological stress on irritable bowel syndrome. Tohoku J Exp Med 151:373–385, 1987.
49. Gatti G, Meluzzi A, Francesetti G, et al: Psychoemotional, cognitive, chronoendocrine, and immune responses to a survival performance in an African desert. Ann NY Acad Sci 650:251–256, 1994.
50. Gerster JC, Hadj–Djilani A: Hearing and vestibular abnormalities in primary fibrositis syndrome. J Rheumatol 11:678–680, 1984.
51. Glaser R, Lafuse WP, Bonneau RH, et al: Stress-associated modulation of proto-oncogene expression in human peripheral blood leukocytes. Behav Neurosci 107:525–529, 1993.
52. Gold PW, Goodwin F, Chrousos GP. Clinical and biochemical manifestations of depression: Relationship to the neurobiology of stress (part 1). N Engl J Med 319:348–353, 1988.
53. Goldenberg DL: Fibromyalgia and its relation to chronic fatigue syndrome, viral illness, and immune abnormalities. J Rheumatol 19:91–93, 1989.
54. Gothe CJ, Molin C, Nilsson CG: The environmental somatization syndrome. Psychosomatics 36:1–11, 1995.

55. Granges G, Littlejohn G: Pressure pain threshold in pain-free subjects, in patients with chronic regional pain syndromes, and in patients with fibromyalgia syndrome. Arthritis Rheum 36:642–646, 1993.
56. Granges G, Littlejohn GO: A comparative study of clinical signs in fibromyalgia/fibrositis syndrome, healthy and exercising subjects. J Rheumatol 20:344–351, 1993.
57. Greenfield S, Fitzcharles MA, Esdaile JM: Reactive fibromyalgia syndrome. Arthritis Rheum 35:678–681, 1992.
58. Hadler NM: Fibromyalgia, chronic fatigue, and other iatrogenic diagnostic algorithms. Do some labels escalate illness in vulnerable patients? Postgrad Med 102:161–177, 1997.
59. Hadler NM: Is fibromyalgia a useful diagnostic label? Cleve Clin J Med 63:85–87, 1996.
60. Hazlett RL, Haynes SN: Fibromyalgia: A time-series analysis of the stressor-physical symptom association. J Behav Med 15:541–558, 1992.
61. Hiltz RE, Gupta PK, Maher KA, et al: Low threshold of visceral nociception and significant upper gastrointestinal pathology in patients with fibromyalgia syndrome. Arthritis Rheum 36:C93, 1993.
62. Hudson JI, Goldenberg DL, Pope HG, Jr, et al: Comorbidity of fibromyalgia with medical and psychiatric disorders. Am J Med 92:363–367, 1992.
63. Hudson JI, Hudson MS, Pliner LF, et al: Fibromyalgia and major affective disorder: A controlled phenomenology and family history study. Am J Psychiatry 142:441–446, 1985.
64. Irwin M. Stress-induced immune suppression: Role of brain corticotrophin releasing hormone and autonomic nervous system mechanisms. Adv Neuroimmunol 4:29–47, 1994.
65. Jacobsen S, Bredkjaer SR: The prevalence of fibromyalgia and widespread chronic musculoskeletal pain in the general population [letter; comment]. Scand J Rheumatol 21:261–263, 1992.
66. Jacobsen S, Jensen KE, Thomsen C, et al: ^{31}P magnetic resonance spectroscopy of skeletal muscle in patients with fibromyalgia. J Rheumatol 19:1600–1603, 1993.
67. Jason L, Taylor R, Wagner L, et al: A pilot study estimating rates of chronic fatigue syndrome from a community based sample. Biol Psychol 59:15–27, 2002.
68. Johnson SK, DeLuca J, Fiedler N, Natelson BH: Cognitive functioning of patients with chronic fatigue syndrome. Clin Infect Dis 18(Suppl. 1):S84–S85, 1994.
69. Katon W, Lin E, von Korff M, et al: Somatization: A spectrum of severity. Am J Psychiatry 148:34–40, 1991.
70. Kellow JE, Eckersley GM, Jones M: Enteric and central contributions to intestinal dysmotility in irritable bowel syndrome. Dig Dis Sci 37:168–174, 1992.
71. Kellow JE, Phillips SF: Altered small bowel motility in irritable bowel syndrome is correlated with symptoms. Gastroenterology 92:1885–1893, 1987.
72. Kendler KS, Eaves LJ, Walters EE, et al: The identification and validation of distinct depressive syndromes in a population-based sample of female twins. Arch Gen Psychiatry 53:391–399, 1996.
73. Kendler KS, Walters EE, Truett KR, et al: A twin-family study of self-report symptoms of panic-phobia and somatization. Behav Genet 25:499–515, 1995.
74. Kiecolt-Glaser JK, Cacioppo JT, Malarkey WB, Glaser R: Acute psychological stressors and short-term immune changes: What, why, for whom, and to what extent? Psychosom Med 54:680–685, 1992.
75. Kirmayer LJ, Robbins JM: Three forms of somatization in primary care: Prevalence, co-occurrence, and sociodemographic characteristics. J Nerv Ment Dis 179:647–655, 1991.
76. Komaroff AL: Clinical presentation of chronic fatigue syndrome. Ciba Found Symp 173:43–54; discussion 54–61, 1993.
77. Kosek E, Ekholm J, Hansson P: Increased pressure pain sensibility in fibromyalgia patients is located deep to the skin but not restricted to muscle tissue. Pain 63:335–339, 1995.
78. Kosek E, Ekholm J, Hansson P: Modulation of pressure pain thresholds during and following isometric contraction in patients with fibromyalgia and in healthy controls. Pain 64:415–423, 1996.
79. Koziol JA, Clark DC, Gittes RF, Tan EM: The natural history of interstitial cystitis. J Urology 149:465–469, 1993.
80. Kroenke K, Mangelsdorf AD: Common symptoms in primary care: Incidence, evaluation, therapy, and outcome. Am J Med 86:262–266, 1989.
81. Kroenke K, Spitzer RL, Williams JB, et al: Physical symptoms in primary care. Predictors of psychiatric disorders and functional impairment. Arch Fam Med 3:774–779, 1994.
82. Krupp L, Mendelson W, Friedman R: An overview of chronic fatigue syndrome. J Clin Psychiatry 52:403–410, 1991.
83. Lane TJ, Manu P, Matthews DA: Depression and somatization in the chronic fatigue syndrome. Am J Med 91:335–344, 1991.
84. Lautenbacher S, Rollman GB: Possible deficiencies of pain modulation in fibromyalgia. Clin J Pain 13:189–196, 1997.
85. Lautenbacher S, Rollman GB, McCain GA: Multi-method assessment of experimental and clinical pain in patients with fibromyalgia. Pain 59:45–53, 1994.
86. Lurie M, Caidahl K, Johansson G, Bake B: Respiratory function in chronic primary fibromyalgia. Scand J Rehabil Med 22:151–155, 1990.
87. Lynn R, Friedman L: Irritable bowel syndrome. N Engl J Med 329:1940–1945, 1993.
88. Manu P, Lane TJ, Matthews DA: Chronic fatigue and chronic fatigue syndrome: Clinical epidemiology and aetiological classification. Ciba Found Symp 173:23–31; discussion 31–42, 1993.
89. Manu P, Lane TJ, Matthews DA, et al: Alpha-delta sleep in patients with a chief complaint of chronic fatigue. South Med J 87:465–470, 1994.
90. Mayer EA, Raybould HE: Role of visceral afferent mechanisms in functional bowel disorders. Gastroenterology 99:1688–1704, 1990.
91. McAllister C, Fielding JF: Patients with pulse rate changes in irritable bowel syndrome. Further evidence of altered autonomic function. J Clin Gastroenterol 10:273–274, 1988.
92. McDonald E, Cope H, David A: Cognitive impairment in patients with chronic fatigue: A preliminary study [published erratum appears in J Neurol Neurosurg Psychiatry 56:1142, 1993]. J Neurol Neurosurg Psychiatry 56:812–815, 1993.
93. McKenzie R, Straus SE: Chronic fatigue syndrome. Adv Intern Med 40:119–153, 1995.
94. Meaney MJ, Bhatnagar S, Larocque S, et al: Individual differences in the hypothalamic–pituitary–adrenal stress response and the hypothalamic CRF system. Ann N Y Acad Sci 697:70–85, 1993.
95. Messinger HB, Spierings ELH, Vincent AJP, Lebbink J: Headache and family history. Cephalalgia 11:13–18, 1991.
96. Mikkelsson M, Latikka P, Kautiainen H, et al: Muscle and bone pressure pain threshold and pain tolerance in fibromyalgia patients and controls. Arch Phys Med Rehabil 73:814–818, 1992.
97. Modolfsky H, Scarisbrick P, England R, Smythe H: Musculoskeletal symptoms and non–REM sleep disturbance in patients with "fibrositis syndrome" and healthy subjects. Psychosom Med 37:341–351, 1975.
98. Morrison L, Behan W, Behan P: Changes in natural killer cell phenotype in patients with post viral fatigue syndrome. Clin Exp Immunol 83:441–446, 1991.
99. Mountz JM, Bradley LA, Modell JG, et al: Fibromyalgia in women. Abnormalities of regional cerebral blood flow in the thalamus and the caudate nucleus are associated with low pain threshold levels. Arthritis Rheum 38:926–938, 1995.
100. Mukerji B, Mukerji V, Alpert MA, Selukar R: The prevalence of rheumatologic disorders in patients with chest pain and angiographically normal coronary arteries. Angiology 46:425–430, 1995.

101. NIH Technology Panel: Integration of behavioral and relaxation approaches into the treatment of chronic pain and insomnia. JAMA 240:313–318, 1996.
102. NIH Workshop Panel: The Persian Gulf experience and health. JAMA 272:391–396, 1994.
103. Ojo-Amaize EA, Conley EJ, Peter JB: Decreased natural killer cell activity is associated with severity of chronic fatigue immune dysfunction syndrome. Clin Infect Dis 18(Suppl. 1):S157–S159, 1994.
104. Pareja JA: Chronic paroxysmal hemicrania: Dissociation of the pain and autonomic features. Headache 35:111–113, 1995.
105. Pellegrino MJ, Van Fossen D, Gordon C, et al: Prevalence of mitral valve prolapse in primary fibromyalgia: A pilot investigation. Arch Phys Med Rehabil 70:541–543, 1989.
106. Pellegrino MJ, Waylonis GW, Sommer A: Familial occurrence of primary fibromyalgia. Arch Phys Med Rehabil 70:61–63, 1989.
107. Pincus T, Callahan LF: Associations of low formal education level and poor health status: Behavioral, in addition to demographic and medical, explanations? J Clin Epidemiol 47:355–361, 1994.
108. Pogacnik T, Sega S, Pecnik B, Kiauta T: Autonomic function testing in patients with migraine. Headache 33:545–550, 1993.
109. Prusinski A, Trzos S, Rozentryt P, et al: [Studies of heart rhythm variability in migraine. Preliminary communication.] Neurol Neurochir Pol 28:23–27, 1994.
110. Qiao ZG, Vaery H, Mrkrid L: Electrodermal and microcirculatory activity in patients with fibromyalgia during baseline, acoustic stimulation and cold pressor tests. J Rheumatol 18:1383–1389, 1991.
111. Quintner JL: Somatisation disorder: A major public health issue [letter; comment]. Med J Aust 163:558; discussion 558–559, 1995.
112. Rasmussen A, Nielsen H, Andersen V, et al: Chronic fatigue syndrome—a controlled cross sectional study. J Rheum 21:1527–1532, 1994.
113. Raspe H, Baumgartner C, Wolfe F: The prevalence of fibromyalgia in a rural German community: How much difference do different criteria make? Arthritis Rheum 36:58, 1993.
114. Reynolds WJ, Moldofsky H, Saskin P, Lue FA: The effects of cyclobenzaprine on sleep physiology and symptoms in patients with fibromyalgia. J Rheumatol 18:452–454, 1991.
115. Romero LM, Plotsky PM, Sapolsky RM: Patterns of adrenocorticotropin secretagog release with hypoglycemia, novelty, and restraint after colchicine blockade of axonal transport. Endocrinology 132:199–204, 1993.
116. Rosenhall U, Johansson G, Orndahl G: Eye motility dysfunction in primary fibromyalgia with dysesthesia. Scand J Rehab Med 19:139–145, 1987.
117. Rosner MJ: Personal communication, 1999.
118. Rowe PC, Bou-Holaigah I, Kan JS, Calkins H. Is neurally mediated hypotension an unrecognised cause of chronic fatigue? Lancet 345:623–624, 1995.
119. Russell IJ, Orr MD, Littman B, et al: Elevated cerebrospinal fluid levels of Substance P in patients with the fibromyalgia syndrome. Arthritis Rheum 37:1593–1601, 1994.
120. Russell IJ, Vaeroy H, Javors M, Nyberg F: Cerebrospinal fluid biogenic amine metabolites in fibromyalgia/fibrositis syndrome and rheumatoid arthritis [see comments]. Arthritis Rheum 35:550–556, 1992.
121. Russo J, Katon W, Sullivan M, et al: Severity of somatization and its relationship to psychiatric disorders and personality. Psychosomatics 35:546–556, 1994.
122. Salit I. Precipitating factors for the chronic fatigue syndrome. Biol Psychol 31:59–65, 1997.
123. Sapolsky RM: Why stress is bad for your brain. Science 273:749–750, 1996.
124. Shorter E: Chronic fatigue in historical perspective. Ciba Found Symp 173:6–16, 1993.
125. Silman A, Schollum J, Croft P: The epidemiology of tender point counts in the general population. Arthritis Rheum 36:59, 1993.
126. Simms RW, Goldenberg DL: Symptoms mimicking neurologic disorders in fibromyalgia syndrome. J Rheumatol 15:1271–1273, 1988.
127. Simms RW, Roy S, Skrinar G, et al: Lack of association between fibromyalgia syndrome and abnormalities in muscle energy metabolism. Arthritis Rheum 37:794–800, 1994.
128. Slotkoff AT, Radulovic DA, Clauw DJ: The relationship between multiple chemical hypersensitivity and fibromyalgia. Arthritis Rheum 37:1117, 1994.
129. Smith GR, Monson R, Ray D: Patients with multiple unexplained symptoms: Their characteristics, functional health, and health care utilization. Arch Intern Med 146:69–72, 1986.
130. Spaccarelli S: Stress, appraisal, and coping in child sexual abuse: A theoretical and empirical review. Psychol Bull 116:340–362, 1994.
131. Stein M, Keller S, Schleifer S: Stress and immunomodulation: The role of depression and neuroendocrine function. J Immun 135:827s–833s, 1985.
132. Stein-Behrens BA, Lin WJ, Sapolsky RM: Physiological elevations of glucocorticoids potentiate glutamate accumulation in the hippocampus. J Neurochem 63:596–602, 1994.
133. Stein-Behrens B, Mattson MP, Chang I, et al: Stress exacerbates neuron loss and cytoskeletal pathology in the hippocampus. J Neurosci 14:5373–5380, 1994.
134. Sternberg EM: Hyperimmune fatigue syndromes: Diseases of the stress response? J Rheumatol 20:418–421, 1993.
135. Stormorken H, Brosstad F: Fibromyalgia: Family clustering and sensory urgency with early onset indicate genetic predisposition and thus a "true" disease. Scand J Rheumatol 21:207, 1992.
136. Straus SE: Studies of herpesvirus infection in chronic fatigue syndrome. Ciba Found Symp 173:132–139; discussion 139–145, 1994.
137. Sutton RE, Koob GF, Le Moal M, et al: Corticotrophin releasing factor produces behavioral activation in rats. Nature 297:331–333, 1982.
138. Turk DC: The role of demographic and psychosocial factors in transition from acute to chronic pain. In Jensen TS, Turner JA, Wiesenfeld-Hallin Z (eds): Proceedings of the 8th World Congress on Pain. Seattle, IASP Press, 1997, pp 185–214.
139. Unwin C, Blatchley N, Coker W, et al: Health of UK servicemen who served in the Persian Gulf War. Lancet 353:169–178, 1999.
140. Urrows S, Affleck G, Tennen H, Higgins P: Unique clinical and psychological correlates of fibromyalgia tender points and joint tenderness in rheumatoid arthritis. Arthritis Rheum 37:1513–1520, 1994.
141. Vaeroy H, Helle R, Forre O, et al: Elevated CSF levels of Substance P and high incidence of Raynaud's phenomenon in patients with fibromyalgia: New features for diagnosis. Pain 32:21–26, 1988.
142. van Denderen JC, Boersma JW, Zeinstra P, et al: Physiological effects of exhaustive physical exercise in primary fibromyalgia syndrome (PFS): Is PFS a disorder of neuroendocrine reactivity? Scand J Rheumatol 21:35–37, 1992.
143. Viau V, Sharma S, Plotsky PM, Meaney MJ: Increased plasma ACTH responses to stress in nonhandled compared with handled rats require basal levels of corticosterone and are associated with increased levels of ACTH secretagogues in the median eminence. J Neurosci 13:1097–1105, 1993.
144. Wallace DJ: Genitourinary manifestations of fibrositis: An increased association with the female urethral syndrome. J Rheumatol 17:238–239, 1990.
145. Walling MK, O'Hara MW, Reiter RC, et al: Abuse history and chronic pain in women: II. A multivariate analysis of abuse and psychological morbidity. Obstet Gynecol 84:200–206, 1994.
146. Waylonis GW, Heck W: Fibromyalgia syndrome. New associations. Am J Phys Med Rehabil 71:343–348, 1992.

147. Waylonis GW, Perkins RH: Post-traumatic fibromyalgia. A long-term follow-up. Am J Phys Med Rehabil 73:403–412, 1994.
148. Welin M, Bragee B, Nyberg F, Kristiansson M: Elevated Substance P levels are contrasted by a decrease in met–encephalin–arg–phe levels in CSF from fibromyalgia patients. J Musculoskel Pain 3:4, 1995.
149. Wessely S, Chalder T, Hirsch S, et al: Psychological symptoms, somatic symptoms, and psychiatric disorder in chronic fatigue and chronic fatigue syndrome: a prospective study in the primary care setting. Am J Psychiatry 153:1050–1059, 1996.
150. White AM, Stevens WH, Upton AR, et al: Airway responsiveness to inhaled methacholine in patients with irritable bowel syndrome. Gastroenterology 100:68–74, 1991.
151. Whitehead WE, Holtkotter B, Enck P: Tolerance for rectosigmoid distension in irritable bowel syndrome. Gastroenterology 98:1187–1192, 1990.
152. Whorwell PJ, Clouter C, Smith CL: Oesophageal motility in the irritable bowel syndrome. Br Med J 282:1101–1102, 1981.
153. Whorwell PJ, Lupton EW, Erduran D, Wilson K: Bladder smooth muscle dysfunction in patients with irritable bowel syndrome. Gut 27:1014–1017, 1986.
154. Wolfe F: The relation between tender points and fibromyalgia symptom variables: Evidence that fibromyalgia is not a discrete disorder in the clinic. Ann Rheum Dis 56:268–271, 1997.
155. Wolfe F, Ross K, Anderson J, Russell IJ: Aspects of fibromyalgia in the general population: Sex, pain threshold, and fibromyalgia symptoms. J Rheumatol 22:151–156, 1995.
156. Wolfe F, Ross K, Anderson J, et al: The prevalence and characteristics of fibromyalgia in the general population. Arthritis Rheum 38:19–28, 1995.
157. Wolfe F, Smythe HA, Yunus MB, et al: The American College of Rheumatology 1990 Criteria for the Classification of Fibromyalgia. Report of the Multicenter Criteria Committee [see comments]. Arthritis Rheum 33:160–172, 1990.
158. Yunus MB: Fibromyalgia syndrome: New research on an old malady. BMJ 298:474–475, 1989.
159. Yunus MB: Towards a model of pathophysiology of fibromyalgia: Aberrant central pain mechanisms with peripheral modulation [editorial]. J Rheumatol 19:846–850, 1992.
160. Yunus MB, Ahles TA, Aldag JC, Masi AT: Relationship of clinical features with psychological status in primary fibromyalgia. Arthritis Rheum 34:15–21, 1991.
161. Yunus MB, Dailey JW, Aldag JC, et al: Plasma tryptophan and other amino acids in primary fibromyalgia: A controlled study. J Rheumatol 19:90–94, 1992.
162. Zigelman M, Appel S, Davidovitch S, et al: The effect of verapamil calcium antagonist on autonomic imbalance in migraine: Evaluation by spectral analysis of beat-to-beat heart rate fluctuations. Headache 34:569–577, 1994.

IMPAIRMENT EVALUATION IN FUNCTIONAL SOMATIC SYNDROMES

STEPHEN L. DEMETER, MD, MPH

The assessment of impairment for the FSS is a challenging prospect. As described by Clauw in this chapter, these diagnoses are controversial and unsupported by definitive objective tests. Yet they attempt to describe medical conditions that can cause impairment as well as disability for individuals who possess the signs and symptoms of these disease processes. Their lack of support in mainstream medicine has, at its heart, the lack of verifiable, objective tests to conclude their presence.

As mentioned by Clauw and delineated in the following list, there are a number of conditions that are considered to be FSS:

1. Fibromyalgia
2. CFS
3. IBS
4. MCSS
5. Sick building syndrome
6. Repetitious stress injury
7. Chronic whiplash
8. Chronic Lyme disease
9. Side effects of silicone breast implants
10. Candidiasis hypersensitivity
11. Gulf War syndrome
12. Food allergies
13. Mitral valve prolapse
14. Chronic carbon monoxide poisoning
15. Chronic mononucleosis
16. Symptoms resulting from exposure to video display terminals, carbonless copy paper, and weak electromagnetic fields

Common threads running through the FSS tapestry are: 1) lack of scientific validity; 2) lack of medical recognition; 3) acceptance by the lay press; 4) confusion on the part of medical caregivers; 5) multiplicity of organ system involvement; 6) multiple Internet sites devoted to these conditions; and 7) reliance by affected persons on nontraditional healers, methods, and medications (usually consisting of herbal preparations, minerals, or massive doses of vitamins). However, as time and science progress, some of these syndromes are yielding to scientific acceptance or nonacceptance as mechanisms of disease are being discovered. Others have gained medical acceptance as more individuals are found to share a commonality of signs and symptoms despite a lack of validating tests. Examples of this medical validity include Barlow syndrome (for mitral valve prolapse), fibromyalgia, and, to some extent, CFS.

SCIENTIFIC VERSUS MEDICAL VALIDITY OF THE FUNCTIONAL SOMATIC SYNDROMES

The three principal diagnoses included under the umbrella term FSS are fibromyalgia, CFS, and MCSS. The most recent listing of the ICDM codes lists both fibromyalgia (729.1; p 136) and CFS (780.71; p 133)[3] as valid diagnoses with codes. MCSS is not listed.[9]

Western medicine has, from its earliest origins, attempted to provide a scientific rationale for medical conditions. (Eastern medicine, in contrast, has adopted a more philosophical approach to disease causation and treatment.) Hippocrates ascribed various medical conditions to the influences of vapors and evil humors. What the ancient Greeks were attempting to describe were the physiologic, biochemical, or microbiological causations of various medical syndromes at a time when medical science was incapable of providing a better answer. As time and science progressed, many of these root causes became known and the "evil humors" were relabeled based on the scientific discoveries that better explained the condition. Thus, we now discuss tuberculosis by its principal cause—*Mycobacterium tuberculosis*—rather than by older terms that implied a lack of scientific understanding, such as consumption, when that understanding was not available. We recognize that the hemoptysis, wasting, and breathing difficulties are caused by the effects of germs on the respiratory tract of the host rather than the influences of "evil humors." The clinical description of the effects of tuberculosis and the medical manifestations caused by this infection were known to the ancient Greeks. The only thing unknown to them was the causation and, hence, the scientific validity of the disease process.

Put in this context, where is the scientific validity of the FSS? Again, as described by Clauw, medical science has attempted to describe and discover the scientific validity of these diagnoses but to little avail as of 2002. That may change in the near future, distant future, or not at all. If there is no current scientific validity, can there be any medical validity? In other words, if medical science cannot prove the existence of a disease process, can that disease process still have validity, can it be accepted as a medical condition by mainstream medicine and/or science, and can it be afforded an "official" diagnostic status sufficient for it to be a credible cause of the disease process and, for the purposes of this book, a sufficient reason for impairment and/or disability?

Again, to turn to the tuberculosis model, sick people have signs and symptoms. The commonality and types of signs and symptoms in people who had tuberculosis led to their being diagnosed with "consumption." Yet there were probably many people with diagnoses of consumption who actually had other diseases. With the advance of medical science, we were able to define, refine, and narrow the causes, condition, symptoms, investigations, diagnosis, and treatment for this particular disease. However, the reason that we can now recognize tuberculosis as a distinct disease entity started with the recognition of the commonality of the signs and symptoms in a certain segment of nonhealthy people. We are at the same point with these three diagnoses: fibromyalgia, CFS, and MCSS. Again, at some point in time, there may be scientific validation for their existence. If not, then the signs and symptoms of these conditions will be ascribed to some other disease process that will have better scientific validation.

Therefore, can we currently accept any of these three diagnoses as valid medical syndromes? Further, can we provide impairment ratings for any of them?

VALIDITY OF THE FUNCTIONAL SOMATIC SYNDROMES AS TRUE MEDICAL SYNDROMES USING PSYCHIATRIC ILLNESSES AS A MODEL

A syndrome is defined as "The aggregate of symptoms and signs associated with any morbid process, and constituting together the picture of the disease; a concurrence of symptoms."[12] Thus, by definition, all three of the FSS are syndromes, notwithstanding their lack of scientific credibility. Each possesses certain diagnostic criteria (see Boxes 42–1 through 42–3). Individuals diagnosed with any of the three will share certain signs and symptoms. A sufficient number of these signs or symptoms allows a physician to make the diagnosis of the syndrome regardless of the medical or scientific acceptance of the diagnosis.

When examined de novo, there are similarities between psychiatric disorders and the FSS. They both describe syndromes that have little scientific validity if one defines scientific validity as possessing anatomic, tissue, biochemical, immunologic, microbiological, or other scientific underpinnings. Medical science is just now beginning to show scientific validation for some, but certainly not all, of the psychiatric disorders. A recent textbook of psychiatry lists several potential causal mechanisms for schizophrenia: genetic factors, neurodevelopmental factors, viral exposures, autoimmune phenomena, and abnormalities in various neurotransmitters.[4,10] Neuroimaging studies have shown several abnormalities of unknown significance, including diminished cortical gray matter (especially in the temporal cortex), decreased volume in the limbic system, and diminished volume of the basal ganglia nuclei.[4] Biological abnormalities in patients with depression include abnormalities in the hypothalamic-pituitary axis (especially with respect to cortisol secretion), GH, serotonin (especially in the brainstem; lower than normal levels of serotonin and its major metabolite 5-hydroxyindoleacetic acid [5-HIAA] can be found in the CSF of suicidal patients and lower levels of both are found in the brains of suicide completers who also have increased postsynaptic numbers of serotonin [5-hydroxytryptamine type 2 {5-HT_2}] receptors in the prefrontal cortex; platelet 5-HT_2 receptors are also increased in subjects with suicidal behavior), and other neurotransmitters.[11,13]

Despite the recent work demonstrating these abnormalities in patients with schizophrenia and depression, the diagnosis of these disorders is still a clinical one. A review of the diagnostic criteria for these diseases in the most recent edition of the Diagnostic and Statistical Manual of Mental Disorders[2] amply demonstrates this point.

Thus we are at a turning point with respect to psychiatric diseases. These diseases have always enjoyed medical validity despite a lack of scientific validity, until recently. Witness the revolution in the understanding and treatment of depression from the days when it was described as melancholia and thought to be a personality defect to the current time when we can demonstrate biochemical deficiencies in certain parts of the neuroanatomy and treat them with medications that replete these chemicals. We have even extended the medications used in the treatment of depression to other psychiatric illnesses such as obsessive-compulsive disorders, with good results, despite the lack of scientific justification. Yet the lack of scientific credibility never stood in the way of the recognition of these disease states, the compartmentalization of various psychiatric diagnoses, or the treatment of these conditions. If recognition and treatment for psychiatric illnesses had waited for scientific validation, we would just now be able to diagnose and treat depression. However, we would only now be able to tentatively diagnose schizophrenia, but not treat it. We would still not be able to even diagnose anxiety disorders, bipolar disorders, delirium, multiple personality disorders, and many others.

Because the psychiatric field depended for so long on clinical diagnoses, many individuals have attempted to place the FSS into this arena (see the discussion by Clauw in the sections on somatoform disorders and their relationship with psychiatric disorders). To do so is to discredit the science of psychiatry whose scientific validity is just now emerging as well as people who have any of the FSS. However, the psychiatric model is useful in understanding the medical validity for the FSS as well as the principles of impairment evaluation for these conditions.

A critical analysis of all psychological tests yields the finding that all are basically based on 1) self-reports of abnormalities in daily functioning, 2) an analysis of self-reports of the patient by a professional observer, 3) stereotypical responses on tests of self-reports by the patient, or 4) supporting observations of the behavior of the patient by those close to him or her (see Chapter 38). These diagnoses are valid and legitimate despite the absence of objective testing. For schizophrenia and depression, gene tests are not sufficiently refined to permit their use in diagnosis. The inheritance potential is merely that—a potential—and not sufficiently useful on its own to permit a validated diagnosis. Radiologic imaging is insufficient to make an unsupported diagnosis. Finally, few patients would submit to a brain biopsy for an analysis of their neurotransmitters in order to establish a diagnosis. Ultimately, psychiatric diagnoses are based on reports of behavioral deviations—whether self-reported, reported by family members, or based on a professional observation or answers on a psychological test.

The FSS share these features with psychological diagnoses, which is not to imply that they are psychological abnormalities. They are based on self-observational data without confirmation by objective testing. They can be supported by observations by friends or family members. They can be typified by professional observers and assessors. They share commonalities with published profiles.

IMPAIRMENT ASSESSMENT IN FUNCTIONAL SOMATIC SYNDROMES

The assessment of impairment for the FSS is not found in the fifth edition of the AMA Guides. There are two reasons for this. First, these are controversial diagnoses, as pointed out by Clauw and in this addendum. Secondly, the Guides tries to avoid rating impairments that are based solely on subjective criteria: "Given the range, evolution, and discovery of new medical conditions, the Guides cannot provide an impairment rating for all impairments. Also, since come medical syndromes are poorly understood and are manifested only by subjective symptoms, impairment ratings are not provided for those conditions."[5(p11)] Also:

> The Guides uses objective and scientifically based data when available and references these sources. When objective data have not been identified, estimates of the degree of impairment are used, based on clinical experience and consensus. Subjective concerns, including fatigue, difficulty in concentrating, and pain, when not accompanied by demonstrable clinical signs or other independent, measurable abnormalities, are generally not given separate impairment ratings. ... The Guides does not deny the existence or importance of these subjective complaints to the individual or their functional impact. The Guides recommends that the physician ascertain and document subjective concerns. Because the presence and severity of subjective concerns varies among individuals with the same condition, the Guides has not yet identified an accepted method with the scientific literature to ascertain how these concerns consistently affect organ or body system functioning.[5(p10)]

In 1999, the American Academy of Disability Evaluating Physicians (AADEP) drafted and published three position papers, after receiving approval by the Fellowship. These were published in the same year and they deal with the three subjects discussed in this addendum: fibromyalgia, CFS, and MCSS.[1] Although based on the fourth edition of the Guides, an examination of the Academy's positions for these three conditions is useful.

For fibromyalgia, the recommendations for assessing impairment provided by the position paper were unclear but are as follows:

> Table 1 shows the usual areas of potential impairment in persons with fibromyalgia. These include the most common areas—generalized pain and/or pain intensification, fatigue, and cognitive difficulties, less common problem areas such as headache and irritable bowel syndrome, and other conditions that are often found in persons with fibromyalgia—arthritis and axial skeletal disorders.[1(p3)]

The position paper then suggests assessing impairment for each of the complicating features:

> Pain can be handled either in the separate pain section or, alternatively for some patients in the mental and behavioral disorders section. There is no listing for fatigue in the AMA Guides, and therefore it must be handled in the mental and behavioral disorders section. Cognitive difficulties are also evaluated in the mental and behavioral disorders section. The musculoskeletal section of the Guides is not appropriate for rating fibromyalgia uncomplicated by other comorbid musculoskeletal conditions.[1(pp3–4)]

The paper then gives a recommended classification scheme for fibromyalgia based on its interference with the activities of daily living (reprinted as Table 42–3).

The confusing aspect of AADEP's approach exists in the duality of approaches to assessment of impairment and the lack of whole person impairment numbers for the separate classes found in Table 42–3.

The same lack of clear direction exists in its position paper on CFS:

> At the present time, impairment rating is best done based upon areas of impairment manifested by the specific individual using known guides and specifically the AMA Guides to the Evaluation of Permanent Impairment (4th Edition). Musculoskeletal ratings are not relevant since there is no apparent musculoskeletal basis for limitation in the CFS patient. If there happens to be a concurrent musculoskeletal or joint abnormality then the appropriate section should be used. The chapter relating to the nervous system, which is Chapter 4, pages 142–143, provides Tables 2, 3, and 6, which include impairments that patients with CFS frequently demonstrate. However, these tables should not be used as a means of impairment rating for chronic fatigue syndrome patients because the Guides state that there have to be neurologic impairments present before using the emotional or behavioral impairment rating tables in Chapter 4. If a sleep disorder is diagnosed, then Table 6 in Chapter 4 may be used.[1(p4)]

In its summary, the position paper states: "Impairment ratings cannot be determined with any single tool at present. They are best determined by detailed review of daily activities and ability to function (performing basic work activities)."[1(p5)]

The paper provides a classification system similar to the one provided for fibromyalgia (although, again, no numbers are suggested) (reprinted here as Table 42–4).

For MCSS, the Academy chose not to provide impairment ratings or rate this syndrome, based on its lack of scientific credibility:

> Based upon a lack of objective permanent clinical findings, MCS should not be rated as a permanent medical impairment. However, individuals with recognized psychiatric conditions, who meet DSM-IV criteria, may be rated according to criteria in the mental and behavioral disorder section in the AMA Guides, or by state or federal guidelines. This committee concludes that the current medical and scientific evidence is inadequate to support an impairment rating for MCS, based on use of the current AMA Guides to the Evaluation of Permanent Impairment. Individuals with MCS who feel disabled as a result of their symptoms need to investigate disability regulations in their state[1(p8)]

As noted, the Academy's position papers were based on the fourth edition of the Guides. However, there are no changes in the fifth edition that have caused the Academy to revise its positions. Notwithstanding the criticisms offered here, the Academy made an important contribution in providing a method, for the first time, for the evaluation of impairment in the FSS.

TABLE 42–3

Classification of Impairments Associated with Fibromyalgia Related Complaints

Problems	Class 1: No Impairment	Class 2: Mild Impairment	Class 3: Moderate Impairment	Class 4: Marked Impairment	Class 5: Extreme Impairment
Pain, fatigue, cognitive dysfunction	No ADL impairment	Impairment levels are compatible with most useful functioning	Impairment levels are compatible with some, but not all useful functioning	Impairment levels significantly impede useful functioning	Impairment levels preclude useful functioning

ADL, activities of daily living.

From American Academy of Disability Evaluating Physicians: Compendium of position papers on impairment and disability issues. Disability 8, 1999, with permission.

TABLE 42-4

Classification of Impairments Associated with Chronic Fatigue Syndrome

Area or Aspect of Functioning	Class 1: No Impairment	Class 2: Mild Impairment	Class 3: Moderate Impairment	Class 4: Marked Impairment	Class 5: Extreme Impairment
Activities of daily living, self care, basic work activities, social functioning, concentration, memory	No impairment is noted	Impairment levels are compatible with most useful functioning	Impairment levels are compatible with some, but not all, useful functioning	Impairment levels significantly impede useful functioning	Impairment levels preclude useful functioning

From American Academy of Disability Evaluating Physicians: Compendium of position papers on impairment and disability issues. Disability 5, 1999, with permission.

RECOMMENDED METHOD OF ASSESSMENT AND RATING FOR THE FUNCTIONAL SOMATIC SYNDROMES

> Given the range, evolution, and discovery of new medical conditions, the Guides cannot provide an impairment rating for all impairments. ... In situations where impairment ratings are not provided, the Guides suggests that physicians use clinical judgment resulting from the unlisted condition to measurable impairment resulting from similar conditions with similar impairment of function in performing activities of daily living. The physician's judgment, based upon experience, training, skill, thoroughness in clinical evaluation, and ability to apply the Guides criteria as intended, will enable an appropriate and reproducible assessment to be made of clinical impairment. Clinical judgment, combining both the 'art' and 'science' of medicine, constitutes the essence of medical practice."[5(p11)]

Thus, the Guides makes provision for clinical conditions that are not specifically addressed in the book. Each of the FSS should be approached in this fashion. If an examinee has an established and supportable diagnosis of one of the FSS based on the history, physical examination, and review of the medical records or if such a diagnosis is suggested de novo by the impairment examination, then the evaluator must decide two important issues—whether he or she believes that the given diagnosis is medically valid and how to rate the claimant.

If the physician does not believe that MCSS is a valid diagnosis, for example, it should be noted in the report. Conversely, if the physician accepts this diagnosis as medically valid, then the report should include a comment to the effect that this diagnosis does not claim current medical legitimacy. The same holds true for the other two syndromes although, as pointed out, their legitimacy is less questioned.

If one chooses not to believe in the medical validity of these diagnoses, the easy answer when rating impairment is to state that no impairment exists because no disease exists. That will, however, leave the physician open to criticism concerning consistency if the physician also rates other conditions that have no scientifically verifiable or objectively verifiable basis, such as pain, tinnitus, psychiatric conditions, and others that are rated by the AMA Guides.

These conditions should be assessed and rated based on their influence and interference in the activities of daily life of the examinee, regardless of their scientific or objective verity. This recommendation is in keeping with the general philosophy of the Guides: "The physician's role in performing an impairment evaluation is to provide an independent, unbiased assessment of the individual's medical condition, including its effect on

TABLE 42-5

Classes of Impairment Due to Mental and Behavioral Disorders

Area or Aspect of Functioning	Class 1 No Impairment	Class 2 Mild Impairment	Class 3 Moderate Impairment	Class 4 Marked Impairment	Class 5 Extreme Impairment
Acitivities of daily living Social functioning Concentration Adaptation	No impairment noted	Impairment levels are compatible with most useful functioning	Impairment levels are compatible with some, but not all, useful functioning	Impairment levels significantly impede useful functioning	Impairment levels preclude useful functioning

From Cocchiarella L, Andersson GBJ (eds): Guides to the Evaluation of Permanent Impairment, 5th ed. Chicago, American Medical Association, 2001, p 363, with permission.

function, and identify abilities and limitations to performing activities of daily living…"[5(p18)] Also, "Impairment percentages or ratings developed by medical specialists are consensus-derived estimates that reflect the severity of the medical condition and the degree to which the impairment decreases an individual's ability to perform common activities of daily living (ADL), excluding work. Impairment ratings were designed to reflect functional limitations and not disability."[5(p4)]

Considering the FSS, they each create an impact on the individual's ADL, regardless of whether they are medically or scientifically verifiable by objective testing, or even medically credible. Therefore, when a psychiatric condition is present, Table 14–1 in the mental and behavioral chapter of the Guides (reprinted here as Table 42–5) can be used as a suggested method of rating the FSS.

References

1. American Academy of Disability Evaluating Physicians: Compendium of position papers on impairment and disability issues. Disability October 1999.
2. American Psychiatric Association: Diagnostic and Statistical Manual of Mental Disorders, 4th ed, rev. Washington, DC, American Psychiatric Association, 2000.
3. Barsky AJ, Borus JF: Functional somatic syndromes. Ann Intern Med 130:910–921, 1999.
4. Buchanan RW, Carpenter WT, Jr: Schizophrenia: Introduction and overview. In Sadock BJ, Sadock VA (eds): Comprehensive Textbook of Psychiatry, 7th ed. Philadelphia, Lippincott Williams & Wilkins, 2000, pp 1096–1110.
5. Cocchiarella L, Andersson GBJ (eds): Guides to the Evaluation of Permanent Impairment, 5th ed. Chicago, American Medical Association, 2001.
6. Cullen MR: The worker with multiple chemical sensitivities: An overview. In Cullen M (ed): Workers with Multiple Chemical Sensitivities. Philadelphia, Hanley & Belfus, 1987, pp 655–662.
7. Fiedler N, Kipen H: Neurobehavioral and psychosocial aspects of multiple chemical sensitivity. In National Research Council: Multiple Chemical Sensitivities. Addendum to Biologic Markers in Immunotoxicology. Washington, DC, National Academy Press, 1992, pp 109–116.
8. Fukuda K, Straus SE, Hickie I, et al: The chronic fatigue syndrome: A comprehensive approach to its definition and study. International Chronic Fatigue Syndrome Study Group. Ann Intern Med 121:953–959, 1994.
9. International Classification of Diseases, 9th rev, vol 2. Chicago, AMA Press, 2001.
10. McClellan JM: Early-onset schizophrenia. In Sadock BJ, Sadock VA (eds): Comprehensive Textbook of Psychiatry, 7th ed. Philadelphia, Lippincott Williams & Wilkins, 2000, pp 2782–2789.
11. Patacki CS: Mood disorders and suicide in children and adolescents. In Sadock BJ, Sadock VA (eds): Comprehensive Textbook of Psychiatry, 7th ed. Philadelphia, Lippincott Williams & Wilkins, 2000, pp 2740–2757.
12. Stedman's Medical Dictionary, 27th ed. Philadelphia, Lippincott Williams & Wilkins, 2000.
13. Thase ME: Mood disorders: Neurobiology. In Sadock BJ, Sadock VA (eds): Comprehensive Textbook of Psychiatry, 7th ed. Philadelphia, Lippincott Williams & Wilkins, 2000, pp 1318–1328.
14. Wolfe F, Smythe HA, Yunus MB, et al: The American College of Rheumatology 1990 criteria for the classification of fibromyalgia. Arthritis Rheum 33:160–172, 1990.

PART

III

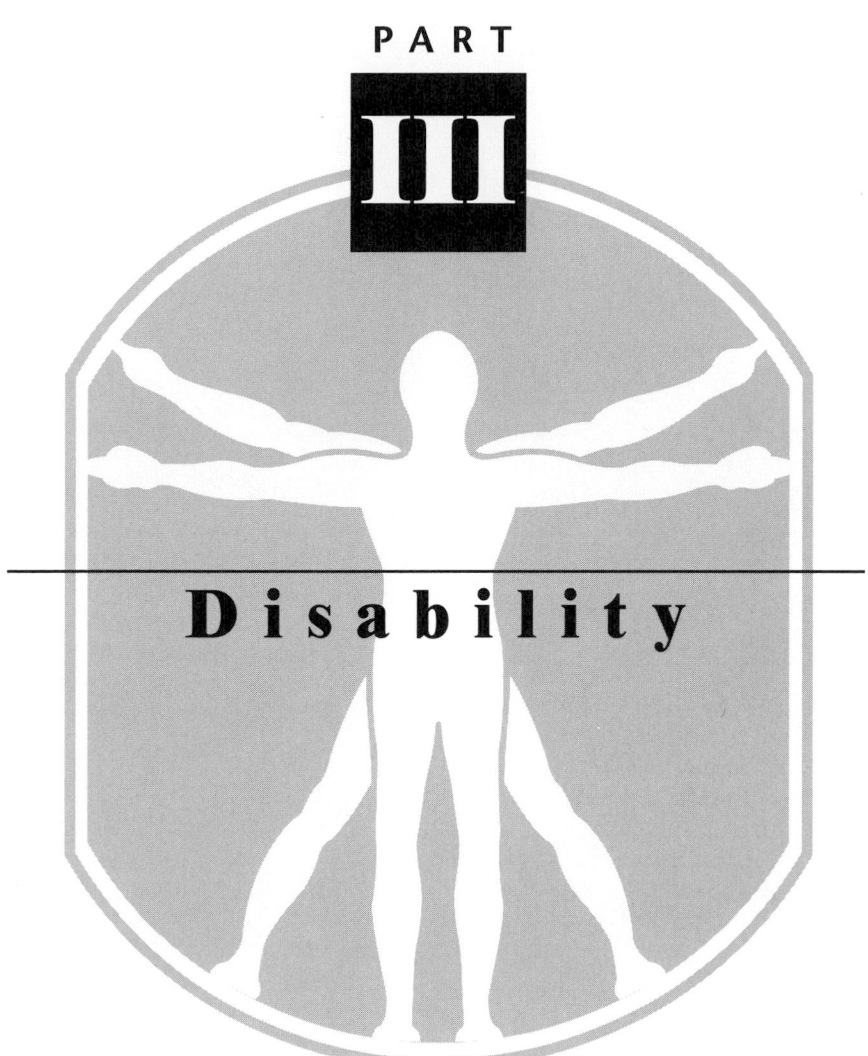

Disability

SECTION

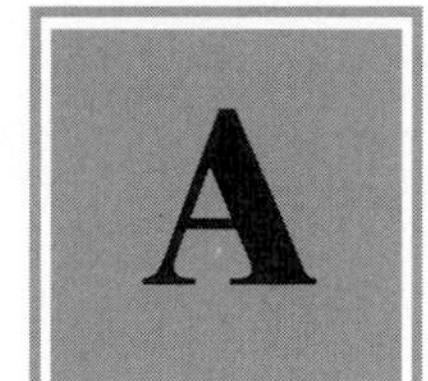

Introductory Concepts

CHAPTER

43

The Disability Evaluation and Report

STEPHEN L. DEMETER, MD, MPH ■ RONALD J. WASHINGTON, MD, FAADEP

As noted in Chapter 11, there are fundamental differences between an impairment evaluation and report and a standard medical evaluation and report. A disability evaluation and report falls in between these two types of examinations.

The purpose of a disability evaluation is to define, measure, and determine an examinee's health status and catalogue that person's impairment(s). The evaluator then takes that information and describes the patient's capabilities or incapabilities with reference to a certain job, function, or task. The disability evaluation is usually (but not always) used by an employer when placing an injured or ill worker back into the workplace following recovery from the injury or illness.

In an impairment evaluation, it is incumbent upon the evaluator to be familiar with the impairment rating system used for a given evaluation. Likewise, the disability evaluator must be knowledgeable of the laws and regulations that touch on this discipline. One of the most important laws that can and will affect an imperfectly recovered worker is the Americans With Disabilities Act. It and other pertinent laws are described in Chapter 47. Another important issue to be aware of is the evaluator's liability when recommending placement in a job situation. If a physician clears a worker to return to work prematurely and the demands of the job exceed the worker's capabilities and further injury occurs, or the worker is returned and, because of poorly described impairments, a coworker suffers harm, then the physician is open to a lawsuit. His or her malpractice insurance may or may not cover the liability incurred in these types of situations. Physicians are urged to discuss these issues with their malpractice carrier or lawyer (see also Chapter 46).

The disability report differs from the impairment report. The goal of an impairment report is to achieve an impairment rating. The goal of the disability report is to describe, to a third party, what a person can or cannot do, as well as to describe methods of overcoming those limitations. The ideal disability report is proactive rather than restrictive. It describes what a person's capabilities are, with and without job modifications, rather than focusing on what the person cannot do or cannot be exposed to.

The disability report may be very short—sometimes, only a notation on a prescription form that a patient may or may not return to work and details of any restrictions that are necessary. The report may also be written on forms provided by the employer. These types of reports or recommendations are usually sufficient for the patient who has completely recovered from an injury or an illness. Various sources describing the expected time for healing from surgical interventions or recovery from medical illnesses exist (see Chapter 1). These issues will not be addressed, except inferentially, in this section.

The forms provided by employers are generally a source of irritation and frustration for the treating physician. Rarely are they specified for the worker's injury or illness. All too often, they are generic forms, which usually contain the Department of Labor's work capability listings (see Chapter 48). The frustration and irritation stem from several sources: 1) the forms may or may not (usually do not) have anything to do with the injured or ill patient's medical problem; 2) the forms may or may not (usually do not) have anything to do with the patient's job; and 3) the forms provide no directions on how to fill them out. For example, does

Parts of this chapter were taken from Chapters 2 and 11 of the first edition of this book which was co-authored by George M. Smith, MD, MPH.

the legal secretary with a low back injury need to have a complete and formal functional capacity assessment to determine her ability to lift 10, 25, or 50 pounds, or her ability to do this 1, 3, 5, or 8 hours per day? Clearly there must be a better way.

This chapter is written for physicians and nonphysicians alike. As discussed in Chapter 1, communication is absolutely necessary for all involved parties to optimally assist the injured or ill patient or worker. Further, a language that all parties can understand must be used.

As noted, disability evaluations and reports span the gamut from very simple to extremely complex. The more complex evaluations are actually easier to perform because the physician and the referring source are usually very clear on each party's roles and expectations of these evaluations and reports. A special problem, however, exists with the very simple return-to-work forms. Unless a patient gives specific consent, the treating physician should be wary of providing medical information (such as diagnoses or treatment), as the inclusion of this material may breach doctor-patient confidentiality.

It is the primary intention of this chapter as well as a recurring goal of this book to address the sources of the problems that exist within the current disability evaluating arena. This chapter offers many generic recommendations and focuses on the extremely complex and detailed evaluation and report, while recognizing that most evaluations will be of lesser complexity and detail. The tables provided may be used as a general background reference or as a checklist depending on the preferences and needs of the physician and the referring source. Lastly, very specific examples of return-to-work forms and how to complete them are found in Appendix B.

COMMUNICATION

The first step the physician takes is to find out what questions are being asked. The second is to determine his or her role. Is it from the perspective of the treating physician or from that of an independent evaluator who acts more as the impairment evaluating physician described in Chapter 12? If active treatment is recommended, will the physician be responsible for that, or simply for re-evaluating the patient after its completion? Is this evaluation used to fulfill legal requirements (such as Americans with Disabilities Act compliance), a post-injury/work placement, or a preretirement evaluation? These issues are addressed in Box 43–1 and should be resolved prior to the evaluation.

The referring source also has a responsibility to communicate with and provide for the needs of the evaluating physician (Box 43–2). The concept of "GIGO" ("garbage in/garbage out") in computer analysis and functions applies equally well for disability evaluations. Unless specific information is provided, specific responses cannot be provided in the report. For example, what is the average candle-watt intensity of lighting in an area for a worker with poor vision? What are the average and maximal decibels in a shop where a worker with a paralyzed vocal cord works? Will that worker pose a threat to coworkers if they cannot hear him? Or will that decibel level pose a threat to a hearing impaired worker's ability to hear in the future? The greater the detail provided by the referring source, the more accurate and precise the evaluator can be.

These issues (preparatory steps by the evaluator and the provisions/recommendations from the referring source) are further refined, again prior to the evaluation, as outlined in Box 43–3. It is critical at this stage to understand what expectations exist and, should further evaluation (especially laboratory investigation or functional capacity assessments) be deemed necessary by the evaluator, to know whether the referring source will be willing to authorize those evaluations. It is far better to be clear on these issues in advance than to produce an incomplete or undesirable report. The issues found in Box 43–4 should be addressed both before and during the evaluation.

THE REPORT

Boxes 43–5, 43–6, and 43–7 provide descriptions of the elements of a comprehensive report and recommendations for the report content and style. If only two principles are adhered to—answering the questions ethically and to the best of one's ability as a health professional and being predominantly proactive rather then restrictive—the disability report will serve the employer, the evaluator, and the employee/patient/examinee well.

In general, the physician preparing the report should keep in mind the four "R"s of a good report (Box 43–8). Less is more. Clear and reasoned thoughts can be lost in excessive verbiage and lose their impact.

BOX 43–1 Steps in Preparing for a Disability Examination, for the Examiner

I. Verify the purpose(s) of the evaluation with the requesting source(s)
  A. Employability determination
    1. Past offer, preplacement medical evaluations (see the section on the Americans With Disabilities Act [ADA], Chapter 47)
    2. Postinjury/illness, return to work
    3. Medically based job modification/accommodation for otherwise eligible employee (see ADA)
    4. Medically based job/environmental restrictions based on injury/illness
    5. Time course for medically based restrictions
  B. Approval of medically based absence
    1. Owing to personal medical condition
    2. In accordance with Family Medical Leave Act (see Chapter 47)
  C. Medical malpractice
  D. Personal injury
  E. Disability insurance
  F. Attainment of maximum medical improvement
II. Obtain specific forms (when applicable)
  A. Review prior to the examination
    1. This may dictate specific choices in the examination methods, testing, etc.
  B. If unclear, communicate with the referring source prior to the evaluation
III. Obtain and review nonmedical records
  A. Job description
    1. Employee's
    2. Employer's (including essential components of job—see ADA, Chapter 47)
  B. Workers' compensation records of present injury
    1. Accident/incident report
    2. Employee's and employer's first report of injury
    3. Employee's and employer's initial claim form
    4. Employee's and employer's supplemental statement
  C. Other workers' compensation records
  D. Other injury, disability, impairment records
    1. Off-work and return-to-work forms by attending or consulting physician(s)
    2. Restrictions on job/environment placed by attending or consulting physician(s)
    3. Records from insurance company or companies
    4. Other independent medical examinations
  E. Legal records
    1. Present case
      a. Deposition(s)
      b. Workers' compensation decisions
      c. Court decisions
    2. Other cases (where applicable)
  F. Personnel records from Human Resources Department
    1. Employment application
    2. Past and present job description(s)
    3. Performance appraisals
    4. Attendance records
    5. Employee relations records
      a. Counseling memos
      b. Written notices and warnings
      c. Termination notices

Box continued on following page

BOX 43–1 Steps in Preparing for a Disability Examination, for the Examiner *Continued*

IV. Obtain and review medical records
   A. Medical office records
   B. Hospital records
   C. Emergency and urgent-care center records
   D. Records of consulting physicians
   E. Reports of other independent medical examinations
   F. Results of testing
      1. Laboratory
      2. Radiological
      3. Psychological
      4. Functional capacity assessments
      5. Others

BOX 43–2 Steps in Preparing for a Disability Evaluation for the Referring Source

I. Be specific about what you are asking for
   A. Is this an impairment or a disability oriented report (or both)?
   B. Do you want to know if the claimant is at maximum medical improvement (MMI)?
      1. If not, do you want to know what is necessary to attain MMI?
         a. Do you want a projected timeline?
         b. Do you want to know the costs?
         c. Do you want an estimate of impairment when the claimant reaches MMI?
   C. Do you want specific forms filled out?
   D. Do you want references to the medical literature?

II. Provide sufficient records for the examiner to review
   A. Material provided by the Human Resources Department, including:
      1. Job description
      2. Essential tasks of the job (Americans With Disabilities Act)
      3. Reports by other personnel, including:
         a. Occupational safety specialists
         b. Industrial hygienists
         c. Dispensary records
   B. Many records will be unnecessary, including those that:
      1. Do not touch on the present case (e.g., a different medical condition)
      2. Are superfluous (e.g., full hospital records of a claimant being assessed for the effects of a particular injury; these may be critical, however, in a malpractice review)
   C. Provide those that will assist the examiner (see the lists under III and IV, Box 43–1)
   D. Communicate with examiner if some materials exist but are not being provided to determine if the examiner needs these documents
   E. Remember that the examiner can prepare an opinion only on the material that is furnished

III. Provide information on how to contact you
   A. Phone and fax numbers
   B. E-mail (if desired)
   C. Hours

IV. Clarify if you want a verbal report prior to anything committed to paper

V. Tell the examiner what to do with the provided material when the case is finished
   A. Return
   B. Keep
      1. For how long?
   C. Dispose
      1. Shred?

VI. Be specific regarding the fee
   A. The agreed price
      1. Hourly
      2. Per case
   B. How and when to bill
   C. How soon to expect payment after receiving the invoice
   D. Your anticipated figure (if necessary)
   E. If research is necessary, do you prefer to do some/all for the examiner?
      1. If not, are you prepared to pay for this service?

VII. Indicate whether you will pay the cost if travel is necessary
   A. Type of transportation
   B. Class of transportation
   C. Hotel/meal reimbursements
   D. Clarify who makes the travel arrangements, hotel reservations, etc.

BOX 43–3 Understanding and Responding to the Needs of the Referral Source in a Disability Evaluation

I. What functions does the medical advisor/consultant/evaluating physician perform for the referral source?
   A. Professional/technical function—Assess and explain the probative value of medical information
   B. Clinical function—Perform an impairment or disability-oriented medical evaluation
   C. Communications function—Analyze and explain, orally and/or in writing, enough about medical issues and their relationship to nonmedical issues so that the referral source feels comfortable with the information and confident in making necessary decisions
II. What critical questions must the medical advisor/consultant/evaluating physician ask of the referral source?
   A. What are the issues of this case?
   B. What is the purpose of the evaluation?
   C. What are you asking me to do?
   D. What questions do you want me to answer?
   E. Will you ask me to help you prepare for and assist in depositions of the claimant's physicians?
   F. Is it likely that I will be deposed?
   G. Will there be a trial if the case is not resolved?
   H. If so, will there be a jury?
   I. Will you ask me to serve as a witness if there is a trial?
   J. If so, will I be a fact witness or an expert witness?
III. What critical question must the medical advisor/consultant/evaluating physician answer personally?
   A. Beyond the information requested, what information does the referral source need?
IV. What information does the evaluating physician need?
   A. Dates
      1. Date of birth
      2. Date of hire
      3. Date of the incident
      4. Date of onset of the medical condition
      5. Date of onset of (alleged) disability
      6. Date of the first medical examination
      7. Critical employment-related dates
   B. Definitions
      1. Impairment—Deviation of an anatomic structure, a physiologic function, an intellectual capability, or the emotional status that the individual possessed prior to an alteration in those structures or functions or from what is expected from population norms
      2. Disability—A medical impairment that prevents an individual from performing specified intellectual, creative, adaptive, social, or physical functions; the inability to successfully complete a specific task that the individual was previously capable of completing or one that most members of society are capable of completing, owing to a medical or psychologic deviation from an individual's prior health status or from the status expected of most members of a society
      3. Workers' compensation/insurance
         a. Medical condition
         b. Temporary/permanent
         c. Partial/complete
      4. Accommodation (Americans with Disabilities Act)—Modification of a job or work situation that enables an individual to meet the same job demands and conditions of employment as any other individual in a similar job
      5. Occupational disability—A medical condition that precludes travel to and from work, being at work, or assignment of appropriate tasks and duties while at work, with or without accommodation
   C. Clear statement of the burden of proof the claimant must meet
      1. Law
      2. Regulations
      3. Insurance policy contract
      4. Employer's policy
      5. Labor management agreement

Box continued on opposite page

BOX 43–3 Understanding and Responding to the Needs of the Referral Source in a Disability Evaluation *Continued*

D. Relevant medical information from primary clinical source documents—Documents containing information obtained or communicated for the purpose of documenting the medical history and clinical findings and for managing a patient's clinical care
   1. Emergency room records or other first encounter records
   2. Medical office records
   3. Hospital inpatient records
   4. Consultation reports
   5. Physical therapy/occupational therapy records
   6. Reports of the results of laboratory tests
   7. Reports of the results of diagnostic tests and procedures
   8. Any other documents related to medical management of the claimant

Note 1—Letters to addressees not involved in managing the clinical management of the claimant (e.g., claims examiners, lawyers, disability evaluating physician) are not medical source documents. They have the quality of testimonial statements only.
Note 2—Reports of independent medical evaluation(s) or disability evaluation(s) by a physician who is not a treating physician are not primary clinical source documents.
Note 3—Unless a physician is a treating physician, the physician's report is not a primary medical source document.

E. Relevant information from the nonmedical primary source documents
   1. Injury report
   2. Employer's first report
   3. Physician's first report
   4. Personnel records
      a. Employment application/employment history
      b. Performance appraisals
      c. Counseling memos/disciplinary actions
      d. Awards and commendations
      e. Dates of changes in employment situation
         (1) Promotion/demotion
         (2) Transfer
         (3) New supervisor
         (4) New work assignment
   5. Legal documents
      a. Complaints
      b. Briefs
      c. Interrogatories
      d. Depositions
      e. Affidavits
   6. Case-related correspondence

Note—If you perform an evaluation:

   1. Verify the examinee's understanding of the purpose of the evaluation
   2. Ensure that it is clinically complete with respect to the medical condition regardless of what is asked for

V. Determination of causality (if requested)
   A. Is condition compatible with an occupational injury?
   B. Is there workplace exposure(s) to potential injurious situation(s)/substance(s)?
   C. Is there a witness, surveillance program, or proper vigilant record-keeping in place?
   D. Is the temporal relationship between the exposure and onset consistent with the type of harm complained of?
   E. Have nonoccupational factors been excluded as causes?
   F. Does the condition improve away from work or on restricted work activity?
   G. Are objective tests consistent with occupational injury?
   H. Has condition been treated by provider prior to workplace exposure?
   I. Clarify the injury-related diagnosis.

BOX 43–4 Components of the Disability Examination

I. Identify the needs/requests of the requesting source
II. Review the reports provided
  A. May assist the focus of the examination
  B. May identify missing parts that need to be explored in greater detail
  C. May identify contentious issues that need particular care
  D. Focus on issue to be addressed in the request; i.e., pre-employment, accommodation need, postinjury placement, etc.
  E. Review documents provided regarding previous issues; for example:
    1. Job description
    2. Injury reports (see Box 43–1)
  F. Communicate with referring source and obtain necessary missing information
    1. May be with specific employer resources (see Chapter 44) such as Human Resources Department, occupational safety specialist, etc.
III. Perform a careful history
  A. Pay specific attention to injury/illness of concern
  B. Full review of systems
  C. Family history
  D. Work history
    1. Past jobs and duties
    2. Accommodation needs (if applicable)
    3. Present job including full job description
    4. Worker's perceived limitations in the job, including:
      a. Performing the specific tasks of that job
      b. Limitations created by the workplace environment but not task-specific for the worker
      c. Problems for the worker in traveling to and from work
    5. Lists of exposures/injuries in prior jobs
  E. Social history
    1. Includes habits such as alcohol use, smoking, and recreational drug use
    2. Includes home environment (heating, humidity, air filtration devices, air conditioning, smokers, animals, stairs/levels of home, site of residence, presence of elevators where applicable)
    3. Travel history (when needed)
    4. Recreational/hobby history
    5. Social circumstances (where needed: education, home life, spouse/children status, income levels)
    6. Home or non-job exposures/injuries mimicking job exposures/injuries (e.g., changing brake shoes on personal automobiles in an asbestos-exposed worker)
    7. Home or non-job exposures/injuries that may influence or alter job exposures/injuries
  F. Present medications
  G. Allergies
  H. Past medical history
    1. Surgeries
    2. Hospital admissions
    3. Significant outpatient treatment (for example, physical therapy, psychological counseling)
    4. Other illnesses/injuries
    5. Complete list of current/past diagnoses
IV. Perform a careful physical examination
  A. Mental status examination
  B. Physical examination
    1. Full/limited based on request from referring source
    2. Specific examinations dictated by impairment system
V. Recommend/perform appropriate laboratory tests
  A. Based on communication with referring source
  B. Based on impairment system
VI. Recommend further medical evaluation as medically warranted and approved by referring source

Box continued on opposite page

BOX 43–4 Components of the Disability Examination *Continued*

VII. Anticipate future needs
  A. Has worker reached maximum medical improvement?
  B. Rehabilitative needs/potential
  C. Effect of further treatment
    1. Drug
    2. Surgical
    3. Rehabilitation
      a. Physical
      b. Occupational
      c. Vocational
  D. Estimate time courses for above
VIII. Prepare a report

BOX 43-5 Structure of the Disability Report

I. Identifying remarks
  A. Purpose of examination
  B. Referring source
  C. Time and place of examination
  D. Attendees (other than the claimant and examining physician)
  E. Time spent with claimant (better—exact time at beginning of interview with claimant and time at the termination of the examination)
  F. Whether the process was recorded for sound/video plus sound
II. List the records available for review
  A. Separate line for each record
  B. Specify the particulars of each record
    1. Prepared by whom
    2. Prepared for whom
    3. Date
    4. Site of report generation
    5. Purpose of the record
  C. (Possibly) list records not available for review
III. Specify purpose of the examination
  A. Attainment of maximum medical improvement (MMI)
  B. Return to work
    1. With or without restrictions
    2. With or without accommodation
IV. Job description
  A. Employee's
  B. Employer's
    1. Total job description
    2. Identify essential duties of job (Americans with Disabilities Act)
V. Present examination
  A. History
  B. Physical
  C. Laboratory
  D. Functional capacity assessment
VI. Summary and analysis of record review
  A. History or histories
  B. Physical examination
  C. Laboratory testing
  D. Functional capacity assessment(s)
VII. Reconciliation of present examination with record review
  A. History
  B. Physical examination
  C. Laboratory testing
  D. Functional capacity assessment
  E. Note congruences and discrepancies for A through D
  F. Cite appropriate historical documents where appropriate
  G. Give reasons for discrepancies
    1. Differences caused by time
    2. Differences caused by different types of tests
      a. Provide analysis of reliability and accuracy of each discrepant test
      b. Cite medical literature where appropriate
    3. Differences caused by different treatments
      a. Medical
      b. Surgical
      c. Rehabilitation

Box continued on opposite page

BOX 43–5 Structure of the Disability Report *Continued*

VIII. Provide assessment
    A. Should contain one paragraph for each issue noted in Part VII
    B. Should summarize all congruences and discrepancies identified in Part VII
    C. References to medical literature
IX. Summary and conclusions
    A. Restate purpose of examination
    B. Provide answer to purpose of examination based on:
        1. Present evaluation
        2. Record review
        3. Identify whether claimant has reached MMI
X. Make recommendations
    A. If claimant has not reached MMI:
        1. Steps necessary to attain MMI
            a. Medical
            b. Surgical
            c. Rehabilitation
        2. Expected time course
        3. Need for further examination once MMI is attained
    B. If claimant has reached MMI:
        1. Environmental restrictions
        2. Workplace restrictions
        3. Workplace accommodations
    C. If further testing is needed to provide more reliable report:
        1. List of tests
        2. (Possible) anticipated cost of those tests
        3. Why these tests are needed
        4. Date of submission of addendum report

BOX 43-6 Content of the Disability Report

I. Introduction
   A. Identifying information
   B. Referral source
   C. Purpose of the evaluation
   D. Date of the initial evaluation and all follow-up visits
   E. Complete list of all information used as the basis of the report (excluding the present examination), including:
      1. All records, reports, x-rays, results of special tests and diagnostic procedures, and laboratory test results, with source and dates for each
      2. All verbal communication with employer/attorneys/others working with or as part of the referring source including dates, times, names, and other appropriate identifying information, including who gave permission for the communication (if necessary)
   F. Presence of attendees at the examination (excluding the physician and the examinee), including:
      1. Family members
      2. Legal representatives
      3. Medical witnesses (e.g., female office staff during an examination between a male physician and a female examinee)
      4. Others

II. Historical evaluation
   A. History of the medical condition(s)
      1. Method by which the history was obtained
      2. Identity of the history taker(s)
      3. Narrative description of the history, including reference to all positive and pertinent negative results:
         a. As extracted from the records and reports
         b. As obtained from the examinee
      4. Comments regarding agreement and discrepancies within and between the sources

III. Physical examination
   A. Ability to dress and undress, get on and off the examining table
   B. Positive and pertinent negative clinical findings
   C. For each body part, system, and function, report observations that are required under the criteria of the disability system of record
   D. Validation signs (as appropriate)
   E. Detect instances of noninjury and/or malingering or symptom exaggeration

IV. Results of medical diagnostic testing
   A. Review all tests
   B. Remark on validity/accuracy of interpretations (if appropriate)
   C. Read radiographic studies (if available)
   D. Comment on whether the claimant could influence the results
   E. Comment on the validity, reliability, accuracy, and appropriateness of the diagnostic studies (provide references if needed)

V. Integration of the results of current medical specialist evaluations provided for this report (other than yours)

VI. Clinical impressions

VII. Assessment of current health status
   A. Explain the basis for a conclusion that the clinical information is or is not sufficient to assess the individual's current health status
   B. Explain whether each medical condition has become static or well-stabilized with reference to past records and current findings to support each conclusion
   C. If improvement or deterioration of any medical condition is expected, explain the basis for the conclusion, the expected course of the condition, and the time frame within which the improvement or deterioration is likely to take place
   D. Explain the influence on the severity of the illness if medical recommendations are/are not adhered to

Box continued on opposite page

BOX 43–6 Content of the Disability Report *Continued*

- E. Performance-related impact
  1. Activities for which performance capacity is called into question based on the medical condition
  2. Activities for which reconditioning would be necessary because of limited strength or endurance
- F. Risk-related impact
  1. Activities that would be likely to result in injury or harm to the examinee or aggravation of the medical condition
  2. The likelihood of sudden or subtle incapacitation
- G. Impact on employability, including whether the medical condition precludes:
  1. Travel to and from work
  2. Being at work
  3. Assignment of tasks and duties
- H. Impact on life activities
  1. Personal activities
     - a. Self-care (personal hygiene, dressing, food preparation and eating, etc.)
     - b. Personal business (maintaining a bank account, paying bills, entering into contracts such as leases, loans, or insurance)
  2. Social activities
  3. Leisure and recreational activities

VIII. Medical management plan (if appropriate)
- A. Recommendations for further diagnostic testing
- B. Referral for medical specialty evaluation
- C. Periodic re-evaluation of active treatment
- D. Rehabilitation/reconditioning
- E. Follow-up disability evaluation
- F. Provide information about unusual conditions or newer trends in medical management
- G. Length of treatment program
- H. Anticipated results of treatment program
- I. Anticipated costs and timeline (if requested)

IX. Synthesis of information
- A. Review and analyze documentation
  1. Note consistency and accuracy of information from various health care providers
  2. Evaluate sufficiency of the information on which diagnosis and medical management plans are based
  3. If the examinee was absent from the job
     - a. Why the examinee stopped working
     - b. Duration
     - c. If still absent from work, why the examinee has not returned to work
- B. Analyze the accumulated medical information
  1. Medical history
     - a. Historical interview, clinical findings, treatment, and response to treatment
     - b. Any conspicuous absence of information
  2. Conclusions
     - a. The examinee's medical condition has or has not become static or well-stabilized
     - b. The examinee is or is not likely to suffer subtle or sudden incapacitation
     - c. The examinee is or is not likely to suffer injury, harm, or aggravation of the medical condition by engaging in specific work-related and nonwork-related activities
     - d. Risk avoidance or therapeutic value associated with restricting the examinee from particular activities, both on and off the job
     - e. The impact of prior work restrictions or workplace accommodations
  3. Life situation factors

Box continued on following page

BOX 43-6 Content of the Disability Report *Continued*

- C. Assess the medical and nonmedical information in relation to the following factors:
  1. Likelihood that the circumstances could have caused or contributed to the onset or aggravation of the medical condition
  2. Consistency or inconsistency in records, reports, history, and previous clinical findings
  3. Validity of the diagnosis with respect to established medical diagnostic criteria
  4. Appropriateness of the treatment with respect to generally accepted medical principles and practices
  5. Assessment of the impact of the medical condition on nonwork-related activities
     - a. Note any discrepancies between nonwork capabilities and workplace incapacities
  6. Likelihood that the examinee will suffer subtle or sudden incapacitation, noting:
     - a. How soon
     - b. How much
     - c. How severe
     - d. The probable consequence(s)
       - (1) Personal injury or harm or aggravation of the medical condition
       - (2) Impact on coworkers
       - (3) Impact on accommodations or workplace restrictions
     - e. The degree to which the medical condition has or has not become static or well stabilized
  7. The need for future treatment and the nature of such treatment
  8. Likelihood that the medical condition will change
  9. Likelihood that job restrictions or accommodations will change
  10. Potential restrictions or job modifications to:
      - a. Enable the examinee to carry out essential job functions
      - b. Reduce to an acceptable level the risk of sudden or subtle incapacitation; injury, harm, or aggravation of the condition; or injury or harm to others

X. Conclusions and recommendations, including a reasoned explanation for their basis
- A. The burden of proof with respect to disability, employability, or accommodation is met
  1. Identify the specific items of information that conform to the specific elements required for proof
  2. Estimate the expected duration of the individual's inability to meet job demands and conditions of employment, personal or social demand, or the requirements of law or regulation
  3. State the medical basis on which to recommend medical follow-up actions, if appropriate and warranted
- B. The burden of proof is not met
  1. Explain what information would have been supportive in relation to the specific elements of the burden of proof and reaffirm their absence or insufficiency in the documentation
  2. Describe necessary testing
  3. Explain sequence of events if the previous information/tests are provided
     - a. Addendum report
     - b. Need for subsequent evaluation of the injured worker

XI. Work recommendations
- A. List capabilities
- B. List incapabilities
- C. List restrictions
- D. List accommodations
- E. Provide return-to-work recommendations

BOX 43–7 Recommendations for Producing a Well-written Disability Report

1. Use short paragraphs.
2. Provide space (two or three lines between headings).
3. Avoid surplus words such as compound prepositions and word-wasting idioms when simple, concise words suffice.
4. Employ active verbs. Passive verbs require a supporting verb (was) followed by a preposition (by).
5. Generally, use short sentences, especially in comparing items. Vary sentence length somewhat for variety, which improves readability.
6. Guide your reader. Begin sentences with names and dates. Place new information or important facts at the beginning of a sentence or paragraph.
7. Arrange your words with care, following the normal English word order of placing the subject first followed by the verb and then the object. Avoid wide gaps among the subject, the verb, and the object.
8. Present material in tables when appropriate. Tables present complicated bits of information clearly and concisely.
9. Use commonly understood English phrases and clearly defined terms. For example, instead of using terms like inspection, palpation, percussion, and auscultation, chose verbs (inspect, palpate, percuss, auscultate). Lay language is preferable: I observe, I see, I feel.
10. Avoid language quirks, habits, current catch phrases, and jargon. Maintain neutrality and objectivity. Make no attempt at humor.
11. Document all sources of information, both medical and nonmedical. Present these materials chronologically, identifying the date, source, recipient, and subject matter.
12. Carefully proofread and edit your report. Typographic errors and other easily corrected mistakes diminish the impact of the report. Rephrase passages that seem unclear on the second reading. Make sure that your report has successfully translated medical language into good English.
13. Use headings, underlining, and boldface print for emphasis and organization. Strive for a professional format that presents information clearly.
14. Be precise.
15. Be terse in the assessment/conclusion parts of your report.
16. Use phrases such as "within a reasonable degree of medical certainty," "more likely then not," and others where and when appropriate.
17. Provide a list of references as needed. If appropriate, enclose a copy of one or two articles with appropriate passages highlighted. This adds power and credibility to your report.

BOX 43–8 The Four "R"s of any Successful Report

1. A *responsive* report fulfills the request of the referring source. The report begins with an introductory statement assuring the requestor that his or her interests will be addressed.
2. *Readable* means that the visual appearance and structure (introduction/body/summary) make the report easy to follow.
3. A *relevant* report provides information that supports or disproves an issue and explains contradictions.
4. The summary ends a well-*reasoned* report and draws impartial conclusions that fit and follow from the reasons offered in the body of the report. These *reasons* flow from established medical science to support or refute specific issues. The results of this analysis are unique to, and specific for, the questions posed by the requesting party.

CHAPTER

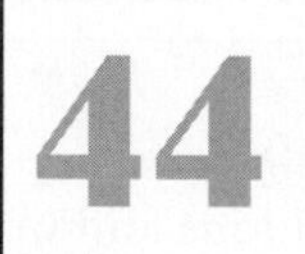

Resource Personnel Used in a Disability Evaluation

JAMES B. TALMAGE, MD

IN IMPAIRMENT AND DISABILITY EVALUATION, WHO ARE THE POTENTIALLY HELPFUL RESOURCE PERSONNEL?

In impairment and disability evaluations, important information may be contributed by individuals from several different disciplines. Such information may already exist in the records, or may be requested by the evaluating physician at the time impairment and disability questions are raised. Such resource personnel include physical therapists, occupational therapists, vocational rehabilitation specialists, industrial hygienists, and human resource managers.

Therapists

Physical and occupational therapists are generally graduates of accredited college programs who are then licensed by state boards. Their training and practice have areas of overlap, especially in treatment and/or evaluation of individuals with impairments or disabilities. Historically, in treatment, the physical therapist would emphasize exercise and movement (stretching), whereas the occupational therapist would emphasize purposeful activity. In current practice, they perform many of the same tasks. Just as spinal surgery is performed by physicians with training as orthopedic surgeons or neurosurgeons, and hand surgery is done by physicians with training as orthopedic surgeons or plastic surgeons, evaluation and treatment of individuals with impairment and disability may have been done by, or may be requested from, individuals with training in either physical therapy or in occupational therapy. Practitioners with either background may have achieved additional certification in subspecialty areas. For example, either a physical therapist or an occupational therapist may become a certified hand therapist.

What Information Might Be in the Medical Record?

The individual being evaluated for impairment and/or disability may have seen a therapist for treatment. The medical record of the therapist will probably contain a detailed evaluation of the individual before the therapist begins treatment, and a similar evaluation at the conclusion of treatment. These evaluations generally contain information about symptoms, physical examination (for example, range of joint motion), and physical capacity. These evaluations can provide the following useful information:

1. Was the examinee compliant with treatment and motivated to improve? The attendance record of the examinee will generally be documented, and reasons (if any) for poor attendance may be recorded. Working with the individual on a repetitive basis allows the therapist to observe behavior. Compliance with assigned home treatment is usually assessed. The evaluator must remember that the therapist's observations about motivation for recovery are, like all such observations, anecdotal and thus potentially biased. No single examination finding or test proves a lack of motivation,[3] but the more signs that are present that might be explained by lack of motivation, the more likely it is that poor motivation for recovery or secondary gain issues are present.

2. Did the examinee improve during the treatment or therapy?
3. Did the therapist feel that the individual was at maximal medical improvement?
4. Since the therapist's final evaluation, has the individual improved (with time and continued home exercise or other treatment), stayed the same (at maximal medical improvement?), or worsened (deteriorated secondary to disuse or disease progression)? To judge these, the physician needs to compare the individual's status on discharge from therapy with the individual's current status. The evaluating physician may be able to measure and compare examination findings (for example, range of motion of a specific joint), or perhaps will need to refer the individual being evaluated back to the therapist for repeat testing (e.g., Purdue Pegboard, a test of dexterity).
5. At the conclusion of treatment, was a formal functional capacity evaluation (FCE) performed? If performed, the FCE may provide useful insights into the individual's capacities. (The value and validity of FCE testing are discussed in Chapter 55.)

WHY MIGHT A REFERRAL TO A THERAPIST BE PART OF AN IMPAIRMENT AND/OR DISABILITY EVALUATION?

After completing a history, physical examination, and record review, a physician may wish to refer the individual being evaluated to a therapist for treatment (if therapy has not been utilized, to see if therapy can decrease the symptoms, impairment, and disability) or evaluation (for formal FCE [see Chapter 55]. These reasons for referral are self-explanatory; however, a third reason—ergonomic evaluation of/intervention at the workplace—may not be a concept familiar to many physicians. Although they are called on to determine whether an individual can return to his or her current employer and do his or her job or another available job for that employer, most physicians do not personally visit the worksite to evaluate the job in question, or other potential jobs, for suitability. Many therapists have acquired the ability to evaluate worksites and suggest job modifications that permit return to work or placement in alternative positions.

In occupational low back pain with disability, there is evidence that participatory ergonomic intervention is effective in decreasing the number of lost work days (disability).[2] In this role, the therapist explains the medical issues to worksite personnel (human resource manager/safety specialist), may recommend reasonable accommodations, and serves as an educator, patient advocate, and dispute mediator/compromise facilitator.

Vocational Rehabilitationists

What Is Vocational Rehabilitation?

Vocational rehabilitation is the process of assisting the individual with disabilities in returning to work. Vocational rehabilitationists have a wide variety of educational backgrounds. They may be employed by state agencies (to serve all citizens, not just workers' compensation patients), by workers' compensation commissions, by rehabilitation facilities, or by insurance companies. In addition, the medical record may contain forensic vocational rehabilitation evaluations requested by either a defense or a plaintiff's attorney.

What Information Might Be in the Medical Record?

If an individual has been evaluated by a vocational rehabilitation professional, the record will probably contain the following:

1. A summary of the individual's preinjury or preillness education, work history, and avocation(s).
2. A summary of the individual's current capacity, and the areas in and extent to which the injury or illness has diminished the premorbid capacity; this is generally documented by testing abilities (intellect, memory, strength, coordination, endurance, etc.).
3. A conclusion that the individual is or is not capable of returning to work in his or her prior career field.
4. A summary of transferable job skills that could be utilized by the individual in different occupations.
5. A listing of jobs the individual would be capable of performing and resources that might assist in job placement "as is."
6. Recommendations of alternative career fields that would be logical options for the examinee, based on interest, retained abilities, and achievable education.
7. Recommendations for additional training to permit work in desired career fields, with consideration of resources for funding the desired training.
8. A summary of known obstacles to re-employment, including motivation and secondary gains.

When Might Referral to a Vocational Rehabilitation Specialist Be Helpful?

Physician referral is not required for an individual to see a vocational rehabilitation specialist. In a treating physician role, referral may be indicated if the ill or injured individual cannot return to work in his or her usual career field, or in another career field for which he or she is qualified by capacity, training, and/or experience. In some administrative situations, vocational rehabilitation evaluation may be mandated (for example, by workers' compensation law in some states).

In an evaluating physician role, if a crucial question is whether an individual is disabled for any occupation, referral for a formal vocational rehabilitation evaluation may occur. If, however, it is obvious to the evaluating physician that the individual being evaluated has the residual capacity for many different jobs, formal vocational rehabilitation evaluation may not be necessary (see also Chapter 45).

Industrial Hygienist

What is Industrial Hygiene?

"Industrial hygiene is the science and practice devoted to the anticipation, recognition, evaluation, and control of those environmental factors and stresses arising in or from the workplace that may cause sickness, impaired health and well-being, or significant discomfort among workers and may also impact the general community."[1] The American Board of Industrial Hygiene offers certification examinations. Earning an appropriate college degree (generally in industrial hygiene; chemistry; physics; chemical, mechanical, or sanitary engineering; or biology), participating in 1 year of full-time professional practice, and passing the core examination permits certification as an industrial hygienist in training. Certification as a certified industrial hygienist requires 5 years of professional practice and successful completion of either the comprehensive practice examination or the chemical practice examination.

What Information Might Be in the Medical Record, and When Might Referral Be Helpful?

The medical record may already contain material safety data sheets (MSDS) on the chemicals to which an employee is exposed at work. In cases where allergy (e.g., occupational asthma or occupational contact dermatitis) or toxicity (e.g., peripheral neuropathy secondary to solvents like n-hexane or methyl n-butyl ketone) is suspected, the MSDS gives the evaluating physician crucial information about chemicals that are known to be present in the workplace, and that therefore may be involved in the employee's illness. Employers are required to maintain a complete set of MSDS covering all chemicals that exist in the workplace.[4] Employers are required by law to provide a copy of the MSDS to employees and to physicians who request an MSDS as part of evaluation or treatment of employees. The MSDS contains several useful pieces of information for the evaluating physician.

The MSDS lists the product name as it appears on the label, which is what the employee will use in describing his or her exposures during history taking. The actual chemical name will also be listed, which permits the physician to consult medical/scientific texts and/or articles as to the health effects of exposure involved.

The MSDS has a section on health hazard data, which lists the organ systems potentially affected and types of problems that are seen frequently enough to be listed by the manufacturer of the chemical.

The MSDS lists the name and phone number of the manufacturer of the chemical. The company may have a medical director with special expertise in the health effects of the chemicals made by that company.

Industrial hygienists or the company's own safety specialist may have already measured the level of employee exposure to agents that may be suspected of causing an employee's symptoms. Examples would include measurement of noise potentially causing hearing loss, and air sampling to measure the level of exposure to cadmium dust potentially causing decreased renal function. Reports from industrial hygienists that contain the results of testing for exposures in the workplace would be kept by, and therefore available from, the human resources department (companies will vary as to whether the reports are kept by the human resource manager, the safety specialist, or someone else). If measurements of potential workplace exposures have not been done, or are in doubt, an industrial hygienist is the appropriate specialist for the physician to request to visit the worksite and measure exposures. Industrial hygienists are the professionals who actually do the sample collection and make the arrangements for laboratory testing of the work environment. Knowing the chemical and/or physical agents to which employees are exposed is crucial. For example, "Asbestosis secondary to working for Company A" is not a viable diagnosis and causation assessment if there is no asbestos at Company A's worksite. Most of the workplace exposures resulting in significant health risk are regulated by Occupational Safety and Health Administration (OSHA) standards.[5] This gives employers an added reason to be certain that workplace exposures do not put employee health at risk. Industrial hygienists may also be consulted by industry to suggest reasonable accommodations to permit an employee to return to work and to prevent problems in other workers.

Human Resource Management, Including Human Resource Manager, Safety Specialist, and Occupational Nurse

What is Human Resource Management?

Human resource manager is a more modern title for the personnel manager. This change in title reflects recognition by industry that employees or people are a valuable resource, just as buildings and equipment are considered, by management, to be resources. In small to medium-sized worksites, the human resource manager may handle all or most of the issues that concern employment. This would include workers' compensation injuries and nonwork-related injuries and illnesses that produce short- or long-term disabilities. The human resource manager is the manager who decides issues such as employability, termination, placement in alternative positions, use of disability benefits, and Family and Medical Leave Act entitlements. In addition, the human resource manager will have significant input into employer decisions on reasonable accommodation or modification of jobs. In large worksites, many of these functions for the worker injured on the job are delegated to a safety specialist, who reports to and thus seeks decision approval from the human resource manager. Some large employers have an occupational nurse as a full-time or part-time employee. The nurse may be a registered nurse or licensed practical nurse. Many of these nurses will have additional training in occupational nursing, and some will have passed certifying examinations as occupational nurses.

What Information Can the Human Resource Manager (or Safety Specialist) Supply?

If the individual being evaluated for impairment and/or disability has resigned from or been terminated by the most recent employer, some human resource managers are reluctant to provide any additional information. If, however, the individual is still an employee of the employer, and if the question to be answered is whether the individual can return to his or her usual job or an alternative job for this employer, then the human resource manager may be able to provide useful information, including the following:

1. A job description listing the essential functions the employee must be able to perform.
2. Whether collective bargaining agreements (union rules) permit modified duty and alternative job placement.
3. An appraisal of the individual's premorbid work status and perhaps motivation; if a preplacement physical examination was performed, if OSHA or the company required annual medical monitoring examinations that were performed, or if medical testing during employee health promotion activities was performed, those results are available on request from the evaluating physician.
4. A list of known barriers to re-employment, including psychosocial issues in the workplace; for example, sometimes the out-of-work individual qualifies for benefits that produce greater after-tax income than he or she would derive by returning to work.
5. Whether a physician or therapist has in the past, or may in the future, visit the worksite to evaluate the job(s) in question and to suggest compromise solutions including job modification and alternative placement.
6. MSDS for chemicals that exist in the workplace.

If the employer has an occupational nurse, the nurse's professional observations and records (medical records) may contain useful information about the presence or absence of objective signs of injury or illness. The nurse may also know about psychosocial factors that may delay recovery and return to work.

Physicians need to remember that a physician can evaluate the individual's physical and mental capacities, tolerance for symptoms, and risk of reinjury or exacerbation if re-employed. Physicians can then make recommendations about return to work. The decision as to whether, from the employee's perspective, the rewards of employment outweigh the symptoms produced by and the risks of re-employment will ultimately be made by the individual. The patient will decide whether he or she will attempt to return to work.

Similarly, the decision as to whether the risks of re-employment outweigh the benefits to the employer, such that the employer will permit re-employment, will ultimately be made by the employer (human resource manager). That decision is subject to review by the court system under the Americans With Disabilities Act and similar state laws.

SUMMARY

The physician charged with evaluating impairment and disability issues can obtain useful information from resource personnel from a variety of disciplines. Thus, similar to health care in general, impairment and disability evaluation is a team project.

References

1. American Industrial Hygiene Association: http://www.aiha.org/AboutAIHA/html/ih-info.htm. June 8, 2002.
2. Frank J, Sinclair S, Hogg-Johnson S, et al: Preventing disability from work-related low-back pain. Can Med Assoc J 158:1625–1631,1998.
3. Lechner DE, Bradbury SF, Bradley LA: Detecting sincerity of effort: A summary of methods and approaches. Phys Ther 78:867–888, 1998.
4. Occupational Safety and Health Administration: http://www.osha.gov/SLTC/hazardcommunications/index.html. June 10, 2002.
5. Occupational Safety and Health Aministration: http://www.osha.gov/comp-links.html.

CHAPTER

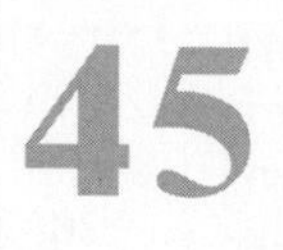

The Role of the Vocational Rehabilitationist

JOHN M. WILLIAMS, DEd

Functional limitations that may appear to allow a person to return to work when viewed outside the context of the functional demands of a particular job or class of jobs may lead to an overestimation of the probability of return to work with the past employer at the same or a new position or with a new employer in a new position. Similarly, other vocational factors such as age, education, acquired skills, work motivation, work performance, and earnings impact the ability to work and earn income following injury or trauma.[16,18] Determination of the probability of a person returning to work and earning substantive income in the future requires understanding of the physical and mental limitations associated with injury or trauma as established by physicians and psychologists, and knowledge of the physical and mental demands of work, the skill and knowledge requirements of the work, availability of work in the labor market, and the hiring practices of employers. It is the vocational rehabilitationist who has the knowledge, skills, and professional experience to make decisions about work and earnings, issues seen as critical to disability determination in civil and administrative law proceedings. Therefore, physicians should be wary about making statements about a person's ability to acquire and perform work. These issues are better left to a vocational rehabilitationist. Transferable skills, adaptation to change, impairment, work, and earnings must be addressed by a vocational rehabilitationist before statements about disability can be made. The following examines how the vocational rehabilitationist addresses these issues and contributes to the understanding of how impairment and functional limitations affect work and disability.

TRANSFERABILITY OF SKILLS ANALYSIS AND WORK

The best and least inferential approach to assessing the impact of functional limitations on ability to work may be a transferability of skills analysis (TSA). Functional limitations, education, age, and acquired skills (based on the materials, products, subject matter, services, machines, tools, equipment, and work aids associated with past relevant work and the job tasks and setting associated with a specific work field) are used to determine what work exists in the labor market that the individual has the capacity to perform.[16] Where injury has resulted in impairment, the effect of limitations on the existence of jobs and the degree to which the limitations have eroded the individual's available labor market before and after the injury can be determined. TSAs offer a viable approach to determining the impact of limitations on ability to work and earn a living following injury and impairment.[17] Such programs can look at the number of jobs in any given labor market that the individual could have performed before and can perform after an injury or event as well as the number of job openings suitable for the person pre- and postinjury/event.[13] In this way a realistic assessment of loss of probability of working can be conducted while maintaining the highest level of scientific precision possible given the nature of the available job and labor market data. Labor market surveys can be used to supplement TSAs to show that specific jobs with specific earnings exist at any given time in the local labor market (a potentially more persuasive argument against total disability).

Social Security Disability Income (SSDI) regulations provide the concept that persons who are over 50 should be expected to make less of an occupational adjustment than younger persons when transferring skills to new jobs (making a "closer" transferability of skills necessary—same or very similar work settings, products, materials, tools, procedures, etc.).[1] Likewise, older persons (50 or older) with no acquired skills and less than a high school (marginal) education are recognized as being sufficiently disenfranchised from the world of work, when they are limited to light or sedentary work, to be considered disabled. Furthermore, someone who has acquired very extensive skills in a narrow area of knowledge (i.e., a skilled craftsperson, scientist, or service professional) may be disabled based on inability to transfer skills that have a very narrow area of application in the labor market to jobs that require similar skills and knowledge but require significant new learning. This is particularly true when mental impairments limit learning ability or when age is seen as a detriment for acquisition of new learning to occur in a timely fashion (i.e., learning would take too long, the years of productive work before retirement would not be sufficient for the employer to make the investment in the older worker, and/or the older worker's knowledge and skills are so dated they are obsolete).

For younger, more educated and highly skilled workers, physical and mental limitations may be overcome through new learning (whether in formal academic or vocational training programs or through on-the-job training). Retraining offers the opportunity for acquisition of current, marketable knowledge and skills that prepare persons with impairments for jobs that require lesser physical exertion (i.e., light or sedentary work). Ability to work and earn income is the test of disability used in administrative law and civil proceedings; therefore, acquisition of marketable knowledge and skills is a paramount concern in assessing the degree of disability.[2] The best vocational rehabilitation alternative is one that enhances knowledge and skills, expands marketability (i.e, the number and types of jobs one can acquire and perform), and increases earnings.[8,17] Understanding physical and mental limitations, the physical and mental demands of work, the nature and availability of work in a given labor market, and the wages associated with individual jobs allows the rehabilitationist to build a viable rehabilitation plan based on the physical, mental, educational, and vocational limitations and capacities of an individual.

ADAPTATION TO CHANGE

Because the success of the vocational rehabilitation process relies to a great extent on an impaired individual's ability to adapt to changed physical and mental capacities (i.e., to identify choice options, determine an appropriate goal, and implement an effective change strategy), it is not surprising that functional limitations in the ability to perform the cognitive and/or behavioral requirements of work could further narrow vocational options for the future. Diminished ability to maintain concentration or attention, understand and follow instructions, deal with customary work stressors, keep a reasonable pace, maintain appropriate behavior when relating to supervisors and coworkers, and adapt to changing work processes, whether resulting from traumatic brain injury or some adverse emotional state (i.e., anxiety, depression, anger, or fear), may also lead to less effective job search and fewer or no job offers. If sufficiently severe cognitive and behavioral limitations are identified by physicians and/or psychologists, disability may occur despite the physical ability to engage in productive work activity. Because how one makes decisions and acts on them helps to determine career path, poor vocational choices and inappropriate actions resulting from lowered cognitive efficiency and/or reduced emotional well-being can have a negative effect on the type of work one performs and on the earnings associated with the chosen job.[3–5] Box 45–1 contains a list of the mental and behavioral capacities required to perform work on a sustained basis. It should be remembered that many of these capacities are also required in order to search for and obtain work on multiple occasions over one's work life.

Self-report or objective documentation of periods of decompensation in the workplace (necessitating taking time off from work, resulting in termination of work, or resulting in frequent job changes) would be given particular attention as an objective indicator of diffi-culty adapting to the physical, mental, and behavioral demands of work. Decline in cognitive and/or behavioral efficiency would be associated with decline in the skill level and pace of work one can perform.[13–15] Inability to sustain performance of skilled tasks (i.e., work requiring considerable judgment; working to specifications; handling multiple, varied tasks) would result from lesser levels of decline in mental and/or behavioral function than would a decline in performance of unskilled tasks (i.e., simple, repetitive work where no judgment is required). Mild to moderate impairment in mental functions would not likely preclude work, but could easily require changing jobs or job duties. The degree to which one sees change as threatening or harmful (a not uncommon perception of persons experiencing depression, anxiety, anger, or fear) could further influence one's ability to adapt successfully to change. For those who are extremely depressed, angry, fearful, or anxious,

BOX 45–1 Mental and Behavioral Capacities Needed to Perform Work

1. Ability to remember locations and work procedures
2. Ability to understand and remember very short and simple instructions as well as detailed instructions
3. Ability to carry out simple and detailed instructions
4. Ability to maintain attention and concentration over extended periods
5. Ability to perform activities within a schedule, maintain regular attendance, and be punctual within customary work tolerances
6. Ability to sustain an ordinary routine without special supervision
7. Ability to work in coordination with and proximity to others
8. Ability to make simple or complex work decisions
9. Ability to complete a normal work day or week without interruption from psychologically based symptoms and to perform in a consistent pace without unreasonable rest periods
10. Ability to interact appropriately with peers and supervisors, including accepting criticism about work performance
11. Ability to respond appropriately to changes in the work setting, including potentially hazardous conditions
12. Ability to travel to and from the workplace or to alternative work settings with private or public transportation

change may not be possible; for those who experience a lesser degree of these emotions, limited change may be handled effectively. Because it is not unusual for mental limitations to be associated with chronic pain, a given person may have both physical and mental impairments and functional limitations, which must be considered in assessing adaptability to change in work capacities. Such interventions as counseling, education, social skills training, job seeking skills training, and job coaching are among the strategies available to a rehabilitationist for promoting successful return to work.[9] Only after these interventions have been tried and their outcomes assessed is it possible to determine if a given individual has reached maximum rehabilitation improvement—the point where maximum physical and mental function, work-related knowledge and skill acquisition, adaptation to change, and work performance are achieved.[15] It should not be surprising that reduction in acquisition of or application of knowledge and skills to work situations would have a dramatic effect on the number of jobs one can perform and the earnings associated therewith. Earnings are often directly proportionate to the educational and skill requirements of the work. Those who retain old learning and/or acquire new learning to a greater degree than others are more likely to earn more money and to remain in the labor force longer than those with lesser education or skill acquisition.[19] Therefore, any change in ability to acquire skills due to injury or trauma may have a profound effect on disability and overall quality of life over the lifespan.[9] For persons with sufficient cognitive abilities and demonstrated ability to learn, education or retraining is a powerful tool to enable them to overcome disability and resume, to the greatest extent possible, a normal career path and overall life development.[15] For those who demonstrate limitations in the ability to learn or do not have a recent history of success precipitated by learning, the rehabilitation goal of restoring the person to full function may be difficult to achieve and acceptance of a lower level of function may be the most realistic outcome of rehabilitation interventions.[7,9]

IMPAIRMENT, WORK, EARNINGS, AND DISABILITY

One's earning capacity following physical and/or mental impairment is best predicted by a rehabilitationist after careful examination of historical and current intellectual function (as indicated by testing, academic performance, or related objective data), skill acquisition (as indicated by completion of specific vocational training or demonstrated work performance), work motivation (as indicated by success in acquiring and sustaining employment), and earnings (as indicated by actual dollars earned). Building on the impairments and functional limitations identified by physicians and psychologists, vocational rehabilitationists can assist individuals, case managers, attorneys, and judges in understanding the impact of changes in functional capacity from before to after an injury or traumatic event on a person's ability to work and earn income. Understanding the implications of specific limitations on a person's ability to perform the physical and mental requirements of work makes disability assessment more accurate and complete.[2] Physicians and psychologists should provide meaningful input within their areas of expertise and should not be asked to be experts in employability (i.e., what jobs one can perform) or placeability (i.e., whether an employer in a given labor market would hire one to perform such a job given one's age, education, acquired skills, and work performance). The rehabilitationist has the unique knowledge and experience to be called an expert in these areas.[10] Using data on the physical and mental demands of work found in the Dictionary of Occupational Titles and the Revised Handbook for Analyzing Jobs, the vocational rehabilitationist can make decisions about whether a person is capable of performing the physical and/or mental demands of given job as it is commonly performed or as it could be modified.[11,12] Jobs that match an individual's knowledge, skills, functional capacities, and aspirations can then be identified by a vocational rehabilitationist through direct contact with employers. If jobs exist in sufficient number, the person can perform them, and there are sufficient openings to suggest that this person can obtain these jobs, then the person is not totally disabled from a vocational perspective. However, earnings may be affected rather dramatically.

SUMMARY

Disability is a complex issue that requires multidisciplinary analysis. This is even more true when the physician, psychologist, and vocational rehabilitationist are asked to render opinions in civil and/or administrative law proceedings under the standard of science applicable to that setting. The vocational rehabilitationist bridges the gap between functional limitations and disability just like the physician or psychologist bridges the gap between impairment and functional limitations. In this way, logic (i.e., chain of cause and effect from injury/trauma to impairment to functional limitations to ability to perform work and perform other important life functions) and empirical data to support the logic (based on objective findings and empirical research in peer-reviewed publications) can be presented in a systematic and persuasive way. Without a persuasive argument that articulates the impact of impairments on function, function on work, and work on earning capacity, lost wages or lost future earnings presented to the court or administrative law judge by an economist become meaningless.[17] Similarly, the cost of future care needs can be tied to the impact of care on functional capacity to perform work and other significant life activities, and thus can demonstrate the true need for and ultimate benefit of care.

Medical, psychological, and vocational rehabilitation experts play critical roles in the disability assessment. However, it is the vocational rehabilitationist who explains the practical implications of impairments and functional limitations on work and disability. A person with a severe injury or trauma may not experience as high a degree of disability as a person with a less severe injury or trauma if this individual has greater personal assets and life accomplishments, greater capacity for adaptation to change, and/or greater drive to succeed. The vocational rehabilitationist, building on the foundation of objective evidence regarding impairment, functional capacity, and anticipated outcomes of future care, can speak to the probability of any given individual's being employed, earning wages, and maintaining a reasonable quality of life in the future.

References

1. Code of Federal Regulations, 20, Parts 400 to 499. Washington, DC, U.S. Government Printing Office, 1996.
2. Dorto AJ, Williams JM: Coordinating rehabilitation efforts and the disability evaluating process. Journal of Back and Musculoskeletal Rehabilitation 8:19–43, 1998.
3. Fabian ES: Supported employment and the quality of life: Does a job make a difference? Rehabilitation Counseling Bulletin 36:84–97, 1992.
4. Ginzberg E: Career development. In Brown D, Brooks L (eds): Career Choice and Development: Applying Theories in Practice. San Francisco, Jossey-Bass, 1984, pp 161–191.
5. Krause JS: Adjustment to life after spinal cord injury: A comparison among three participant groups based on employment status. Rehabilitation Counseling Bulletin 35:218–229, 1992.
6. Krumboltz JD, Mitchell AM, Jones GB: A social learning theory of career selection. The Counseling Psychologist 6:71–81, 1976.
7. Matkin RE: Insurance Rehabilitation. Austin, TX, Pro–Ed, 1985.
8. Murphy PA, Williams JM: Assessment of Rehabilitative and Quality of Life Issues in Litigation. Boca Raton, Fla, CRC Press, 1998.
9. Roessler RT: A conceptual framework for return to work interventions. Rehabilitation Counseling Bulletin 32:98–107, 1988.
10. Rogers R: Role of the expert witness. In Petersen RA (ed): The Vocational Expert's Testimony. Topeka, Kan, American Board of Vocational Experts, 1991, pp 1–13.
11. U.S. Department of Labor: Dictionary of Occupational Titles, 4th ed. Washington, DC, U.S. Government Printing Office, 1991.
12. U.S. Department of Labor: Revised Handbook for Analyzing Jobs. Washington, DC, U.S. Government Printing Office, 1991.
13. Williams JM: Transferability of skills methodologies used in computerized job matching systems: Sufficient or insufficient control of methodologically induced error variance. Journal of Forensic Vocational Assessment 1:29–41, 1998.
14. Williams JM, Burlew L: Dealing with catastrophic injury: A developmental perspective on rehabilitation care planning. Adultspan 9:4–8, 1995.

15. Williams JM, Fidanza NS: Ensuring the success of industrial rehabilitation program: The role of the rehabilitation counselor in return to work. NARPPS Journal and News 5:67–71, 1990.
16. Williams JM, Maze M: The Role of the Rehabilitation Expert in Administrative Law and Civil Proceedings. Iowa City, ACT, 1994.
17. Williams JM, Reavy G: Effective use of rehabilitation and economic experts in personal injury litigation: An integrated approach. In Stein D (ed): Vocational Expert Monograph Series. Topeka, Kan, American Board of Vocational Experts, 1993, pp 16–27.
18. Williams JM, Sawyer H, LaBuda J: Forensic rehabilitation. In Thorson R (ed): CIRS Self-Study Guide. Rolling Meadows, Ill, Certified Insurance Rehabilitation Specialist Commission, 1993, pp 69–88.
19. Wright GN: Total Rehabilitation. Boston, Little, Brown, 1980.

CHAPTER

46

Legal Issues of Off-Work

CHARLES G. ATKINS, JD

THE LEGISLATIVE SEA AND REGULATORY CHARYBDIS

A Physician's Odyssey

The perilous sea of federal and state legislative and regulatory constraints in which the physician must practice the science and art of medicine is formidable. It is of increasing concern that the physician, through no lack of medical knowledge or application of craft, may violate unwittingly the most fundamental precept in all of medicine, *primum non nocere.*[1]

Intellectual and physical resources of the physician are tested daily—seeing office patients, making hospital rounds, managing an office in one degree or another, having conferences with other physicians regarding patient care, attending committee meetings, dictating letters to the specialist or to the referring physician, responding to patient telephone calls, reviewing laboratory reports and diagnostic studies, updating patient files and charts, writing medical certifications for patient-employees—and on it goes.

There is probably no study that demonstrates the discrepancy between the role of the physician and the bureaucratic imposition to "fill in the boxes" or "select the most appropriate coding number to describe the diagnosis and treatment plan." These impositions aside, in the overwhelming number of patient-employee medical evaluations dealing with medical leave or return to work issues, the physician, with the consent of the patient, will be able to supply to the third party the required medical evaluation of the patient-employee.

The many federal regulatory directives and requirements, with respect to the Family Medical Leave Act (FMLA), the Americans With Disabilities Act (ADA), and the Social Security Act (Disability Chapter) (SSA), occasionally suffer from an inherent lack of clarity. Regulatory variation and overburden can frustrate the physician's compliance with the relevant legislation. How is the physician to determine the nature and extent of the information required? Commonly, the physician's frustration when providing certification of medical condition is brought about by obfuscating regulatory details. Fortunately, most of the administrative regulations of concern are reasonably comprehensible.

It is the intent of this chapter to provide helpful, useful information that the reader can appreciate and understand in a single reading.

FEDERAL LAW

This chapter considers the physician's "short list" of commonly encountered federal and state legislation, and to some extent private disability insurance contracts and the various corresponding requirements and obligations, that regulate the relationship between the patient-employee seeking eligibility for benefits and the third-party[2] benefit provider.

The following discussion should enable the physician to assist the governmental agency or private insurance company where there is to be a determination by such third party of patient-employee eligibility for benefits under the applicable program or insurance policy. Eligibility determinations are strongly influenced by the physician's relevant medical opinion that certifies to the third party the medical condition of the patient-employee.

A GENERAL OVERVIEW

Family Medical Leave Act

The FMLA[3] is federal legislation that primarily provides for and regulates employee eligibility, rights, and job protection in matters of absence from and return to work. The implementing federal regulations[4] may be obtained from the U.S. Government Printing Office (GPO) upon request and also via GPO access.[5]

Americans With Disabilities Act

The ADA[6] is primarily concerned with equal opportunity for employment where the employee, prospective or actual, has a physical or mental condition that may constitute an impairment but that does not prevent such employee from performing relevant job requirements.[7]

Social Security Act

Long the most comprehensive of federal social programs, SSA[8] provisions pertinent to this chapter are scattered throughout 20 CFR Part 416 (Supplemental Security Income For the Aged, Blind and Disabled). The Act's definition of disability and the physician's role are contained in Regulation Subparts I and J.[9]

STATE LAW

Workers' Compensation

Workers' compensation benefits are creatures of state legislative action. The various provisions found in 50 state statutes are a challenge to summarize in any but the most general terms. For the current purposes a general summary will do. It is the common premise in all such state statutes and accompanying administrative regulations that eligibility for benefits must arise from an injury or disabling condition sustained by the employee while performing a work-related activity. The particular state legislation is available through the U.S. Department of Labor.[10]

PRIVATE INSURANCE

Union Contracts

Group Plans

Single Coverage

Each of these subgroups of private insurance will have a defined eligibility for "the covered person" as well as specifying the condition and duration of coverage between the insurer and the insured. This "bargained for" scope of coverage is the common denominator in all private sector employee disability insurance contracts. A state legislature will occasionally enact public policy oversight legislation covering the scope and terms of private disability coverage. Such public policy is usually enacted under the constitutional mandate to provide for health, safety, and welfare. Occasionally, public policy is recognized through judicial pronouncement. In general, considerations of worker eligibility and benefits among the states are not as fundamentally disparate in social philosophy as are other matters of individual state public policy, such as whether to permit gambling.

STATUTORY RIGHTS OF THE PATIENT–EMPLOYEE VIS-À-VIS THIRD PARTIES

Matters of Privilege

Physicians, as well as other health care professionals, are aware that statements made to them in confidence by the patient-employee for the purposes of diagnosis and treatment are deemed privileged communications under state and federal law.[11] The physician-patient relationship creates a privilege that protects the confidentiality of such statements and substantially limits disclosure of their content to third parties without consent of the patient. Privilege in the present context is fundamentally a statutory protection[12] of the patient's privacy and nondisclosure in matters of a personal nature disclosed confidentially by the patient to the physician for purposes of diagnosis or treatment relating to the physical or emotional health of the patient.

The physician should obtain from the patient a written consent to disclose confidential medical information and keep the signed consent in the patient's office file. The information to be disclosed should be specifically identified in the consent form, which should authorize disclosure of the described information, either orally or in writing, and only to the third party therein designated.

The most basic position for the physician to take is as follows: "No disclosure of patient confidential medical information to any third party unless there is relevant prior or contemporaneous written consent by the patient." Technically, this is correct, but at times it is unworkable, as in the following instances:

1. The patient is physically unable or mentally incapable of giving consent and the confidential medical information sought by a qualified health

care provider is important or enabling for the necessary and immediate treatment of the patient.

2. The treating physician, with the consent of the patient (or without such consent in an emergent situation), finds it medically advisable to contract another physician or other health care professional in consultation and perhaps for collaborative treatment.
3. The patient has previously consented to the disclosure of specific information and a later disclosure requested by this previously designated third party is merely a timely request for the physician to update the initial treatment and the specific confidential information initially disclosed.

In every jurisdiction there appears to be either an express or implied legislative exemption or a judicially recognized exception to disclosure of the patient's confidential medical information by the physician without prior patient consent where any one or more of these conditions exist at the time of the needed disclosure.

The physician must be guided by the express terms of the patient's written authorization or consent to disclose the relevant confidential medical information. Disclosure of a patient's confidential medical information may be authorized by the patient in its scope and directed to be disclosed only to designated third parties. Occasionally the physician may be confronted with a demand for disclosure of confidential medical information beyond or regardless of the patient's consent. In such instances, the patient should be notified and any subsequent disclosure by the physician should be in response to a subpoena of a governmental agency or court order. In the absence of patient authorization, unless the physician is under direct order by a court of competent jurisdiction or under subpoena from a legally empowered agency, the disclosure of such confidential medical information by the physician is tantamount to disclosure without the consent of the patient.

When a third party requests a patient's confidential medical information, the physician's disclosure should err on the side of strict relevance to the medical information concerning the condition about which inquiry is made. In certain situations, such as a "serious health condition" as described under FMLA, the physician (or office staff) can best avoid disclosure of unrelated confidential medical information when the physician keeps a separate medical file related only to that serious health condition. This way, the patient's confidential disclosures to the physician about domestic situations, recurring fears, states of minor depression, and such matters that may not be the focus of the serious health condition, are kept confidential and prevent the third party from becoming privy to information about the patient that is irrelevant to a determination of eligibility for benefits.

Frequently, in matters of workers' compensation, the disclosure sought will be presumed to have been consented to by the patient-employee as part of the state's enabling legislation or regulations. Most often, however, the workers' compensation request for disclosure of medical information, in contrast to requests from governmental agencies or private insurance companies, will relate specifically and only to the on-the-job injury or the alleged condition of a job-acquired impairment then under consideration.

CONTENT OF PHYSICIAN CERTIFICATION

For the physician who is asked to write a certification of the patient-employee's medical condition, the fundamental questions are "What am I being asked to certify?" "Why am I being asked to give the certification?" and "How do I give the certification in proper form?" The answers depend upon the particular federal or state legislation (or private disability insurance contract) under which the certification is sought. Often the definition of "medical condition" or "impairment" is contained within the legislation or the private contract of insurance. The enabling legislative regulation may require specific physician certification or assessment about the level of impairment (usually as defined in the legislation or the implementing regulations). Many times the physician will be asked also to opine concerning the prognosis or the duration of the relevant medical condition. Summarily, the "what," "why," and "how" must be considered with respect to each of the referenced acts, statutes, or private disability insurance contracts.

FMLA (see Appendix I and Chapter 49)

What

The physician is being asked to evaluate the medical condition of the patient-employee to assist the agency in its determination whether the patient-employee has the requisite serious health condition.[13]

Why

A serious health condition is the prerequisite for a subsequent administrative determination of the patient-employee's eligibility for benefits and job protection provided by the FMLA. The usual circumstances are as follows:

1. The patient-employee claims to have an impairment, whether in the form of an illness, injury, or physical or mental condition (none of which is required to be work-related) that involves inpa-

tient care (an overnight stay) in a hospital or medical facility, including any period of related and/or continuing treatment of more than three consecutive days that also involves at least one related treatment by a health care professional and a regimen of continuing treatment for various specified periods; such a condition is defined as a "serious health condition."[14]
2. Due to the serious health condition, the patient-employee must be absent from work to receive medical treatment and "unable to perform the functions of employment."
3. Once the serious health condition can be medically managed, such that the patient-employee is again able to perform the functions of employment, the job protection provided by FMLA will enable the patient-employee to return without penalty to the same or equivalent job held before the "covered" leave of absence.[15]

How

The physician has several optional methods to provide certification of the serious health condition:

1. The medical information indicated on the Department of Labor optional form (Form WH–380, as revised; see Appendix A) or a similar form used by the employer (however, the employer form may not require any additional information that is not on Form WH–380);
2. Another option is to provide a less formal statement of certification; however, every physician certification of the patient-employee's serious health condition must contain the following data:
   A. Certification as to which part of the definition of serious health condition, if any, applies to the patient's condition and the medical facts that support the certification, including a brief statement that explains the medical facts related to the criteria of the definition;
   B. The approximate onset date of the serious health condition; the probable duration of incapacity to work; and
   C. Various other facts regarding whether additional treatments will be necessary, whether the incapacity will be intermittent, the patient's prognosis, and related matters.

ADA (see also Chapter 47)

The declared purpose of the Act is to implement equal employment opportunities for qualified individuals with disabilities. Disabilities are defined in the Act as physical or mental impairments[16] that substantially limit the person's ability to perform one or more of the major life functions, such as taking care of one's self, performing manual tasks, walking, seeing, hearing, speaking, breathing, learning, and working. Not surprisingly, the ability to engage in sexual intercourse (but not on the job, of course) is judicially recognized as a major life function.[17]

What

The physician is being asked to evaluate the patient medically and to report facts and render opinions to the employer concerning any impairment that will prevent present performance of work in the context of specific job requirements. Does the patient have a physical and/or mental condition, pre-employment or on return to work, which constitutes a disability as defined, and that either substantially limits or prevents such performance of the job requirements? The physician must consider whether the patient can perform the specific job requirements without presenting a present, direct threat to the safety of the patient or fellow workers.[18]

Why

Numerous patients may have one or more impairments. Those impairments may have no substantial compromising effect on the patient-employee's ability to perform the specific job requirements. In context of the specific job requirements, the physician is being asked to evaluate the patient's medical condition, whether physiologic or mental. This evaluation is appropriate under the Act only as a condition of a patient-employee's beginning employment duties after being hired or as part of an employee's later job-related evaluation. An impairment that does not prevent the patient's present performance of the specific job requirements, with reasonable accommodation[19] of the job conditions by the employer, cannot be the basis for the covered employer[20] to refuse to hire or thereafter to refuse the patient-employee's right to return to the specific job.[21]

How

An understanding and appreciation of the job description and the particular requirements and conditions of the job are essential if the physician is to be able to assess whether an impairment is significant within the context of the job description. The employer must furnish these job data to the physician and the physician should require them in written form. The description should be clear, definite, and readily understandable. The employer's description of the job requirements and conditions should be retained by the physician in the patient's chart.[22] The physician should also discuss the employer's statement of the job description with the patient. If the physician is still in doubt about the job requirements or working environment, written clarification from the employer should be obtained before the medical opinion is rendered.

The opinion need not be on any official form or in any prescribed format, but it must contain the following:

1. A prefacing statement, literally restating or adopting by identifiable reference the employer's written job description sent to the physician;
2. Whether the physician's examination of the employee has disclosed a physical or mental impairment that substantially limits the patient's ability to perform a major life activity and whether such impairment significantly restricts or prevents the employee's ability to perform the particular job, or alternatively, whether such impairment significantly restricts the employee's ability to perform a broad range of jobs[23];
3. A specific factual statement, and test results if applicable, relative to the job description and requirements to substantiate the bases for the medical opinion.

After reviewing the physician's report, if the employer determines the employee is unable to perform the essential requirements of the specific job without threat to the employee or others, even with reasonable accommodation, the employer need not retain or rehire the employee. To the extent that the patient-employee disagrees and claims discrimination prohibited by the Act, there is recourse available to the patient-employee against the employer.[24]

SSA (see also Chapter 6)

SSA disability benefits and workers' compensation benefits can be coextensive. There are instances where the injured patient-employee, within certain limitations, may be eligible to receive benefits from both programs at the same time, and for the same or different disabilities or injuries.

What

The physician is being asked by the SSA to provide medical evidence to support the claim of disability made upon application by the patient-employee to the SSA. (See Appendix II for the SSA form for authorization of power to release information to the SSA.)

Why

In order to be determined eligible for Social Security disability (SSD) benefits the patient-employee must present medical evidence of a medically determinable physical or mental condition sufficient to constitute disability, as defined in the Act.[25]

How

Physicians, osteopathic physicians, and certain other specifically listed licensed health care professionals[26] are acceptable medical sources to establish whether the patient-employee (or applicant) has a medically determinable condition.[27] The medical report of the primary care physician and the treating physician (or other treating health care professional) is of particular relevance and is accorded substantial weight in the agency's determination of disability.[28] The contents of the physician's or other medical source's medical report is given in detail in the Regulations[29] and should include the following:

1. Medical history
2. Clinical findings (such as the results of physical or mental status examinations)
3. Laboratory findings (blood pressure, x-ray reports)
4. Diagnosis (statement of disease or injury based on signs and symptoms)
5. Treatment prescribed with response and prognosis
6. A statement about what the patient can still do despite the impairment(s) based on the above data (except in the case of blindness)

The conditions (impairments) can be considered in their totality under Social Security and need not be work related.[30] There is another somewhat related program available under the broad provisions of Social Security protection and benefits. Supplemental Security Income is a program for the impoverished and is based on need only. No former or present employment is required. The determination of disability is judged by the same criteria used for the SSD patient-employee.

WORKERS' COMPENSATION (see also Chapter 5)

There are 50 separate state statutes defining and regulating the eligibility and benefits available for the injured worker. A useful comparison is beyond the scope of this chapter, but there are certain threshold considerations common to most if not all workers' compensation statutes.

What

The physician (or other specified, treating health care professional) is being asked to provide medical information about a specific mental or physical condition of the patient-employee and any related treatment provided to the patient-employee.

Why

Eligibility for worker benefits is dependent on the injury or acquired condition being work related and having happened on the job or acquired over time while in the performance of the actual or contemplated scope of work of the patient-employee.[31]

How

In the majority of states, the physician can provide the relevant medical information by using (or following the topical outline) of the forms provided by the state's Workers' Compensation Bureau. These forms will usually be specific and focused on the following particulars:

1. When did the injury occur?
2. Is there a prior medical history of this injury?
3. Is the claimed injury an aggravation of a pre-existing condition?
4. Was the pre-existing condition work related? Has there been a previous determination of work-related injury with respect to the present condition?
5. When was medical treatment or diagnosis first sought by the worker?
6. If the injury is one acquired over time through a necessary work-related activity, when were the first signs or symptoms noticed, or reported to the physician?
7. What is the medical diagnosis?
8. Is the claimed injury permanent or temporary?
9. What is the expected duration of the treatment?
10. What is the prescribed treatment?

Often, it is convenient and sufficient for the physician to use the forms provided by the state when expressing a requested medical opinion, treatment regimen, and prognosis. Rarely, if ever, does the agency (or bureau) require disclosure by the physician of the patient-employee's comprehensive past medical history when there is an acute injury on the job resulting from a work-related activity. Therefore, the likelihood of inadvertent disclosure of irrelevant confidential medical information by the treating physician, particularly the primary care physician, is substantially lessened.

In many states, workers' compensation statutes provide that the patient-employee, by making a claim for benefits due to a work-related injury or work-acquired medical condition, thereby irrevocably consents to a continuing disclosure to the agency of otherwise confidential medical information relating to the specific injury or condition. Even where the statute provides for such irrevocable consent, it is good and prudent practice for the physician to obtain written consent from the patient-employee before disclosing the relevant information requested to the bureau.

PRIVATE INSURANCE

The provisions of the contract of insurance determine private insurance eligibility for covered person disability benefits. This is true whether the contract involves a labor union on behalf of its members, a group health plan under any number of employer-employee arrangements, or individual or single family coverage. In most instances, where substantial numbers of employees are being insured privately, the union or the group health plan usually has enough negotiating strength to obtain advantageous disability benefit provisions and conditions. The benefits are closely correlated to the number of potential enrollees in the private insurance disability contract.

These contracts will require some sort of certification, usually physician certification, of a medical condition that prevents the covered person from performing the usual work in the course of employment. There is usually a preliminary period of time that must elapse before eligibility for benefits begins. After the preliminary qualifying days of incapacity have passed and the disability persists, the disability benefits are activated. In such instances, the private insurer has forms that will be specific concerning the information to be supplied by the physician. In many cases, it is necessary to fill in the blanks and mark the appropriate boxes in the form. The covered person usually must sign a "consent to release" medical information provision contained within the form. When that provision is absent, the physician should obtain written consent from the patient before supplying the relevant medical information to the third party.

OFF-WORK AND BACK-TO-WORK PRESCRIPTIONS

"Doctor, I need a note." Off-work and back-to-work prescriptions are familiar medical services the physician provides for the patient. Here, the physician fills the additional role of the impartial medical evaluator, ostensibly for the purpose of initiating or continuing a regimen for the treatment of the patient's medical condition within the context of continuing employment. This prescription may be the only potentially safe passage visa for the patient's leaving and returning to the job without penalty or loss of position.[32]

The good news is that no particular form is required for the off-work or the back-to-work prescriptions. The bad news is that no one knows in either instance how to write the perfect one-size-fits-all prescription. If the physician bears in mind the sometimes competing interests of the patient-employee vis-à-vis the employer,[33] and also takes into account the pertinent provisions and comments in the previous sections, there are some reliable touchstones for the physician when writing such a prescription.

There are degrees of explanation that may be required of the physician when writing the prescription. To whom will the prescription be addressed and who will assess the bona fides of the medical reason for the patient-employee being off work or the limitations of the patient-employee upon return to work? Will the assessment be made in the first instance by a plant physician or will the assessment be made by a lay supervisor who may have little appreciation for the regimen of treatment or the health maintenance of the patient-employee?

A good first principle for the treating physician is to write the prescription with the level of explanation appropriate to the level of medical sophistication that the intended recipient is likely to possess. If the prescription is addressed "To Whom It May Concern," as many are, then the appropriate level of such sophistication is probably unknown. On the other hand, if the intended recipient-evaluator is a physician retained by the employer, the level of sophistication when explaining the diagnosis and regimen might differ from that where the intended recipient is a lay person not trained to evaluate the patient-employee medical bona fides, except within the context of the treating physician's prescription.

In every instance the prescription should be well thought out and calculated to make sense to the intended recipient. Particularly helpful to include as a preamble to the prescription would be 1) a short statement that the patient-employee is currently being evaluated/treated for difficulties in swallowing (or shortness of breath, kidney function, headaches, or such other plain descriptions that are noncommittal and suggestive of signs or symptoms that may be related to any number of causes)[34]; 2) a statement defining work-related physical activities that must be limited, modified, or avoided for a specific period of time; 3) a statement concerning the time anticipated to make a diagnosis and to complete the treatment plan; and 4) the probable exacerbating potential if literal compliance with the prescription is prevented by the employer.[35] A potential advantage to this approach is the limited initial disclosure of personal confidential patient-employee information until such time as more specific information may or must be disclosed, with the prior consent of the patient-employee, to the employer or other relevant third party.

In every instance, the physician should avoid the inadvertent disclosure to third parties of the patient-employee's confidential medical information. To that end, it is good practice to have the patient sign a consent form as a prerequisite for the physician's off-work or back-to-work prescription and to discuss or review the prescription with the patient before sending it to the third party employer.

The physician will have to find the middle path between the following two extremes of prescription disclosure:

1. "Francis is ill and must be off work for 5 days."
2. "Francis presents with clinical evidence suggestive of advanced restrictive cardiomyopathy, which may be the result of an underlying cardiac amyloidosis, a condition with near term potentially fatal prognosis. The expected time for the completion of diagnostic testing will require the patient-employee's absence from work for 5 days."

The first disclosure amounts to an unconvincing non-disclosure (perhaps suggestive to the employer of a naive physician, or worse yet, a benign complicity in the suspected scheming of the employee). The second disclosure contains information meaningful only to another physician but wholly unnecessary in any event to explain that a cardiovascular assessment involving various tests over several days is necessary in order to diagnose the patient-employee's condition. These examples are overdrawn solely for illustrative purposes. To the extent that the physician has complied with the requirements of FMLA or ADA, the patient-employee is protected against retributive firing or demotion in job pay/advancement by these federal laws.[36] This subject is also covered, more graphically, in Appendix B at the end of the book.

FORMS

The reader may refer to the Appendices I and II as well as Appendix B at the end of the book for examples of forms and Appendix III for an algorithm designed to assist in the preparation of the physician's medical certification.

SUMMARY

The best medicine is first to understand what the physician or other qualifying health care professional is being asked to do. Understand what and why the report or information is sought and how to provide it. In all instances, bearing in mind the previous admonitions concerning information produced in response to a subpoena or court order, obtain the written consent of the patient-employee for the disclosure of confidential medical information to the third party requesting or requiring such information. The consent should specify the condition about which the physician will provide the relevant medical information. Offer to supplement or clarify any part of the report upon written request directed specifically to the points to be addressed. Keep a copy of the report in the patient's chart. It is good practice also to send a copy to the patient, unless there is a strong medical contraindication. Above all, the physicians' off-work and back-to-work prescriptions should contain only confidential medical information about the patient-employee that is relevant, necessary, and clearly stated in language free of unnecessary medical jargon and in the first instance, appropriate for the probable medical sophistication of the anticipated evaluator.

APPENDICES

Appendix I: U.S. Department of Labor Certification of Health Care Provider (WH-380)

Certification of Health Care Provider
(Family and Medical Leave Act of 1993)

U.S. Department of Labor
Employment Standards Administration
Wage and Hour Division

(When completed, this form goes to the employee, ***not to the Department of Labor****.)*	OMB No.: 1215-0181 Expires: 06/30/02

1. Employee's Name	2. Patient's Name *(If different from employee)*

3. Page 4 describes what is meant by a **"serious health condition"** under the Family and Medical Leave Act. Does the patient's condition[1] qualify under any of the categories described? If so, please check the applicable category.

   (1) ________ (2) _______ (3) _______ (4) ________ (5) _______ (6) _______ , or None of the above _______

4. Describe the **medical facts** which support your certification, including a brief statement as to how the medical facts meet the criteria of one of these categories:

5. a. State the approximate **date** the condition commenced, and the probable duration of the condition (and also the probable duration of the patient's present **incapacity**[2] if different):

   b. Will it be necessary for the employee to take work only **intermittently or to work on a less than full schedule** as a result of the condition (including for treatment described in Item 6 below)?

   If yes, give the probable duration:

   c. If the condition is a **chronic condition** (condition #4) or **pregnancy**, state whether the patient is presently incapacitated[2] and the likely duration and frequency of **episodes of incapacity**[2]:

[1] Here and elsewhere on this form, the information sought relates **only** to the condition for which the employee is taking FMLA leave.

[2] "Incapacity," for purposes of FMLA, is defined to mean inability to work, attend school or perform other regular daily activities due to the serious health condition, treatment therefor, or recovery therefrom.

Form WH-380
Revised December 1999

Continued on opposite page

APPENDIX I *Continued*

6. a. If additional **treatments** will be required for the condition, provide an estimate of the probable number of such treatments.

   If the patient will be absent from work or other daily activities because of **treatment** on an **intermittent** or **part-time** basis, also provide an estimate of the probable number of and interval between such treatments, actual or estimated dates of treatment if known, and period required for recovery if any:

   b. If any of these treatments will be provided by **another provider of health services** (e.g., physical therapist), please state the nature of the treatments:

   c. **If a regimen of continuing treatment** by the patient is required under your supervision, provide a general description of such regimen (*e.g.*, prescription drugs, physical therapy requiring special equipment):

7. a. If medical leave is required for the employee's **absence from work** because of the **employee's own condition** (including absences due to pregnancy or a chronic condition), is the employee **unable to perform work** of any kind?

   b. If able to perform some work, is the employee **unable to perform any one or more of the essential functions of the employee's job** (the employee or the employer should supply you with information about the essential job functions)? If yes, please list the essential functions the employee is unable to perform:

   c. If neither a. nor b. applies, is it necessary for the employee to be **absent from work for treatment**?

Continued on following page

APPENDIX I *Continued*

8. a. If leave is required to **care for a family member** of the employee with a serious health condition, **does the patient require assistance** for basic medical or personal needs or safety, or for transportation?

   b. If no, would the employee's presence to provide **psychological comfort** be beneficial to the patient or assist in the patient's recovery?

   c. If the patient will need care only **intermittently** or on a part-time basis, please indicate the probable **duration** of this need:

Signature of Health Care Provider

Type of Practice

Address

Telephone Number

Date

To be completed by the employee needing family leave to care for a family member:

State the care you will provide and an estimate of the period during which care will be provided, including a schedule if leave is to be taken intermittently or if it will be necessary for you to work less than a full schedule:

Employee Signature

Date

Continued on opposite page

APPENDIX I *Continued*

A **"Serious Health Condition"** means an illness, injury impairment, or physical or mental condition that involves one of the following:

1. Hospital Care

   Inpatient care (*i.e.*, an overnight stay) in a hospital, hospice, or residential medical care facility, including any period of incapacity[2] or subsequent treatment in connection with or consequent to such inpatient care.

2. Absence Plus Treatment

   (a) A period of incapacity[2] of **more than three consecutive calendar days** (including any subsequent treatment or period of incapacity[2] relating to the same condition), that also involves:

   (1) **Treatment**[3] **two or more times** by a health care provider, by a nurse or physician's assistant under direct supervision of a health care provider, or by a provider of health care services (*e.g.*, physical therapist) under orders of, or on referral by, a health care provider; or

   (2) **Treatment** by a health care provider on **at least one occasion** which results in a **regimen of continuing treatment**[4] under the supervision of the health care provider.

3. Pregnancy

   Any period of incapacity due to **pregnancy**, or for **prenatal care**.

4. Chronic Conditions Requiring Treatments

   A **chronic condition** which:

   (1) Requires **periodic visits** for treatment by a health care provider, or by a nurse or physician's assistant under direct supervision of a health care provider;

   (2) Continues over an **extended period of time** (including recurring episodes of a single underlying condition); and

   (3) May cause **episodic** rather than a continuing period of incapacity[2] (*e.g.*, asthma, diabetes, epilepsy, etc.).

5. Permanent/Long-term Conditions Requiring Supervision

   A period of **Incapacity**[2] which is **permanent or long-term** due to a condition for which treatment may not be effective. The employee or family member must be **under the continuing supervision of, but need not be receiving active treatment by, a health care provider**. Examples include Alzheimer's, a severe stroke, or the terminal stages of a disease.

6. Multiple Treatments (Non-Chronic Conditions)

   Any period of absence to receive **multiple treatments** (including any period of recovery therefrom) by a health care provider or by a provider of health care services under orders of, or on referral by, a health care provider, either for **restorative surgery** after an accident or other injury, **or** for a condition that **would likely result in a period of Incapacity**[2] **of more than three consecutive calendar days in the absence of medical intervention or treatment**, such as cancer (chemotherapy, radiation, etc.), severe arthritis (physical therapy), and kidney disease (dialysis).

This optional form may be used by employees to satisfy a mandatory requirement to furnish a medical certification (when requested) from a health care provider, including second or third opinions and recertification (29 CFR 825.306).

Note: Persons are not required to respond to this collection of information unless it displays a currently valid OMB control number.

---

[3] Treatment includes examinations to determine if a serious health condition exists and evaluations of the condition. Treatment does not include routine physical examinations, eye examinations, or dental examinations.

[4] A regimen of continuing treatment includes, for example, a course of prescription medication (*e.g.*, an antibiotic) or therapy requiring special equipment to resolve or alleviate the health condition. A regimen of treatment does not include the taking of over-the-counter medications such as aspirin, antihistamines, or salves; or bed-rest, drinking fluids, exercise, and other similar activities that can be initiated without a visit to a health care provider.

Public Burden Statement

We estimate that it will take an average of 10 minutes to complete this collection of information, including the time for reviewing instructions, searching existing data sources, gathering and maintaining the data needed, and completing and reviewing the collection of information. If you have any comments regarding this burden estimate or any other aspect of this collection of information, including suggestions for reducing this burden, send them to the Administrator, Wage and Hour Division, Department of Labor, Room S-3502, 200 Constitution Avenue, N.W., Washington, D.C. 20210.

DO NOT SEND THE COMPLETED FORM TO THIS OFFICE; IT GOES TO THE EMPLOYEE.

Appendix II: SSA Authorization for Source to Release Information to the Social Security Administration (SSA-827)

TO BE COMPLETED BY SSA

NUMBER HOLDER

SOCIAL SECURITY NUMBER

EMPLOYEE/CLAIMANT/BENEFICIARY *(If other than Number Holder)*

AUTHORIZATION FOR SOURCE TO RELEASE INFORMATION TO THE SOCIAL SECURITY ADMINISTRATION (SSA)

INFORMATION ABOUT MEDICAL OR OTHER SOURCE-PLEASE PRINT, TYPE, OR WRITE CLEARLY

NAME AND ADDRESS OF SOURCE *(Include Zip Code)*	RELATIONSHIP TO DISABLED PERSON

INFORMATION ABOUT DISABLED PERSON-PLEASE PRINT, TYPE, OR WRITE CLEARLY

NAME AND ADDRESS *(If known)* AT TIME DISABLED PERSON HAD CONTACT WITH SOURCE *(Include Zip Code)*	DATE OF BIRTH	DISABLED PERSON'S I.D. NUMBER *(If known and different than SSN) (Clinic/Patient No.)*

APPROXIMATE DATES OF DISABLED PERSON'S CONTACT WITH SOURCE *(e.g., dates of hospital admission, treatment, discharge, etc.)*

TO BE COMPLETED BY DISABLED PERSON OR PERSON AUTHORIZED TO ACT IN HIS/HER BEHALF

GENERAL AND SPECIAL AUTHORIZATION TO RELEASE MEDICAL AND OTHER INFORMATION IN ACCORDANCE WITH THE PROVISIONS OF THE SOCIAL SECURITY ACT; THE PUBLIC HEALTH SERVICE ACT, SECTIONS 523 AND 527; AND TITLE 38 U.S.C. VETERANS BENEFITS, SECTION 4132.

I hereby authorize the above-named source to release or disclose to the Social Security Administration or State agency the following information for the period(s) identified above:

1) All medical records or other information regarding my treatment, hospitalization, and/or outpatient care for my impairment(s), including psychological or psychiatric impairment(s), drug abuse, alcoholism, sickle cell anemia, human immunodeficiency virus (HIV) infection (including acquired immunodeficiency syndrome (AIDS) or tests for HIV), or sexually transmitted diseases;
2) Information about how my impairment(s) affects my ability to complete tasks and activities of daily living;
3) Information about how my impairment(s) affected my ability to work.

I authorize the use of a telefax or photocopy of this form for the release or disclosure of the information described above.

I understand that this authorization, except for action already taken, may be voided by me at anytime. If I do not void this authorization, it will automatically end when a final decision is made on my claim. If I am already receiving benefits, the authorization will end when a final decision is made as to whether I can continue to receive benefits.

READ IMPORTANT INFORMATION ON REVERSE BEFORE SIGNING FORM BELOW.

SIGNATURE OF DISABLED PERSON OR PERSON AUTHORIZED TO ACT IN HIS/HER BEHALF	RELATIONSHIP TO DISABLED PERSON (If other than self)	DATE
STREET ADDRESS	TELEPHONE NUMBER (Area Code)	
CITY	STATE	ZIP CODE

The signature and address of a person who either knows the person signing this form or is satisfied as to that person's identity is requested below. This is not required by the Social Security Administration, but without it the source may not honor this authorization.

SIGNATURE OF WITNESS	STREET ADDRESS	
CITY	STATE	ZIP CODE

Form SSA-827 (1-97) Use Prior Editions EF-FF (1-97) (OVER)

Continued on opposite page

APPENDIX II *Continued*

Explanation of Form SSA-827, Authorization For Source to Release Information to the Social Security Administration (SSA)

We are requesting that you authorize the release of information about your impairment to us. Sources usually require this authorization before releasing information to us. Also, the law requires this authorization for release of information about certain conditions.

You can provide this authorization by signing a Form SSA-827, Authorization For Source to Release Information to the Social Security Administration (SSA), for each source identified during your disability interview or during the processing of your claim. We must inform you that because of various Federal disclosure laws, SSA cannot give an absolute pledge of confidentiality regarding information submitted in connection with your claim.

PRIVACY ACT NOTICE

The Social Security Administration is authorized to collect the information on this form under sections 205(a), 223(d) and 1631(e)(1) of the Social Security Act. The information on this form is needed by Social Security to make a decision on your claim. While giving us the information on this form is voluntary, failure to provide all or part of the requested information could prevent an accurate or timely decision on your claim and could result in the loss of benefits. Although the information you furnish on this form is almost never used for any purpose other than making a determination on your disability claim, such information may be disclosed by the Social Security Administration as follows:

(1) To enable a third party or agency to assist Social Security in establishing rights to Social Security benefits and/or coverage;

(2) To comply with Federal laws requiring the release of information from Social Security records (e.g., to the General Accounting Office and the Department of Veterans Affairs);

(3) To facilitate statistical research and audit activities necessary to assure the integrity and improvement of the Social Security programs (e.g., to the Bureau of the Census and private concerns under contract to Social Security).

We may also use the information you give us when we match records by computer. Matching programs compare our records with those of other Federal, State, or local government agencies. Many agencies may use matching programs to find or prove that a person qualifies for benefits paid by the Federal government. The law allows us to do this even if you do not agree to it.

Explanations about these and other reasons why information you provide us may be used or given out are available in Social Security offices. If you want to learn more about this, contact any Social Security office.

Form SSA-827 (1-97) Use Prior Editions EF-FF (1-97)

Appendix II. *Continued*

Appendix III: Algorithm

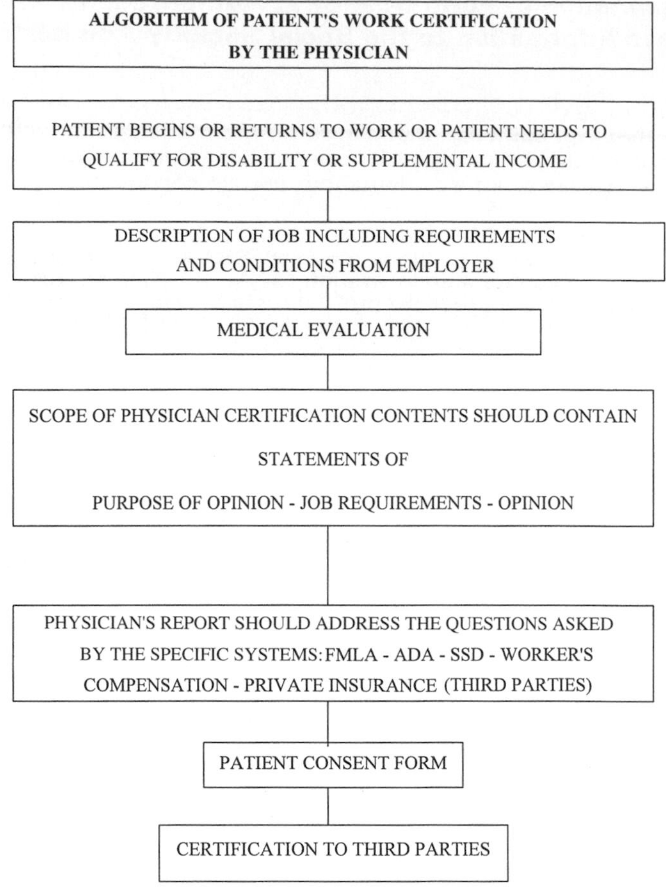

References

1. There is a potential for unwitting harm done when the patient-employee applies for benefits due to an alleged impairment that compromises the ability to work. The problem for the physician is to determine what relevant confidential medical information must be provided in the application process and how best to present it to the agency or other third party. It can be a confusing and often daunting task to comply precisely and efficiently with the numerous, divergent requirements of governmental regulations and private insurance contract provisions that require a physician's certification concerning the physical and/or mental condition of the injured, the impaired, or the handicapped patient-employee's anticipated fitness to perform job requirements, return to work, or application for other benefits.
2. Throughout this chapter, "third party" is intended to mean one or more of the following: state agencies, federal agencies, and/or private insurance companies.
3. Family and Medical Leave Act, 29 USC §§ 2601–2619 (rev. July 1, 2000). FMLA also includes certain benefits that are tangential to the primary focus of this chapter, such as up to 12 weeks' leave for eligible employees during any 12-month period for birth of a child. The FMLA is implemented through Regulations, Dept. of Labor Wage and Hour Division: Family and Medical Leave Act Interim Regulations, 29 CFR § 825 (rev. July 1, 2000). USC and CFR are the abbreviations commonly used, respectively, for the United States Code and for the Code of Federal Regulations.
4. 29 CFR § 825.305, et seq.
5. One of the more comprehensive current Web addresses is the following: http://www.access.gpo.gov/nara/cfr/
6. Americans With Disabilities Act of 1990, 42 USC §§ 12101–12113 (rev. July 1, 2000); the ADA is implemented through Regulations, Equal Employment Opportunity Commission: Regulations to Implement the Equal Employment Provisions of the Americans With Disabilities Act, 29 CFR § 1630 (rev. July 1, 2000). See also Equal Employment Opportunity Commission: Technical Assistance Manual to Title 1 of the Americans With Disabilities Act, 2000.
7. See fn. 5, supra.
8. See Social Security Act, 42 USC §§ 301–1395 (as amended through April 7, 2000). The regulations that implement the provisions of the Social Security Act relevant to this chapter are Employees Benefits, Social Security Administration: Federal Old-Age, Survivors And Disability Insurance, Determining Disability and Blindness, 20 CFR § 416.20 et seq. and especially, in present context, §416.913 (as amended, June 2000).
9. 20 CFR Part 416 (as amended through June 30, 2000); see §§ 416.901–416.1018, passim; see also fn. 5, supra.
10. U.S. Department of Labor, Employment Standards Administration. Office of Workers' Compensation Programs: State Workers' Compensation Laws. See fn. 5, supra. One may also consult the separate publications from each state's workers' compensation law.
11. The federal law, aside from specific provisions within the particular legislation or Act, generally considers the statutory law of the relevant state to be definitive and controlling in the scope of the

physician-patient relationship and the manner by which such confidential, privileged information may be (or can compelled to be) disclosed to third parties. See Federal Rules of Evidence FRE 501 and corresponding state rules of evidence.

12. Many rights at common law, as we have come to consider them, find their genesis in the largely uncodified laws and ancient customs existing in England from the time of William the Conqueror and as developed significantly in the reign of Henry III (1216–1272) and thereafter by the crown, the parliament, and the English Courts of record. See, passim, Pollock F, Maitland FW: The History of English Law, vols. 1 and 2, 2nd ed. Cambridge at University Press. Boston, Little, Brown, 1899; and Holmes OW Jr: The Common Law. Boston, Little, Brown, 1881. However, the common law did not recognize on the basis of ancient custom a right of privacy against unauthorized disclosure to third parties of confidential communications by the patient to the physician. In the common law there was no recognized physician-patient privilege. Whatever privilege there is against such unauthorized disclosure to third parties, it is created and codified in the various legislations of the respective states.
13. See fn. 14, infra.
14. A serious health condition, as defined in the Act, may also include work leave of the patient-employee to care for a seriously ill spouse, child, or parent. In such instances, the physician must be able to certify medically that such family member is seriously ill and describe the nature and extent of the illness and its probable duration.
15. See 29 CFR § 825.214 (a), which in pertinent part provides " ... an employee is entitled to be returned to the same position ... or an equivalent position with equivalent benefits, pay and other conditions of employment." But see also § 825.310, which recognizes that although the employer may request a "fitness-for-duty" certification before returning the employee to work, such certification must be "only with regard to that particular health condition that caused the employee's need for FMLA leave."
16. Disability is defined in the Act as a physical or mental impairment that substantially limits one or more of the major life activities of the individual. See 29 CFR §1630.2 (g), which defines disability as 1) a physical or mental impairment that substantially limits one or more of the major life activities of such individual; 2) a record of such an impairment; or 3) being regarded as having such an impairment. All references to the CFR applicable to ADA are as amended July 1, 2000.
17. Bragdon v Abbott, 141 L Ed 2d 540, 118 S Ct 2196 (1998, US).
18. A direct threat is defined as a significant risk of substantial harm, considering the present ability of the employee to perform safely the essentials of the job requirements. See 29 CFR §1630.2(r).
19. See 29 CFR §1630.2(o)(2); reasonable accommodation basically means making the job condition capable of being performed by the employee without creating an undue hardship upon the employer. The determination of what is an undue hardship is not the responsibility of the physician. Generally, only politicians, bureaucrats, and lawyers have the genetic predisposition for such self-inflicted mental flagellation.
20. A covered employer, quite generally, is one who has 25 or more employees working per day for 20 or more weeks per year. See 29 CFR 1630.02 (e).
21. See 29 CFR §1630.10, which makes it unlawful to use screening tests or other criteria that tend to screen out an individual with a disability, unless the disability is shown to be job related for the position in question. Consider, for example, the acrophobic steeple jack applicant.
22. It is highly advisable for the physician to require a written job description from the employer and to retain it in the patient's medical chart. If, when performing the explicit job requirements, the patient is injured or injures another employee, the physician will have kept the necessary data. This also has potential importance in the event of litigation where the physician, who may be one of the defendants, will be able to offer the job description to show that at the time the medical evaluation was made, the impairment did not pose a direct threat to the patient-employee or to others. An ounce of proof is worth a pound of accusation.
23. See 29 CFR §1630.2(j).
24. See 42 USC §12117.
25. Disability is defined as the inability to do any substantial gainful activity because of any "medically determinable physical or mental condition" which is terminal or has a duration of a year or more. Whether the patient-employee is disabled by the condition(s) is an administration determination. See 20 CFR 416.950 (rev. April 20, 2000).
26. See 20 CFR § 416.913 (a) (as amended June 1, 2000).
27. In general, the physician diagnoses and defines an impairment or condition while the third party subsequently determines whether such impairment or condition constitutes a disability that makes the patient-employee eligible for benefits. The impairment or condition must be the result of an anatomic, physiologic, or psychological abnormality that can be demonstrated by medically acceptable clinical and laboratory diagnostic techniques. See 20 CFR § 416.908, 1991.
28. See 20 CFR § 416.920.
29. See 20 CFR § 416.913.
30. The physician may wish to consult the American Medical Association's "A Medical and Legal Transition to the Guides to the Evaluation of Permanent Impairment, 5th ed" (September 2001). It is important to remember that the physician determines whether an impairment exists, while the third party determines whether the impairment constitutes a disability.
31. In many instances, for example, carpal tunnel syndrome has been determined to be a work-related acquired injury.
32. See fn. 3, 15, 18, 21, 24, supra.
33. The tension that sometimes exists between the employer and the off work or returning to work employee is often created by the employer's underlying suspicion, sometimes with good and sufficient reason, that employee malingering and/or mendacity are principal motivating factors for being off work or returning to less rigorous physical work. In some instances, the employer may show an intractable, near phobic suspicion of even the most obvious and legitimate limiting medical condition of the employee. Such conditions may portend an employer-employee impasse. Here, the clinical evaluating skills of the physician, coupled with a straightforward, jargon-free prescription, will in many instances temper and place in perspective the patient-employee's complaints and demonstrable work-related medical limitations to the reasonable satisfaction of both employer and employee.
34. The point here is simply that at this juncture the physician is well advised not to list all the potential conditions that a differential diagnosis would take into account.
35. In such instances, the employer's support for and compliance with the prescription may be engendered by economic self interest to avoid the potential of a later work-related claim caused by the employer's unwillingness to permit compliance with the prescription. Economic self interest can be considered an adjuvant social therapy, so to speak, regardless of the employer's otherwise compassionate and altruistic accommodation for the employee's medical condition.
36. See fn. 32, supra.

CHAPTER

47

Overview of the Americans With Disabilities Act and the Family and Medical Leave Act

CHRISTOPHER BELL, JD, WITH UPDATES BY BARBARA JUDY, RN, MA

Since 1990, Congress has enacted two major pieces of legislation prohibiting discrimination on the basis of disability and providing for family and medical leave. The Americans With Disabilities Act of 1990 (ADA) and the Family and Medical Leave Act of 1993 (FMLA) radically affect the practice of occupational medicine as well as both the medical and nonmedical aspects of managing employment-related disability matters.

The ADA protects persons with disabilities from discrimination and mandates accommodations for disabled employees, customers, clients, and patients. The ADA affects the provision of health care in many ways, including architectural design of a health care provider's office; how the health care provider communicates with patients with impaired cognitive or communication skills; the scope and timing of a medical examination requested for an employee by an employer; and the timing and nature of the medical information an employer may require of a treating physician.

The ADA has also spawned a considerable volume of claims of disability discrimination. For example, from July 1992 through December 2000, 149,615 charges of employment discrimination have been received by the Equal Employment Opportunity Commission (EEOC), the federal agency that enforces the ADA. Approximately 17% of these charges were filed by individuals claiming to have a disabling back impairment and another 20% of the charges were filed by persons with some other form of impairment not administratively catalogued by the EEOC.

The FMLA is not quite so sweeping in its impact on health care providers. The FMLA provides unpaid time off for eligible employees of a covered employer for up to 12 weeks for a variety of family and medical reasons. These employees are guaranteed job restoration and the continuation of health benefits while on leave. Leave may be taken because of a serious health condition of an employee that prohibits him or her from doing his or her job for more than 3 days; the care of a spouse, child, or parent with a serious health condition; and the birth, adoption, or placement in foster care of a child. Employers are provided only certain limited rights of access to medical information by the FMLA with respect to authorizing employee absences and return to work.

This chapter briefly explores the impact of the ADA and the FMLA on the business and practice of medicine. In particular, the chapter discusses how these two laws affect health care providers in their obligations to patients and the nature and timing of medical input an employer may obtain to comply with these legal mandates.[1]

THE ADA

This section provides a general overview of the ADA and explores the patient's rights vis-à-vis the doctor, the patient's employer, and the employer's relationship with the doctor.

Overview of the ADA

The ADA is a civil rights law that prohibits discrimination in public and private employment, governmental services, public accommodations, public transportation, and telecommunication. Its prohibitions apply to employers

"Disability" in this chapter is used in the context of the Americans With Disabilities Act, rather than in the context used throughout this text.

with 15 or more employees and to state and local governments and public services of any size. The ADA's protections apply to an individual with a disability. A disability is defined by the ADA as a mental or physical impairment that currently substantially limits an individual in any major life activity including working, that did so at some documented time in the past, or that is now perceived by the employer as doing so. The ADA's employment provisions protect an applicant or an employee with a disability if the employee is a "qualified individual with a disability." A qualified individual is defined by the ADA as a person with a disability who satisfies certain job prerequisites such as knowledge, skills, abilities, education, and experience and who has the capacity to perform the "essential functions" of a job with or without reasonable accommodation.[2] The ADA prohibits discrimination against a qualified individual with a disability in all aspects of the employment relationship including recruitment, hiring, compensation, training, discharge, and benefits.[3]

An employer is required to provide a reasonable accommodation to enable a qualified individual with a disability to perform the essential functions of the job and to otherwise meet the demands of the job and conditions of employment, unless the specific accommodation would impose an undue hardship on the employer's business.[4]

The essential functions of a job are the fundamental rather than the marginal duties of a position, considering factors such as the job description, the time spent doing a function, the number of people available to do the function, and the consequences if the function is not performed.[5] A reasonable accommodation is a modification or adjustment to the work environment or to the manner or circumstances under which a job is customarily performed that enables a qualified individual with a disability to perform the essential functions of that position, to be considered for employment, or to receive equal benefits provided to other similarly situated employees.

The ADA's definition of disability is, at once, both broader and narrower than traditional definitions of disability used in benefits systems (see Chapter 1). The ADA adopts a functional approach to disability but also recognizes that societal attitudes may define when a particular medical condition is considered to be disabling. A person with a disability is defined in three ways by the ADA:

1. Any person who has a physical or mental impairment that substantially limits one or more of the individual's major life activities.[6]
2. Any person who has a record of a substantially limiting impairment.[7]
3. Any person who is regarded as having a substantially limiting impairment, regardless of whether the person is in fact disabled.[8]

Major life activities include caring for oneself, performing manual tasks, walking, seeing, hearing, speaking, learning, and working.[9] Other common daily activities such as sitting, standing, bending, reaching, grasping, concentrating, reasoning, and basic socialization skills would also be included.

Minor, nonchronic impairments of short duration with little or no permanent or long-term impact do not constitute an ADA-covered disability.[10] This includes common workplace injuries such as a broken leg or sprained joints.[11]

However, according to the EEOC, even a temporary condition, such as a broken leg, can become a disability when the recovery period is significantly longer than normal and if, during the healing period, the individual is unable to walk, or if the impairment heals but leaves a permanent residual impairment, such as a limp, that substantially limits the individual's ability to walk.[12]

An applicant or employee may also be protected because of a record of a disability. An injured worker has a record of a disability when that employee has recovered in whole or in part from an impairment that is documented as having substantially limited a major life activity in the past. For example, according to the EEOC, an injured worker who had been unable to work for 1 year because of a personal injury or workplace injury would probably have a record of a disability. If an employer refused to hire or return this person back to work because of this record alone, this action would violate the ADA if the worker were otherwise qualified for the position sought. Note, however, that a mere record of having filed a workers' compensation claim or a claim for other disability benefits does not automatically give a person a record of a substantially limiting impairment.[13]

An applicant or employee also may be regarded as disabled; that is, he or she may have no current or past disability but still be protected by the ADA because of the subjective perception of an employer that the individual is disabled. When an employer perceives that an individual is significantly restricted in the ability to perform manual tasks or any other major life activity, the individual is thereby regarded as disabled by the employer.[14] This is true regardless of whether the individual is, in fact, substantially limited by the impairment.

The "regarded as" part of the ADA's definition of disability is expansive and depends upon the attitude of the employer, not the nature of the medical condition. Many injured workers may potentially be protected by the ADA as a result of an employer's fears concerning the risk of future injury, increases in workers' compensation premiums, or the cost of accommodation. These common employer concerns about an injured worker create ADA coverage when it can be shown that the employer took an adverse employment action because it regarded the individual as being substantially limited in a major life activity such as performing manual tasks or performing a class of jobs.[15]

Physicians may unwittingly provide a trigger for ADA coverage by recommending broad work restrictions without addressing an applicant's or employee's ability to perform particular job functions with or without a reasonable accommodation. If a physician recommends work restrictions by simply focusing on what he or she believes an employee is unable to do and does not relate these restrictions to the particular functions of the job at issue, and if the employer accepts the restrictions, it will be easier for an employee or applicant to claim that he or she was regarded as a person with a disability by the employer.

Suppose, for example, an employer accepts and implements a doctor's recommended work restrictions permanently prohibiting repeated bending and stooping, sitting for more than 2 hours at a time, and standing for more than 1 hour at a time. Even if the employer had no way of knowing that the restrictions were not medically warranted, it may be difficult for the employer to successfully argue that it did not regard the applicant or employee as having a disability under the terms of the ADA. Accordingly, to avoid inadvertently creating a potential ADA liability, it is important for both the physician and the employer to review critically the physician's recommendations, to verify that there is in fact a medical basis for recommending restrictions, and to verify the expected duration of the restrictions.

Case law developed under the ADA and its precursor, the Rehabilitation Act of 1973, however, continues to be more favorable to employers in limiting claims by persons who profess to have a disability. Courts are interpreting both laws to exclude from disability status persons who merely are unable to perform or are regarded by an employer as being unable to perform one job for one particular employer.[16] Rather, to be covered by the ADA because of a medically related limitation in working, an individual must be disabled from a class of jobs or broad range of jobs in many classes.[17]

In addition, because a growing number of courts are interpreting that the ADA and the Rehabilitation Act do not cover temporary or perceived temporary disabilities,[18] many more injured workers will be excluded from ADA protection.

Qualified Individual With a Disability

Operationally, the ADA requires that an applicant or employee be simultaneously disabled and qualified. These twin standards put a potential ADA claimant in a different "Catch-22"; if the claimant emphasizes the severity of limitations resulting from disability, the claimant is likely to prove not to be qualified for the job. On the other hand, if the claimant emphasizes ability, this may defeat the claim of being disabled. However, being simultaneously disabled yet qualified is not necessarily an insurmountable burden. For example, an individual is protected from discrimination based on a past record of a disability, such as a history of severe back problems, and also on being perceived as being more disabled than one actually is. The impediments for employment for such a qualified person are addressed by the ADA without that individual being caught in the law's Catch-22 when the person has recovered from a disability or when the disability is in the perception of an employer. Reasonable accommodation also can turn an unqualified person with a disability into a qualified individual with a disability by reducing or eliminating the effects of the individual's functional limitation on the job by changing some features of the job, without affecting the person's disability status. However, when an individual cannot be effectively accommodated and the job's essential functions require the use of physical or mental functions that the individual cannot perform because of impairments, the individual is not likely to be qualified.

The tension between being disabled and qualified is increased when an employee files for disability benefits. A current employee who files for permanent total disability benefits is claiming an inability to perform on the job but might, at the same time, seek reasonable accommodation. A claim of permanent and total disability, however, may undercut that employee's claim of being a qualified individual with a disability, and thus able to perform the essential functions of a job in spite of a disability. Courts have used the sworn factual statements on an application for long-term disability benefits as a basis for finding that an employee is not qualified to perform the essential functions of a job.[19]

To avoid this problem, some individuals with disabilities have asserted that their only disability stems from an employer's perception that they are not qualified for a position because of an impairment. This emphasis on being qualified rather than disabled also has doomed claims for workers because some courts have concluded that such individuals are not truly disabled.[20]

Accordingly, health care providers need to be aware that their statements attesting to a disability claimant's inability to perform a job may well be used against the claimant, if the claimant later pursues a claim of disability discrimination. Health care providers should recognize that the eligibility requirements for most disability benefits do not take into account either an employee's essential job functions or the possibility that the employee might be somehow accommodated to perform in the original job or in another job to which an employee might be reassigned. Overly broad assertions regarding an employee's inability to work or perform in the customary occupation without regard to these ADA refinements may not be in the employee's or employer's best interest.

Restrictions on Medical Examinations and Inquiries

The employment provisions of the ADA severely restrict disability-related medical inquiries and examinations in ways that affect medical practice. Before a job offer is made, an employer may not inquire about an applicant's impairment or medical history. Inquiries concerning past on-the-job injuries or workers' compensation claims are expressly prohibited.[21] This includes inquiries to third parties about an applicant's workers' compensation history.

An employer may, however, conditionally offer a position based on the satisfactory completion of a medical examination or medical inquiry, but only if such examination or inquiry is made of all applicants for the same job category and the results are kept confidential with a few narrow exceptions.[22] For example, an employer may choose to require all postoffer candidates to complete a medical history questionnaire and to selectively require medical examinations of those candidates whose medical history justifies a more thorough medical evaluation concerning a particular issue.[23] Postoffer medical examinations and inquiries do not have to be job-related; questions concerning recent medical treatment, hospitalization, prescription drug use, past workers' compensation claims, and on-the-job injuries are expressly permitted.

A job offer may be withdrawn only if the findings on the medical examination, when reviewed in conjunction with a job's essential functions, support a conclusion that an individual 1) is unable to do the essential functions of a job, even with reasonable accommodation or 2) would pose a direct threat to his or her own health or safety or the health or safety of others that cannot be eliminated or acceptably reduced by reasonable accommodation .[24]

Medical examinations and inquiries of current employees are required to be job-related and consistent with business necessity.[25] Accordingly, in connection with current employees, an employer may not require a medical examination or make inquiries to determine if an employee has an impairment or to ascertain the nature or severity of an impairment unless the employer can demonstrate that there is a substantive basis for such an inquiry or examination. For example, a medical inquiry, including medical examination, when warranted, may be carried out if medical issues arise when an employee is having difficulty performing on the job or an employer has reason to believe that an employee may pose a risk to the health or safety of the employee or others in the workplace.

The postemployment medical examination also is narrower in scope than the postoffer, preemployment medical examination. Although an employer is permitted to require a full medical examination during the postoffer stage, it may not require a general medical examination once an employee has commenced work. Rather, the examination must focus on ascertaining whether and to what degree an employee has a medical condition impacting the ability to perform, safely and satisfactorily, the essential functions of the position the employee occupies. Thus, for example, a hospital employee whose essential functions include lifting and transferring patients and who is complaining of back pain could be evaluated to determine the employee's current capacity to continue safely lifting and transferring patients. However, that medical examination cannot include bloodwork for human immunodeficiency virus (HIV) disease because this would not relate to the employee's essential job functions.

Finally, return-to-work medical evaluations, in addition to addressing the capacity of the employee to perform the essential duties of the job, must also consider the possibility that an employee may return to work with a reasonable accommodation.

Direct Threat to Health or Safety

In order to withdraw a job offer or restrict the return to work on health or safety grounds, an employer must show that the individual poses a high probability of causing substantial harm to his or her health or safety and that the risk of substantial harm cannot be eliminated or reduced below the direct threat level by reasonable accommodation.[26] This is a very stringent standard that employers rarely will be able to meet when attempting to screen for potential future injury. In fact, medical science will rarely have the data to demonstrate that there is a high probability that something bad will happen. Moreover, such claims cannot be speculative or based on potential future risk. Only the current abilities of the individual to perform essential job functions safely can be assessed.

The following examples were derived from the EEOC's Technical Assistance Manual (TAM). They demonstrate how the direct threat standard applies to common scenarios.

1. An applicant for a laborer job has had no back pain or injuries in his previous jobs that required heavy lifting, but a back x-ray reveals a back anomaly. The patient has no medical history or clinical findings that indicate a current back problem, but the company doctor worries that, because of the x-ray finding, there is a slight chance that the applicant could develop back

problems in the future. The threat of future back injury in such a case is too slender to meet the direct threat standard, according to the EEOC.
2. A significant risk would exist for an individual with a back anomaly who has a history of repeated back injuries in similar jobs, and whose back condition has been aggravated further by injury, and where there are no accommodations that would eliminate or reduce the risk.
3. A physician's evaluation indicates that an employee has a disc condition that might worsen in 8 to 10 years. This is not a sufficient indication of imminent potential harm.[27]

Reasonable Accommodation

Unlike most disability benefit systems, the ADA requires an employer to make reasonable accommodations for the known physical or mental limitations of an individual with a disability who is qualified for a job in all respects except for limitations imposed by the disability. The concept underlying reasonable accommodation is a deceptively simple one. Making adjustments in the job structure, work space, work schedule, or tools used on the job can enable a person with medically based functional limitations to perform a job successfully. Of necessity, however, reasonable accommodation must be tailored to the specific abilities and limitations of the individual as well as the particular demands of the job. To this end, the ADA provides a list of nonexclusive examples of reasonable accommodations.

Reasonable accommodation under the ADA means:

1. Modifications or adjustments to a job application process that enable a qualified applicant with a disability to be considered for the position such qualified applicant desires; or
2. Modifications or adjustments to the work environment, or to the manner or circumstances under which the position held or desired is customarily performed, that enable a qualified individual with a disability to perform the essential functions of that position; or
3. Modifications or adjustments that enable a covered entity's employee with a disability to enjoy equal benefits and privileges of employment as are enjoyed by its other similarly situated employees without disabilities.[28]

The statute and regulations provide the following nonexclusive list of examples:

1. Making existing facilities used by employees readily accessible to and usable by individuals with disabilities; and
2. Job restructuring; part-time or modified work schedules; reassignment to a vacant position; acquisition or modification of equipment or devices; appropriate adjustment or modifications of examinations, training materials, or policies; the provision of qualified readers or interpreters; and other similar accommodations for individuals with disabilities.

Good communication among employer, employee, physician, and various occupational specialists (including industrial hygienists, safety specialists, and plant engineers) is essential to the provision of reasonable accommodation. Providing reasonable accommodation is an interactive process between an employer and the person with a disability requesting it. The EEOC has suggested that the following steps be taken when an employee is unable to suggest a reasonable accommodation that an employer is willing to provide:

1. Identify the purpose and functions of the job the individual is seeking to perform.
2. Identify barriers to employment by consulting with the individual with a disability to ascertain abilities and limitations as they relate to performance of the job's essential functions.
3. Identify possible accommodations by consulting with the individual and, where necessary, seek technical assistance.
4. Select a reasonable accommodation that is effective, and that provides an equal employment opportunity.[29]

Moreover, should an employer not grant a request for accommodation, the employer's failure to make an effort to identify possible accommodations in consultation with the person with a disability who requested accommodation results in denial of an employer's "good faith" defense to liability for compensatory and punitive damages.[30]

Medical input may be critical in any accommodation decision, and an employer has a right to medical information necessary to determine the nature and extent of a medical impairment and its expected duration, and to information regarding the impact of the impairment on an individual's daily life activities. The accommodation requested must be medically warranted and the employer is entitled to sufficient medical information to understand the medical basis for the accommodation. An employer has a legitimate interest in knowing, for example, the specific medical reasons for which an individual with diabetes could be expected to suffer injury, harm, or aggravation of the condition when precluded from rotating shifts. In addition, the employer may be entitled to obtain copies of medical records of an employee seeking reasonable accommodation in circumstances where the individual's disability status and need for accommodation are not obvious. An employer is not limited to accepting a treating physician's "doctor's note" as the only proof of the disability status or the medical necessity for the accommodation requested by the employee, and employers are allowed to seek guidance from an independent medical advisor.

Undue Hardship

An employer does not have to provide a reasonable accommodation that would impose "significant difficulty or expense" on the employer in relation to its business and the resources available to provide the accommodation.[31] An accommodation is not required if it is "unduly costly, extensive, substantial, or disruptive, or that would fundamentally alter the nature or operation of the business."[32] In determining whether the cost of an accommodation would pose an undue hardship, the EEOC has apparently instructed its investigators to consider the cost of making the accommodation and the amount of money an employer would save in workers' compensation related expenses if an injured worker is returned to work with reasonable accommodations as opposed to the amount spent if that employee remained out of work and received benefits.[33]

Role of Physicians in ADA-related Determinations

From the foregoing brief summary, it should be clear that medical input of various kinds can be critical to both an employee or applicant and an employer in making ADA-compliant employment decisions. Medical input may be necessary in assessing whether an individual has a physical or mental impairment and whether that impairment "substantially limits" the individual's major life activities. Medical input also may be needed to determine whether an applicant has the physical or mental capacity to perform a job and to do so safely without posing significant risk to the individual or others. In addition, an employer may need to understand how an individual's medical condition limits an employee's ability to perform essential job functions or otherwise meet job demands, so that the employer can consider possible reasonable accommodations.

Physicians can only provide medical information and give recommendations. The quality of the information and recommendations is, of necessity, influenced by the quality of the questions asked by the employer, as well as by the knowledge and experience of the physician. Physicians do not make the employment decision. This is the employer's responsibility. Using this input, an employer can decide, consistent with applicable law and company policy, whether to hire, return to work, or accommodate a particular person. The ultimate decision is a management one, not a medical one. The EEOC makes this point clear in its ADA Technical Assistance Manual:

> A doctor who conducts medical examinations for an employer should not be responsible for making employment decisions or deciding whether or not it is possible to make a reasonable accommodation for a person with a disability. That responsibility lies with the employer.
>
> The doctor's role should be limited to advising the employer about an individual's functional abilities and limitations in relation to job functions, and about whether the individual meets the employer's health and safety requirements.[34]

However, whereas physicians play a significant role in many aspects of ADA compliance, the nature of the needed medical input may differ from the information a physician has provided to an employer.

It will sometimes be necessary for an employer to know the diagnosis of the physical or mental impairment in order to determine whether an individual has a disability or to determine whether a requested accommodation is medically necessary. For example, suppose an applicant requests that an employer provide extra time for an employment test because of difficulty with reading. This could be a reasonable accommodation if the employee's need for accommodation is due to a medical condition such as dyslexia. On the other hand, it the employee simply never learned to read well, such an extension of time would not be required.

Patients' Rights to Equal Access to Medical Services

Physicians, in the private and public practice of medicine, have new obligations toward patients with disabilities under the ADA. These obligations can be summarized as follows: 1) provision of accessible facilities, 2) provision of effective communication for patients with communication impairments, and 3) nondiscrimination in the provision of medical services on the basis of disability.

Providing Accessible Facilities

A physician or other health care provider in private practice has an obligation to ensure that patients with disabilities, including patients with mobility impairments, have physical access to the health care facilities. Narrow doorways, steps, deep pile carpeting, and furniture-cluttered waiting rooms may prove obstacles to a person using a wheelchair or crutches. The ADA imposes an obligation on health care providers who provide services from a place of public accommodation, including a doctor's office, to take steps to remove architectural and communication barriers in existing facilities. After January 26, 1992, architectural barriers were to be removed if it was readily achievable to do so. This means if the barrier can be removed without significant difficulty or expense. The Department of Justice provides the following examples of barrier removal[35]:

1. Installing ramps
2. Making curb cuts in sidewalks and entrances
3. Repositioning shelves
4. Rearranging tables, chairs, vending machines, display racks, and other furniture
5. Repositioning telephones
6. Adding raised markings on elevator control buttons
7. Installing flashing alarm lights
8. Widening doors
9. Installing offset hinges to widen doorways
10. Eliminating a turnstile or providing an alternative accessible path
11. Installing accessible door hardware
12. Installing grab bars in toilet stalls
13. Rearranging toilet partitions to increase maneuvering space
14. Insulating lavatory pipes under sinks to prevent burns
15. Installing a raised toilet seat
16. Installing a full-length bathroom mirror
17. Repositioning the paper towel dispenser in a bathroom
18. Creating designated accessible parking spaces
19. Installing an accessible paper cup dispenser at an existing inaccessible water fountain
20. Removing high pile, low density carpeting
21. Installing vehicle hand controls

However, in an existing facility, the ADA does not require extensive ramping of a flight of stairs or the installation of an elevator, because such extensive renovations would be burdensome and expensive to undertake and therefore would not be readily achievable. The ADA also does not require a health care provider to lease only accessible space. However, once space is leased, the obligation to undertake readily achievable barrier removal applies to both landlord and tenant.[36]

Greater accessibility modifications are required once a health care provider makes alterations to a facility. The alterations must be done in compliance with the ADA's Accessibility Guideline (ADAAG). Put simply, the altered space must be designed to be fully accessible.[37] This obligation covers a wide range of items too numerous to mention here. In addition, if a health care provider alters patient service or work areas, there is an additional obligation that there be an accessible path of travel leading from the outside of the building through to the altered area of the facility. Along this accessible path of travel, various amenities, including bathrooms, drinking fountains, and public telephones, also may have to be altered to make them accessible and usable to persons with disabilities. A sufficient number of accessible parking spaces also would have to be provided if parking is made available for patients or employees. However, expenses associated with providing an accessible path of travel are capped at 20% of the cost of the original renovation.[38]

The greatest degree of accessibility is required of buildings designed for first occupancy after January 26, 1993. These buildings must be designed and built to be fully accessible in accordance with ADAAG.[39] There is no cost defense applicable to the construction of new public accommodations or commercial facilities. In some cases, an elevator may be required in order to provide accessible vertical access to health care facilities and providers.[40]

Providing Effective Communication

Patients or clients with communication impairments may have a right to an auxiliary aid or service from the health care provider to facilitate effective communication. Auxiliary aids or services include qualified interpreters or other effective methods of making aurally delivered materials available to individuals with hearing impairments; qualified readers, taped texts, or other effective methods for making visually delivered materials available to individuals with visual impairments; acquisition or modification of equipment or devices; and other similar services and actions.[41] For example, in the past, a patient with a severe hearing impairment might have brought a relative who knew sign language when visiting a doctor. With the enactment of the ADA, the doctor may have an obligation to provide and pay for a sign language interpreter when requested.[42]

In some cases, effective communication is satisfied when the health care provider and a hearing- impaired patient communicate by passing written notes. However, when the complex interchange of medical information occurs, such as the patient's detailed description of symptoms or a physician's discussion of potential side effects of proposed medication, passing notes may not be sufficient. In addition, a physician may be required to read aloud a consent form to a visually impaired patient.

Nondiscrimination in the Provision of Medical Services

A health care provider is prohibited from discrimination on the basis of disability in providing health care. One area that is spawning litigation is the denial of medical or dental treatment to patients with HIV disease.[43] The ADA does not require a physician to expand into other areas of medical specialty. Whereas the ADA would prohibit an ear, nose, and throat (ENT) specialist from denying treatment to a patient with acquired immunodeficiency syndrome with a throat infection, it would not require the ENT physician to treat the patient's broken leg. The ADA only requires equal access to the medical services provided by the physician to other patients.

THE FMLA[44]

The FMLA requires an employer of 50 or more employees to make provision for up to 12 weeks of unpaid leave, within a 52-week period, to FMLA eligible employees for the birth and subsequent care of a child; for the placement of a child for adoption or foster care; for care of an employee's seriously ill spouse, child, or parent; and for care of a serious health condition that makes an employee unable to perform a job.[45] An employee is entitled to the continuation of employer-provided health care benefits for the duration of the FMLA leave and must be restored to the same or equivalent position if able to return to work within the leave entitlement period.

Health care providers are being called upon to provide medical input concerning certain leave authorizations mandated by the FMLA. An employer may require an employee to provide medical certification when requesting leave because of the employee's or employee's spouse's, child's, or parent's serious health condition.[46] The FMLA defines a serious health condition as one that requires either inpatient care or continuing treatment by a health care provider.[47] The term "serious health condition" is intended to cover conditions or illnesses affecting one's health to the extent that inpatient care is required, or absences are necessary on a recurring basis or for more than a few days for treatment or recovery. When inpatient care is not involved, the interim regulations require that the absence from work, or from school, or incapacity in performing other daily activities in the case of a family member, be for a period of more than 3 days in addition to requiring the continuing treatment of a health care provider.[48]

The health care provider may be a doctor of medicine or osteopathy licensed to practice medicine, podiatrist, dentist, clinical psychologist, or optometrist; certain chiropractors, nurse practitioners, nurse midwives, and Christian Science practitioners are also included.[49]

The information that an employer may require an employee to provide includes explaining the reasons for which the employee is needed to care for the serious health condition of a covered family member, or for which the employee is unable to work at all or unable to perform at least one essential function of the position. The regulations anticipate that the employer will provide the health care provider with a list of the employee's essential job functions. If no such job description is provided by the employer, then the health care provider is to identify those functions through discussion with the employee.

If the employee requests intermittent or reduced leave, the health care provider will be asked to certify as to the medical necessity for such leave. In addition, an employer may obtain the practitioner's name and type of medical practice or specialty, the date the serious health condition commenced, and the health care provider's best medical judgment concerning the probable duration of the condition; the diagnosis[50]; a brief statement of the regimen of treatment, including the estimated number of visits and the nature, frequency, and duration of treatment, including treatment by another provider of health services on referral; and indication of whether inpatient hospitalization is required.

The U.S. Department of Labor, the agency that enforces the FMLA, has provided an optional certification form for employers to use. However, an employer is prohibited from seeking further medical information or from contacting the health care provider directly (see Appendix B).

If an employer has reason to believe that a medical certification provided by an employee is not valid, the employer may invoke the law's procedure for contesting medical certifications. This procedure permits the employer to refer an employee to a second health care provider, of the employer's choosing, but not in the employer's regular employ or under contract with the employer, for issuance of a second medical certification. If the second certification disagrees with the employee's initial certification, the employer and employee may mutually agree upon a third health care provider whose certification is binding on both the employer and employee.[51]

Significantly, the FMLA's restrictions on an employer's access to medical information apply only to authorization of FMLA leave and job restoration after an FMLA leave. The FMLA does not restrict an employer's access to medical records for determining benefit eligibility or processing a workers' compensation claim.

Interestingly, the FMLA establishes a leave entitlement that is not abrogated if an employer is willing and able to provide an employee with a serious health condition with reasonable accommodation or light duty that would enable the employee to return to work.[52] Although the employer is not obligated to pay the employee during the period of FMLA leave, the employer cannot require the employee to report to work.

An employer may adopt a uniformly applied policy requiring an employee out on leave for a serious health condition to present a physician's certification stating that the employee is able to return to work.[53] As with the ADA, the medical certification must be related only to the employee's ability to perform, safely and effectively, essential job functions.

CONCLUSION

The ADA and FMLA pose challenges for health care providers. The definition of disability used in many public and private benefit systems is not congruent with the ADA's concept of disability and a qualified individual with a disability. Health care providers are being required to focus more closely on an applicant's or employee's abilities, as well as medically based inabilities or risks; to take into account the essential functions of a job; and to consider the consequences and benefits of reasonable accommodation that the employer may be required to offer, including reassignment of an employee to a different job.

The FMLA, which imposes another demand for medical input, ironically does not permit consideration of the possibility of reasonable accommodation. Health care providers will need to become familiar with these two laws in order to assist patients and employers in assessing how a medical condition impacts an applicant's or employee's employability.

References

1. Portions of this chapter have been previously published.
2. 42 USC § 12111 (8); 29 CFR § 16 3 0.2 (m).
3. 42 USC § 12112(a); 29 CFR § 1630.4.
4. 42 USC § 12112(b)(5)(A); 29 CFR § 1630.9.
5. 1630.2 (n).
6. 42 USC § 12102 (2) (A); 29 CFR § 1630.2(g)(1).
7. 42 USC § 12102 (2) (B); 29 CFR § 1630.2(g)(2).
8. 42 USC § 12102(2) (C); 29 C. F. R. § 1630.2(g)(3).
9. 29 CFR § 1630.2(i).
10. 29 CFR § 1630.2(j) App.
11. 29 CFR § 1630.2(j) App.
12. See EEOC, Technical Assistance Manual (TAM) on the Employment Provisions (Title 1) of the Americans With Disabilities Act (TAM), January 1992, p IX2.
13. TAM, p IX-2.
14. See, e.g., Cook v Rhode Island; E. E. Black, Ltd, v Marshall, 497 F. Supp. 1088 (D. Haw. 1980).
15. TAM, p IX-3.
16. See, e.g., Welsh v City of Tulsa, 977 F.2d 1415 (10th Cir. 1992); Byrne v Board of Educ., School District of West Allis-West Milwaukee, 979 F.2d 560 (7th Cir. 1992); Maulding v Sullivan, 961 F.2d 694 (8th Cir. 1992); Dailey v Koch, 892 F.2d 212 (2d Cir. 1989); Forrisi v Bowen, 794 F.2d 931, 934 (4th Cir. 1986); Jasany v United States Postal Service, 755 F.2d 1244 (6th Cir. 1985); Fuqua v Unisys Corp., 716 F. Supp. 1201 (D. Minn. 1989); Elstner v South Western Bell Telephone Co., 659 F. Supp. 1328 (S.D. Tex. 1987) aff'd, 863 F.2d 881 (5th Cir. 1988); and Tudyman v United Airlines, 608 F. Supp. 739 (D. Cal. 1984).
17. Id. 1630.2(j)(3).
18. See, e.g., Evans v Dallas, 861 F.2d 846, 852-853 (5th Cir. 1988); Grimard v Carlston, 567 F.2d 1171, 1174 (1st Cir. 1978); Paegle v Dept. of Interior, No. 91-1075 (D. D.C. Feb. 8, 1993); Visarraga v Garrett, No. C-88-2828, 1992 U.S. Dist. LEXIS 9164 at *13 (N.D. June 16, 1992); Saffer v Town of Whitman, No. 85-4470, 1986 WL 14090 at *1 (D. Mass. Dec. 2, 1986); Stevens v Stubbs, 576 F. Supp. 1409 (D. Ga. 1983).
19. August v Offices Unlimited, Inc., 2 AD Cases 401 (1st Cir. 1992); Reigel, M.D. v Kaiser Foundation Health Plan of North Carolina, No. 93-556-CIV-5-F (June 29, 1994), slip op. at 24 ("[R]equiring the Medical Group to either permanently assign an existing physician assistant to work with plaintiff to perform the physical aspects of her position or hire a new assistant to do the same cannot be considered a reasonable accommodation. The [ADA] does not require an employer to hire two individuals to do the tasks ordinarily assigned to one."); Johnston v Morrison, Inc., 849 F. Supp. 777, 780 (N.D. Ala. 1994) (Restaurant not required to assign another employee to help food server during her panic attacks as this would eliminate essential job functions); see also Gilbert v Frank, 949 F.2d 637, 644 (2d Cir. 1991) (Employer not required to assign coworker to do physically demanding tasks employee no longer able to do); Treadwell v Alexander, 707 F.2d 473, 478 (11th Cir. 1983) (Assigning additional employees to cover plaintiff's physically demanding duties was an undue hardship); Coleman v Darden, 595 F.2d 533, 540 (10th Cir.), cert. denied, 444 U.S. 927 (1979) (Under the Rehabilitation Act, an employer may be required to have someone assist the disabled individual to perform the job, but the employer is not required to have someone perform the job for the disabled individual).
20. Jasany v U.S. Postal Service, 755 F.2d 1244 (6th Cir. 1985); Forrisi v Bowen, 794 F.2d 931 (4th Cir. 1986).
21. 42 USC § 12112(d); 29 CFR § 1630.13.
22. 42 USC § 12112(d)(3); 29 CFR § 1630.14.
23. EEOC, Enforcement Guidance: Preemployment Disability-Related Inquiries and Medical Examinations Under the Americans With Disabilities Act of 1990, May 19, 1994.
24. 42 USC § 12112(d)(3); 29 CFR § 1630.14(b) and .15.
25. 42 USC § 12112(d)(4); 29 CFR § 1630.14(c) and 1630.15.
26. 42 USC § 12113(b); 29 CFR § 1630.15(b)(2).
27. See generally, TAM, Chapter IV, "Establishing Non-discriminatory Qualification Standards and Selection Criteria."
28. 29 CFR § 1630.2(o)(1).
29. 29 CFR § 1630.9 App.
30. 42 USC § 198la(a)(3).
31. 42 USC § 12111(10); 29 CFR § 1630.2(p).
32. 29 CFR Part 1630, App. at 413.
33. Letter from Evan J. Kemp, Jr., Chairman, EEOC to Christopher G. Bell.
34. EEOC, Technical Assistance Manual on Title I of the Americans With Disabilities Act, § 6.4.
35. 28 CFR § 36.304(b).
36. The ADA's prohibition of discrimination in public accommodation applies to private entities who lease, own, or operate a place of public accommodation. 42 USC § 12182(a); 28 CFR § 336.201 (b).
37. 42 USC § 12183.
38. 28 CFR §§ 36.402-36.404.
39. 42 CFR § 12183.
40. Id.
41. 42 USC § 12102(1).
42. Mayberry v Von Valtier, 3 AD Cases 39 (E.D. Mich. 1994); Aikens v St. Helena Hospital, 3 AD Cases 29 (N.D, Cal. 1994).
43. U.S. v Morvant, 2 AD Cases 51769 (E.D. La. 1994).
44. The definition of a "serious health condition" and other aspects of the Department of Labor's interim final regulations have been under review. Final regulations were issued by the Department of Labor on January 6, 1995. The reader is encouraged to consult an attorney or the final regulations directly when FMLA issues arise.

45. The FMLA applies to employers with 50 or more employees. It took effect on August 5, 1993, for nonunionized employers and no later than February 5, 1994, for employers with collective bargaining agreements. An individual must be an "eligible employee" in order to take FMLA leave. An employee must have at least 1 year of service with the employer, have worked 1,250 hours in the 12 months preceding the request for leave, and work at a worksite with 50 or more employees within a 75 mile radius.
46. 29 CFR § 825.304.
47. 29 CFR § 825.114.
48. 29 CFR § 825.306.
49. 29 CFR § 825.118.
50. Note that under the final FMLA rules issued January 6, 1995, an employer is not entitled to receive the diagnosis of an employee's medical condition.
51. 29 CFR § 825.307.
52. 29 CFR § 825.792(b).
53. 29 CFR § 825.310.

CHAPTER

48

Department of Labor Guidelines for Job Categorization

ANTHONY J. DORTO, MD

Physicians are asked to make decisions regarding return to work (RTW) parameters. These parameters include when a worker can return to work, physical demands of work—i.e., sedentary, light, medium, heavy, or very heavy—and issues of work intensity, such as occasionally, frequently, and constantly, as pertains to task repetitions with various weights and activities performed. Many times physicians complete RTW forms without having a good understanding of the physical requirements behind the classifications.

This chapter is intended to give the reader an understanding of the various work classifications and what physical demands are included within them. Extensive research has been done over the years by many respected authors addressing a multitude of work issues.[2,7,8,10] It is not within the scope of this chapter to do an extensive review of work issues. Work takes into consideration many factors—e.g., medical, psychological, and vocational. Assessment and intervention methodologies are tied to their impact on work options. This chapter deals primarily with the medical aspects of work and focuses on the functional limitations associated with impairment rather than impairment alone when assessing disability. We recognize that there is no direct correlation between the impairment rating and disability.[1,11] Individuals with high impairment ratings may be able to do their prior work with or without accommodation or do another, completely different job and stay in the labor market. Other persons may have relatively small impairment ratings and be completely disabled from their prior work, require extensive retraining to re-enter the labor force, or are determined to be permanently and totally disabled due to various psychosocial issues including limited educational achievement, language restrictions, appearance, or availability of jobs within the demographic area. Many times, medical, psychological, and vocational assets and limitations must be assessed in order to determine if an individual has the capacity to engage in work activities on a sustained basis.

The ability to perform the physical and/or mental demands of work of which one is capable given one's age, education, and acquired skills and that is available in the labor market is the most recognized criterion for determining whether one is disabled.[12]

One's ability to sit, stand, and walk as well as one's ability to lift and carry are critical to establishing the exertion level of work suitable for a person with identified impairments. A person who can only sit for 3 hours per day and can stand only 4 hours per day, as seen in Table 48–1, cannot perform a full range of light or sedentary work even if this individual can lift 20 pounds occasionally. This person would need a job that allows a sit/stand option. A person who cannot walk more than 30 minutes per day would not be able to perform most medium exertion work because of the need to do extensive walking even if the person could lift 50 pounds occasionally. Because the vast majority of sedentary jobs involve some work at a desk and typically the use of a computer or other office machines, inability to use both upper extremities for bimanual, fine finger activities such as typing at a keyboard might result in disability despite the ability to sit or stand for prolonged periods and the ability to lift/carry. If an individual can return to light duty according to a physician, but cannot stand or walk in combination more than 4 hours per day (despite being able to lift 20 pounds), a vocational rehabilitation expert is left with the dilemma of pointing out that the person is limited to sedentary work, an opinion that may appear on first impression to be inconsistent with the doctor's statement about light duty. Inability to stand at least 5 hours in an 8-hour day (more than 33% and up to 100% of the day), as required to meet the definition of light work contained in the Dictionary of Occupational Titles (DOT)[4] and the Revised Handbook for Analyzing Jobs (RHAJ),[5] would eliminate the vast majority of light work, but would allow performance of a full range of sedentary occupations (defined as work that requires sitting from 5 to 8 hours per 8-hour day [more than 33% and up to 100% of the day] and standing 0 to 3 hours [33% of the day or less] even if the individual was able to lift and carry 20 pounds [the weight restriction associated with light work]).[3,9] Similarly, stating that an individual cannot sit for more than 3 to 4 hours per day, but is restricted to sedentary work, means that the person can work at best on a part-time basis and cannot perform any full-time sedentary work. Suggesting the need for a sit/stand option for a person with a severe back injury may result in inability to perform work normally done in a seated position or in a standing position without bending (a function commonly restricted to occasionally or none for persons with severe back pain). Work normally performed in a standing position may not easily be performed in a seated position unless a high stool could compensate for standing.

The risk of using global categories like sedentary or light work without understanding that the number of repetitions of lifting or carrying affect overall expenditure of energy over time (a concept rooted in the National Institute of Occupational Safety and Health [NIOSH] research) is overestimation of the types of work a person can perform. If one must grasp and move negligible weights constantly then one is performing light and not sedentary work based on the number of repetitions. If one must work more than 4 hours per day, one is performing medium and not light work even if one lifts and carries 20 pounds. Also, it should be remembered that if a person works more than 8 hours a day, the amount of exertion required to perform job tasks will exceed the level of exertion associated with 8 hours per day of work. For example, a nurse working 12-hour shifts where she is required to stand 50% of the time and walk 50% of the time, even if she is not required to lift more than 20 pounds, would be engaging potentially in medium work. Total energy expenditure over the working day and not just the amount of weight lifted or carried determines functional capacity to perform work.

NIOSH is part of the Department of Health and Human Services. It is charged with research and education, in contrast to the Occupational Safety and Health Administration (OSHA), which is part of the Department of Labor and is charged with enforcement. In 1981, NIOSH published The Work Practices Guide

TABLE 48–1

Lifting/Carrying and Postural Demands of Work

Physical Demand (Except Strength)	Occasionally*	Frequently*	Constantly*
% Of the time	0–33% of Day	34–66% of Day	67–100% of Day
Approximate repetitions	1–100 per 8-hr day	101–500 per 8-hr day	500+ per 8-hr day
Strength			
Lifting/carrying and position			
Sedentary†	Lift/carry up to 10 lbs Sit 6–8 hours Stand/walk 0–2 hours	Negligible	Negligible
Sedentary-Light†	Lift/carry up to 15 lbs	Up to 7 lbs	Negligible
Light†	Lift/carry up to 20 lbs Stand 4–8 hours Walk 0–4 hours	Up to 10 lbs	Negligible
Light-medium‡	Lift/carry up to 35 lbs	Up to 18 lbs	Up to 9 lbs
Medium†	Lift/carry up to 50 lbs Stand/walk 8 hours	Up to 20 lbs	Up to 10 lbs
Medium-heavy‡	Lift/carry up to 75 lbs	Up to 30 lbs	Up to 15 lbs
Heavy†	Lift/carry up to 100 lbs Stand/walk 8 hours	Up to 50 lbs	Up to 20 lbs
Very heavy†	Lift/carry over 100 lbs Stand/walk 8 hours	Over 50 lbs	Over 20 lbs

* Occasional, frequent, and constant are terms defined by the Dictionary of Occupational Titles that refer to the frequency of "exerting a force," and including lifting, carrying, pushing, pulling, or any other physical activity.

† U.S. Department of Labor: Dictionary of Occupational Titles, 4th ed, supplement, appendix. Washington, DC, U.S. Government Printing Office, 1986, pp 101–102.

‡ Extrapolated taken in part from Blankenship KL: Industrial Rehabilitation. Atlanta, Georgia, American Therapeutics, 1990, and Matheson LN, Niemeyer ND: Work Capacity Evaluation: Systematic Approach to Industrial Rehabilitation. Anaheim, Calif, Employment and Rehabilitation Institute of California, 1986.

for Manual Lifting (the "NIOSH Lifting Equation"). This initial equation was designed to assist safety and health practitioners to evaluate lifting demands in the sagittal plane. This equation provided an empirical method for computing a weight limit for manual lifting tasks. This limit proved useful for identifying certain lifting tasks that posed a risk for developing low back pain. This equation proved to have its limitations. It was revised and expanded in 1991 to apply to a larger percentage of lifting tasks (see Chapter 52).

The revised 1991 lifting equation provides methods for evaluating asymmetric lifting tasks and objects with less than optimal hand-container couplings, and presents new procedures for evaluating a larger range of work durations and lifting frequencies than the initial 1981 equation. The objective of both the 1981 and 1991 equations was to prevent or reduce the occurrence of lifting-related industrial low back pain among workers. The equation also has the potential to reduce the incidence of other musculoskeletal injuries that may cause shoulder or arm pain. Although there are many limitations to this guideline, it serves as the basis for industrial use of appropriate weight lifting standards that are more useful than simplistic weight limits presented previously, which overlooked many of the crucial variables in lifting.[2] However, the NIOSH formula has only limited value in terms of assessing "real world" physical demands of work. It is more useful for a clinician to understand the lifting demands of actual work as identified by the U.S. Department of Labor in the DOT and RHAJ, as reflected in Table 48–1.[4,5]

The NIOSH lifting equation provides an added degree of empiricism to the assessment of low back pain (a common precursor to impairment, functional limitation, and disability). However, lifting is only one of the causes of low back pain and disability. Other causes believed to be risk factors include whole body vibration, prolonged sitting, static postures, and direct trauma to the back. The revised NIOSH lifting equation is based on the assumption that manual handling activities other than lifting are minimal and do not require significant energy expenditures, especially when repetitive lifting tasks are performed. Nonlifting tasks include holding, pushing, pulling, carrying, walking, and climbing.[2]

The revised NIOSH lifting equation was established using well-defined parameters pertaining to stability of the load being lifted, secured coupling, work surface friction, height, distance of lift, and other factors. The revised NIOSH lifting equation does not apply if any of the following occur:

- Lifting/lowering with one hand
- Lifting/lowering for over 8 hours
- Lifting/lowering while seated or kneeling
- Lifting/lowering in a restricted work space
- Lifting/lowering unstable objects
- Lifting/lowering while carrying, pushing, or pulling
- Lifting/lowering with wheelbarrows or shovels
- Lifting/lowering with high speed motion (faster than about 30 inches/second)
- Lifting/lowering with unreasonable foot/floor coupling (<0.4 coefficient of friction between the sole and the floor)
- Lifting/lowering in an unfavorable environment (i.e., temperature significantly outside 66 to 79 °F (19 to 26 °C) range; relative humidity outside 35 to 50% range)

Table 48–1 represents the lifting and carrying requirements of work only and is the most commonly used method for categorizing the functional demands of work. Notice the task repetitions from occasionally (1 to 100) to frequently (101 to 500) to constantly (500+). The clinician must know what the physical demands of the job are including task repetitions and duration of the workday performing the repetitions. Table 48–1 clearly defines this.

References

1. Dorto AJ, Williams JM: Coordinating rehabilitation efforts and the disability evaluating process. Journal of Back and Musculoskeletal Rehabilitation 8:19–43, 1998.
2. Legg SJ: Maximum acceptable repetitive lifting workloads for an 8-hour work-day using psychophysical and subjective rating methods. Ergonomics 24:218–229, 1981.
3. Snook S, Ciriello V: The design of manual handling tasks: Revised titles of maximum acceptable weights and forces. Ergonomics 34:1197–1213, 1991.
4. U.S. Department of Labor: Dictionary of Occupational Titles, 4th ed. Washington, DC, U.S. Government Printing Office, 1991.
5. U.S. Department of Labor: Revised Handbook for Analyzing Jobs. Washington, DC, U.S. Government Printing Office, 1991.
6. Waters T, Anderson V, et al: Revised NIOSH equation for the design and evaluation of manual lifting tasks. Ergonomics 36:749–776, 1993.
7. Williams JM: Transferability of skills methodologies used in computerized job matching systems: Sufficient or insufficient control of methodologically induced error variance. Journal of Forensic Vocational Assessment 1:29–41, 1998.
8. Williams JM, Burlew L: Dealing with catastrophic injury: A developmental perspective on rehabilitation care planning. Adultspan 9:4, 1995.
9. Williams JM, Fidanza NS: Ensuring the success of industrial rehabilitation program: The role of the rehabilitation counselor in return to work. NARPPS Journal and News 5:67–71, 1990.
10. Williams JM, Reavy G: Effective use of rehabilitation and economic experts in personal injury litigation: An integrated approach. In David Stein (ed): Vocational Expert Monograph Series. Topeka, Kan, American Board of Vocational Experts, 1993, pp 16–27.
11. Williams JM, Sawyer H, LaBuda J: Forensic rehabilitation. In Thorson R (ed): CIRS Self-Study Guide. Rolling Meadows, Ill, Certified Insurance Rehabilitation Specialist Commission, 1993, pp 69–88.
12. Wright GN: Total Rehabilitation. Boston, Little, Brown, 1980.

CHAPTER

49

Disability under the Federal Aviation Administration

ARNOLD A. ANGELICI, JR., MD ■ STANLEY R. MOHLER, MD, MA

The purpose of the airman's medical examination is to ensure that the applicant meets the medical standards specified by the Federal Aviation Administration (FAA). The examination of an airman or the applicant by a physician who is an FAA designated Aviation Medical Examiner (AME) is a rather unique situation in the field of medicine. The AME is designated by the Regional Flight Surgeon (RFS) of the FAA and is trained at a 5-day basic seminar at the Civil Aerospace Medicine Institute (CAMI) in Oklahoma City. Follow-up 3-day seminars sponsored by CAMI at various locations around the country are required to retain this designation.

The examination of the pilot by the AME is performed on behalf of the FAA. The pilot is the one who pays the AME for this examination. The materials of the examination, including the FAA Form 8500-8 and all other accompanying forms that may be required to complete this examination, are the property of the FAA. Since October 1999, the examination is a combination of hard copy paper as well as a Web-based, electronic document that is transmitted to CAMI in "real time." The paper original with the airman's and the AME's signatures is forwarded to CAMI. The system is expected by some to eventually become completely paperless, with electronic records and signatures.

THE FEDERAL AVIATION REGULATIONS CONCERNING MEDICAL CERTIFICATION

There are three separate classes of Airman Medical Certificates specified in the Federal Aviation Regulations (FAR). The requirements and duration of the medical certificates are described in FAR Part 61.23. The medical standards and certification are found in FAR Part 67.101–115, 201–215, and 301–315. The three classes are referred to as First Class, Second Class, and Third Class.

First Class Medical Certificates are required for pilots who are operating as pilot-in-command of an airline transport aircraft. Second Class Medical Certificates are for pilots who are airline transport copilots, or flight engineers, corporate pilots, and other pilots who fly for hire. Third Class Medical Certificates are for general aviation private pilots, as well as recreational pilots. The exception to this regulation is that the pilots of unpowered aircraft and ultra light aircraft are self-certified.

In the past, other sanctioning bodies, such as auto racing and scuba diving, have sought these examinations. The pilot who holds a First Class Medical Certificate requires an electrocardiogram at age 35 and one each year after age 40. The holder must be re-examined every 6 months by an AME for the certificate to stay current. The Second Class Medical Certificate holder must be examined every year to stay current. Should the holder of the Second Class Medical Certificate not undergo an examination by an AME, the medical certificate becomes a Third Class Medical Certificate for an additional year if the holder is over 40 years of age. If the holder is under 40 years of age the Third Class Medical Certificate is good for an additional year. Third Class Medical Certificates are good for 3 years for airmen under 40 years of age and for 2 years for pilots over 40 years of age. There is no maximum age limit on any FAA medical certificate class.

There are several disqualifying conditions, which are outlined in Table 49–1. Groupings cover the body systems as they appear in the FARs.

EYES

Eye standards for medical certificates are covered under Part 67.103, .203, and .303. For the First and Second Class Airman Medical Certificate, distance visual acuity of 20/20 or better in each eye separately is required, with or without corrective lenses; if corrective lenses, spectacles, or contact lenses are necessary for 20/20 vision, a person may be eligible only on the condition that lenses are worn while exercising the privileges of the airman. For the Third Class Airman Medical Certificate, the visual acuity may be 20/40 or better in each eye separately, with or without corrective lenses. If corrective lenses are needed for 20/40 vision, the person may be eligible on the condition that the corrective lenses are worn while exercising the privileges of the airman.

Pilots applying for First or Second Class certificates must have near vision of 20/40 or better, Snellen equivalent, at 16 inches in each eye separately, with or without corrective lenses. If the pilot is age 50 or older, near vision of 20/40 or better, Snellen equivalent at 16 inches (near vision) and 32 inches (intermediate vision), each eye separately, with or without corrective lenses, must be demonstrated at the time of the examination. For a Third Class Medical Certificate, the requirement is for 20/40 or better vision, Snellen equivalent, at 16 inches, each eye "with or without corrective lenses."

The reason for the two distances of 16 and 32 inches has to do with the design of the cockpit and the ability to read charts, approach plates, and the operating manuals that are in each aircraft flown by the pilot.

TABLE 49–1

Disqualifying Conditions for Civil Airmen (Federal Aviation Regulations Part 67)

Neurologic
- Transient loss of neurologic function
- Unexplained loss of consciousness
- Epilepsy
- Alzheimer's disease

Psychiatric
- Substance dependence
- Substance abuse
- Bipolar disorder
- Psychosis
- Personality disorder

Endocrinologic
- Diabetes requiring hypoglycemic medications

Cardiac
- Angina pectoris
- History of myocardial infarction
- Clinically significant arterial disease
- Permanent cardiac pacemaker
- Cardiac valve replacement
- Heart transplant

Additional requirements for the eyes include normal fields of vision and no acute or chronic pathologic condition of either eye or adnexa that interferes with the proper function of an eye that may reasonably be expected to progress to a significant degree or that may reasonably be expected to be aggravated by flying.

The FAA Part 67.103(f) addresses bifoveal fixation vergence-phoria relationship sufficient to prevent a break in fusion under conditions that may be reasonably expected to occur in performing airman duties. The limitations here are no more than one prism diopter of hyperphoria and six prism diopters of esophoria, or six prism diopters of exophoria. If these values are exceeded, the FAS may require that a qualified eye specialist examine the person, and if there is bifoveal fixation in an adequate vergence-phoria relationship, the AME may issue a medical certificate pending the results of this examination if the airman being examined is otherwise eligible.

EAR, NOSE, THROAT, AND EQUILIBRIUM

Under the FAR 67.105, .205, and .305, the applicant shall demonstrate acceptable hearing by at least one of the three following tests. The first is to demonstrate an ability to hear an average conversational voice in a quiet room, using both ears at a distance of 6 feet from the AME, the applicant's back turned toward the AME. Also, it is necessary that the applicant demonstrate acceptable understanding of speech, determined by audiometric speech discrimination testing to a score of at least 70% obtained in one ear or sound field environment. The third method is to provide acceptable results on pure tone audiometric testing of unaided hearing acuity according to Table 49–2, where the worst acceptable threshold is noted, using the calibration standards of the American National Standards Institute.

Also, no disease or condition of the middle or internal ear, nose, oral cavity, pharynx, or larynx that interferes with or is aggravated by flying, or that may reasonably be expected to do so, or that interferes with or may reasonably be expected to interfere with clear and effective speech communication, and no disease or condition manifested by or that may reasonably be expected to be manifested by vertigo or a disturbance of equilibrium, may be present. The diseases that can manifest symptoms of vertigo, hearing loss, or a disturbance of equilibrium are listed in Table 49–3.

TABLE 49–2

Worst Acceptable Thresholds for Pure Tone Audiometric Testing (Unaided Hearing Aquity)

Frequency (Hz)	500 Hz	1000 Hz	2000 Hz	3000 Hz
Better ear (dB)	35	30	30	40
Poorer ear (dB)	35	50	50	60

TABLE 49–3

Causes of Vertigo

Peripheral causes of vertigo
- Benign paroxysmal positional vertigo
- Ménière disease (endolymphatic hydrodrops)
- Inflammatory labyrinthitis
  - Syphilis (similar to Ménière disease except the vertigo is not episodic and is reversible with treatment)
  - Vasculitis
- Drug ototoxicity (vestibulotoxic)
- Peripheral vestibulopathy
  - Acute labyrinthitis
  - Vestibular neuronitis
  - Acute and recurrent peripheral vestibulopathy
- Focal peripheral disease
  - Acute and chronic otitis media
  - Other middle ear diseases (vertigo accompanied by hearing loss or tinnitus)
  - Perilymph fistula (from barotrauma)
  - Malignant or benign tumors of the external or middle ear, inner ear, base of skull, carotid body, or infratemporal fossa
- Lesions of the cerebellopontine angle
  - Acoustic neuroma (primary symptom is unilateral hearing loss)
  - Cholesteatoma (epidermoid cyst)
  - Arachnoid cyst
  - Glomus jugulare tumor
  - Metastatic tumor
  - Plasmacytoma of the petrous bone
  - Vascular malformations
- Post-traumatic vertigo
  - Temporal bone fracture
  - Labyrinthine concussion
  - Traumatic perforation of the tympanic membrane
- Motion sickness
- Temporolmandibular joint neuralgia

Central causes of vertigo
- Cerebrovascular disease (infrequent cause of dizziness)
- Vertebral-basilar artery insufficiency ← vertigo ← drop attacks
- Demyelinating diseases
  - Multiple sclerosis (vertigo is the presenting symptom in 10% of patients)
- Intrinsic brainstem lesions
  - Arteriovenous malformation
  - Ischemia and infarction
- Intracranial aneurysms
- Migraine headaches
- Seizure disorder (temporal lobe epilepsy)
- Hereditary disorders
  - Spinocerebellar degeneration: Friedreich ataxia
  - Olivopontocerebellar atrophy

Systemic causes of vertigo
- Medications (alcohol, analgesics, anticonvulsants, antihypertensives, hypnotics, tranquilizers)
- Endocrine disease (diabetes, hypothyroidism)
- Hyperventilation
- Vasculitis (systemic lupus erythematosus, giant cell arteritis, drug induced vasculitis)
- Infectious diseases
  - Herpes zoster oticus (Ramsay Hunt syndrome: viral inflammation of the geniculate ganglion in the petrous portion of the temporal bone, with or without tinnitus and deafness)
  - Bacterial meningitis
  - Systemic infection
- Miscellaneous disorders
  - Orthostatic hypotension
  - Cataracts
  - Cardiac arrhythmia

From Adams RD, Victor M: Viral infections of the nervous system. Principles of Neurology, 5th ed, chap 33. New York, McGraw Hill, 1993, p 646; and Yarington CT, Hanna HH: Otolaryngology in aerospace medicine. In DeHart RL (ed): Fundamentals of Aerospace Medicine, 2nd ed, chap 17. Baltimore, Williams & Wilkins, 1996, with permission.

MENTAL

Mental standards for airmen under FAR Parts 67.107, .207, and .307 state that the airman must have no established medical history or clinical diagnosis of the following:

1. A personality disorder severe enough to have repeatedly manifested itself by overt acts;
2. A psychosis, defined by the FAA as a condition that has caused or may reasonably be expected to cause the pilot delusions, hallucinations, grossly bizarre or disorganized behavior, or other commonly accepted symptoms of this condition; or
3. Additional diagnoses such as a bipolar disorder, or substance dependence, except where there is established clinical evidence satisfactory to the FAS of recovery, including sustained total abstinence of substance(s) in the preceding 2 years (note: this period may be shorter for airline pilots and flight engineers). The term "substance," as defined by the FARs, includes alcohol, other sedatives and hypnotics, anxiolytics, opioids, central nervous system stimulants such as cocaine, amphetamines and similarly acting sympathomimetics, hallucinogens, phencyclidine or similarly acting arylcyclohexylamines, cannabis, inhalants, and other psychoactive drugs and chemicals.

Substance dependence is defined by the FAA for medical certification purposes as a condition in which a person is dependent on a substance (other than tobacco or ordinary xanthine-containing beverages, later defined as caffeine-containing beverages), as evidenced by increased tolerance, manifestation of withdrawal symptoms, impaired control of use, or continued use despite damage to health or impairment of social, personal, or occupational functions. The FAA defines no substance abuse within the preceding 2 years as follows:

1. The use of a prohibited substance in a situation where the use was physically hazardous, or if there has been at any other time an instance of the use of a prohibited substance. Also the situation where use was hazardous to the user;
2. A verified positive drug test result acquired under an antidrug program or internal program of the U.S. Department of Transportation or any other Administration within the U.S. Department of Transportation;
3. Misuse of a substance that the FAS, based on case history and appropriate, qualified medical judgment relating to the substance involved, finds that, owing to its use, the medical certificate holder or applicant:
   a. Is unable to safely perform the duties or exercise the privileges of the airman certificate applied for or held; or
   b. May reasonably be expected, for the maximum duration of the Airman Medical Certificate applied for or held, to be unable to perform those duties or exercise those privileges.

The applicant also may not have a personality disorder, neurosis, or other mental condition that the FAS, based on the case history and appropriate, qualified medical judgment relating to the condition involved, finds that:

1. Makes the person unable to safely perform the duties or exercise the privileges of the airman certificate applied for or held; or
2. May reasonably be expected to make the person unable to perform those duties or exercise those privileges of the Airman Medical Certificate applied for or held.

NEUROLOGIC

Neurologic standards for airman medical certification for FAR Parts 67.109, .209, and .309 are as follows:

(a) There is no established medical history or clinical diagnosis of any of the following:
   1. Epilepsy;
   2. A disturbance of consciousness without satisfactory medical explanation of the cause; or
   3. Transient loss of control of nervous system function(s) without satisfactory medical explanation of the cause.

(b) There can be no medical history or clinical diagnosis of other seizure disorder, disturbance of consciousness, or a neurologic condition that the FAS, based on the case history and appropriate, qualified medical judgment relating to the condition involved, finds that:
   1. Makes the person unable to safely perform the duties or exercise the privileges of the airman certificate applied for or held; or
   2. May reasonably be expected to make the person unable to undertake these duties or exercise the privileges of the certificate applied for or held.

Conditions that may be classified here include Alzheimer disease; cerebral vascular disease, which includes transient ischemic attacks and other cerebrovascular diseases that lead to neurologic deficits; and tumors, whether they are primary, metastatic, or of unknown origin, to the brain tissue.

CARDIOVASCULAR

The cardiovascular standards for an Airman Medical Certificate, according to the FAR Parts 67.111, .211, and .311, are that:

(a) No established medical history or clinical diagnosis of any of the following must exist:
   1. Myocardial infarction;
   2. Angina pectoris;
   3. Coronary heart disease that has required treatment or, if untreated, that has been symptomatic or clinically significant;
   4. Cardiac valve replacement;
   5. Permanent cardiac pacemaker implantation; or
   6. Heart replacement.

If the pilot develops or undergoes any of the above, he or she is grounded and the medical certificate is not valid until cleared by the FAA. The FAA, through the "discretionary" process, may, on recovery, issue the pilot a medical certificate.

Where the Federal Aviation Regulations differ between classifications of airmen, under Part 67.113(b), a person applying for first-class medical certification must demonstrate an absence of myocardial infarction and other clinically significant abnormality on electrocardiography examination:

(a) at the first application after reaching the 35th birthday; and
(b) on an annual basis after reaching the 40th birthday.

Subparagraph (c) of this section describes the electrocardiogram that will satisfy the requirement of paragraph (b) of this section. It states that the electrocardiogram cannot be dated earlier than 60 days before the date of the application it is to accompany and must be performed and transmitted according to acceptable standards and techniques. The FAA requires that the electrocardiogram be transmitted to CAMI in a "real-time" fashion. This requires a specific setup with an electrocardiograph machine and a specific digital modem. This requirement does not apply to the granting of Second and Third Class Medical Certificates.

GENERAL MEDICAL CONDITION

The general medical standards for airman medical certification refer to body systems not included in the above-mentioned sections. A history or clinical diagnosis of diabetes mellitus that requires insulin or any other hypoglycemic control is disqualifying at the time of physical examination. Also, there may be no other organic, functional, or structural disease, defect, or limitation that the FAS finds, based on the case history and appropriate, qualified medical judgment relating to the condition involved, that may render the person unable to safely perform the duties or exercise the privileges of the airman certificate applied for or held or may reasonably be expected, for the maximum duration of the Airman Medical Certificate applied for or held, to make the person unable to perform those duties or exercise those privileges.

The FAS has determined that the applicant must not be taking any medication or other treatment that, based on the case history and appropriate, qualified medical judgment relating to the medication or other treatment involved, makes the person unable to safely perform the duties or exercise the privileges of the airman certificate applied for or held.

DISCRETIONARY ISSUANCE

A person who does not meet the provisions of FAR Parts 67.101–115, .201–215, and .301–315, as these are applicable, may apply for the discretionary issuance of a certificate under FAR Part 67.401. The authorization for special issuance of a medical certificate is at the discretion of the FAS and is valid for a specified period. A Special Issuance may be granted to a person who does not meet the provisions of subparts (b), (c), or (d) of Part 67. This may be accomplished if the person shows to the satisfaction of the FAS that the duties authorized by the class applied for may be performed without endangering public safety during the period in which the authorization would be in force. The FAS may authorize a special medical flight test, practical test, or medical evaluation. Upon expiration of the current authorization, a new authorization may be granted if the pilot demonstrates to the satisfaction of the FAS that the duties authorized by the class of medical certificate applied for can be performed without endangering public safety during the period the authorization would be in force. The authorizations are not necessarily renewable but must be issued after re-evaluation of the applicant's medical status. The authorization expires at the time of the applied-for medical certificate. If the applicant has a disqualifying condition that is static or not progressive and has been found capable of performing airman duties without endangering public safety, a Statement of Demonstrated Ability (SODA) may be granted instead of an authorization. The SODA does not expire and authorizes the designated AME to issue a medical certificate of the specified class if the examiner finds that the condition described on the SODA has not adversely changed. In granting an authorization or SODA under Part 67.401, the FAS specifies the class medical certificate to be issued, may limit the duration of the authorization, and may make the granting of the new authorization conditional on results of subsequent medical examinations, tests, or evaluations. These are stated on the authorization or SODA. Any medical certification based on operational limitations needed for safety or made conditional; the continued effect of the SODA; or authorization of any Second or Third Class Medical Certificate must be in compliance with a statement of functional limitations issued to the pilot in coordination with the Director of Flight Standards, or the Directors designee. The FAS has the discretion of withdrawing the authorization, or SODA, granted under the provisions of this section. Conditions for the above withdrawal can be based on a change in the holder's medical condition, or if the holder fails to comply with the statement of functional limitations or operational limitations issued as a condition of certification under this certification. If the person was granted an authorization or SODA under the above section based on a special medical flight test or practical test, the person may not need to take the flight test again during the later physical examinations, unless the FAS determines or has reason to believe, that the physical deficiency has or may have degraded to a degree to require another flight test or practical test. If the holder of an authorization or SODA has this authorization withdrawn for any of the above reasons, the holder will be served with a letter of withdrawal, stating the reasons for the action and that the holder has 60 days after the service of the letter of withdrawal to appeal for a review of the withdrawal. The appeal must be accompanied by supporting medical evidence.

CONCLUSION

The FARs stipulate who may give physical examinations, under Part 67.405. Only an AME who is specifically designated by the FAA RFS for the purpose of giving the examination for the First Class Medical Certificate may issue a First Class Medical Certificate. Second and third class examinations may be given by any AME. The AME has the discretion to deny or defer issuance of a medical certificate, although most AMEs will defer the issuance of the medical certificate when in doubt of the applicant's health status. Therefore, the Manager, Aeromedical Certification Division, or the RFS reviews the applicant's examination, and if either of these two denies an issuance, the Administrator of the FAA considers this a denial, and the pilot or applicant must refrain from exercising the privileges of the certificate held.

With respect to medical records, whenever the Administrator determines that additional medical information is necessary to determine whether the applicant or holder of a medical certificate meets the medical standards, the Administrator may request that the applicant furnish the necessary medical information to the FAA. This information includes all pertinent clinic, hospital, and physician records. If sufficient information is not released to the Administrator, the Administrator may suspend, modify, or revoke all medical certificates the airman holds, or may deny the applicant an Airman Medical Certificate. If this is a suspension or modification, it will remain suspended or modified until the requested information, history, or authorization is provided to the FAA. The FAS will then determine whether the person meets the medical standards under this part.

References

1. Adams RD, Victor M: Viral infections of the nervous system. Principles of Neurology, 5th ed, chap 33. New York, McGraw Hill, 1993, p 646.
2. Federal Aviation Regulations Part 67, Title 14 of the Code of Federal Regulations (14 CFR). U.S. Department of Transportation, 2001.
3. Hickman JR, Tolan GD, Gray GW, Hull DH: Clinical aerospace cardiovascular and pulmonary medicine. In DeHart RL (ed): Fundamentals of Aerospace Medicine, 2nd ed, chap 15. Baltimore, Williams & Wilkins, 1996.
4. Jordan JL, Hark WH, Salazar GJ: Aviation medicine in the Federal Aviation Administration. In DeHart RL (ed): Fundamentals of Aerospace Medicine, 2nd ed, chap 26. Baltimore, Williams & Wilkins, 1996.
5. Moser R: Additional medical and surgical conditions of aeromedical concern. In DeHart RL (ed): Fundamentals of Aerospace Medicine, 2nd ed, chap 19. Baltimore, Williams & Wilkins, 1996.
6. Yarington CT, Hanna HH: Otolaryngology in aerospace medicine. In DeHart RL (ed): Fundamentals of Aerospace Medicine, 2nd ed, chap 17. Baltimore, Williams & Wilkins, 1996.

RESOURCE

Federal Aviation Administration, Office of Aviation Medicine, Civil Aeromedical Institute, Aeromedical Certification Web page: http://www.cami.jccbi.gov/AAM-300/index.html.

CHAPTER

50

Fitness to Work for Commercial Drivers

NATALIE P. HARTENBAUM, MD, MPH

In determining whether an individual is able to return to his or her job after an illness or injury, in general, health care providers base their determinations on the patient's subjective complaints and physical findings. If an individual appears to be able to perform the required job tasks, it is often assumed that he or she is able to return to work. In many occupations, the concern with an employee returning to work is whether he or she is likely to cause damage to him- or herself; but for many in the transportation industries, the concern is with public safety. Prior to providing documentation that the patient may work, health care providers should be certain that individuals are not covered by federal medical standards. Many employees in the transportation industry are required to meet certain medical criteria. Individuals who work as commercial drivers must meet the medical criteria of the Federal Motor Carrier Safety Administration's (FMCSA) Safety Regulations.

These standards first became effective in 1970 and have undergone minor modifications since then. They cover drivers involved in interstate (between state) commerce only. Many states have adopted the federal standards for their intrastate drivers, although some will grant exemptions under certain circumstances. Whereas motor carriers are required to comply with the requirements of the Americans With Disabilities Act (ADA), the ADA does not override federal medical standards if meeting these standards is an essential function of that individual's job.[1] Although courts have found that public safety is a significant consideration in ADA cases based on commercial driver fitness, a carrier is still required to determine if the employee is able to perform other positions that may be available. Decisions in suits against the Federal Highway Administration have been inconsistent in lower courts and courts of appeal with the majority upholding the importance of the medical standards.[2–4] Three cases that have been decided at the Supreme Court level relevant to the federal medical standards have upheld an employer's right to have medical criteria that exceed the federal standards, provided they are not based on a disability which significantly impairs an individual in activities of daily living. The cases also narrowed the definition of "covered individual" under the ADA by indicating that a person is not covered if he or she is not excluded from a broad range of jobs, not just one specific position.[5–7]

Potential physician liability in determining whether a driver meets federal medical standards can be difficult to assess. Where a driver clearly does not meet an absolute requirement such as vision, and an accident occurs, in some situations the examiner has been held responsible.[8] Since a major accident in New Orleans on Mother's Day 1999, more attention has been paid to the importance of a driver's medical status. Increasingly, suits are being filed against companies where a driver's medical condition may be a proximate or potential cause of injury. There are also cases where an injured party or related party has filed against the examiner or the carrier.[9] With the medical determination of fitness being the responsibility of the medical examiner, third party cases against examiners may be seen in the future. Many of these cases are recent and have been settled out of court or are still in litigation. Cases filed under the ADA are also pending against examiners who have determined that a driver does not meet the medical standards and the company based its hiring decision on the medical examiner's determination.

A physician or other health care professional who indicates that the driver is safe to drive should be aware that he or she is required by statute to be aware of not only the regulations but also the supporting and guidance material. These examinations may be performed by any licensed health care provider permitted by his or her state license to perform examinations. This includes physicians (MD or DO), and in some states, physician's assistants, advanced practice nurses, or chiropractors. Additional guidance material from the FMCSA is available in the form of the medical advisory criteria, now included on the Medical Examination Report Form, regulatory guidance,[10] and conference reports[11–14] recommendations. Handbooks and newsletters are also available as additional resources.[15,16] The examination must be completed "substantially in accordance" with the form published in the Federal Register on October 5, 2000.[17] In addition to the physical qualifications, this form includes general information to the examiner on the driver's role and medical advisory criteria. Prior to indicating that a commercial driver is able to perform his or her job, it is essential that at a minimum, this document be reviewed and understood. The assumption that the company is responsible for ensuring that its driver meets these standards is only partially correct. In general, the carrier should not have detailed medical information and should not be assumed to understand medical issues. The medical examiner is the one responsible for the medical determination; however, the carrier should ensure that the examiner has, and understands the standards and the driver's job tasks. In the current system, an examiner cannot place restrictions on a driver other than requiring corrective lenses or a hearing aid, or indicating that the driver requires a skill performance evaluation certificate for certain limb abnormalities. If a personal physician indicates to his or her patient that return to work is acceptable and either the company or an examiner with an understanding of the federal guidelines determines that medical standards are not met, an avoidable adversarial situation is produced.

There are 12 medical standards that the examiner must consider (Box 50–1). All but four leave discretion to the medical examiner. The examiner must consider not only the current risk of sudden inability to operate the commercial vehicle safely, but also whether sudden incapacitation may occur during the duration of the certification. This is not a decision of high likelihood but must be based on acceptable risk. The adverse event that is of concern is not to the individual but to the general public, who do not knowingly accept being on the road with a driver with medical problems. The Canadian Cardiovascular Society has indicated that for commercial drivers, an annual risk of sudden incapacitation of greater than 1% would be too great a risk to which to expose the driving public.[18] Commercial motor vehicle accidents with resultant injury or death to passengers or other drivers are being found in both civil and criminal courts and increasing attention is being paid to the role of medical problems in motor vehicle accidents. This chapter covers the basic requirements, but additional information should be sought for final determinations. The longest duration of a commercial driver medical certificate is 2 years. For those conditions that may not preclude safe driving at the time of the examination but may not be stable for 2 years, the examiner is encouraged to certify for a shorter period of time. It is also important for any health care provider certifying that the driver can meet the medical standards that he or she has not just looked a single medical problem but at how conditions and the treatments may interact. An assessment of the individual's compliance and the course of any disease should be a factor in the qualification decision as well as the duration of the certification. Additional testing may also be indicated.

ORTHOPEDIC—49 CFR 391.41(B)(1) AND (2)

The driver is not only required to be able to get into and out of his or her vehicle and drive but is also required to perform other job tasks. Although it may seem that inspecting the vehicle, loading freight, and properly tying down transported material do not have public safety implications, an improperly prepared run could result in accidents. The driver with an impairment or loss of a limb is eligible to apply for an exemption from the standards in the form of a skill performance evaluation certificate. Prior to applying for this, the driver must demonstrate that he or she meets all other medical requirements and present information from an orthopedist or physiatrist documenting that he or she is able to safely perform any required tasks. A road test to demonstrate ability is also required.

DIABETES—49 CFR 391.41(B)(3)

Owing to unstable and unpredictable mealtimes and work schedules, drivers who require insulin for control of diabetes are not permitted to operate commercial vehicles in interstate commerce. The medical examiner is unable to restrict a driver's duties and once a certificate is signed as qualified, a mechanism does not exist to ensure that irregular schedules are not assigned. There previously was a waiver study program open to drivers who met certain criteria. Drivers who were in the program and have continued to meet criteria can continue to drive but no new applications are being

BOX 50–1 Federal Motor Carrier Safety Regulations—Physical Qualifications for Drivers

49 CFR 391.41

§391.41 Physical qualifications for drivers

(a) A person shall not drive a commercial motor vehicle unless he/she is physically qualified to do so and, except as provided in 391.67, has on his/her person the original, or a photographic copy, of a medical examiner's certificate that he/she is physically qualified to drive a commercial motor vehicle.

(b) A person is physically qualified to drive a commercial motor vehicle if that person—

(b) (1) Has no loss of a foot, a leg, a hand, or an arm, or has been granted a skill performance evaluation certificate pursuant to 391.49;

(b) (2) Has no impairment of:

(b) (2) (i) A hand or finger which interferes with prehension or power grasping; or

(b) (2) (ii) An arm, foot, or leg which interferes with the ability to perform normal tasks associated with operating a commercial motor vehicle; or any other significant limb defect or limitation which interferes with the ability to perform normal tasks associated with operating a commercial motor vehicle; or has been granted a skill performance evaluation certificate pursuant to 391.49.

(b) (3) Has no established medical history or clinical diagnosis of diabetes mellitus currently requiring insulin for control;

(b) (4) Has no current clinical diagnosis of myocardial infarction, angina pectoris, coronary insufficiency, thrombosis, or any other cardiovascular disease of a variety known to be accompanied by syncope, dyspnea, collapse, or congestive cardiac failure;

(b) (5) Has no established medical history or clinical diagnosis of a respiratory dysfunction likely to interfere with his/her ability to control and drive a commercial motor vehicle safely;

(b) (6) Has no current clinical diagnosis of high blood pressure likely to interfere with his/her ability to operate a commercial motor vehicle safely;

(b) (7) Has no established medical history or clinical diagnosis of rheumatic, arthritic, orthopedic, muscular, neuromuscular, or vascular disease which interferes with his/her ability to control and operate a commercial motor vehicle safely;

(b) (8) Has no established medical history or clinical diagnosis of epilepsy or any other condition which is likely to cause loss of consciousness or any loss of ability to control a commercial motor vehicle;

(b) (9) Has no mental, nervous, organic, or functional disease or psychiatric disorder likely to interfere with his/her ability to drive a commercial motor vehicle safely;

(b) (10) Has distant visual acuity of at least 20/40 (Snellen) in each eye without corrective lenses or visual acuity separately corrected to 20/40 (Snellen) or better with corrective lenses, distant binocular acuity of at least 20/40 (Snellen) in both eye with or without corrective lenses, field of vision of at least 70° in the horizontal meridian in each eye, and the ability to recognize the colors of traffic signals and devices showing standard red, green, and amber;

(b) (11) First perceives a forced whispered voice in the better ear at not less than 5 feet with or without the use of a hearing aid or, if tested by use of an audiometric device, does not have an average hearing loss in the better ear greater than 40 decibels at 500 Hz, 1,000 Hz, and 2,000 Hz with or without a hearing aid when the audiometric device is calibrated to American National Standard (formerly ASA Standard) Z24.5 1951;

(b) (12) (i) Does not use a controlled substance identified in 21 CFR 1308.11 Schedule I, an amphetamine, a narcotic, or any other habit-forming drug;

(b) (12) (ii) Exception. A driver may use such a substance or drug, if the substance or drug is prescribed by a licensed medical practitioner who:

(b) (12) (ii) (A) Is familiar with the driver's medical history and assigned duties; and

(b) (12) (ii) (B) Has advised the driver that the prescribed substance or drug will not adversely affect the driver's ability to safely operate a commercial motor vehicle; and:

(b) (13) Has no current clinical diagnosis of alcoholism.

accepted. Those drivers are required to maintain a logbook of glucose measurements before driving and every 4 hours while driving. An examiner should review this log to ensure that there are no episodes of hypo- or hyperglycemia. Those drivers not controlled on oral hypoglycemic agents should not be certified to drive commercial vehicles. Poor diabetic control can affect vision and cognition and lead to potentially impairing end organ damage. Risk of hypoglycemia is also found with some oral hypoglycemic agents. Individuals who have hypoglycemic unawareness present a danger as they may be unaware when their sugar has dropped to impairing levels. It has been demonstrated that hypoglycemia will impair driving performance and drivers are often slow to respond to hypoglycemia.[19] One study showed an increased risk of accidents in diabetic drivers not using insulin.[20]

CARDIAC—49 CFR 391.41(B)(4)

One area where there appears to be a correlation between medical conditions and accidents is cardiac disease.[21] In an attempt to decrease risk of sudden incapacitation to an acceptable degree, the regulations state that if the driver's condition may lead to congestive heart failure, shortness of breath, or loss of consciousness, he or she should not be certified to drive a commercial vehicle. Those drivers with a history of ischemic heart disease should be free of evidence of ischemia and have adequate cardiac reserve to safely perform tasks. Electrocardiogram (EKG) abnormalities have been observed in drivers under stressful conditions. Normal resting and stress EKGs are advised prior to returning to work after an ischemic event or cardiac procedure and periodic repeats are also recommended. For drivers with arrhythmias, the severity and control of the arrhythmia must be assessed as well as any potential impairment caused by the treatment.[22] For any cardiac abnormality a reasonable waiting period should occur to ensure stability. Pacemaker use should be evaluated on an individual basis and permitting drivers with implantable cardioverter defibrillators to operate commercial vehicles is generally not considered advisable.

PULMONARY—49 CFR 391.41(B)(5)

Drivers with borderline lung function may do well under normal circumstances; however, commercial drivers are required to operate in various environmental conditions and under stressful situations. Decreased oxygen saturation or carbon dioxide retention can result in decreased alertness and decrements in performance. Chronic cough or cough syncope can result in a sudden inability to drive safely. Accidents have been attributed to these and to the side effects of many medications used as cough suppressants or antihistamines.[23] Impairment associated with the use of some antihistamines has been found to be greater than that found with alcohol use.[24]

Many studies have indicated that commercial drivers do not obtain sufficient sleep.[25] Others have found that there is an increased risk of motor vehicle accidents in patients with sleep disorders such as sleep apnea.[26,27] Questions were recently added to the medical examination reporting form regarding this condition. Normal sleep studies such as maintenance of wakefulness test or a multiple sleep latency test should be obtained to ensure a minimal risk of accidents. Annual repeat of testing and follow-up evaluations were recommended by pulmonary conference participants.[14]

HYPERTENSION—49 CFR 391.41(B)(6)

Complications from uncontrolled hypertension can lead to cardiomyopathy, nephropathy, or retinopathy, any of which can produce impairment. Severe hypertension can be the cause of transient ischemic attacks or stroke. Detailed guidance has been provided by the FMCSA (Fig. 50–1) on the certification process in hypertensive commercial drivers. It is recommended that those drivers with hypertension who are controlled on medication be re-evaluated on at least an annual basis for blood pressure control, evidence of end organ damage, and to ensure that there are no side effects from the medication(s).

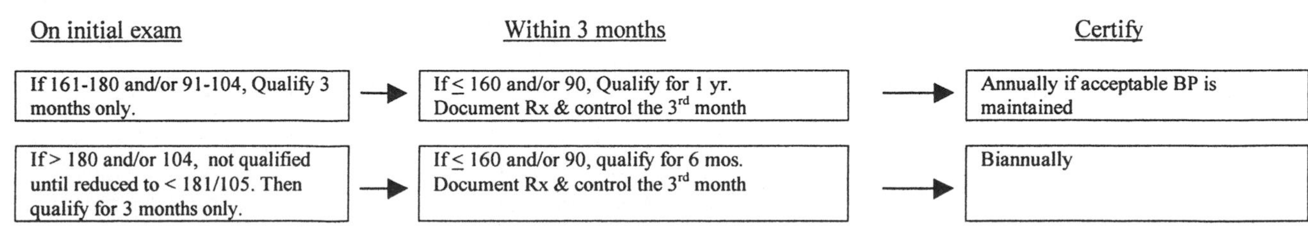
On initial exam
Within 3 months
Certify
If 161-180 and/or 91-104, Qualify 3 months only.
If ≤ 160 and/or 90, Qualify for 1 yr. Document Rx & control the 3rd month
Annually if acceptable BP is maintained
If > 180 and/or 104, not qualified until reduced to < 181/105. Then qualify for 3 months only.
If ≤ 160 and/or 90, qualify for 6 mos. Document Rx & control the 3rd month
Biannually

Figure 50–1. Guidelines for blood pressure evaluation.

RHEUMATIC, ARTHRITIC, ORTHOPEDIC, MUSCULAR, NEUROMUSCULAR, OR VASCULAR DISEASE—49 CFR 391.41(B)(7)

Diseases such as rheumatoid arthritis, multiple sclerosis, and Parkinson's disease may have variable courses with the possibility of progressive and unpredictable limitations. A driver with decreased range of motion or strength will have difficulty safely performing many of the essential tasks of the commercial driver. Current limitations and the likelihood of progression must be considered. Workers with conditions where the degree of impairment has the potential to be severe or sudden should not be considered safe to drive commercial vehicles.

EPILEPSY OR LOSS OF CONSCIOUSNESS—49 CFR 391.41(B)(8)

States have various regulations for the duration of driving limitation after a seizure. For commercial driving, the driver may not have a "current clinical diagnosis" of a seizure disorder or to be taking antiseizure medication. No discretion is left to the examiner for this prohibition and no waiver is currently available. Neurologists and others knowledgeable about the risks and responsibilities of commercial drivers recommended at a conference sponsored by the Federal Highway Administration[11] that a driver be seizure free and off medication 10 years with an established history of a seizure disorder and 5 years off medication and seizure free for a single seizure. Those drivers who have a loss of consciousness of unknown etiology should have a complete neurologic evaluation to ensure that the risk of recurrence is minimal. At least a 6-month waiting period is recommended prior to returning to work.

MENTAL DISORDERS—49 CFR 491.41(B)(9)

Commercial driving is recognized to be stressful with work conditions, long periods away from home, and pressure to meet delivery requirements. Many drivers are paid by the mile or load and not by the time on duty, adding financial pressures to the equation. Weather conditions, pressure to arrive on time, and irregular schedules, as well as drivers of other vehicles, can result in a driver with a personality disorder or other mental health problem being unsafe. Aggressive, paranoid, or depressed behavioral patterns may cause the driver to not appreciate a hazard or act appropriately in stressful situations. Equally important are the medications used to treat these medical conditions. Common side effects of centrally acting agents are sedation or decreased alertness. Participants in the conference on Psychiatric Disorders and Commercial Drivers[12] recommended that use of and reliance on certain medications be considered grounds for disqualifying a commercial driver.

VISION—49 CFR 391.41(B)(10)

The vision requirement is one of the absolute requirements for commercial drivers with the examiner having no discretion. The drivers must have 20/40 or better in each eye, with or without corrective lenses. Neither monocular vision nor use of monovision contact lenses is acceptable in commercial drivers. Drivers are not required to have normal color vision, but must be able to correctly identify the colors of the traffic signals. A number of drivers who did not have the required visual acuity were entered into a waiver program similar to that for insulin-taking diabetics. Currently the FMCSA is accepting applications and granting exemptions under certain circumstances for those drivers who do not meet the standards.[28] In general the driver must have at least 3 years of safe commercial driving with the visual deficiency. The application must include how the level of safety would not be any less than if the driver had the required visual acuity.

HEARING—49 CFR 391.41(B)(11)

The driver must be able to pass a forced whisper test at 5 feet or not have an average hearing loss of greater than 40 dB in the better ear, with or without a hearing aid. There is no exemption available for this requirement at this time.

DRUG USE—49 CFR 391.41(B)(12)

Commercial drivers are not only prohibited from using illegal substances but should also not be using narcotics or other habit-forming substances. If the treating health care provider is aware of the tasks, responsibilities, and risks of that driver and is convinced that the driver is not likely to be impaired, then legal medications could be used. The examiner must also be assured that the driver is taking the medication as prescribed. According to the FMCSA's advisory criteria, a driver on methadone should not be medically qualified. A driver who has a history of drug use or who has had a positive drug test should be carefully evaluated by a substance abuse professional before being cleared to drive. Drug and alcohol testing are required for commercial drivers but this is not a part of the medical examination.

ALCOHOLISM—49 CFR 391.41(B)(13)

A driver who is under the influence of alcohol clearly presents a danger on the highway. Drivers with alcoholism should not be permitted to drive commercial vehicles. Evaluation by a substance abuse professional could aid in identifying those who are currently not drinking and are unlikely to relapse.

OTHER TRANSPORTATION MODES

Commercial drivers are not the only workers in transportation who are required to meet federal medical standards. There are also federally mandated standards for pilots, railroad engineers, and employees covered by the Coast Guard. When determining if these patients can return to work, it is important to explore whether they are required to meet specific standards.

CONCLUSION

For health care providers who are tasked with determining whether an individual is able to perform his or her normal job, it is essential to not only consider physical ability. A consideration of the potential risk of impairment and possible subsequent harm is necessary. The Federal Motor Carrier Safety Regulations are in place to guide health care professionals as to those medical conditions that may carry an unacceptable risk. Review of the regulations and supporting material must occur prior to stating that the driver may return to work. Drivers with underlying medical conditions will often require more than just a cursory examination; reviewing medical records and at times additional diagnostic studies to ensure the stability of the disease are needed. For a driver who may be safe to drive in the short term, but longer term status is unknown, a shorter certification period must be entertained.

References

1. EEOC Technical Assistance Manual, ADA Technical Assistance Manual.
2. Parker v U.S. Department of Transportation, No. 98-4, 2000, Sixth Circuit, March 17, 2000.
3. Anderson v Department of Transportation, Federal Highway Administration, 213 F. 3d 422, U.S. Court of Appeals, Eighth Circuit, May 1, 2000.
4. Rauenhorst v U.S. Department of Transportation, Federal Highway Administration, 95 F. 3d 715, C.A. 8, 1996. Decided September 12, 1996.
5. Sutton v United Air Lines, Inc., 119 S. Ct. 2139, 144 L. Ed. 2d 450, 9 A.D. Cases (U.S. 06/22/1999), U.S. Supreme Court (no. 97-1943, June 22, 1999v1).
6. Murphy v United Parcel Service, Inc., 119 S. Ct. 2133, U.S., 1999. Decided June 22, 1999.
7. Albertson's Inc v Kirkinburg, 119 S. Ct. 2162, U.S. Or., 1999. Decided June 22, 1999.
8. Wharton Transport v Bridges, 606 S.W. 2d 521, July 7, 1980.
9. Gates v Riley ex rel. Riley, 723 N.E. 2d 946, Ind. App, 2000, February 10, 2000.
10. U.S. Department of Transportation, Federal Highway Administration: Regulatory Guidance for the Federal Motor Carrier Safety Regulations. Federal Register 62(65):16370–16431, 1997.
11. U.S. Department of Transportation, Federal Highway Administration: Conference on Neurological Disorders and Commercial Drivers (Pub. No. FHWA-MC-88-042). Washington, DC, Office of Motor Carriers, 1988.
12. U.S. Department of Transportation, Federal Highway Administration: Conference on Psychiatric Disorders and Commercial Drivers (Pub. No. FHWA-MC-91-006). Washington, DC, Office of Motor Carriers, 1991.
13. U.S. Department of Transportation, Federal Highway Administration, Office of Motor Carriers: Conference on Cardiac Disorders and Commercial Drivers (Pub. No. FHWA-MC-88-040). Washington, DC, Office of Motor Carriers, 1987.
14. U.S. Department of Transportation, Federal Highway Administration, Office of Motor Carriers: Conference on Respiratory/Pulmonary Disorders and Commercial Drivers (Pub. No. 1991 FHWA-MC-91-004). Washington, DC, Office of Motor Carriers, 1991.
15. Hartenbaum NP (ed): The DOT Medical Examination: A Guide to Commercial Driver Medical Certification, 2nd ed. Beverly, Mass, OEM Press, 2000.
16. American College of Occupational and Environmental Medicine: CDME (Commercial Driver Medical Examiner) Review. Arlington Heights, Ill, American College of Occupational and Environmental Medicine.
17. U.S. Department of Transportation, Federal Motor Carrier Safety Administration: Physical Qualification of Drivers: Medical Examination: Certificate–Final Rule. Federal Register 65(194):59363–59379, 2000.
18. Anonymous: Assessment of the cardiac patient for fitness to drive: 1996 update. Can J Cardiol 12:1164–1170,1996.
19. Cox DJ, Gonder-Frederick LA, Kovatchev BP, et al: Progressive hypoglycemia's impact on driving simulation performance: Occurrence, awareness and correction. Diabetes Care 23:163–170, 2000.
20. Laberge-Nadeau C, Dionne G, Ekoe J, et al: Impact of diabetes on crash risk of truck-permit holders and commercial drivers. Diabetes Care 25:612–617, 2000.
21. National Transportation Safety Board: Fatigue, Alcohol, Other Drugs and Medical Factors in Fatal-to-driver Heavy Truck Crashes (PB90-917992, NTSB/SS-90/01:1990). Washington, DC, National Transportation Safety Board, 1990.
22. Epstein AE, Quyyumi AA, Bonow RO, et al: Personal and public safety issues related to arrhythmias that may affect consciousness: Implications for regulation and physician recommendations. Circulation 94:1147–1166, 1996.
23. Kay GG: The effects of antihistamines on cognition and performance. J Allergy Clin Immunol 105(Suppl.):S622–S627, 2000.
24. Weiler JM, Bloomfield JR, Woodworth GG, et al: Effects of fexofenadine, diphenhydramine, and alcohol on driving performance: A randomized, placebo-controlled trial in the Iowa driving simulator. Ann Intern Med 132:354–363, 2000.
25. Mitler MM, Miller JC, Lipsitz JJ, Walsh JK: The sleep of long-haul drivers. N Engl J Med 337:755–761, 1997.
26. Moore-Ede M, Campbell S, Baker T: Falling asleep behind the wheel: Research priorities to improve driver alertness and highway safety. Proceedings of the Federal Highway Administration Symposium on Truck and Bus Driver Fatigue, Washington, DC, November 1998.
27. Teran-Santos J, Jimenez-Gomez A, Cordero-Guevara J: The association between sleep apnea and the risk of traffic accidents. N Engl J Med 340:847–851, 1999.
28. U.S. Department of Transportation, Federal Highway Administration: Federal Motor Carrier Safety Regulations, Waivers, Exemptions, and Pilot Programs: Rules and Procedures. Federal Register 63(235):67600–67612, 1988.

CHAPTER

51

The Generic Functional Capacity Assessment

STEPHEN L. DEMETER, MD, MPH ■ GERALDINE T. DEMETER, MA

As the name implies, a functional capacity assessment (FCA) assesses, tests, or addresses the ability of someone to perform a specific task. When used in disability medicine, FCA refers to the spectrum of tests that allow one to test an organ or organ system in performance of its basic function. FCA could refer to a test of visual acuity, of creatinine clearance, or of the ability to lift an object. Each organ or organ system has its own functions and, therefore, its own set of tests of functions. This chapter addresses the concept of an FCA from a generic standpoint. Principles are given and the specifics of the assessments are found in the chapters on organ systems in this book.

The easiest and most natural way to approach a return-to-work (RTW) decision is using a simplistic approach. A patient injures his or her back or experiences a myocardial infarction. The physician of record is asked if that injured worker may safely return to the workforce. By measuring that individual's capacity to perform labor—whether sustained, peak, or intermittent—and considering this capacity in light of the physical requirements of the job, the physician can decide if the patient can or cannot perform the functions of that job. Unfortunately, real life and the practice of medicine preclude such a simplistic approach. RTW recommendations involve numerous decisions based on a variety of data, most of which are unique to a given worker or patient. Many of these issues are found in Table 51–1.

Some of this material was taken from "Back to Work, Functional Capacity Assessment, Work Accommodation," presented at The American Academy of Disability Evaluating Physicians International Disability Medicine Synopsis, May 4, 1997, with permission of the American Academy of Disability Evaluating Physicians.

The practicing physician, regardless of specialty, can create a RTW prescription using the principles found in Table 51–1. Points 1 through 4 relate to the job, 5 through 10 relate to the injured or ill worker, and 11 through 15 relate to the Americans With Disabilities Act

TABLE 51–1

Points for Consideration in a Return-to-Work Recommendation by the Physician

I. The Job Requirements
   1. What are the physical and psychological requirements of the job?
   2. How are these requirements determined?
   3. Who has measured/described these requirements?
   4. How valid, reliable, and complete are these measurements?

II. The Injured or Ill Worker
   5. What were the worker's preinjury capabilities?
   6. How did the injury or illness change these capabilities?
   7. How long are the changes in capability expected to exist (maximum medical improvement [MMI])?
   8. What is the resultant performance level, for the injured or ill worker, at MMI?
   9. How is the performance level measured?
   10. What are the resultant restrictions for a particular worker?

III. Ability to Function in a Specific Job Setting
   11. What are the essential tasks of the job?
   12. Are accommodations possible?
   13. Do the effects of the injury or illness, or do the residual effects after recovery has been completed, create an enhanced risk to the worker owing to work exposures/functions and/or do these residuals make the worker a risk to coworkers?
   14. Is there a problem with traveling to and from work?
   15. Can the worker be at the workplace for the required work shift?

(ADA) and peripheral issues affecting a person's ability to function in the job setting.

THE JOB REQUIREMENTS

What Are the Physical and Psychological Requirements of the Job?

A job is defined as an activity that one performs that produces an item of value in the marketplace for which the worker receives compensation. That item may be the result of manual or intellectual labor requiring the expenditure of a certain amount of physical or mental energy. In many circumstances, these requirements are known, however crudely. This is especially true for manual labor. To produce manual labor, the worker calls upon various parts of the body to perform muscular work that requires the coordinated functioning of many body parts, including the lungs and gastrointestinal tract, for energy substrate acquisition and excretion; the cardiovascular system, for delivery and removal of these substrates to and from the muscles; and an intact and functioning musculoskeletal system, to actually perform the work.

The levels of energy expenditure, measured in $\dot{V}O_2$ (oxygen uptake) or METS (metabolic equivalents), have been measured for a variety of activities ranging from sedentary to heavy manual labor (see Chapters 22 and 24). Although these measurements have been made, they are fairly generic and may not be applicable to a particular job.

The field of ergonomics has arisen in the past several decades to the level of a science. It describes the muscular strength necessary to perform various tasks and the stresses imposed on the muscular and skeletal systems. Many variables have been analyzed by ergonomists, including horizontal, vertical, and other planes of movement; torque; load; frequency of performance; duration; and others. Flexibility or range of motion (ROM) is another important aspect (see Chapter 53).

Other aspects of the job that are knowable or measurable include the ambient temperature, humidity, air quality, noise, lighting, presence of toxins, presence of hazards (chemicals, physical, and others), and functions of coworkers.

To say that these variables of a job are known or are knowable is not to say that they have been described in detail for a given job or job setting. Many times one can extrapolate from the body of literature to a given job setting. Other means of determining the physical or psychological requirements of a particular job include job descriptions (from generic, as in the Dictionary of Occupational Titles,[2] to specific, as in written descriptions by company personnel), observations (plant tours, videotapes), verbal reports (patients, supervisors), and listings of protective equipment (lists, discussions with plant safety specialists, perusal of Material Safety Data Sheets).

How Are These Requirements Determined?

As discussed, are the requirements available to the evaluator generic or actual? If actual, who gave these requirements? Bias may be an important factor. In some circumstances it is to the advantage of one of the involved parties to make the requirements seem greater or lesser than they actually are. If the descriptions are generic, then the source needs to be identified. This leads to the following two categories in this section.

Who Has Measured/Described These Requirements? How Valid, Reliable, and Complete Are These Measurements?

Most people who work with computers are familiar with the concept of "garbage in, garbage out," or "GIGO." If the job requirements are extrapolations from generic formulae, will they accurately predict a specific job in terms of its physical or psychological requirements, and are the generic predictions correct in the first place? In other words, are back-to-work recommendations being based on faulty assumptions?

In many respects, the generic issues are fairly well standardized. This applies especially to the fields of ergonomics and energy production. It is not the purpose of this chapter to produce a meta-analysis of the various papers written on these subjects or to comment on their validity, reliability, or use as extrapolation models. Various references are provided in the list of suggested readings. The chapters in this section are also excellent sources of specific information. What is known has been found to be fairly reliable. However, any science is always in a state of flux and what appears reasonable today may be changed and modified, or discarded and replaced, in the future.

There are still large gaps in our knowledge regarding job requirements. Perhaps the largest gaps involve psychological issues, where questions such as the following arise: How much stress is involved in a job? How much emphasis does the job place on social interactive skills? What type of personality is best suited for a particular job? Because these issues are fairly job-specific and their measurements lie in the domain of a "soft" science (rather than a "hard" science such as ergonomics or energy production), these issues may never be explained as rationally, objectively, and scientifically as the medical/legal/occupational communities would like.

THE INJURED OR ILL WORKER

What Were the Worker's Preinjury Capabilities?

This issue is addressed by the same measuring paradigms as noted for the generic models. Thus one could take a worker and measure his or her capabilities with respect to joint and extremity integrity, function, flexibility, and strength. A person's peak $\dot{V}O_2$ could be measured by a cardiopulmonary stress test. (It is assumed that a person can work, on a sustained basis, at a level of 40% of peak $\dot{V}O_2$.) Performance of almost any part of the body could be measured in terms of anatomy and physiology (e.g., testing liver and kidney function; testing cardiac performance by stress testing, echocardiograms, and cardiac catheterization; testing strength by various machines; testing flexibility by measuring ROM). We could also measure a person's mental, emotional, and interactive skills.

To address preinjury function, one would need realistic measurements of these functions. These are rarely performed or known precisely, but in many circumstances they can be inferred. A worker who develops occupational asthma owing to a toxic inhalation (reactive airways dysfunction syndrome [RADS]) may have had prior pulmonary function tests performed as part of a respirator certification program. A worker exposed to a hepatotoxin may have had liver function tests performed as part of a prior routine physical examination. Further, these factors may have previously been unmeasured but there may be indirect proof of performance capability by the successful premorbid achievement of various intensities of work. For example, if before an illness, a worker withstood the psychological stresses involved in a job (as corroborated by discussions with family, coworkers, etc.) or if a worker performed at a certain level of manual labor without undue restrictions, then it can be inferred that the worker possessed those capabilities.

How Did the Injury or Illness Change These Capabilities?

In order to assess the issue of change created by an injury or illness, it is necessary to know the results of that injury or illness. Anatomic changes are perhaps the easiest to assess. For example, if a person had a traumatic amputation of a foot or an arm or if a nerve injury produced paralysis of a body part, the extrapolation becomes relatively simple. Physiologic changes (breathing ability, cardiac output, liver and kidney function, or partial functioning of a nerve) are also measurable and, to some degree, predictable in terms of alterations of work ability and job performance. Psychological issues are more difficult areas to test reliably. These changes caused by injury or illness must be defined individually, rather than on a more generic basis as seen with alterations in anatomy and physiology.

In order to measure the change in capability created by an injury or illness, the worker can be assessed in a variety of ways by methods similar to those discussed. If the premorbid function is unknown, it will be necessary to use population norms to assess pre- to postinjury change. There are two important issues that must be remembered when using population norms. The first is that population norms use the concept of standard deviations. In order to serve the dual concepts of sensitivity and specificity, norms are devised to include the majority of healthy people and to exclude the majority of unhealthy people. Ideally, a level of two standard deviations is chosen, meaning that 97.5% of healthy people are included and 97.5% of unhealthy people are excluded. However, unless one knows the sensitivity/specificity, positive/negative predictive values, and standard deviations of a given test, then one cannot accurately interpret a test result. (Realistically, how many clinicians include this analysis of test results in their analyses? For example, if the upper limit of a liver function test is 45 mg/dL, how many healthy/unhealthy people are above/below that cutoff?) Also implicit in the concept of standard deviations is the idea that a healthy person will always have a chance of having a test result above or below the cutoff level or that an unhealthy person will have a value in the "normal range." Some tests have very little separation between normal and not normal (Fig. 51–1*A*); others have a fairly large overlap, with normal and not normal ranges possessing similar values (Fig. 51–1*B*); and other tests will have such a large separation that the boundaries between normal and not normal are discreet (Fig. 51–1C) (for example, it is normal to have 4 limbs—not 3, 3.5, or even 3.98). These are depicted in the graphs seen in Figure 51–1.

The other important issue is normality for the individual. For example, assume the predicted forced expiratory volume in 1 second (FEV_1) for a person of a given height, sex, race, and age is 3.00 L. If the measured value for that individual is 3.00 L, then he is at 100% of predicted. If, postinjury or illness, FEV_1 falls to a value of 2.40 L, the patient is still in the normal range for the test (see Chapter 22). However, owing to injury/illness, his FEV_1 dropped by 20%. If his normal FEV_1 was 3.60 L (20% above the normal but still in the "normal range") and the FEV_1 dropped to 2.40 L (also still in the "normal range"), there would be a 50% reduction in the FEV_1—hardly an insubstantial value. Unless the normal for an individual is known, using population norms is risky.

How Long Are the Changes in Capability Expected to Exist (Maximum Medical Improvement [MMI])? What is the Resultant Performance Level, for the Injured or Ill Worker, at MMI?

The issues of MMI are based on a knowledge of the injury or illness; its treatment; the expected effect of the

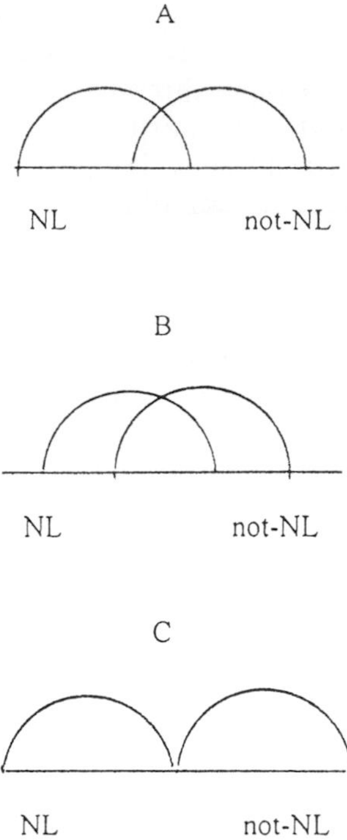

Figure 51–1. *A* refers to the separation found in most clinical tests where the value for sensitivity and specificity overlap to some degree. However, the value chosen for the upper limits of "normal," while including some "not-normal" value, is still high enough to include many of the "normal" while excluding many of the "not-normal." *B* refers to a selection of sensitivity/specificity values which do not clearly separate the "normal" from the "not-normal." These values are not chosen to reduce the reliability of a test but, rather, reflect the imprecision that the data generated during the test allows for. *C*, There is a clear separation between the "normal" and "not-normal" population. This is the ideal test and one which is rarely found. See also Appendix A for a more complete explanation.

treatment; the time course of the illness, treatment, and expected recovery time based on that treatment; the adherence to a treatment protocol by the patient; and personal factors such as the level of effectiveness of a treatment for an individual as well as the side effects and complications. Only by mastering a particular field of specialization (e.g., cardiology, orthopedics, psychiatry) can a physician feel competent to address these issues. If one possesses no such mastery, then a review of the pertinent medical literature or a referral to a specialist will be necessary. Although in many circumstances these issues are known, especially on a generic basis, they are often unknown or unknowable when referenced to a particular person. For example, how long after a myocardial infarction will a specific person take to reach MMI? How long after a discectomy? How long after a carpal tunnel release or rotator cuff surgery?

How is the Performance Level Measured?

Performance levels are measured by the same means as discussed previously. Diminished performance levels can be estimated by inferential means but are best when measured. Measurements are best made at MMI or when the injury or illness results are static and well stabilized and when no further changes are likely. Some impairment/disability systems place artificial time limits on this time course. For example, the Social Security system uses 1 year. For some injuries or illnesses, this is appropriate. For others, it is too long or too short. Additionally, the effects created by the unwillingness of a patient to conform to recommended treatment guidelines will severely hamper the ability to utilize, at any given time, the concept of MMI. For example, is a patient with a back injury, who has undergone appropriate physical therapy and work hardening programs, at MMI at 1 year if he or she did not undergo the recommended discectomy? Or what of the individual who is 1 year post myocardial infarction but continues to smoke?

In some circumstances, postinjury measurements are not sufficiently reliable. This is most apparent in the areas of psychological assessment but can also be seen when a person voluntarily (or involuntarily) diminishes his or her peak anatomic or physiologic performance. The advantage of anatomic or physiologic testing, as opposed to psychological testing, is that, by the very nature of these tests, one can appreciate and make note of suboptimal performance; unfortunately, the question will still remain of what that person is actually capable of doing.

What are the Resultant Restrictions for a Particular Worker?

To address this issue one needs to start with the present capabilities of the injured or ill worker, regardless of the time point in the injury or illness. Thus, an RTW recommendation will vary depending on the nature of the injury or illness, the natural time course of that injury or illness, the type of treatment (including issues such as adherence by the worker), complications and side effects (particularly with regard to medications and extraneous effects such as seen in surgery), the presence of MMI, and others.

Restrictions can be approached either generically or specifically. If specific, they are listed according to a predetermined listing of the job requirements.

Capabilities/restrictions are, in many circumstances, best be approached from a prospective standpoint. Physicians need to remember that many of their patients are active members of the workforce. Many injuries or illnesses interfere with the patient's normal activities in the workplace. These interferences and their anticipated time course should be communicated to both the worker and the employer. Further, when a referral is made to a physician who practices a different specialty (e.g., a surgeon, internal medicine subspecialist, psychiatrist) or to a therapeutic center (e.g., physical therapy), these issues should be addressed in the referral request. Thus a cover letter may include standard elements such as the nature of the concern and reason for the referral, pertinent aspects of the patient's medical history, and suspicions and diagnoses, as well as a request for RTW information as detailed previously.

Although the tenor of this chapter has centered on restrictions—what a patient cannot do—the practicing physician needs to be aware that information concerning what patients can do—their capabilities (vis-à-vis the injury or illness, treatment, time course, etc.)—is just as important to identify, quantify, and report on as restrictions. In many cases, it is even more important. Thus, RTW recommendations need to be viewed positively (capabilities) as well as negatively (restrictions).

Whereas some factors are measurable, many are not. Much is known about the physical requirements of jobs on a generic basis but much is unknown regarding specific jobs. Less is known, from a generic standpoint, about mental requirements. Usually one can measure a person's mental and physical capabilities and, at times, can document a deviation created by an injury or illness by comparing pre- to postmorbid functioning from pre- to postmorbid test results, extrapolations, or deviations from the norm. At times, a predicted timing for MMI can be given on a generic basis for a given injury or illness, but individual factors greatly alter this concept for an individual patient or worker.

The physician now takes the worker capabilities, as imprecise as they are, and applies them to the specific workplace to which his or her injured or ill patient will return.

ABILITY TO FUNCTION IN A SPECIFIC JOB SETTING

What Are the Essential Tasks of the Job? Are Accommodations Possible?

In order to address these two issues, one must understand the totality of a person's job. Various resources are available, including interviews with the injured worker or patient, interviews with supervisors, interviews with human resource personnel, the Dictionary of Occupational Titles,[2] videotapes, and written job descriptions. Since the passage of the ADA, it has become important for the employer to provide written job descriptions that detail the essential components of a job.

Accommodation involves three essential issues:

1. What is the nature of a person's injury or illness? What restrictions are placed on the individual because of the injury or illness? At what stage in the injury or illness is the worker? Does the prescribed treatment of the injury or illness create additional restrictions?
2. What are the essential/nonessential components of the job?
3. Does the job need to be modified to accommodate the restrictions imposed on the injured or ill worker? Can the job be modified? Is the employer ready, willing, and able to make these modifications?

Communication is critical in making appropriate recommendations, including between the physician and the employer representative (e.g., human resources personnel, supervisor, occupational safety specialist), physician and patient/worker, physician and union representative (at times), and others including worker–union, worker–employer representative, and union–employer representative. The issue of job accommodation is job-specific, worker-specific, and injury/illness-specific. It cannot be generalized.

Do the Effects of the Injury or Illness, or Do the Residual Effects After Recovery Has Been Completed, Create an Enhanced Risk to the Worker Owing to Work Exposures/Functions and/or Do These Residuals Make the Worker a Risk to Coworkers?

This is basically an extension of the discussion on the restrictions imposed by the injury or illness and the nature of the job. However, it is more proactive than the previous discussion, and is based on a thorough understanding of not only the job but also the work environment, including the concept of fellow workers as part of the work environment. For example, for a person who developed asthma as a result of workplace exposures, do the fumes or dust create a risk where none previously existed? Does the worker with low back pain and sciatica pose a risk to a coworker who is responsible for lifting heavy, bulky objects with him or her?

Is There a Problem With Traveling To and From Work?

For example, if a person with two fractured and casted legs has a desk job, he may have no difficulty in performing the essential components of the job, but may not be able to get there by car, bus, or train.

Can the Worker be at the Workplace for the Required Work Shift?

Treatments can and do modify a person's ability to work and to be physically present at the worksite. At times a physician will recommend that a person be present for only a certain number of hours. Some treatments (e.g., dialysis, physical therapy) can only be scheduled during work hours. These factors need to be assessed when writing a RTW prescription.

RETURN TO WORK PRESCRIPTIONS/RECOMMENDATIONS

(see also Appendix B)

RTW recommendations require information about the job, the worker, the nature of the injury or illness, treatment potential and duration, and the residual effects of the injury or illness. It would seem that a written recommendation given by a knowledgeable and experienced physician, produced after a discussion with the patient and employer, would be the ideal RTW form. However, there is another confounding factor: the premade RTW forms. Most physicians have seen them and many have become frustrated by their questions.

RTW forms can be generic or specific. These basically ask whether the injured or ill worker can return to his or her prior job. The critical information needed prior to completing these forms is what the job entails in terms of physical and/or mental capabilities. Usually this information is not provided—only the RTW form with several questions (e.g., Can the worker return to the former position? If not, what is the medical reasoning/proof preventing such a return? Can the worker return to the former position if specific accommodations are met? If so, what are these job modifications? How long are they expected to last? What is the medical reasoning/proof behind these job changes/this duration of change? Can the injured or ill worker sustain any remunerative employment?). Again, it seems obvious that, in order to address these issues, the physician needs a complete job description, but one is not always provided. Usually the physician relies on the interview with the injured or ill worker to obtain this information. The alternative is to request that the employer provide the job description in writing. The latter is greatly preferred for several reasons: a written job description is almost always available, is more complete than the worker's description, and is usually more reliable than the worker's description, will be used as the basis for incorporating the physician's recommendations, and requesting the documentation makes the physician seem more competent.

The generic forms are harder to complete. These forms ask many questions that may or may not have anything to do with what the injured or ill worker previously did in his or her job. Questions are generally broken down into two main categories: physical capabilities and psychological issues. The physical capabilities are usually divided into three major categories: strength, agility, and endurance. The psychological issues consider topics related to stress, competency, and interactive skills. Occasionally, environmental issues are raised. The physician, faced with the task of completing these forms, needs to have some rational basis for checking the appropriate boxes. How is this done?

The psychological issues are fairly easy to address. In the course of a physician's dealings with the patient, he or she must decide whether there are any psychological constraints for that worker. If so, then he or she can complete the form, refer the worker to someone else for psychological testing prior to completing the form, or state, on the form, that the issues were not examined and that a specialist referral is recommended.

Environmental restrictions are necessary in only a handful of medical conditions. These usually relate to problems with the senses, such as vision (where restrictions caused by poor lighting in the work environment may be necessary), hearing (where restrictions caused by excessive noise or need for normal or near normal hearing arise; for example, one must consider whether a person with a hearing loss has an enhanced risk for future loss created by noise levels in the work environment or if there is an enhanced risk to fellow workers due to an inability to hear sufficiently well on the part of the hearing-impaired worker), and smell (does the worker place him- or herself at risk by not being able to discriminate between nonharmful and noxious or toxic fumes in the working environment?). Fumes or dust or smoke in the working environment are generally an issue only in patients with asthma (either as the sole respiratory condition or as part of another respiratory condition, such as chronic obstructive pulmonary disease, bronchiectasis, or hypersensitivity pneumonitis; inhalants such as fumes, dust, and smoke are disease- and worker-specific). Temperature may be an important environmental issue when extremes of cold (in asthma, Raynaud's phenomenon, and other circulatory disorders) or heat (in cardiovascular disease or with the use of certain medications, peripheral vasodilation caused by high temperatures or wearing an excessive amount of protective clothing may create circulatory collapse) are found.

Probably the most vexing issue relates to strength, especially lifting strength. This is a difficult problem to solve for orthopedists, ergonomists, and occupational medicine specialists (as well as occupational safety specialists, employers, and human resource personnel). How much normal labor (lifting, carrying, and performing manual labor with a variety of tools such as shovels, axes, and sledgehammers) a noninjured worker can safely perform has never been satisfactorily addressed. It is no surprise, then, that physicians sometimes have trouble when completing forms that create RTW recommendations for the injured or ill worker. If what was safe before an injury is unknown, how can a physician reliably state what is safe after the injury?

In many circumstances, physicians, when faced with this dilemma, ask the injured worker what he or she feels he or she can do safely and use the answer as the sole basis for the RTW recommendation. This is a poor approach. First, it does not take into account actual performance levels. It merely lends credence to what the injured worker states that he or she can do and legitimizes a nonprofessional opinion. For a variety of reasons, not all injured or ill workers are willing to return to the workplace. For example, Bigos et al[1] found that in patients with low back pain, the second most important factor associated with the recurrence of back injuries (after a history of prior back injuries) was the degree of satisfaction that the worker had with the job. In addition, legitimizing nonprofessional assessments runs counter to a physician's responsibilities when making RTW recommendations, which include recommending a working environment and level that is within the capability of the patient and that, hopefully, will not create unacceptable levels of risk.

When approaching this problem area, three approaches can be used: becoming familiar with the National Institute for Occupational Safety and Health (NIOSH) formula;[6,7] becoming familiar with the U.S. Department of Labor categorization of work based on strength and endurance; and measuring strength, flexibility, and endurance, as discussed previously and in the following (see also Chapter 48).

In 1981, after working with a panel of experts, NIOSH proposed a means of predicting safe lifting loads. This became known as the NIOSH formula.[6] An excellent discussion of the development of this formula is found in reference 4. This formula was developed to permit employers to assess the workplace and identify jobs that needed to be modified. It was derived from cadaveric studies of lumbar vertebrae to determine compressive forces required to produce osseous injury. It was never developed as a paradigm to be applied to individual workers, nor did it concern itself with soft tissue injuries to the low back or to joints other than the low back. A review of this formula's development illustrates the primitive nature of our abilities to recommend prescriptions or restrictions for activities involving muscular strength. This not only applies to young and healthy workers but especially to older, unfit, injured, or ill workers.

The U.S. Department of Labor has divided work by the amount of strength needed to lift/carry into five categories: sedentary, light, medium, heavy, and very heavy.[2] These categories are found in Table 51–2.

The major problem with filling out the forms is reliably and accurately predicting what a worker is capable of doing and what will be safe for that worker. In the past several years, a variety of machines have entered the marketplace that can test for strength, flexibility, and ability to perform manual labor in a variety of body positions. These machines are often used for testing or are incorporated into a work-hardening program where testing is performed at various times in the training. The advantages of using these machines include objectivity and a numerical result. The disadvantages are imperfect replication of job-specific tasks, expense, limited availability, and unknown application of the results (see Chapter 56).

Flexibility can be measured by standard ROM techniques. How these relate to concepts of stooping, crawling, climbing, and bending is unknown. Perhaps it is best to address these issues as a blending of the clinical condition with the measured ROM.

TABLE 51–2

U.S. Department of Labor Table of Work Activity Levels for Lifting/Carrying

Physical Demand Level	Occasional (0 to 33% of the Workday)	Frequent (34 to 66% of the Workday)	Constant (67 to 100% of the Workday)	Typical Energy Required
Sedentary	10 lbs	Negligible	Negligible	1.5–2.1 METS
Light	20 lbs	10 lbs and/or walk/stand/ push/pull of arm/leg controls while seated.	Negligible and/or push/pull of arm/leg controls	2.2–3.5 METS
Medium	20 to 50 lbs	10 to 25 lbs	10 lbs	3.6–6.3 METS
Heavy	50 to 100 lbs	25 to 50 lbs	10 to 20 lbs	6.4–7.5 METS
Very heavy	Over 100 lbs	Over 50 lbs	Over 20 lbs	Over 7.5 METS

The last issue of concern is related to endurance. This issue is addressed by the concept of "all of the time, some of the time, part of the time, none of the time" or various fractions of an 8-hour day. However, endurance is also implicit in the concept of strength. Whether due to cardiac or pulmonary disease, protein-losing disease states (malabsorption, cancer, chronic infection), or chronic poor health, if muscle mass is lost, endurance will be diminished and so will peak performance. Endurance can be measured by assessing the $\dot{V}O_2$, as discussed earlier in this chapter (see also Chapter 24).

RECOMMENDATIONS

As can be seen throughout this chapter, RTW recommendations can be very simple or very complex. How does the physician approach the recommendation for an injured or ill worker who is capable of returning to the workforce, although not to the degree that that worker was capable preinjury?

First, the 15-point checklist should be assessed for each worker. Recommendations are then given based on the checklist. The broad issues of psychological and environmental restrictions were discussed earlier. Again, these issues either belong to the domain of specialists and/or are disease-specific.

Second, for the issue of manual labor capabilities, one of two approaches can be used. The physician may simply guess. There is nothing wrong with guessing, as long as the physician is aware of two important issues: he or she may have to justify a guess and that the physician is liable, from a legal standpoint, for guesses. (A malpractice charge can be entered for overly liberal or conservative RTW recommendations based on possible adverse outcomes. Interested physicians should contact their malpractice carrier or attorney.) The physician's estimations (or guesses) are based on skill, experience, and training. In other words, these are educated guesses and the more skill, training, and experience that the physician possesses, the more likely it is that his or her educated guesses will be accurate and appropriate. If the physician is unwilling to guess, then the only other approach is to measure. Flexibility can be measured by ROM techniques. Strength can be measured by various isokinetic machines. Endurance can be measured by a cardiopulmonary exercise stress test.

The following is a suggested approach to making an educated guess. Strength can be measured and once it is known, no significant modifications will ordinarily be needed for flexibility unless the specific ROM restriction was not tested in the strength measurement. For example, if isokinetic strength is tested for the biceps and brachioradialis groups, generally, disease-induced restrictions caused by elbow ROM abnormalities will be included in the diminished strength capacity. However, if pronation/supination of the forearm is restricted and the job entails some forearm twisting, and only strength in the elbow flexors is tested, then appropriate modifications created by the altered ROM in the forearm may be necessary. If a person has normal strength in the legs and normal ROM of the knee joint but disease precludes repetitive squatting activities, then modifications, measured by abnormal ROM in the hip, are necessary. A simplistic approach would be to use the diminished ROM as found in the AMA Guides[3] and use the percent diminution, expressed as either the upper or lower extremity impairment, as a modifier. If, for example, the evaluee exhibited a muscular or strength ability to lift 30 pounds with the forearm but there was a 10% impairment for diminished ROM due to restricted pronation/supination, then the 30 pounds would be reduced by 10% to produce a level of 27 pounds of maximal expected strength capability. Sometimes the Guides give impairment ratings for joints based on disease processes (e.g., the spine and lower extremities) without necessarily referring to diminished ROM, also known as the DRE (diagnosis related estimate) method. The impairment value for the diminished ROM is preferred over the latter method for modifying the strength of capabilities.

In 1994, Johns et al[5] described a method of detailing diminished lifting ability by applying the NIOSH formula and using an additional modifier, namely, prior low back disease. They suggested three criteria—1) high risk (three or more episodes of low back pain in the preceding 5 years entailing loss of work/medical treatment), 2) moderate risk (one to two episodes in the preceding 5 years), and 3) low risk (no prior episodes)—and recommended a 50%, 25%, or 0% reduction in physical capabilities based on these criteria, respectively. To this modifier, a further restriction can be introduced based on anticipated reductions in endurance. The AMA Guides use a four-point categorization for pulmonary disease, coronary artery disease, and congestive heart failure (for the congestive heart failure categorization, see section 3.5 on Cardiomyopathies).[3] These can be measured by a variety of techniques but all may be measured using a cardiopulmonary exercise stress test deriving the $\dot{V}O_2$ for a person. Regardless of the means of categorization, if any worker/patient has a disease placing him or her into one of these four categories for those three conditions, he or she should have his or her strength recommendations reduced by 0%, 25%, 50%, 75%, or 100% based on his or her ranking. For example, if 30 pounds of lifting strength is recommended based on the NIOSH formula and the worker is in Category 2 from a cardiac or pulmonary standpoint, then the 30 pounds should be reduced to 22.5

pounds (30 × 25% = 7.5 pounds; 30 – 7.5 = 22.5). If that worker had a history of two episodes of low back pain in the preceding 5 years involving time away from work, then the maximum lifting would be 17 pounds (30 × 25% = 7.5 pounds; 30 –7.5 = 22.5 pounds; 22.5 × 25% = 5.6; 22.5 – 5.6 = ~17). As with the modifications in the NIOSH formula between 1981 and 1991,[6,7] research should be performed to validate this approach.

Third, the report/RTW recommendation should be positive as well as negative. Capabilities as well as restrictions should be detailed. Remember that a RTW recommendation is being written. It is not the physician's job to define which job in the workplace his or her patient will be performing. That is the employer's role. The job in which the employer places the patient will be dictated by a number of factors, one of which is the physician's recommendation of capabilities/restriction.

Fourth, a time limit should be placed on any restrictions that are necessary. Again, the report should be positive and proactive. The physician's recommendations and restrictions may need to be shortened, altered, or extended as he or she monitors the patient during the treatment phase of an illness. It is better to modify the RTW prescription over time than to be dogmatic about specific time frames, such as 6, 12, or 18 months in the future.

Fifth, whenever possible, the employer or employer representative should be asked for a written job description, and the physician should base the RTW recommendation on that job description.

Finally, as in any other branch of medicine, it is the physician's responsibility to keep current on recent research. Just as it is inappropriate to recommend operative or medical interventions that were the standard of care 20 or 30 years ago but that have been superseded by newer, more effective forms of treatment, so, too, should a physician make great effort to be current with up-to-date information regarding the effects of a patient's injury or illness on his or her ability to function in the workforce.

References

1. Bigos SJ, Battie MC, Spengler DM, et al: A prospective study of work perceptions and psychosocial factors affecting the report of back injury. Spine 16:1–6, 1991.
2. Department of Labor: Dictionary of Occupational Titles, 4th ed, rev, vols 1 and 2. Washington, DC, Department of Labor, 1991.
3. Cocchiarella L, Andersson GBJ (eds): Guides to the Evaluation of Permanent Impairment, 5th ed. Chicago, American Medical Association, 2001.
4. Erdil M, Dickerson OB, Chaffin DB: Biomechanics of manual materials handling and low back pain. In Zenz C, Dickerson OB, Horvath EP (eds): Occupational Medicine. St. Louis, Mosby, 1994, pp 239–257.
5. Johns RE, Bloswick DS, Elegante JM, et al: Chronic, recurrent low back pain. A methodology for analyzing fitness for duty and managing risk under the Americans with Disabilities Act. J Occup Med 36:537–547, 1994.
6. U.S. Department of Health and Human Services, National Institute for Occupational Safety and Health: NIOSH 1981, Work Practices Guide for Manual Lifting (NIOSH Technical Report No. 81-122). Cincinnati, Ohio, NIOSH, 1981.
7. Waters TR, Putz-Anderson V, Garg A, et al: Revised NIOSH equation for the design of manual lifting tasks. Ergonomics 36:749–776, 1993.

Suggested Readings

1. Chaffin DB, Andersson GBJ, Pope MH, et al: Workplace evaluation. In: Occupational Low Back Pain: Assessment, Treatment and Prevention. St. Louis, Mosby–Year Book, 1991, pp 217–239.
   Discusses various aspects of the workplace, utilizes the NIOSH formula, and describes changes that can be made in the workplace to accommodate the NIOSH formula.
2. Frymoyer JW, Haldeman S, Andersson GBJ: Impairment rating—the United States perspective. In: Occupational Low Back Pain: Assessment, Treatment, and Prevention. St. Louis, Mosby–Year Book, 1991, pp 279–295.
   Discusses low back injury, impairment, and disability, as well as the pathoanatomic correlates behind an inability to work.
3. U.S. Departm.ent of Labor, Employment and Training Administration: Dictionary of Occupational Titles, 4th ed, rev, vols 1 and 2. Washington, DC, US Government Printing Office, 1991.
   Describes the physical and intellectual demands of more than 20,000 jobs.
4. McArdle WD, Katch FI, Katch VL: Exercise Physiology. Philadelphia, Lea and Febiger, 1981.
   Has excellent tables of the energy costs of a variety of occupational and recreational activities.

CHAPTER

52

Can Joe Work?

JAMES B. TALMAGE, MD

Physicians are often asked by patients, employers, and insurance companies to complete forms that describe a patient's work abilities or work restrictions. Because physicians can perform scientific wonders, the public perception is that physicians must know how to scientifically fill out forms that ask, "How long can he or she stand?" or "How much weight can he or she lift?" Ironically, there is little science available to guide decisions on these questions, and most physicians have not received any training in how to make these decisions.

Physicians are sometimes asked to perform impairment ratings on patients, usually "according to the AMA Guides."[3] One key concept is that, in workers' compensation, an impairment rating helps determine compensation to the injured worker, but has no relationship to whether the individual can do a specific job or any class of jobs. For example, some workers who strain their backs end up at maximal medical improvement with persisting back pain symptoms but no objective findings, and thus their impairment is rated by the injury method (diagnosis related estimate method) as 0% whole person impairment. Despite no objectively definable impairment, some do not work because of pain. In contrast, other injured workers sustain severe spinal fractures with resulting paraplegia, and yet work despite considerable pain and handicaps. Their impairment ratings are greater than 90% whole person, and yet they work.

KEY TERMS: CAPACITY, TOLERANCE, AND RISK

In deciding on an appropriate level of work restrictions, physicians must consider the situation of each patient by considering three concepts: capacity, tolerance, and risk. The term capacity refers to concepts like strength and endurance. These are measurable with a fair degree of scientific precision. Actually, the word capacity indicates that training to maximal ability has already occurred, like an athlete ready for competition. Current ability is a more accurate term for what physicians estimate. Current ability can increase with training and exercise, and sometimes with further medical treatment. Strength, flexibility, and endurance are measurable, but can increase with exercise or decrease with inactivity. This principle is embodied in the aphorism "Use it or lose it." Physicians, employers, and insurance carriers all tend to substitute the word capacity for the term current ability.

The second concept physicians must consider when prescribing work restrictions is tolerance. Tolerance is a psychophysiologic concept. It means the ability to tolerate sustained work at a given level. Symptoms like pain or fatigue are what limit performance. In functional capacity or exercise testing, or during a trial of work, the patient can declare a level of work that is his or her maximal tolerance for the activity being tested, but this is not scientifically verifiable. Tolerance depends on the rewards available for doing the activity or work. Tolerance is generally less than either capacity or current ability.

The third concept physicians use in setting work restrictions is risk. Unfortunately, there are few scientific studies on the risk of work for someone who has recently been treated for significant musculoskeletal symptoms. One frequently quoted study is the Boeing Aircraft prospective study on the risk of future workers' compensation back injury claims.[7] In that study, current employees (who were at work) were assessed for factors that would correlate with a subsequent workers' compensation low back pain or injury claim. A total of 3020 employees were evaluated and then followed for 4 years.

The risk of a future claim was found to correlate with few factors (see Table 52–1).

Many published studies on risk are retrospective. Retrospective studies can generate hypotheses for further testing, but because of confounding by biases, they cannot establish or prove causation.[13] Most epidemiologic studies on the risk of work, other than studies on exposure to toxins, are retrospective. Again, retrospective studies do not prove causation, they merely prove associations and generate hypotheses for future, prospective studies (see also Appendix A).

Epidemiologic studies apply to populations, not to individuals. For example: If cigarette smoking increases the risk of myocardial infarction by 2.5 times the baseline risk of an individual, and if 10,000 individuals who smoke and a matched control group of nonsmokers are followed, some of the smokers will sustain a myocardial infarction. There is no way to predict which smokers will have a heart attack, and once the heart attacks have occurred, there is no way to know whether smoking caused the heart attack in a particular individual or whether that heart attack occurred unrelated to the smoking as part of the baseline rate of heart attacks in the population.

Similarly, suppose a control group of 10,000 normal workers and a study group of 10,000 workers, being sent back to work after an absence due to back pain, are followed for a year. The rate of workers' compensation back claims in general industry is 2 claims per 100 employees per year. Multiplying 2 claims/100 employees/year times 10,000 control employees yields a total of 200 back injury claims in the control group.

From the previously mentioned Boeing study,[7] in the study group with current or recent back pain, we would expect an increase in the rate of claims of 1.7 times compared to the control group. We would expect the control group to have 1.7 times 200 claims, or 340 workers' compensation back claims.

There is no way to predict which workers in the study group will experience a subsequent back episode. Once a new episode of back pain or injury has occurred, there is no way to know whether a single individual's back injury occurred as one of the 200 expected claims that represent the baseline rate of injury in the control group, or whether that individual's claim is one of the 140 claims that represent the increased rate of claims due to re-employment. Again, epidemiologic studies apply to populations rather than individuals.

In the United States, risk assessment in return to work situations is affected by the Americans With Disabilities Act (ADA). The implementation instructions for this Act indicate that the employer may require that the employee not pose a direct threat to self or others. (Per a recent case in the 9th Federal Circuit, on appeal in 2002, employers may only require that employees not pose a risk to others.[22])

TABLE 52–1

Risk of Future Workers' Compensation Back Pain Claim: "Boeing Study"

Variable	Relative Risk	95% Confidence Interval
Current or prior back pain	1.7	1.17–2.46
Employee does not enjoy the job	1.7	1.31–2.21
MMPI, scale 3	1.37	1.11–1.68

MMPI = Minnesota Multiphasic Personality Inventory.

If there is a high probability of substantial harm (not merely an increase in pre-existing symptoms) that is imminent (not in the distant future) based on objective medical evidence related to the particular individual, and if the employer cannot make reasonable accommodations that permit continued employment, the employer may terminate the employment relationship. Physicians are the principal source of information for the employee and employer on the employee's probability of risk, imminence of risk, and the nature of the potential harm. Decisions on whether reasonable accommodation can be accomplished are the employer's.

In talking with patients, and in reporting to employers and insurance carriers, physicians commonly use undefined terms to quantitate risk, such as mild, moderate, and high risk. This risk assessment is rarely based on published scientific studies (because there are not many). The assessment is occasionally based on published consensus documents, but is usually based on the anecdotal experience of the physician.

In terms of the ADA, when a physician declares high risk, this will usually meet the direct threat test, assuming that significant harm is imminent. When a physician uses the terms moderate risk or low risk, the ADA definition of direct threat will not usually be met.

In this chapter, we use the examples of coronary artery disease and low back pain because these two conditions are the most frequent reasons for individuals to be considered disabled. When studies are done to evaluate the risk of working despite these two conditions, objectively verifiable, serious, single incidents such as myocardial infarction and disk herniation permit scientific study of their rate of occurrence, and thus risk. Unfortunately, subjective, nonverifiable symptoms often limit an employee's work tolerance. If a study is done and employees limit their performance because of an increase in previous back pain or exertional chest pain that may or may not be angina, this confounds scientific study. This many times is due to somatization.

Somatization is not a diagnosis listed in the Diagnostic and Statistical Manual of Mental Disorders, fourth edition (DSM-IV).[4] It is rather an ego defense, as are humor and rationalization. Somatization is defined as somatic symptoms with no pathophysiologic basis. Somatization is a common reflection of emotional or psychosocial stressors and explains physical symptoms not caused by known disease or injury. Somatization is so common that 25% to 50% of patients in primary care practices complain of symptoms that have no serious cause, and psychosocial factors appear to play a role. In addition, of primary care patients with a diagnosable DSM-IV disorder, 50% to 70% initially present to the health care system with somatic symptoms, and these symptoms often obscure the underlying psychiatric distress from the physician's view.[6] This process of somatization is so common that there is an English idiom reflecting it: "My neighbor is a pain in the neck" can be reworded as "My neighbor's obnoxious behavior makes my neck hurt."

Thus somatization can explain some of the causes of nonspecific pain in the low back, neck, hand, and chest. It explains many of the situations in which physical or organic factors fail to explain disabling symptoms, and it confuses return to work assessments, both for individuals and for groups (scientific studies of risk).

Following both myocardial infarction and myocardial revascularization, symptomatic and functional recovery correlate poorly with the return to work status. Psychosocial factors such as adequate nonwork income, older age, anxiety or depression, and the perception of coronary disease as job-related are negative predictors of return to work.[17] Similarly, psychosocial factors are more important than physical factors in affecting symptoms, response to treatment, and long term outcomes, including return to work in adults with chronic low back pain problems.[8]

This conundrum has been summarized well by Marcia Scott, MD, a medical director at Prudential Insurance Company:

> It is difficult to make decisions about an individual's ability to function based solely on the medical diagnosis. This is especially true early in the course of a chronic illness. In the past, diagnosis of illness like diabetes or multiple sclerosis was rarely made early in its course. Patients presented for compensation only when the illness was obvious. By that time, the disability was clear and the course was often brief and brutal because of ineffective treatment. Today, through earlier diagnosis and more effective treatment, many of these disorders are now chronic illnesses. Individuals can work in the face of a relapsing illness and have longer life spans. More chronically ill people perform high function, well-compensated jobs. *Medical issues no longer suffice to explain the failure to function* (emphasis added).[29]

Thus, current ability can be estimated by measurement, although it may be increased up to capacity through exercise or training. Risk of objectively definable serious events can be rated as mild, moderate, or high, but usually with little scientific basis. Tolerance involving psychosocial factors and nonverifiable end points like pain is what in the real world usually determines whether an individual will work at a particular job. Employers and third parties usually ask physicians about current ability (using the term capacity), expecting scientific answers. The art of medicine is to guess the individual's tolerance.

CORONARY ARTERY DISEASE

Assessing the work capacity in the individual with known coronary artery disease involves the concepts of capacity, tolerance, and risk. Capacity, or current ability, may be determined by the event that led to the diagnosis of coronary artery disease.

If angina without infarction was the presenting symptom, there is usually normal pump function and the capacity for at least sedentary, light, and/or moderate work (by Dictionary of Occupational Titles criteria). More severe disease would probably already have been treated with revascularization, due to risk. If angina is ongoing, exertional chest pain or true angina may limit current ability. Unfortunately, nonanginal chest pain due to psychosocial factors (tolerance) may be what limits performance. Separating anginal pain from nonanginal chest pain is difficult in many cases.

If work ability assessment is being performed following myocardial infarction, there may be some degree of cardiac failure limiting current ability. The risk of chronic exercise (work)–induced myocardial remodeling is still poorly understood. The presence of scarring in the ventricle increases the risk of an exercise-induced arrhythmia. A myocardial infarction is an emotional event, with many patients choosing disability despite adequate current ability and an acceptably low risk with return to work.

Heavy physical exertion precipitates only 10% to 15% of myocardial infarctions, and regular exercise appears to be protective, preventing infarction and sudden cardiac death. Occupational physical activity or exertion is the most protective exercise, probably because it is performed regularly and for many hours each week.[2]

In a study of 1048 patients[32] whose myocardial infarctions were precipitated by exertion, factors that would have predicted the infarction were as shown in Table 52–2. The most important risk for infarction was being sedentary. Work involving exercise would thus be protective. A different study[27] looked at 216 consecutive patients who had sustained a myocardial infarction. They were all evaluated at the same occupational medicine clinic in Israel for return to work prescriptions. A total of 168 of the 216 patients attempted to return to work. Of the 150 who did return to work, 6 sustained a second infarction during the 2-year study. Of the six infarctions, two occurred at work. If 25% of an individual's time is spent at work (40 hours per week out of a 168-hour week), by chance alone 1.5 of the six infarctions would be expected to occur while the individual happened to be at work. Thus work that the physician believed was reasonable for the individual and that the individual was willing to perform did not appear to raise the rate of reinfarction (1.5 infarctions expected, two observed).

In evaluating a patient's return to work status, the first question for the physician to consider is "Does this person meet the definition of total disability?" In the United States, this usually means the Social Security Administration's definition of an inability to engage in any gainful employment. The book the Social Security Administration publishes for physician evaluators[35] can be consulted to determine if the severity of the disease or condition meets or exceeds the listing. If the patient's disease meets or exceeds the listed anatomic or physiologic severity criteria, the physician should explain that fact to the patient, as he or she may wish to apply for disability. If, however, the disease severity is well below the level required for the determination of total disability, the examining physician must then determine reasonable work restrictions or work abilities. This is most often done using a treadmill or similar type of exercise testing.

The exercise test can characterize the individual's exercise ability in METs (one MET or metabolic equivalent is the amount of oxygen expenditure required at rest, with activity or exercise described in multiples of this unit). The measured exercise ability in METs can then be compared to the job demands to see if the job in question is or is not appropriate. Patients should have an exercise performance free of significant cardiac problems (ischemia, arrhythmia) that is at least twice the average energy requirement and 20% more than the expected peak energy requirement of the job.[30]

TABLE 52–2

Cardiac Risk Factors Identified in Patients whose Myocardial Infarction was Precipitated by Physical Exertion

Factor	Odds Ratio
Low/very low activity level	3.35
Male sex	3.26
Hyperlipidemia	2.27
Current smoking	2.15
Obesity (BMI ≥ 30)	1.87

BMI = body mass index.

The job demands or the energy cost of doing the particular job in question need to be determined. Very rarely will an employer-supplied job description list the metabolic demands of a job in METs. One way to estimate the difficulty of the job is to use published studies that list the oxygen consumption required to perform multiple jobs.[30,33] This permits a comparison of the average METs required to do a job, but not necessarily the peak MET requirement. Also, although these references cover almost 500 jobs or activities, they may not apply to the particular job the patient must perform.

One method of dealing with this is to evaluate the job in question. A healthy coworker who is acclimated to the job can be asked to do the job while wearing a heart rate recorder (Holter monitor, for example). The healthy coworker's highest heart rate is then known for the peak energy expenditure tasks, and a computer can calculate an average heart rate for the time spent working. The healthy coworker then needs to perform a treadmill exercise test. If a Balke protocol is used for this testing, the treadmill workload changes every minute, permitting graphing of the healthy coworker's METs of exertion versus his or her heart rate at multiple different workloads. This graph will reveal how many METs the healthy coworker was exercising at any heart rate. This graph then permits looking at the healthy coworker's Holter monitor report and changing peak heart rate to peak METs, and similarly changing average heart rate to average METs expended in the job in question. The physician can then compare the METs at peak exercise from the treadmill test of the patient with coronary heart disease to the job requirements (see also Chapters 22, 24, and 25).

■ Example: Mr. Jones, a patient believed to be ready to return to work after myocardial infarction, can exert to 10 METs on a treadmill with no adverse consequences (ischemia, arrhythmia, or falling blood pressure).

A healthy coworker, Mrs. Smith, wears a Holter monitor for an 8-hour work day doing the job Mr. Jones used to do and to which he now wants to return. Mrs. Smith completes a standard treadmill test. Her maximal heart rate at work was 130 beats per minute, and from her treadmill test it is determined that she was exerting at 6 METs when her heart rate was 130. Mr. Jones can exert safely to 10 METs. He is thus safe using the "20% more than the expected peak energy requirement"[30] test (6 METs + 20% = 7.2 METs, which is less than 10 METs).

Similarly, Mrs. Smith's average heart rate doing the job in question was 100 beats per minute. From her treadmill test graph of METs versus heart rate, it can be determined that her average METs expended was 4. Mr. Jones can safely exert to 10 METs. He is thus safe using the "at least twice the average energy expenditure"[30] test (4 METs doubled is 8 METs, which is less than 10 METs). Thus his physician can reasonably predict that Mr. Jones should be able to do the job in question. ■

For heart conditions other than coronary artery disease, the consensus document entitled "26th Bethesda Conference Recommendations for Determining Eligibility for Competition in Athletes with Cardiovascular Abnormalities"[33] is a useful reference. This document provides activity recommendations for patients with known cardiovascular disease. There are sections on congenital heart disease, acquired valvular disease, cardiomyopathies, hypertension, coronary artery disease, and arrhythmias. Although the document is written to address sports participation by athletes, in the introduction it recognizes that some will utilize the recommendations for nonathletes whose jobs require strenuous exertion.

If analysis of work ability and job difficulty suggests that the individual is not capable of doing the job in question, one option would seem to be cardiac rehabilitation. Cardiac rehabilitation is supervised, medically safe exercise, generally performed with a peer group to help overcome anxiety. It has been shown to improve exercise capability and to decrease both total and heart disease mortality. Symptoms like angina develop at higher workloads. Although this may seem to suggest that cardiac rehabilitation should help return patients to appropriate levels of work, when studied, it does not.[34] The Agency for Health Care Policy and Research review concluded that cardiac rehabilitation is not recommended to facilitate return to work. Cardiac rehabilitation should logically improve the patient enough that work might then be possible, but psychosocial factors, not physical factors, are the more important determinants of return to work after infarction. This is why studies fail to find that cardiac rehabilitation improves the return to work rate. Thus tolerance, not capacity or current ability, is what determines return to work.

Medical assessment of cardiac impairments and return to work ability is hindered by several factors[26]:

1. Tolerance or subjective complaints are what limits performance.
2. Differences in motivation exist among persons with similar cardiac abnormalities.
3. There is frequent discrepancy between subjective complaints and objective findings.
4. Difficulties exist in transferring measurements made under controlled testing situations to the uncontrolled workplace.
5. The progressive nature of coronary disease renders invalid assessments made at an earlier point in time.

LOW BACK PAIN

Low back pain is extremely common. Approximately 80% of adults experience back pain at some time during life.[38] In less than 10% of these cases, physicians are able to state with certainty why the patient has back pain (what structure generates the pain or what disease is present). Over 90% of the time, physicians use a nonspecific label as a diagnosis. Examples are shown in Table 52–3.

TABLE 52–3

Non-Specific Labels Used by Physicians as Diagnoses in Patients with Low Back Pain

Diagnosis	ICD-9 Code
Back pain	724.5
Lumbago	724.2
Low back strain	847.2

ICD = International Classification of Diseases.

Low back pain with or without sciatica is a common reason for adult disability. To assess whether a patient with back pain can work, the physician must consider the same three terms: capacity, tolerance, and risk.

The first consideration is capacity. Few individuals function at maximal capacity. Current ability can be increased with exercise. Exercise may mean formal work conditioning or work hardening in a physical therapy program. Alternatively, exercise may mean returning to work in a modified duty status, with progressively decreasing work restrictions. As lighter work results over time in improved strength, flexibility, and endurance, the restrictions are progressively decreased.

Current ability may be approximated by functional capacity assessment testing, although these examinations are a better measure of tolerance than of capacity or even current ability. Unfortunately, their real world validity remains unproven.[20,26] Tolerance, or ability to work despite subjective symptoms, like pain, is what usually determines whether a patient with back pain will work at a particular job.

Risk assessment is difficult for patients with low back pain when return to work limitations are to be evaluated, as there is very little scientific literature on this subject. The patient with back pain who returns to work may claim that the pre-existing back pain increased upon return to work, but that is not a new injury. Almost all painful musculoskeletal conditions have pain that increases with activity and decreases with rest. This history is expected with back pain. If a patient says that pain in the region of the back does not increase with activity or decrease with rest, but rather the pain is constant and unaffected by activity, this is a red flag to the physician to evaluate the patient for abdominal or retroperitoneal pathology. If the patient is not willing to tolerate the pain (tolerance) for the rewards available, either the physician needs to provide better analgesia[5] or the patient will choose another job.

The patient with back pain who returns to work may claim a work task reinjured the back and made him or her worse. Again, at least 90% of the time physicians will not be able to objectively detect a new injury to account for the complaint of pain.

The complications that physicians fear are disk herniation and fracture. There is no literature on return to work with low back problems, the difficulty of the job involved, and the incidence of spinal fracture on the job. Work-related spinal fractures are almost always due to major trauma, like falls from a height. Patients with severe osteoporosis, who are thus at significantly increased risk of fracture, usually have their osteoporosis detected by imaging studies during the pre-return to work treatment phase. Their return to work status will be determined to a significant degree by the severity of the osteoporosis.

Similarly, there is no literature on return to work with low back pain problems, the difficulty of the job involved, and the risk of disk herniation. The largest prospective study of the risk of subsequent workers' compensation low back pain/injury claim was the Boeing Aircraft study by Bigos et al.[7] In that 4-year study of over 3000 workers (already working), current back pain or a history of prior back pain increased the risk of a future back claim by 1.7 times. This risk was the same for workers with current pain as it was for workers with a history of prior pain. The risk was the same for workers in light jobs as it was for workers in heavy jobs. Again, the relative risk was small (1.7).

As previously discussed if the general industry rate of low back workers' compensation claims is two claims per 100 employees per year, and if having prior or current pain increases the risk of a future claim by a factor of 1.7, few employees would be reinjured by returning to work. Two back claims will occur among 100 normal employees in a year. If a group of 100 employees is returning to work after a back pain episode/injury, then two multiplied by 1.7 means that 3.4 claims should occur in the next year, instead of the expected two. Thus, over 98 of every 100 employees returning to work after an absence due to back pain will return successfully. This would be an example of very low risk under the ADA.

The highest risk situation in return to work with back problems would be the patient who returns to work after lumbar discectomy (surgery). The surgeon leaves a hole in the disk annulus that has already proven to be aimed at the nerve root. If any additional material from the nucleus of the disk extrudes, it will leave the disk headed directly toward the nerve root, where it can cause recurrent sciatica. Historically, most spine surgeons have given patients who had surgical discectomy permanent activity restrictions, hoping to prevent reherniation. Historically, with these restrictions, the rate of reherniation has been 5% to 8%.[11] Based on the observation that many patients ignored their surgeon's advice (restrictions), and following discectomy returned to unlimited activity at home and at work, recent studies have given no restrictions to discectomy patients. These patients returned to full, unrestricted activity as soon as possible after surgery (generally in 8 weeks or less). The rate of reherniation in these studies is 5% to 6%, or identical to the rate during the historic practice of permanently restricting these patients.[9,10]

How, then, does a physician decide what restrictions to place on a patient returning to work after a back injury or back pain episode? One solution might be to determine the job demands from the employer's job description, usually by looking only at the lifting requirement. The patient's lifting ability, estimated from a functional capacity evaluation, can be consulted to see if the patient's lifting ability meets or exceeds the job demands (see also Chapters 53 to 56).

Unfortunately, there are problems with this method. First, many times the employer's written job descriptions are not accurate. Second, a recent review of spinal biomechanics concluded that there is much more literature to indicate that static postures, repetitive bending, twisting, and whole body vibration put the spine at risk for injury than there is to indicate that lifting is a risk.[25] Whether ergonomic factors put the individual at risk for back problems is controversial, with many reviews stating that this relationship is not proven.[14,24,36,37] Third, as mentioned earlier, the validity of functional capacity evaluation remains unproven. The study reported by Hall et al[16] is pertinent. In this study workers with on the job back injury were rehabilitated in a work conditioning program. When it was time for the physician to write return to work restrictions for the workers, the control group was sent back to work with restrictions based on their pain and functional capacity assessments. The study group patients were instead sent to full duty (no restrictions), ignoring the functional capacity assessments, which many times said they were not capable of doing the job in question. In the 4-month follow up, the study group, sent to full duty ignoring the functional capacity assessments, did considerably better than the control group in which the functional capacity assessments guided return to work restrictions.

Tolerance often determines whether an individual with back pain will work. An interesting and not uncommon anecdote is of the injured worker with back pain who cannot tolerate the pain and work at his usual job. While off work, he applies for, and is hired for, a much more physically strenuous job with a different employer. The same physician, who has been certifying that this individual could not work at the low paying easy job for company A because of back pain, is now asked by the patient to certify that he can now do the high paying but strenuous job for company B, with no observable change in the symptoms or examination. In accordance with the ADA, the physician must certify that this individual may work full duty for company B, as the increase in pain in a previously painful condition does not constitute objective evidence of substantial harm.

What science is there on which to base return to work restrictions? When the United States Government Agency for Health Care Policy and Research published its monograph on adult acute back problems, they had reviewed 10,317 articles, and found none that addressed this question adequately. They stated that eight articles provided some useful information, permitting their conclusion that work restrictions that progressively decreased over time were perhaps logical for up to 90 days, but there was no apparent benefit beyond 3 months.[8]

Since this 1994 document was published, there have been several studies to indicate that physicians should encourage return to normal activity, including work, as soon as possible after back injury or back pain episodes. Malmivaara et al[21] studied employees of a city government seen at the city's occupational health center for acute back injury. The group sent back to usual activity (including work) did better than the groups treated with either bed rest for 2 days or with extension exercises.

Indahl et al[19] looked at patients off work for 8 to 12 weeks for subacute back pain/injury. Compared to a control group that received usual care, the study group had an extensive consultation with a spine specialist who explained in detail why it was more likely than not that light activity would enhance, rather than hinder, the repair process. Over 6 months later there was a dramatic improvement in the return to work rate in the study group that received this reassurance. Indahl et al looked back at the original subjects 5 years later[18] and found that the study group still had a statistically significant increase in being at work. Hagen et al repeated Indahl et al's study with a different cohort of patients and came to the same conclusions.[15]

Moffett et al randomized patients with 1 to 6 months of back pain disability to either usual care or to physical therapist–led exercise classes with a cognitive-behavioral therapy component to discourage the patients from viewing themselves as invalids and to discourage letting pain be a guide for activity restriction. At 6 weeks, 6 months, and 12 months, the exercise/cognitive/behavioral group had significantly less distressing pain and disability (work loss), but no change in total pain.[23] Thus the program did not cure their pain, but the patients learned to view their pain as no longer distressing, and learned that they could function (work) despite their pain.

Thus consensus groups now recommend that patients with low back problems return to work as quickly as possible, despite ongoing symptoms. These include the British Royal College of General Practitioners,[28] The London Faculty of Occupational Medicine,[12] and the International Paris Task Force on Back Pain.[1]

The Canadian Medical Association has a policy statement: "Prolonged absence from one's normal roles, including absence from the workplace, is detrimental to a person's mental, physical, and social well being. Physicians should therefore encourage a patient's return to function and work as soon as possible..."[31] By this standard, a physician who does not wish to harm her or his patient must return the patient to work as soon as possible.

CONTESTED CASES

Sometimes the return to work decision is highly contested. The employer wants the employee/patient back at work, while the employee does not feel comfortably capable of doing the job in question. In these contested cases, the treating physician will generally agree with one or the other of these two alternatives, but, because the case is contested, each side gets a second opinion from an independent medical examiner (IME). The scenario then usually plays out like this:

The patient (Joe)'s attorney says, "Joe, go see Dr. A."
The employer's attorney says, "Joe, go see Dr. B."

Dr A. sees Joe and says, "I usually declare patients like Joe 'disabled.' They usually do not go back to work or get better, so I must be correct."

Dr B. sees Joe and says, "I usually declare patients like Joe fit to work. They usually go back to work and do fine, so I must be correct."

Both doctors make the decision based on anecdotal experience, rather than on science. The reasoning involved is Gestalt, or based on intuition. The decision is a response to a complete and unanalyzable whole. This leaves the ultimate decision maker (trial judge, employer, disability insurer) with a persisting dilemma.

One problem with this scenario is the source of each IME's anecdotal clinical experience. Many times the doctor's experience actually comes from lawyers. The IME only sees the examinee one time. The plaintiff's lawyer will tell Dr. A to follow up on the cases in which the doctor's prediction was correct, but not on the cases in which the doctor's predictions were incorrect. Similarly, the defense lawyer will tell Dr. B to follow up on the cases in which the doctor's prediction was correct, but not on the cases in which the doctor's predictions were incorrect. Each lawyer has a vested interest, whether conscious or unconscious, in telling the doctor about cases in which the doctor's prediction was correct and was also in the lawyer's financial interest (which is also in the lawyer's client's financial interest).

Thus these two, well-trained, competent, and honest physicians have diametrically opposed positions on the same question: "Can Joe do this job?" This process of decision making based on anecdotal experience explains why judges, lawyers, administrators, and claims managers, believing that doctors should answer this question scientifically, sometimes conclude that doctors' testimony is for sale. Unfortunately, physicians have not done a good job of educating these other professionals that their opinions are biased and anecdotal, and not based on science.

CONCLUSIONS

- Physicians need to think through return to work decisions using the terms capacity (or current ability), tolerance, and risk.
- Capacity is rarely achieved.
- Current ability can be measured with some degree of validity. It can be increased by exercise or by work.
- Risk assessment is rarely based on scientific studies.
- Most risk assessment is done based on the anecdotal, and thus biased, experience of the physician.
- Tolerance is what in the real world determines whether the individual will work at a particular job.
- Third parties inquire about the patient's capacity (or actually current ability) expecting scientific answers.
- Guessing a reasonable level of activity or tolerance for a patient is part of the art of medicine.
- Motivating (or cognitively restructuring) the patient to improve tolerance is part of the art of medicine.
- As Tom Landry, the late coach of the Dallas Cowboys football team, is reported to have said: "Motivation is the art of helping people achieve what they want to achieve by making them do what they don't want to do."

References

1. Abenhaim L, Rossignol M, Valat JP, et al: The role of activity in the therapeutic management of back pain: Report of the International Paris Task Force on Back Pain. Spine 25:1S–33S, 2000.
2. American Heart Association: Advanced Cardiac Life Support. Dallas, American Heart Association, 1997, p 9–3.
3. Cocchiarella L, Andersson GBJ (eds): Guides to the Evaluation of Permanent Impairment, 5th ed. Chicago, American Medical Association, 2001.
4. American Psychiatric Association: Diagnostic and Statistical Manual of Mental Disorders, 4th ed. Washington, DC, American Psychiatric Association, 1994.
5. Aronoff G: Opioids in chronic pain management: Is there a significant risk of addiction? Curr Rev Pain 4:112–121, 2000.
6. Barsky AJ, Borus JF: Somatization and medicalization in the era of managed care. JAMA 274:1931–1934, 1995.
7. Bigos SJ, Battie MC, Spengler DM: A prospective study of work perceptions and psychosocial factors affecting the report of back injury. Spine 16:1–6, 1991.
8. Bigos SJ, Bowyer OR, Braen GR, et al: Acute Low Back Problems in Adults. Clinical Practice Guideline Number 14, Agency for Health Care Policy and Research Publication 95–0642. Rockville, Md, Agency for Health Care Policy and Research, 1994.
9. Carragee EJ, Han MY, Yang B, et al: Activity restrictions after posterior discectomy: A prospective study of outcomes in 152 cases with no postoperative restrictions. Spine 24:2346–2351, 1999.
10. Carragee EJ, Helms E, O'Sullivan GS: Are postoperative activity restrictions necessary after posterior lumbar discectomy? A prospective study of outcomes in 50 consecutive cases. Spine 21:1893–1897, 1996.
11. Errico TJ, Fardon DF, Lowell TD: Contemporary concepts in spine care: Open discectomy as treatment for herniated nucleus pulposus of the lumbar spine. Spine 20:1829–1833, 1995.
12. The Faculty of Occupational Medicine of the Royal College of Physicians: Occupational health guidelines for the management of low back pain at work: Evidence review and recommendations. www.facoccmed.ac.uk/Publications%20list.htm. Accessed on June 21, 2002.
13. Guyatt G, Rennie D: User's Guide to the Medical Literature: Essentials of Evidence-Based Clinical Practice. Chicago, AMA Press, 2002, pp 133–135.
14. Hadler N: Occupational Musculoskeletal Disorders, 2nd ed. Philadelphia, Lippincott Williams & Wilkins, 1999, p 266.
15. Hagen EM, Eriksen HR, Ursin H: Does early intervention with a light mobilization program reduce long-term sick leave for low back pain? Spine 25:1973–1976, 2000.
16. Hall H, McIntosh G, Melles T, et al: Effect of discharge recommendations on outcome. Spine 19:247–258, 1994.
17. Hurst JW: The Heart, 9th ed. New York, McGraw Hill, 1998, p 1628.
18. Indahl A, Haldorsen EH, Holm S, et al: Five-year follow up study of a controlled clinical trial using light mobilization and informative approach to low back pain. Spine 23:2625–2630, 1998.
19. Indahl A, Velund L, Reikeraas O: Good prognosis for low back pain when left untampered. Spine 20:473–477, 1995.
20. King PM, Tuckwell N, Barrett TE, et al: A critical review of functional capacity evaluations. Phys Ther 78:852–866, 1998.
21. Malmivaara A, Hakkinen U, Aro T, et al: The treatment of acute low back pain—Bed rest, exercises, or ordinary activity? N Engl J Med 332:351–355, 1995.
22. Mario Echazabal v. Chevron. No. 98-55551. U.S. Court of Appeals (9th Cir., May 23, 2000).
23. Moffett JK, Torgerson D, Bell-Syer S, et al: Randomised controlled trial of exercise for low back pain: Clinical outcomes, costs, and preferences. Br Med J 319:279–283, 1999.
24. Nachemson AL, Jonsson E: Neck and Back Pain. Philadelphia, Lippincott Williams & Wilkins, 2000, p 118.
25. Pope MH, DeVocht JW: The clinical relevance of biomechanics. Neurol Clin 7:17–41, 1999.
26. Pransky G: Functional capacity evaluations and disability. The Guides Newsletter March/April:4–5, 1998.
27. Referral to occupational medicine clinics and resumption of work after myocardial infarction. J Occup Environ Med 41:943–947, 1999.
28. Royal College of General Practitioners: Clinical Guidelines for the Management of Acute Low Back Pain. London, Royal College of General Practitioners, 1996. Available at: www.rcgp.org.uk.
29. Scott M: Subjective illness and disability. The Guides Newsletter May/June:6, 1998.
30. Task Force II: Determination of occupational working capacity in patients with ischemic heart disease. J Am Coll Cardiol 14:1025–1034, 1989.

31. The physician's role in helping patients return to work after illness or injury. Can Med Assoc J 156:680A–F, 1997.
32. Thompson GS, Clive FJ, Hirst JA, et al: Clinical and angiographic characteristics of exertion-related acute myocardial infarction. JAMA 282:1731–1736, 1999.
33. Twenty-sixth Bethesda conference recommendations for determining eligibility for competition in athletes with cardiovascular abnormalities. J Am Coll Cardiol 24:845–899, 1994.
34. U.S. Agency for Policy and Research, Cardiac Rehabilitation Publication No. 96–0672, October 1995, p 76. Washington, DC.
35. U.S. Department of Health and Human Services, Social Security Administration: Disability Evaluation Under Social Security (SSA Publication No. 64–039, ICN No. 468600). Washington, DC, U.S. Department of Health and Human Services, Social Security Administration, 1994.
36. Videman T, Battie MC: Spine update: The influence of occupation on lumbar degeneration. Spine 24:1164–1168, 1999.
37. Waddell G: The Back Pain Revolution. Toronto, Churchill Livingstone, 1998, p 93.
38. Walker BF: The prevalence of low back pain: A systematic review of the literature from 1966 to 1998. J Spinal Disord 13:205–217, 2000.

SECTION

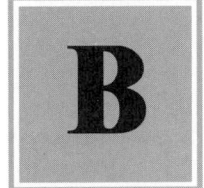

Musculoskeletal Disability

CHAPTER

53

Introduction to Fitness for Duty

RICHARD E. JOHNS, JR., MD, MSPH ■ ALAN L. COLLEDGE, MD ■ EDWARD B. HOLMES, MD, MPH

Medical capability statements are often required from providers by patients, employers, governmental agencies, and insurance carriers to determine if an employee is fit for duty. Those who make or suggest ability statements are legally obligated to carefully justify such fitness statements for the placement of employees, in the or exclusion of employees from, the workplace. The Americans With Disabilities Act (ADA) mandates that health care providers use objective medical criteria and rational thought when determining the capability and risk of an employee. This chapter describes the medical components providers should consider in making fitness for duty (FFD), or ability, statements. Also included is an objective methodology by which health care professionals and employers can mitigate discrimination liability when making FFD decisions within the context of the ADA. Although determining FFD is a process that continues to evolve, the methods listed here have been developed in various medical and administrative settings and are applicable situations where employability decisions must be made to prevent discrimination under the ADA.

Irrespective of medical specialty, physicians and other allied health care personnel are frequently asked to determine a person's physical, mental, and social abilities, for either temporary or permanent conditions. Such requests typically originate from governmental agencies (Social Security, State Welfare, Employment Security, Labor Commissions, Vocational Rehabilitation, Driver's License Divisions), employers, insurance payers (workers' compensation, short and long term disability), Family Medical Leave Act (FMLA) qualifications, and/or loan deferment plans. These capability statements are usually requested during the recovery period and at maximum medical improvement (MMI) as shown in Figure 53–1. MMI is defined as a point when a person's medical condition is well stabilized and unlikely to change substantially in the next year with or without medical treatment.[2] Once MMI has been reached, permanent physical ability and risk assessment

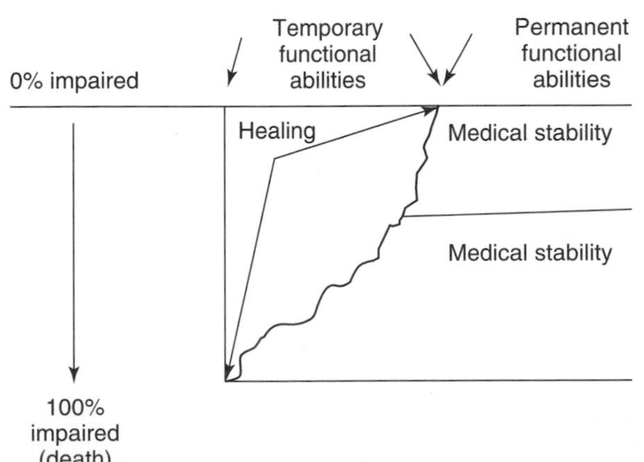

Figure 53–1. Healing and recovery spectrum.

statements become the first step toward the final administrative disposition as to whether a person is determined fit or unfit for duty. Assisting impaired people back to work requires the combined efforts and effective interaction among medical providers, the employee/patient, and administrative actions by an employer to carefully evaluate the person's ability and then, if necessary, to consider efforts to provide reasonable accommodations.[3]

Provided with capabilities information from physicians and the essential job functions for which an employee was hired, an employer can make defensible employability decisions, under the provisions of the ADA, as to whether an individual is a "qualified employee." A mismatch can cause employee–employer stress, which can unfavorably affect productivity and potentially lead to unnecessary job-related injuries or illness claims. Epidemiologic studies reveal significant relationships among anxiety, injury claims, and the associated claims costs, both direct and indirect.[4,12,20,30,32,64,65,92,116,123,126] Today, the average cost of a workers' compensation claim is $13,182,[76] while a lost-time claim can be more than $20,000.[22] Also problematic to workers' compensation programs is the fact that the claim itself can inherently prolong recovery,[34,45,94] increase disability cost,[36,49,57,70] and decrease the potential to return to work.[28,35] This employee-job fit can be simply portrayed as making certain the functional abilities of the individual are at least equal to or greater than the job requirements (essential functions of the job), as illustrated in Figure 53–2.

When the essential functions or job requirements are less than the capabilities of the employee, job-related stresses are minimized. However, when the essential job functions exceed the capabilities of the employee, job-related stresses increase along with the potential for injury claims. An acceptable match between the job functions and worker abilities may be facilitated by "reasonable accommodation,"[3] by increasing the capabilities of the patient/employee through physical conditioning, by employee and/or coworker training, or by decreasing the physical requirements of the essential functions through task analysis and/or engineering redesign.

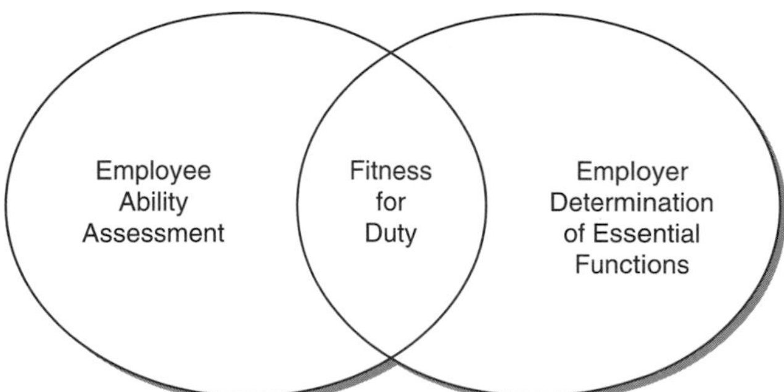

Figure 53–2. Matching worker abilities to essential job functions.

Ability or inability statements or opinions carry heavy legal and ethical responsibilities, as FFD decisions are often directly related to the patient's/employee's earning capacity and/or disability benefits. The status of current employment law dictates that any attempt to limit a patient's/employee's employability involves the need for a legal and ethical approach that protects the medical provider, the worker, the employer, and the general public as well.[3] Unfortunately, the medical literature contains very little research or epidemiologic models that can predict what type of patient/employee or condition would lead to disability. Each FFD disposition is the product of complex medical, psychosocial, and administrative factors. Currently, most FFD statements are intuitive opinions offered by medical providers.[10,74,102,130] Generally, medical providers rendering ability statements cannot be sued for their opinions concerning an patient's/employee's ability to work unless their statement is proven false or made with recklessness. However, medical providers can be sued for negligent assignment or interference with the worker's contractual relationship.[86] For these reasons, all individuals involved in interpreting or managing physical ability decisions must realize that medical providers determine ability, not disability. It is not the medical practitioner's responsibility to determine the essential functions of the job, devise accommodations for the patient/employee, or determine the reasonableness of any accommodation proposed by the employer. Employability, accommodation, and disability decisions are, by definition, administrative in nature.

Medical providers who make injured worker ability statements should be aware that returning individuals to gainful employment is one of the most potent therapeutic and rehabilitative modalities available to them. Work promotes independence and is essential to a person's self-respect and quality of life.[82] Resumption of work has also been shown to be a significant part of the treatment for an injury or illness, even benefiting patients suffering from chronic pain.[21,23,69,72] Conversely, prolonged time away from work makes recovery and eventual return to work progressively less likely.[26,103] American industry has come to appreciate W. Edwards Demming's philosophy that the "individual worker is the company's most important asset and respect for individuals is paramount for business success."[122] Studies have shown that workers who return to work for their original employers are usually better off financially than workers who choose other options, such as alternative vocational rehabilitation plans that include retraining or new job placement.[33,106] For these reasons it is recommended that employers sponsor modified or transitional work programs before full duty activities can be resumed. Since the advent of the ADA, and consistent with the

Act's purpose, there has been a significant reduction in lost workday cases and a greater willingness to accommodate workers. From 1990 to 1998, the number of workers losing time has been reduced from 4.1/100 workers to 3.1/100 workers, while for the same period of time, there has been an increase in workers involved in restricted workday activities from 0.7/100 workers to 1.2/100 workers.[112]

HISTORY OF FFD EVALUATIONS

Historically, investigators in various occupational settings have pioneered creative systems to assist practitioners and employers in performing FFD evaluations. In 1974, Koyl[55] devised a method for charting the worker's physical and environmental requirements for performing a specific task. The old idea of matching the worker to the job was objectified using a seven-category scale (GULHEMP) to organize and rate the data coming from a medical history and physical examination. The same scale is used to rate and profile the requirements of a specific job. The outcome produces objective criteria for matching the two. Approximately 10 years later, Nylander and Carmean, working for the County of San Bernadino, published the Medical Standards Project.[79] This work promoted a method by which an organization could implement a complete and comprehensive job-related medical screening program based on assessing the physical demands of jobs and a physical abilities analysis. Further improvements in this system are now proprietary and must be obtained through consulting agreements with the original authors. The U.S. Department of Labor (DOL) and Social Security Administration[117] have, for many years, classified jobs in terms of exertional level, skill level, and other categories. All jobs in the U.S. economy have been classified into the following five levels of exertion: sedentary, light, medium, heavy, and very heavy work. The DOL model is widely accepted and used in making legal determinations of disability and fitness for duty. A representative form used by the DOL system is shown in Table 53–1. Although not a specific FFD model, Himmelstein and Pransky[42] coedited a significant work on the medical, legal, and ethical aspects of patient/worker fitness and risk assessment evaluations.

Building on the excellent work of our predecessors and the authors' previous publications on this subject,[17,18,51,52] we suggest that the following legal background form the framework for the medical and administrative components of any FFD determination in order to maintain compliance with the ADA.

LEGAL BACKGROUND RELATED TO FFD DETERMINATIONS

FFD Under ADA

Assessment of pre- or post-hire medical abilities may be illegal if not performed within the guidelines established under the ADA and the implementing regulations of the Equal Employment Opportunity Commission (EEOC).[3,113] The ADA is a civil rights law that prohibits discrimination in public and private employment, governmental services, public accommodations, public transportation, and telecommunications. ADA prohibitions apply to employers with 15 or more employees and to state and local governments and public services of any size. The ADA specifically protects all individuals with "a physical or mental impairment that substantially limits one or more of the major life activities of such individuals, or has a record of such impairment or is being regarded as having such an impairment." This law protects injured employees, those who acquire various diseases, and those who have lifetime disabilities and may have never worked. The ADA is also designed to assist employers in managing the

TABLE 53–1

United States Department of Labor—Physical Demand Characteristics of Work Chart

Physical Demand Level	Occasional (0 to 33% of Workday)	Frequent (34 to 66% of Workday)	Constant (67 to 100% of Workday)	Typical Energy Required
Sedentary	10 lbs	Negligible	Negligible	1.5–2.1 METS
Light	20 lbs	10 lbs and/or walk/ stand/push/pull of arm/leg controls	Negligible and/or push/pull of arm/leg controls while seated	2.2–3.5 METS
Medium	20 to 50 lbs	10 to 25 lbs	10 lbs	3.6–6.3 METS
Heavy	50 to 100 lbs	25 to 50 lbs	10 to 20 lbs	6.4–7.5 METS
Very heavy	Over 100 lbs	Over 50 lbs	Over 20 lbs	Over 7.5 METS

effects of patients' disabilities and places very specific requirements on employees, employers, and their medical advisors to determine the conditions under which patients can work.[3]

The ADA closely regulates medical inquiries for pre- and post-employment issues. At the pre-offer stage, however, there can be no inquiry as to any underlying disability, whether visible or hidden. Physical examinations cannot be designed to screen out the disabled unless the disability tested for results in exclusion of individuals because of business necessity and job-related reasons. There can be no questions as to how the applicant became disabled, although questions about previous worker's compensation claims can be presented. Where a post-offer medical examination discloses a medical condition that may be protected as a disability under the ADA, the results of the examination cannot be a reason for rejection unless the rejection is job-related and justified by business necessity. At this stage, however, the examining physician may probe without limit to determine and define the history and severity of any medical condition and the extent of the conditional employee's ability to perform the essential functions of the job offered. Under the ADA, it is no longer sufficient for a medical provider simply to determine if a person is disabled. Capability must first be ascertained before other employee motivation or administrative issues such as "reasonable accommodation," "undue hardship," or "direct threat"[3] can be addressed. At any stage of employment, an employer may also inquire as to an applicant's ability to perform the essential functions of the job offered or held. Failure to comply with the ADA may result in costly litigation. Medical providers can unwittingly provide a trigger for ADA coverage by recommending work restrictions simply focused on what he or she believes an patient/employee is unable to do and not relating these restrictions to the specific essential functions of the job in question.[9]

ADA: Direct Threat

In order for an employer to determine that an employee is unfit for his or her current job, or that a job offer should be withdrawn based on a medical provider's recommendations, it must be shown that the patient/employee poses a "high probability" of causing substantial harm to him- or herself or others. It must also be shown that the risk of substantial harm cannot be eliminated or reduced below the direct threat level by reasonable accommodation.[1] Probability is a term that refers to the likelihood or chance that an injury or illness was caused or aggravated by a particular factor. Possibility is used to imply a likelihood of 50% or less; probability is used to imply the likelihood of occurrence at a level of 51% or greater.[2] This is a very stringent standard that most employers and medical providers will rarely be able to meet when attempting to screen for potential future injury, in that medical science can rarely produce data that demonstrate a high probability of an adverse occurrence or outcome. Moreover, such "at risk claims" cannot be speculative or based on potential or future risk. Only the current abilities of the patient to perform essential job functions safely can be assessed (see also Chapter 52).

ADA: Undue Hardship

Given appropriate medical abilities information, an employer's administrative responsibility is to determine whether reasonable accommodations can be made. If the employer feels that accommodations represent an undue hardship or that the employee is considered a threat to him- or herself or others, an employability decision by management of the patient/employee being unfit for duty will have to be made. Such actions require significant documentation and appropriate legal review if a termination decision is eventually reached. An employability decision may depend on a number of variables, including the size of the employer's organization, available resources, and nature of the operation.[3,113] Whether a particular accommodation will impose an undue hardship must be determined on a case-by-case basis.[3,113] An accommodation that poses an undue hardship for one employer at one particular time may not pose an undue hardship for another employer or for the same employer at another time. Factors to be considered in determining whether an accommodation would create an undue hardship on a particular business are reviewed in greater detail in the ADA Technical Assistance Manual.[113]

Confidentiality of Information

Medical providers and employers alike must remember that all medically related information must be kept confidential at the worksite and limited only to what is necessary for an appropriate job assignment or for making a reasonable job accommodation. In certain instances, an employer may have a need to know the medical diagnosis. However, specific information about the nature of the medical condition must be kept confidential in the employee's personal medical record. The employer is only entitled to know what functional ability limitations exist. By using the methodology described in this chapter, the nature of a worker's problem is not revealed and the ADA requirements for confidentiality are met. This also permits the employer to act in a prudent and reasonable fashion when making

FFD and employability decisions. Exceptions to preserving confidentiality include the following: 1) supervisors and management must be informed about necessary work restrictions; 2) first aid and safety personnel should be informed if the disability may require emergency treatment or if any specific procedures are needed in the case of fire or other evacuations; 3) government officials can investigate compliance with ADA; 4) relevant information must be provided to state workers' compensation offices or second injury funds; and 5) relevant information must be provided to insurance companies for cases in which the company requires a medical examination in order for health or life insurance to be provided.

EMPLOYEE ABILITY ASSESSMENT

Variability of Employee Ability Statements

The variability that can be found with different ability statements on the same patient/employee is attributed to several nonmedical factors, such as the methodology utilized, the examiners and examiner training, and varying medical reports. A certain skill level and experience are necessary to accurately and consistently determine capability. These skills are seldom taught as part of the curriculum training for physicians. As a result, most examiners are left to interpret, at times erroneously, existing guidelines as they see fit. There currently is a need to improve the accuracy of capability assessments and reduce variability. It is believed that improving and standardizing the criteria physicians are required to use and interpret could lessen variability for an ability or fitness assessment.

Who Is Qualified to Make Employee Ability Statements?

Contributing to this variability is the controversy as to who is qualified to provide fitness statements. Within the medical profession, physicians of various specialties argue that their field of medicine best qualifies them for this process. Added to this are capability statements given by other health care providers, including chiropractors, physical therapists, exercise physiologists, athletic trainers, and physician extenders. Such individuals bring to the process widely varying backgrounds and underlying clinical philosophies. We believe that the attending physician is the person most knowledgeable regarding the patient's/employee's condition, progress, and final status, and is therefore encouraged to render the capability statement. If, for any reason, the attending physician prefers not to make this evaluation, the requesting party should be notified on a timely basis. The treating physician may then refer the patient/employee to another physician, or ask the requesting party to refer the patient/employee to a physician experienced in determining capability and risk. This should eliminate medical providers who are only marginally interested, allowing the patient/employee to be seen by more qualified examiners for the evaluation.

Medical Components of Employee Ability Assessments

Physicians, in arriving at a final determination of medical capability, should consider a number of medical components. These can include the diagnosis, history, literature-based medical outcome studies, current consensus guidelines, impairment ratings, functional capacity evaluations (FCEs), and effort determination.

A clear, accurate, and complete report is essential to support FFD statements. The medical capability report is a comprehensive report prepared either during recovery or when the patient has reached MMI. MMI is defined as a point in the patient's medical condition when it is well-stabilized and unlikely to change substantially in the next year with or without medical treatment.[2]

With report writing, various assumptions are generally required based on reasonable medical probability, rather than opinions based on surmise, speculation, or conjecture.[2,107] To arrive at the most valid conclusion, the physician must have available all applicable information that can be obtained. Assessing conclusions on incomplete data should be avoided, unless complete data are unobtainable. If one believes additional data may alter the conclusions, this should be stated. As this is both an administrative as well as a legally discoverable document, the report of the physician should include the following information:

1. A history of the medical condition with the onset and course of the condition, symptoms, findings on previous examinations, treatment, and responses to treatment, including adverse effects. Information should be included that may be relevant to onset, such as an occupational exposure or injury. Historical information should refer to any relevant investigations. A detailed list of prior evaluations should be included in the clinical data section.
2. A work history with a detailed, chronological description of work activities; specific type and duration of work performed; materials used in the workplace; any temporal associations with the medical condition and work frequency, intensity, duration of exposure, and activity; and any protective measures should be noted. Additional questions regarding absenteeism, job satisfaction, etc., should be explored.

3. An assessment of current clinical status, including chief complaints, history of present illness, psychosocial history, review of symptoms, physical examination, and a list of contemplated treatments, rehabilitation strategies, and anticipated dates for re-evaluation should be presented.
4. A list of diagnostic study results and outstanding pertinent diagnostic studies should be provided. These may include laboratory tests, electrocardiograms, exercise stress studies, radiographic and other imagining studies, rehabilitation evaluations, mental status examinations, and other tests or diagnostic procedures.[2]
5. A discussion of the medical basis for determining whether the person is at MMI should be included. If MMI has not been reached, the physician should estimate and discuss the expected date of full or partial recovery.
6. The examiner should clearly state the diagnosis as substantiated from the medical record. If this is a compensation claim, the examiner should also define, as clearly as possible, the causal relationship of the diagnosis (within reasonable medical probability) to a specific illness or injury. It is recognized that, in many cases, specific pathologic diagnoses are not clearly evident. The examiner has the responsibility to provide a diagnostic impression that is correlated to the clinical findings.
7. If applicable, using valid, standardized criteria, the examiner, if requested, may calculate an impairment rating, based on objective clinical findings, testing, and information found in the medical records. The fifth edition of the American Medical Association Guides to the Evaluation of Permanent Impairment includes most of the commonly encountered conditions. Because this edition encompasses the most current criteria and procedures for impairment assessment, it is recommended that physicians use the fifth edition of the Guides and/or local and state guidelines when rating permanent impairment.[2]
8. Finally, th e physician should make a definitive statement regarding the current fitness capacity or ability of the patient/employee using one or more of the suggested methods described in the following.

Medical History: Severity Indexing

The medical history is one of the most important factors a medical provider or employer can rely on to identify a worker's future risk. Recurrent episodes of low back pain (LBP) appear frequently to be a precursor of future LBP. Rowe[93] found that 83% of those with LBP had recurrent attacks. Patients with sciatica had a recurrence rate of 75%.[71] Other investigators have reported similar recurrence rates.[83,110] In determining the significance of the history, a number of factors must be considered. These include ongoing treatment, the number of visits received for an injury to the same region, objective testing to the same region, work restrictions because of problems in the same area, the duration since the last episode, the number of episodes in the same region, and time lost from work because of symptoms in the same region.

These factors have been severity indexed in Table 53–2 (Prior History Severity Indexing and Recommendations), which allows evaluators a consistent and logical approach to improve uniformity and reliability in determining risk from prior occurrences. Further outcome studies will need to be performed to validate this process.

Literature-based Medical Outcome Studies

With the current exponential knowledge explosion and easy access to the Internet, all individuals making FFD statements have unprecedented access to current outcome studies by which to make sound, objective medical statements. One of the best locations to begin an Internet search is at the National Library of Medicine's Web site, PubMed.[115]

Clinical Practice Guidelines

Clinical practice guidelines are systematically developed statements to assist practitioner and patient decisions about appropriate health care for specific clinical circumstances.[47] Using the Internet, physicians making FFD statements have access to the most updated and comprehensive evidence-based clinical guidelines that can be found by searching the Web site of the National Guideline Clearinghouse (NGC).[75] Updated weekly with new and changed guidelines by the Agency for Healthcare Research and Quality (AHRQ) (formerly the Agency for Health Care Policy and Research [AHCPR]), in partnership with the American Medical Association (AMA) and the American Association of Health Plans (AAHP), the NGC mission is to provide physicians, nurses, health care providers, health plans, integrated delivery systems, purchasers, and others an accessible mechanism for obtaining objective, detailed information on clinical practice guidelines.

Impairment Ratings

Impairment is defined by the AMA in its Guides to the Evaluation of Permanent Impairment as a loss, loss of use, or derangement of any body part, organ system, or organ function.[2] Since 1950, all 50 states have some form of workers' compensation law, which awards compensation for residual permanent physical impairment from a

TABLE 53-2

Prior History Severity Indexing and Recommendations

Severity Indexing for Determining Future Risk

Severity Index the History for Treatment/Testing to the Same Anatomic Region by the Following Schedule:

Score	0	1 point	2 points
A: Time lost from work in the last 12 months because of symptoms in the same region	0	1–3 days	>3 days
B: Number of prior episodes in the same region	0	1–3	>3
C: Duration since last episode	0	1–3 years	<1 year
D: Prior work restrictions because of problems in the same region	None	Temporary	Permanent
E: Prior objective testing to the same region (EMG-NCV, x-ray, MRI-CT, bone scan)	>3 years	If taken prior to 2 years	If taken within the last 2 years
F: Prior to latest claim, what ongoing medical, physical therapy, chiropractor, etc, visits were received for an injury to the same region	0–2 times in last 3 years	3–6 times in last 3 years	>6 in last 3 years

Total Points	Risk	Recommendations
0–3	Minimal risk for future recurrence	
3–6	Moderate risk for future recurrence	Administrative or ergonomic/engineering considerations to reduce future risk of recurrence
>7	High risk for future recurrence	Individual being evaluated should not return to work at prior work level or forces

EMG-NCV = electromyography–nerve conduction velocity; MRI-CT = magnetic resonance imaging–computed tomography.

Note: A significant predictor of future problems in any given area is the patient's past medical history. For this reason above model procedes reasonable and logical approach from an evaluator to improve uniformity and reliability in determing risk from prior occurrences.

work-related injury (i.e., scars, disfigurement, amputation, etc.) according to a defined compensation schedule.[111] This schedule ranges from 0% to 100%, with 0% whole person impairment rating being assigned to a person with no significant organ or body system functional consequences and no limitations on the performance of the common activities of daily living. A 90% to 100% impairment indicates a very severe organ or body system loss requiring the person to be fully dependent on others for self-care, or even approaching death.[2]

Although the AMA or various state impairment rating systems have supposedly been derived from a well structured set of thorough observations, most do not convey specific information about the person or impact of the impairment on the person's capacity to meet personal, social, or occupational demands or statuary or regulatory requirements because of an impairment, referred to as disability.[2] Thus, disability is more accurately defined according to the following equation:

Impairment + Impact on life = Disability

(see also Chapter 1 for definitions)

As with the other benefits, there are significant differences between states on the methodology utilized to calculate permanent partial disability benefits.[14] Currently, the AMA Guides is the most widely used instrument worldwide to estimate adult permanent impairment. A survey completed in 1999 indicates that in the United States, 40 of 51 jurisdictions (50 states and the District of Columbia) require some utilization of the different editions of the AMA Guides.[131] Originally published as a series of articles in JAMA, the Guides has been revised periodically since its initial publication as a single volume in 1971.[2] The Guides is a tool to convert medical information about permanent impairments into numerical values. Each chapter focuses on a single organ system and description of the diagnostic and evaluative methods for assessing specified impairments. Each impairment is assigned a rating, expressed as a percentage of whole person loss of function for that system.

Studies suggest a relationship to an individual's assigned impairment and future performance. The state of Texas found that 83% of injured workers receiving impairment ratings in the range of 1% to 14% reported experiencing future personal hardships,[27] and that those who received impairment ratings had a less favorable chance of returning to work. This probability of not returning to work was dependent on the amount of the rating awarded. For workers who received an 8% rating, 11% never returned to work, whereas 22% of workers with a 14% rating did not return to work.[91] A study of the California's workers' compensation system found that workers who suffer workplace injuries resulting in a permanent impairment experienced large and sustained wage losses.[84] Although studies are limited, some suggest that for measuring spinal range of motion (ROM), which can be strongly influenced by pain and technique, impairment and disability ratings among examiners can be inconsistent and unreliable.[16,19,63,68,77,87,95,105] To try and improve standardization of ROM measurements, the AMA published a manual on proper techniques for measurement of ROM with the intent of having greater reproducibility among examiners.[132]

Although an evolving idea, if impairment has been awarded in the past or can be calculated at present, it should be considered as part of current and future capability determinations. As listed in the report writing section, the consistent listing of a rating on a FFD statement will help provide additional information for administrators and further improve both impairment and capability methodology through future research.

Functional Capacity Evaluations

The FCE is another component that physicians may consider reviewing or ordering when determining capability (see also Chapters 51, 53, 55, and 56). The FCE is an extensive set of physical tests, either job-specific or generic, that purports to assess a patient's/employee's ability to perform present as well as future work.[104] A review of the medical literature reveals concern about the absence of formal standards, specific guidelines, and validity for these assessments. The way in which FCEs are currently conducted varies in the number of measurements obtained, degree of standardization, clarity of the concepts, and underlying theories. They also vary in choice of measuring instruments, adequacy of measurement for certain injury groups, use and availability of normative data, and ability to predict return to work or recurrence of injury. Issues of inter-rater reliability, intra-rater reliability, report writing, qualifications of examiners, examiner training, projection of findings to an 8-hour day, and safety need to be addressed. Few assessments, however, have demonstrated levels of reliability sufficient for clinical (or legal) purposes.[46] For over a decade, numerous authors have identified insufficient evidence of reliability, validity, and predictive value of most work-related assessments as a major problem that requires further research and development.[56,59,109,125] These studies leave open the question of whether "FCEs are acceptable."[54] At present, the FCE is not a stand-alone test, but part of a wide variety of subjective tests that can be utilized with other criteria listed in this section in determining a fitness profile.

Motivation Determination—APGAR Performance Model

The amount of motivation a patient/employee extends to improve his or her condition is an essential component in determining performance level in FFD evaluations. Motivation and effort can conceivably be plotted along a continuum with the physiologic bone ligament complex responses to loading conditions[127,128] and with psychosocial factors determining how close one performs to his or her physiologic limits (Fig. 53–3). Elite athletes perform much closer to their physiologic limits than most persons (see also Chapter 52).

Motivation can be influenced by multiple factors, including the illness or injury, the patient's personality, coping style, self-esteem, associates, environment, and self-confidence.[2] Owing to the intrinsic intertwined nature of the mental, social, and physical demands of work, the assessment of effort and motivation is a difficult task. This is particularly true for patients/employees who are receiving compensation to get well or perceive themselves entitled to compensation.[38,44] For such individuals, research has demonstrated a more prolonged recovery,[34,45,94] increased disability,[36,49,57,70] and decreased potential to return to work.[28,35,70]

Considerable energy and resources are spent in determining a person's motivation. Those whose efforts are not sincere during rehabilitation or testing may overuse treatment, have a prolonged recovery, have increased cost of care, or receive unwarranted disability payments.[8,53] On the other hand, evaluators who draw unwarranted conclusions about an examinee's motiva-

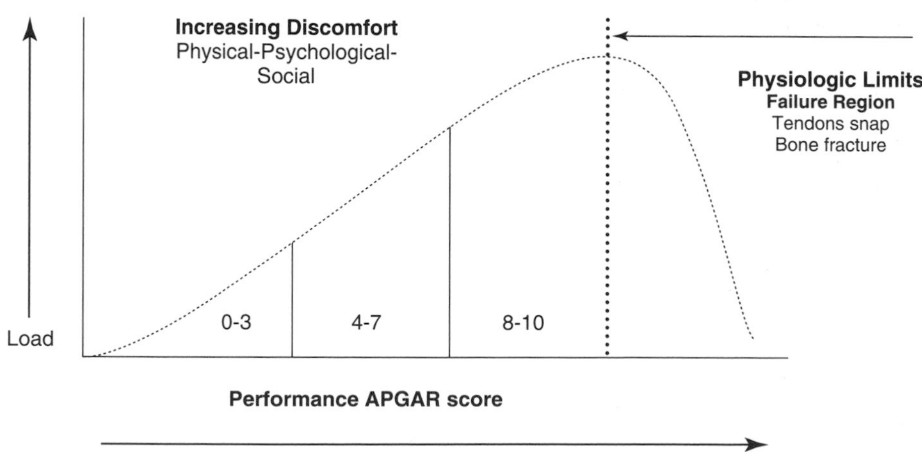

Figure 53–3. Effort determined by physiological, psychological, and social limits.

tion, may be "violating the rights of the person being tested," with the potential for the report to be emotionally and financially devastating.[58] This is particularly true when an undiagnosed medical condition is later discovered that was significantly limiting performance. It is recommended that the examiner qualify capability statements with an opinion as to whether the performance might be due to the physical impairment or to secondary gain.

Currently, a number of procedures are promoted for a clinician to objectify motivation, including Waddell's nonorganic signs,[121] dynometric grip strength variation,[85] bell-shaped force curves,[101] and rapid exchange grip.[60] Other evaluations include the correlation between musculoskeletal evaluation and FCE,[48] documentation of pain behaviors,[99] documentation of symptom magnification,[66] and the ratio of heart rate to pain intensity.[13]

An attempt to develop a comprehensive performance model that considered the above components was recently published as the BICEPS model.[17] After further review and consultation, the BICEPS model provided a rational basis for a proposed "Performance APGAR Model" in a FFD setting. Like the infant APGAR, developed by Virginia Apgar in 1952, which is given at birth, the Performance APGAR is a composite summary of methods used to determine patient motivation level and is rated on a scale of 1 to 10. A score of 8 to 10 is consistent with what is optimally expected from a motivated person, a score of 4 to 7 indicates concern about issues affecting performance, and a score of 0 to 3 suggests poor motivation to improve functional abilities. Although best suited for objective musculoskeletal disorders, the APGAR scores can be used for many different types of impairments. Performance APGAR scores can be given at each visit or over a series of visits and provide an indication of the motivation a patient is currently expending to improve his or her condition.

A worksheet for the comprehensive APGAR performance score is shown in Table 53–3, along with descriptors for each variable. Each of the five categories of the APGAR can be given a value of up to 2, making the maximum composite score of 10 consistent with acceptable motivation and effort. The following describes the five components of the APGAR: acceptance, performance, grimacing, appearance, and resolution.

Acceptance

Accepting of Condition

Most patients, as they reach MMI, have an understanding of their condition and what they need to do to control their symptoms. Unfortunately, many patients who have pain persisting after the tissue has healed will be left with some residual discomfort. To some patients, this is seen as an acceptable part of living[5,11,118]; others see this discomfort as unacceptable. How the patient responds to the question "If this just doesn't get any better, what will you do?" helps identify where the patient is, either consciously or subconsciously, on the Kubler-Ross continuum of acceptance.[78,81] Research has shown that acceptance is a very legitimate goal for intervention in patients with chronic pain. Patients who have learned to live with their pain are more accepting of their condition, have reduced levels of unrealistic thinking, have less pain-related distress, have higher activity levels, have higher levels of internal orientation, and require fewer medications.[62,90] Those patients who are unaccepting of their condition often express anger, denial, or statements reflective of bargaining, and feel anxiety or depression. Unfortunately, these patients often resort to more medical opinions, treatments, alternative health care therapies, or aggressive surgeries, with marginal chance for improvement.[6,81] The evaluator rates the examinee's response to the previous question and he or she is given one point if he or she is accepting of his or her current condition.

Compliance

In order to improve the quality of life with most conditions that are chronic, the patient must be compliant with recommended medical treatment. This includes medications, exercises, medical appointments, weight reduction, smoking cessation, etc. The examinee's effort to comply is rated by the evaluator with one point given if the evaluator feels he or she is making good efforts to comply.

Performance

Consistency With Distractions

Most medical practitioners are aware of various methods by which to observe a patient while he or she is distracted. One might observe a patient walking into and out of the office, the parking lot, or the examination room during questioning. If the patient's behavior is consistent, even when distracted, he or she is awarded one point.

Performance of Actual Testing Maneuvers

This would include a measurement of grip strength,[67] or perceived exertion as measured by the Borg RPE Pain Scale, comparing the perceived psychophysical with actual.[13] For grip strength, the reviewer is to note the repeated maximal grip strength testing. If the grip strength varies greatly between attempts, this inconsistency is noted. More detailed grip consistency testing

TABLE 53-3

Performance APGAR Measurement of the Sincerity of Effort an Individual Puts Forth

			Scoring Options			Score up to 2 points
			0	1	2	
A	Acceptance (choose best test or average)	If this just does not get any better, what will you do?	I can't live like this	I am going to have some problems	I will live with it	A
		Are you satisfied with your job?	Not satisfied	Partially satisfied	Satisfied	= ____
P	Pain (choose best test or average)	Pain drawing	Non-Physiologic	Some of it physiologic	Physiologic	
		Pain behaviors score AMA Guides Table 18–5	Exaggerated or non physiologic	Mixed or ambiguous	Appropriate and confirm clinical findings	P = ____
G	Gut (intuition) (choose best test or average)	Credibility tool (see AMA Guides Table 18–2)	Not credible	Partially credible	Credible	G
		Intuition of effort	Poor effort	Partial effort	Excellent effort	= ____
		Duration	Much longer than expected	Longer than expected	As expected	
A	Acting (choose best test or average)	Consistency with distractions	Poor consistency	Partial consistency	Excellent consistency	
		Waddell signs	More than 2 Waddell signs	2 Waddell signs	0 to 1 Waddell sign	A = ____
		Grip strength testing	Unreliable grip strength (high variance, etc.)	Partial validity	Reliable grip strength	
R	Reimbursement	Comprehension/Litigation	Someone else liable WC, PI, Disability Application Attorney Representing	Someone else liable WC, PI, Disability Application	No one liable	R = ____

Total *Performance APGAR Score* = ____
(Add A, P, G, A, R sections for a maximum of 10)

Under each letter (APGAR) choose the most applicable test for the particular patient or more than one test can be done and the scores averaged for that section. A total score of 8–10 is consistent with what is optimally expected from a motivated patient, a score of 4–7 indicates concern about motivation, and a score of 0–3 suggests poor motivation to improve their functional abilities.

can involve calculation of the coefficient of variation,[85] the bell-shaped curve,[101] or the rapid exchange grip.[60] If the examinee's performance is consistent, he or she is given one point.

Grimacing

Pain Behaviors[99]

Pain behaviors may be viewed as indicating symptom magnification,[66] especially when they grossly exceed what might be expected from experience with a similar diagnosis. Pain behaviors include the following: sitting with a rigid posture, moaning, moving in a guarded or protective fashion, frequent shifting of posture or position, facial grimacing, using a cane, cervical collar,, or other device, limping or distorted gait, extremely slow movements, or stooping while walking. The experienced evaluator will make a judgment regarding the pain behaviors and award one point if the behaviors are considered reliable and consistent with the known diagnosis.

Waddell's Nonorganic Signs[31,73,121]

Waddell's nonorganic signs were described and standardized in 1980 and are the physical examination findings most widely used in studies in which patients with low back pain are evaluated, for both acute and chronic pain.[24,29,37,39,43,107,119–121,124] These eight behavioral signs are believed to be overt inappropriate physical examination manifestations that signify the patient is coping poorly with the pain and is showing psychological distress out of proportion to the organic back disorder. Their presence can interfere with medical interventions and cause delayed recovery and failure to return to work. Waddell's tests should be performed and scored. The presence of zero or one Waddell's signs translates to one point on the APGAR. More than one Waddell's sign is given an APGAR score of zero for this section.

Appearance

Intuition

Experts working with different conditions have extensive experience with a wide spectrum of patients, from the motivated elite athlete to the elderly patient, thereby developing an intuitive sensitivity of a patient's motivation to improve. This intuition has been objectively described as a sensitive indicator of effort.[40,41,50] The evaluator uses judgment, experience, and intuition in giving one point if it is felt the examinee's activity was consistent and genuine.

Pain Drawing Score[88]

The examinee should have been given a pain drawing on which to describe his or her symptoms. Symptom patterns of the drawing are to be compared to known anatomic distributions. The person who provides drawings that are physiologically and anatomically consistent is given one point.

Resolution

Duration

By comparison with national published guidelines[75,89,129] and the medical literature,[115] if the time required for healing appears acceptable, then one point is awarded (see also Chapter 1).

Compensation-Litigation

Paradoxically, compensation programs that are designed to facilitate a worker back to gainful employment have been shown to inherently prolong recovery,[34,45,94] increase disability,[36,49,57,70] and decrease the potential to return to work.[28,35,70] The majority of compensation-related litigation is directly related to the frustration, ignorance, anxiety, unrealistic expectations, and/or fear level of the injured worker.[15] These nonbiological factors have an even greater negative impact on motivation when the entitled individual retains an attorney and becomes a legal claimant.[45,61] Once this happens the person is obligated to prove and preserve an alleged injury or illness. To improve physically jeopardizes the ability to prevail in a suit. Additionally, the worker's own credibility is placed at risk. Hence, the disability continues throughout the litigation process, even in the absence of any objective medical basis for the disability. This is not to say that the pain or disability is non-existent, only that it cannot be objectified, and could therefore be attributable to secondary gain factors.[19] If the individual is not expected to enter litigation or has not retained an attorney, one point is given.

Hopefully, further research will validate and refine the usefulness of the proposed Performance APGAR score. In the next section of this chapter, we discuss methods to determine the credibility of alleged limitations. The credibility assessment lends itself well to more "subjective" impairments. The authors are currently creating a model, for publication, that incorporates the objective measures of the APGAR and the subjective measures of credibility into one model to measure patient/employee motivation.

Patient Credibility Assessment

Credibility Issues

Physicians involved in the evaluation of impairment, disability determination, and FFD regularly make judgments regarding the veracity and reliability of a person's alleged symptoms. It is a difficult process to attempt to determine whether he or she is reporting the truth. The determination becomes even more difficult as the amount of potential secondary gain increases. Experienced clinicians are generally skilled in the art of distinguishing between real and fabricated allegations. The level of skill involved varies by practitioner. There is little if any training on the subject in standard American medical school curriculums. The process may seem subjective and judgmental, but experienced physicians, working with the multifaceted issues involved in functional limitation determination, are keenly aware of the need to make a judgment regarding the credibility of the allegations.

It should be noted that the credibility assessment involves experience, instinct, and a thorough analysis of the history. There are some specific factors that can be considered in order to make a determination about the credibility of a person's alleged limitations.

It should also be noted that a credibility assessment is not to be thought of as a judgment about a person or patient's character. What a credibility determination is meant to do, for FFD determination purposes, is to make an informed judgment about the truthfulness of the alleged symptoms or limitations being evaluated. The current symptoms and limitations may be entirely credible in an otherwise historically dishonest individual. For example, there may be a politician who has been plagued with corruption, found to have lied on television to his constituents, and to have committed perjury in court. However, this same politician, when applying for disability, may have absolutely truthful and accurate allegations of symptoms and limited function regarding lumbar spine impairment. One needs to exercise caution and avoid jumping to conclusions.

Credibility Determination Process

It is generally accepted that one should use caution in determining the existence of functional permanent impairment on the basis of symptoms alone. For example, Social Security Administration (SSA) rules state, "Under no circumstances may the existence of an impairment be established on the basis of symptoms alone."[98] Furthermore, with regard to a disability evaluation, the SSA states that regardless of how many symptoms a person alleges, or how genuine his or her complaints may be, impairment cannot be established in the absence of objective medical abnormalities. This guidance not only applies to all types of impairment but also helps provide guidance in the determination of credibility for FFD and ability determinations. If there are clinically accepted medical signs and laboratory findings of an impairment or a diagnosis that could reasonably cause the alleged symptoms or limitations, it is then necessary to further evaluate the alleged limitations. One initially makes a professional assessment of the extent to which the symptoms can reasonably be accepted as consistent with the objective and other evidence available in the case file. Next, a determination regarding the extent to which the alleged limitations truly limit function is made using a two-step process: first, determining whether the symptoms alleged are reasonably attributable to an established impairment or diagnosis; second, evaluating the extent to which these symptoms produce work capacity limitations.

Credibility Factors

In making the determination of the effect of the alleged symptoms on true functional capacity, the examining physician should consider the intensity and persistence of the symptoms and their association with examination findings. There is much information that can be useful in determining the true impact of the alleged symptoms on function, including prior work record, employer contact, treating physician opinion, examining/consulting physician opinion, and observation by nursing, clerical, and physician staff.

When performing FFD evaluations or making medical ability statements, it is useful to consider guidance provided by the SSA.[97] The SSA disability determination process closely evaluates the credibility of symptoms and their true effect on function. In this guidance the SSA lists several factors to consider before making a final judgment about the limiting effects of the alleged symptoms. Some factors to consider are as follows:

- Activities of daily living: How are they reporting their functioning with regard to shopping, cooking, self-care, housework, yard work, etc.?
- Location, duration, frequency, and intensity of pain or symptoms: Is it consistent with the known diagnosis?
- Precipitating factors and aggravating factors: Will these factors prevent or limit ability to return to work?
- Type, dosage, effectiveness, and side effects of medications: Are they requiring large doses or multiple medications to relieve discomfort? Is the medication addicting? Is there evidence of narcotic drug seeking behavior? Are there legitimate side effects to required medication that will limit functional ability in a work setting?
- Treatment sought and received: Has the individual sought relief for the alleged symptoms from professionals? Has there been extensive searching for relief by attempting multiple treatments or unconventional treatment?
- What measures are used to relieve the pain or symptom? Must the person find relief by lying flat? Must he or she frequently alternate their position, thereby preventing stationary work?
- Opinions about function given by treating and examining sources.
- Inconsistencies or conflicts in the allegations, statements, or medical evidence in the file.

Other considerations in the overall assessment of credibility are the findings on certain tests, such as Waddell's signs or the Rey 15-Item Test for Malingering.[96]

Inconsistencies and conflicting statements make a significant contribution to the overall credibility assessment. Consistency is very important in determining credibility; however, it obviously is not the only measure. A strong indication of credibility is given by the degree to which the allegations are consistent with the objective evidence. Another area where consistency is important is in the history given at different examinations. For example, the history of the injury or illness, its onset, duration, symptoms, and functional effects should be fairly consistently reported to various sources of medical evidence. The initial history and physical should be reasonably consistent with independent medical evaluations (IMEs) for workers' compensation and these should be consistent with other specialist consultations in the file. Furthermore, the longitudinal medical record should be consistent in demonstrating the attempts to treat the condition. One may also make some inferences about the overall credibility of the allegations based on the frequency of treatment. If the allegation is quite severe, yet no medical treatment has been sought, the credibility of the allegation comes into question. One would then need to consider whether there were financial or other impediments to obtaining the appropriate level of treatment for the diagnosis.

Weighing Source Opinions

A key component of the overall credibility determination is the weight given to the opinions of treating and examining physicians in the file. It is not uncommon to perform a FFD examination on a person who has been off work for an extended period of time, seen several physicians, including specialists, and had notes written from the various specialists regarding his or her functional capacity. The opinions of other physicians in the file regarding the examinee's functional ability can vary significantly based on the physician's role in the patient's care. Many treating physicians inadvertently become inappropriate advocates for their patient by prolonging the disability period or assuming causal relationships to work without obtaining details from the employer's investigation of the alleged claim. How does the physician evaluating functional ability for a FFD examination determine which recommendation to follow? This process is called weighing the source opinions. In this process, the evaluating physician reviews all the information regarding credibility listed previously and then compares that information with the treating/examining physician opinions in the file. One must remember that other sources may give opinions on the examinee's functional abilities. These other sources might include chiropractors, physical therapists, optometrists, etc. Such sources can be valuable in determining the true extent of limitations and thereby assist in the overall credibility determination. In general, when differing opinions about function are in the file, the opinion most consistent with the evidence will be given the most weight. Other factors to consider in making a determination about which source opinion to follow include the following:

- Examining sources: The opinions of those who have examined the individual would be given greater weight than the opinions of those who have not (insurance company file reviews, etc.).
- Treating sources rather than one-time examiners: A medical provider with a longstanding relationship would likely be more familiar with his or her limitations than would a one-time consultant.
- Supporting evidence: A source that provides supporting evidence to substantiate the opinion about functional ability would be given more weight than one without supporting evidence.
- Consistency with the record: Obviously, those opinions most consistent with the preponderance of evidence will be given greater weight.
- Specialty: The opinion of a specialist in the field may be given greater weight than a generalist, even if the length of treatment was much less.

Many sources will write opinions such as "light duty," "moderate lifting," or "sedentary work." These generalized, nonspecific statements of functional ability are inherently unreliable and meaningless for making appropriate FFD and ability statements. There is no consistency among physicians as to the definition of "light work" or "sedentary work." Further confusion can come when a treating physician writes a note into a file that states "This patient is disabled." Again, there is not a specific level of impairment, known by all physicians, to equate with "disabled." To one physician the inability to lift more than 50 pounds may make the person disabled. To another examining physician this same person may be felt capable of performing the essential functions of his or her current job. The important thing to remember is that the opinion of the physician who knows the patient/employee best and has the most knowledge about the specific limiting condition should be weighed carefully in a FFD evaluation. In some cases where the treating physician makes a generalization regarding functional ability, further contact with the physician may be required in order to clarify the specific functional restrictions and the true residual capacity. Once the weight to be given is determined, it should be addressed in the report, giving the specific reasons why more weight was given to one opinion over another.

The experienced clinician will make the appropriate objective medical assessment of the FFD evaluee and then consider all the factors of credibility, weigh the source opinions, and then make a final determination of his or her functional ability.

Credibility Conclusions

Finally, when evaluating the credibility of a person's allegations in a written report, the specific findings on examination, in the history, or in the test results that led to a specific finding of credibility should be cited. There are three main possible credibility determinations:

1. Allegations are credible: If you make a finding that the allegations are largely credible and consistent with the diagnosis and the objective evidence, you are essentially giving those allegations such great weight that they are guiding your ultimate determination of functional ability.
2. Allegations are partially credible: In this case you have analyzed the data as outlined in this section and determined that the allegations of pain and/or limitation are not as severe as alleged. You should cite specific reasons and evidence upon which you made this determination in your report.
3. Allegations are not credible: This, hopefully, is a rare circumstance where every allegation of pain or limitation is found to be entirely unfounded.

Of course, with the determination comes a written rationale describing how the accumulated evidence supports such a determination.

Functional Ability Profiles

Unified Fitness Report

To facilitate the collection and reporting of the medical diagnosis and capabilities, a novel interdisciplinary approach referred to as the unified fitness report (UFR) has been developed by the Utah Medical Association (UMA).[108] Originally published elsewhere,[17,18,51,52] this model continues to expand toward a goal of providing a comprehensive and defensive methodology for determining medical capability. The guidelines were developed by a consensus of 28 specialists of the UMA, with consideration to the ethical and legal liabilities of physicians, ergonomists, attorneys, business managers, and supervisors who must balance the patient/employee and societal interests as required under ADA. For the past 5 years, data have been compiled, and were recently updated by the Utah Driver's License division.[25,100] The specific purposes of the UFR are to:

1. Assist workers who develop health problems to return to the appropriate levels of work that they can do.
2. Assist those who have health problems and who have not worked to gain employment at tasks they can accomplish effectively.
3. Help employers by providing guidelines for appropriate levels of work as determined by the employee's health condition.
4. Offer employers suggestions as to possible accommodations to consider in determining if an employee might accomplish the essential functions of a job.

The term "unified fitness" was used to focus on what a person can do with a specific diagnosis, not on what one cannot do. Whereas many of the functional ability categories are concerned with specialized capabilities, such as vision, hearing, or learning, others are related primarily to physical demands for lifting or carrying. As described in Table 53–1, the U.S. DOL and SSA have classified all jobs into five levels of exertion and skill.[114] The DOL model is widely accepted and used in making legal determinations of disability and FFD. The UMA's medical specialists have indexed severity, using the DOL work profiles, each of the 21 different categories of health concerns as shown in Figure 53–4. This categorization scheme, established with the consensus of medical specialists, provides a uniform standard necessary to meet the ADA's direct threat definition of "reasonable medical judgment that relies on the most current medical knowledge and/or the best available evidence."

A profile severity level of one indicates no present or past limitation for that category of health concern; level 10 indicates a condition in which work of any sort does not appear to be indicated, as shown in Figure 53–4 ("Summary of Profile Levels and Work Activities"). The UFR's unique value lies in assessing a person when more than one medical diagnosis exits simultaneously. Physicians have found the UFR Medical Report Form, as shown in Figure 53–5, quick and easy to use. An "x" placed in the appropriate severity profile of each medical category along with a notation as to hours of work and stability will suffice. As the condition improves or deteriorates, a simple change in the profile level will modify work activity level. There is room to add additional comments in unusual circumstances. In more complex cases or in special situations, a full profile of all categories may be needed. The severity profile of each medical category is recorded, with the most severe profile level indicating the patient's/employee's maximum safe work capability.

Limitations of the musculoskeletal category profiles for upper extremity conditions have been identified as not being sufficiently specific, for which there continues to be ongoing updates and improvements. Because the 21 categories of health concerns involve comprehensive medical knowledge, a doctor of medicine or osteopathy should make the final capability for duty statement, with input from the examinee and other allied health sources as described previously. The medical disposition should be limited to advising the employer about a person's current functional abilities and limitations in relation to essential job functions and about whether he or she meets the employer's health and safety requirements.[3]

Further detailed information on use of the UFR and the 21 health categories is provided in the UFR's documentation guidelines, which can be obtained for a nominal fee by writing the Utah Medical Association, 540 E. 500 So., Salt Lake City, UT 84102.

A simplified version of a generic functional ability profile is noted in Figure 53–6. This type of profile can also be easily completed by a treating or evaluating physician and reviewed by the employer who can quickly compare ability statements to the essential job functions when making FFD determinations and employability decisions.

EMPLOYER DETERMINATION OF ESSENTIAL JOB FUNCTIONS

An employer faced with a disabled or potentially disabled employee with a likely direct threat risk or undue hardship has a distinct legal responsibility under the ADA. In order to successfully meet this challenge, decisions must be made in accordance with all ADA guidelines, as described previously. By creating a system that brings medical, employee, and employer interests together, difficult risk assessment and FFD decisions can be successfully managed to produce legally defensible conclusions.

Category		Profile Levels 1	2	3	4	5	6	7	8	9	10
A-U	Musculoskeletal — Upper Extremity	All work activities	All work activities	Infrequent heavy lifting — affected extremity	Medium lifting — affected extremity	Light lifting— affected extremity	No lifting — affected extremity	No lifting — either extremity	According to special circumstances — depends upon nature of problem	Temporary adjustment — under evaluation — depends on situation	No work activity appropriate
A-H	Musculoskeletal — Hand			Minimal loss of skill/lifting — one hand	Slight loss of skill/lifting — one hand	Medium skill/lifting — one hand	Minimum skill/light tasks — bilateral	Substitute for all hand functions			
A-L	Musculoskeletal — Lower Extremity			Heavy: May Lift — Occasional - 100 lbs. Frequent - 50 lbs. Constant - 20 lbs.	Medium: May Lift: Occasional - 50 lbs. Frequent - 20 lbs. Constant - 10 lbs.	Light: May Lift: Occasional - 20 lbs. Frequent - 10 lbs. Constant - Negligible	Sedentary: May Lift - Occasional - 10 lbs. Frequent - Negligible Constant - Negligible	Limited sedentary			
A-S	Musculoskeletal — Spine							Limited sedentary			
B-G	Neurology — General						Limited tasks or sedentary	Limited sedentary or substitute functions			
B-E	Epilepsy/Other Episodic Disorders			Moderately high risk tasks	Moderate risk tasks	Slight risk tasks	Slight risk or special limits	Sedentary or ground-level tasks			
C	Pulmonary (Lung)			Heavy, not sustained	Medium	Light or intermittent medium	Sedentary, without oxygen	Sedentary, with oxygen			
D	Cardiovascular (Heart/Blood Vessels)			Heavy	Medium	Light	Sedentary	No risk to others			
E	Hematology/ Immunology/Oncology			Heavy	Medium	Light	Sedentary or decreased standing	Limited sedentary			
F	Ophthalmology (Eye)			No commercial driving	No undue risk - moving equipment/power tools	Desk/bench work	Sound/light signals	No allergens/irritants			
G	Otolaryngology (E.N.T.)			No special hearing skills	Limited hearing	No hearing required	Limit noise exposure	No allergens/irritants			
H	Gastroenterology (Digestive)			Heavy, except at intervals	Medium	Medium — less work load	Sedentary	Selected facilities			
I-G	Genitourinary- General (G.U.– Male or Female)			Heavy	Medium	Light	Sedentary	Selected facilities			
I-W	Genitourinary — Women/Pregnancy			Heavy	Heavy, with adjustment	Medium	Light	Sedentary			
J	Diabetes			Allowance for access to snacks/meals and regular work schedules Heavy	Heavy, with injections	Minimal risk tasks	Limited risk tasks	Sedentary/limit standing			
K	Dermatology (Skin)			Limit exposure to allergens/irritants	Minimize irritants	Eliminate allergens	No exposure to irritants	No exposure to allergens			
L-M	Memory/Learning/ Communication			Learn new, complex tasks	Complex tasks; usual supervision	Previous complex tasks with assistance	New, simple tasks with supervision	Simple tasks with supervision			
L-P	Psychiatric/ Psychological/Emotional			All — with monitoring	Select tasks; monitoring	Medium tasks; close supervision	Limited tasks/risks; close supervision	Highly selected tasks/ risks; close supervision			
L-S	Substance Use Disorders			Moderately high risk tasks; normal supervision[a]	Moderate risk tasks; intermediate supervision[a]	Slight risk tasks; increased supervision[a]	Limited risk tasks; close supervision[a]	No risk to self; close supervision[a]			
M-M	General Medical			Heavy; may reduce hours	Medium	Light	Sedentary	Limit exposure to others			
M-S	General Surgery			Heavy; may reduce hours	Medium	Light	Sedentary	Depends on type of problem			

Figure 53–4. Unified fitness report: Summary of profile levels and work activities.

Name ______________________ **Phone** __________

last first middle

Home Address ______________________

I hereby authorize my physician or other health care provider to release to ______________________ information about my health condition as it may relate to the appropriateness and wisdom of beginning or returning to work.

Signature **Birthdate** **Current date**

To Whom It May Concern: This report is being made to facilitate the beginning or return to modified or full-duty work by the above-named individual. I have checked any and all categories of which I am aware that may affect work status, as outlined in the Workplace Functional Ability Medical Guidelines.

Nature of health problem(s): ______________________

(In general terms, such as "back", "heart", etc.)

X = Functional Ability Profile with use of personal compensating device(s), such as glasses, hearing aids, braces, or prostheses, etc.

Profile Category		Functional Ability Profile Level									
		1	2	3	4	5	6	7	8	9	10
A-U	Musculoskeletal - Upper Extremity										
A-H	Musculoskeletal - Hand										
A-L	Musculoskeletal - Lower Extremity										
A-S	Musculoskeletal - Spine										
B-G	Neurology - General										
B-E	Epilepsy/Other Episodic Disorder										
C	Pulmonary (Lung)										
D	Cardiovascular (Heart/Blood Vessels)										
E	Hematology/Immunology/Oncology										
F	Ophthalmology (Eye)										
G	Otolaryngology (Ear/Nose/Throat)										
H	Gastroenterology (Digestive)										
I-G	Genitourinary (Kidney/Bladder-M or F)										
I-W	Genitourinary (Women's/Pregnancy)										
J	Diabetes										
K	Dermatology (Skin)										
L-M	Memory/Learning/Communication										
L-P	Psychiatric/Psychological/Emotional										
L-S	Substance Use Disorders										
M-M	General Medical										
M-S	General Surgical										

May begin or return to work activity appropriate to the above profile: ❐ as of current date, or ❐ approx.____________.

Hrs. of work: ❐ Full time
❐ Less than full time-approximately _____hrs/day; approx. _____days/week
❐ Gradually increase to full time by _____________.

Stability: ❐ Medical stability has been reached (little change expected). Date stability reached _______________.
❐ Not fully stable. Should be reviewed in approximately ______ weeks or _______ months.

Possible workplace accommodation(s) other than impled by the profile level:
(This and the possible adaptations for various profile levels are suggestions for employers to consider in determining if the essential functions of a job may be accomplished within the scope of limitations indicated by the profiles.)

Comments/treatment recommendations/suggestions, etc.:

Printed name of health care provider **Address**

Phone

Signature **Date** **Degree/ Title**

Figure 53–5. Unified fitness report: Medical report form.

Patient/Employer Information (to be filled out by referring location)

Employee Name: ______________________ Company Location: ______________________

Job Title: ______________________ Company Contact: ______________________

Date of Injury: ______________________ Company Phone No. ______________________
or Illness Fax No. ______________________

Physician Information (to be filled out by treating/evaluating physician or therapist)

Note: The following Essential Functional Ability Report is required to assist Company health care professionals and management personnel in making job placement and reasonable accommodation decisions for this employee.

Current Work Status:

❑ FULL DUTY as of: ______________________ ____________ (date)
❑ TEMPORARILY OFF WORK through: ______________________ (date)
❑ MODIFIED DUTY through: ______________________ (date)
  ❑ Temporary
  ❑ Permanent
❑ MAXIMUM MEDICAL IMPROVEMENT reached (not expected to significantly improve over next 12 months)
❑ MEDICAL DISABILITY RECOMMENDED (The patient has a physical or mental condition that substantially limits a major life activity. The medical condition(s) prevents this individual from returning to his/her current job)

Essential Job Function Review : (to be completed by treating/evaluating physician or therapist after reviewing attached list of Essential Job Functions - please check each category according to estimated medical ability)

Essential Function Category	No Limitations (✓)	Limitations (✓ and specify below)
1. Leadership (only if applicable)		
2. Reasoning (cognitive) Ability		
3. Mathematical Ability		
4. Language Ability		
5. Physical Demands (general)		
6. Physical Demands (specific)		
7. Visual Demands		
8. Hearing Demands		
9. Environmental Demands		

Specific Essential Job Function Limitations or Restrictions

Physician: ______________________ ______________________
Printed Name Signature

Date: ______________________

Figure 53–6. Sample Functional Ability Profile Report.

The following administrative functions must be documented and managed appropriately in order to prevent costly discriminatory actions from arising out of difficult and complex FFD and employability decisions. Specific activities and forms are described for each function in order to complete the proposed FFD model proposed in this chapter.

Documenting Essential Job Functions

EEOC regulations and guidance[3,113] that implement the ADA recommend that the following considerations be made by an employer when identifying the essential functions of a job:

1. Whether employees in the position actually are required to perform the function
2. Whether removing that function would fundamentally change the job
3. Whether the position exists to perform the function
4. Whether there are a limited number of other employees available to perform the function, or among whom the function can be distributed
5. Whether a function is highly specialized, and the person in the position is hired for special expertise or ability to perform it

Other relevant factors could ultimately be considered, and although the ADA leaves to the employer the judgment as to which functions are essential, the burden of proof remains on the employer to defend the requirements of a job as truly being essential in a contested disability case. In doing so, we have used the following system to define essential job functions.

Essential Function Review List

The essential function review (EFR) list (Table 53–4) consists of nine different categories, which describe progressive ability statements that could reasonably be required of an employee to perform the essential functions of any job. Ability statements range from basic or entry level and progress to more advanced or technical level requirements. An employer can simply review the list and determine what ability level for each category is required to perform the essential functions of a specific job. Ideally, each major job classification within a company should have its own list of essential functions developed from this or a similar list. Many business software programs are also available to accomplish this important FFD task. The EFR list is to be used as a guide for managers and supervisors to decide which ability statements truly constitute an essential function. Guidance from individuals who are knowledgeable

TABLE 53–4

Essential Function Review List

Notice:

1.	The following categories and "ability statements" are to be used in completing an Essential Function Review Form. Choose the most appropriate statement(s) that corresponds to the essential functions of the job being reviewed. Management and employees are encouraged to work together to ensure the essential function profile accurately characterizes the job.
2.	This Essential Function Review in no way states or implies that these are the only tasks to be performed by the employee occupying this position. He or she will be required to follow any other instructions and to perform any other job-related duties requested by his or her supervisor.
3.	Essential function requirements are representative minimum levels of knowledge, skills, and/or abilities. To perform this job successfully, the incumbent will possess the abilities and aptitudes to perform each task proficiently.
4.	Ability means to possess and apply *both* knowledge and skill.
5.	A review of essential functions intentionally excludes marginal or peripheral functions of the position that are incidental to the performance of primary job functions. All tasks and requirements listed on the Essential Function Review Form must be essential job functions.
6.	This document lists various categories and essential function criteria that describe minimum requirements to qualify or remain qualified for a given position. However, promotion and other employment decisions are also based on company needs, being in good standing (including lack of disciplinary actions), fully competent performance, and other non-discriminatory issues.
7.	All essential functions are subject to possible modification to reasonably accommodate individuals with objectively defined disabilities.
8.	The company is not required to make accommodations for individuals if the accommodations pose a direct threat or significant risk to the health and safety of the individual or other employees or undue hardship on the company.
9.	Completion of an Essential Function Review Form does not create an employment contract, implied or otherwise, other than an "at will" employment relationship.

Table continued on opposite page

TABLE 53–4
Essential Function Review List *Continued*

1. **GENERAL EDUCATION—REASONING ABILITY: The ability to apply common sense or logic to a problem-solving situation. Describes the MINIMUM (not optimum) reasoning ability for the successful completion of the position. This ability is generally acquired through formal education prior to occupying this position. (Choose one statement for Essential Function Review Form)**
   a. Ability to apply common sense understanding to carry out simple one-or two-step instructions; to deal with standardized situations with occasional or no variables in or from these situations encountered on the job.
   b. Ability to apply common sense understanding to carry out detailed but uninvolved instructions; to deal with problems involving a few concrete variables in or from standardized situations.
   c. Ability to apply common sense understanding to carry out detailed, involved instructions; to deal with problems involving several concrete variables in or from standardized situations.
   d. Ability to apply principles of rational systems to solve practical problems and deal with a variety of concrete variables in situations where only limited standardization exists; to interpret a variety of complex instructions.
   e. Ability to apply principles of logical or scientific thinking to define problems, collect data, establish facts, and draw valid conclusions; to interpret an extensive variety of technical instructions in mathematical or other form; to deal with several abstract and concrete variables.
   f. Ability to apply principles of logical or scientific thinking to a wide range of intellectual and practical problems; to deal with nonverbal symbolism (formulas, scientific equations, graphs, etc.) in its most difficult phases; to deal with a variety of abstract and concrete variables; to comprehend the most abstruse classes of concepts.

2. **GENERAL EDUCATION—MATHEMATICAL ABILITY: The LEVEL of ability to understand mathematical concepts and apply them to problem solving situations. Describes the MINIMUM (not optimum) math ability for the successful completion of the position. This ability is generally acquired through formal education prior to occupying this position. (Choose one statement for Essential Function Review Form)**
   a. Ability to add and subtract two-digit numbers; to multiply and divide 10's and 100's by 2, 3, 4, 5; to perform the four basic arithmetic operations with coins as part of a dollar; to perform operations with units such as inch, foot, and yard, and ounce and pound (and their metric counterparts).
   b. Ability to add, subtract, multiply, and divide all units of measure; to perform the four operations with like or common decimal fractions; to compute ratio, rate, and percent; to draw and interpret bar graphs; to perform arithmetic operations involving all American monetary units.
   c. Ability to compute discount, interest, profit, and loss; commission, markup, and selling price; ratio and proportion, and percentage; to calculate surfaces, volume, weights, and measures. Using Algebra, to calculate variables and formulas; monomials and polynomials; ratio and proportion variables; and square roots and radicals. Using Geometry, to calculate plane and solid figures; circumference, area, and volume; to understand kinds of angles, and properties of pairs of angles. Using Advanced Shop Math: Ability to use practical application of the essentials of trigonometry.
   d. Using Algebra: Ability to deal with system of real numbers; linear, quadratic, rational, exponential, logarithmic, angle and circular functions, and inverse functions; related algebraic solution of equations and inequalities; limits and continuity, and probability and statistical inference. Using Geometry: Ability to perform deductive axiomatic geometry, planer and solid; and rectangular coordinates.
   e. Using Algebra: Ability to work with exponents and logarithms, linear equations, quadratic equations, mathematical induction and binomial theorem, and permutations. Using Calculus: Ability to apply concepts of analytic geometry, differentiation and integration of algebraic functions with applications. Using Statistics: Ability to apply mathematical operations to frequency distributions, reliability and validity of tests, normal curve, analysis of variance, correlation techniques, chi-square application and sampling theory, and factor analysis.
   f. Using Advanced Calculus: Ability to work with limits, continuity, real number systems, mean value theorems, and implicit function theorems. Using Modern Algebra: Ability to apply fundamental concepts of theories of groups, rings, and fields; to work with differential equations, linear algebra, infinite series, advanced operational methods and functions of real and complex variables.
   g. Using Statistics: Ability to work with mathematical statistics, mathematical probability and application, experimental design, statistical inference, and econometrics.

Table continued on following page

regarding the ADA and employment law should help management distinguish between essential and marginal functions before proceeding to complete the EFR form, described in the following section. OSHA's continued interest in promulgating an Ergonomics Standard suggests close scrutiny when employers define the physical demand characteristics of essential job functions.[80]

Essential Function Review Form

The EFR form (Table 53–5) is the final result of the EFR process. The job title, location, person completing the form, date, and other pertinent information about the job is completed on the form. It is recommended that job descriptions used for recruiting and hiring purposes be kept separate from the list of essential job functions.

TABLE 53-4

Essential Function Review List *Continued*

3. GENERAL EDUCATION—LANGUAGE ABILITY: The LEVEL of ability to deliver, understand, and apply language to problem solving situations. Language ability is measured and illustrated in terms of reading by sight, writing (to inscribe by whatever means), and communicating (by voice or sign). Describes the MINIMUM (not optimum) language ability for the successful completion of the position. This ability is generally acquired through formal education prior to occupying this position. (Choose one statement for Essential Function Review Form)

a. Ability to recognize the meaning of 2500 (two and three syllable) words; to read by sight at a very slow rate; to compare similarities and differences between words and between series of numbers.
Ability to print (to inscribe by whatever means) simple sentences containing subject, verb, and object; series of numbers, names, and addresses. Ability to express or exchange ideas by means of the spoken word. Ability to communicate in simple sentences, using normal word order and present and past tenses.

b. Ability to use a passive vocabulary of 5000 to 6000 words; to read by sight at a slow rate; to read by sight adventure stories and comic books; to define unfamiliar words in dictionaries for meaning, spelling, and pronunciation; to read by sight instructions, safety rules, etc.
Ability to write (to inscribe by whatever means) compound and complex sentences, using cursive style, proper end punctuation, and employing adjectives and adverbs.
Ability to communicate in complex sentences; using normal word order with present and past tenses; using a good vocabulary.

c. Ability to read by sight a variety of books, novels, magazines, instructions, atlases, and encyclopedias.
Ability to prepare memoranda, reports, and essays, using proper format, punctuation, spelling, and grammar.
Ability to communicate distinctly with appropriate pauses and emphasis; correct pronunciation (or sign equivalent) and variation in word order; using present, perfect, and future tenses.

d. Ability to read by sight periodicals, journals, poems, manuals, dictionaries, thesauruses, and encyclopedias.
Ability to prepare business letters, proposals, summaries, and reports; using prescribed format and conforming to all rules of punctuation, grammar, diction, and style; using all parts of speech.
Ability to conduct training; to communicate at panel discussions and to make presentations with poise and control.

e. Ability to read by sight literature, scientific and technical journals, abstracts, financial reports, and legal documents.
Ability to prepare articles, abstracts, editorials, journals, manuals, and critiques.
Ability to make comprehensive presentations; participate in formal debate; communicate extemporaneously; communicate before an audience with poise, using correct English or other language.

4. PHYSICAL DEMANDS—TYPE: The physical activity of this position. (Choose appropriate statements for Essential Function Review Form)

a. Ability to ascend or descend ladders, scaffolding, and the like with agility.
b. Ability to maintain body equilibrium to prevent falling from precarious situations.
c. Ability to (stoop or crawl) lower the body to floor level and move about with agility.
d. Ability to (reach) extend out and retrieve objects outside immediate range.
e. Ability to (stand) support oneself and stay in an upright position.
f. Ability to (push) press against something with substantial steady force in order to thrust forward, downward, or outward.
g. Ability to (pull) exert a considerable force in order to draw, drag, haul, or tug objects in a sustained motion.
h. Ability to raise substantial objects from a lower to a higher position or moving objects horizontally from position-to-position.
i. Ability to (pinch or pick) maneuver small objects precisely by whatever means.
j. Ability to (grip) seize an object by applying considerable force.
k. Ability to (feel) detect attributes of objects, such as size, shape, temperature, texture, tension or force by tactile means.
l. Ability to be subject to substantial repetitive motions of the body or its parts.
m. Ability to work rotating shifts, including weekends, with crews of size (specify number).

Table continued on opposite page

However, during the interview and selection process it is appropriate to ask applicants if they can perform the essential job functions and to document the response. Each of the nine categories from the EFR list is shown with the most appropriate ability statement(s) profiled for that category. Frequently, management will need to add specific essential functions that are unique to the job but not mentioned on the generic EFR list. Ability statements such as "ability to work rotating shifts" or "ability to be subject to stressful management responsibilities" may be added to accurately describe the position. Once the EFR form and list have been electronically created, simple cut-

TABLE 53–4
Essential Function Review List *Continued*

5. PHYSICAL DEMANDS—Requirements (Choose appropriate statement(s) for Essential Function Review Form)

a. Standing
(1) Hours at one time
(a) 8
(b) 7
(c) 6
(d) 5
(e) 4
(f) 3
(g) 2
(h) 1
(i) 0

(2) Total hours during day
(a) 8
(b) 7
(c) 6
(d) 5
(e) 4
(f) 3
(g) 2
(h) 1
(i) 0

b. Sitting
(1) Hours at one time
(a) 8
(b) 7
(c) 6
(d) 5
(e) 4
(f) 3
(g) 2
(h) 1
(i) 0

(2) Total hours during day
(a) 8
(b) 7
(c) 6
(d) 5
(e) 4
(f) 3
(g) 2
(h) 1
(i) 0

c. Walking—(distance)
(1) Hours at one time
(a) 8
(b) 7
(c) 6
(d) 5
(e) 4
(f) 3
(g) 2
(h) 1
(i) 0

(2) Total hours during day
(a) 8
(b) 7
(c) 6
(d) 5
(e) 4
(f) 3
(g) 2
(h) 1
(i) 0

d. Lifting maximum pounds (one person)
(1) Frequently (34 to 66%)
(a) 80 lbs or above
(b) 70
(c) 60
(d) 50
(e) 40
(f) 30
(g) 20
(h) 10

(2) Infrequently (0 to 33%)
(a) 80 lbs or above
(b) 70
(c) 60
(d) 50
(e) 40
(f) 30
(g) 20
(h) 10

e. Carrying maximum pounds (one person)
(1) Frequently (34 to 66%)
(a) 80 lbs or above
(b) 70
(c) 60
(d) 50
(e) 40
(f) 30
(g) 20
(h) 10

(2) Infrequently (0 to 33%)
(a) 80 lbs or above
(b) 70
(c) 60
(d) 50
(e) 40
(f) 30
(g) 20
(h) 10

Table continued on following page

TABLE 53–4
Essential Function Review List *Continued*

f. Required movements
   (1) Bend—frequently ________ occasionally ________ not at all ________
   (2) Reach—frequently ________ occasionally ________ not at all ________
   (3) Squat—frequently ________ occasionally ________ not at all ________
   (4) Kneel—duration at one time ________
   frequently ________ occasionally ________ not at all ________
   (5) Climb—on ________________________________ (specify)
   frequently ________ occasionally ________ not at all ________
   (6) Push/pull—lbs
   frequently ________ occasionally ________ not at all ________
   (7) Twist—body part ________________________________ (specify)
   frequently ________ occasionally ________ not at all ________
   (8) Rotate—body part ________________________________ (specify)
   frequently ________ occasionally ________ not at all ________
   (9) Crawl—distance ________
   frequently ________ occasionally ________ not at all ________

6. **VISUAL DEMANDS: The visual acuity requirements including color, depth perception, and field of vision. (Choose appropriate statement[s] for Essential Function Review Form)**
   a. MACHINE OPERATORS (including inspection), INSPECTION, CLOSE ASSEMBLY: This is a minimum standard for use with those whose work deals largely with visual inspection involving small defects, small parts, operation machines (including inspection), using measurement devices, assembly or fabrication of parts at distances close to the eyes.
   b. MACHINE OPERATORS (without inspection), MECHANICS, SKILLED TRADESPEOPLE: This is a minimum standard for use with those whose work deals with machines such as lathes, mills, power saws where the seeing job is at or within arm's reach. (If the machine operator also inspects, use "A" standard, which requires more acuity.) Also mechanics and skilled tradespeople and those who do work of a nonrepetitive nature such as carpenters, technicians, service people, plumbers, painters, mechanics, etc.
   c. MOBILE EQUIPMENT OPERATORS: This is a minimum for use with those who operate cars, trucks, forklifts, cranes, and high lift equipment.
   d. OTHER: This is a minimum standard based on the criteria of accuracy and neatness of work for janitors, sweepers, etc.

7. **HEARING DEMANDS: Hearing requirements including ability to discriminate verbal commands and environmental safety sounds. (Choose one statement for Essential Function Review Form)**
   a. Ability to hear well enough for any type of position (e.g., normal hearing and audiogram including normal noise and speech discrimination).
   b. Ability to hear well enough to be employed where hearing acuity is not the reason for employment (e.g., able to hear fine changes in motors, steam valves, bearings, etc. Should not have difficulty hearing over loud noise, etc.)
   c. Ability to be employed where moderate degrees of hearing loss are unimportant (e.g., able to converse without strain, talk and make notes in meetings, hear warning bells/sounds, tone of running motors, answer phone over high noise levels, etc.)
   d. Ability to hear well enough to work where severe hearing impairment is not a handicap (e.g., able to hear warning noises with or without a hearing aid, able to be in contact with coworkers and receive and transmit information, able to hear verbal instructions, etc.)
   e. Ability to perform any type of work where complete deafness with ability to read lips allows contact with other workers or environment where hearing is of no importance or unnecessary to perform essential job functions.

Table continued on opposite page

and-paste functions can build the essential function form in a matter of minutes. It is important that top management reviews, signs, and dates the form. This ensures individuals involved in FFD evaluations that the essential functions of the job are accurate, are valid, and have not recently been manipulated by anyone within the organization in an attempt to disqualify employees from the job.

FFD DETERMINATION PROCESS

Objective ability statements about a specific person should be derived from the medical history, examination, laboratory, radiographic, psychological, or functional ability tests or evaluations as described in "Medical Components of Employee Ability Assess-

TABLE 53–4
Essential Function Review List *Continued*

8. **ENVIRONMENTAL DEMANDS: The conditions the worker will be subject to in this position. (Choose appropriate statement(s) for Essential Function Review Form)**
   a. The worker is subject to Inside Environmental conditions: Protection from weather conditions but not necessarily from temperature changes.
   b. The worker is subject to Outside Environmental conditions: No effective protection from weather.
   c. The worker is subject to Both Environmental conditions: Activities occur inside and outside.
   d. The worker is subject to Extreme Cold: Temperature below 32° for periods of more than 1 hour.
   e. The worker is subject to Extreme Heat: Temperatures above 100° for periods of more than 1 hour.
   f. The worker is subject to Noise: There is sufficient noise to cause the worker to shout in order to be heard above the ambient noise level.
   g. The worker is subject to Vibration: Exposure to oscillating movements of the extremities or whole body.
   h. The worker is subject to Hazards: This category includes a variety of physical conditions, such as proximity to moving mechanical parts, electrical current, working on scaffolding and high places, exposure to high heat, or exposure to chemicals (airborne and/or skin exposure).
   i. The worker is subject to Atmospheric conditions: One or more of the following conditions that affect the respiratory system or the skin: fumes, odors, dusts, mists, gases, or poor ventilation.
   j. The worker is subject to Oils: There is air and/or skin exposure to oils and other cutting fluids.
   k. The worker is required to wear Respirator.
   l. None: The worker is not substantially exposed to adverse environmental conditions (such as in typical office administrative work).

ments." A method of accurately reporting this information to the employer, such as the UFR or other type of functional ability report, is important so that legally defensible administrative decisions can be made.

Matching Essential Job Functions to Patient/Employee Functional Abilities

The administrative process of matching the abilities of an employee to the essential functions of a job forms the heart of the proposed FFD model in this chapter. One of the chapter authors has developed the following methodology in a corporate setting that has applicability to virtually all FFD and employability decisions regardless of employer size or circumstances. The use of a job accommodation team (JAT) and the documentation strategies and forms used in this model are described in the following sections and in Tables 53–5, 53–6, and 53–7.

Job Accommodation Team

When a person, due to a medical condition, is given a questionable functional ability profile or placed on permanent restrictions by a treating and/or evaluating physician, a FFD question is raised and a potential ADA case is created. In these situations, an objective review of the physical or mental capabilities of the patient/employee must be compared to the essential job functions in order to prevent potential ADA discrimination. A JAT best accomplishes this purpose. The JAT is a multidisciplinary team consisting of the employee in question, company and treating physicians (or written opinions) if available, human resources personnel, key managers responsible for accommodation decisions, union representation (if applicable), and legal counsel or vocational rehabilitation specialists if the employee may no longer be considered a qualified employee after FFD decisions have been made. Accurate documentation of each JAT meeting (of which there may be many) is kept by human resource or other administrative personnel. Medical records are maintained separately under ADA requirements; however, a JAT Documentation Form, as shown in Table 53–6, can be maintained in personnel files to describe the employee's input, the accommodation review process, considerations of direct threat, concerns over undue hardship, and final management decisions regarding employment status.

Essential Function/Physical Abilities Review

When the JAT identifies that the current or other available positions should be reviewed for potential accommodations, the essential function/physical abilities review

TABLE 53–5

Essential Function Review (EFR) Form

Job classification or title: ❑ **New EFR** ❑ **Updated EFR** **Person completing this form:**	**Work Area:** **Date Completed:**
General Category	**Ability Statements:**
1. ***Leadership ability***: (ability to lead, guide direct, positively influence, etc.)	
2. ***Reasoning ability***: (ability to apply common sense or logic to problem solving situation)	
3. ***Mathematics ability***: (level of ability to understand mathematical concepts and apply to problem solving situations)	
4. ***Language ability***: (level of ability to deliver, understand, and apply language to problem solving situations)	
5. ***Physical demands***: (type of physical activity requirements of this position)	a. b. c. etc.
6. ***Physical demands***: (specific physical requirements of this position)	a. b. c. etc.
7. ***Visual demands***: (visual requirements including color, depth perception, and field of vision)	
8. ***Hearing demands***: (hearing requirements including ability to discriminate verbal commands and environmental safety sounds)	
9. ***Environmental demands***: (environmental conditions to which workers will be subject)	a. b. c.
Signature: ________ Date: ________ Approved (Supervisor):	Signature: ________ Date: ________ Approved (Manager):

form (Table 53–7) or a similar method should used to objectively document the FFD decision. The employer, usually through the immediate supervisor of the employee in question, is provided with the medical restrictions/limitations or other objective medical information such as that contained in the UFR functional ability profile (column 1). The supervisor must then analyze each essential job function (column 2) and note which functions are impacted by the limitation (column 3). The supervisor then notes what if any reasonable accommodations might be made (column 4) to allow the employee to return to the job without creating a direct threat risk (column 5) or undue hardship (column 6).

Final Employability or Reassignment Decisions

All members of the JAT provide input to this process and suggest both positions and/or accommodations that could be considered to maintain the individual's employability at the current location. It should be noted, however, that the ADA does not require an employer to create a new job or displace an able-bodied employee to create an accommodation. When dealing with employees represented by a collective bargaining unit, a unique legal dilemma may be created. This is based on the union seniority system, which might allow a senior "disabled" employee to displace a junior able-bodied employee. The supervisor completing the form has the responsibility to determine if any suggested accommodation creates a direct threat or undue hardship. If neither exists, the employee may be reasonably accommodated in the current position. If, in the supervisor's opinion, a direct threat risk or undue hardship does exist, he or she must validate and explain the rationale that led to the non-accommodation decision. This process is repeated until either a vacant position is found within the company for which reasonable accommodations can be matched to the employee's abilities or inabilities, or no position can be

TABLE 53-6

Job Accommodation Team (JAT) Documentation Form

Date: ______________________ Job Title/Area: ______________________

Employee: Ext. ______________ Home: ______________

JAT Members Present: Representing:

HR Generalist Introduction:

Medical Restriction Review:

Employee Response:

Accommodations Requested to Current Job: Qualified Vacant Positions:

Actions: JAT Signatures:

Next JAT Scheduled for: ______________________

found and the employee is granted available benefits and terminated.

Providing Transitional Support

Once a non-accommodation decision has been reached and legally validated for current, alternate, or vacant positions the employee may be qualified to hold, the employer may initiate termination proceedings. However, due to the complexity of the ADA, and employment law in general, we strongly recommend that the company's decision and documentation be reviewed by legal counsel familiar with employment law. We have also found that, in contested disability/non-accommodation situations, the earlier a vocational rehabilitation specialist can be involved

TABLE 53–7

Essential Function/Physical Abilities/Performance Review Form

Employee Name:	*Date:*
Position Being Reviewed:	*Work Area:*
Person Completing Review:	

Restrictions/Inabilities/Performance Issues: (per attached documentation, use other side if necessary)
1.
2.
3.
4.
5. etc.

Applicable Essential Job function (EJFs) (use other side if necessary)	*Applicable Restrictions/ Inabilities/Performance Issues*	*Suggested Accommodations per Management & Employee Input*	*Direct Threat**	*Undue H'ship**
1.				
2.				
3.				
4. etc.				

Direct Threat/Undue Hardship Explanation:

EJF No.	*Explanation*
etc.	

Conclusions/Recommendations (check box that applies):

	Able to Accommodate in Above Position
	Unable to Accommodate in Above Position

______________________ / ____________ / ______________________ / ____________

Signatures: (Supervisor) Date Area Manager Date

with the case, or as a member of the JAT, the better the chances are for resolution without discrimination charges being filed. The employee should have all short and long-term disability benefits, pensions, outstanding vacation pay, etc., made available by the company. We have also found it useful, in some cases, to assist disabled employees facing termination in filing for Social Security benefits and have written supportive letters in their behalf. Based on our experience with this model, employees feel that a fair and objective method has been used to "hear their case." Although they may not agree with the final employer decision for non-accommodation they have, nevertheless, been involved with the decision-making process from the beginning. Union officials have been supportive of this model and have, in many cases, assisted in bringing the case to a nonadversarial conclusion. In multiple cases over the past 10 years, discrimination claims for non-accommodation or employment discrimination were dismissed at the resolution conference or administrative hearing levels based on the FFD documentation from the described model.

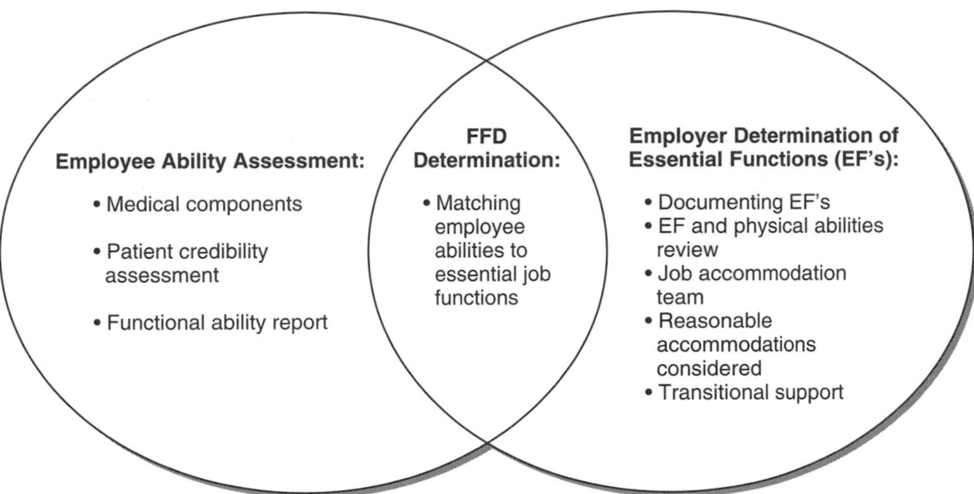

Figure 53–7. Comprehensive fitness for duty determination process.

CONCLUSIONS

Whether an applicant for a position or a worker seeking to continue employment, a person whose medical condition limits a major life activity, thus rendering him or her a disabled person, is protected by the ADA with respect to employment decisions. Professionals such as management, health care providers, attorneys, and ergonomic experts should work together by applying the methodology outlined here for FFD determinations. Legal counsel experienced in ADA law should always review contested reassignment or termination actions. A coordinated individual, medical, and administrative approach significantly reduces potential employer liability for increased risk of workers' compensation actions as well as discriminatory violations of the ADA. The original methodology described in Figure 53–2 is now more completely described in Figure 53–7.

Special acknowledgment is given to Dr. Madison Thomas, Task Force Chairman, and the 28 members of the Utah Medical Association who contributed to the UFRs. Copies of the Unified Fitness Report Guidelines Booklet and the Report Forms can be obtained at a reasonable cost from the Utah State Department of Health, 288 North 1460 West, P.O. Box 15680, Salt Lake City, UT 84116-1580. All or part of the Unified Fitness Report Guidelines Booklet may be duplicated freely by individuals or organizations for their use, but not for purposes of sale or profit.

References

1. 26.42 USC § 12113(b); 29 CFR § 1630.15(b)(2).
2. Cocchiarella L, Andersson GBJ (eds): Guides to the Evaluation of Permanent Impairment, 5th ed. Chicago, American Medical Association, 2001, p 2.
3. Americans With Disabilities Act 42 USC § 12101 (1991).
4. Anderson GJB, Svensson HO, Oden A: The intensity of work recovery in low back pain. Spine 3:880–884, 1984.
5. Anderson RT: An orthopedic ethnography in rural Nepal. Medical Anthropology 8:46–59, 1984.
6. Astin JA: Why patients use alternative medicine: Results of a national study. JAMA 279:1548–1553, 1998.
7. Atlas SJ, Singer DE, Keller RB, et al: Application of outcomes research in occupational low back pain: The Maine Lumbar Spine Study. Am J Ind Med 29:584–589, 1996.
8. Baker JC: Burden of proof in detection of submaximal effort. Work 10:63–70, 1998.
9. Bell C: Overview of the Americans With Disabilities Act and the Family and Medical Leave Act. In Disability Evaluation. St. Louis, Mosby, 1996, pp 582–591.
10. Berkowitz E: Disabled Policy: America's Programs for the Handicapped. New York, Cambridge University Press, 1987.
11. Biddle J, Roberts K, Rosenman KD, Welch EM: What percentage of workers with work-related illnesses receive workers' compensation benefits? J Occup Environ Med 40:325–331, 1998.
12. Bigos SJ, Battie MC, Fisher LD, et al: A prospective study of work perceptions and psychosocial factors affecting the report of back injury. Spine 16:1–6, 1991.
13. Borg G, Holmgren A, Lindblad I: Quantitative evaluation of chest pain. Acta Med Scand Suppl 644:43–45, 1978.
14. Burton JF: Workers' compensation benefits paid to workers. John Burton's Workers Compensation Monitor 9, 1996.
15. California Workers' Compensation Institute: Report to the Governor and Legislature, July 1985.
16. Clark WL, Haldeman S, Johnson P, et al: Back impairment and disability determinations: Another attempt at objective, reliable rating. Spine 12:332–341, 1988.

17. Colledge AL, Johns RE Jr: Unified fitness report for the workplace. Occup Med 15:723–739, 2000.
18. Colledge AL, Johns RE Jr, Thomas MH: Functional abilities assessment: Guidelines for the workplace. J Occup Environ Med 41:172–180, 1999.
19. Colledge AL, Johnson HI: SPICE—A model for reducing the incidence and costs of occupationally entitled claims. Occup Med 15:723–739, 2000.
20. Craufurd DIO, Creed F, Jayson MIV: Life events and psychological disturbances in patients with low back pain. Spine 15:480–493, 1990.
21. Dent GL: Curing the disabling effects of employee injury. Risk Manage 30, 1985.
22. Department of Labor and Industries: Attending Doctor's Handbook. Olympia, Wash, Department of Labor and Industries, 1999, p 4.
23. Derebery VJ, Tullis WH: Delayed recovery in the patient with a work compensable injury. J Occup Med 25:829–835, 1983.
24. Deyo RA, Rainville J, Kent DL: What can the history and physical tell us about low back pain? JAMA 268:760–765, 1992.
25. Diller E: Evaluating the Existing System of Drivers With Medical Conditions in Utah. Salt Lake City, Mountain Injury Control Research Center, University of Utah, 1999.
26. Dworkin RH, Handlin DS, Richlin DM, et al: Unraveling the effects of compensation, litigation, and employment on treatment response in chronic pain. Pain 23:49–59, 1985.
27. Economic Outcomes of Injures: Workers With Permanent Impairment. Austin, TX Texas Workers' Compensation Research Center, 1995, p 1.
28. Fredrickson BE, Trief PM, Van Beveren P, et al: Rehabilitation of the patients with chronic back pain: A search for outcome predictors. Spine 3:351–353, 1988.
29. Frymoyer JW: An international challenge to the diagnosis and treatment of disorders of the lumbar spine. Spine 18:2147–2152, 1993.
30. Frymoyer JW, Rosen JC, Clements J, Pope MH: Psychologic factors in low back pain disability. Clin Orthop 195:178–184, 1985.
31. Gaines WG Jr, Hegmann KT: Effectiveness of Waddell's nonorganic signs in predicting a delayed return to regular work in patients experiencing acute occupational low back pain. Spine 24:396–400, 1999.
32. Gallagher RM, Rauh V: Determinants of return-to-work among low back pain patients. Pain 39:55–67, 1989.
33. Gice J, Tomokins K: Cutting costs with return to work programs. Risk Manage 35:62–65, 1988.
34. Greenough CG, Fraser RD: The effect of compensation on recovery from low back injury. Spine 14:947–955, 1989.
35. Guck TP, Meilman PW, Skultery FK, Dowd ET: Prediction of long-term outcome of multidisciplinary pain treatment. Arch Phys Med Rehabil 67:233–236, 1986.
36. Guest GH, Drummond PD: Effect of compensation on emotional state and disability in chronic back pain. Pain 48:125–130, 1992.
37. Hadjistavropoulos H, Craig K: Acute and chronic low back pain: Cognitive, affective, and behavioral dimensions. J Consult Clin Psychol 62:341–349, 1994.
38. Hadler NM: Comments on the "Ergonomics Program Standard" proposed by the Occupational Safety and Health Administration. J Occup Environ Med 42:951–969, 2000.
39. Hayes B, Solyom CA, Wing PC, Berkowitz J: Use of psychometric measures and nonorganic signs testing in detecting nomogenic disorders in low back pain patients. Spine 18:1254–1259, 1993.
40. Hazard RG: Isokinetic trunk and lifting strength measurements: Variability as an indicator of effort. Spine 13:54–57, 1988.
41. Hazard RG, Reeves V, Fenwick JW, et al: Test-retest variation in lifting capacity and indices of subject effort. Clin Biomech 8:20–24, 1993.
42. Himmelstein JS, Pransky GS: Worker fitness and risk evaluations. In Occupational Medicine, State of the Art Reviews. Philadelphia, Hanley & Belfus, 1988.
43. Hirsch G, Beach G, Cooke C, et al: Relationship between performance on lumbar dynamometry and Waddell score in a population with low-back pain. Spine 16:1039–1043, 1991.
44. Hoogendoorn WE, van Poppel MNM, Bongers PM, et al: Systematic review of psychosocial factors at work and private life as risk factors for back pain. Spine 25:2114–2125, 2000.
45. Hunter SJ, Shaha S, Flint DF, et al: Predicting return to work: A long term follow-up study of railroad workers after low back injuries. Spine 23:2319–2328, 1998.
46. Innes E, Straker L: Reliability of work-related assessments. Work 13:107–124, 1999.
47. Institute of Medicine: Clinical Practice Guidelines: Directions for a New Program. Washington, DC, National Academy Press, 1990, p 38.
48. Isernhagen SJ: Isernhagen Work Systems Functional Capacity Evaluation. Duluth, Minn, Isernhagen Work Systems, 1996, pp 52a–52b, 83.
49. Jamison RN, Matt DA, Parris WCV: Effects of time, limited vs. unlimited compensation on pain behavior and treatment outcome in low back pain patients. J Psychosom Res 32:277–283, 1988.
50. Jay MA, Lamb JM, Watson RL, et al: Sensitivity and specificity of the indicators of sincere effort of the EPIC lift capacity test on a previously injured population. Spine 25:1405–1412, 2000.
51. Johns RE Jr, Bloswick DS, Elegante JM: Chronic, recurrent low back pain, a methodology for analyzing fitness for duty and managing risk under the Americans With Disabilities Act. J Occup Med 36:537–547, 1994.
52. Johns RE Jr, Elegante JM, Teynor PD, et al: Fitness for Duty: Disability Evaluation. St. Louis, Mosby, 1996, pp 592–604.
53. King PM: Analysis of approaches to detection of sincerity of effort through grip strength measurement. Work 10:9–13, 1998.
54. King PM, Tuckwell N, Barrett TE: A critical review of functional capacity evaluations. Phys Ther 78:852–866, 1998.
55. Koyl L: Employing the Older Worker: Matching the Employee to the Job, 2nd ed. Washington, DC, National Council on the Aging, 1974.
56. Krefting LM, Bremner A: Work evaluation: Choosing a commercial system. Can J Occup Ther 52:20–24, 1985.
57. Leavitt F: The physical exertion factor in compensable work injuries: A hidden flaw in previous research. Spine 17:307–310, 1992.
58. Lechner D, Bradbury SF, Bradley LA: Detecting sincerity of effort: A summary of methods and approaches. Phys Ther 78:867–888, 1998.
59. Lechner D, Roth D, Straaton K: Functional capacity evaluation in work disability. Work 1:37–47, 1991.
60. Lister G: The Hand: Diagnosis and Indications, 3rd ed. New York, Churchill Livingstone, pp 162–163, 1984.
61. Litigation and Workers' Compensation: A Report to Industry. Report to the Governor and California Legislature, 1979.
62. Lorig KR, Mazonson PD, Holman HR: Evidence suggesting that health education for self-management in patients with chronic arthritis has sustained health benefits while reducing health care costs. Arthritis Rheum 36:439–446, 1993.
63. Madson TJ, Youdas JW, Suman VJ: Reproducibility of lumbar spine range of motion measurements using the back range of motion device. J Orthop Sports Phys Ther 29:470–477, 1999.
64. Magora A: Investigation of the relation between low back pain and occupation. V. Psychological aspects. Scand J Rehabil Med 5:191–196, 1973.
65. Magnusson M, Granqvist M, Jonson R, et al. The loads on the lumbar spine during work at an assembly line. The risks for fatigue injuries of vertebral bodies. Spine 15:774; 1990.

66. Matheson LN: Use of the BTE Work Simulator to screen for symptom magnification syndrome. Ind Rehabil Q 2:5–31, 1989.
67. Mathiowetz V: Role of physical performance component evaluations in occupational therapy functional assessment. Am J Occup Ther 47:225–230, 1993.
68. Mayer RS, Chen IH, Lavender SA, et al: Variance in the measurement of sagittal lumbar spine range of motion among examiners, subjects, and instruments. Spine 20:1489–1493, 1995.
69. Mayer TG, Gatchel RJ, Kishono N, et al: Objective assessment of spine function following industrial injury: A prospective study with comparison group and one year follow up. Spine 10:483–493, 1985.
70. Milhous RL, Haugh LD, Frymoyer JW, et al: Determinants of vocational disability in patients with low back pain. Arch Phys Med Rehabil 70:589–593, 1989.
71. Nachemson AL: Back problems in childhood and adolescence (in Swedish). Lakartidningen 65:2831–2842, 1968.
72. Nachemson AL: Work for all. Clin Orthop 179:77, 1983.
73. Nachemson AL, Bigos SJ: The low back. In Cruess RL, Rennie WRJ (eds): Adult Orthopaedics. New York, Churchill Livingstone, 1984, pp 843–937.
74. Nagi S: An epidemiology of disability among adults in the United States. Milbank Mem Fund Q 54:439–468 1976.
75. National Guideline Clearinghouse. Available at: http://www.guidelines.gov/index.asp.
76. National Safety Council: Accident Facts. Itasca, Ill, National Safety Council, 1998.
77. Nitschke JE, Nattrass CL, Dissler PB, et al: Reliability of the American Medical Association Guides' model for measuring spinal range of motion. Its implication for whole-person impairment rating. Spine 24:262–268, 1999.
78. Noyes R Jr, Clancy J: The dying role: Its relevance to improved patient care. Psychiatry 40:41–47, 1977.
79. Nylander A, Carmean G: Medical standards project—Final report, vols 1 and 2, 2nd rev ed. San Bernadino County, Calif, Office of Personnel Management, 1983.
80. OSHA Ergonomics Programs Standard, 29 CFR 1910, Subpart W, November 2000.
81. Walker J, Holloway I, Sofaer B: In the system: the livid experience of chronic back pain. Pain 80:621–628, 1999.
82. Panzarella JP: The nature of work, job loss, and the diagnostic complexities of the psychologically injured worker. Psych Ann 21:10–15, 1991.
83. Pedersen PA: Prognostic indicators in low back pain. J R Coll Gen Pract 31:209–216, 1981.
84. Peterson MA, Reville RT, Steen RK, et al: Compensating Permanent Workplace Injuries: A Study of the California System (RAND MR-920-ICJ). Institute for Civil Justice, 1998.
85. Portney LG, Watkins MP: Foundations of Clinical Research: Applications to Practice. East Norwalk, Conn, Appleton & Lange, 1993, p 680.
86. Postal L: Medical–Legal Interference: Disability Evaluation. St. Louis, American Medical Association, 1996, p 59.
87. RAND: Findings and Recommendations on California's Permanent Partial Disability System: Executive Summary (Rachel Kaganoff Stern, Mark A. Peterson, Robert Reville, Mary E. Vaiana). Santa Monica, CA, RAND, 1997.
88. Ransford AO, Cairns D, Mooney V: The pain drawing as an aid to the psychological evaluation of patients with low back pain. Spine 1:127–134, 1976.
89. Reed P: The Medical Disability Advisor, 4th ed. Boulder, CO, Reed Group, 2001.
90. Reitsma B, Meijler WJ: Pain and patienthood. Clin J Pain 13:9–21, 1997.
91. Return to work patterns for permanently impaired workers. Texas Monitor 1:1–12, 1996.
92. Romano JM, Turner JA: Chronic pain and depression: Does the evidence support a relationship? Psych Bull 97:18, 1985.
93. Rowe ML: Preliminary statistical study of low back pain. J Occup Med 5:336–341, 1963.
94. Sander RA, Meyers JE: The relationship of disability to compensation status in railroad workers. Spine 11:141–143, 1986.
95. Shirley FR, O'Connor P, Robinson ME, MacMillan M: Comparison of lumbar range of motion using three measurement devices in patients with chronic low back pain. Spine 19:779–783, 1994.
96. Simon MJ: Rey 15-item test to assess malingering. J Clin Psychiatry 50:913–917, 1994.
97. Social Security Administration: Program Operations Manual System, Part 04, Disability Insurance, Chapter 245, Subchapter 15, paragraph 061C3, Federal Register, 65 FR 34950.
98. Social Security Administration: Program Operations Manual System, Part 04, Disability Insurance, Chapter 245, Subchapter 15, paragraph 065A, Federal Register, 65 FR 34950.
99. Solomon PE: Measurement of pain behavior. Physiotherapy Canada 48:52–58, 1996.
100. State of Utah Functional Ability in Driving: Guidelines Standards for Health Care Professionals. Utah State Driver's License Medical Advisory Board. Oct 2000 Edition. PO 30560, Salt Lake City, UT 84130–0560.
101. Stokes HM: The seriously uninjured hand: Weakness of grip. J Occup Med 25:683–684, 1983.
102. Stone D: The Disabled State. Philadelphia, Temple University Press, 1984.
103. Stung JP: The chronic disability syndrome. In Aronoff GM (ed): Evaluation and Treatment of Chronic Pain. Baltimore, Urban & Schwarzenberg, 1985.
104. Suesterhaus MP: Orthopedic Physical Therapy, Functional Capacity Evaluation Study Course, Orthopedic Section. American Physical Therapy Association, 1998, pp 1–14.
105. Sullivan MS, Dickinson CE, Troup JD: The influence of age and gender on lumbar spine sagittal plane range of motion. A study of 1126 healthy subjects. Spine 19:682–686, 1994.
106. Taylor T: Working around workers' injuries. Nation's Business 76:39–40, 1988.
107. The Industrial Commission of Utah: Utah's 1997 Impairment Guides. Salt Lake City, Utah, The Industrial Commission of Utah, 1997.
108. Thomas MH: Work place Functional Ability Guidelines. Salt Lake City, Utah, Utah Medical Association, 1994.
109. Tramposh AK: The functional capacity evaluation: Measuring maximal work abilities. Occup Med 7:113–124, 1992.
110. Troup JDG, Martin JW, Lloyd DCEF: Back pain in industry. A prospective survey. Spine 6:61–69, 1981.
111. U.S. Chamber of Commerce: 1997 Analysis of Workers' Compensation Laws. Washington, DC, U.S. Chamber of Commerce, 1997.
112. U.S. Department of Labor: Bureau of Labor Statistics, Workplace Injuries and Illnesses in 1998. Washington, DC, U.S. Department of Labor, 1999, p 3.
113. U.S. Equal Employment Opportunity Commission: A Technical Assistance Manual on the Employment Provision (Title I) of the Americans With Disabilities Act (Section VI-7). Washington, DC, US Equal Employment Opportunity Commission, 1992.
114. U.S. Employment Service: Dictionary of Occupational Titles, 4th ed. Washington, DC, U.S. Government Printing Office, 1991, p 1013.
115. U.S. National Library of Medicine, www.nlm.nih.gov.
116. Vallfors B: Acute, subacute and chronic low back pain: Clinical symptoms, absenteeism and working environment. Scand J Rehabil Med 11(Suppl.):1–98, 1985.

117. Vocational Services Bureau: Appendix C—Physical demands. In The Classification Of Jobs According To Worker Trait Factors: Addendum of Occupational Titles. Roswell, Ga, Vocational Services Bureau, 1977.
118. Waddell G: The Back Pain Revolution. New York, Churchill Livingstone, 1998, pp 4–5.
119. Waddell G, Bircher M, Finlayson D, Main CJ: Symptoms and signs: Physical disease or illness behavior? Br Med J Clin Res Educ 289:739–741, 1984.
120. Waddell G, Main C, Morris E, et al: Chronic low back pain, psychologic distress, and illness behavior. Spine 9:209–213, 1984.
121. Waddell G, McCulloch JA, Kummel E, Venner RM: Nonorganic physical signs in low-back pain. Spine 5:117–125, 1980.
122. Walton M: The Demming Management Method. New York, Putnam, 1986.
123. Weinstein MR: The concept of the disability process. Psychosomatics 19:94–97, 1978.
124. Wernecke MW, Harris DE, Lichter RL: Clinical effectiveness of behavioral signs for screening chronic low back pain patients in a work-oriented physical rehabilitation program. Spine 18:2412–2418, 1993.
125. Wesolek JS, McFarlane FR: Perceived needs for vocational assessment information as determined by those who utilize assessment results. Vocational Evaluation & Work Adjustment Bulletin 24:55–60, 1991.
126. Westin CG: Low back sick-listing: a nosological and medical insurance investigation. Scand J Soc Med (Suppl. 7):1–116, 1973.
127. Woo SL, Vogrin TM, Abramowitch SD: Healing and repair of ligament injuries in the knee. J Am Acad Orthop Surg 8:364–372, 2000.
128. Woo SLY, An KN, Arnoczky SP, et al: Anatomy, biology, and biomechanics of tendons, ligament, and meniscus. In Simon SR (ed): Orthopedic Basic Science. Rosemont, Ill, American Academy of Orthopedic Surgeons, 1994, pp 45–87.
129. Work-Loss Data Institute: Official Disability Guidelines, 3rd ed. Corpus Christi, TX, Work-Loss Data Institute, 1998.
130. Yuker HE: The Disability Hierarchies: Comparative Reactions to Various Types of Physical and Mental Disabilities. Hempstead, NY, Hofstra University Press, 1987.
131. Cocchiarella L, Lord SJ Master the AMA Guides Fifth: A Medical and Legal Transition to the Guides to the Evaluation of Permanent Impairment, Fifth Edition. First Edition. Chicago, American Medical Association, 2001.
132. Gerhardt JJ, Cocchiarella L, Lea RD: The Practical Guide to Range of Motion Assessment, First Edition. Chicago, American Medical Association, 2002.

CHAPTER

54

Ergonomic Basis for Job-related Strength Testing

DON B. CHAFFIN, PhD

Impairment evaluations are performed by physicians. These examinations provide information about a patient's health status. Disability determinations use the impairment evaluation as one of the criteria in assessing a work-related injury. One of the goals of a disability determination is to determine a person's ability to return to work. This ability is evaluated according to the worker's capabilities and the particular job demands. Capabilities are determined by measuring an individual's total medical impairments, including the degree (total or partial), organ system involved, and the time course (temporary or permanent), as well as an individual's psychosocial capabilities, such as pain tolerance, adaptability, and level of training. The demands of the job are assessed by methods including biomechanics, energy expenditure (see Chapter 24), and time and motion study.

The combination of the worker's capabilities and the demands of the job results in a functional capacity analysis (see Chapters 51 and 54 through 56). These determinations not only establish whether an impaired worker can return to his or her former job, but also can help indicate what type of alternate job or job modification would be appropriate. This chapter introduces one of the available job evaluation topics—ergonomics.

Ergonomics is a word derived from two Greek words: "ergo," meaning work, and "nomos," meaning principles or laws. Within industry, ergonomics methods and principles are used to evaluate and design tools, equipment, tasks, and procedures to assure the highest human performance possible while minimizing errors and hazards. Clearly, in application, ergonomics requires an eclectic philosophy and knowledge from different disciplines rooted in the life, behavioral, and engineering sciences.

In recent years the occupational applications of ergonomics have emphasized biomechanics as one primary science.[5] This focus on the physical aspects of worker-hardware systems in industry has arisen due to:

1. The increasing recognition that people's musculoskeletal systems are vulnerable to a variety of overstress syndromes that are caused, or at least aggravated by, common manual exertion in jobs.
2. The ability to measure objectively human musculoskeletal exertion capabilities, which has produced a realization that normal, healthy workers vary greatly in their performance capabilities (e.g., approximately 10:1 difference in functional strength capabilities).
3. The emergence of computerized biomechanical models that allow the study and prediction of normal human performance capabilities in different work settings.
4. The development of methods to quantify the physical stresses associated with many different types of manual tasks.

WHY PERFORM BIOMECHANICAL JOB EVALUATIONS?

The ability to allow a person to return to work, or to be classified as permanently disabled, depends a great deal on the types of jobs available to that person. As summarized by Feuerstein,[12] there are multiple factors that affect return-to-work decisions. Some of these are depicted in Figure 54–1.

In essence, returning a person to productive work after injury to the musculoskeletal system requires a comprehensive and well-managed program. Information from many experts is needed at different times in the rehabilitation and return-to-work process. This information often will vary greatly as the person's functional capabilities change and as the employer's work requirements are altered by new production and technical conditions or by attempts to modify the work to accommodate the person's limitations. The acquisition and effective use of this information is not easy. As Sandler[27] wrote:

> The difficulty in predicting the eventual outcome of a patient's injury helps fuel to a great extent the costs and abuses in worker's compensation. Additionally, once . . . impairment has been declared by a medical practitioner, it is rarely removed no matter what happens down the road. It is often difficult to know exactly how much a stabilized injury will limit function. Careful functional capacity evaluations against job-specific medical standards will provide fair, consistent, and predictable assessments for such injuries.

The question is not as much about whether specific job information should be considered in a return-to-work or disability decision, but rather what type of job information should be considered and how can it be acquired. Because human strength performance varies so greatly in a healthy population, and is affected by injury and resulting pain-related performance inhibition, knowing a job's strength performance requirement relative to population norms is often critical. If the job strength requirements are well documented, these can not only provide the basis for job-related functional evaluations of individuals who wish to return to gainful employment, but also provide the information necessary to justify the need for specific assistive technologies, such as pallet lifts so people do not have to bend to lift from near floor level or balance hoists and articulated arms to move heavy objects. In essence, by combining information from both population and job attributes related to human strength performance, a better match is achieved, as indicated in Figure 54–2.

USE OF STRENGTH TESTING IN INDUSTRY

Although it is difficult to say when strength testing per se first became popular in industry, Frederick W. Taylor[29] advocated selection of the best workers for each particular task in his now-famous book *Principles of Scientific Management*, published in 1929. The armed forces have since formally recognized that strength and endurance are required in most combat duties. In this latter regard, "Liftest" was advocated for Air Force personnel selection by Kroemer.[19] Liftest consists of a set of handles that slide in a vertical track. These are lifted by the person being evaluated from near the floor to overhead reach. With repeated trials additional weight is added to the handles until the person can no longer perform the lift. This procedure is reported to simulate many different common lifting tasks in the Air Force, thus having content validity.

Human strength as measured in Liftest and other such tests is defined as the ability to perform a maximum volitional exertion for a few seconds, with adequate rest between trials to avoid fatigue. Performance in such strength tests is measured as either the peak or average force (or moment) displayed by the person for a few seconds of exertion.[3] The person may apply the force against a stationary load-measuring device in which case static or isometric strength is measured. A formal protocol for this type of testing has been devel-

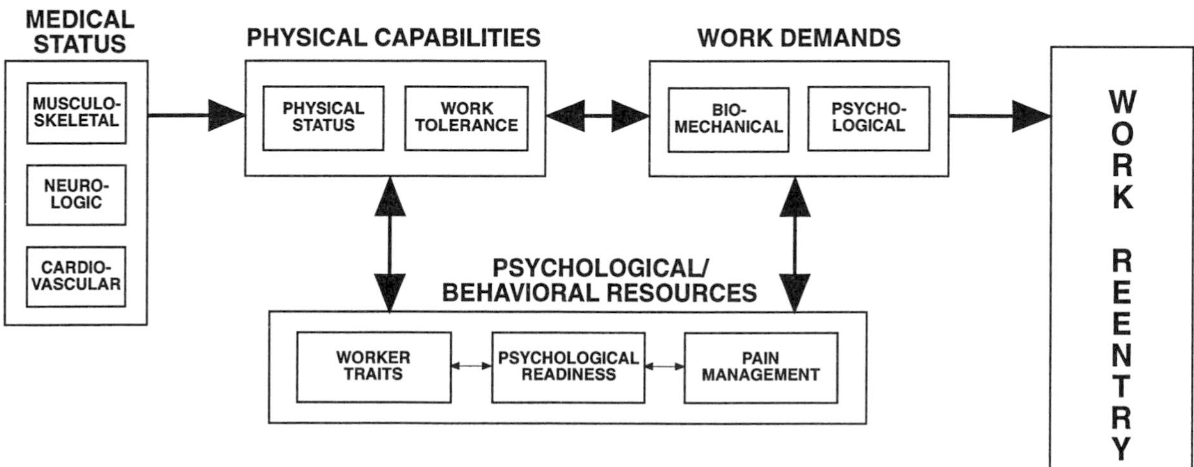

Figure 54–1. Multiple factors potentially affecting return to work following occupational musculoskeletal injury/illness. Conceptual model of work disability. (From Feurestein M: Workers' compensation reform in New York State: A proposal to address medical, ergonomic, and psychological factors associated with work disability. J Occup Rehab 3:125–135, 1993.)

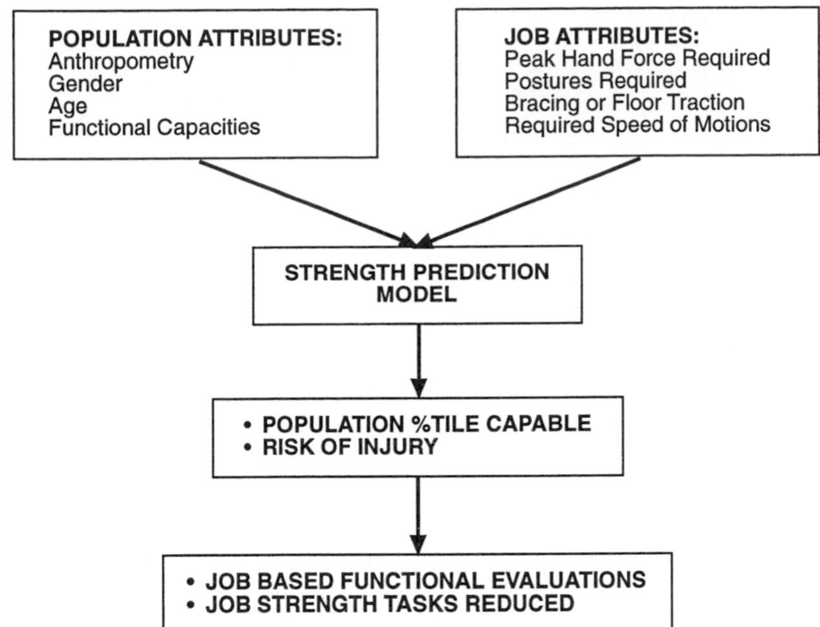

Figure 54–2. Logic used to guide job strength–based functional evaluations of patients and ergonomic assistive technologies to accommodate injured workers.

oped by the American Industrial Hygiene Association (AIHA).[3] If movement occurs, as in the Liftest, then the test is a measure of dynamic strength. If the load applied is moved at a constant velocity, which is possible for only a limited part of the motion and for one body segment, then it is referred to as isokinetic strength (i.e., near constant velocity). The latter type of test requires expensive equipment to control the velocity. In general, the faster the speed of motion, the lower the resulting dynamic strengths. Figure 54–3 depicts a comparison of dynamic back- and arm-lifting strengths performed at various speeds. The result of this phenomenon is that when an object to be lifted approximates the lifting strength of a person performing the lift, the slower the lift will become (i.e., less dynamic stress is created).

Isokinetic tests have been developed primarily for clinical use, wherein a designated strength-speed evaluation involving a specific joint is needed to assess treatment effectiveness. A 1994 study by Wheeler et al[31] has shown that in a laboratory, carefully performed isometric and isokinetic trunk-extension strength tests can predict simple lifting capacities ($r^2 > 0.88$). A critical review of such applications by Newton and Waddell,[25] however, indicates a lack of good empirical evidence for use of standardized trunk testing to predict risk of low-back injury. These same investigators confirmed, as have others, that isolated dynamic trunk strengths are lower in patients with low back pain when compared to healthy individuals, but the overlap in strength distributions between the two groups is so large as to negate the practical use of such tests for prediction of future risk or status of low back injury.[24]

The Liftest described earlier is a form of dynamic, whole-body strength test. Because the load being moved is constant with each trial, it is referred to as an isoinertial (constant mass) type of test. By incrementally increasing the loads between trials, the testing procedure is referred to as a psychophysical protocol (i.e., the physical stress is increased until the person perceives he or she can no longer tolerate it). This type of testing is becoming standard for functional strength performance evaluations. When careful protocols are used, very good test-retest values are achieved.[9,28] The ability of a standardized isoinertial or isometric lifting test to predict general lifting capability has been shown by Jiang et al[13] and Aghazadeh and Ayoub[1] to be excellent, with $r^2 > 0.77$ for isoinertial tests and $r^2 > 0.72$ for isometric tests. The ability of various types of tests to predict on-job exertion capability accurately is essential to meet the requirements of the Americans With Disabilities Act (ADA) (see Chapters 47 and 54). Such a requirement has further stimulated the development of whole-body work capacity types of strength evaluations.[11]

Whether these newer whole-body work capacity strength tests can predict who is at risk of future musculoskeletal injury remains in question. Isokinetic and isometric testing using standardized (non–job specific) lifting postures have not been able to predict low-back injury.[2,10,23] Earlier studies by Chaffin et al[6] and Keyserling et al[16] using job-specific isometric tests indicated that workers who could not demonstrate the strength to perform specific high-strength elements in their jobs were about three times more at risk than their stronger counterparts. The difference in the outcome of these studies appears to be how well the functional strength tests replicated the high-strength elements in the workers' jobs.

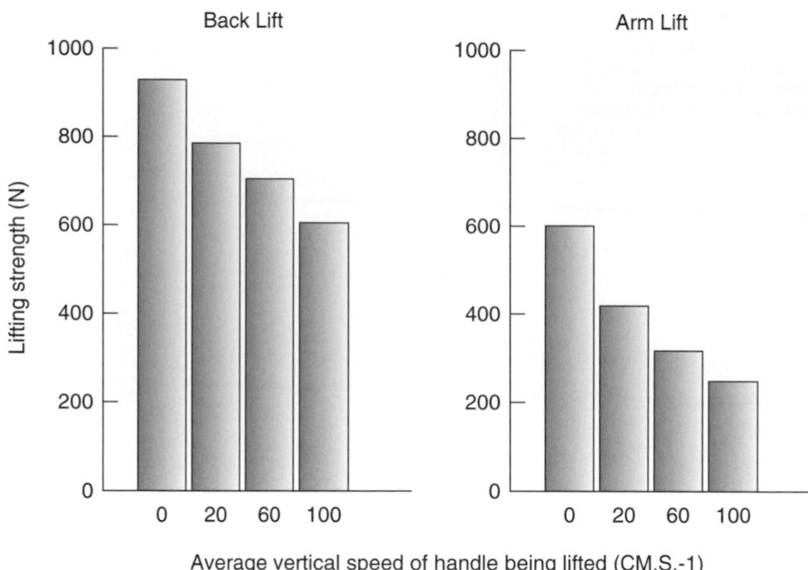

Figure 54–3. Typical dynamic lifting strength test mean results for 10 healthy men performing maximum isokinetic lifts at different lift speeds. (From Kumar S, Chaffin DB, Redfern M: Isometric and isokinetic back-and-arm-lifting strengths: Device and measurement. J Biomech 21:35–44, 1988.)

IDENTIFYING HIGH-STRENGTH ELEMENTS IN A JOB

Given that ADA and occupational health and safety outcomes depend on the data used to define job strength demands, how can such data be acquired? Traditionally, industrial engineers and work methods practitioners in companies have been held responsible for the following, which can become useful in this quest[5].

1. Developing a preferred work method (sequence of motions) to be used by a worker to minimize the time required to perform a manual job
2. Documenting the preferred method and any conditions that would affect a person's performance
3. Determining the standard time for the job to be performed by a healthy, normal worker
4. Preparing training materials and aids to assure a general understanding of the preferred work method

Detailed studies by time and motion study personnel in many different industries for over 70 years have resulted in formalized classifications for different types of elemental reaches, moves, grasps, and positions. The time that a well-trained worker would require to perform each of these elemental motions also has been determined and is well predicted. These predetermined times are used by time and motion analysis to predict job performance times.[17]

The procedure for such analyses requires a time and motion study analyst to identify through reference to published tables similar time values for the following standardized elemental motions:

1. Reach—a motion of the unloaded hands or fingers
2. Position—small motion necessary when aligning object to be released at end of motion
3. Release—either a distinct motion of fingers or the release of an object at the end of a motion without such an overt motion
4. Disengage—an involuntary (rebound) motion often required when two objects suddenly come apart under exertion
5. Grasp—an overt motion necessary to gain control of an object
6. Eye focus travel—the time required for the eyes to move and accommodate to provide visualization of an object
7. Turn apply pressure—the manipulation of controls, tools, and objects necessary to turn an object by rotation of the hand about the long axis of the forearm
8. Body, leg/foot motion—the motion of transporting the body with values given per step for varied conditions
9. Simultaneous motions—rules are given so that some motions can be performed together (for example, both the right and left hand reach to an object); therefore only the greater of these two time values is used in standard time prediction

As one can imagine from this list, a great deal of detailed job information is available from such a job analysis. Although widely used in many industries for estimating production capacities and labor costs, some important biomechanical information still needs to be added for ergonomic purposes. For instance, although the load a person moves may be noted, only the average load is needed for time prediction purposes. Biomechanically, the peak load handled is normally the most strength required, but often only average loads or weights being handled frequently are documented in traditional time-and-motion studies. A second limitation arises in that extreme work postures are not delineated in traditional time-and-motion studies. The reality is that when a person must reach down to the floor or to the side or overhead while applying large forces to lift, push, or pull on an object, high biomechanical strength is required. Finally, traditional time-and-motion study only documents those work elements that comprise at least 95% of the job content (i.e., the time-related productive activities). Unfortunately, many peak biomechanical strength requirements are created but go undocumented when a worker performs auxiliary tasks (e.g., replaces stock, lifts and moves defective parts, and performs machine maintenance).

In essence, traditional time-and-motion study information provides an excellent beginning for a biomechanical job strength analysis. Too often this valuable information is neglected because ergonomics or health and safety experts will use simple checklists to document the frequency and types of lifting, stooping, walking, or carrying in a job.[5] Such general checklists may suffice for rapid identification of potential exertion-related problems in many different jobs, but they rarely contain enough information to discriminate exposures to specific peak biomechanical stresses.[15]

Perhaps because of such deficiencies, a third approach to job strength evaluation has emerged recently. This approach uses videotaping of incumbent workers performing the tasks reported by them and their supervisors to require high levels of exertion to perform. This direct observation method was found to be more accurate than self-reporting alone of high manual-stress job conditions.[32] If care is taken to ensure that the video data can be scaled—that is, size of objects and their orientation is known in each frame—adequate postural data can be acquired for subsequent biomechanical analyses.[26]

It should be noted that in addition to the postural requirements of a job provided from the videotapes, hand force data must be acquired with particular emphasis on the peak hand forces incurred, especially when the exertion is performed while a person is in an awkward posture. Normally these hand loading data are obtained either by weighing objects that are lifted or by using a hand-held force gauge for measuring push-and-pull forces.[5] Care must be taken to ensure that both the direction of the hand force as well as its magnitude is determined. As shown in Figure 54–4, in unencumbered lifting the hand force vector at the beginning of the lift is toward the body. As the lift proceeds, after about 200 to 300 msec when the load is closer to the body, the hand force vector becomes more vertical. It is at this latter location that the peak acceleration of the object often causes the hand forces to be the largest (perhaps 30% to 50% larger than the static weight of the object if the load is well below a person's lifting strength). It is at this point in the lift that the biomechanical analysis should be performed to determine the peak strengths required for a population or person who may be assigned such a task.

NATIONAL INSTITUTE OF OCCUPATIONAL SAFETY AND HEALTH (NIOSH) LIFTING GUIDE JOB EVALUATION METHOD

If a job's most physically stressful elements are believed to be caused by two-handed lifting tasks, then the NIOSH revised equation for manual lifting evaluation should be consulted.[30] The purpose of the NIOSH analysis procedure is to combine analytically several physical workspace and task factors into the prediction of a recommended weight limit (RWL). The six job factors that must be considered for each lift being performed are:

1. The horizontal (H) distance from the object being lifted to the person's ankles.
2. The vertical (V) distance of the object from the floor at the beginning of the lift.
3. The distance (D) the object is moved vertically.
4. The asymmetry (A) of the object location relative to the person's lower body and legs when beginning a lift. If the object is directly in front of a person, it would be symmetrically located.
5. The degree of hand grip coupling (C) with the object.
6. The frequency (F) of lifts per minute during 1-, 2-, or 8-hour periods.

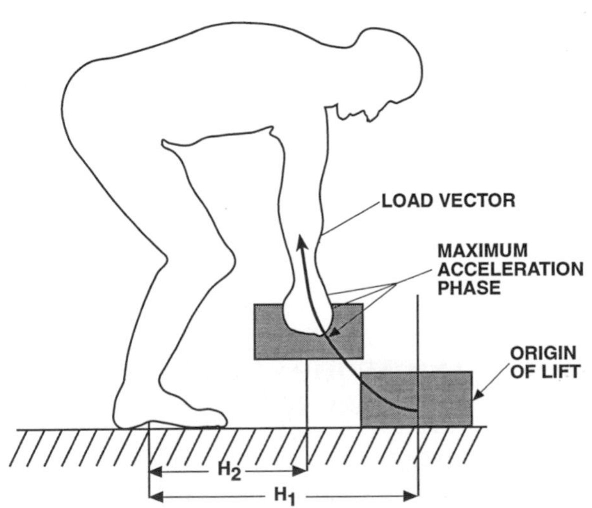

Figure 54–4. Example of typical load lifting trajectory during an unconstrained floor lift.

Given job data that describe each of the above factors, simple algebraic equations or tables are provided by NIOSH to estimate the amount of discounting due to each factor. In other words, if one knows the horizontal distance (H) at the beginning of a lift, a table, graph, or equation is provided that gives a modified HM value (which ranges from 0 to 1.0). The resulting modifiers are then used in the following multiplicative equation for computing the RWL (in pounds) for each lift:

RWL = 51 (HM) (VM) (DM) (AM) (CM) (FM)

If all of the job conditions are optimal, then each modification factor would equal 1.0, and the RWL would equal 51 pounds. This would only occur when a worker is standing erect, the load lifted is about 30 inches from the floor, it is compact and lifted close to the body and directly in front of the body, it is lifted only a couple of inches for a few seconds, and it is lifted less than once every 5 minutes. Clearly, this is not a very common task. Because the discounting modifiers often have values less than 1.0, it is not uncommon for a typical job that requires lifting of objects from the floor to have an RWL of 15 pounds or less.

NIOSH proposes that the RWL value for a lifting task represents the magnitude of weight that can be lifted by about 90% of normally healthy men and women in industry, and creates an L5/S1 spinal disc compression force of less than 770 pounds (3400 N [newtons]). If a weight being lifted on a job exceeds the RWL computed for the lift, then excessive musculoskeletal injuries would be expected, according to Waters et al.[30]

In essence, the NIOSH lifting analysis is a comprehensive lifting task evaluation process. It is based on a large amount of published human biomechanical, psychophysical, and physiologic data, and thus has good construct validity. For this reason it has been used by many different industries and government agencies to rank or rate the risk of injury in lifting jobs. In this context, it provides a rigorous method for identifying those types of lifts that would be most difficult and potentially hazardous to perform. It does not, however, provide a means to evaluate one-handed lifting, nor does it apply to any other types of manual tasks than two-handed lifting (e.g., pushing or pulling exertions are excluded).

BIOMECHANICAL JOB STRENGTH AND LOW-BACK EVALUATION

Because the NIOSH Work Practices Guide for Manual Lifting applies only to lifting with two hands, a more comprehensive job physical stress analysis scheme may be necessary to provide the basis for job-related strength testing. One such scheme relies on a computerized static-strength prediction model described in Chaffin et al.[5] This model compares the load moments produced at various body joints when a person performs manual exertions. Population norms obtained from tests of over 2000 workers in the United States are then used for comparison. By performing this comparison at each body joint, the static-strength model predicts the proportion of the population capable of performing the exertion, as well as predicting compression forces that may be acting on the lower lumbar discs during the simulated exertions.

This computerized strength-prediction methodology provides the means to evaluate a variety of manual exertion data obtained from direct observations of workers. The job analysis procedure is generally the same as that adopted by NIOSH in that a job is first described as a series of physical exertions. What is different, however, is that the analyst must also identify the load vector direction operating on each hand (i.e., "lift" is a vertical plane, downward load vector; "push" is a sagittal plane, horizontal load vector toward the body; and "pull" is a sagittal plane, horizontal load vector away from the body). In addition, for each task the posture of the torso and extremities at the time of a peak exertion of interest are recorded, usually from measuring body segment angles obtained from stop-action videos or photographs. These postural images are simultaneously compared to a computer-generated human form, which can be easily manipulated to replicate the video images of interest.

An example of the use of this method is shown in Figure 54–5 for the lifting of a 44-pound (200-N) stock reel. The input and output screens from the 3D Static Strength Prediction Program (3DSSPP) developed at The University of Michigan are displayed. The input data required are 1) load magnitude and direction (example: 44 pounds [200 N] acting downward at −90°), 2) whether one or two hands are involved (example: two hands are lifting the stock reel), 3) general anthropometry of people to be analyzed (example: average weight and stature of men and women are assumed), and 4) the body postural angles relative to a horizontal reference axis. The latter is shown as a silhouette from a photograph in Figure 54–5, with the reference angles superimposed. Given these input data, the program then outputs several results, shown at the bottom of Figure 54–5. First is a stick figure drawing of the human kinematic linkage being analyzed along with a solid 3D hominoid. Comparison of these computer images with a photograph, video image, or drawing board manikin provides a qualitative check on the postural-input angles. Also, the vertical and horizontal coordinates of the load or hand center, relative to the ankle, and the L5/S1 disc horizontal to load center distance provide quantitative checks on the postural and anthropometric input values (i.e., is the load located where one expects it to be relative to that measured from the person being analyzed?).

If the input data are appropriate, the logic described in Chaffin et al[5] and outlined in Figure 54–6 is executed, and the program displays 1) a graphical and tabular prediction of the percentage of the male or female populations expected to have sufficient static strength at each major joint, 2) a graphical and tabular prediction of the L5/S1 disc compression forces for men or women, 3) the required static coefficient-of-friction required to not slip, and 4) a statement as to whether the task being performed would result in loss of balance.

In this context, the stock reel lifting analysis depicted earlier in Figure 54–5 shows that:

1. The moment strength requirements are greatest at the hips, with only 83% of men having the expected hip extensor strengths. A separate analysis for women (not shown) indicated that only 54% of women had sufficient hip extensor strengths.
2. The large H distance and stooped posture cause the predicted compression forces on the L5/S1 disc to be high, over 900 pounds (4375 N), which is above the NIOSH spinal limit of 770 pounds (3400 N).
3. Because it is a vertical lift, the required floor static coefficient-of-friction is 0, and no forward or backward balance problem exists for the posture analyzed.

Further analysis with the 3DSSPP™ model of successive postures required to lift the 44-pound stock reel up to the stock holder (63 inches above the floor) revealed an interesting trade-off between excessive back stress and shoulder strength demands. Both of these biomechanical outcomes are plotted in Figure 54–7, with predicted L5/S1 compression forces at the top and the predicted percent of men and women with enough strength shown in the bottom graph. Inspection of the graphs shows that when the load is in the middle position the spinal compression force is at its lowest value and the greatest percent of the population could perform such an exertion. As the load is lifted higher to the stock holder, spinal-compression forces approach (or slightly exceed) the suggested NIOSH hazard level and fewer than 40% of women and only about 80% of

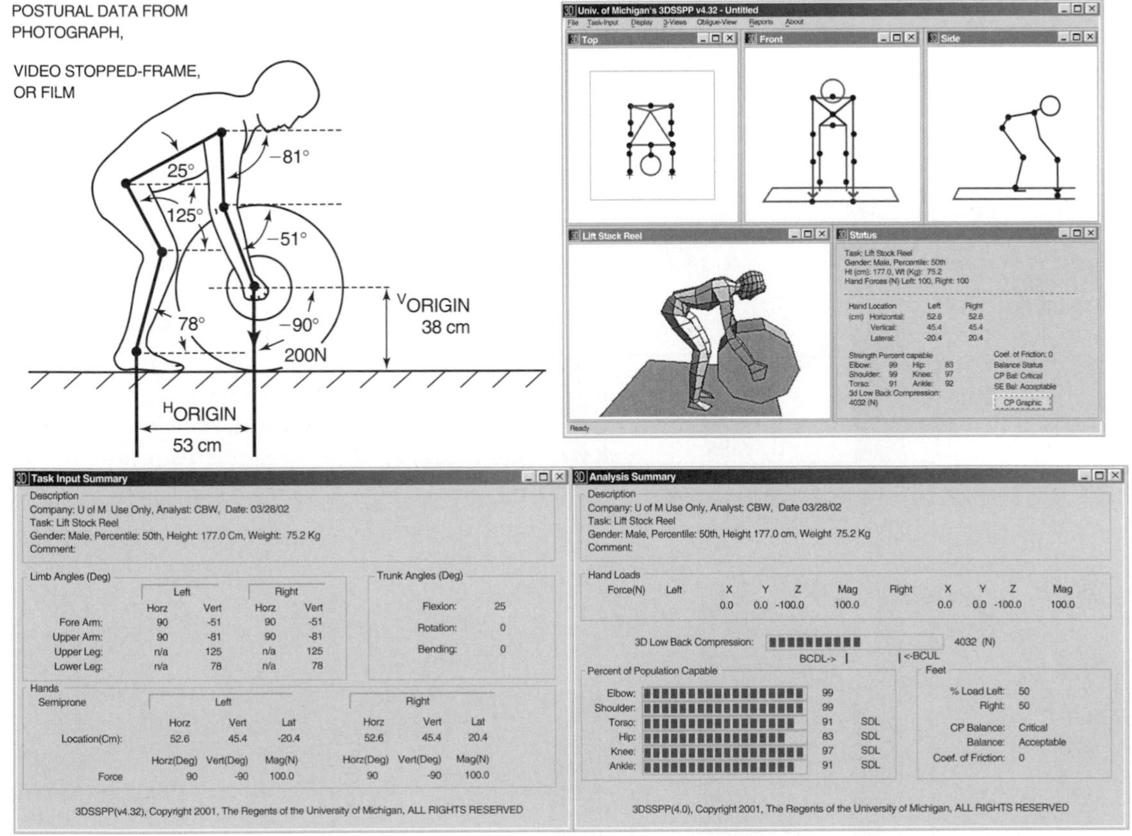

Figure 54–5. The University of Michigan 3D Static Strength Prediction Program with the input conditions for evaluating the stock reel lifting task displayed at top and the resulting output screen displayed at bottom. (Courtesy of The Regents of the University of Michigan.)

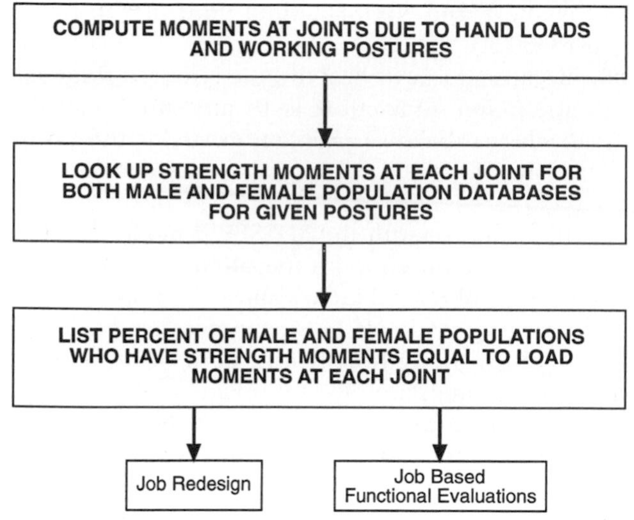

Figure 54–6. Logic used in 3D Static Strength Prediction Program. (From Chaffin DB, Anderson GBJ, Martin BJ: Occupational Biomechanics, 3rd ed. New York, John Wiley & Sons, 1999, with permission.)

men have the shoulder strengths required for such a high lift.

Although the static strength prediction program provides a powerful tool for determining the various conditions on a job that demand a great deal of strength, it is only a static simulation of an exertion. Marras et al[22] have shown that not only is it important to know what the peak low-back moment requirements are to assign a risk level to a job but that the velocity of the person's torso motion can be a separate risk factor. Indeed, when young, healthy men were asked to lift a load from the floor to a table, they chose a maximal acceptable weight and lifted it dynamically in such a way that peak spinal compression forces were actually double the NIOSH hazard level for a more heterogenous population.[7] In other words, static biomechanical analyses may not be enough to understand all of the complex stresses in a particular exertion. Although dynamic biomechanical analysis models exist, they either require attaching electronic goniometers to workers or require sophisticated video processing tools to measure the motion dynamics. For these reasons their use in industry has been limited to studies of low back pain risk assessments.

SUMMARY

Given that most experts agree with the concept that disability should be determined by how well a person's functional capability matches required job demands, it is surprising that so many studies attempt to quantify the former with little or no attention given to the latter. In fact, it would appear that a large proportion

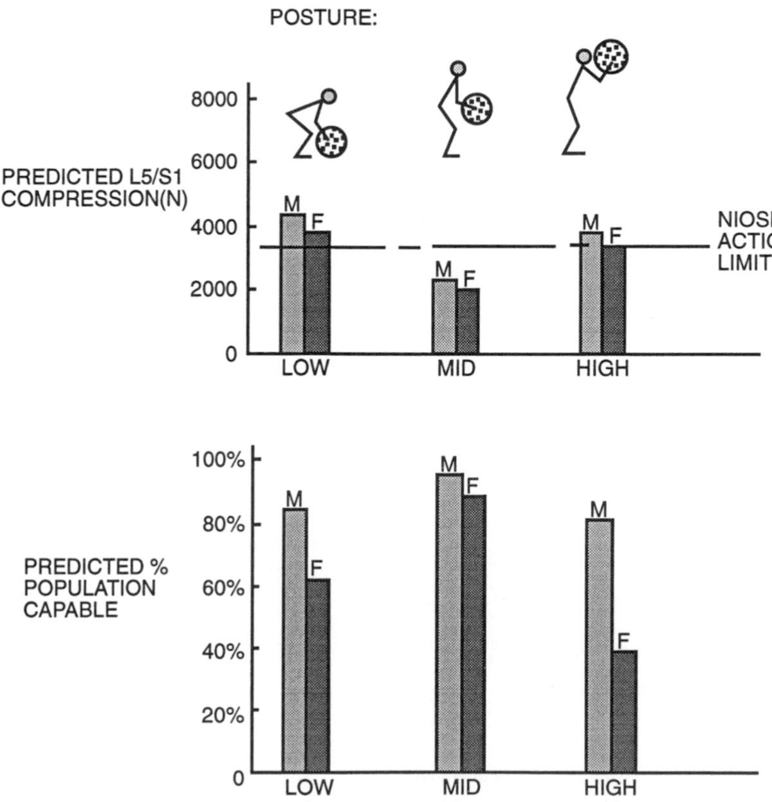

Figure 54–7. Lifting a 44-pound stock reel using UM-3DSSPP software with three different lift postures being evaluated. (From Chaffin DB: A biomechanical strength model for use in industry. Appl Ind Hyg 3:79–86, 1988.)

of the medical community would like to neglect job demand information altogether in determining an individual's capacity to work. A 1993 review by Clark and Haldeman[8] of factors used in rating impairment levels for neck and back injuries disclosed 37 factors believed to be important by a group of California Industrial Medical Examiners. Surprisingly, none of the 37 factors included the need to evaluate the patients' capabilities to perform specific manual jobs. In other words, rating work capacity in clinical practice seems to require only knowledge about the patient, not the job, despite continual recognition by rehabilitation experts regarding the importance of the work environment in disability determinations.[14,18] As long as the medical community ignores the fact that job demands vary greatly, their ability to make a fair and rational decision about a person's work status will be greatly compromised.

As Lehmann et al[21] have noted, "Patients must be encouraged to return to work, and employers encouraged to modify injured workers' job tasks to lighter duties until they have recovered sufficiently to return to normal duties." This is the essence of affirmative action. Only by knowing both the person's capabilities and the corresponding job demands can real progress be made. To accomplish this, those that know about people and those that know about the physics of jobs must work together to manage better the injured worker. Not only will the injured worker benefit from such a team approach but perhaps job biomechanical risk factors will be identified and reduced, thus benefiting all workers in the future.

References

1. Aghazadeh F, Ayoub MM: A comparison of dynamic and static strength models for prediction of lifting capacity. Ergonomics 28:1409–1417, 1985.
2. Battie MC, Bigos SJ, Fisher LD, et al: Isometric lifting strength as a predictor of industrial back pain reports. Spine 14:851–856, 1989.
3. Caldwell LS, Chaffin DB, Dukes-Dobos FN, et al: A proposed standard procedure for static muscle strength testing. Am Ind Hyg J 35:201–206, 1974.
4. Chaffin DB: A biomechanical strength model for use in industry. Appl Ind Hyg 3:79–86, 1988.
5. Chaffin DB, Andersson GBJ, Martin BJ: Occupational Biomechanics, 3rd ed. New York, John Wiley & Sons, 1999.
6. Chaffin DB, Herrin GD, Keyserling WM: Preemployment strength testing. J Occup Med 20:403–408, 1978.
7. Chaffin DB, Page GB: Postural effects on biomechanical and psychophysical weight lifting limits. Ergonomics 37:663–676, 1994.
8. Clark W, Haldeman S: The development of guideline factors for the evaluation of disability in neck and back injuries. Spine 18:1736–1745, 1993.
9. Dales JL, Macdonald EB, Anderson JAD: The Liftest strength test—an accurate method of dynamic strength assessment? Clin Biomech 1:11–13, 1986.
10. Dueker JA, Ritchie SM, Knox TJ, Rose SJ: Isokinetic trunk testing and employment. J Occup Med 36:42–48, 1993.
11. Dusik L, Menard MR, Cooke C, et al: Concurrent validity of the ERGOS work simulator versus conventional functional capacity evaluation techniques in a workers' compensation population. J Occup Med 35:759–767, 1993.
12. Feurestein M: Workers' compensation reform in New York state: A proposal to address medical, ergonomic, and psychological factors associated with work disability. J Occup Rehabil 3:125–135, 1993.
13. Jiang BC, Smith JL, Ayoub MM: Psychophysical modeling of manual materials-handling capacities using isoinertial strength variables. Hum Factors 28:691–702, 1986.
14. Johns RE Jr, Bloswick DS, Elegante JM, Colledge AL: Chronic, recurrent low-back pain. J Occup Med 36:537–547, 1994.
15. Keyserling WM, Brouwer M, Silverstein BA: A checklist for evaluating ergonomics risk factors resulting from awkward postures of the legs, trunk, and neck. Int J Industrial Ergonomics 9:283–301, 1992.
16. Keyserling WM, Herrin GD, Chaffin DB: Isometric strength testing as a means of controlling medical incidents on strenuous jobs. J Occup Med 22:332–336, 1980.
17. Konz S: Work Design. Columbus, Ohio, Grid Publishing, 1979.
18. Krause N, Ragland DR: Occupational disability due to low back pain: A new interdisciplinary classification based on a phase model of disability. Spine 19:1011–1020, 1994.
19. Kroemer KHE: Development of LIFTEST: A dynamic technique to assess individual capacity to lift material. NIOSH Report 210–79–0041. Cincinnati, Ohio, NIOSH, 1982.
20. Kumar S, Chaffin DB, Redfern M: Isometric and isokinetic back-and-arm-lifting strengths: Device and measurement. J Biomech 21:35–44, 1988.
21. Lehmann TR, Spratt KF, Lehmann KK: Predicting long-term disability in low-back-injured workers presenting to a spine consultant. Spine 18:1103–1112, 1993.
22. Marras WS, Lavender SA, Leurgans SE, et al: The role of dynamic three-dimensional trunk motion in occupationally related low back disorders. Spine 18:617–628, 1993.
23. Mostardi R, Noe DA, Kovacik MW, Porterfield JA: Isokinetic lifting strength and occupational injury. Spine 17:189–193, 1992.
24. Newton M, Thow M, Somerville D, et al: Trunk-strength testing with iso-machines—Part 2. Spine 18:812–824, 1993.
25. Newton M, Waddell G: Trunk-strength with iso-machines—Part 1. Spine 18:801–811, 1993.
26. Paul JA, Douwes M: Two-dimensional photographic posture recording and description: A validity study. Appl Ergonomics 24:83–90, 1993.
27. Sandler HM: ADA and occupational health: A status report. Occupational Hazards 55:55–56, 1993.
28. Snook SH: The design of manual handling tasks. Ergonomics 21:973–985, 1978.
29. Taylor W: The Principles of Scientific Management. New York, Harper, 1929.
30. Waters TR, Putz-Anderson V, Garg A, Fine LJ: Revised NIOSH equation for the design and evaluation of manual lifting tasks. Ergonomics 36:749–776, 1993.
31. Wheeler DL, Graves JE, Miller GJ, et al: Functional assessment for prediction of lifting capacity. Spine 19:1021–1026, 1994.
32. Wiktorin C, Karlqvist L, Winkel J: Stockholm Music I study group: Validity of self-reported exposures to work postures and manual materials handling. Scand J Work Environ Health 19:208–214, 1993.

CHAPTER

55

The Functional Capacity Evaluation

LEONARD N. MATHESON, PhD

In recent years, there has been an increased emphasis on the development of the scientific basis of the functional capacity evaluation (FCE). This has been stimulated by a growing awareness of its utility, and supported by major investments in research by large insurance providers and by state, provincial, and federal governmental agencies such as the United States Social Security Administration.[36] The most important development has been the application of a taxonomic approach to FCEs to organize and focus this research.[72] This chapter employs this taxonomic approach, using it to organize both conceptual and applied information. The material presented in this chapter is formed by findings from a research project that was funded by the Social Security Administration (SSA) to develop methods to use information about the patient's functional limitations to improve the SSA disability determination system. In order to render the task manageable within the limitations of a textbook format, this chapter is focused on FCEs with persons who have musculoskeletal impairments.

This chapter emphasizes the evidentiary basis of FCEs, in which results and opinions derived from FCE measures must be qualified in terms of science. It is clear today that FCEs must be based on standardized FCE measures that have acceptable psychometric properties.[6,7] Further, to be accepted as evidence in courts in the United States, FCE data must be based on the "existence and maintenance of standards controlling the technique's operation,"[23] including administration by trained and qualified personnel, using tests that have been demonstrated to be scientifically valid. This chapter presents the basic framework for the scientific practice of FCE, including a model of work disability and definitions of major terms and concepts.

DEFINITION

A FCE is a systematic method of measuring an individual's ability to perform meaningful tasks on a safe and dependable basis.[144] A FCE includes all impairments, not just those that result in physical functional limitations.[127] In general, the purpose of a FCE is to collect information about the functional limitations of a person with medical impairment. Beyond this general purpose, FCEs have three specific purposes:

1. To improve the likelihood that the patient/employee will be safe in subsequent job task performance.[83,157] Routinely, the comparison of a patient's/employee's abilities to a job's demands is made in an attempt to diminish the risk of reinjury that is associated with a mismatch. Shortfalls in the relationship between the worker's resources and the environment's demands result in stress[224] or increased risk for injury.[8,11,12,35] Numerous researchers point to the importance of properly matching the worker's capacity to the job's demands.[1,13,62,65,68,203,225]
2. To assist the patient/employee in improving role performance through identification of functional decrements so that they may be resolved or worked around.[95,154,177] Health care professionals use this information to triage patients into proper treatment programs and to measure treatment progress.

The studies presented here were supported in part by Contract No. 600-97-32018 from the Social Security Administration to the American Institutes for Research, Washington Research Center, Washington, DC. Washington University, St. Louis, served as a subcontractor. The views expressed in this article reflect those of the author and do not necessarily represent those of the U.S. government, Social Security Administration, American Institutes for Research, or Washington University.

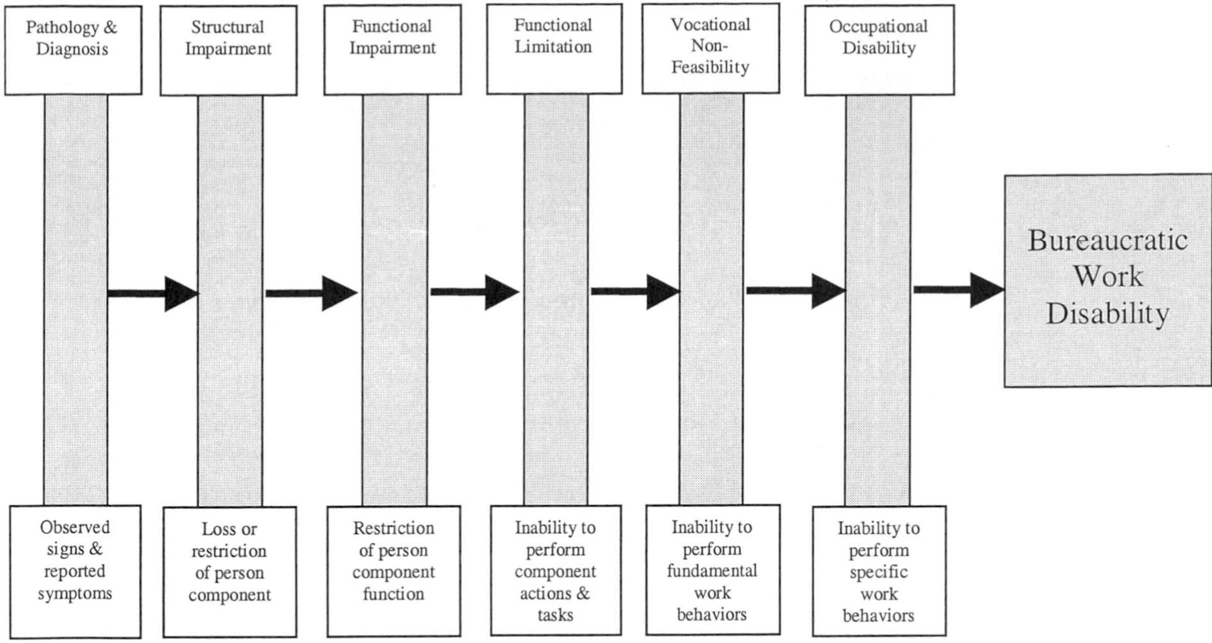

Figure 55–1. Conceptual model of bureaucratic work disability.

3. To determine the presence (and, if present, the degree) of disability so that a bureaucratic or juridical entity can assign, apportion, or deny financial and medical disability benefits.[5,155]

The term functional connotes performance of a purposeful, meaningful, or useful task that has a beginning and an end with a result that can be measured. Functional limitations are the effect of the individual's impairment on his or her ability to perform meaningful tasks. Function is the focus of this type of evaluation process because functional limitations translate the effect of impairment on disability.[144] Functional limitations are the proximal cause of disability. Several authors have described models of disablement.[107,166,167, 169,171,227,233,234] Models of disability have been developed that focus on the person as a worker.[42,131] A model of disability for industrial rehabilitation has been proposed,[154] as has a model to measure work disability for benefit entitlement as it is defined by the U.S. SSA.[72] A composite model, depicted in Figure 55–1, is used as a schematic for this chapter, employing the definitions presented in Table 55–1.

TABLE 55–1

Definitions Used in the Conceptual Model of Bureaucratic Work Disability

Stage	**Definition**	**Measured by or in terms of . . .**
Pathology and diagnosis	Medical abnormality	Observed signs and reported symptoms
Structural impairment	Loss or restriction of the organic or psychological component	Loss or restriction of the organic or psychological component compared to normal
Functional impairment	Loss or restriction of the organic or psychological component's ability to perform	Loss or restriction of the organic or psychological component's performance compared to normal
Functional limitation	Restriction of ability to perform simple observable behaviors that share a common purpose	Inability to perform actions and tasks
Vocational nonfeasibility	The acceptability of the patient as an employee in the most general sense	Inability to perform fundamental work behaviors
Occupational disability	Any restriction of ability resulting from functional limitation to perform an activity within the range considered normal for the occupation	Inability to perform specific work behaviors

This is a deterministic model with six related stages, across which causality is posited. Although the author recognizes that unidirectional causality is too simplistic for general use,[29,171,234] this model is designed to address bureaucratic needs for causal links between diagnosis and work disability, in which each succeeding stage is dependent on all preceding stages. This simple system is an example of those employed by most entities that administer disability determination systems to provide disability benefits, including the U.S. SSA. Disregarding the context of the individual's environmental and personal resources, this model describes pathology and impairment as factors that are the precursors of functional limitation, and thereby disability. It is silent on the issue of proportional linearity and the degree of impairment does not necessarily dictate the degree of functional limitation or disability; this hotly debated issue[45,47,108] is unresolved.[38] To implement this model of work disability, the physician uses a medical diagnostic evaluation to address pathology and impairment. If the structural or functional impairment is sufficiently severe, functional limitations can result. Beyond the evaluation of impairment, functional limitations are measured by physicians, occupational therapists, physical therapists, vocational evaluators, kinesiologists, psychologists, and exercise physiologists in a FCE. If the functional limitations are sufficiently severe and are pertinent to role tasks, disability with regard to that role can result. Disability can be described in terms of the role consequences of functional limitations.[53,107,169,171] Disability can be operationally defined as the patient's uncompensated shortfalls in responding to role demands.[144] Figure 55–2 represents this definition in graphic terms.

The FCE of disability is based on the measurement of the functional consequences of impairment in tasks that are pertinent to the particular role under consideration. In order to evaluate disability, one must measure functional limitations in terms of a particular role. Individuals assume several roles in society, such as spouse, parent, or worker. Functional limitations that are measured in terms of, for example, parental role tasks, are not as useful in determining whether a patient can return to work as are functional limitations that are measured in terms of worker role tasks. The emphasis in this chapter is on determining the presence or degree of work disability. In order to do so, it will focus on tasks in the worker role found within the work environment.[218] There are several contexts of measurement outside of the worker role focus that medical professionals are often concerned about, including measurement of the patient's ability to participate in activities of daily living and the patient's perception of his or her quality of life. Only if the functional consequences of the medical impairment are significant and occur in tasks that are critical to the performance of the job can the patient be described as having a work disability.[154]

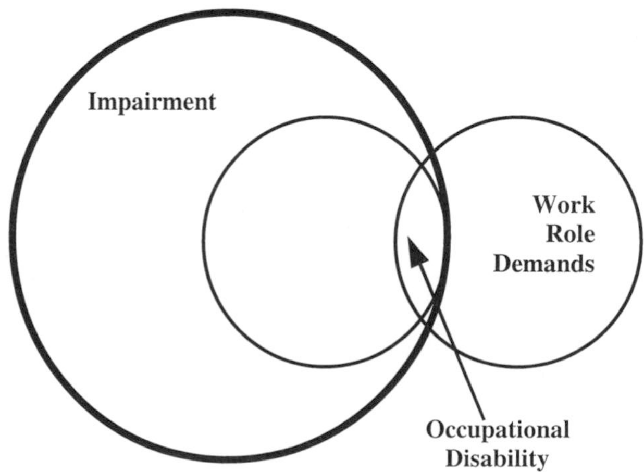

Figure 55–2. Assessment of work disability requires knowledge about the demands of the work role and the functional limitations of the worker.

The term capacity connotes the maximum ability of the individual, beyond the level of tolerance that is measured. Capacity is the patient's potential. The use of this term in the phrase "functional capacity evaluation" can be somewhat confusing because capacity is rarely measured in a performance task unless a person is highly trained to perform that particular task. Examples of maximum task performance are found when experienced athletes compete. When a person is an injured worker, functional capacity usually is inferred from the evaluation of task performance. Even when the evaluation task is designed to measure the individual's maximum performance level, this is achieved rarely. The maximum level of performance that usually can be measured is termed the person's tolerance for the demands of that task.[66] Further, the maximum dependable ability of the person usually is less than his or her tolerance. Finally, many FCEs are concerned only with adequacy for task performance rather than the person's maximum dependable ability in that task. That is, if the patient/examinee is under consideration for a particular job, the task demands of that job may be substantially less than his or her potential level of demonstrated ability. In this circumstance, as the evaluation progresses with increasing loads placed on that person, the evaluation will conclude when the job demand is reached. This may be at a lower performance level than the person's maximum dependable ability, which is lower than his or her tolerance, which is lower than his or her capacity.

The term evaluation describes a systematic approach to measuring ability that requires the evaluator to administer a test, collect data, interpret the data, and report the patient's ability to perform a task.[83] FCE includes many different modalities of measurement, including performance tests,[25,98,115,125,215] expert ratings from observation,[43,77,88,123,130,164,179] collateral ratings or reports,[76] and the patient's self-report.[47,52,55,150] A recent study[146] identified more than 800 FCE instruments and devices, including structured performance protocols using test equipment, simulated activities to measure functional performance, and structured behavior rating scales to rate observations or self-perceptions.

FUNCTIONAL CAPACITY EVALUATION STANDARDS OF CARE

Professionals who use FCE measures to evaluate work disability must meet criteria for performance tests that are found in professional guidelines, state and federal legislation, and case law. Guidelines for testing have been developed and published by the American Psychological Association,[6] American Physical Therapy Association,[190] American Academy of Physical Medicine and Rehabilitation,[109] and American College of Sports Medicine.[3] Federal guidelines for employment testing are found in the Uniform Guidelines for Employee Selection,[53] while in Daubert v Merrill Dow,[23] the rules of evidence for scientific opinions based on tests were established. When the testing procedure involves a qualified individual with a disability, the Americans With Disabilities Act of 1990[214] is pertinent. Taken together, these guidelines and laws create a framework for the standard of care for FCE. These criteria can be summarized in a simple hierarchy:

1. Safety—Given the known characteristics of the patient, proper administration of the FCE measure should not be expected to lead to injury.
2. Reliability—The score derived from the FCE measure should be dependable within the test trial and across evaluators, patients, and the date or time of test administration.
3. Validity—The decision based on interpretation of the score derived from the FCE measure should reflect the patient's true ability.
4. Practicality—The cost of administration, interpretation, and reporting of the FCE measure should be reasonable.

These criteria provide the underpinnings for the utility of FCE measures. The most important characteristic of a measure is its utility. Utility represents the overall value of the measure to its users. Utility is difficult to achieve and is threatened by many factors.[7,142,181,182] In disability evaluation, the most serious threats to utility are posed by problems with reliability of the instrument that will put a ceiling[40] on the instrument's validity for all applications, thereby decreasing its utility. Mathematically, the validity coefficient of a score cannot exceed the square of the reliability coefficient of the measure multiplied by the reliability coefficient of the criterion.[69] To the degree that there are limitations on the safety, reliability, validity, or practicality of the instrument, utility will be limited.[45,83]

IMPORTANT THREATS TO RELIABILITY

Excellent reviews of the reliability and validity of work-related assessments recently have been published,[93,94] to which the reader is referred. Although a full explication of the many potential threats to reliability in FCE is beyond the scope of this chapter, two specific threats that are of particular importance, test reactivity and less than full effort performance, are addressed briefly.

Test Reactivity

The threat to the reliability of a measure having to do with the instrument's reactivity is the effect of the measurement process on the evaluee's response to testing.[181] A test instrument is said to have reactivity when the evaluee's experience of taking the test affects test performance. This can occur in the absence of change due to treatment effect, directly affecting the measurement of both clinical validity[45] and prescriptive validity.[109] For example, a patient who participates in functional testing on two occasions may perform better on the second occasion simply because the first test resulted in skill development or addressed safety concerns that limited performance on the first occasion of testing. If a therapeutic intervention were administered between the two occasions of testing, apparent improvement on the second test could not be allocated to either the intervention or to the reactivity of the test. The effect of reactivity on the test is to limit its temporal stability. This limit on its reliability places a ceiling on its validity as a measure of therapeutic effect. It is becoming increasingly important to measure therapeutic effect in terms of the functional consequences of impairment.[171,205] Serial testing prior to treatment and after treatment can be a useful strategy to measure the effect of therapeutic intervention only if the test's reactivity is taken into account. Unfortunately, reactivity is rarely addressed in the rehabilitation literature. Reactivity is not listed as a consideration in the selection of either performance tests or self-report instruments in medical rehabilitation.[44,46,109,190] In the medical literature, issues such as sensitivity to change and reactivity are rarely studied or referenced,[45,47,153] although they are widely recognized as important aspects of reliability[6,7,181] In vocational rehabilitation, the situation is somewhat better,[26] in that several widely used functional performance tests have adjustments for reactivity that allow the test to be used on a serial basis.[215]

Less Than Full Effort Performance

The patient's full effort performance during the FCE is receiving increasing attention.[37,51,87,105,111,117,124,148,184,186] Full effort is important for the reliability of the score[155] and thereby a necessary underpinning of the validity of the assessment decision. It is imperative that the patient gives his or her best effort, and that less than full effort is identified when it occurs. Failure to identify less than full effort performance may result in exaggeration of disability findings and a false positive determination of disability. There are many reasons for less than full effort performance, some of which are components of medically determined impairments and thus should be considered as legitimate factors contributing to valid performance.[142] Other reasons for less than full effort performance are contaminants of the disability determination process; their effects must be minimized. Still other reasons are fraudulent attempts to circumvent the disability determination process and must be identified for subsequent legal action. A comprehensive literature review[4] identified 11 causes for less than full effort performance during the disability determination process:

1. Malingering syndrome
2. Factitious disorder
3. Learned illness behavior
4. Conversion disorder, pain disorder, or other somatoform disorders
5. Depressive disorders
6. Test anxiety
7. Fear of symptom exacerbation or injury
8. Fatigue
9. Medication and psychoactive substance effects
10. Lowered self-efficacy expectations
11. Need to gain recognition of symptoms

Often, several these causes of less than full effort performance are found to occur simultaneously. Some of these are transient and, once addressed properly, will not recur. Some are, not surprisingly, consequences of mismanagement of the disability experience by the patient, professionals, and bureaucrats that will be less prevalent as the healthcare system becomes better attuned to needs of the person with a disability. Others are more insidious and require sophisticated processes to identify and ameliorate.

It is important to note that there are other causes than lack of full effort for the test performance to be less than optimal. These include the patient's misunderstanding of instructions, poor test administration technique, and the use of poorly calibrated equipment. This chapter focuses on causes of less than optimal performance that are related to less than full effort.

There are several methods to identify persons who are unusually symptomatic or for whom symptoms are unusually disruptive that are not addressed here.[141,180,221–223] These methods are used to screen persons for symptom behaviors that may lead to less than full effort performance due to concern about, fear of, or attention to symptoms. In contrast, focusing directly on identification of less than full effort during a FCE, two principal themes characterize the methods that have been developed:

1. Intra-test inconsistency that exceeds normal error values is assumed to be an indicator of less than full effort, if a well-designed test has been administered properly.
2. Absence of expected relationships among related measures. Identification of several dependable measures of related attributes has allowed rational standards for inter-test comparisons to be developed as indicators of less than full effort.

There have been many rational implementations of these strategies. This important topic has been a focus of research in the neuropsychological literature for many years.[17,20,101,128,189] As a consequence, methods that are used to identify less than full effort in cognitive tests and self-report measures have been more thoroughly investigated than those that are used with persons who have musculoskeletal impairments. Although scientists in neuropsychology have made notable progress, it must be emphasized that most of the current tests have been adopted without being studied empirically. In particular, many of the physical performance measures continue to be used without any attempt to confirm that they possess adequate psychometric properties.[124,148] This has occurred for several reasons, chief of which is the professional community's undisciplined adoption of procedures that address this issue. There are many procedures in popular use that unfairly identify patients who are not performing at maximum as malingerers. An opinion such as this, rendered by a professional, has tremendous negative consequence for a person with a disability, including loss of access to necessary medical services and loss of financial support. Such an opinion should not be rendered without a clear idea of the sensitivity and specificity of the test that is used to support this opinion. Unfortunately, a central problem with scientific study of this topic is that empirical testing is quite difficult because the base rate of less than full effort behavior is unknown. Without knowledge of the base rate, the sensitivity and specificity of identification methods cannot be determined, nor can we determine positive predictive values or negative predictive values. (The sensitivity and specificity of a test are measures of its validity. In this case, sensitivity is the probability that a person who is performing at less than full effort will test positive. Specificity is the probability that a person

TABLE 55–2
Different Types of Functional Capacity Evaluation

Type	Question	Compared to . . .	Example Output	Duration
Functional goal setting	Ability to perform key task	Preinjury ability	"Limited ability to lift from knuckle to shoulder level"	30 minutes
Disability rating	Loss of work capacity	Normal values	"35% loss of work capacity"	90 minutes
Job matching	Adequacy for job	Specific job demands	"Adequate for demands of Fitter at ACME, Inc."	3–6 hours
Occupation matching	Adequacy for occupational group	General occupational demands	"Inadequate for demands of Fitter occupational group"	4–8 hours
Work capacity evaluation	Maximum dependable ability	Competitive employment standards	"Feasible for competitive employment at the Medium PDC level"	2–8 days

who is performing at full effort will test negative. Positive predictive value is the likelihood that a person who tests positive will be identified and negative predictive value is the likelihood that a person who tests negative will be identified.

Randomized and blinded studies of less than full effort assessment that use persons with a disability as subjects are almost nonexistent. Although the scientific community has urged caution and restraint in this area,[124,148] the pressure from some stakeholders in the disability determination system is so great that current practices in most areas include wholesale adoption of unproven tests. This places individual professionals, their employers, and to a significant extent, the whole enterprise of FCEs at risk of legal and societal censure.

It is important to recognize that almost any indicator of less than full effort can be volitionally defeated, and that some tests are more robust than others. The ease with which a person can misrepresent ability varies with the volitional control and transparency of the attribute being measured and with the method of measurement. The easiest method to contravene is one that is most transparent, such as a grip strength test or pulmonary function measure.[37,73,90,117,121,172,184–186,201] Those that are more difficult to contravene are more complex, subtle, and depend on nonvolitional responses, such as blood pressure and heart rate. There are a few performance tests that have been designed to be sensitive to less than full effort, with reasonable utility. In the only randomized blind study of persons with a disability to date,[105] evaluators who were blinded to the status of the subjects (performing at full effort or less than full effort) were able to identify volitional less than full effort performance with 94% positive predictive value and 80% negative predictive value. Other widely used tests that have been promoted as effective in identifying less than full effort have been much less successful[148] and should be considered of limited utility.

TYPES OF FUNCTIONAL CAPACITY EVALUATIONS

There are five different types of FCE processes, defined by the purpose to which the information derived from the evaluation will be put. The primary issues that differentiate among the types of FCEs are presented in Table 55–2. Each of the five types of FCEs is described in the following, arranged along a hierarchy of increasing complexity, time, and expense.

Functional Goal Setting

If the patient's medical impairment is sufficiently severe to warrant referral to therapy, measurement of the functional status of the component(s) affected by the impairment in order to set recovery goals is useful. This type of FCE measures the usual functional consequences of the impairment at the component level. For example, in the case of a musculoskeletal impairment, joint range of motion or segmental strength could be measured.[85,86,129,168] The information that is collected is used in consultation with the patient to set functional goals.[157] It is also used to provide objective indices of performance to gauge the progress of therapy.

Disability Rating

If the functional consequences of a person's impairment are sufficiently severe to potentially result in limitation of ability to work, measurement of the loss of ability in key functional areas of work can be used as an estimate of disability.[118,131] This method is analogous to the measurement of percent impairment of the whole person described in the Guides to the Evaluation of Permanent Impairment.[5] This method is used frequently in forensic evaluations to provide an estimate of

TABLE 55–3
Sample Disability Ratings Using the California Workers' Compensation Model

Occupation	Age at injury, yr	Diagnostic or Impairment Category	Disability Category	Standard Rating	Occupational Group	Occupational Adjustment	Age Adjustment	Disability Rating
Carpenter	60	Amputation of arm at or above elbow, not above shoulder joint, reasonably satisfactory use of prosthesis possible, major arm	7.121	70%	380	75%	6%	81%
Medical front office clerk	45	Low back injury, resulting in disability precluding heavy work, contemplating the individual has lost approximately 50% of preinjury capacity for bending, stooping, lifting, pushing, pulling, and climbing	12.1	30%	212	28%	2%	30%
Elementary school teacher	36	Hand injury resulting in limited motion of the thumb and index finger of the major hand	9.2111	25%	214	30%	–2%	28%
Carpenter	36	Hand injury resulting in limited motion of the thumb and index finger of the major hand	9.2111	25%	380	33%	–1%	32%
Judge	36	Hand injury resulting in limited motion of the thumb and index finger of the major hand	9.2111	25%	370	25%	–1%	24%
Parking lot attendant, booth	36	Hand injury resulting in limited motion of the thumb and index finger of the major hand	9.2111	25%	370	23%	–1%	22%

the effect of the injury or illness on an individual's lifetime earning capacity. In the workers' compensation arena, most state and provincial systems have adopted the Guides' rating of permanent impairment as an ersatz disability rating in spite of the official position of the American Medical Association that this is inappropriate.[5] This has created problems with the validity of the Guides, given validity's dependence on the context within which a measure is applied.[7]

In a rare but important exception, the State of California[235] uses a bona fide disability rating procedure, invoking an algorithm that includes impairment, a constant that is related to functional loss, and an "occupational variant." The components of this model are shown in Table 55–3, as they are applied to typical case examples. In this approach, physician-generated data are used with occupational and age data to develop a percent disability rating. This method is based on collection of information about the examinee's diagnosis, medical impairment, and prophylactic work restrictions obtained through a medical examination. (An important assumption for disability rating is that the functional limitations are a consequence of the impairment. This assumption requires substantial judgment on the part of the physician that can be obtained by data collected during an FCE. Without confirmation of this assumption, attribution of measured functional limitations to a particular impairment is difficult to achieve.) Using this information, a tabular algorithm is employed to derive the disability rating, presented as a percent of total disability, which determines the amount of disability indemnity that is to be paid. The treating physician is permitted to base opinions about work restrictions on inference, without formal functional testing, although this practice is coming under increasing scrutiny and on an individual basis is often successfully challenged. In two studies in which the author has participated,[138,155] a substantial minority of California workers' compensation disability claimants who were provided benefits based on physician's opinions without benefit of FCE were found, based on subsequent FCE, to not be valid. The benefits had been awarded unnecessarily. As the scientific basis of FCE develops, and functional data are used in these decisions more often, rational allocation of workers' compensation benefits will be commonplace.

Job Matching

Matching the adequacy of the worker's abilities to the essential functions of the job is the next most complex type of FCE. Information concerning the physical demands of a particular job is obtained through a job analysis, whereas information concerning the worker's impairment is obtained through a medical examination. A comparison of these two sets of information leads to the identification of the physical abilities that require an evaluation of functional adequacy. This FCE usually employs a standardized test battery, although the new taxonomic FCE approach allows selection of only those tests that are necessary. The performance targets of this standardized test battery are different from the Occupation Matching FCE test battery (following) in that the level of demand of the job is more specific (and usually lower) than the demand level of the occupational group.

Occupation Matching

Matching of the examinee's functional capacity to the demands of an occupational group is a separate type of FCE. Information concerning the physical demands of an occupation is obtained from a source such as the United States Department of Labor's Dictionary of Occupational Titles[212] or the O*NET system[81] for typical jobs in the occupational group. The FCE tests and level of demand are based on this information. The physical demand level is often described in terms of the system used by the Dictionary of Occupational Titles, as depicted in Table 55–4.

This type of FCE is more complex than Job Matching because the occupational classification contains all job tasks that might be required in the variety of jobs that are found within the classification. It is usually more physically demanding than the Job Matching FCE because the full range of job demands within the occupational classification must be considered.

Work Capacity Evaluation

Matching the examinee's functional capacity to the demands of all occupations in the competitive labor market is the most comprehensive type of FCE. Because there is no occupational target, the focus of the Work Capacity Evaluation is very broad, encompassing all of the frequently encountered task demands and worker behaviors. Behaviors are assessed through observation of performance in a simulated work environment. This type of evaluation uses structured work simulations that often can be constructed based on descriptions found in published resources.[30,137,177] The duration of the Work Capacity FCE is very broad because it is possible to quickly determine that a person is unable to meet basic criteria, such as workplace tolerance and sustained activity tolerance. Conversely, if the examinee is able to meet these criteria, it is difficult and time consuming to determine which vocational assets the patient should subsequently use to enter the labor market.

FCE Test Batteries versus the Focused Test Approach

Triage into the FCE that is appropriate for the examinee is guided by joint consideration of the probable functional limitations that are naturally consequent to the examinee's impairment and the performance demand targets that are contemplated. In recent years, most FCEs have been conducted through the use of a standardized FCE test battery, several of which are available within each FCE type described. Although the administration of complete test batteries is generally regarded as not being the most efficient approach, it is employed by all but a small number of the more experienced evaluators who select to evaluate only those specific functional assessment constructs that are pertinent to the case at hand. The focused test approach is preferred over the test battery approach as long as the safety, reliability, and validity guidelines presented previously are addressed adequately. However, the focused test approach requires an evaluator who is usually more experienced; this approach is beyond the ability of most test battery administrators. Research conducted recently[70–72,146] is likely to make the focused test approach more available, with the advent of expert systems that employ the taxonomic approach.

TABLE 55–4

Dictionary of Occupational Titles System for Classifying the Strength Demands of Work

Physical Demand Level	Occasional, 0 to 33% of the Workday	Frequent, 34% to 66% of the Workday	Constant, 67% to 100% of the Workday	Typical Energy Required
Sedentary	10 lbs	Negligible	Negligible	1.5–2.1 METS
Light	20 lbs	10 lbs and/or walk/stand/push/pull of arm/leg controls	Negligible and/or push/pull of arm/leg controls while seated	2.2–3.5 METS
Medium	20 to 50 lbs	10 to 25 lbs	10 lbs	3.6–6.3 METS
Heavy	50 to 100 lbs	25 to 50 lbs	10 to 20 lbs	6.4–7.5 METS
Very heavy	Over 100 lbs	Over 50 lbs	Over 20 lbs	Over 7.5 METS

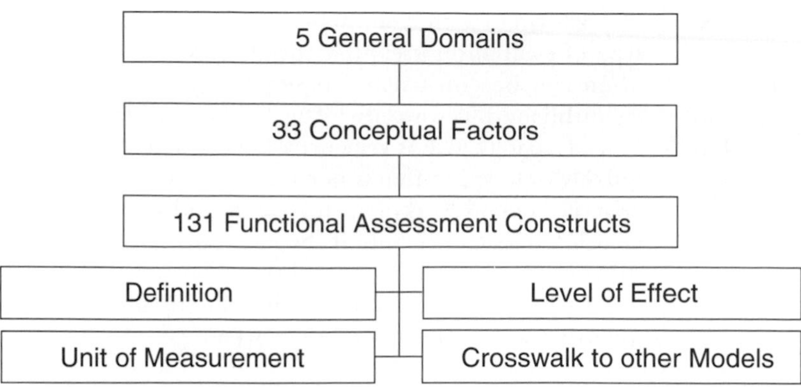

Figure 55–3. Organizational hierarchy of the Functional Assessment Constructs Taxonomy.

TAXONOMY OF FUNCTIONAL ASSESSMENT CONSTRUCTS

In the most generic sense, the FCE considers the consequences of numerous impairments on numerous work demands. As a consequence, the interface between impairment and work demands is broad and complex. More than 800 FCE measures used to evaluate the work disability of adults have been identified. A database of these measures organized through the use of the functional assessment constructs taxonomy[72] has been developed.[146] The "FAC Taxonomy" includes 131 constructs that have been grouped into 33 conceptual factors, which themselves have been grouped into five domains. Each construct has been cross-referenced in terms of impairment, functional limitation, vocational feasibility, and occupational disability. In addition, each construct has been defined in terms of level of effect, reflecting ability factors along a continuum of increasing complexity. Figure 55–3 describes these relationships.

The constructs in this taxonomy represent attributes of the person that are pertinent to the demands of work. Initial development of the taxonomy was based on a thorough literature review of constructs that are currently measured by professionals who evaluate disability. This was followed by an expert judgment exercise in which assessment professionals considered a matrix of approximately 18,000 combinations of constructs to identify factors, groupings, and voids. This was followed by a focused literature review designed to resolve inconsistencies and voids. Finally, the taxonomy was edited while being used to organize information on approximately 800 instruments containing more than 3000 scales. Each scale was linked to one or more constructs, conceptual factors, or domains in the taxonomy.

The FAC Taxonomy includes constructs that originated in various taxonomies of human performance and job demands. Prominent sources were those provided by the United States Department of Labor in the Dictionary of Occupational Titles and the O*NET system, as well as the recognized human performance taxonomies described in Fleishman and Quaintance.[63] The relationships between the five domains and the 32 conceptual factors are presented in Table 55–5.

As noted earlier, the taxonomy focuses on "work disability" as a subset of disability, using the model described in Figure 55–1. It is remarkable that, even with this narrowed focus, 131 distinct constructs were identified that currently are measured to determine disability. A review of all of these constructs is beyond the scope of this chapter, which will focus on several of the constructs that are encountered when evaluating persons with musculoskeletal impairment (additional information about the Functional Assessment Measures database is available at FAMdatabase.com). This chapter addresses 13 of the 32 physical domain constructs that would normally be of concern with impairments of this type, focusing on those in the Hand Use and Manual Material Handling Conceptual Factors (constructs related to pain and other symptoms are considered in the Vocational Behavior domain and will not be presented here). The constructs are presented with comparisons to constructs found in the taxonomies of various systems in the United States, Great Britain, and The Netherlands.

The data in Table 55–6 are of interest because they depict the incomplete nature of the systems that are reviewed. No one system currently includes all constructs in the FAC taxonomy, although every construct in the taxonomy is addressed by at least one system. The absence of uniformity across systems is also noteworthy.

REPRESENTATIVE FUNCTIONAL ASSESSMENT MEASURES

The functional assessment constructs taxonomy was used in the development of a database of more than 800 functional assessment measures[146] that are currently used to determine disability. Data about the measures' psychometric properties and other pertinent issues were

TABLE 55–5

Relationship Between Domains and Conceptual Factors in the Functional Assessment Constructs Taxonomy

Domain	Conceptual Factor	Ability Within the Worker Role and Work Environment
Sensory–Perceptual	Hearing	Ability to clearly perceive spoken and other sounds
	Vision	Ability to clearly perceive visual stimuli
	Cutaneous discrimination	Ability to discriminate light touch, pressure, vibration, pain, and temperature
	Proprioceptive discrimination	Ability to discriminate the position of the body in relation to the environment
	Body reactivity	Ability to tolerate the effect on the body of contact with the environment
	Psychomotor speed/reaction time	Ability to react quickly to a stimulus
	Visuospatial abilities	Ability to identify, generate, retain, and manipulate visual images
Physical	Digestive control	Ability to control nourishment and elimination of body wastes
	Lower extremity use	Ability to use legs and feet in coordinated and purposeful movement
	Upper extremity use	Ability to use shoulders and arms in coordinated and purposeful movement
	Head and trunk use	Ability to use the head and trunk to perform coordinated and purposeful movement
	Hand use	Ability to use the wrists and fingers in coordinated and purposeful movement
	Whole body postural maintenance	Ability to maintain the body in a standing or sitting position
	Whole body change of position	Ability to transition to and from lying, standing, or sitting positions
	Whole body mobility	Ability to move oneself across space
	Manual material handling	Ability to lift, handle, and transport objects of various weights and sizes
Cognitive–Intellectual	Consciousness	Ability to be awake and alert
	Orientation	Ability to identify oneself in relation to location and time
	Attention concentration	Ability to focus on task to completion, managing symptom distractions
	Numerics	Ability to understand and apply numerical concepts
	Language and communication	Ability to communicate using language and alternate modes
	Memory	Ability to store and retrieve information
	Learning	Ability to develop conceptual, abstract, and practical knowledge, skills, and abilities
Interpersonal and Emotional	Interpersonal interaction	Ability to interact constructively with others in the workplace
	Behavior modulation	Ability to modulate behavior associated with affective experience
	Tolerance for distractions	Ability to maintain activity despite distractions
	Adaptability	Ability to adapt to changes within the workplace
Vocational	Task performance	Ability to begin, follow through, and complete goal-directed activities
	Planning and organizing work	Ability to plan, sequence, prioritize, and organize tasks
	Problem saving and decision making	Ability to adjust one's behavior according to changing contingencies
	Dependability	Ability to adhere to a structured work schedule
	Work safety	Ability to perform work in a manner that is safe for self and others
	Travel	Ability to travel to and from work and around workplace

collected. This research confirmed the findings of an earlier study[192] that there was no standard procedure to evaluate functional limitations. The recent study found that this stems in part from the fact that, while some FCE procedures have been developed specifically for medical practice, many have been borrowed from the fields of education, psychology, or vocational rehabilitation. The confusion in the professional literature about how the attributes of the person should be organized led to development of the model of work disability (Fig. 55–1), the units of analysis system (Table 55–1), and to the functional assessments constructs taxonomy. These will be useful in future efforts in the United States and elsewhere to develop scientific methods to determine disability.

In order to develop a database of functional assessment measures, the development of definitions to assist the project scientists to distinguish among test batteries, test instruments, test scales, test protocols, and test equipment was necessary. Measurement of functional assessment constructs typically is performed at the scale level. Most instruments have several scales; five to six scales were found in each of the approximately 620 instruments that could be studied closely. Every scale was measured through the use of a test protocol. Some of the test protocols meas-

TABLE 55-6

Comparison of the Disability Determination Systems in the United States, Great Britain, and The Netherlands in Terms of Constructs in the Physical Domain of the Functional Assessment Constructs Taxonomy

Conceptrial Factor	Construct	Definition	United States DOT*	United States SSA†	Great Britain	The Netherlands
Hand use	Hand range of motion	Ability to move the hands through a full range of motion	Handling	Lift and carry	Manual dexterity	Hand finger dexterity
	Hand sensitivity	Ability to use the hands to sense by touch and temperature	Feeling	Lift and carry	Manual dexterity	Hand-finger dexterity
	Hand speed	Ability to use the hands in rapid movement	Handling	Lift and carry	Manual dexterity	Hand-finger dexterity
	Hand coordination	Ability to use the hands in a coordinated manner	Handling	Lift and carry	Manual dexterity	Hand-finger dexterity
	Hand dexterity	Ability to use the hands for fine coordinated movement	Handling	Lift and carry	Manual dexterity	Hand-finger dexterity
	Hand strength	Ability to use the hands in a forceful manner	Handling	Lift and carry	Lifting and carrying	Lifting
	Hand endurance	Ability to use the hands in a sustained or repetitive manner	Handling			
	Eye-hand coordination	Ability to coordinate fine movements using visual information	Handling		Manual dexterity	Hand-finger dexterity
	Manipulating objects	Ability to seize, hold, grasp, or turn objects with hands and fingers	Fingering	Lift and carry	Manual dexterity	Hand-finger dexterity
Manual material handling	Reaching	Ability to stretch arms and trunk in a coordinated manner to grasp or manipulate objects	Reaching	Lift and carry	Reaching	Reaching
	Lifting and lowering	Ability to lift and lower objects	Strength	Lift and carry	Lifting and carrying	Lifting
	Pushing and pulling	Ability to push and pull objects	Strength			Pushing and pulling
	Carrying objects	Ability to carry objects while ambulating	Strength	Lift and carry	Lifting and carrying	Carrying

* Dictionary of Occupational Titles job analysis factors.
† Social Security Administration residual functional capacity factors.

ured several scales. Some of the protocols required test equipment, often composed of mechanical or electronic devices. Many of the test protocols used only a test booklet and required only paper and pencil to record either the examinee's own responses or observations made by others, including both professionals and family members. Confusion often occurs when both the test protocol and test equipment are not specified in reports and scientific papers. For example, it is common to read that "hand strength was measured by the Jamar Hand Dynamometer." The Jamar dynamometer is test equipment with which isometric hand strength is measured, using one of several test protocols. In this example, static force can be measured in terms of one handle position, two positions, or all five positions, providing different spans of grip, using single trials, three repeated trials, based on a mean score, or the highest of the repeated scores. The protocol endorsed by the American Society of Hand Therapists[160] is the most broadly adopted test protocol, but by no means the only protocol in use. It is necessary to specify the test protocol and equipment. Confusion also occurs when the mode of testing is inaccurately linked to the functional assessment construct. For example, it is common to read that "lift capacity was determined by isometric testing."

Isometric strength testing is not a mode of lift capacity measurement. Lift capacity is predicted by isometric strength measurement only under very special circumstances.[149,151,226]

In the sections that follow, global test batteries and functional assessment measures that are used with two clusters of constructs, those having to do with hand use and those having to do with manual material handling, are presented. These measures are grouped according to constructs that share common characteristics. This is a representative list that is not exhaustive. The functional assessment measures and test batteries that are presented in the following are in widespread use.

Global Test Batteries

In the research to compile the functional assessment measures database, a small number of FCE global test batteries were identified, each comprised of one dozen to three dozen scales, using a combination of scales and instruments. Some of the scales and instruments in these batteries can be used on a stand-alone basis, with prior studies identifying the psychometric properties of each. However, confusion occurs when psychometric properties derived for individual scales or instruments are applied to a test battery as a whole, rather than to the scales and instruments that comprise the battery. It is important to differentiate the psychometric properties of the scales and instruments from the psychometric properties of the test batteries. See Table 55–7.

Functional Group: Hand Use

Definition: Ability to use the wrists and fingers in coordinated and purposeful movement.

This group of functional assessment constructs has a wide variety of strategies that are used to measure performance, with some of the measures developed in the 19th century. Many of the best developed tests in this area, those supported by the greatest amount of research, were used and studied extensively immediately before and during World War II to select recruits for training positions in the armed forces. In the last 30 years, several work sample tests have been developed to measure these constructs in persons with a disability. See Tables 55–8 through 55–12.

Functional Group: Manual Material Handling

Definition: Ability to lift, handle, and transport objects of various weights and sizes.

Most of the tests that are used to measure these functional assessment constructs have been developed in the last 30 years, often specifically for use with persons who have medical impairments. These tests usually were developed with reference to ergonomic standards, especially those developed by the National Institute of Occupational Safety and Health.[174] Additionally, tests of this type often were developed with reference to the U.S. Department of Labor stan-

TABLE 55–7

Representative Global Test Batteries That are Frequently Used in Functional Capacity Evaluation

Battery or Instrument	Source or Developer	References
Blankenship Functional Capacity Evaluation	Blankenship, Inc.	24, 25, 111, 127
BTE Work Simulator	Baltimore Therapeutic Equipment, Inc.	18, 21, 22, 32, 54, 84, 114, 116, 117, 127, 173, 228, 230
California Functional Capacity Protocol (Cal-FCP)	Mooney & Matheson	155
DOT Residual Functional Capacity Battery	Fishbain & Abdel-Moty	57, 58
ERGOS Work Simulator	Work Recovery, Inc.	39, 50, 149, 200
Isernhagen Functional Capacity Evaluation	Isernhagen Work Systems, Inc.	96, 97, 99, 100
Key Method Functional Capacity Assessment	Key Functional Assessments, Inc.	115
LIDO WorkSET Work Simulator	Baltimore Therapeutic Equipment, Inc.	64, 147, 195, 231
Matheson Work Capacity Evaluation	RMA, Inc.	137, 139, 140
Physical Work Performance Evaluation	ErgoScience, Inc.	125, 126
Valpar Component Work Sample System	Valpar, Inc.	15, 33, 78, 110, 188, 193, 194, 215
WorkAbility Mark III	Heyde & Shervington	197–199
WorkHab	Roberts & Bradbury	28

TABLE 55–8

Eye-hand Coordination Functional Capacity Evaluation Scales

Representative Scale	Battery or Instrument	Disability Model Level	Source or Developer	References
Eye Hand Coordination	APTICOM—Eye Hand Foot Coordination	Functional limitation	Vocational Research Institute	82
Screws	Crawford Small Parts Dexterity Test	Functional limitation	The Psychological Corporation	19, 178
Coordination	Flanagan Aptitude Classification Test	Occupational disability	National Computer Systems, Inc.	60, 165
Coordination	Flanagan Industrial Test	Occupational disability	National Computer Systems, Inc.	61, 229
Copy Geometric Form	Loewenstein Occupational Therapy Cognitive Assessment	Occupational disability	Western Psychological Services	34, 112, 113
Placing	MESA System 2000	Functional limitation	Valpar International Corporation	27, 102–104, 207
Soldering and inspection	Valpar 12—Soldering and Inspection	Functional limitation	Valpar International Corporation	215
Eye Hand Foot Coordination	Vocational Interest Temperament and Aptitude System	Occupational disability	Jewish Employment & Vocational Service	2
Use of compass and circle Template	Valpar 16—Drafting	Functional limitation	Valpar International Corporation	215

TABLE 55–9

Finger Dexterity Functional Capacity Evaluation Scales

Representative Scale	Battery or Instrument	Disability Model Level	Source or Developer	References
Assembly	Purduce Pegboard Test	Occupational disability	Science Research Associates Inc.	134, 219
Fine Finger Dexterity	Valpar 204—Fine Finger Dexterity	Functional limitation	Valpar International Corporation	215
Finger Dexterity	General Aptitude Test Battery	Occupational disability	U.S. Department of Labor	16, 122, 208, 220
Manual Speed and Dexterity	Career Ability Placement Survey	Occupational disability	Educational & Industrial Testing Service	89, 120
O'Connor Finger Dexterity Test	O'Connor Finger Dexterity Test	Occupational disability	O'Connor & Johnson	75
Pins and Collars	Crawford Small Parts Dexterity Test	Functional limitation	The Psychological Corporation	19, 135, 178
Sequential Occupational Dexterity Assessment	Sequential Occupational Dexterity Assessment	Functional limitation		216, 217

TABLE 55–10

Hand Coordination Functional Capacity Evaluation Scales

Representative Scale	Battery or Instrument	Disability Model Level	Source or Developer	References
Aiming	Comprehensive Ability Battery	Occupational disability	Institute for Personality & Ability Testing	79, 80, 119
Hand Dexterity	Valpar 4	Functional limitation	Valpar International Corporation	215
Hand Tool Dexterity Test	Bennett Hand Tool Dexterity Test	Functional limitation	The Psychological Corporation	132
Motor Coordination	General Aptitude Test Battery	Occupational disability	U.S. Department of Labor	16, 49, 122, 208, 220
Grasp	Action Research Arm Test	Functional limitation	Lyle	41, 56, 59, 67, 91, 92, 133
One Hand Turning and Placing Test	Minnesota Rate of Manipulation Test	Functional limitation	American Guidance Service	14, 170
Rods and Caps	Roeder Manipulative Aptitude Test	Occupational disability	Lafayette Instruments Co.	187

TABLE 55–11

Hand Strength and Endurance Functional Capacity Evaluation Scales

Representative Scale	Battery or Instrument	Disability Model Level	Source or Developer	References
Continuous Torque	WEST 4A	Functional limitation	Work Evaluation Systems Technology	9, 230
Isometric Grip Strength Test	JAMAR Hand Dynamometer	Occupational disability	Therapeutic Equipment Corp.	48, 74, 158, 160
Isometric Grip Test	ARCON Grip	Functional limitation	Applied Rehabilitation Concepts, Inc.	48, 74, 158, 160
Isometric Pinch Test	Hanoun Medical Pinch	Functional limitation	Hanoun Medical, Inc.	156, 158, 160, 202, 232
Key Pinch	B & L Isometric Pinch Gauge	Functional impairment	B and L Engineering	156, 158, 160, 202, 232

TABLE 55–12

Hand Speed Functional Capacity Evaluation Scales

Representative Scale	Battery or Instrument	Disability Model Level	Source or Developer	References
Alphanumeric Speed and Accuracy	CRT Skills Test	Occupational disability	National Computer Systems, Inc.	10, 175
Both Hands	Purdue Pegboard Test	Occupational disability	Science Research Associates Inc.	134, 159, 183, 210, 219
Card Turning	Jebsen Hand Function Test	Functional impairment	Jebsen	31, 106, 196, 204, 206
Manual Speed and Accuracy	Employee Aptitude Survey	Occupational disability	Psychological Services, Inc.	191
Precision	Flanagan Aptitude Classification Test	Occupational disability	National Computer Systems, Inc.	60, 165
Precision	Flanagan Industrial Test	Occupational disability	National Computer Systems, Inc.	61, 229
Turning Test	Minnesota Rate of Manipulation Test	Functional limitation	American Guidance Service	14, 170

TABLE 55–13

Manual Material Handling Functional Capacity Evaluation Scales

Representative Scale	Battery or Instrument	Disability Model Level	Source or Developer	References
Carrying & Climbing Balance	WEST EPIC 5	Functional limitation	Work Evaluation Systems Technology	143
Dynamic Physical Capacities	Valpar 19—Dynamic Physical Capacities	Functional limitation	Valpar International Corporation	15, 215
Dynamic Strength	Valpar 201—Physical Capacities and Mobility Screening Evaluation	Functional limitation	Valpar International Corporation	215
Lift Capacity	ARCON Lift Capacity	Functional limitation	Applied Rehabilitation Concepts, Inc.	
Lift Capacity	EPIC Lift Capacity	Functional limitation	Employment Potential Improvement Corporation	105, 145, 152, 153
Lift Capacity	Hanoun EPIC Lift Capacity	Functional limitation	Employment Potential Improvement Corporation	105, 145, 152, 153
Lift Capacity	Progressive Isoinertial Lifting Evaluation	Functional limitation	Mayer et al	161–163
Range of Motion Under Load	WEST Standard Evaluation	Functional limitation	Work Evaluation Systems Technology	136, 138, 176, 209

dards for strength demands of work as described in the Handbook for Analyzing Jobs.[211,213] See Table 55–13.

THE FUTURE OF FUNCTIONAL CAPACITY EVALUATION

Driven by both market demands and the needs of large insurance carriers and governmental agencies, the scientific basis of FCEs will continue to develop. Organizational tools such as the Model of Work Disability and the Functional Assessment Constructs Taxonomy that have been presented in this chapter will facilitate this development. Although the future is always difficult to predict, several issues seem clear and readily predictable:

- Given the wide variety of functional assessment measures already available, it is unlikely that many new measures will be developed. Currently available measures will be more extensively studied and the psychometric properties will be improved and formally demonstrated, with results published in peer reviewed scientific journals.
- Interdisciplinary standards that are as technical as those offered by the American Psychological Association[6] and as clinically applicable to this type of assessment as those offered by the American Academy of Physical Medicine and Rehabilitation[109] will be developed.
- Certification of health care professionals who provide FCE services will become widespread, supported by several of the major universities, and demanded by underwriters.
- Development of expert triage systems to guide the selection of functional assessment constructs that should be measured, accompanied by catalogs of tests that are appropriate for each construct, will become available.
- The FCE process will be supported by expert administrative systems that are available online with built-in monitoring so that professionals with lower levels of skill who have received appropriate training will be able to work as evaluators and test technicians.
- New FCE administrative systems will identify patterns of performance that indicate less than full effort through dynamic monitoring of test performance, and will trigger follow-up testing to confirm or deny less than full effort. This will increase the reliability and, thereby, the validity and utility of FCE results.
- FCE will be used much more often as practicality improves. The advent of focused test systems will assist evaluators to select only those constructs that are necessary to evaluate, and not include those that are unnecessary.

Through these improvements, the value of the FCE to industrialized societies throughout the world will continue to improve, so that FCEs will become indispensable to the process of disability determination.

SUMMARY

This has been a review of FCE as it is used in rehabilitation, with a focus on its use in the determination of work disability. A new model of work disability has been presented and a taxonomic structure of functional assessment constructs has been introduced and briefly described. The taxonomy was used to organize several hundred functional assessment measures into a database that was tapped to provide representative instruments that are used to measure constructs in two areas: hand use and manual material handling. The chapter concludes with predictions of likely improvements in FCEs that will be developed through the application of the new taxonomic method.

References

1. Abdel-Moty E, Fishbain D, Khalil T, et al: Functional capacity and residual functional capacity and their utility in measuring work capacity. Clin J Pain 9:168–173, 1993.
2. Abrams M: A new work sample battery for vocational assessment of the disadvantaged: VITAS. Vocational Guidance Quarterly 28:35–43, 1979.
3. American College of Sports Medicine: Guidelines for Exercise Testing and Prescription, 4th ed. Philadelphia, Lea & Febiger, 1991.
4. American Institutes for Research: Synthesis of research and development of prototypes for a new disability determination methodology: Measurement concepts and issues relevant to the Social Security Administration's disability determination process. Washington, DC, American Institutes for Research, 1999.
5. Cocchiarella L, Andersson GBJ (eds): Guides to the Evaluation of Permanent Impairment, 5th ed. Chicago, American Medical Association, 2001.
6. American Psychological Association, Association AER, Education NcoMi: Standards for Educational and Psychological Testing. Washington, DC, Author, 1999.
7. Anastasi A, Urbina S: Psychological Testing, 7th ed. Upper Saddle River, NJ, Prentice-Hall, 1997.
8. Andersson G: Epidemiologic aspects on low back pain in industry. Spine 6:53–60, 1981.
9. Author: WEST 4A Work Capacity Evaluation Device User Manual. Ft. Bragg, CA, Work Evaluation Systems Technology, 1989.
10. Author: CRT Skills Test Examiner's Manual. Rosemont, Ill, National Computer Systems, 1990.
11. Ayoub M: Control of manual lifting hazards: I. Training in safe handling. J Occup Med 24:573–577, 1982.
12. Ayoub M: Control of manual lifting hazards: II. Job redesign. J Occup Med 24:668–676, 1982.
13. Ayoub M: Problems and solutions in manual materials handling: The state of the art. Ergonomics 35:713–728, 1992.
14. Bain G, Pugh D, MacDermid J, Roth J: Matched hemiresection interposition arthroplasty of the distal radioulnar joint. J Hand Surg [Am] 20:944–950, 1995.
15. Barrett T, Browne D, Lamers M, Steding E: Reliability and validity testing of Valpar 19. Proceedings of the 19th National Conference of the Australian Association of Occupational Therapists, 1997, 2, pp 179–183.
16. Baydoun R, Neuman G: The future of the general aptitude test battery for use in public and private testing. Journal of Business and Psychology 7:81–91, 1992.
17. Beaber J, Marston A, Michelli J, Mills M: A brief test for measuring malingering in schizophrenic individuals. Am J Psychiatry 142:1478–1491, 1985.
18. Beaton D, O'Driscoll S, Richards R: Grip strength testing using the BTE work simulator and the Jamar dynamometer: A comparative study. J Hand Surg 20A:293–298, 1995.
19. Berger Y: Does the Crawford Small Parts Dexterity Test require new norms? Percept Mot Skills 60:948–950, 1985.
20. Bernard L, Houston W, Natoli L: Malingering on neuropsychological memory tests: Potential objective indicators. J Clin Psychol 49:45–53, 1993.
21. Bhambhani Y, Esmail S, Britnell S: The Baltimore Therapeutic Equipment work simulator: Biomechanical and physiological norms for three attachments in healthy men. Am J Occup Ther 48:19–25, 1994.
22. Blackmore S, Beaulieu D, Baxter-Petralia P, Bruening L: A comparison study of three methods to determine exercise resistance and duration for the BTE work simulator. J Hand Ther 1:165–171, 1988.
23. Blackmun J: Daubert v Merrell Dow Pharmaceuticals. Washington, DC, United States Supreme Court, 1993.
24. Blankenship K: The Blankenship FCE system behavioural profile: A four year retrospective study. Proceedings of the 1996 National Physiotherapy Congress of the Australian Physiotherapy Association, 1994, pp 111–112.
25. Blankenship K: The Blankenship system functional capacity evaluation procedure manual. Macon, Ga, The Blankenship Corporation, 1994.
26. Bolton B (ed): Handbook of Measurement and Evaluation in Rehabilitation, 3rd ed. Gaithersburg, Md, Aspen, 2001.
27. Bordieri J, Musgrave J: Client perceptions of the Microcomputer Evaluation and Screening Assessment. Rehabil Couns Bull 32:342–345, 1989.
28. Bradbury S, Roberts D: WorkHab Australia Functional Capacity Evaluation Workshop Manual. Bundaberg, Qld, WorkHab Australia, 1996.
29. Brandt E, Pope A: Enabling America: Assessing the Role of Rehabilitation Science and Engineering. Washington, DC, National Academy Press, 1997.
30. Brown C, McDaniel R, Couch R, McClanahan M: Vocational Evaluation Systems and Software: A Consumer's Guide. Menomonie, WI, Materials Development Center, Stout Vocational Rehabilitation Institute, School of Education and Human Services University of Wisconsin–Stout, 1994.
31. Carlson J, Trombly C: The effect of wrist immobilization on performance of the Jebsen Hand Function Test. Am J Occup Ther 37:168–175, 1983.
32. Cathey M, Wolfe F, Kleinheksel S: Functional ability and work status in patients with fibromyalgia. Arthritis Care Res 1:85–98, 1988.
33. Cederlund R: The use of dexterity tests in hand rehabilitation. Scand J Occup Ther 2:99–104, 1995.
34. Cermak S, Katz N, McGuire E, et al: Performance of Americans and Israelis with cerebrovascular accident on the Loewenstein Occupational Therapy Cognitive Assessment. Am J Occup Ther 49:500–506, 1995.
35. Chaffin D, Andersson G: Occupational Biomechanics. New York, John Wiley & Sons, 1984.
36. Chater S: Plan for a New Disability Claim Process. Washington, DC, Social Security Administration, 1994, p 70.
37. Chengalur S, Smith G, Nelson R, Sadoff A: Assessing sincerity of effort in maximal grip strength tests. Am J Phys Med Rehabil 69:148–153, 1990.
38. Cocchiarella L, Turk M, Andersson G: Improving the evaluation of permanent impairment. JAMA 283:532–533, 2000.
39. Cooke C, Dusik L, Menard M, et al: Relationship of performance on the ERGOS Work Simulator to illness behavior in a

workers' compensation population with low back versus limb injury. J Occup Med 36:757–762, 1994.
40. Cronbach L: Essentials of Psychological Testing, 3rd ed. New York, Harper & Row, 1970.
41. Dekker J, Wagenaar R, Lankhorst G, de Jong B: The painful hemiplegic shoulder: Effects of intra articular triamcinolone. Am J Phys Med Rehabil 1997;76:43–48.
42. Demeter S, Andersson G, Smith G: Disability evaluation. N Engl J Med 335:1245–1246, 1996.
43. Depoy E: A comparison of standardized and observational assessments. J Cogn Rehabil Jan/Feb:30–33, 1992.
44. Deyo R: Comparative validity of the sickness impact profile and shorter scales for functional assessment in low-back pain. Spine 11:951–954, 1986.
45. Deyo R: Measuring the functional status of patients with low back pain. Arch Phys Med Rehabil 69:1044–1053, 1988.
46. Deyo R, Centor R: Assessing the responsiveness of functional scales to clinical change: An analogy to diagnostic test performance. J Chron Dis 39:897–906, 1986.
47. Deyo RA, Andersson G, Bombardier C, et al: Outcome measures for studying patients with low back pain. Spine 19(18 Suppl.):2032S–2036S, 1994.
48. Dodrill C: The hand dynamometer as a neuropsychological measure. J Consult Clin Psychol 46:1432–1435, 1978.
49. Droege R: Is Age a Moderator of GATB Validity? Paper presented at the Annual Meeting of the American Psychological Association, August 26–30, 1983, Anaheim, CA.
50. Dusik L, Menard M, Cooke C, et al: Concurrent validity of the ERGOS Work Simulator versus conventional capacity evaluation techniques in a workers' compensation population. J Occup Med 35:759–767, 1993.
51. Dvir Z: Differentiation of submaximal from maximal trunk extension effort: An isokinetic study using a new testing protocol. Spine 22:2672–2676, 1997.
52. Edwards M: The reliability and validity of self report activities of daily living. Can J Occup Ther 57:273–278, 1990.
53. EEOC: Uniform guidelines on employee selection procedures (1978). Federal Register July 1:212–239, 1993.
54. Esmail S, Bhambhani Y, Britnell S: Gender differences in work performance on the Baltimore Therapeutic Equipment work simulator. Am J Occup Ther 49:405–411,1995.
55. Falconer J, Hughes S, Naughton B, et al: Self report and performance-based hand function tests as correlates of dependency in the elderly. J Am Geriatr Soc 39:695–699, 1991.
56. Feys H, DeWeerdt W, Selz B, et al: Effect of a therapeutic intervention for the hemiplegic upper limb in the acute phase after stroke: A single blind, randomized, controlled multicenter trial. Stroke 29:785–792, 1998.
57. Fishbain D, Abdel-Moty E, Cutler R, et al: Measuring residual functional capacity in chronic low back pain patients based on the Dictionary of Occupational Titles. Spine 19:872–880, 1994.
58. Fishbain DA, Cutler RB, Rosomoff H, et al: Validity of the Dictionary of Occupational Titles residual functional capacity battery. Clin J Pain 15:102–110, 1999.
59. Fisher AG, Liu Y, Velozo CA, Pan AW: Cross-cultural assessment of process skills. Am J Occup Ther 46:876–885, 1992.
60. Flanagan J: SRA Flanagan Aptitude Classification Test Manual. Rosemont, Ill, NCS, 1964.
61. Flanagan J: SRA Flanagan Industrial Tests Manual. Rosemont, Ill, NCS, 1975.
62. Fleishman E: Evaluating physical abilities required by jobs. The Personnel Administrator June:82–87, 1979.
63. Fleishman E, Quaintance M: Taxonomies of human performance: The description of human tasks. Orlando, Fla, Academic Press, 1984.
64. Ford D, Kwak A, Wolfe L: Grip strength decrease and recovery following isotonic exercise. J Hand Ther 3:36, 1990.
65. Fraser T: Fitness for Work. Bristol, Pa, Taylor & Francis, 1992.
66. Fry R, Botterbusch K (eds): VEWAA glossary: A collection of terms and definitions of special importance to vocational evaluation and adjustment services personnel. Menomonie, Wis, University of Wisconsin-Stout, Materials Development Center, Stout Vocational Rehabilitation Institute, 1988.
67. Garcy P, Mayer T, Gatchel RJ: Recurrent or new injury outcomes after return to work in chronic disabling spinal disorders: Tertiary prevention efficacy of functional restoration treatment. Spine 21:952–959, 1996.
68. Garg A: Ergonomics and the older worker: An overview. Dev Aging Res 17(S3):143–155, 1991.
69. Gatewood R, Feild H: Human Resource Selection, 3rd ed. Fort Worth, Tex, The Dryden Press, 1994.
70. Gaudino E, Mael F, Matheson L: A Literature Review: Functional Assessment and Related Construct Taxonomies. Washington, DC, American Institutes for Research, 1999.
71. Gaudino E, Mael F, Matheson L: Synthesis of Research and Development of Prototypes for a New Disability Determination Methodology: A Literature Review of Functional Assessment and Related Construct Taxonomies. Washington, DC, American Institutes for Research, 1999.
72. Gaudino E, Matheson L, Mael F: Development of the functional assessment taxonomy. J Occup Rehabil 11:155–175, 2001.
73. Gilbert C, Knowlton R: Simple method to determine sincerity of effort during a maximal isometric test of grip strength. Am J Phys Med 62:135–144, 1983.
74. Gill D, Reddon J, Renney C, Stefanyk W: Hand dynamometer: Effects of trials and sessions. Percept Mot Skills 61:195–198, 1985.
75. Gloss D, Wardle M: Use of a test of psychomotor ability in an expanded role. Percept Mot Skills 53:659–662, 1981.
76. Granger C, Gresham G (eds): Functional Assessment in Rehabilitation Medicine. Baltimore, Williams & Wilkins, 1984.
77. Granger C, Gresham G (eds): New Developments in Functional Assessment. Philadelphia, WB Saunders, 1993.
78. Growick B, Kaliope G, Jones C: Sample norms for the hearing impaired on select components of the Valpar work sample series. Vocational Evaluation and Work Adjustment Bulletin 16:56–57, 68, 1983.
79. Hakstian A, Bennet R: Validity studies using the Comprehensive Ability Battery (CAB): I. Academic achievement criteria. Educational and Psychological Measurement 37:425–437, 1977.
80. Hakstian A, Woolsey L: Validity studies using the Comprehensive Ability Battery (CAB): IV Predicting achievement at the University Level. Educational and Psychological Measurement 45:329–341, 1985.
81. Hanson M, Matheson L, Borman W: The O*NET Occupational Information System. In Bolton B (ed): Handbook of Measurement and Evaluation in Rehabilitation, 3rd ed. Gaithersburg, Md, Aspen, 2001, pp 281–309.
82. Harris J: Innovations in vocational evaluation and work adjustment. APTICOM: A computerized multiple aptitude testing instrument for cost and time effective vocational evaluation. Vocational Evaluation and Work Adjustment Bulletin 15:161, 1982.
83. Hart D, Iserhagen S, Matheson L: Guidelines for functional capacity evaluation of people with medical conditions. J Orthop Sports Phys Ther 18:682–686, 1993.
84. Harvey P, Gench B: A comparison of static grip strength measurements taken on the Jamar dynamometer and the BTE. J Hand Ther 6:53–54, 1993.
85. Hasten D, Johnston F, Lea R: Validity of the Applied Rehabilitation Concepts (ARCON) system for lumbar range of motion. Spine 20:1279–1283, 1995.
86. Hasten D, Lea R, Johnston F: Lumbar range of motion in male heavy laborers on the Applied Rehabilitation Concepts (ARCON). Spine 21:2230–2234, 1996.

87. Hazard R, Reeves V, Fenwick J: Lifting capacity: Indices of subject effort. Spine 17:1065–1070, 1992.

88. Heinemann A, Linacre J, Wright B, et al: Measurement characteristics of the functional independence measure. Topics in Stroke Rehabilitation 1:1–15, 1994.

89. Herdmann J: An exploratory factor analysis of the Career Ability Placement Survey (CAPS) with the WAIS-R and the WRAT with a referral population. Dissertation Abstracts International 47 (4-B):1783–1784, 1986.

90. Hildreth D, Breidenbach W, Lister G, Hodges A: Detection of submaximal effort by use of the rapid exchange grip. J Hand Surg 14A:742–745, 1989.

91. Holden MK, Gill KM, Magliozzi MR: Gait assessment for neurologically impaired patients. Standards for outcome assessment. Phys Ther 66:1530–1539, 1986.

92. Hsieh C, Hsueh I, Chiang F, Lin P: Inter-rater reliability and validity of the action research arm test in stoke patients. Age Ageing 27:107–113, 1998.

93. Innes E, Straker L: Reliability of work-related assessments. Work 13:107–124, 1999.

94. Innes E, Straker L: Validity of work-related assessments. Work 13:125–152, 1999.

95. Isernhagen S: Functional capacity evaluation and work hardening perspectives. In Mayer TG, Mooney JV, Gatchel R (eds): Contemporary conservative care for painful spinal disorders. Philadelphia, Lea & Febiger, 1991, p 328–345.

96. Isernhagen S: Contemporary issues in functional capacity evaluation. In Isernhagen S (ed): The Comprehensive Guide to Work Injury Management. Gaithersburg, Md, Aspen, 1995, pp 410–429.

97. Isernhagen S, Hart D, Matheson L: Reliability of independent observer judgments of level of lift effort in a kinesiophysical functional capacity evaluation. Work 1999, pp 145–150.

98. Isernhagen SJ: Functional capacity evaluation. In Isernhagen SJ (ed): Work Injury: Management and Prevention. Rockville, Md, Aspen, 1988.

99. Isernhagen SJ: Return to work testing: Functional capacity and work capacity evaluation. Orthopaedic Physical Therapy Clinics/Industrial Physical Therapy 1:83–97, 1992.

100. Isernhagen Work Systems: Reliability and validity of the Isernhagen Work Systems Functional Capacity Evaluation. Duluth, Minn, Author, 1996.

101. Iverson G, Franzen M: Detecting malingering memory deficits with the Recognition Memory Test. Brain Inj 12:275–282, 1998.

102. Janikowski T, Berven N, Bordieri J: Validity of the Microcomputer Evaluation Screening and Assessment aptitude scores. Rehabil Couns Bull 35:38–51, 1991.

103. Janikowski T, Bordieri J, Musgrave J: Construct validation of the academic achievement and general educational development subtests of the Microcomputer Evaluation Screening and Assessment (MESA). Vocational Evaluation and Work Adjustment Bulletin 23:11–16, 1990.

104. Janikowski T, Bordieri J, Shelton D, Musgrave J: Convergent and discriminant validity of the Microcomputer Evaluation Screening and Assessment (MESA) interest survey. Rehabil Couns Bull 34:139–149, 1990.

105. Jay M, Lamb J, Watson R, et al: Sensitivity and specificity of the indicators of sincere effort of the EPIC Lift Capacity test on a previously injured population. Spine 25:1405–1412, 2000.

106. Jebsen R, Taylor N, Trieschmann R, et al: An objective and standardized test of hand function. Arch Phys Med Rehabil 50:311–319, 1969.

107. Jette A: Physical disablement concepts for physical therapy research and practice. Phys Ther 74:380–386, 1994.

108. Jette A, Cleary P: Functional disability assessment. Phys Ther 67:1854–1859, 1987.

109. Johnston M, Keith R, Hinderer S: Measurement standards for interdisciplinary medical rehabilitation. Arch Phys Med Rehabil 73:S3–S23, 1992.

110. Jones C, Lasiter C: Worker-non-worker differences on three Valpar component work samples. Vocational Evaluation and Work Adjustment Bulletin 10:23–27, 1997.

111. Kaplan G, Wurtele S, Gillis D: Maximal effort during functional capacity evaluations: An examination of psychological factors. Arch Phys Med Rehabil 77:161–164, 1996.

112. Katz N, Champagne D, Cermak S: Comparison of the performance of younger and older adults on three versions of a puzzle reproduction task. Am J Occup Ther 51:562–568, 1997.

113. Katz N, Itzkovich M, Averbuch S, Elazar B: Loewenstein Occupational Therapy Cognitive Assessment battery for brain-injured patients: reliability and validity. Am J Occup Ther 43:184–192, 1989.

114. Kennedy L, Bhambhani Y: The Baltimore Therapeutic Equipment work simulator: Reliability and validity at three work intensities. Arch Phys Med Rehabil 72:511–516, 1991.

115. Key G: Functional capacity assessment. In Key G (ed): Industrial Therapy. St. Louis, Mosby-Year Book 220–253, 1995.

116. King J, Berryhill B: A comparison of two static grip testing methods and its clinical applications: A preliminary study. J Hand Ther 1:204–207, 1988.

117. King J, Berryhill B: Assessing maximum effort in upper-extremity functional testing. Work 1:65–76, 1991.

118. Kirkpatrick J: Evaluation of grip loss: A factor of permanent partial disability in California. Indust Med Surg 26:285–289, 1957.

119. Kline P, Cooper C: The factor structure of the Comprehensive Ability Battery. British Journal of Educational Psychology 54:106–110, 1984.

120. Knapp RR, Knapp L, Michael WB: Stability and concurrent validity of the Career Ability Placement Survey (CAPS) against the DAT and the GATB. Educational and Psychological Measurement 37:1081–1085, 1977.

121. Krombholz H: On the association of effort and force of handgrip. Percept Mot Skills 60:161–162, 1985.

122. Kujoth R: The validity of the GATB for the educationally deficient. Journal of Employment Counseling 10:44–48, 1973.

123. Laver A: Structured observational test of function: Clinical and research applications. Presented at the 1995 annual conference of the American Occupational Therapy Association, Denver, Colo.

124. Lechner D, Bradbury S, Bradley L: Detecting sincerity of effort: A summary of methods and approaches. Phys Ther 78:867–888, 1998.

125. Lechner D, Jackson J, Roth D, Straaton K: Reliability and validity of a newly developed test of physical work performance. J Occup Med 36:997–1004, 1994.

126. Lechner D, Jackson J, Straaton K: Interrater reliability and validity of a newly developed FCE: The physical work performance evaluation. Phys Ther 73:S27, 1993.

127. Lechner D, Roth D, Straaton K: Functional capacity evaluation in work disability. Work 1:37–47, 1991.

128. Lee G, Loring D, Martin R: Rey's 15-item visual memory test for the detection of malingering: Normative observations on patients with neurological disorders. Psychological Assessment 4:43–46, 1992.

129. Leggett S, Pollock M, Graves J, et al: Quantitative assessment of full range-of-motion lumbar extension strength. Med Sci Sports Exerc 20:S87, 1988.

130. Light K, Purser J, Rose D: The functional reach test for balance: Criterion related validity of clinical observations. Issues on Aging 18:5–9, 1995.

131. Luck J, Florence D: A brief history and comparative analysis of disability systems and impairment rating guides. Orthop Clin North Am 19:839–844, 1988.

132. Ludlow G, Pollard G: The Bennett Hand-Tool Dexterity Test: Normative data for a hearing-impaired/deaf secondary student population. Vocational Evaluation and Work Adjustment Bulletin 17:62–64, 1984.
133. Lyle R: A performance test for assessment of upper limb function in physical rehabilitation treatment and research. Int J Rehabil Res 4:483–492, 1981.
134. Mack J: Validity of the Purdue Pegboard as screening test for brain damage in a psychiatric population. Percept Mot Skills 28:832–834, 1969.
135. Maddox T: A Comprehensive Reference for Assessments in Psychology, Education, and Business. Austin, Tex, Pro-Ed, 1997.
136. Matheson L: WEST Standard Evaluation Examiner's Manual. Huntington Beach, Calif, Work Evaluation Systems Technology, 1980.
137. Matheson L: Work Capacity Evaluation for Occupational Therapists. Trabuco Canyon, CA, Rehabilitation Institute of Southern California, 1982.
138. Matheson L: Evaluation of lifting and lowering capacity. Vocational Evaluation and Work Adjustment Bulletin 19:107–111, 1986.
139. Matheson L: Integrated work hardening in vocational rehabilitation: An emerging model. Vocational Evaluation and Work Adjustment Bulletin 22:71–76, 1988.
140. Matheson L: Work capacity evaluation. In: Tollison C, Kriegel M (eds): Interdisciplinary Rehabilitation of Low Back Pain. Baltimore, Williams & Wilkins, 1989, pp 323–342.
141. Matheson L: Symptom magnification syndrome structured interview: Rationale and procedure. J Occup Rehabil 1:43–56, 1991.
142. Matheson L: Basic requirements for utility in the assessment of physical disability. APS Journal 3:193–199, 1994.
143. Matheson L: Manual Material Handling Examiner's Manual. Wildwood, Mo, Employment Potential Improvement Corporation, 1995.
144. Matheson L: Functional capacity evaluation. In Andersson G, Demeter S, Smith G (eds): Disability Evaluation. Chicago, Mosby Yearbook, 1996.
145. Matheson L: Relationships among age, body weight, resting heart rate, and performance in a new test of lift capacity. J Occup Rehabil 6:225–237, 1996.
146. Matheson L, Kaskutas V, McCowan S, et al: Development of a database of functional assessment measures related to work disability. J Occup Rehabil 11:177–199, 2001.
147. Matheson L, Anzai D, Niemeyer L, et al: Lido WorkSET Cookbook. Sacramento, Calif, Employment and Rehabilitation Institute of California, 1991.
148. Matheson L, Bohr P, Hart D: Use of maximum voluntary effort grip strength testing to identify symptom magnification syndrome in persons with low back pain. J Back Musculoskel Rehabil 10:125–135, 1998.
149. Matheson L, Danner R, Grant J, Mooney V: Effect of computerized instructions on measurement of lift capacity: Safety, reliability, and validity. J Occup Rehabil 3:65–81, 1993.
150. Matheson L, Matheson M, Grant J: Development of a measure of perceived functional ability. J Occup Rehabil 3:15–30, 1993.
151. Matheson L, Mooney V, Caiozzo V, et al: Effect of instructions on isokinetic trunk strength testing variability, reliability, absolute value, and predictive validity. Spine 17:914–921, 1992.
152. Matheson L, Mooney V, Grant J, et al: A test to measure lift capacity of physically impaired adults. Part 1: Development and reliability testing. Spine 20:2119–2129, 1995.
153. Matheson L, Mooney V, Holmes D, et al: A test to measure lift capacity of physically impaired adults. Part 2: Reactivity in a patient sample. Spine 20:2130–2134, 1995.
154. Matheson L, Ogden L, Violette K, Schultz K: Work hardening: Occupational therapy in industrial rehabilitation. Am J Occup Ther 39:314–321, 1985.
155. Matheson LN, Mooney V, Grant JE, et al: Standardized evaluation of work capacity. J Back Musculoskel Rehabil 6:249–264, 1996.
156. Mathiowetz V: Reliability and validity of grip and pinch strength measurements. Phys Rehabil Med 2:201–212, 1991.
157. Mathiowetz V: Role of physical performance component evaluations in occupational therapy functional assessment. Am J Occup Ther 47:225–230, 1993.
158. Mathiowetz V, Kashman N, Volland G, et al: Grip and pinch strength: Normative data for adults. Arch Phys Med Rehabil 6:69–74, 1985.
159. Mathiowetz V, Rogers S, Dowe-Keval M, et al: The Purdue Pegboard: Norms for 14- to 19-year-olds. Am J Occup Ther 40:174–179, 1986.
160. Mathiowetz V, Weber K, Volland G, Kashman N: Reliability and validity of grip and pinch strength evaluations. J Hand Surg 9A:222–226, 1984.
161. Mayer T, Barnes D, Kishino N, et al: Progressive isoinertial lifting evaluation. I. A standardized protocol and normative database. Spine 13:993–997, 1988.
162. Mayer T, Gatchel R, Mooney V: Safety of the dynamic progressive isointertial lifting. Spine 15:985–986, 1990.
163. Mayer TG, Barnes D, Nichols G, et al: Progressive isoinertial lifting evaluation. II. A comparison with isokinetic lifting in a disabled chronic low-back pain industrial population [published erratum appears in Spine 15:5, 1990]. Spine 13:998–1002, 1988.
164. McDaniel L, Anderson K, Bradley L, et al: Development of an observation method for assessing pain behavior in rheumatoid arthritis patients. Pain 24:165–184, 1986.
165. Muchinsky P: Validation of intelligence and mechanical aptitude tests in selecting employees for manufacturing jobs. Journal of Business and Psychology 7:373–382, 1993.
166. Nagi S: Disability concepts and prevalence. Paper presented at Mary Switzer Memorial Seminar, National Rehabilitation Association, Cleveland, Ohio, 1975.
167. Nagi S: Disability concepts revisited: Implications for prevention. In Pope A, Tarlov A (eds): Disability in America. Washington, DC, National Academy Press, 1991, pp 309–327.
168. Nattrass C, Nitschke J, Disler P, et al: Lumbar spine range of motion as a measure of physical and functional impairment: An investigation of validity. Clin Rehabil 13:211–218, 1999.
169. NCMRR: Research plan for the National Center for Medical Rehabilitation Research. Washington, DC, National Institutes of Health, 1993.
170. Needham W, Eldridge L: Performance of blind vocational rehabilitation clients on the Minnesota Rate of Manipulation Tests. Journal of Visual Impairment & Blindness 84:182–185, 1990.
171. NIDRR: National Institute on Disability and Rehabilitation Research: Correction for final long-range plan for fiscal years 1999–2003; Notice. Washington, DC. Federal Register 64:68575–68614, 1999.
172. Niebuhr B, Marion R: Detecting sincerity of effort when measuring grip strength. Am J Phys Med 66:16–23, 1987.
173. Niemeyer L, Matheson L, Carlton R: Testing consistency of effort: BTE Work Simulator. Industrial Rehabilitation Quarterly 2:5,12–13,27–32, 1989.
174. NIOSH: Work Practices Guide for Manual Lifting. Cincinnati, Ohio, Division of Biomedical and Behavioral Science, NIOSH, 1981.
175. Nueman F, Nomoto J: Personnel selection tests for computer professional and support technicians. Journal of Business and Psychology 5:165–177, 1990.
176. Ogden-Niemeyer L: Procedure Guidelines for the West Standard Evaluation. Ft. Bragg, Calif, Work Evaluation Systems Technology, 1989.
177. Ogden-Niemeyer L, Jacobs K: Work Hardening: State of the Art. Thorofare, NJ, Slack, 1989.

178. Osborn R, Sanders W: The Crawford Small Parts Dexterity Test as a time-limit test. Personnel Psychol 9:177–180, 1956.
179. Ottenbacher K, Hsu Y, Granger C, Fiedler R: The reliability of the functional independence measure: A quantitative review. Arch Phys Med Rehabil 77:1226–1232, 1996.
180. Pilowsky I, Spence N, Cobb J, Katsikitis M: The Illness Behavior Questionnaire as an aid to clinical assessment. General Hospital Psychiatry 6:123–130, 1984.
181. Portney L, Watkins M: Foundations of Clinical Research. Applications to Practice. East Norwalk, Conn, Appleton & Lange, 1993.
182. Portney L, Watkins M: Foundations of Clinical Research: Applications to Practice, 2nd ed. Upper Saddle River, NJ, Prentice-Hall, 2000.
183. Reddon J, Gill D, Gauk S, Maerz M: Purdue Pegboard: Test-retest estimates. Percept Mot Skills 66:503–506, 1988.
184. Robertson L, Brodowicz G, Swafford A: Improved detection of submaximum effort in upper extremity strength and strength-endurance performance testing. J Occup Rehabil 7:83–96, 1997.
185. Robinson M, Geisser M, Hanson C, O'Connor P: Detecting submaximal efforts in grip strength testing with the coefficient of variation. J Occup Rehabil 3:45–50, 1993.
186. Robinson M, Sadler I, O'Connor P, Riley J: Detection of submaximal effort and assessment of stability of the coefficient of variation. J Occup Rehabil 7:207–215, 1997.
187. Roeder W: Roeder Manipulative Aptitude Test. Lafayette, IN, Lafayette Instruments, 1967.
188. Rondinelli R, Dunn W, Hassanein K, et al: A simulation of hand impairments: Effects on upper extremity function and implications toward medical impairment rating and disability determination. Arch Phys Med Rehabil 78:1358–1363, 1997.
189. Rose F, Hall S, Szalda-Petree A: A comparison of four tests of malingering and the effects of coaching. Arch Clin Neuropsychol 13:349–363, 1998.
190. Rothstein J, Campbell S, Echternach J, et al: Appendix: Standards for tests and measurements in physical therapy practice. In Rothstein J, Echternach J (eds): Primer on Measurement. Alexandria, Va, American Physical Therapy Association, 1993, p 3–47.
191. Ruch F, Ruch W: Employee Aptitude Survey. Los Angeles, Calif, Psychological Services, 1963.
192. Rucker K, Wehman P, Kregel J: Analysis of functional assessment instruments for disability/rehabilitation programs. Richmond, Va, Virginia Commonwealth University,; 1996.
193. Saxon J, Spitznagel R, Shelhorn-Schutt P: Intercorrelations of selected Valpar Component Work Samples and General Aptitude Test Batter scores. Vocational Evaluation and Work Adjustment Bulletin 16:20–23, 1983.
194. Schult M, Soderback I, Jacobs K: Swedish use and validation of Valpar work samples for patients with musuloskeletal neck and shoulder pain. Work 5:223–233, 1995.
195. Shackleton T, Harburn K, Noh S: Pilot study of upper-extremity work and power in chronic cumulative trauma disorders. Occup Ther J Res 17:3–24, 1997.
196. Sharma SH, Schumacher R, McLellan AT: Evaluation of the Jebsen Hand Function Test for use in patients with rheumatoid arthritis. Arthritis Care Res 7:16–19, 1994.
197. Shervington J, Balla J: Screening workplace capabilities for competitive employment: Report on workplace feedback. Industrial engineering in occupational health. ANAMA Seminars 3:31–65,1994.
198. Shervington J, Balla J: WorkAbility Mark III: Functional assessment of workplace capbilities. Work 7:191–202,1996.
199. Shervington J, Lam A, Ganora A: Functional testing with WorkAbility Mark III. Paper presented at the twelfth annual scientific meeting of the Australasian College of Rehabilitation Medicine, Melbourne, Victoria, Australia, 1992.
200. Simonsen J: Coefficient of variation as a measure of subject effort. Arch Phys Med Rehabil 76:516–520, 1995.
201. Smith G, Nelson R, Sadoff S, Sadoff A: Assessing sincerity of effort in maximal grip strength tests. Am J Phys Med Rehabil 68:73–80, 1989.
202. Smith R, Benge M: Pinch and grasp strength: Standardization of terminology and protocol. Am J Occup Ther 39:531–535, 1985.
203. Snook S: Psychophysical Assessments of Material Handling Efforts. Proceedings of the 12th Triennial Congress of the International Ergonomics Association, Hopkinton, Mass, 1994.
204. Spaulding SJ, McPherson JJ, Strachota E, et al: Jebsen Hand Function Test: Performance of the uninvolved hand in hemiplegia and of right-handed, right and left hemiplegic persons. Arch Phys Med Rehabil 69:419–422, 1988.
205. Spieler E, Barth P, Burton J, et al: Recommendations to guide revision of the Guides to the Evaluation of Permanent Impairment. JAMA 283:519–523, 2000.
206. Stern E: Stability of the Jebsen-Taylor Hand Function Test across three test sessions. Am J Occup Ther 46:647–649, 1992.
207. Stoelting C: A study of the construct validity of the MESA. Vocational Evaluation and Work Adjustment Bulletin 23:85–91, 1990.
208. Swarthout D, Synk D: The Effect of Age, Education, and Work Experience on General Aptitude Test Battery Validity and Test Scores. Washington, DC, USES Employment and Training Administration, 1987, p 65.
209. Tan H, Barrett T, Fowler B: Study of the Inter-rater, Test-retest Reliability and Content Validity of the WEST Standard Evaluation. Proceedings of the 19th National Conference of the Australian Association of Occupational Therapists, Perth, Australia, 1997, 2, pp 245–251.
210. Tiffin J, Asher E: The Purdue Pegboard: Norms and studies of reliability and validity. J Appl Psychol 32:234–247, 1948.
211. U.S. Department of Labor: Handbook for Analyzing Jobs. Washington, DC, Manpower Administration, 1972.
212. U.S. Department of Labor: Dictionary of Occupational Titles, 4th ed. Washington, DC, Author, 1991.
213. U.S. Department of Labor: The Revised Handbook for Analyzing Jobs. Washington, DC, Author, 1991.
214. U.S. Department of Justice CRD, Office on the Americans With Disabilities Act: The Americans With Disabilities Act: Title II Technical Assistance Manual. Washington, DC, Author, 1992.
215. Valpar International Corporation: Valpar Component Work Sample Series. Tucson, Ariz, Author, 1996.
216. Van Lankeveld W: Sequential occupational dexterity assessment: A new test to measure hand disability. J Hand Ther 91:27–32, 1996.
217. Van Lankveld W: Predictors of changes in observed dexterity during one year in patients with rheumatoid arthritis. Br J Rheumatol 37:733–739, 1998.
218. Velozo C: Work evaluations: Critique of the state of the art of functional assessment of work. Am J Occup Ther 47:203–209, 1993.
219. Verdino M, Dingman S: Two measures of laterality in handedness: The Edinburgh Handedness Inventory and the Purdue Pegboard test of manual dexterity. Percept Mot Skills 86:476–478, 1998.
220. Vevea J, Clements N, Hedges L: Assessing the effects of selection bias on validity data for the general aptitude test battery. J Appl Psychol 78:981–987, 1993.
221. Waddell G, Bircher M, Finlayson D, Main C: Symptoms and signs: Physical disease or illness behavior? Br Med J 289:739–741, 1984.
222. Waddell G, McCullock J, Kummel E, Venner R: Nonorganic physical signs in low-back pain. Spine 5:117–125, 1980.
223. Waddell G, Pilowsky I, Bond M: Non-anatomical symptoms and signs: A response to critics. Pain 42:260–261, 1990.

224. Waters T, Putz-Anderson V, Garg A (eds): Applications Manual for the Revised NIOSH Lifting Equation. Cincinnati, Ohio, U.S. Department of Health & Human Services, 1994.
225. Waters T, Putz-Anderson V, Garg A, Fine L: Revised NIOSH equation for the design and evaluation of manual lifting tasks. Ergonomics 36:749–776, 1993.
226. Wheeler D, Graves J, Miller G, et al: Functional assessment for prediction of lifting capacity. Spine 19:1021–1026, 1994.
227. Whitten E: Pathology, impairment, functional limitation and disability—Implications for practice, research, program and policy development and service delivery. Cleveland, Ohio, National Rehabilitation Association, 1975.
228. Wilke N, Sheldahl L, Dougherty S, et al: Baltimore Therapeutic Equipment Work Simulator: Energy expenditure of work activities in cardiac patients. Arch Phys Med Rehabil 74:419–424, 1994.
229. Winkler R: Validation of a test battery for manufacturing machine operators. Journal of Business and Psychology 7:137–149, 1992.
230. Wolf L, Klein L, Cauldwell-Klein E: Comparison of torque strength measurements on two evaluation devices. J Hand Ther 2:24–27, 1987.
231. Wolf L, Matheson L, Ford D, Kwak A: Relationship among grip strength, work capacity, and recovery. J Occup Rehabil 6:57–70, 1996.
232. Woody R, Mathiowetz V: Effect of forearm position on pinch strength measurements. J Hand Ther 1:124–126, 1988.
233. World Health Organization: International Classification of Impairments, Disabilities and Handicaps. Geneva, World Health Organization, 1980.
234. World Health Organization: ICIDH-2: Towards a Common Language for Functioning and Disablement: The International Classification of Impairments, Activities, and Participation. Geneva, World Health Organization, 1998.
235. Young C: Schedule for Rating Permanent Disabilities. Sacramento, Calif, State of California Department of Industrial Relations, Division of Workers' Compensation, 1997.

CHAPTER

56

Work Hardening

SUSAN J. ISERNHAGEN, PT

Musculoskeletal injuries create a perceived or actual inability for a worker to continue working. With the filing of a claim, the injured worker enters an arena that may include medical diagnosis, therapist diagnosis, immediate care, palliative care, restorative care, or even benign neglect. Regardless of the medical interventions and the outside attempt by employers to reduce workers' compensation costs, the system that an injured worker enters creates a milieu that often leads to prolonged absence from work.

Experts have agreed, disagreed, and debated the reason for prolonged absence of work after reported industrial injury. Regardless of the debate, and notwithstanding the many components experts identify (e.g., back strains, psychosocial problems, cumulative traumas, poor relationships between worker and management, absence of safe ergonomic work in the workplace), it is a fact that many injured workers are off work for a period of time. This creates a financial disadvantage to employers through workers' compensation, questioning in the medical communities regarding work progress of the patient, and various responses in the injured worker that range from frustration at being hurt to anger at "the system."

Matheson was one of the first professionals to recognize that an injured worker's productive role could be restored with a complex system that included the following:

- Physical restoration
- Psychological support
- Strong functional goals

He first described his work hardening program at Rancho Los Amigos Hospital.[11] He continued to define and publish on work hardening, which he described as a "work oriented treatment program that has an outcome which is measured in terms of improvement in the client's productivity."

Dr. Matheson further defined work hardening perspectives:

> Unlike conventional programs, it does not focus on such goals as symptom reduction or increased physical capacity. Through graded work simulations conducted in a realistic industrial or office setting, a multidisciplinary team rebuilds physical and psychological fitness to work. Injured workers also receive counseling to help them compete effectively with other workers. The program has helped to transform many participants who viewed themselves as disabled back into employable workers.

As many professionals and payers began to look at the efficacy of restoring work function, more pressure was generated to make the outcome not only "functional" but actually resulting in a return to work.

Thus work rehabilitation programs became one of the first medical based programs to focus on cost effectiveness and outcomes as a means of proving their worth. Professionals recognized the need for structure and the need for return to work outcome measurement in conjunction with the programs. Since then, the following concepts have been utilized:

- Recognition that each individual has both physical and psychosocial elements regarding the work injury and the relationship with the workplace.
- Recognition that physical deficiencies such as loss of strength or endurance or identification of specific pathologies are only part of the picture. Human beings function despite pathologies. It is the attention to the functional aspect, not the pathological aspect, that allows work rehabilitation to succeed.

- Recognition of the importance of the combination of goal orientation among worker, employer, and rehabilitation professional. Because the physical goals must actually be attained by the worker and the outcome goals of return to work are often in the hands of the employer, the rehabilitation professional can become the facilitator of both these processes.
- Use of a reality check, such as work simulation and functional capacity evaluation as part of the program to avoid work rehabilitation becoming just another "treatment."

HISTORY: CLINICAL

King postulates that in order for work hardening centers to compete, they must define the service and for whom it is best suited.[7] Measuring and evaluating outcomes as related to the amount of time and money spent will lead to opportunities for improvement. King delineates program evaluation that determines how efficient and effective a work hardening program is. One should expect performance of the program to be congruent with its expectations. "Program evaluation information is the basis on which to make decisions regarding performance."

Practitioners recognized the mandate toward outcome beyond discharge. "Functional capacity rehabilitation is not only hardening or strengthening of the body, but also includes rehabilitation to a safe, productive work level."[3] The issue of safety was integrated into the return to work process to begin to focus on avoiding injury recurrence.

Barriers to full treatment go beyond mere physical impairments. Ambrosius et al indicate that external factors, including high cost of treatment, can prevent some people from getting the care they need.[1] Internal factors such as self-image damage may be additionally disabling.

Beyond workers' compensation costs, the social costs, such as human suffering, loss of self-esteem, and reduced income, are significant problems that cannot be calculated. Graly et al state that work hardening can fix a body and technique through education, but sometimes more than that is needed to return a worker to work.[4] Lack of social support is linked with lower outcome of return to work. Their study also indicated that perceived pain is a large factor in predicting which work rehabilitation clients will return to work and/or stay at work. High pain scores were linked with the non-working group after the work hardening program.

Outcome studies have been performed in order to understand whether these rehabilitation programs affect disability. Lechner[8] indicated that 12 studies of work hardening and work conditioning programs in the United States showed that a work conditioning program may be more useful in producing a higher percentage of return to work than in an untreated population. One reported study demonstrated that a work hardening program increased the rate of return to work by 52%. Positive results in outcome studies overall are reported in individual research and also in this collected research.

These findings are compatible with those of King,[7] which indicated that of 22 work programs in Wisconsin, most clients were treated and discharged within the 3-week period and more than half of these clients had returned to their full and customary jobs.

HISTORY: PROFESSIONAL GUIDELINES

In 1986, the American Occupational Therapy Association (AOTA) Commission on Practice published work hardening guidelines.[13] The AOTA Commission defined work hardening as "an individualized work oriented activity process that involves a client in simulated or actual work tasks. These tasks are structured and graded progressively to increase psychological, physical and emotional tolerance and improve endurance in work feasibility." One these guidelines were promulgated, insurance companies and other professionals began to see the benefit of defining a field that was beginning to see significant growth.

The Commission for Accreditation of Rehabilitation Facilities (CARF) in 1988 appointed a multidisciplinary advisory committee to develop concepts including definitions and descriptions that would then be made available to payers and regulatory bodies. In 1999, CARF described Occupational Rehabilitation as an individualized program "focused on return to work, and designed to minimize risk to and optimize the work capability of the persons served. An Occupational Rehabilitation Program identifies, addresses and reduces, when possible, risks of injury, re-injury, disease and illness. The program may be provided at a hospital-based program, a free-standing program, or a private or group practice, or it may be provided in a work environment (at the job site)."

The American Physical Therapy Association created definitions and descriptions for work conditioning and work hardening. Through a 4-year field review process, it developed and published "Guidelines for Programs for Injured Workers."[2]

> Workers who have been injured benefit from (physical therapy) services from the onset of injury through their return to work. Early ... intervention consists of treatment for acute musculoskeletal problems and other injuries. Many clients who receive appropriate early care return to their jobs without additional rehabilitation services.
>
> ... For those who are not able to return to work because of unresolved physical problems following acute care, treatment focus changes to restoration of function. Defined as

"work conditioning" these programs address the physical issues of flexibility, strength, endurance, coordination and work related function with a goal of return to work. For the limited number of clients with behavioral and vocational dysfunction, "work hardening" may be indicated. Work hardening programs are interdisciplinary and address the physical, functional, behavioral and vocational needs of the injured worker, with the goal of returning to work.

WORK REHABILITATION: DEFINITION AND DESCRIPTION

Definitions

1. Work rehabilitation: A work-oriented, structured treatment program that utilizes the restorative philosophy of rehabilitation for the goal of a safe and functional return to work. A work rehabilitation program utilizes a "whole person" approach to improve the functional ability of a potential worker to match the physical demands of gainful employment. The process is entitled "work rehabilitation."
2. Participants: Participants in work rehabilitation are workers or potential workers who have physical conditions that preclude them from full or partial gainful employment. The physical problems are medically based but may have additional components of psychological or vocational overlay.

Clients

Work rehabilitation is utilized for the following:

1. An injured worker whose physical abilities do not match the physical requirements of an intended job
2. A worker with progressive disease-based physical impairment whose physical capacity has diminished
3. An applicant who does not have the physical abilities to do the job intended
4. A currently employed worker moving to a job that requires higher physical abilities

As defined both by CARF and APTA, a potential work rehabilitation client also must demonstrate willingness to comply with terms of the program and must have a personal goal of return to work.

Team Members

Professionals with a scientific base in neuromusculoskeletal diagnoses and functions form the core of the team. If work rehabilitation addresses psychosocial or vocational conditions, professionals with expertise in those backgrounds are also included. Professionals evaluate, manage, and provide ongoing supervision and discharge evaluation for workers in the program.

TABLE 56–1

Competencies Required in Work Rehabilitation

Client centered	Positive, firm client interaction Knowledge of the work client required to do Knowledge of the team at worksite
Professional skill	Supervision of support staff Differentiating normal function from dysfunction Medical-physiologic safety Goal setting for functional return to work

Competencies for professional staff should include the ability to interact in a positive yet constructively firm manner with clients, skill in supervising the safe and correct restorative treatment program designed by the professional, ability to identify deviations from expected or safe performance, scientific background knowledge of the pathologies/dysfunctions of the clients, skill in evaluating and differentiating normal function from dysfunction, aptitude in the evaluation of functional status with goal-setting, and knowledge of work, worksites, and specific employer requirements (see Table 56–1).

Settings

Settings for work rehabilitation have evolved as the needs have changed. Originally, work rehabilitation was designed for the most chronic populations and many settings were focused on clinic work with simulation equipment. With the advent of more focused physical rehabilitation, clinics with strength and endurance training were more commonly utilized. Today, the worksite is a desired option for on-the-job conditioning monitored by professionals. It is preferred as the ideal setting for at least the end stage of work rehabilitation.

SPECIFIC CHARACTERISTICS OF WORK REHABILITATION

Rehabilitation differs from acute care in a number of ways (see Table 56–2).

When work rehabilitation begins, acute hands-on therapy should be essentially finished. The client should have plateaued in his or her medical progress or healing stage so that the restorative focus is on increasing function rather than changing the structure of a person (see Table 56–2). Work rehabilitation should be started when there is a plateau in acute progress (and return to work has not been accomplished).

TABLE 56-2

Return to Work Treatment Flow

I	Stay at work modified duty with active treatment	50%	→	Return
II	Active acute treatment	↓ 40%	→	To
III	Work rehabilitation	↓ 9%	→	Work
	Disability	↓ 1%		

If the treatment level does not result in return to work, the next level of care is an option. All three treatment levels are return to work oriented. Percentages are estimated.

- If active healing is not finished, heavier activities of work rehabilitation may exacerbate the dysfunction or reinjure the healing part. Therefore, the musculoskeletal system should be stable before beginning the intensive rehabilitation progression.
- There is a difference in patient relationships between the medical management and the rehabilitation phase. In healing (acute or subacute hands-on care), the worker realizes that some of the healing process is taking place through the effort of the medical practitioner or treater. Therefore, there is a joint effort in getting past this healing phase. Also, the patient has the feeling that the treater is at least partially responsible for the increased function.
- Conversely, in the rehabilitation phase, the medical practitioner no longer "heals or fixes" the patient. Rather, the focus is on self-management and self-rehabilitation. If one tries to mix the message "I will help you" with the message "you are in charge of your own self-management," it is confusing to the patient. Therefore, there should be a clear understanding at the inception of the work rehabilitation phase that unless circumstances are very unusual, there will be no hands-on treatment. Patient self-management will be the focus.
- The term "plateau" does not mean that maximum healing has necessarily taken place. It rather means that the patient has reached a point in the healing or acute care phase where no further rapid changes are being made. In this plateau, if a person has not yet returned to work, active effort at the rehabilitation process should be made.

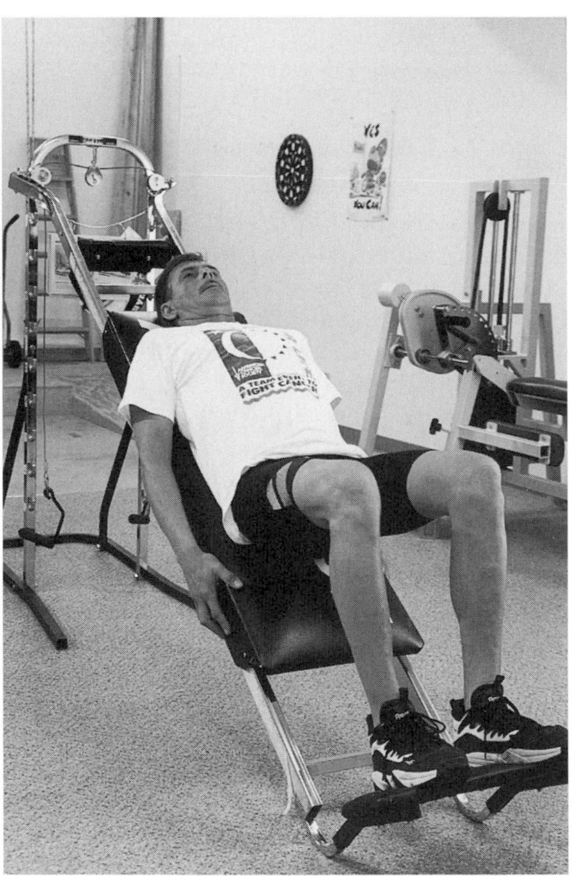

Figure 56–1. Performing leg extensions. This, as well as other exercises, is done to build muscle strength and endurance, as a precursor to work activity.

WORK REHABILITATION USES REHABILITATION PRINCIPLES

The Worker Becomes the Rehabilitator

Rehabilitation utilizes the facilitation of a medical/rehabilitation professional but the actual rehabilitation takes place through the efforts of the worker. No one can strengthen a person except the person doing his or her own exercise. No one can practice safe body mechanics except the person using his or her back in the correct manner. The medical/rehabilitation practitioner designs the most effective program but the worker is his or her own rehabilitator. This self-responsibility and awareness of self-management must be made clear at the entry point of work rehabilitation. The worker must agree to self manage.

The Goals are Functional

The initial evaluation will clearly define both the functional capacity of the worker and the functional demands of work. The work rehabilitator then documents where the discrepancy between the current status and the needed status lies. Functional goals are then written and a step-by-step plan of increasing function to the point of return to work is identified.

The true functional goals will lie in the plan as return to work aspects. For example:

- Ability to lift 40 pounds from 6 inches to 50 inches on an occasional basis

- Ability to sit at 1-hour intervals to do hand coordination work
- Ability to climb 6 flights of stairs in 4 minutes
- Ability to carry a 50-pound toolbox 100 feet

The rehabilitation program combines knowledge and treatment of the physical injury with functional activity. Examples are as follows:

- If discomfort in the low back is a limiting factor, methods of increasing spinal stability, changing the ergonomic position of the work, or taking rest and stretch breaks appropriate for work will be identified so that the functional goal can be met.
- If the heart rate goes above 80% of the maximum predicted heart rate, this is a limiting factor in stair climbing. Both aerobic capacity and muscle strength improvements will be identified and gained on a slow basis toward the functional goal. The client will understand how to monitor his or her own heart rate to determine when it is safe to progress an activity.
- If symptoms of increased irritation (such as in carpal tunnel syndrome or epicondylitis) become an issue, the client will learn to identify these symptoms early, change activities, and avoid aggravating the part. This does not mean activity must stop, but rather that it needs to be changed so that the affected part is not stressed with work continuing in another manner. Resumption of activity in the stressed part will happen when the symptoms abate. Thus, the symptoms become something to be controlled and the function becomes something to be developed. The mere presence of a symptom will not stop the program. Rather, it will start a process of problem solving.

This is an important concept because the goal of a "perfect body" cannot be attained and it derails the practitioner from the goal that can be attained. The goal of perfect body also gives the wrong message to the worker as he or she believes he or she will be somehow restored to a former capability level (which may be impossible) or that he or she may be restored to a pain-free existence (which also may be impossible).

The Whole Body is Involved

In workers' compensation there are reimbursement arguments such as "the degenerative knee condition was not the result of work, rather it was the result of an old football injury." Workers' compensation is more concerned about the low back condition that has been identified as being the work injury. In true rehabilitation, however, it is impossible to allow this injured worker to progress in lifting, carrying, or climbing unless the whole body is addressed. In many cases, a previous knee injury has even been the cause of a back injury as the worker has protected the old injury (knee) and utilized improper body mechanics (bending and twisting at the low back) to create a new problem.

Because the employer needs a "whole" worker back at work and the worker must be productive from a whole body aspect, it is impossible to rehabilitate without considering whole body function.

FOUR COMPONENTS OF WORK REHABILITATION

Work rehabilitation is not segmented treatment. It is comprised of components that interact. Each component has its own purpose. When all are combined, the whole person has improved in general function and, more importantly, in work outcome[5] (see Table 56–3).

Exercise

Exercise addresses neuromusculoskeletal issues. Exercise can be grouped into three broad categories:

- Stability/mobility
- Strength/endurance
- Coordination/balance

Stability/Mobility

Stabilization is that aspect of movement that provides a solid base of support that allows coordinated free motion to the other end. Examples are as follows:

- If the spine is stable, the extremities can move in all possible patterns.

TABLE 56–3
Work Rehabilitation

Musculoskeletal exercise	Stability–mobility Strength–endurance Balance–coordination
Aerobic training	Equipment based Aerobic classes Functional activities
Education	Principles Technique training Problem solving
Work activity	Simulated activity Actual equipment Actual work

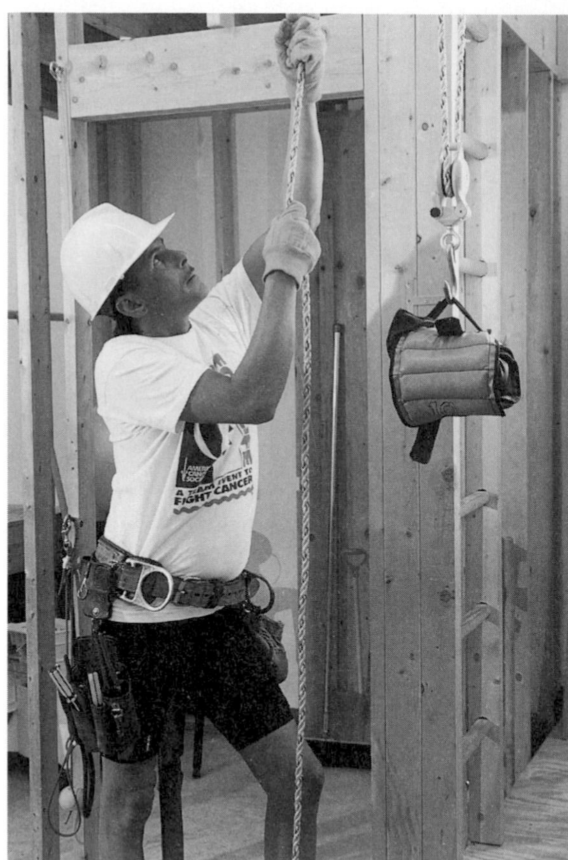

Figure 56–2. Man working with pulley simulating the work experience in the clinic builds job specific abilities and confidence.

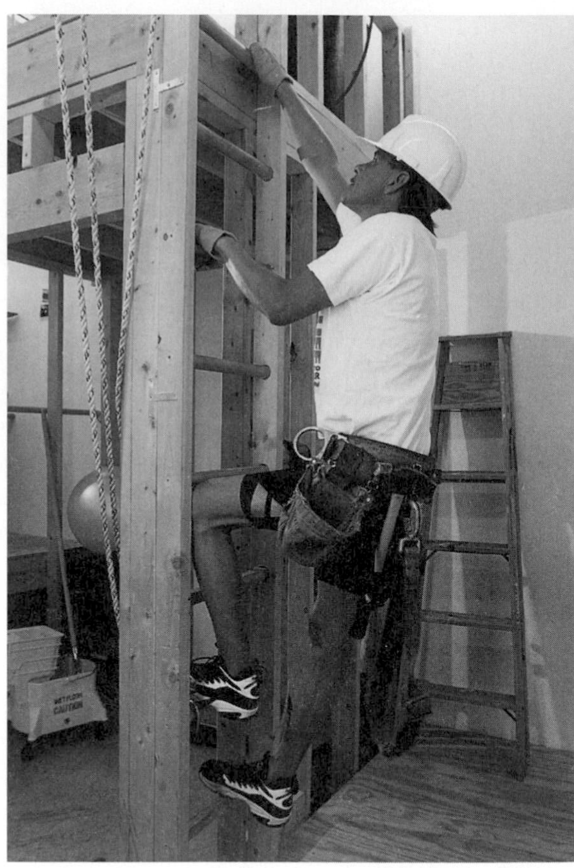

Figure 56–3. Climbing ladder. Balance and coordination in work-related activity are superior to basic exercise because of whole body training.

- If the spine is not stable at the body, the extremity movement loses control.
- If the low back is unstable and the legs begin a lift activity, this may result in loss of control in the lift and a movement-related injury to the lumbar spine.[9,10]

Spine

The movement patterns of manual material handling utilize small interlocking muscles of the spine to control proximal stability while powerful leg muscles or arm muscles produce the manual handling motion.

Sample equipment/methods of improving spinal stabilization are the following:

- Gymnastic ball with gymnastic ball routine.
- Pulley systems or free weight equipment or movement activity such as body blade

Upper Extremity Joints

The upper spine stabilizes so the shoulder can move; the shoulder stabilizes the upper arm so the elbow and lower joints can move. The wrist stabilizes the proximal wrist–hand so the fingers can freely move. The stability-mobility concept is important to recognize and evaluate in a client. Instability created through weakness, poor technique, or unexpected forces can occasionally result in fractures.

Sample Equipment/Methods of Extremity Mobility

- A pulley system with multiple attachments for its pulleys. The direction of the pull can be matched to the work activities of the client.
- Isolated muscle group exercisers selected for strengthening the correct muscle groups. The actual exercise should take place in as close to the plane used in the worksite as possible.
- Free weights are also excellent as they can work against gravity and in free movement patterns that can simulate work. It is extremely important for the progression of weights to be done in a safe progressive manner.

Strength/Endurance

When particular muscle groups are selected for strength and endurance training, similar equipment and activities can be utilized. Difference in application of the exercise regime will target short, strong muscle bursts for strengthening or a slower, lighter activity for endurance.

Strength

This is the production of maximum effort utilized at work. For example, lifting 40 pounds from the floor to 36 inches would be a typical activity. The worker is evaluated upon entry to the program for current maximum strength. The discrepancy between current function and job goals is noted. During the work rehabilitation program, specific goals should be set for increasing the maximum strength on a regular basis to match the highest level needed for the job.

Endurance

This is the ability of the neuromuscular system and the aerobic system to support repetitious activity. Endurance itself is built through repetitious activity in low weight sequences. Activities done in a "circuit" are often utilized as they replicate repetitious activity at less than maximum weight for the purpose of building endurance and coordination in specific work tasks. It is also notable that, over time, endurance is built through an increase in blood supply and strength of supporting structures and in aerobic capacity. Therefore, endurance itself must be built over time and maintained through work activity.

Balance/Coordination

A worker's capacity requires balance, particularly in:

- Climbing
- Frequent moving and twisting
- Walking over rough surfaces or outdoors
- When quick foot movement is necessary for sudden reactions at the workplace
- When the surface itself may be moving (such as working on a ship or train)

Workers who have had injuries that also damage their joints or muscle joint connections (necessary for proprioception), or who have mild neurologic injuries, may have impaired balance that has not been previously identified. Integrity of the balance and reaction systems must be evaluated. Balance should be incorporated into the exercise and work simulation.

Coordination, when impaired, is linked with work injury as well as caused by work injury. Poor work "technique" may have been an underlying cause of the initial injury. Attention to the following is specifically important so that the worker not only goes back to work with generalized balance and coordination, but utilizing the specific best "technique" of the job.

- Body mechanics must be evaluated as ability and understanding of keeping the spine stable while doing heavy activities will prevent the stresses on the spinal structures that can lead to injury.
- Utilizing weights and objects with good body sense will also be necessary. For example, for a nurse, the ability to use his or her own weight as a counterbalance to the patient's weight when doing a transfer is critical.
- Rolling and sliding objects is always preferable to lifting. An untrained worker at a new worksite may lift bags and products more than necessary when doing manual materials handling. The ability to slide, roll, and shift objects through proper "technique" will reduce the stresses on the body.

Because specific fine motor coordination of the hands is necessary in many jobs, hand coordination testing identifies skill level or differences in aptitude between one side and the other. To prevent upper extremity cumulative traumas, positioning of the neck, back, and all joints of the upper extremities is also important. Particular attention should be paid to optimizing the most relaxed and efficient position in which to gain the necessary hand coordination. Ergonomic positioning and aids are brought into the rehabilitation regime and incorporated upon return to work (Figs. 56–2 and 56–3).

Aerobic Training

Prior to aerobic training, the rehabilitation staff should have a procedure for the entry of workers into the program. Risk factors that require further medical evaluation should be identified.

Monitoring of heart rate is performed to inform evaluator and client of heart rate during activity, teach clients about their own heart rate and its response to activity, and as an objective measure of progress.

Equipment types utilized in aerobic training are treadmills, upper body ergometers, ergometer bicycles, and stair steppers. Aerobic movement classes are also amenable to group participation. Specific patterned activities can be designed for improvement of aerobic capacity and flexibility. Free movement activities such as walking or jogging produce a feeling of well-being and an increase in aptitude and daily living as well as work. Because these activities utilize no equipment, they are particularly adaptable to usefulness as home exercise programs.

Functional activities such as lifting training can become an aerobic activity if done in a "circuit." Large muscle groups are used in conjunction with walking and whole body movement. Functional activities, such as lifting and carrying, can also be dual activities for increasing aerobic endurance and improving muscular strength/endurance.

Education

There is no difference in principle between a lift at work and a lift at home. Lifting properly will maintain spinal safety. Cumulative trauma injuries from overuse of gripping and pinching can be problematic at home as well as at work. Therefore, education is targeted not only to the whole person, but also to the person's total environment. The worker should leave work rehabilitation with an empowered feeling of understanding his or her own body, his or her specific reaction to body mechanics and stressful physical activities, and a plan on how to moderate his or her own behaviors to improve safety and prevent injury.

Technique training reduces stresses on the body. It is a critical part of both return to work and training for new jobs. It will require either actual work production or excellent simulation.

Problem solving incorporates information learned with practical application. Group settings work effectively. The discussion and interactive portion is pivotal. Each worker must have an opportunity to discuss his or her own issues, needs, and questions in order to maximize benefit from the education program. Workers hear from group participants that there is a "buy-in" to the concepts being discussed and can be carry-over into the world of work.

Work Simulation or Actual Work

There are three primary methods of providing work simulation in work rehabilitation (see Table 56–4).

The first emphasizes simulated motions, forces, and stresses when actual equipment cannot be used. For example, a welder who will do welding on the job cannot bring in masks and welding equipment and do hot welds in the clinic. Therefore, the therapist will identify the positions the welder must attain, heaviness of the materials that will be utilized, sustained positions that the welder must hold, and work "techniques." Weights, forces, and body positions will be simulated on an increasing basis to allow the worker's body to tolerate positions, stresses, and the amount of time needed to do the work to the point that when he or she ends the program he or she will have the strength, endurance, and technique ability to hold and use the welding equipment.

In the second form, the worker utilizes the actual equipment that he or she handles at work. For example, a worker in a tire building plant may be able to have the tires available to handle, move, and throw even though the conveyor belts are not available. A city maintenance worker who must handle manhole covers can bring in such equipment even though the clinic will not have the sewer tunnels to utilize. The welder may be able to bring in welding equipment. In this way, the worker becomes able to perform the motions, positions, and hold times needed and the actual equipment becomes the weight and activity against which the worker works. This also may facilitate technique in a better way as the worker becomes more able to again "roll and throw tires" or position and hold the welding equipment. This type of simulation also works well with an "on the job" discharge as the actual work being done is the final outcome and the proof that the worker can do the work safely and functionally.

In the third method, the actual activity with actual equipment can be done either at the worksite or when the work can be simulated in the clinic. Those most amenable to this would be office workers, simple material handlers, or workers in light manufacturing.

INTEGRATION WITH FULL RETURN TO WORK

During or at the end of the rehabilitation phase, integration with work takes place on site in industry. Not only does this increase the worker's capacity in the components of specific work strength, endurance, aerobic capacity, and safety education, but it also allows work techniques to be practiced in a real setting. It is desired by workers and employers because it maintains the connection with the worker and the workplace and coworkers. This allows the worker to maintain identity in the workplace and allows the coworkers and supervisor to see that the worker is, in fact, willing to come back to work and participate on a productive level.

The benefits of on-site work rehabilitation over clinical work rehabilitation are work-specific activity, regular work hours, credit to the worker for productive work, ability to modify work as needed, and progression of the worker through the higher levels of work until full work, or the highest functional level, is accomplished.

TABLE 56–4

Sites for Work Rehabilitation

Site	Pros and Cons	
At the worksite	Pros:	Productive work Work bond continues
	Cons:	Safety issues Little exercise equipment
Clinic and worksite combination	Pros:	Best of real world and clinical rehabilitation monitoring
	Cons:	Difficult for some employers to approve
Clinic	Pros:	Control of safety Full equipment Little distraction
	Cons:	Not real Lost bond with work

The employer can provide administrative controls that allow the injured worker to return to his or her level at the workplace. Some of the options available are full job with fewer hours of work, full job will additional assistive equipment or change in work method, modified job, or different job with a physical demand level that meets the worker's capacity.

All of these can be productive work. They are combined with the rehabilitation plan, which begins with matching the work level at which they begin with a specific plan for timelines and progress anticipated. This is monitored and progressed by the therapist until either full work is accomplished or the highest functional level has been reached. There is formal evaluation through the process and this appears in the medical records. Physicians are involved according to state regulations and as the treating physician in understanding and directing medical case management. The records for on site work rehabilitation continue to be medical records and should have the same confidentiality as any medical record within an industry. The therapist will keep the main patient record.

An advantage of the therapist being on site, interacting with the worker and work rehabilitation, is the ability to recognize flare-up or need for additional modifications. This allows a timely solution to take place. Also, the worker is reassured that he or she can work because any problems that may arise will be addressed. In addition, the coworkers are able to identify the level that the worker is reaching and know that full capacity of the worker is reached each day. Modified duty programs should be explained to the entire workforce so that when a worker comes back on this plan, he or she is supported. All workers could have this need, so all workers cooperate to make the program successful. This interaction of the therapist, worker, and coworker team is important so that the worker does not get labeled as someone who desires easy work.

If the on-site therapist has also developed functional job descriptions for the company, targeting of goals for the rehabilitation program will increase effectiveness. If the therapist has not developed formal functional job descriptions, the job should be analyzed so that job/worker matching continues throughout the process.

The worker is discharged from on site work rehabilitation when he or she meets the goals that were set. This is identical to the process of discharge from clinical work rehabilitation. The benefit is that actual work is being done at that time and there is no opportunity for a gap to be created.

There are several levels of work return (see Table 56–5).

Light Duty

"Light duty" is the lightest level and is generally in an area of the workplace where easy work (often paperwork or inspection) is carried out. The concept of light duty may have negative tones in the workplace because it is perceived as a place where real work is not done. If the light work area has a negative reputation among workers, two things will happen. First, workers will view the injured workers who participate in light duty as getting off very easy from their actual work duties. There can even be negative attitudes toward those in light duty. Secondly, the workers, perceiving that these attitudes are held by their coworkers, often do anything to avoid this light duty area. This often forces them back into their regular job before they are fully ready.

Transitional Work

An option that adds productivity to lighter work is transitional work. Transitional work is structured, progressive, and functional. It has a beginning and an endpoint and it time limited. It is productive work even if it is light, and the knowledge that actual productive work is being done must be shared throughout the entire workplace.

It is productive work because there is a financial benefit to the company for having it done. This transitional work is not the worker's regular work, and it must be time limited to ensure that the worker, coworkers, and employer understand that it is really a transition into a regular duty job.

Modified Duty

Modified duty is a job in the plant that is a similar job to the one the worker did, but one that eliminates the physical demands that the worker cannot perform. The modified duty is clearly related to the original job and the work is done in the former work team so the

TABLE 56–5

Work Options

Light duty	Not regular job Not highly productive work
Transitional work	Not regular job Productive work Time limited
Modified duty	Similar job Productive work
Regular work modified	Original job–partially productive work
Regular work, modified hours	Original job–fully productive work Less than full hours

coworkers are part of the productive group. For example, someone who operates machines may be moved to the fork truck because that job meets his or her physical abilities. He or she is still in the same group, but temporarily operating the fork truck in the area rather than performing the manufacturing process. On a daily basis, he or she is with his or her team and it is understood that full duty will be returned as soon as possible.

Regular Job, Modified

In this case, the job is the original job, but a modification has been made to allow the worker to be able to do the job while a physical dysfunction is present. This could be a manufacturing or warehouse job where the lifting is assisted by a vacu-hoist, a pulley, or teamwork. This allows all of the other functions of the original job to be done, but the modification only takes place in the specific physical areas where the worker has difficulty.

Full Job, Part Hours

This implies that the worker has the capacity to do all of the essential functions of the original job, but his or her endurance and tolerance has not yet built to the point where he or she can tolerate an 8-, 10-, or 12-hour day. This allows the worker to be with the work group doing full work during a portion of the time. The other portion of the time would be in a type of modified or transitional duty.

PROGRAM ISSUES

Compliance

Work rehabilitation, because it often involves workers who have been off work for a substantial period or who have had a chronic condition, may involve issues of compliance with a program. The following methods are utilized in a work rehabilitation program:

1. An entry conference in which the goals and rules of participation in a work rehabilitation program are discussed. At this time the worker often signs a contract to have the work behaviors necessary for compliance with this program.
2. Specific work-like requirements are designated:
   A. Being on time or early for the work rehabilitation sessions.
   B. Taking breaks only as designated.
   C. Completing the required number of hours each day.
   D. Calling in with medical information if there is a medical reason for failure to appear (such as sickness). If this sickness persists more than 2 days, a doctor's approval will be necessary.
   E. No unauthorized excuses for work conditioning if there is a second day of absenteeism without a medical excuse. The client will be discharged for noncompliance.
   F. Work behaviors must be positive. There must be no negative talk regarding other clients, current employer, former work experiences, or rehabilitation personnel. If any negative talk occurs, there will be a conference with the client and this will be addressed. If the worker continues to use negative behaviors, this will be a reason for discontinuance of the program.
   G. Full effort must be utilized in the program. If full effort is not given or the full program is not done during the day, a conference will be held and this will be discussed. Not following the program guidelines without medical reasons is reason for discontinuance.
   H. If the worker has unusually increased abilities or decreased abilities concurrent with increased symptoms, he or she is to notify the functional rehabilitation professional immediately. This allows early recognition of any problems and seeking appropriate help. All changes from the progressive program must be made by the functional rehabilitator.

Compliance in the program with good "work" behavior is important. If one or more workers begin to have poor work behaviors, this will affect the entire work rehabilitation group. Therefore, not only will this have a negative effect on the individual client but it can make the entire rehabilitation program stressful for all professionals and clients involved. This is why immediate attention to nonpositive work behaviors is addressed.

If for any reason noncompliance surfaces, a conference will be held, the particular issue discussed, and the client given another chance. If noncompliance continues, a quick discharge from the program is necessary. A report will be written that will explain the reason for discharge and this will be sent to all parties involved in case resolution.

Progression

The program will be designed to progress in a slow and realistic fashion each day so that the functional goals are met by the projected end of the program. Therefore, each day there is generally some increase in physical activity intensity for the worker. This may be increase of weight, repetition, or difficulty of the activity.

It is best to begin the progression in a slow and steady process. Work rehabilitation programs become problematic if the progression begins too fast. There is a natural inclination to soreness at the beginning of work rehabilitation. Muscle soreness associated with safe increase in exercise will be explained to the client. Other symptoms such as swelling in the joint or exacerbation of a cumulative trauma will be appropriately treated and the activity modified so the progress can be made without creating a physical exacerbation. Therefore, the soreness must be reported to the functional rehabilitator so that there can be a differentiation between structural problems and normal soreness that accompanies increased functional levels.

Another phenomenon occurs often in the last week of a program. With discharge imminent, the worker has a flare-up in his or her condition. Whether this is physical, psychological, or a combination is not known. The functional work rehabilitator must expect that this may happen and be prepared to deal with it in an objective way.

Because it may be expected, the best approach is to evaluate quickly, modify the work rehabilitation to allow progress but not increase exacerbation, and reassure the client. Work rehabilitation goals will be met by the end of the program and the transition to actual return to work can still take place.

OUTCOME MEASUREMENTS

Outcome of work rehabilitation has been suggested by the American Physical Therapy Association and other professionals who have identified the variables that should be measured (see Table 56–6).

As costs of work-related injury are detrimental to both employer and worker, measurement of cost-effectiveness can demonstrate efficiency. In addition, valuable workers returning to work present opportunities for loyalty, experience, and teamwork to be enhanced in the workplace.

MAXIMUM MEDICAL IMPROVEMENT

Maximum medical improvement (MMI) is a medical/legal designation. The work rehabilitation program is pivotal in identifying whether a person can continue to improve from his or her original injury or illness. The establishment of MMI in a person who has not had the benefit of work rehabilitation is often premature. Merely determining MMI by impairments or healing times does not take into account that the debilitation of a person from time off work and aspects due to injury or illness may impact functional ability.

The rehabilitation focus allows work function to be raised to the highest possible level. The following will be identified:

- Whether the person is capable of returning to his or her full preinjury job, at which time rehabilitation will be ended.
- The highest functional level that the person is able to reach.
- Job matching using objective functional capacity evaluation matched to validated functional job demands will provide the work-related match for the MMI evaluator.
- Regarding impairment and healing, functional testing measurements at the end of the work rehabilitation program will identify the musculoskeletal aspects of the worker as well. Both prior to work rehabilitation and at the end of work rehabilitation the evaluations will provide impairment measurements of range of motion, muscle strength, etc., which can also help determine endpoints for those aspects of MMI.

CONCLUSION

Work rehabilitation is a structured program with goals of returning an injured worker to work. Professionals working in the field must have knowledge of the neuromusculoskeletal aspects of the injured worker, ergonomic conditions in the workplace, and physical requirements necessary for productive work.

TABLE 56–6

Outcome Study

Demographics	Age Sex Length of employment Length of time at specific job DOT categorization of job heaviness
Treatment	Hours per day Location of rehabilitation Total days in program Total hours of program Total cost of program
Outcome	Return to work • Full duty, regular job • Modified, regular job • New job, same employer • Different job, different employer
Follow-up study	Ability to perform job Reinjury/new injury Final job
Financial	Lost days Modified duty days Medical costs of injury Replacement costs Other costs of injury Disability costs

The ultimate goal of work rehabilitation is to safely and productively match a worker with a physical dysfunction with productive work. The optimum level of return is to the same job and same employer in as short and safe a time as possible. Other options include return to productive work in different jobs, with different employers and in other capacities.

Work rehabilitation bonds the value of productive work with physiologic-based rehabilitation. It is a humanitarian approach that benefits both the injured worker and the employer. In meeting its initial goals, it benefits the social environment by reducing workers' compensation costs, increasing industrial productivity, and maintaining the positive bond between the worker and the workplace.

Because work is involved with many of the same functional aspects as life, work rehabilitation not only facilitates productive work, but also produces a healthier human in a living environment.

Ongoing values are as follows:

- Empowerment of the worker to understand his or her own body and how functional implications of the injury/illness can be minimized.
- Encouragement of the worker to value maximized productivity as a benefit to him- or herself.
- Enhancement of the worker's work ethic regarding timeliness, productive work, and positive work behaviors as important in the psychosocial construct of work.
- Knowledge of safety practices so that further injury can be prevented.
- Ability to identify places and types of intervention if new symptoms arise.
- Ability to carry out a specific exercise program in daily living and at home to maintain general and specific health.
- Knowledge that "teamwork" of employer, employees, and medical practitioner is an effective means of solving problems.

Work rehabilitation is a concept that is broad and embraces principles that do not restrict it from change. Programs will change, but the principles of work rehabilitation, to match the work to the worker, will not change. Workers, employers, and medical professionals are able to reduce the effects of work illness or injury and optimize productivity for the benefit of the individual worker and the employer.

References

1. Ambrosius FM, Rounds BK, Herkner PB, et al: Reactivation of injured workers involved in a work-hardening program. Work 4:28, 1994.
2. American Physical Therapy Association: Guidelines for Programs for Injured Workers. Alexandria, Va, APTA 1, 1995.
3. Darphin LE, Smith RL, Green EJ: Work conditioning and work hardening. Orthopaedic Physical Therapy Clinics 1:105, 1992.
4. Graly JM, Yi S, Jensen GM, et al: Factors influencing return to work for clients in a work-hardening center. Work 4:9, 1994.
5. Isernhagen SJ: Exercise technology for work rehabilitation programs. Orthopaedic Physical Therapy Clinics 1:361, 1992.
6. Isernhagen SJ: Immediate care delivery systems. In Isernhagen SJ (ed): Work Injury Management and Prevention. Gathersburg, Md, Aspen, 1988, p 115.
7. King PM: Outcome analysis of work-hardening programs. Am J Occup Ther 47:595, 1993.
8. Lechner DE: Work hardening and work conditioning interventions: Do they affect disability? Phys Ther 74:471, 1994.
9. Marras WS, Lavender SA, Leurgans SE, et al: The role of dynamic three-dimensional trunk motion in occupationally-related low back disorders: The effects of work place factors, trunk rotation, and trunk motion characteristics on risk of injury. Spine 18:617,1993.
10. Marras WS, Mikra GA: Trunk strength during asymmetric trunk motion. Human Factors 31:1, 1989.
11. Matheson LN: Work hardening for patients with back pain. J Musculoskel Med September:53, 1993.
12. Wyrick JM, Niemyer LO, Ellexson M, et al: Occupational therapy work-hardening programs: A demographic study. Am J Occup Ther 45:109, 1991.

Bibliography

Isernhagen S (ed): Comprehensive Guide to Work Injury Management. Gaithersburg, Md, Aspen, 1995.

Isernhagen S (ed): Work Injury: Management and Prevention. Gaithersburg, Md, Aspen, 1988.

Commission on Accreditation of Rehabilitation Facilities: Occupational Rehabilitation Programs. Tucson, Ariz, Commission on Accreditation of Rehabilitation Facilities, 1989.

CHAPTER

57

Orthopedic Disability

The Joints

ROBERT H. HARALSON III, MD, MBA

The goal in treatment of a workers' compensation injury is to get the patient back to work and there is increasing evidence that the sooner that is accomplished, the better. A number of studies have shown that the longer a person remains off work from a work-related injury, the less likely he or she is to ever return to work. Over the years, the treatment of musculoskeletal injuries has changed. Previously, the treatment for back pain was bed rest for long periods of time. That is no longer true. The treatment now is to keep the patient up and going as much as possible. Instead of requiring several weeks of strict bed rest after disc surgery, we now have the patient walking the day of surgery and many surgeons are performing disc surgery on an outpatient basis. The same is true for other joint conditions. The gentle motion of a joint in its normal planes and arc is thought to be beneficial. The synovial fluid nourishes the articular cartilage and gentle motion enhances that nourishment.

There is good evidence that most joint problems respond better to exercise than to immobilization. The study from West Point proved that sprained ankles responded better to exercise than to casting and the study by Egol et al showed that fractured ankles requiring open treatment rehabilitated faster when splinted with mobile ankle braces rather than casting.[7] The most difficult sprained ankles to treat are the ones that are seen 3 days after the patient has been to the emergency department, placed in an ace wrap, given crutches, and told to be nonweight bearing. The swelling resulting from the dependant, nonweight bearing position makes rehabilitation much more difficult. The best way to treat a sprained ankle is to allow protected weight bearing and start a gentle active and passive exercise program.

Knee ligament injuries are no longer immobilized in casts, even when they require surgery. Houston and colleagues have determined that the more rigidly one immobilizes a ligament injury, the worse the result.[13] Proper healing requires gentle motion. Today, even anterior cruciate ligament reconstructions are not immobilized in casts.[20] Some physicians use movable braces and many orthopedists do not use any immobilization at all. A possible exception to this approach may be certain conditions in the shoulder. Surgery for instability of the shoulder is directed at tightening loose shoulder joint capsule and stretching this capsule too early may be detrimental.[12] This does not mean that the patient cannot return to work but the work prescription should include limitations that prevent stretching of the reconstructed capsule and ligaments.

The decision to return a worker to work then becomes one of deciding what accommodations are necessary and which of these accommodations the employer is willing to provide. The question is: "When is the patient able to travel to and from work and be at work?"[25] It is then a matter of when the employer is willing to pay for the worker to be at work and do whatever he or she can do. There are very few conditions that will prevent early return to work with the proper accommodations. Mayer has published suggestions for how one-handed workers can reasonably function in a two-handed world.[17]

Pain may be the most confounding factor. There is no doubt that joint injuries, including surgery, cause pain. Pain is impossible to accurately assess. We cannot qualify or quantify pain. We cannot tell whether is present or to what degree. Therefore it falls on the shoulders of the physician to interpret how much pain the patient is having. Patients may return to work while taking mild pain medications but there is concern about patients driving and being around machinery if they are under the influence of narcotics.

The decision to return a patient to work and the restrictions that will be placed on the worker hinge on the factors that might cause more injury. There have been few studies on how much a person can tolerate without injury. However, there have been studies that suggest how much repetition and how much lifting are likely to cause injury. When writing a return to work prescription, the physician must be cognizant of this information. The usual procedure is to limit the activities to below levels that are known to cause injury. According to the comprehensive study by the Occupational Safety and Health Administration, there are seven basic biomechanical risk factors.[3,8] These are force, awkward posture, static posture, repetition, dynamic factors, compression, and vibration. Modifying factors include intensity, duration, temporal profile, and cold temperature. Each of these factors must be taken into consideration when making these decisions.

Many studies have demonstrated that early return to work is essential for a successful return to work. Studies by Weisel et al and Hall et al demonstrated that returning a patient to work without restrictions was more likely to result in a successful return to work than placing restrictions on a patient.[11,28] Ash and Goldstein have published a treatise on the predictors of returning to work.[1] Talmage, in an unpublished meta-analysis of return to work literature, found that there is no scientific evidence that placing back pain patients on work restrictions had any benefit and there was no evidence that returning to full duty led to further injury (see Chapter 52).[26] On the contrary, the restrictions actually decreased the incidence of successful return to work. The best results were obtained when the patient was allowed to restrict him- or herself within the limits of pain. Unfortunately, many employers will not allow this approach for fear that the employee will not perform.[4]

Perry showed that paying an employee full wages, even if he or she was sent to a rehabilitation facility remote from the workplace, was less expensive in the long run than allowing the individual to be off work until he or she was "ready" to return to work.[21] Millstein et al reported successful return to work by amputees.[19] Crook et al reported that men returned to work 1.5 times as often as women, successful return to work was twice as high in individuals who were returned to modified jobs than those with no such accommodation, and there was a 20% decease in return to work with each decade of increasing age.[5]

Wexler et al reported a series of 22 workers' compensation patients with anterior cruciate ligament reconstructions and all 22 were successfully returned to work.[29]

A number of authors have suggested that fear of reinjury is commonplace among injured workers and an important part of a return to work program is for the treating physician to counsel the patient and to convince him or her that return to work is not punishment but rather rehabilitation and that the likelihood of reinjury is no greater at work than at home. Indahl et al demonstrated that information provided the worker about the nature of his or her injury was important in returning the worker.[14] In addition, many workers are depressed about the injury and the possibility of inability to earn a living wage and as a result, treatment of depression may be a necessary component of the return to work effort. Communication by upper management of the company is also important. Someone from upper management should immediately go to the injured worker and explain that the company will provide the best medical care available, that the worker's job will be waiting when he or she is ready to return, and that if the worker is unable to do his or her job, another within his or her capabilities will be available. This approach leads to far less lost time and indemnity payments. Upper management seems to understand this concept but it is infrequently communicated to the supervisor level. Once the employee is accused of impropriety associated with an injury, the worker begins to believe all the adverse advice he or she has received from well meaning but uninformed coworkers. This starts the never-ending cycle of pain behavior that leads to "workers' compensation-itis". Atcheson et al have demonstrated that early referral to a musculoskeletal specialist rather than to a discounted fee clinic resulted in earlier return to work and lower total cost.[2] Fleeson has published a book for the injured worker that helps guide the worker through the morass of the workers' compensation system.[10]

There are two resources that give guidelines for the length of time a person might stay off work after certain conditions. The first is by Reed and is based on procedures; the second is from the Work Loss Data Institute and is based on diagnosis.[6,23] When writing a return to work prescription the physician might rely on the 30-second rule of Putz-Anderson.[22] Although his rules were devised for cumulative trauma disorders, they serve as good guidelines for upper extremity joint conditions. He assumes 420 minutes in an 8-hour day. He defines low repetitions as 840 30-second intervals or parts in a day or 120 parts per hour. Moderate repetition is 1260 30-second intervals or parts in a day, or 180 parts per hour, and high repetition as 1680 15-second intervals or parts per hour or 240 per hour. Mayer et al have published a comprehensive text on occupational musculoskeletal disorders.[18] They and Robinson et al have pointed out that industrial medicine is a specialty in and of itself.[24]

We have provided sample return to work forms that may be used by the reader (see Tables 57–1 through 57–6). They may be copied and altered as the user sees fit and as further scientific evidence becomes available. These forms were developed by studying the Occupational Safety and Health Administration (OSHA) guidelines to determine levels of activity that frequently cause injury and then extrapolating down to an acceptable level.[3] These forms were developed for the Foothills Occupational Health Association in Maryville, Tenn, by Baron Johnson, PT, of Appalachian Physical Therapy, also in Maryville. We print the forms as three sheets in three different colors, using National Cash Register (NCR) paper. One form is given to the patient, one to the employer, and one is retained in the patient's chart. We have found that a white form is best for the chart copy as that color can be faxed more successfully.

DEFINITIONS

A few definitions are appropriate. A ligament is a structure that attaches one bone to another. A tendon is a structure that attaches a muscle to a bone. A sprain is a tear or a partial tear of a ligament. A strain is a tear of a tendon or muscle unit. Both sprains and strains occur in three degrees. A first-degree sprain or strain is a stretch

TABLE 57-1

Patient Work Restrictions Shoulder

PATIENT NAME: ______________________________ DATE: _____ /_____ /_____

DIAGNOSIS: ______________________________

DISPOSITION:
PATIENT SHOULD BE OFF WORK UNTIL _____ /_____ /_____
PATIENT MAY RETURN TO WORK _____ /_____ /_____ WITHOUT RESTRICTIONS
PATIENT MAY RETURN TO WORK _____ /_____ /_____ WITH RESTRICTIONS

(CIRCLE ONE)

LEVEL 1–JOINT PROTECTION
No reaching activities or use of the involved extremity.
Uninvolved single arm lifting.

LEVEL 2–JOINT MOVEMENT, NO STRAIN
Reaching 12 inches in front of body below chest height.
Reaching 6 inches to the side.
Overhead reaching limited to 20/day.
No static positions of reach.
No lifting.
50 or less shoulder movements/hour and 800 or less body movements/hour.

LEVEL 3–FULL JOINT MOTION WITH PROTECTED STRAIN
Reaching 18 inches to the front and overhead but less than 45 degrees flexion.
Reaching 12 inches to the side, but less than 45 degrees abduction.
Static positions to 10 seconds.
Lifting to 3 pounds shoulder height.
75 or less shoulder movements/hour or 1200 body movements/hour.

LEVEL 4–INCREASED STRAIN, TENSION
Full reaching activities but recommend less than 45 degrees of flexion or abduction at all times.
Lifting overhead to 5 pounds.
Lifting to shoulder height 15 pounds.
Normal static positions.
100 or less shoulder movements/hour or 1500 or less body movements/hour.

LEVEL 5–NORMAL ACTIVITIES
No limitations.

NEXT APPOINTMENT: _____ /_____ /_____ PHYSICIAN'S SIGNATURE ______________________________
_____ DAYS _____ WEEKS

TABLE 57–2

Patient Work Restrictions Elbow

PATIENT NAME: ______________________________ DATE: _____ /_____ /_____
DIAGNOSIS: ______________________________

DISPOSITION:
PATIENT SHOULD BE OFF WORK UNTIL _____ /_____ /_____
PATIENT MAY RETURN TO WORK _____ /_____ /_____ WITHOUT RESTRICTIONS
PATIENT MAY RETURN TO WORK _____ /_____ /_____ WITH THE FOLLOWING RESTRICTIONS

(CIRCLE ONE)

LEVEL 1–JOINT PROTECTION
No use of the involved extremity.
Uninvolved single arm tasks.
Paper and pencil tasks acceptable but break frequently 5 to 10 minutes per hour.

LEVEL 2–JOINT MOVEMENT, NO STRAIN
Reaching activities with no lifting.
No grasping, gripping or pinching.
No hand tool use and no rapid forearm movements of supination or pronation.
300 or less elbow movements/hour and 800 or less body movements/hour.

LEVEL 3–FULL JOINT MOTION WITH PROTECTED STRAIN
Full reach with lifting less than 2 pounds, 1 lift in 20 seconds.
Partial reach with lifting less than 5 pounds, 1 lift every 20 seconds.
No manual hand tool use.
Grasping, gripping and pinching for less than 3 seconds every 20 seconds or more.
Elbows bent less than 60 degrees when carrying objects.
450 or less elbow movements/hour and 1200 or less body movements/hour.

LEVEL 4–INCREASED STRAIN, TENSION
Full reach with lifting less than 5 pounds, 1 lift in 20 seconds.
Partial reach with lifting less than 10 pounds, 1 lift every 20 seconds.
Grasping, gripping and pinching for less than 3 seconds every 20 seconds.
No manual screwdrivers.
Elbows less than 90 degrees when carrying objects.
550 or less elbow movements/hour and 1500 or less body movements/hour.

LEVEL 5–NORMAL ACTIVITY
Recommend less than 600 elbow movements, 2000 body movements/hour.

NEXT APPOINTMENT: _____ /_____ /_____ PHYSICIAN'S SIGNATURE ______________________________
_____ DAYS _____ WEEKS

of the structure that does not disrupt any significant amount of the structural integrity. Therefore, activities within limits of pain are acceptable, because the structure is no weaker than it was before the injury. A second-degree injury is one that partially disrupts the structure and therefore the structure is weaker and must be protected from stress for a period of about 6 weeks. A third-degree injury is one in which the structure is completely disrupted and obviously requires more aggressive treatment and protection, from 6 to 12 weeks. Some third-degree sprains and strains require operative repair of the involved structure.

GENERAL TREATMENT

Sprains and Strains

Sprains and strains are usually treated with protected and gentle range of motion. They are associated with inflammation and thus anti-inflammatory medication will often shorten the period of pain and swelling. In addition, most anti-inflammatories are analgesic. Some third-degree sprains and strains require surgery and, if so, may require immobilization, although the tendency is for early motion.

TABLE 57-3

Patient Work Restrictions Wrist/Hand

PATIENT NAME: ______________________________ DATE: _____ /_____ /_____
DIAGNOSIS: ______________________________

DISPOSITION:
PATIENT SHOULD BE OFF WORK UNTIL _____ /_____ /_____
PATIENT MAY RETURN TO WORK _____ /_____ /_____ WITHOUT RESTRICTIONS
PATIENT MAY RETURN TO WORK _____ /_____ /_____ WITH THE FOLLOWING RESTRICTIONS:

(CIRCLE ONE)

LEVEL 1–JOINT PROTECTION
No use of the involved extremity.
Single arm tasks with non-involved extremity.

LEVEL 2–JOINT MOVEMENT, NO STRAIN
Finger, hand and wrist movement OK, such as twisting and turning.
No static activities with involved extremity such as holding an object in the hand with or without reaching activities.
No handling objects greater than 1 pound.
No lifting, pushing or pulling greater than 1 pound.
No lifting while the arm is reaching.
No manual hand tool use, only counterbalanced suspended tool can be used that is electric, pneumatic and has low torque.
Grip and pinch with pencil, pen and clipboard OK.
No ulnar or radial deviation of the wrist positions allowed.
300 or less wrist movements/hour–800 body movements or less/hour.
6000 or less finger movements/hour with data entry 10 minute break/hour.

LEVEL 3–FULL JOINT MOTION WITH PROTECTED STRAIN
Normal hand movements.
Static positions to be avoided, especially ulnar and radial deviation.
No handling objects greater than 5 pounds.
No lifting, pushing or pulling greater than 5 pounds.
No static grip and pinch activities.
Counterbalanced suspended hand tools with no vibration, heavy torque or single finger trigger.
450 or less wrist movements/hour and 1200 or less body movements/hour.
8000 finger movements/hour with data entry 10 minute break/hour.

LEVEL 4–INCREASED STRAIN, TENSION
Normal reaching, handling, fingering and feeling activities.
Lifting, pushing and pulling limited to 15 pounds.
Static grip and pinch limited to 3 seconds duration, 1 every 20 seconds.
Normal hand tool use with no wrist deviations for prolonged periods.
550 or less wrist movements/hour, 1500 or less body movements/hour.
1000 finger movements/hour with data entry 10 minute break/hour.

LEVEL 5–NORMAL ACTIVITIES
No limitations.

NEXT APPOINTMENT: _____ /_____ /_____ PHYSICIAN'S SIGNATURE ______________________________
_____ DAYS _____ WEEKS

Fractures can be treated closed or open. The tendency now is to operatively fix most fractures, especially those in and around joints, except for those that are completely undisplaced. This minimizes immobilization and allows early motion. Closed treatment may require casting but in the upper extremity, single extremity activities are permissible if the proper accommodations are available. In the lower extremity, patients can usually ambulate with ambulatory aids, whether they are non-weight bearing or full weight bearing. Open fractures

TABLE 57–4

Patient Work Restrictions Hip

PATIENT NAME: ______________________________ DATE: _____ /_____ /_____
DIAGNOSIS: ______________________________

DISPOSITION:
PATIENT SHOULD BE OFF WORK UNTIL _____ /_____ /_____
PATIENT MAY RETURN TO WORK _____ /_____ /_____ WITHOUT RESTRICTIONS
PATIENT MAY RETURN TO WORK _____ /_____ /_____ WITH THE FOLLOWING RESTRICTIONS:

LEVEL 1–JOINT PROTECTION
Sedentary activities.
Non-weight bearing ambulation with crutches or walker.
No excessive motion of hip joint.

LEVEL 2–JOINT MOVEMENT
Sedentary activities.
Partial weight bearing with crutches or walker.
No excessive motion of hip joint.

LEVEL 3–PROTECTED STRAIN
Full weight bearing (may use cane for pain control).
Ambulation 1/4 mile in 1 hour.
Stand 30 minutes/hour.
May squat.
No lifting from squat.
No lifting or carrying over 25 pounds.

LEVEL 4–INCREASED STRAIN
Ambulation without support.
Full weight bearing.
Ambulation 1/2 mile per hour.
Stand 50 minutes per hour.
Full range of motion (may squat).
Lift and/or carry 50 pounds.

LEVEL 5–NORMAL ACTIVITIES
No limitations.

NEXT APPOINTMENT: _____ /_____ /_____ PHYSICIAN'S SIGNATURE ______________________________
_____ DAYS _____ WEEKS

can lead to infections if not treated properly and as a result, multiple trips to the operating theater for repeated debridement may be indicated and many patients require extended periods of intravenous antibiotics. These sometimes may be administered by home infusion therapists but are often required several times daily and this regimen will preclude return to work until it has been completed.

Dislocations result in ligament compromise but most are stable after reduction, except at the extremes of motion, and are best treated by very short periods of immobilization, if any, followed by range of motion activities.

Overuse syndromes are best treated by anti-inflammatories, either orally or by injection into the affected area, rest, and stretching and strengthening exercises, but most workers should be able to remain at work with temporary modifications of their jobs. Many workers have trouble ever returning to the same activity that caused the original problem and permanent activity modifications may be indicated.

SPECIFIC JOINTS, UPPER EXTREMITY

Shoulder

Bursitis and tendonitis and overuse strains make up the majority of workers' compensation shoulder problems. Rotator cuff tears, fractures, and instability problems

TABLE 57-5

Patient Work Restrictions Knee

PATIENT NAME: ____ DATE: _____ /_____ /_____
DIAGNOSIS: ____

DISPOSITION:
PATIENT SHOULD BE OFF WORK UNTIL _____ /_____ /_____
PATIENT MAY RETURN TO WORK _____ /_____ /_____ WITHOUT RESTRICTIONS
PATIENT MAY RETURN TO WORK _____ /_____ /_____ WITH THE FOLLOWING RESTRICTIONS:

(CIRCLE ONE)

LEVEL 1–JOINT PROTECTION
Sedentary activities.
Non-weight bearing ambulation with crutches or walker.
No excessive motion of knee joint (may wear splint or cast).

LEVEL 2–JOINT MOVEMENT
Sedentary activities.
Partial weight bearing with crutches or walker.
No excessive use of knee joint (may wear splint or cast).

LEVEL 3–PROTECTED STRAIN
Full weight bearing (may use cane).
Ambulation 1/4 mile in 1 hour.
Stand 30 minutes/hour.
Partial squatting.
No lifting from squat.
No lifting or carrying over 25 pounds.

LEVEL 4–INCREASED STRAIN
Ambulation without support.
Full weight bearing.
Ambulation 1/2 mile per hour.
Stand 50 minutes per hour.
Full range of motion (may squat).
Lift and/or carry 50 pounds.

LEVEL 5–NORMAL ACTIVITIES
No limitations.

NEXT APPOINTMENT: _____ /_____ /_____ PHYSICIAN'S SIGNATURE ____________________
_____ DAYS _____ WEEKS

make up most of the others. Multidirectional instability can be a unique problem. The overuse syndromes usually respond to anti-inflammatories, including steroids orally or by injection and specific exercises. Because the external rotators are also strong depressors of the humeral head, exercises to strengthen this group of muscles are often beneficial. Activities that repeatedly press the humeral head underneath the coracoacromial arch, such as overhead lifting, tend to aggravate these conditions and should be avoided. Therefore, overhead activities should be discouraged at first. Arthroscopic surgical correction of overuse syndromes involves subacromial decompression and, except in the cases of rotator cuff tears that require repair, there is no disruption of critical structures and progressive range of motion activities are encouraged as soon as pain will allow, usually within 1 week. If the rotator cuff requires repair, either open or arthroscopically, a full passive range of motion can be encouraged immediately but active arm elevation against resistance should not be undertaken for at least 6 weeks. Activities that involve motions below shoulder level, even when associated with moderate force, are usually acceptable except in the case of fractures.

A rather new entity that has been discovered since the advent of arthroscopy is the superior lateral anterior posterior (SLAP) lesion. This is a disruption of the labrum from the glenoid at the level of the insertion of

TABLE 57–6

Patient Work Restrictions Ankle and Foot

PATIENT NAME: ______________________________ DATE: _____ /_____ /_____
DIAGNOSIS: ______________________________

DISPOSITION:
PATIENT SHOULD BE OFF WORK UNTIL _____ /_____ /_____
PATIENT MAY RETURN TO WORK _____ /_____ /_____ WITHOUT RESTRICTIONS
PATIENT MAY RETURN TO WORK _____ /_____ /_____ WITH THE FOLLOWING RESTRICTIONS:

(CIRCLE ONE)

LEVEL 1–JOINT PROTECTION
Sedentary activities.
Non-weight bearing ambulation with crutches or walker.
No excessive motion of ankle joint (may wear splint or cast).

LEVEL 2–JOINT MOVEMENT
Sedentary activities.
Partial weight bearing with crutches or walker.
No excessive motion of ankle joint (may wear splint or cast).

LEVEL 3–PROTECTED STRAIN
Full weight bearing (may use cane for pain control, may be in cast or splint).
Ambulation 1/4 mile in 1 hour.
Partial squatting.
No lifting from squat.
May lift or carry up to 25 pounds.

LEVEL 4–INCREASED STRAIN
Ambulation without support.
Full weight bearing.
Ambulation 1/2 mile per hour.
Stand 50 minutes per hour.
Full range of motion (may squat).
Lift and/or carry 50 pounds.

LEVEL 5–NORMAL ACTIVITIES
No limitations.

NEXT APPOINTMENT: _____ /_____ /_____ PHYSICIAN'S SIGNATURE ______________________________
_____ DAYS _____ WEEKS

the biceps tendon into the glenoid. The involvement of the biceps tendon insertion is variable. The lesion is frequently repaired or debrided arthroscopically and postoperative management is similar to repair of the torn rotator cuff and recurrent dislocations.

Early fracture treatment normally includes gentle range of motion below shoulder level but with minimal force and after 6 weeks or so, when early consolidation of the fracture fragments has occurred, even overhead range of motion activities and progressive resistance exercises are encouraged. Activities close to the body put less stress on the shoulder because the further from the body a weight is, the longer the lever arm and the more the force required to move the weight.

Hawkins has shown that early stretching out of surgical repairs of multidirectional instability leads to frequent recurrence of the instability, and as a result, he recommends avoidance of overhead stretching exercises for 6 weeks.[12] For the first 6 weeks, below shoulder level range of motion and strengthening activities are encouraged.

Dislocation and subluxation (a partial dislocation that reduces spontaneously) is fairly common and at times difficult to treat. Eighty percent or so of those patients 20 to 50 years of age who dislocate their shoulders will develop a recurrent dislocation. This is because dislocation of a shoulder in a young healthy patient usually requires a tear of the capsule as it attaches to the glenoid labrum (the Bankhart lesion). Because of the architecture of the shoulder joint, the tear frequently cannot heal. Treatment of the first dislocation should be treated with 3 to 6 weeks of immobilization, but after the second, it is probably not advantageous to immobilize the shoulder and conservative treatment should include avoidance of the statue of liberty position and a specific exercise program to strengthen muscles that stabilize the shoulder. Most recurrent dislocations require surgical correction to prevent further dislocations.

Acromioclavicular Joint

Acromioclavicular joint injuries usually involve first-, second-, or third-degree strains of the ligament complex that stabilizes the joint. The injury is caused by a fall on the tip of the shoulder that drives the acromion distally and forces the distal clavicle cephalad. First- and second-degree strains can be treated with a short course of anti-inflammatories and exercises. Because very few activities result in downward pressure on the distal clavicle, restrictions are within the limits of pain, which should disappear in 1 to 2 weeks. Third-degree strains result in a dislocation of the joint. This results in a bump at the level of the distal clavicle. Some surgeons feel that surgical repair is necessary but many recommend no treatment at all. The end result is a permanent bump at the end of the clavicle but because it is usually not a functional problem, it is usually an acceptable and satisfactory alternative to a surgical procedure and a scar. If the bump is unsightly, or if in a few instances it is painful, it can be resected with minimal loss of function to the shoulder. If surgery is performed, it usually involves some form of metal fixation of the joint and limitation of overhead motion is necessary for 6 to 12 weeks.

Biceps Tendon Rupture

Rupture of the long head of the biceps tendon usually occurs at the musculotendinous junction and as a result repair is unsuccessful. The rupture results in "bunching up" of the belly of the biceps muscle in the mid arm. Most surgeons treat the condition with exercises. The functional deficit is minimal despite the unsightly mass on the front of the arm. No activity restrictions are required except for a short period of time for pain relief.

Elbow

By far the most common problems in the elbow are the overuse syndromes. Tendonitis of the wrist extensors (lateral epicondylitis or tennis elbow) or of the wrist flexors (medial epicondylitis or golfer's elbow) make up the majority of these conditions. These usually respond to anti-inflammatories by mouth or injection and an exercise program to stretch and strengthen the effected muscle tendon unit. Patients need not be taken off work but may be advised to avoid repetitive activities that use the affected muscle group for 6 weeks while the muscles are strengthened. These conditions frequently become chronic and a change of job may be indicated. An innovative approach by employers is to rotate repetitive jobs among employees so that no one activity is performed by each employee more than 2 hours per day. Surgical correction now involves release of the tendinous attachment to the bone and, because no major structures need to heal, range of motion and strengthening activities are encouraged immediately.

Return to work after fractures can be successful and need not be delayed if the employer will make accommodations. As with fractures in and around any joint, the goal of open treatment is to stabilize the fracture adequately to allow early motion. Immobilization in these fractures invariably leads to stiffness of the joint. Although early range of motion is encouraged frequently, the timing and amount of force placed through the joint will be dependant on the fracture architecture and the confidence in the fixation by the surgeon. If the fracture is immobilized, as is occasionally necessary, single arm activities will be necessary until the immobilization is removed. Light use of the fingers in the immobilization is therapeutic as it will help avoid swelling.

Dislocations are no longer treated with long periods of immobilization and gentle range of motion activities, avoiding full extension but encouraging flexion, are encouraged. Moderate flexion forces may even be beneficial, but patients should avoid activities that cause passive extension.

Arthroscopic treatment of a number of intra-articular conditions is becoming commonplace. Most of these involve removing loose bodies, debridement of synovium, or shaving of chondral defects. None require immobilization and activities that encourage range of motion are encouraged immediately, even those that require moderate force.

Hand and Wrist

Filan as well as Kasdan and June have published guidelines for return to work after hand injuries.[9,15,16] By far the most common and perplexing problem in the wrist is carpal tunnel. There is an increasing body of evidence that carpal tunnel is not the result of an injury but actually an anatomic variant. Whatever the etiology, there are apparently some people who cannot perform repetitive activities with the wrist. Conservative treatment of carpal tunnel syndrome includes anti-inflammatories, splinting of the wrist in a neutral position, and temporary avoidance of the activity that causes the condition. Because there is evidence that birth control hormones can cause swelling in the carpal canal, these medications should be discontinued. Strengthening exercises for the wrist flexors has proven beneficial. After symptoms have been relieved, an attempt to return the patient to the original job is appropriate. If the attempt is unsuccessful, there is no choice but to change the job. Surgery for correction of carpal tunnel syndrome has been unpredictable in the workers' compensation setting, especially if the patient is returned to the job that supposedly caused the problem in the first place, and should be undertaken with caution and only in those whose symptoms persist after a job change.

Dislocations of finger joints are usually associated with second- or third-degree injuries to the ligaments and thus require protection. However, complete immobilization ultimately leads to stiffness and thus most physicians encourage range of motion exercises within the normal arc of the joint, possibly avoiding full extension. Three weeks of protection is usually enough and after that full range of motion is encouraged.

Activities after fractures of the wrist depend on the architecture of the fracture and the stability of the immobilization. Casts used for closed treatment are usually left in place for 6 to 8 weeks and while these are in place, single arm activities are possible. As with other upper extremity fractures, finger motion against minimal resistance is encouraged to help prevent swelling. Open treatment of wrist fractures, especially those that involve the joint surface, is much more common today and as a result, earlier mobilization is encouraged.

Phalangeal and metacarpal fractures can be treated open or closed but the goal is to allow as early motion as possible. For 3 to 6 weeks, motion against resistance should be avoided.

Overuse syndromes are common in workers who perform repetitive activities. These usually involve tendons that slide through sheaths or around pulleys. Treatment includes anti-inflammatories, splinting, and temporary avoidance of the offending activity. Like carpal tunnel syndrome, surgical treatment is unpredictable in those workers who return to the same repetitive activity and if return to work after relief of the symptoms is unsuccessful, a change in job description should be considered.

THE LOWER EXTREMITY

Unlike the upper extremity, where the main function is to place the hand in the proper position, a function that does not necessarily require force, the function in the lower extremity is to bear weight and that has significant implications in return to work philosophy. Regaining range of motion and strength are paramount in the upper extremity but stability, even at the cost of range of motion and strength, is acceptable in the lower extremity. Because axial loading of the lower extremity is an inevitable consequence of weight bearing, the rehabilitation of lower extremity injuries must take that phenomenon into account. In addition, as protection from full weight bearing and axial loading require the use of ambulation aids, such as walkers, crutches, or canes, the combination of concomitant upper and lower extremity injuries may be one of the few conditions that dictates total abstinence from work. Lack of strength and fatigue of the upper extremities may inhibit long periods of protected ambulation.

Hip

Injuries to the hip are the same as in other joints; that is, sprains, strains, overuse syndromes, fractures, and dislocations occur. Arthritis, although occasionally seen in the upper extremity, is much more common in the lower extremity. Avascular necrosis in the hip may be a consequence of trauma, certain medications such as cortisone and immunosuppressive drugs, and of chronic alcoholism. It is occasionally seen in the humeral head but is much more common in the hip and the knee.

Sprains and strains in and around the hip are usually treated successfully with anti-inflammatories and stretching and strengthening exercises and normally require only a short period of avoidance of repetitive motion activities. Sedentary activities or jobs that do not require ambulation may be considered for a short period of time.

Dislocation of the hip usually requires significant trauma and the treatment used to be bed rest and non-weight bearing, but most surgeons now only limit weight bearing to the painful period, about 1 to 2 weeks. Most dislocations not associated with fractures are very stable after reduction and it is not necessary to avoid motion except for the extremes of flexion, adduction, and internal rotation.

Most fractures about the hip, including those of the acetabulum, are now treated with open reduction and internal fixation and individuals in the working age population can nearly always withstand ambulation with partial weight bearing. For this reason, the presence of one of these fractures is not in and of itself a reason to be off work if appropriate accommodations are possible. In the absence of proper accommodations, fracture healing to allow full weight bearing may require as much as 3 to 4 months.

Arthritis can be treated with anti-inflammatories but most patients with significant arthritis in the hip should avoid activities that require frequent and continued ambulation. Although weight bearing by itself should not lead to further degeneration of the hip, weight bearing ambulation might. In addition, long periods of sitting in the same position can be uncomfortable so the patient should be allowed to move intermittently. The use of a cane in the hand opposite the arthritic hip for ambulation significantly relieves the forces across the hip and will often reduce the pain enough to allow a comfortable existence. Steroid injections offer temporary relief. Viscosupplementation is being used experimentally in the hip and holds some promise, especially in the earlier stages of the disease.

Arthroplasty of the hip is very common today and many of these workers can be successfully returned to active employment. Partial weight bearing is usually allowed immediately after arthroplasty but the patients are required to avoid the extremes of motion for at least 3 months. Therefore, return to work with ambulatory aids is permitted but the patient/employee cannot be required to bend over or squat to retrieve objects from the floor and must avoid sitting in low chairs, as arising from a low seat often requires bending forward at the hips. Unfortunately, arthroplasties last a finite period of time and there is good evidence that the more an arthroplasty is used, the shorter a period of time it lasts. Therefore, individuals with hip arthroplasties should not be required to ambulate for long periods of time and should avoid activities that require high degrees of impact loading.

As a cautionary note, it is often difficult to differentiate hip pain from back pain referred to the hip area. We have observed a number of total hips being done for disc pathology and a number of discs excised for arthritis of the hip. The physician must be cognizant of the similarity in the symptom complex.

Knee

Tendonitis, bursitis, and other overuse syndromes about the knee are usually treated with anti-inflammatories and a short period of avoidance of repetitive activities. Medial collateral ligament injuries are normally treated nonsurgically and, although partial weight bearing is required, range of motion activities are encouraged. Lateral collateral ligament tears still often require surgery. Postinjury swelling can be a problem and so the patient may need to be able to elevate the extremity for several hours per day. The length of time is dependent on the particular structures involved and the severity of the sprain.

Intra-articular injuries, including those to the anterior cruciate ligament, are treated arthroscopically. Meniscal excisions do not disrupt any structures and as a result do not require activity limitation except to relieve pain. We have had football players playing football again within 2 weeks of arthroscopic menisectomy. Anterior cruciate ligament reconstructions require a period of protected weight bearing, but most surgeons now allow nearly full weight bearing if the patient keeps the knee in full extension while bearing weight. Some surgeons use movable and removable braces postoperatively for up to 6 weeks, but many are using no immobilization.[20]

Since the advent of arthroscopy, we have discovered a new entity in the young adult, that being traumatic injuries to articular cartilage. Treatment for this previously devastating injury is controversial and includes microfracture, mosiacplasty, cultivated autologous cartilage transplantation, and allographic osteocartilaginous transplantation. The jury is not in on the most efficacious of these procedures but all require a long period of minimal weight bearing to allow reconstitution of the cartilage defect. These patients need nonweight bearing range of motion but cannot bear weight for periods of up to 6 to 12 weeks.

Fractures in and around the knee, like those in the hip, are normally treated with internal fixation and usually do not require complete immobilization. Usually, range of motion is encouraged, although weight bearing is often limited. Elevation of the extremity to prevent swelling is often necessary so if the patient is returned to work in the immediate postoperative period, the proper accommodations are required.

Arthroplasties of the knee, like the hip, are commonplace and the patient can be successfully returned to work. Range of motion is encouraged immediately and weight bearing to tolerance is the norm. Contrary to this, however, patients who have uncemented tibial components may require a period of protected weight bearing for up to 3 months. As in the hip, they last a finite period of time, and these individuals should avoid constant ambulation and impact loading.

Ankle and Foot

The ankle and foot are at a major disadvantage as far as healing are concerned. They are the most dependent structures in the human body and as a result, the circulation is often compromised. Additionally, swelling, increased by the dependent position, can further compromise the circulation. The ankle and foot are at the bottom of the pile and each time a human takes a step, the full weight of the body is transmitted through these structures. For these reasons, protected weight bearing and elevation are the hallmarks of rehabilitation of the ankle/foot complex.

Sprains and strains are common, especially of the lateral ankle ligaments. The air cast has revolutionized the treatment of the sprained ankle. Previously, ankle sprains were treated with nonweight bearing and/or casting. Now we apply air casts and encourage weight bearing and range of motion. Protected weight bearing may be necessary for a few days for pain control but is not necessary to protect the ligament integrity. Early return to work should be the goal. Other sprains and strains can be treated with protective shoes and protected weight bearing but should not necessitate being off work. It may be necessary for the patient/employee to elevate the foot for periods of time during the work day.

Fractures that are treated closed can be immobilized with braces or casts but most will allow partial weight bearing. Removable fracture braces are now commonplace and allow removal for range of motion exercises. Fractures that are opened and fixed with internal fixation may require less immobilization but may also require protected weight bearing. A common and unfortunate fracture is the fracture of the calcaneus. Controversy remains about the best way to treat these fractures. Displaced, intra-articular fractures are probably best treated by open reduction, but even with anatomic reductions, the rehabilitation is long and arduous. A study by Tufescu and Buckley suggested that men, multiply injured patients, and heavy laborers did better with open treatment, whereas women and non-workers' compensation patients did better with non-operative treatment. Because every time a person takes an unsupported step all of his or her weight is transmitted through the calcaneus, it is not surprising that the results of treatment of this fracture are less than satisfactory.[27] Several studies have shown that it may take up to 2 years to reach maximum medical improvement. Many will eventually require arthrodesis of at least the subtalar joint and that is so common that some surgeons prefer to perform the fusion at the time of the initial operative treatment in fractures that are significantly displaced. Any form of open treatment will require 6 to 12 weeks of cast immobilization.

Whichever treatment is undertaken, a period of limited weight bearing of 6 to 12 weeks is necessary for fracture healing. Intermittent elevation to prevent swelling will be necessary for the first several weeks. Return to work can be accomplished within a few weeks if the employer can provide appropriate accommodations. Full weight bearing and activities that require considerable ambulation may not be possible for many months.

Fractures of the talus are a problem similar to that of calcaneus with the additional problem of avascular necrosis. Because of the anatomy of the blood supply to the talus, it is frequently disrupted in severe fractures and dislocations of the talus. This may lead to death of part or all of the talus. Return to work issues are similar to those in the calcaneus; that is, it may take an extended period of partial weight bearing to allow for pain to subside but with protected weight bearing, there is no reason not to return the patient/employee to work as soon as accommodations can be arranged.

There are two nerve entrapment syndromes in the ankle/foot area: the posterior tibial nerve in the tibial tunnel and the deep branch of the peroneal nerve as it passes under the extensor retinaculum. Both problems are usually treated conservatively but either may require operative management. Neither surgery disrupts a supportive structure so postoperative treatment is limited to pain control and early return to work, maybe with ambulation support as indicated. A third neurologic condition more common in the foot is interdigital neuroma. Although this is uncommonly a workers' compensation problem, surgical excision of the neuroma is often recommended for definitive treatment. Postoperative protected weight bearing is indicated for pain control but because there are no supportive structures disrupted in the surgery, the protection is for pain control only and rapid return to work with limitations on ambulation should be possible.

SUMMARY

In many cases, return to work is limited only by the ability of the employer to provide appropriate accommodations and the employer's willingness to pay the employee to be at work but not producing at full capacity. There is increasing evidence that early return to work, even with limitations, leads more often to an eventual successful return to full work. Conversely, the longer an individual remains off work, the less likely that there will be a successful return to work. Providing proper accommodations may be troublesome, expensive, and even impossible in certain situations, but doing so routinely will result in a much higher rate of successful return to work. In addition, paying wages to a worker while he or she attends a required rehabilitation program instead of remaining sedentary at home will result in decreased costs, despite the lack of production.[21]

References

1. Ash P, Goldstein SI: Predictors of returning to work. Bull Am Acad Psychiatry Law 23:205–210, 1995.
2. Atcheson SG, Brunner RL, Greenwald EJ, et al: Paying doctors more: Use of musculoskeletal specialists and increased physician pay to decrease workers compensation costs. J Occup Environ Med 43:672–679, 2001.
3. Biomechanical Risk Factors and Modifiers in the Etiology of Musculoskeletal Disorders: OSHA guidelines. Available at: www.osha-slc.gov.
4. Brooker AS, Cole DC, Hogg-Johnson S, et al: Modified work: Prevalence characteristics in a sample of workers with soft tissue injuries. J Occup Environ Med 43:267–284, 2001.
5. Crook J, Moldofsky H, Shannon H: Determinants for disability after work related musculoskeletal injury. J Rheumatol 25:1570–1577, 1998.
6. Denniston P (ed): Official Disability Guideline 2001, 6th ed. Corpus Christi, Tex, Work Loss Data Institute, 2001.
7. Egol KA, Dolan R, Koval KJ: Functional outcome of surgery for fractures of the ankle. A prospective comparison of management

in a cast or a functional brace. J Bone Joint Surg [Br] 82:264–269, 2000.

8. Ergonomics Standard: Occupational Safety & Health Administration, U.S. Department of Labor. Available at: www.osha-slc.gov.
9. Filan SL: The effect of workers' or third-party compensation on return to work after hand surgery. Med J Aust 165:80–82, 1996.
10. Hall H, et al: Going on Comp: How to Get Through a Workers' Compensation Injury Without Losing Your Cool. Duluth, Minn, Med-Ed Books, 1991.
11. Hall H, McIntosh T, Holowachuk B, Wai E: Effect of discharge recommendations on outcome. Spine 19:2033–2037, 1994.
12. Hawkins R: Update on shoulder surgery. Presented at the Tennessee Orthopaedic Society, White Sulphur Springs, WVa, 2001.
13. Houston J: Personal communication, 1980.
14. Indahl A, Haldorsen EH, Holm S, et al: Five year follow-up study of a controlled clinical trial using light mobilization and an informative approach to low back pain. Spine 23:2625–2630, 1998.
15. Kasdan ML, June LA: Returning to work after a unilateral hand fracture. J Occup Med 35:132–135, 1993.
16. Kasdan ML: Occupational Hand Injuries in Occupational Medicine, vol 4, no 3. Philadelphia, Henley & Belfus, 1989.
17. Mayer TG: One-handed in a Two-handed World. Boston, Prince-Gallison, 1996.
18. Mayer TG, Gatchel RJ, Polatin PB (eds): Occupational Musculoskeletal Disorders: Function, Outcomes and Evidence. Philadelphia, Lippincott Williams & Wilkins, 2000.
19. Millstein SG, Hunter GA: A review of employment patterns of industrial amputees: Factors influencing rehabilitation. Prosthet Orthot Int 9:69–78.
20. Noyes FB, Barber-Westin SD: Reconstruction of the anterior and posterior cruciate ligaments after knee dislocation. Use of early protected postoperative motion to decrease arthrofibrosis. Am J Sports Med 25:769–778, 1997.
21. Perry MC: REACH: An alternative early return to work program. AAOHN J 44:294–298, 1966.
22. Putz-Anderson V: Cumulative Trauma Disorders: A Manual for Musculoskeletal Disease of the Upper Limbs. Bristol, Pa, Taylor & Francis, 1992.
23. Reed P: The Medical Disability Advisor, 4th ed. Boulder, Colo, Reed Group, 2001.
24. Robinson JP, Rondinelli RD, Scheer SJ, Weinstein SM: Industrial rehabilitation medicine. 1. Why is industrial rehabilitation medicine unique? Arch Phys Med Rehabil 78(3 Suppl.):3–9, 1997.
25. Smith G: Personal communication, 1982.
26. Talmage JB: Unpublished meta-analysis.
27. Tufescu TV, Buckley R: Age, gender, work capability, and workers' compensation in patients with displaced intra-articular calcaneal fractures. J Orthop Trauma 15:275–279, 2001.
28. Weisel SW, Boden SD, Feffer HL: A quality-based protocol for management of musculoskeletal injuries. A ten-year prospective outcome study. Clin Orthop 301:164–176, 1994.
29. Wexler G, Bach BR Jr, Bush-Joseph CA, et al: Outcomes of anterior cruciate ligament reconstruction in patients with workers compensation claims. Arthroscopy 16:49–58, 2000.

CHAPTER

58

Orthopedic Disability

The Spine

GUNNAR B.J. ANDERSSON, MD, PhD

Decisions about when to return a patient to work and whether to impose restrictions are common for physicians in all specialties. During this process we weigh the risk of making a disease or injury worse against the implicit goal of returning a patient to normal function and activities, which can be enhanced by work return.[1] In the workers' compensation and personal injury arena, economic, social, and legal factors influence these decisions, and because the decisions are often made by the patient and physician together, patient-physician relationships are also an important influence. This has led to the use of second opinions and independent medical evaluations (IMEs) to eliminate this bias, with advantages and disadvantages discussed elsewhere in this book. A major obstacle in the process is the lack of well-supported evidence-based guidelines on which to base decisions about work return and disability. This is perhaps more true in the area of back pain than in many other disease and injury areas because there may be no visible evidence of an injury or disease and often the patient's complaints are the only available information on which to base work return and activity level decisions.

A variety of guidelines have developed over time, mostly based on experience and consensus.[14] For the most part they are supported by basic science and epidemiologic research. These guidelines are used by a variety of professionals including claims and case managers, rehabilitation and vocational specialists, and health care professionals. They also provide useful information to patients, who legitimately need to know what to expect in this regard.

At least four sources of guidelines exist for back pain and other conditions: the Official Disability Guidelines,[13] the Medical Disability Advisor—Workplace Guidelines for Disability Duration,[16] the Healthcare Management Guidelines,[4] and the American College of Occupational and Environmental Medicine (ACOEM) Guidelines.[8] In addition, proprietary guidelines have been produced by utilization review organizations, third-party payers, disability management companies, and private companies.

The Official Disability Guidelines[13] is organized by ICD-9 codes and based on a database of 3 million cases, usually from the Annual National Health Interview Survey. Every diagnosis is covered. The Medical Disability Advisor[16] has more information about conditions and procedures, which are listed alphabetically. It covers about 1000 conditions (or 10% of ICD-9 codes). The Health Management Guidelines[4] is organized by body parts, covering about 300 different diagnoses. Finally, the ACOEM Guidelines[8] covers 54 different diagnoses organized in eight sections by body parts including neck and upper back and lower back separately.

Little is known about the natural history of treated and untreated spinal conditions as they relate to the activities of an individual. This has led to large differences in return to work decisions and restrictions. Over the past 20 years or so, considerable consensus has been reached that rest is worse than activity and that work return offers more advantages than risks. The purpose of this chapter is to provide further thoughts on the disability issues relating to a variety of spinal conditions. Because these conditions are fundamentally different, they are separated by etiology. Spinal fusions present a particular biomechanical situation and are therefore described separately.

BACK STRAINS AND SPRAINS

Most back injuries are soft tissue injuries affecting muscles and ligaments. A strain is defined as a muscle disruption caused by an indirect trauma such as excessive stretch or tension. Strains can theoretically occur as a result of physical activities or indirect trauma. Depending on severity, a strain is graded as Grade I (microscopic disruption of fibers), II (macroscopic disruption with preserved structural integrity), or III (complete disruption). Grade III is rare. Most strains occur at the myotendinous junctions, not in the substance of the muscle. Animal research suggests a very rapid healing of a partial tear, with almost normal function of a rabbit muscle after 7 days.[12] Mobilization and activity enhances healing and reduces scar tissue formation. Human experience suggests that return to full muscle performance may take several weeks (3 to 6), but rarely longer. Muscles can be expected to fully recover from contraction-induced injuries.[2,5,6] Patients with a strain/sprain can typically perform modified or clerical type work, often without any work loss. In severe cases, a few days off work may be indicated. A medium workload (lifting up to 50 pounds occasionally) should be possible after 2 to 3 weeks with return to heavy manual work after 4 to 6 weeks in most cases.

DISC HERNIATIONS

A herniated disc is a common finding even in asymptomatic individuals. Myelograms, discograms, computed tomography scans, and magnetic resonance imaging studies of asymptomatic individuals show disc herniations in 25 to 35% of cases, with increasing percentages in older populations.[3,9–11,17,19] The fact that these individuals have no symptoms in spite of performing widely different work activities suggests that a finding of a herniation, as such, is not a reason for disability. Impingement of nerve tissue by a herniation can be extremely painful, sometimes disabling. This disability is temporary, however, as demonstrated by the classical study by Weber.[18] In this study, Weber followed 126 subjects who were randomly assigned to operative and nonoperative care for 10 years. At 1 year, 60% of nonoperated patients did well (versus 90% of surgically treated), and at 4 and 10 years, results were similar in both groups, with excellent return of function irrespective of treatment. Other studies show similar good results with respect to work return and activities in patients who have had no specific treatment.[7,15]

In the acute stages, a disc herniation causing radiculopathy may prevent any type of work. This is typically only for a short period, but lifting, twisting, bending, and walking may be influenced for months. Thus, sedentary work may be possible after 2 to 3 days, provided there is opportunity to change work posture at will. At 4 weeks, light to medium work should be possible in most patients responding to nonoperative care, with return to regular work within 12 weeks. When there is no result or a poor response to treatment, surgery becomes an option, typically between 6 and 12 weeks. A discectomy does not preclude returning to manual work. Usually 3 to 4 weeks is sufficient for tissue healing, after which modified work return and physical therapy can proceed, with the goal of returning the patient/employee to unrestricted work in another 4 to 6 weeks. Individuals with recurrent disc herniations may require modest accommodations.

SPINAL STENOSIS

Spinal stenosis is very common in the elderly, and not infrequently associated with degenerative spondylolisthesis. Stenosis, as such, is not disabling. The effect of the stenotic process on the neural tissues is what may cause disability. These individuals may lose their ability to extend the spine, while flexion usually relieves symptoms. Walking is also often affected (spinal or neurogenic claudication), as is standing. These activities may be impossible to perform when the symptoms are acute. Fortunately, the natural history is often benign and stenosis is not a progressive disorder in most individuals. Further, because stenosis is age related, most individuals with these symptoms are already retired. Most individuals with stenosis are pain free when sitting and thus sedentary work is almost always an option. The stenosis as such does not worsen because of work activities and is not caused by injury except when a fracture or dislocation reduces the size of the spinal canal.

DISC DEGENERATION

Disc degeneration is part of aging. By age 30, most people have early degenerative changes; by age 50, everyone does. Thus, as such, disc degeneration is normal. Further, disc degeneration is not a traumatic event but rather a slow development over years and decades. Trauma can temporarily aggravate degeneration but unless it is so severe that it disrupts the integrity of the motion segment, aggravation lasts for a few weeks to a month only. During this period, clerical or modified work is appropriate, perhaps in severe cases after an initial 1 to 3 days off work. At 4 weeks, manual work can safely resume.

The degenerative process may have secondary effects causing symptoms and disability. Except in childhood and adolescence, disc herniations do not occur unless the disc is degenerative. Occasionally, therefore, an individual with disc degeneration will have a traumatically induced herniation—not only because of the trauma but also because the disc was already degenerative. The clinical manifestations of such an event are immediate with radicular symptoms and associated findings clinically and on imaging studies. When clinical symptoms of radiculopathy do not occur following an accident, the relationship of an imaging finding to an accident is unlikely. As discussed in the section on disc herniation, disability may result for a limited time period from a traumatically induced herniation.

Another consequence of the degenerative process is a weakening of the disc structure. This can cause minor instability and make the back mechanically sensitive. Again, this is not an injury-related problem, but may permanently prevent a person from performing heavy manual work. Sedentary or light duty jobs, however, should always be possible. In the acute stages a few days' rest may be appropriate followed by a gradual work return.

SPINAL FUSION

Fusing a motion segment, whether from the front, the back, or both, changes the biomechanics of the spine. When one or more motion segments are fused, most of the compensation for the fairly minor loss of motion occurs at the hip joints. The remaining lumbar motion segments will be the focus of increased stress, however, which can result in accelerated degeneration of particularly the adjacent motion segments. For those reasons, patients with a fusion are at some increased risk in the future. This risk is higher when the back is severely stressed as in jobs requiring frequent heavy lifting, bending, and twisting. Some permanent modification of work is therefore reasonable in these individuals, particularly when the fusion spans several motion segments. Bone healing following fusion often takes 6 months or so. Individuals can often return to sedentary work activities after 4 to 6 weeks and to light duty work after 12 weeks. As the fusion heals and therapy is initiated, typically after 12 to 16 weeks, the person can gradually resume normal labor, perhaps with a 50-pound work restriction. A fusion by itself is not a permanent reason not to return to work.

DISCUSSION

Disability following a back injury or as a result of back pain is rare. Specific conditions affecting the nervous system or the load-bearing and movement characteristics of the spine will cause disability, however. Typically, this is temporary, often short in duration and limited. Almost never should a back problem cause permanent inability to work. Permanent modifications, as discussed in this chapter, may sometimes be necessary. In providing guidelines, I have tried to be fair and believe the opinions expressed are defensible. Disability duration guidelines will always be controversial, and are often challenged by the involved parties. The type of treatment and response to therapy, the severity of injury, and the type of job are factors influencing the duration of the disability. Economic, social, and legal factors also influence recovery. Much of the information about a back pain complaint is from the patient. This creates problems related to verification and can result in disputes and distrust, which are always negative with respect to recovery. Chronic back syndrome is a special symptom entity discussed in Chapter 21. The difficult balance of over- or underprotecting patients with respect to work return and restrictions should not prevent physicians from making these necessary decisions.

References

1. Abenhaim L, Rossignol M, Valat JP, et al: The role of activity in the therapeutic management of back pain. Spine 25:1S–33S, 2000.
2. Armstrong RB, Warren GL III, Lowe DA: Mechanisms in the initiation of contraction-induced skeletal muscle injury. In Gordon SL, Blair SJ, Fine LJ (eds): Repetitive Motion Disorders of the Upper Extremity. Rosemont, AAOS, 1995, pp 339–350.
3. Boden SD, Davis DO, Dina TS, et al: Abnormal magnetic resonance scans of the lumbar spine in asymptomatic subjects. J Bone Joint Surg [Am] 72:403–408, 1990.
4. Bruckman RZ, Rasmussen H: Healthcare Management Guidelines: Volume 7, Workers' Compensation. Seattle, Milliman & Robertson, 1996.
5. Fielding RA: The role of inflammatory processes in exercise-induced muscle injury: implications for changes in skeletal muscle protein turnover. In Gordon SL, Blair SJ, Fine LJ (eds): Repetitive Motion Disorders of the Upper Extremity. Rosemont, AAOS, 1995, pp 323–338.
6. Friden J, Lieber RL: Biomechanical injury to skeletal muscle from repetitive loading: eccentric contractions and vibrations in repetitive motion disorders of the upper extremity. In Gordon SL, Blair SJ, Fine LJ (eds): Repetitive Motion Disorders of the Upper Extremity. Rosemont, AAOS, 1995, pp 301–312.
7. Hakelius A, Hindmarsh J: The significance of neurological signs and myelographic findings in the diagnosis of lumbar root compression. Acta Orthop Scand 43:239, 1972.
8. Harris JS, et al: Occupational Medicine Practice Guidelines: Evaluation and Management of Common Health Problems and Functional Recovery in Workers. Beverly Farms, Mass, OEM Health Information Press, 1997.
9. Hitselberger WE, Witten RM: Abnormal myelograms in asymptomatic patients. J Neurosurg 28:204–208, 1968.
10. Holt EP: The question of lumbar discography. J Bone Joint Surg [Am] 50:720–726, 1968.
11. Jensen MC, Brant-Zawdzki MN, Obuchowki N, et al: Magnetic resonance imaging of the lumbar spine in people without back pain. N Engl J Med 331:69–73, 1994.

12. Nikolaou PK, MacDonald BL, Glisson RR, et al: Biomechanical and histological evaluation of muscle after controlled strain injury. Am J Sports Med 15:9–14 1987.
13. Official Disability Guidelines, 6th ed. Corpus Christi, Tex, Work Loss Data Institute, 2001.
14. Prezzia C, Dennison P: The use of evidence-based duration guidelines. The Journal of Workers' Compensation 10:43–53, 2001.
15. Saal JA, Saal JS: Nonoperative treatment of herniated lumbar intervertebral disc with radiculopathy: An outcome study. Spine 14:431–437, 1989.
16. The Medical Disability Advisor, 3rd ed. Boulder, Colo, The Reed Group, 1997.
17. Walsh TR, Weinstein JN, Spratt KF, et al: Lumbar discography in normal subjects. A controlled, prospective study. J Bone Joint Surg [Am] 72:1081–1088, 1990.
18. Weber H: Lumbar disc herniation: A controlled, prospective study with ten years of observation. Spine 8:131–140, 1983.
19. Wiesel SW, Tsourmas N, Feffer HL, et al: A study of computer-assisted tomography. I. The incidence of positive CAT scans in an asymptomatic group of patients. Spine 9:549–551, 1984.

SECTION

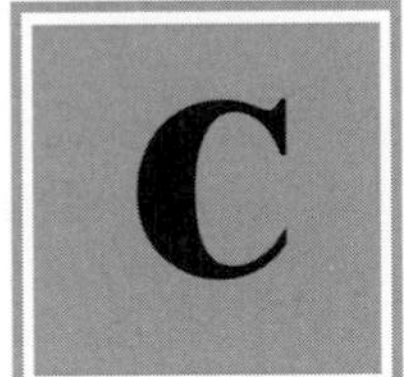

Internal Medicine Disability

CHAPTER

59

Pulmonary Disability

STEPHEN L. DEMETER, MD, MPH

Pulmonary diseases are frequent causes of both impairment and disability. The Disability Statistics Report, published by the National Institute on Disability and Rehabilitation Research, stated that in 1992 in the total U.S. noninstitutionalized population, 15% (37.7 million people) reported some activity limitation due a chronic health condition. In the working age population (18 to 69 years), 11.6% (19.0 million people) had some degree of limitation in working at a job owing to a chronic health condition. Of these people, 278,000 are limited by chronic bronchitis, 904,000 by emphysema, 2.6 million by asthma, 53,000 by other obstructive airway diseases, 66,000 by pneumoconioses, and 470,000 by "other." The total figure for respiratory diseases is 4.8 million. Of all medical conditions causing disability, pulmonary problems ranks fourth.[32] This applies for males as well as females.[29] In 1996, respiratory diseases were responsible for 5.6% of conditions limiting a person's ability to work.[56]

In the Social Security System, in 1999, there were a total of 4.9 million disabled workers who were receiving pay benefits. Of these, 3.7% were for pulmonary diseases, representing the sixth largest group.[55]

Thus, pulmonary problems represent one of the larger categories of diseases creating work disability. Chapter 43 stated that the purpose of a disability evaluation is to define, measure, and determine an examinee's health status and catalogue a person's impairments. This information is then used to describe capabilities or incapabilities with reference to a certain job function or task. There are two essential components to the disability evaluation, one that focuses on the examinee/worker and one that centers on the job/work environment.

This chapter explores these concepts with reference to pulmonary diseases. Not all pulmonary diseases or work exposures can be covered in a chapter such as this and, many times, certain principles will be described that will have broad application for a variety of pulmonary disorders or work environments. Five areas of pulmonary diseases will be presented (asthma and obstructive pulmonary diseases, chronic obstructive pulmonary disease [COPD], hypersensitivity pneumonitis, interstitial lung disease [ILD], and sleep apnea). Textbooks of pulmonary diseases or occupational medicine should be consulted for more specific conditions (e.g., work environments/exposures that could be hazardous to the patient with a history of bronchogenic carcinoma).

ASTHMA AND OBSTRUCTIVE PULMONARY DISEASES

Before explaining workplace restrictions, it will be useful to have an understanding of asthma and obstructive airway diseases. Over time, asthma has been defined in many ways based on our understanding of its scientific origins and pathophysiology. Asthma has been known from antiquity but in 1917 it was defined as "a form of paroxysmal dyspnea, the characteristic feature of which is marked diminution or arrest of the respiratory movements with prolonged expiration."[31] In 1920, Osler's Textbook of Medicine described it as "a reaction of an anaphylactic nature in sensitized persons, in others possibly a reflex neurosis characterized by swelling of the nasal or respiratory mucous membrane, increased secretion, and ... spasm of the bronchial muscles with dyspnea, chiefly expiratory."[46] In 1962, the American Thoracic Society stated that it is "a disease characterized by an increased responsiveness of the trachea and bronchi to various stimuli and manifested by a widespread narrowing of the airways that change in severity either spontaneously or as a result of therapy."[10]

During the 1970s and 1980s, asthma research focused on the inflammatory nature of asthma relegating the cardinal defining component of asthma (bronchospasm) to a manifestation of airways inflammation that can also include other features such as mucous gland hypersecretion, smooth muscle hyperplasia, and others. This work culminated in a 1989 definition wherein asthma was defined as "an eosinophilic inflammatory disorder of the airways."[2] Greater emphasis has been given to the inflammatory concept of asthma for two major reasons: the development of new drug treatments (and the reassessment of older ones) and the concept of "airways remodeling" (permanent airways obstruction—i.e., nonreversible—due to chronic, unrelieved airway inflammation).

However important these issues are for the proper understanding and treatment of asthma, this chapter views asthma and obstructive airways diseases from a different perspective. It is this change in perspective that will enable the evaluator to have a working paradigm for a pulmonary disability evaluation.

The Rheostat Concept of Asthma*

It has been said that "Everything in biology, and medicine, can be described on a bell-shaped curve." Although oversimplistic, this is a useful concept when addressing asthma. Asthma testing was described in Chapter 22. What must be appreciated is that if airflow rates were measured before and after the inhalation of acetylcholine (the neurally mediated smooth muscle stimulator in the bronchial system liberated from parasympathetic nerve endings), all people would have a normal, physiologic response. This response is a reduction in airflow rates caused by smooth muscle contraction (or bronchospasm). Various constrictive agents can be used in an asthma test (as described in Chapter 22), including methacholine (a chemical surrogate for acetylcholine), histamine (a chemical mediator liberated in the inflammatory reaction producing, among other responses, bronchospasm), cold air, exercise, and others. All these mediators will produce the same response in all people—bronchospasm or contraction of the bronchial smooth muscle. This can be assessed, indirectly, by measuring airflow rates. This is the principle behind the spirometric assessment of airways disease. What must be further appreciated is that, although all people will respond to those agents, the degree of response will be different.

The concept of stimulus/response is familiar to those who have studied biological sciences. In the bronchoconstrictive test, the stimulus is an agent (acetylcholine, methacholine, histamine, etc.) and the response is smooth muscle contraction in the airways. The stimulus could just as easily be a workplace agent such as dust, smoke, a specific chemical agent such as isocyanate, or others. The response could just as easily be another response created by the inflammatory reaction such as cough or mucus secretion. For ease of demonstration and testing, the response that is traditionally chosen is bronchospasm/airflow reduction.

If a population is studied in this stimulus/response model, a range of quantitative responses is seen. If one applies an identical stimulus to these individuals, variable degrees of airflow reductions are seen. Conversely, if the same response is desired in these individuals, the stimulus will need to be varied. These concepts underlie the principles of asthma testing. Again, all people will respond to acetylcholine (or methacholine) with smooth muscle contraction in the bronchial walls creating a reduction in airflow rates. It is the amount of reduction that underlies all asthma testing (or the amount of dilation that occurs in a bronchodilator test). Those individuals who are hyper-responders are those who are diagnosed with asthma.

Figure 59–1 represents this range of biological responses. The + refers to the exaggerated or "hyper" response; the – represents a minimal or "hypo"-responsive state. Everything in between represents the range of "normal" responses. Point 1 is the average response to a standard dose of a constrictive agent. Point 2 is defined as the cutoff point for hyper-responsiveness. Approximately 6 to 8% of the population has asthma and an arbitrary cutoff point was determined based on the sensitivity and specificity of this point in diagnosing asthmatics (see Chapter 22). It should be understood, however, that this response to a bronchoconstrictive agent is a continuum and not all people who have clinical features of asthma will be to the right of Point 2 nor will all those individuals to the right of Point 2 have features of asthma. (Again, the model of asthma being used in this chapter utilizes simplistic concepts. It is presented because of its utility. However, this model is valid from a scientific perspective as well. From a strictly scientific viewpoint, the distribution is not bell shaped but more unimodal. The distinguishing feature in dose/response curves for asthmatics is one of continuous response whereas plateaus are seen in nonasthmatics. Further, not all asthmatics will respond to a methacholine challenge. Not all asthmatics respond to every single stimulus [or bronchoprovocative agent] nor will there be a uniform response to each stimulus. In other words, one asthmatic may have a different quantitative response to histamine or exercise then to methacholine. Further, the difficulty in assessing the value of these tests rests upon the clinical concept of asthma [including disease severity] and reconciling this with physiologic findings. The medical literature is particu-

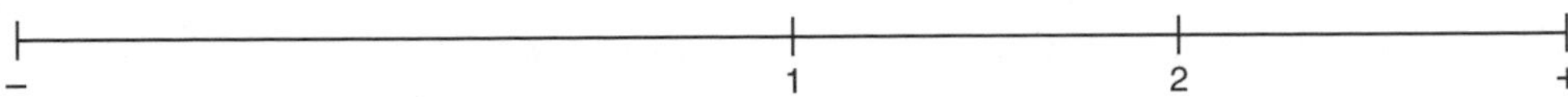

Figure 59–1. "Rheostat" Model of asthma.

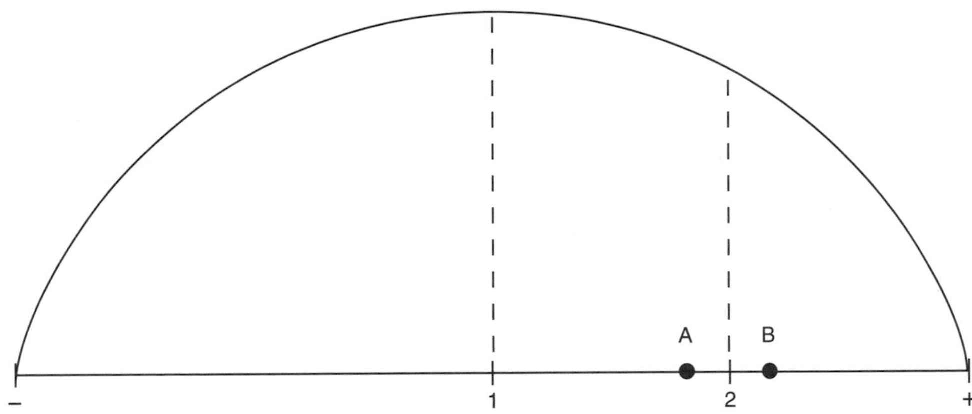

Figure 59–2.

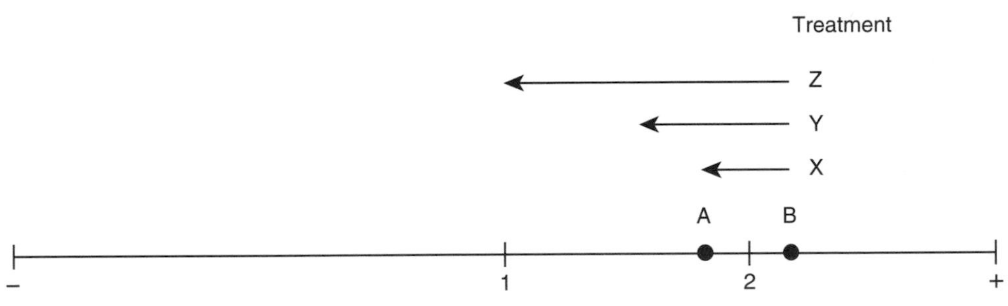

Figure 59–3.

larly rich in describing the above issues and references 7, 9, 13, 20, 21, 24, 28, 33, 37, 40, 41, 43, 44, 45, 47, 49–51, 54, 59, 60, and 64 are recommended for background reading.)

Returning to this simplistic model, consider Patients A and B (Fig. 59–2). Patient A by definition does not have asthma whereas Patient B does. Is there a significant difference between these two individuals in their bronchial hyper-responsiveness or in their clinical presentations? Probably not, yet a line had to be drawn somewhere and again it was arbitrarily defined as Point 2 in Figure 59–1.

What effect does therapy have on asthma? Clearly, one would like to see a reduction/control of symptoms. If the baseline in Figure 59–3 represents symptoms (as opposed to the bronchial response to bronchoconstriction agents), then the clinical response can be appreciated. Bronchodilators or anti-inflammatory agents used in the treatment of asthma will push the patient to the left, at least temporarily. Therefore the cardinal symptoms of asthma (bronchoconstriction, cough, and mucus production) will lessen.

There is scientific evidence that asthma treatment, especially with potent anti-inflammatory medications such as steroids, can actually accomplish the same change if the baseline is kept as the degree of bronchial hyper-responsiveness. In other words, patients chronically treated with inhaled steroids can actually decrease their response to a methacholine challenge test.[3] The more medication used (either in terms of dosage or different agents), the further to the left the patient becomes symptomatically (Fig. 59–3X,Y,Z). The opposite effect could, of course, be seen in the treated asthmatic who had medications progressively removed (Fig. 59–4) or in the person who is exposed to greater and greater amounts of a bronchoconstrictive stimulus (R,S,T).

Thus, when the examinee is approached, the issues that need to be decided are as follows: 1) What is the amount of hyper-responsiveness that the person has at the current time (where on the rheostat is that person)? 2) What medications is that person receiving (factors pushing his or her position to the left)? 3) What stimuli does the individual encounter (factors pushing his or her position to the right)? In some circumstances, asthma medications are synergistic, in others they are additive, and there may be a plateau in the effects of increased numbers of medications. The amount of asthmatic signs and symptoms will be a reflection of where on the rheostat the individual is (based on his or her intrinsic responsiveness and the usage of medications) and his or her exposure to varying degrees of stimuli.

This concept also helps the evaluator in making return to work (RTW) recommendations. As an example, in Figure 59–5, Patients A and B have similar degrees of hyper-responsiveness (i.e., the same degree of pulmonary impairment; Points A1 and B1), but Patient B is on four medications and Patient A is only on two medications (Points A2 and B2). Both are asymptomatic at home (low to moderate environmental stimuli) but both work in a dusty, smoky foundry. Patient A will have more symptoms than Patient B when exposed to these asthmogenic stimuli. Patient A may not be capable of working in that occupational setting (i.e., disabled) given the present level of medication usage. Both patients, however, would be capable of working in a more restricted environment. Therefore, if Patient A is incapable of taking more medication (lack of effect/ side effects), then a recommendation for environmental restrictions would be appropriate. To summarize, both Patients A and B are equally impaired. Patient A is disabled for the foundry whereas Patient B is not. Patient A may be able to work in the foundry if he receives more medications (moves further to the left), works in an environmentally restricted part of the foundry (decreased stimuli), or wears a protective device (respirator). The latter two issues are examples of workplace accommodations and handicaps (see Chapter 1).

Asthmogenic stimuli can be specific or nonspecific. Examples of nonspecific stimuli include temperature extremes, dust, fumes, and smoke. Examples of specific stimuli include substances that the patient has an allergic response to (IgE mediated) or other types of individual intolerance. In some instances these stimulus/response biochemical pathways are known; in others it is not. For example, a person may develop an antibody reaction that does not involve the IgE pathway (e.g., IgG or IgM antibodies to platinum salts[15]).

Workplace Restrictions for the Asthmatic

The physician recommending workplace restrictions should go through a mental checklist with components similar to those found in Table 59–1. As discussed in multiple preceding chapters, disability is task specific. In order to recommend workplace restrictions, the physician must know what the workplace is like. This information is available. It may or may not be complete, but it is available. By law, employers must submit material safety data sheets to physicians upon request (see Chapter 44). These forms will identify specific workplace exposures. Ambient levels of dust, fumes, and smoke can be obtained through the Human Resources Department, if they have been measured by an Industrial Hygienist (see Chapter 44). The same holds true for workplace temperatures, although the Occupational Safety Specialist may

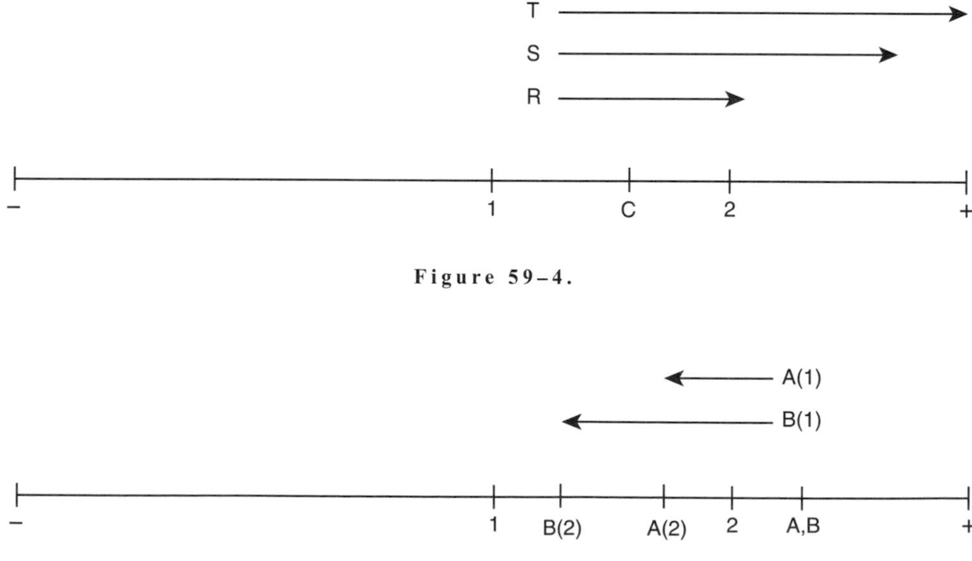

Figure 59–4.

Figure 59–5.

TABLE 59–1

Steps in Preparing a Restriction List for the Patient With Asthma

1. Determine location on the "rheostat"
2. Review job description
   - A. Tasks
   - B. Level of physical/emotional stress
   - C. Work environment
     1. Levels of dust
     2. Levels of fumes
     3. Levels of smoke
     4. Specific exposures
3. Assess need for intervention. Possible steps:
   - A. Increase medication
   - B. Environmental restrictions (see Table 59–2)
     1. General
     2. Specific
   - C. Personal protective devices
   - D. Workplace accommodations

be the person responsible for this measurement. (See also reference 8 for an excellent discussion of occupational asthma that also identifies other potential sources/resources for information concerning the workplace.) Table 59–2 provides a generic checklist for categories of workplace restrictions for an asthmatic.

Workplace accommodations are always preferable to personal protective devices. Thus, if an exhaust fan, vacuum system, environmental hood, or other types of engineered worksite modifications can be used, there may be a sufficient reduction in the nonspecific asthmogenic stimuli that might allow the asthmatic patient to work in that job environment. If the patient has an asthmogenic response to a specific chemical or other stimulus in the work environment, then job shifting may be all that is necessary. If all else fails, the use of personal protective devices (such as masks and respirators) can be considered although the asthmatic (or workers with other pulmonary diseases such as COPD) may not be the ideal candidate for these devices.[25,38]

There are over 200 workplace-specific asthmogenic substances known.[15] Occupational asthma is the most common nonacute occupational lung disease in many industrialized countries including the United States.[8]

TABLE 59–2

Workplace Restrictions in the Patient with Asthma

General	Specific
1. Dust	1. Allergens
2. Fumes	2. Others
3. Smoke	
4. Temperature extremes	
5. Physical stress, including exercise	
6. Emotional stress	

Occasionally, specific bronchoprovocative testing will elucidate the cause/effect relationship but, although this is a very specific test and offers compelling evidence that a person is reacting to a specific workplace exposure, it is rarely performed due to inconvenience, cost, lack of testing facilities, and inherent danger. (Reference 8 provides details of bronchoprovocative testing protocol.) Occasionally serologic or skin testing will be of value. In most circumstances, the history alone is sufficient,[15] although it has been suggested that the clinical history is more reliable in excluding occupational asthma than in confirming its presence.[8] Various criteria have been proposed for the diagnosis of occupational asthma and were published as consensus statements by the American College of Chest Physicians.[8] This reference addresses the variety of tests that can be used (peak flow monitoring, bronchodilator and bronchoconstriction tests, bronchoprovocation testing, and others) and is highly recommended. Reference 39 is a similar report published by the European Academy of Allergy and Clinical Immunology.

Asthma in the workplace exists as one of three types of problems: 1) asthma created by workplace exposures in a previously healthy individual (this usually develops insidiously over time [measured in weeks to years]; an example is isocyanate-induced asthma), 2) asthma aggravated by occupational exposures (i.e., a prior asthmatic encounters factors in the workplace that either precipitates an asthmatic reaction or makes the asthma worse), or 3) asthma as a result of a sudden, brief toxic exposure (reactive airways dysfunction syndrome [RADS]).[15] RADS is a sequela of a toxic exposure and that toxic exposure can cause not only lower airway problems (asthma) but also upper airways disease (chronic rhinosinusitis) and systemic responses with disease states in other organ systems.[16,17] In a retrospective review of 609 claims submitted to the Ontario Workers' Compensation Board for occupational asthma between the years 1984 and 1988, 39% were found to be workplace induced and 39% were for workplace aggravation of pre-existing asthma.[58]

As noted in Chapter 25, occupational asthma has become the most frequent type of workplace pulmonary disease.[8] In the 18- to 44-year-old group, asthma is second only to back disease as a cause of work disability.[5] The diagnosis of asthma carries a serious risk to the patient as well as to the employer. It is not infrequent that job restrictions or modifications are necessary. In a survey of California pulmonary and allergy specialists, 7% of the survey group had to leave work completely with another 10% having a partial work disability. (Complete work disability was defined as total work cessation due to asthma and partial work disability was defined as a change in job, duties, or a reduction in work hours because of the asthma.) Overall, the group had asthma of only a moderate intensity. As would be expected, the more severe the asthma, the greater the risk of disability. Higher educational status was associated with less complete disability but no difference was found in partial work disability rates.[5]

In asthmatics, workplace exposures can worsen symptoms. The estimated frequency lies between 5 and 16%.[36,57] This number is lower than might be expected for a variety of reasons, including the "healthy-worker effect" (people self-select themselves out of jobs that make them sick) and because not all jobs have asthmogenic stimuli present in the work environment. In a study of 56 patients with asthma (42 available for follow-up at 2 years), Blanc et al found that 19% of these patients had to change their duties, 17% reported a reduction in pay, 20% had a change in job or work status, and 36% had at least one of these changes in their work status. As expected, the greater the severity of the asthma, the greater the impact on the work status.[6]

In summary, asthma is a frequent cause of pulmonary disability (the most frequent pulmonary disease associated with disability and second only to low back problems among all medical conditions) that can impact upon a person's ability to participate in specific job/work environments, with significant financial impact on the worker.

COPD

As discussed in Chapter 25, COPD encompasses varying degrees of emphysema and chronic bronchitis. Chapter 25 introduced the concept of a continuum of COPD patients with "pink puffers" (pure emphysematics) on one end of the spectrum and "blue bloaters" (chronic bronchitics) on the other end. Patients with chronic bronchitis also display a continuum with one end being those individuals with a larger degree of response to bronchodilators and those on the other end having more fixed obstruction.

In the occupational setting, there is a condition called "occupational bronchitis." It is defined as a wholly reversible airflow obstruction, of a temporary nature, caused by workplace irritants. It is a manifestation of the diseased or nondiseased airway's reaction to nonspecific stimuli. It is completely reversible upon cessation of exposure and its presence and severity depend on the amount of stimuli present in the work environment. The history and the absence of a positive asthma testing make this diagnosis.

Workers with occupational bronchitis will have signs and symptoms of airway inflammation while in the work environment. Their symptoms include cough, mucus expectoration, and dyspnea. Wheezing can be heard and flow rates are depressed while in the working environment. The rheostat model is useful in understanding this problem. These are nonasthmatic patients who have a temporary "asthmatic" reaction due to the intensity of the stimulus. Figure 59–4 most closely shows this relationship. The worker at Point C does not, by definition, have asthma, but he or she is more hyperresponsive then the average person. He or she can be pushed into the asthmatic symptom range by progressively greater and greater degrees of stimuli yet remain free of symptoms when not exposed to these stimuli or to lesser degrees as might be found in the home environment. Stimulus reduction (engineering changes, job transfers, or personal protective devices) are the preferred approach for this type of worker as opposed to medication usage.

In the patient with pure emphysema, the cardiopulmonary exercise stress test (CPEST) best assesses disability and impairment (see Chapters 22, 24, and 25). The closer the COPD patient is to the emphysematous end of the spectrum (leftward; see Fig. 25–1), the greater will be the reliance on this test. These patients can, of course, have a dual problem creating workplace disability if airflow obstruction is also present (moving to the right in Fig. 25–1). Their ventilation/perfusion (V/Q) mismatch may be profound enough to limit their exercise capacity. The presence of airflow obstruction may magnify the V/Q mismatch by further limiting ventilation. Medication trials (measuring pre- and post-bronchodilator FVC, FEV_1, or other air flow parameters) may be very helpful in determining the place of treatment of the airway obstructive problems. It is only after the airflow obstruction has been eliminated (as much as possible) that the CPEST should be performed. These patients may also benefit from the same type of work restrictions as in the asthmatic patient although the use of personal protective devices becomes more problematic in the severer forms of these diseases.[25]

HYPERSENSITIVITY PNEUMONITIS (EXTRINSIC ALLERGIC ALVEOLITIS)

Interstitial lung diseases are caused by over 150 factors. Many of these factors are agents that cause hypersensitivity pneumonitis (HP). HP is an immunologically driven disease (IgG, IgM, or IgA but, importantly, not IgE) that creates a systemic reaction to an inhaled agent. The pulmonary responses include an interstitial pneumonitis causing dyspnea and occasionally hypoxemia with fine basilar rales heard on examination. The chest x-ray may show interstitial infiltrates. A harsh cough is usually present although wheezing is rare. Systemic features include chills, fever (as high as 104 to 106 degrees), malaise, headache, and myalgias.

The exact criteria required to make a diagnosis of HP are not entirely agreed upon. Various methods have been proposed.[22,26] Most of the offending agents are found in the workplace but some are found in the home environment. There are at least 50 known causes of HP[22,26] with many being fungal species. Animal proteins can also cause HP. Nonorganic causes include cobalt, beryllium, gold salts, di-isocyanates, and plastic dust.[22,26] Many of these causes are associated with a variety of exotic names.

The diagnosis of HP, as noted previously, consists of the presence of a variety of clinical, serologic, pathologic, and radiologic factors. In many, but by no means all cases, a serologic test will be positive. Again, this is an immunologic disease relying on T-cell hyper-reactivity with antibodies of the IgG, A, or M type.[12] This hyper-reactivity can be identified with a bronchoalveolar lavage,[12,22,23,26] by the presence of granuloma formation in a biopsy specimen,[12,22,23,26] and by the presence of antibodies against the offending agent.[12,22,23,26] The interstitial changes in established (i.e., nonreversible) HP include combinations of bronchiolitis and alveolitis with granuloma formation.[12,22,23,26] Granulomatous changes in intrathoracic lymph nodes can also be found,[26] although hilar lymphadenopathy is unusual in most forms of HP.[26] Granulomas can also be found in the spleen in patients with active disease.[26]

The presence of precipitating antibodies is helpful in arriving at a diagnosis.[12] However, by itself, this is not a test that can either rule in or out a diagnosis or even provide a risk assessment.[12] Reference 26 reviews a number of studies of HP. In farmer's lung, approximately 90% of patients had precipitating antibodies to thermophilic actinomycetes in one referenced study, with approximately 50% of patients with chronic disease and 100% of patients with acute disease being positive. Some patients with farmer's lung will have precipitating antibodies to fungal species other than thermophylic actinomycetes (the traditional agent that causes farmer's lung). In biopsy specimens, positive immune fluorescent studies are demonstrated in bronchial walls and alveolar septae, again more commonly in acute versus chronic cases.[26]

The difficulty, as noted, is not in understanding the immunopathogenesis but in understanding why all individuals do not develop an immunologic reaction/disease. Fink et al, when describing pigeon breeder's disease, stated: "(I)n a population similarly exposed to potential sensitizing antigens, only 5% to 15% develop illness. Yet approximately 50% of exposed asymptomatic individuals in similar environments have detectable humoral or cellular immune responses to the antigen without clinical evidence of disease" (in reference 22, p 207; similar statements are also found in reference 23). Thus the presence of serum precipitins proves that the individual was exposed and had an immune reaction, but does not prove the presence of a disease.[12]

Other than the tests mentioned, HP could be diagnosed by a bronchoprovocative maneuver similar to that done for occupational asthma. A positive response consists of the development of fever, dyspnea, and leukocytosis 4 to 6 hours after the inhalation of the suspected agent; transient interstitial infiltrates on the chest x-ray and hypoxemia can also be seen. As with specific bronchoprovocative testing in occupational asthma, this can be a dangerous maneuver and should be restricted to research laboratories.[12,23] The sensitivity and specificity of this type of testing is about 80%.[26] Skin testing is of little benefit in the diagnosis of HP.[23]

The serial chest x-ray is a useful test in assessing workers with intermittent symptoms (acute phase and possibly some cases of subacute HP). However, not all patients with acute or subacute HP will have a positive radiograph, with an estimated positivity rate of 80 and 90%, respectively.[26]

HP is separated into three forms: acute, subacute, and chronic. The acute response is characterized by the above symptoms that occur within 4 to 8 hours of exposure. These symptoms usually resolve spontaneously over several hours (rarely days). The chronic form may have an insidious onset and can totally bypass the acute phase. The subacute form is characterized by repeated exposures and repeated responses although the amount of response is markedly less than in the acute form. HP is characterized by progressive pathology dependent on repeated exposures. The ultimate expression is granulomatous ILD (see references 5, 6, 36, 57, and 58 for a more complete discussion of HP; see also Chapters 22 and 25). Airflow obstruction may or may not be present.[6]

The treatment of HP consists of 1) avoidance of exposure, 2) corticosteroids to diminish the inflammatory response in acute and subacute cases, 3) bronchodilators (if needed and if shown to be effective), and 4) oxygen in more severe cases of chronic HP. The chronic from of HP is a disease characterized by high morbidity with an overall mortality rate of 9 to 17% although the overall mortality from all forms of HP is considerably lower.[22,26] The most effective form of treatment, however, is avoidance of further exposure, especially earlier in the disease. Curtis and Schuyler state that if "exposure persists, some patients (proportion unclear, but probably 10%–30%) will progress to diffuse fibrosis with resultant cor pulmonale and premature death."[12(p404)]

Thus, HP can be an impairing disease (permanent pulmonary pathophysiology) but is always a disabling disease. (There are reports, however, of individuals with HP who continued their exposures with no further pathophysiologic declines. Obviously this confuses the comments regarding disability and avoidance of exposure. However it is still the recommended approach that all further exposures be eliminated as much as possible [engineering changes, personal protective devices] or eliminated [job transfer].[11,12,51] Additionally, at this time, it is unknown how to predict the response that an individual may have; i.e., which person with acute disease will have only that—an isolated episode of acute HP—and which person will go on to develop more permanent manifestations of this disease.) The use of corticosteroids is much more effective with acute disease than with chronic disease.[22,23] In more chronic cases, the use of corticosteroids may merely delay but not change the eventual outcome.[30] Additionally, there is a concern that corticosteroids may favor the occurrence of recurrent attacks of farmer's lung.[30]

The sequelae of HP depend on the stage of presentation and the recurrence of exposures. Symptomatic chronic bronchitis (not attributable to smoking) is seen in approximately 25% of patients with HP.[12] Most of the clinical improvement occurs within the first month, with or without treatment, if the person is removed from the offending agent/environment.[26]

Organic Dust Toxic Syndrome (ODTS)

ODTS is a syndrome that often is mistaken for HP. It occurs in the same occupational settings and has many of the same presenting features. Yet it is a disease that is self-limited without the progression to a chronic form as seen in HP. The parallel between this and industrial bronchitis/asthma (see previous) is striking.

The clinical features include dry cough, fever, malaise, dyspnea, myalgias, chest tightness, and headache that begin 4 to 12 hours after exposure (reference 63 is excellent and highly recommended for further reading on this topic). It usually lasts less than 24 hours but can linger for up to 5 days. Rales, interstitial infiltrates, and hypoxemia can all be seen although the incidence and severity is much less than with HP.[48,53,63] Fungal elements and alveolitis can be seen on biopsy specimens[63] but many believe that this is a reaction to preformed endotoxins found in grain dust as opposed to a systemic response to the inhaled fungal organisms.[63]

This disease is much more frequent than HP. The estimated frequency[63] is 10 to 190/10,000 versus 2 to 30/10,000 for HP. Others have found much higher incidences (36/100).[62] Treatment is avoidance of the precipitating dust or the use of airway protective devices.[4] It is not a progressive disorder and there is no chronic form of the disease. Again, its relationship to HP can be thought of in the same way that "industrial bronchitis" relates to asthma.

INTERSTITIAL LUNG DISEASE

As noted, of the more than 150 causes of ILD, the etiologies with the greatest number of causative factors are those caused by either HP or drug-induced interstitial disease.[12,14,19] Twenty to forty-five percent of all cases of ILD are due to idiopathic pulmonary fibrosis.[27,52] There exist others, however, that are created by a variety of occupational exposures.

A pneumoconiosis is an ILD created by inhalation of an organic or inorganic dust. In the patient with a pneumoconiosis, an inflammatory reaction ensues after exposure and inhalation of a dust resulting in ILD. Examples of pneumoconioses include those caused by the inhalation of inorganic materials such as silica, asbestos, talc, mica, lead, aluminum, and titanium. Other dust-induced interstitial lung diseases are caused by the inhalation of organic materials such as coal dust or dusts known to cause HP (especially the chronic phase) such as cotton dust, tobacco dust, and grain dust (as discussed perviously). Other occupational causes of ILD include inhalations of pesticides, fly ash, and oil mists.[34]

ILD is both an impairing and disabling disease. ILDs present with a V/Q mismatch with variable degrees of airflow obstruction. The primary pathophysiologic consequence in this group of diseases is with gas transfer. This can be caused by the V/Q mismatch or by the thickened alveolar-capillary membrane that limits gas exchange, especially during exercise. Thus the best test to assess the degree of impairment from ILD is the CPEST (as noted in Chapter 25).

When assessing disability due to ILD, two issues must be addressed: 1) Is this an occupationally/environmentally acquired disease (if so, are occupational/environmental restrictions required)? 2) What are the exercise demands of the job? The first issue is assessed by the history, a perusal of the job description, and occasionally by testing such as a serology or biopsy. Restrictions are then recommended. The second issue is determined by an analysis of a person's exercise capacity with the CPEST and estimating the demands of the job (see Chapters 22 and 24).

OBSTRUCTIVE SLEEP APNEA

As discussed in Chapters 22 and 25, obstructive sleep apnea (OSA) is a syndrome characterized by disrupted sleep with apneas and hypopneas and daytime somnolence. It is present in an estimated 2 to 4% of the U.S. adult population.[46] The respiratory disturbance index (RDI) or apnea/hypopnea index (AHI) alone, although associated with increased morbidity, is insufficient in making this diagnosis.

Impairment due to OSA is characterized by cardiovascular complications (hypertension, pulmonary hypertension, cardiac arrhythmias, congestive heart failure, acute myocardial ischemia, and stroke), neurocognitive abnormalities, and excessive somnolence. Successful treatment of OSA is associated with a diminished risk in many if not all of these complications (see Chapter 25).

Disability due to OSA is primarily due to the cognitive problems. The exact role of OSA in the cardiovascular complications, independent of simultaneous cardiovascular disease, is unclear but it probably plays only a small role in the disability due to this condition. Affective disorders and cognitive functions, best determined by a psychiatric and/or neurologic evaluation, may be amenable to treatment.[1,46] They may limit the ability to travel to and from work (uncontrolled somnolence creating traffic accidents), limit the ability to perform work (intellectual/creative functions), create a disruptive work environment (affective changes), and pose a danger to the worker (especially in jobs requiring a high degree of intellectual performance and/or attention) or to coworkers (for the same reasons). Therefore, in some circumstances, OSA may be a totally disabling disease (e.g., in an aircraft pilot with uncontrolled daytime somnolence).

In assessing disability due to OSA, tests of neurocognitive function dominate. They may be performed in the untreated state, in the treated state, or in a before/after fashion. Disability will then be assessed by the test results and knowledge of the job specifications. Chapter 69 covers psychiatric disability in more depth.

It should be noted, however, that not all patients with OSA can be treated. There are a variety of treatment modalities (see Chapter 25), each with its own success rate. Of equal concern is that many patients, regardless of their level of cooperation, are intolerant to many of the treatments. Thus each individual with OSA needs to be assessed after treatment, specifying the degree of success, frequency of use, and impact on his or her health status. Consensus statements on the indications for treatment of OSA have been published.[1,35]

References

1. American Thoracic Society: Indications and standards for use of nasal continuous positive airway pressure (CPAP) in sleep apnea syndrome. Am J Respir Crit Care Med 150:1738–1745, 1994.
2. Barnes PJ: A new approach to the treatment of asthma. N Engl J Med 321:1517–1527, 1989.
3. Bel EH, Timmers MC, Zwinderman AH: The effect of inhaled corticosteroids on the maximal degree of airway narrowing to methacholine in asthmatic subjects. Am Rev Respir Dis 143:109–113, 1991.
4. Blanc PD, Cisternas M, Smith S, et al: Asthma, employment status, and disability among adults treated by pulmonary and allergy specialists. Chest 109:688–696, 1996.
5. Blanc PD, Jones M, Besson C, et al: Work disability among adults with asthma. Chest 104:1371–1377, 1993.
6. Blanc PD: Husker days and fever nights. Counting cases of organic dust toxic syndrome. Chest 116:1157–1158, 1999.
7. Bramen SS, Corrao WM: Bronchoprovocation testing. In Mahler DA (ed): Clinics in Chest Medicine, vol 10. Philadelphia, WB Saunders, 1989, pp 165–176.
8. Chan-Yeung M: Assessment of asthma in the workplace. Chest 108:1084–1117, 1995.
9. Cockroft DW, Berscheid BA, Murdock KY: Unimodal distribution of bronchial responsiveness to inhaled histamine in a random human population. Chest 83:751–754, 1983.
10. Committee on Diagnostic Standards for Non-Tuberculous Diseases: American Thoracic Society's definitions and classifications of thoracic bronchitis, asthma, and pulmonary emphysema. Am Rev Respir Dis 85:762–768, 1962.
11. Cornier Y, Belanger J: Long term of physiologic outcome after acute farmer's lung. Chest 87:796–800, 1985.
12. Curtis JL, Schuyler M: Immunologically mediated lung disease. In Baum GL, Crapo JD, Celli BR, Karlinsky JB (eds): Textbook of Pulmonary Diseases, 6th ed. Philadelphia, Lippincott–Raven, 1998, pp 367–406.
13. Dales RE, Spitzer WO, Tousignant P, et al: Clinical interpretation of airway response to a bronchodilator. Epidemiologic considerations. Am Rev Respir Dis 138:317–320, 1988.
14. Demeter SD, Cordasco EM, Guidotti T: Permanent respiratory impairment and upper airway symptoms despite clinical improvement in patients with reactive airways dysfunction syndrome. Sci Tot Env 270:49–55, 2001.
15. Demeter SL, Ahmad M, Tomashefski JF: Drug-induced pulmonary disease. Part 1. Patterns of response. Cleve Clin Q 46:89–99, 1979.
16. Demeter SL, Cordasco EM: Occupational asthma. In Zenz C, Dickerson DB, Horvath EP (eds): Occupational Medicine, 3rd ed. St. Louis, Mosby, 1994, pp 213–228.
17. Demeter SL, Cordasco EM: Reactive airways dysfunction syndrome: a subset of occupation asthma. J Disability 1:23–29, 1990.
18. do Pico GA: Hazardous exposure and lung disease among farm workers. Clin Chest Med 13:311–328, 1992.
19. Dweik RA, Ahmad M, Demeter SL: Drug-induced pulmonary disease. In Baum GL, Crapo JD, Celli BR, Karlinsky JB (eds): Textbook of Pulmonary Diseases, 6th ed. Philadelphia, Lippincott–Raven, 1998, pp 477–490.
20. Enarson DA, Vedal S, Schulzer M, et al: Asthma, asthmalike symptoms, chronic bronchitis, and the degree of bronchial hyperresponsiveness in epidemiologic surveys. Am Rev Respir Dis 136:613–617, 1987.
21. Filuk RB, Serrette C, Anthonisen NR: Comparison of responses to methacholine and cold air in patients suspected of having asthma. Chest 95:948–952, 1989.
22. Fink JN, Lindesmith LA, Horvath EP: Hypersensitivity pneumonitis. In Zenz C, Dickerson OB, Horvath EP (eds): Occupational Medicine, 3rd ed. Mosby, St. Louis, 1994, pp 205–212.
23. Fink JN, Zacharisen MC: Hypersensitivity pneumonitis. In Middleton E, Reed CE, Ellis EF, et al (eds): Allergy: Principles & Practice, 2nd ed. St. Louis, Mosby, 1998, pp 994–1004.
24. Heaton RW, Henderson AF, Costello JF: Cold air as a bronchial provocation technique. Reproducibility and comparison with histamine and methacholine inhalation. Chest 86:810–814, 1984.
25. Hodous TK: Screening prospective workers for the ability to use respirators. J Occup Med 28:1074–1080, 1986.
26. Inhalation of organic dust. In Fraser RS, Muller NL, Colman N, et al (eds): Diagnosis of Diseases of the Chest, 4th ed. Philadelphia, WB Saunders, 1999, pp 2361–2385.
27. Interstitial pneumonitis and fibrosis. In Fraser RS, Muller NL, Colman N, et al (eds): Diagnosis of Diseases of the Chest, 4th ed. Philadelphia, WB Saunders, 1999, pp 1584–1626.
28. Jackson LK: Functional aspects of asthma. In Bailey WC (ed): Clinics in Chest Medicine, vol 5. Philadelphia, WB Saunders, 1984, pp 573–587.
29. Jans L, Stoddard S: Chartbook on Women and Disability in the United States. An InfoUse Report. Washington, DC, U.S. Department of Education, National Institute of Disability and Rehabilitation Research, 1999.

30. Kokkarinen JI, Tukiainen HO, Terho EO: Effect of corticosteroids treatment in the recovery of pulmonary function in farmer's lung. Am Rev Respir Dis 145:3–5, 1992.
31. Landis HRM: Bronchial asthma. In Norris GW, Landis HRM (eds): Diseases of the Chest and Principles of Physical Diagnosis. Philadelphia, WB Saunders, 1917.
32. LaPlante M, Carlson D: Disability in the United States: Prevalence and Causes, 1992. Disability Statistics Report (7). Washington, DC, U.S. Department of Education, National Institute of Disability and Rehabilitation Research, 1996.
33. Lemire TS, Hopp RJ, Bewtra AK, et al. Comparison of ultrasonically nebulized distilled water and cold air hyperventilation challenges in asthmatic patients. Chest 95:958–961, 1989.
34. Levy SA: Pulmonary reactions to other occupational dusts and fumes. In Zenz C, Dickerson OB, Horvath EP (eds): Occupational Medicine, 3rd ed. St. Louis, Mosby, 1994, pp 194–204.
35. Loube DI, Gay PC, Strohl KP: Indications for positive airway pressure treatment of adult obstructive sleep apnea patients. A consensus statement. Chest 115:863–866, 1999.
36. Malo JL, Pineau L, Cartier A, et al: Reference values of the provocative concentrations of methacholine that cause 6% and 20% changes in forced expiratory volume in one second in a normal population. Am Rev Respir Dis 128:8–11, 1983.
37. Malo JL: How much adult asthma can be attributed to occupational factors (revisited)? Chest 118:1232–1234, 2000.
38. McLellan RK, Schusler KM: Guide to the Medical Evaluation for Respirator Use. Beverly Farms, Mass, OEM Press, 2000.
39. Moscato G, Gudnic-Cvar J, Maestrelli P: Statement on self monitoring of peak expiratory flows in the investigation of occupational asthma. Eur Respir J 8:1605–1610, 1995.
40. O'Connor G, Sparrow D, Taylor D, et al: Analysis of dose-response curves to methacholine. Am Rev Respir Dis 136:1412–1417, 1987.
41. O'Connor GT, Sparrow D, Weiss ST: Normal range of methacholine responsiveness in relation to prechallenge pulmonary function. The normative aging study. Chest 105:661–666, 1994.
42. Osler W, McCrea T: Hay fever and bronchial asthma. In The Principles and Practice of Medicine. New York, Appleton, 1920.
43. Palmeiro EM, Hopp RJ, Biven RE, et al: Probability of asthma based on methacholine challenge. Chest 101:630–633, 1992.
44. Pattemore PK, Asher MI, Harrison AC, et al: The interrelationship among bronchial hyperresponsiveness, the diagnosis of asthma, and asthma symptoms. Am Rev Respir Dis 142:549–554, 1990.
45. Perpina M, Pellicer C, de Diego A, et al: Diagnostic value of the bronchial provocation test with methacholine in asthma. A Bayesian analysis approach. Chest 104:149–154, 1993.
46. Piccirillo JF, Duntley S, Schotland H: Obstructive sleep apnea. JAMA 284:1492– 1494, 2000.
47. Popa V, Singleton J: Provocation dose and discriminant analysis in histamine bronchoprovocation. Chest 94:466–475, 1988.
48. Von Essen S, Fryzek J, Nowakowski B, Wampler M: Respiratory symptoms and farming practices in farmers associated with an acute febrile illness after organic dust exposure. Chest 116:1452–1458, 1999.
49. Pratter MR, Irwin RS: The clinical value of pharmacologic bronchoprovocation challenge. Chest 85:260–265, 1984.
50. Rijcken B, Schouten JP, Weiss ST, et al: The distribution of bronchial responsiveness to histamine in symptomatic and in asymptomatic subjects. Am Rev Respir Dis 140:615–623, 1989.
51. Rose C, King TE: Controversies in hypersensitivity pneumonitis (editorial). Am Rev Respir Dis 145:1–2, 1992.
52. Saag KG, Kline JN, Hunninghake GW: Interstitial lung disease. In Baum GL, Crapo JD, Celli BR, Karlinsky JB (eds): Textbook of Pulmonary Diseases, 6th ed. Philadelphia, Lippincott–Raven, 1998, pp 341–365.
53. Selman-Lama M, Perez-Padilla R: Airflow obstruction and airway lesions in hypersensitivity pneumonitis. Clin Chest Med 14:699–714, 1993.
54. Sherrill DL, Martinez FD, Sears MR, et al: An alternative method for comparing and describing methacholine response curves. Am Rev Respir Dis 148:116–122, 1993.
55. Social Security Administration: Social Security Bulletin, Annual Statistical Supplement. Washington, DC, Social Security Administration, 2000.
56. Stoddard S, Jans L, Ripple J, et al: Chartbook on Work and Disability in the United States, 1998. An InfoUse Report. Washington, DC, U.S. National Institute of Disability and Rehabilitation Research, 1998.
57. Tarlo SM, Leung K, Broder I, et al: Asthmatic subjects symptomatically worse at work. Prevalence and characterization among a general asthma clinic population. Chest 118:1309–1314, 2000.
58. Tarlo SM, Liss G, Cozey P, et al: A workers' compensation claim population for occupational asthma. Comparison of subgroups. Chest 107:634–641, 1995.
59. The International Clinical Respiratory Group: Assessment of therapeutic benefit in asthmatic patients. Chest 103:914–916, 1993.
60. Toren K, Brisman J, Jarvholm B: Asthma and asthma-like symptoms in adults assessed by questionnaires. Chest 104:600–608, 1993.
61. Townley RG, Hopp RJ: Measurement and interpretation of nonspecific bronchial reactivity. Chest 94:452–453, 1988.
62. Von Essen S, Fryzek J, Nowakowski B, et al: Respiratory symptoms and farming. In Baum GL, Crapo JD, Celli BR, Karlinski JB (eds): Textbook of Pulmonary Diseases, 6th ed. Philadelphia, Lippincott–Raven, 1998, pp 477–490.
63. Von Essen S, Robbins RA, Thompson AB, et al: Organic dust toxic syndrome: An acute febrile reaction to organic dust exposure distinct from hypersensitivity pneumonitis. Clin Toxicology 28:389–420, 1990.
64. Zamel N: Threshold of airway response to inhaled methacholine in healthy men and women. J Appl Physiol 56:129–131, 1984.

CHAPTER

Cardiac Disability

HARVEY L. ALPERN, MD

In cardiac disability, the physician measures cardiac impairment. Disability is addressed by taking into account the needs of the workplace. This is usually done by vocational experts or administrative individuals. The physician may estimate what an individual can do at work by the same testing used for impairment ratings. Cardiac testing can be thought of as a functional capacity evaluation for cardiac disability rating.

The physician must decide if any present impairment is severe. It is also customary for the physician to determine how long the impairment has been present based on the history and findings. The physician also will determine what functional limitations, both exertional and nonexertional, would be present and have an effect on the individual's ability to work as a result of the impairments that have been identified.

The physician must also decide if the side effects of medications cause an effect on the impairments and whether a past or present history of use of alcohol or other drugs had a material effect on the impairment. This is important in some Social Security decisions.

The physician must also identify any conditions that might improve in the foreseeable future even though they are sufficient to meet the concept of maximal medical improvement (MMI) at the time that the person is being evaluated for disability. An example of this would be a situation where an individual refuses therapy and thus is at MMI; but frequently, the physician will be asked what the likelihood of improvement would be if the therapy were given, and when it should be evaluated.

The physical demands of exertional efforts are described in Chapters 22 and 24. In addition to the exertional limitations, the physician is typically asked to indicate whether postural limitations are present because of the impairment, or limitations based on hearing or vision or communication. Environmental limitations are frequently addressed in cardiac and pulmonary conditions such as restrictions from fumes or dust.

CORONARY ARTERY DISEASE

If an exercise test done to evaluate a person with coronary artery disease were stopped due to angina, there would be an endurance restriction. If the test were stopped due to arrhythmia, there may be a restriction from heights and dangerous machinery and also possibly an endurance restriction.

Most insurance companies looking at long-term or short-term disability in cardiac patients utilize the results of an exercise test to see the limits or the impairment of the condition in objective terms. The physician needs to indicate for short-term disability the length of time of the temporary disability and how long it will be before recovery to a higher level occurs. At this point the individual may return to work or may be considered for long-term disability if the improvement is not sufficient. The disability rating would be applied when the individual is at MMI.

In each of these steps the level of exertion required is usually determined by doing an exercise study where results are expressed in peak oxygen uptake ($\dot{V}o_2max$) or in metabolic energy units (METs). This level of exertion is then compared to the work requirements.

Tables of MET requirements for most jobs in the job market are available (see Chapters 22 and 24). One can simply compare the individual's ability to these levels. Unfortunately, these tables of required exertion in METs are to do a specific job and are not always accurate as they usually do not take into account peak effort and effort to get to and from work.

One can estimate what an individual can do in an 8-hour workday by looking at the MET level for a specific job. The person should be able to work an 8-hour work day if the MET level of a job is 40% or less of the examinee's measured peak MET level.

In a similar manner, short-term maximum work can be estimated. Short-term maximum work is less then 15 minutes once a day. In an individual with heart disease who is not currently symptomatic, one would take 80% of the maximal achieved MET level, assuming the end point of the exercise is the target heart rate and not symptoms. This figure of 80% of the maximum MET level would be the amount of work the individual could do in a short period less than 15 minutes once a day. However, should cardiac symptoms be the reason the exercise test was stopped, then one would use a figure of 70% of that MET level to consider how much maximum short-term work the individual can achieve.

Coronary ischemia, congestive heart failure, cardiomyopathy, congenital heart disease, and some valvular heart diseases may all be evaluated for functional status by doing an exercise study, preferably using METs to describe peak achievement.

The reason for using METs is so that one physician can communicate with another no matter what type of exercise study was done. A MET is a resting energy unit that represents 3.5 cc of oxygen consumption per kilogram per minute. Impairment ratings using Vo_2max or peak METs generally consider a range of 2.5 METs to 7 METs as the range of activity where there would be impairments. These ratings can also be used for disability whereby 2.5 METs or less results in total disability and greater then 7 METs suggests that there is little disability. This rating system for disability is satisfactory for most cases as long as there are no cardiac symptoms of ischemia at peak METs. Thus, if there were angina at a certain MET level, then the individual would probably be considered disabled at a lower level.

In coronary artery disease, disability is considered to be present in Social Security systems when the individual is unable to exert to beyond 5 METS and has symptoms of heart disease at that level whether it be angina or heart failure. One would expect that an individual with significant coronary disease would have restrictions from walking and this, again, is based on the exercise testing and MET level. Standing and sitting usually is not a restriction in these cases. There would also be a restriction from extreme temperatures because of the coronary disease. Individuals would typically be restricted from very heavy lifting because this type of activity could increase afterload and increase the blood pressure. If there is evidence of cardiac decompensation from chronic hypertension with heart failure then the walking, lifting, and exertional restrictions would commensurably be more strict and would be based again on functional testing.

HYPERTENSION

In hypertension, an individual who is rated according to AMA Guides as Class II for impairment might be totally disabled. If the individual had elevated blood pressure poorly controlled by medication at the rating level, that individual may be totally disabled. If the individual had an impairment rating of Class II and had markedly elevated blood pressure with stress, a different level of disability may result. In a hypertension disability evaluation, one may want to monitor an individual with a blood pressure monitor and do a simulated work situation to determine if the activities of work, including stress, would result in dangerous elevation of blood pressure. Thus the impairment ratings for hypertension would not be correlated directly with disability and a functional test of blood pressure monitoring would be more valuable.

If one cannot actually test the individual in the work situation then a functional capacity center should be able to simulate the type of work and monitor the blood pressure during that exertion.

In hypertension there would usually be restriction from extreme temperatures and there may also be restrictions from concentrated exposure to noise as this has been associated with hypertension as well (see also Chapter 61). There would also be restrictions from undue emotional stress because of the association of emotional stress with hypertension, especially where the emotional stress is of the type of chronic high demand with low control. An objective technique to determine blood pressure reactivity to emotional stress consists of obtaining an impedance hemodynamic study where, with emotional stress, one can determine how high the blood pressure goes and whether it is due to increased cardiac output or peripheral vascular resistance.

ARRHYTHMIAS

Cardiac arrhythmias that are rated for permanent impairment according the AMA Guides give a fairly clear description of the individual's status.

A Class IV individual would probably be disabled for all work. However, individuals in Class I through III probably would have some work restrictions depending on the specifics of the individual symptoms and findings. Here, Holter monitoring during either actual work or simulated work would be very helpful in determining the type and frequency of arrhythmia during specific types of work. In general, there are usually work restrictions at heights or working with dangerous equipment because of the possibly of lightheadedness or loss of consciousness in these individuals. However, this is not always the case and again needs to be looked at on an individual basis.

SOCIAL SECURITY

The Social Security Administration has specific criteria for listings of disability although the physician is given leeway in that if a specific situation does not match the listings then the physician may indicate that even though the listing does not match, there is an impairment present that would be equivalent in severity or at least equal to one of the listings. A physician must decide if the individual has a medically determinable impairment even though it is not listed or the combination of impairments, not one of which meets a listing, which will meet the medical equivalents determination. Even though an individual may not meet a listing he or she may not have the residual functional capacity to engage in sustained gainful activity (see Chapter 6 and Appendix B).

Social Security looks at chronic heart failure of whatever cardiac origin as manifested by evidence of pulmonary or systemic congestion and symptoms of limited cardiac output such as weakness, fatigue, dyspnea, or decreased physical activity.

In chronic heart failure, a listing is said to be met if there is cardiac enlargement demonstrated on x-ray or echocardiography, a clinical picture consistent with heart failure, findings of an ejection fraction of 30% or less, or evidence clinically of heart failure as manifested by abnormal wall motion or third heart sound. If an exercise test is done, a workload of 5 METs or less would be consistent with the listing for heart failure. Other criteria are exercise testing limited by runs of ventricular tachycardia or drops of 10 mm or more of the blood pressure with exercise. Any clinical findings of decreased perfusion of the head or extremities would also be significant.

In ischemic heart disease the criteria for disability are findings of exercise endurance limited to 5 METs or less with a positive exercise test and/or failure of systolic blood pressure to increase (or a decrease), or an abnormal perfusion study. Ejection fractions of 30% or less or an abnormal wall function are also utilized. Coronary angiography is generally not authorized by Social Security, but if done, an individual with 50% or more narrowing of the non-bypassed left main vessel, 70% or more narrowing of another non-bypassed coronary artery, 50% or more narrowing in a long segment of greater than 1 cm of a non-bypassed artery, 50% or more narrowing of two non-bypassed vessels, or total occlusion of a graft would meet a listing.

In those individuals who do not meet a listing of heart disease in Social Security, a functional capacity evaluation is helpful to determine what the functional capacities are for an individual. They may also be estimated based on the activities of daily living and the type of disease. Functional capacity examinations generally determine the strength for lifting tasks based not just on the physical lifting but also on exercise endurance using $\dot{V}O_2$max and MET and heart rate. Generally, functional capacity evaluations are done with walking or step tests rather then formal treadmill tests because of the cost and logistical factors of testing. Testing is also done to take into consideration whether the individual can lift above the shoulder or only to the waist level or below the knuckles and this is done by observation and testing with weights. The $\dot{V}o_2$max and MET levels are used as part of the National Institute of Occupational Safety and Health recommendation for endurance during an 8-hour workday as outlined previously. The full functional capacity evaluation addresses lifting and carrying in all positions and strength.

SUMMARY

Cardiac disability is determined by taking information from impairment testing and functional capacity testing and applying it to the specifics of work. It is not always able to be done only by a physician and frequently requires a functional capacity evaluation by the appropriate clinics and the input of a vocational rehabilitation counselor.

Bibliography

Alpern HL: Cardiac disability. In Brodwin MG, Tellez FA, Brodwin SK: Medical, Psychosocial and Vocational Aspects of Disability, 2nd ed. Athens, Ga, Elliott & Fitzpatrick, 2002.

Cocchiarella L, Andersson GBJ (eds): Guides to the Evaluation of Permanent Impairment, 5th ed. Chicago, American Medical Association, 2001.

Industrial Medical Council: Guideline for Evaluation of Cardiac Disability. San Francisco, State of California, California Code of Regulations, 1998.

Social Security Administration: Disability Evaluation Under the Social Security Department. Baltimore, Social Security Administration, U.S. Government Printing Office, 1998.

CHAPTER

61

Peripheral Vascular Disability

STEPHEN L. DEMETER, MD, MPH ■ DENNIS J. WRIGHT, MD

Chapter 1 defines the concepts of impairment and disability. Impairment of the peripheral vascular system reflects deviations from normal. Disease states, congenital malformations, and anatomic abnormalities can all be considered impairments. The impact of these conditions on activities of daily living was considered in Chapter 27 (Peripheral Vascular Impairment). The subject of this chapter is the effect of these conditions on an individual's ability to participate in the workplace.

The diagnosis, treatment, natural history, and impairment evaluation of the conditions covered in this chapter were covered in Chapter 27 and are not repeated here. Certain etiologic considerations that were not covered in that chapter are discussed, especially when they refer to workplace exposures or conditions. Cerebrovascular diseases are covered in separate chapters (34 and 67) and are not covered in this chapter.

Finally, the format of Chapter 27 is used. Arterial diseases are discussed first followed by venous diseases. Lymphatic diseases are considered with venous diseases as their presentations and job restrictions are essentially identical. Diseases of the upper extremity follow diseases of the lower extremities.

Central diseases (disease of the aorta and the arteries arising from the abdominal aorta) are not discussed. By and large, these diseases will have either no impact on a person's ability to participate in the workplace or, depending on the extent and location of the pathology, they may have such a devastating impact on a person's life, that issues of whether a person can perform work are meaningless. For example, a person who has had a mesenteric thrombosis and has a short gut may be unable to eat, function, or perform any activities of daily living due to severe cachexia. Lesser forms may present with lesser physiologic consequences and can be assessed by the appropriate chapter (the gastrointestinal chapter for splanchnic vascular disease, the genitourinary chapter for renovascular disease, etc.). Finally, intrinsic diseases of the aorta rarely present with any reasons for work restrictions unless they affect the proximal ascending aorta. In those situations, there may be significant aortic regurgitation but this condition may be assessed under the principles discussed in Chapter 60 (Cardiac Disability). The only exceptions to this rule would be Ehlers-Danlos syndrome and Marfan syndrome, diseases characterized by defects in connective tissue that cause aortic and arterial disease and other connective tissue abnormalities wherein the musculoskeletal abnormalities may preclude certain types of work activities. Finally, the concept of aortoiliac disease is considered with the lower extremities.

ARTERIAL DISEASES

General Concepts

The common symptoms of arterial disease are ischemic pain (claudication) and fatigue in a limb. The loss of vascular supply may lead to ulceration, neuropathies, and amputations. All of these may cause a person to be disabled, depending on the desired activity. Each case must be decided based on knowledge of the job requirements. It is not enough to know that a person is engaged in moderate manual labor only. The specific job requirements must be thoroughly detailed so that a physician may make a recommendation during a fitness-for-duty assessment. If a person has extensive lower extremity disease, and his or her job requires him or her to be seated but perform multiple lifts of objects weighing 3 to 8 pounds from an assembly line to a bench and back to an assembly line, then that person may be capable of performing that job. The person with upper extremity disease, however, will not, owing to muscle fatigue caused by the inadequate arterial supply under the conditions of exertion as specified in this particular job description.

The job description must be known for a person with an amputation. It must also be determined how adequate the amputee's abilities are with a prosthesis. It is not enough to know, for example, that a person has a lower or upper limb prosthesis. It must be known by the assessing physician how well the amputee is able to use and function with the prosthesis, whether it can be worn comfortably, how long it can be worn, what the level of exertion with the prosthesis is (this will differ significantly with an upper versus a lower limb prosthesis), whether there are sores on the stump, etc. The assistance of a physical or occupational therapist may be invaluable in making these determinations.

Individuals with neuropathies caused by vascular disease may have job limitations. The individual with disease in the upper extremity may have difficulty with fine manipulations. The individual with lower extremity disease may have limitations in walking owing to the possibility of damage to the feet caused by poor awareness of subtle injuries or pain caused by excessive pressure on the feet.

Patients with poor circulation are more prone to superficial infections caused by poor wound healing. Certain occupations may place a person at risk owing to frequent, minor skin irritation or wounds. Again, a thorough job description is essential.

Individuals with peripheral arterial disease will have a diminished ability to perform motor activities. Certainly pain will be a limiting factor. The development and causation of pain (claudication) is a function of the severity of the vascular insufficiency and this has been correlated with the ankle brachial index (ABI). Additionally, there is a loss of muscle fibers in the affected muscle groups. Both type 1 and type 2 muscle fibers are lost, although the specific proportions are dependent on the muscle studied.[4]

Lower Extremity Diseases

Claudication is the most frequent disabling condition affecting the lower extremities in the patient with lower extremity vascular disease. This symptom can be variable and is dependent on the level of exertion needed by the job. The degree of exertion necessary to produce symptoms can be assessed by treadmill testing as described in Chapter 27. This degree can be matched with the job description or can be assessed in a modified functional capacity assessment where the symptom-limiting variable is claudication rather than strength, flexibility, or endurance, as in the more traditional tests.

The normal ABI is considered to be 0.8 or above. At any level below this, symptoms of claudication may be seen. Disabling claudication usually occurs with an ABI = 0.5 or if it takes > 10 minutes to return to baseline levels.

Medical or surgical therapies may modify the job restrictions. Following aortic surgery, most patients can return to previous levels of activities. If the procedure was performed for occlusive disease, postoperative physiologic testing can determine the degree of functional return. These results should also be compared to the preoperative or pretreatment levels to assess the degree of improvement. Full recovery usually takes about 1 month or less following endovascular procedures. More standard operative techniques often require up to 3 months before a patient is ready to return to work. Complications that relate to the cardiac, respiratory, renal, gastrointestinal, and musculoskeletal systems will need to be individually addressed. Most medical therapies for arterial diseases take as long a 3 months to become effective. If these treatments are not sufficient in providing symptomatic relief, more aggressive interventions may be necessary.

A note should be made with regard to the dynamic, progressive nature of vascular disease. There may be steady and gradual worsening or the disease may become suddenly worse. Noninvasive testing with waveforms and segmental pressures can be invaluable when attempting to evaluate a sudden change in symptoms. These tests are readily available and without significant risk. They often help identify when a patient has progressed from a well-compensated disease state to a point that will not allow him or her to perform many of his or her normal daily activities.

In its most advanced state, arterial insufficiency can cause some degree of tissue loss. After revascularization, many patients will have limited areas of amputation at the forefoot level and full rehabilitation may be possible. More advanced cases may require below the knee amputations regardless of whether revascularization has been performed. In these situations, the disability may be similar to that encountered by patients who have had a traumatic amputation. However, owing to the bilateral nature of vascular disease, a patient may have significant disease in the opposite leg that limits his or her ability to rehabilitate completely.

Diabetes mellitus is a well-known cause of vascular disease. It classically produces disease in small arteries and arterioles. The role of small vessel disease in the development of hypertension and renal failure in the kidney, the effects of microvascular disease on cerebral function (especially in the elderly), and its effects on the heart (syndrome X) have been the subject of numerous medical reports over recent years. Another subject, germane to this discussion, is the effect of diabetes on the microvasculature of the lower extremities, especially the feet. The small vessels in the arterial system of patients with diabetes show patchy pathology with not all vessels affected evenly. Basement membrane thickening is the hallmark of diabetic microangiopathy. This appears to be an early lesion and the pathologic abnormalities can precede the diagnosis of diabetes in some patients. Hypertrophy of the endothelial layer impairs oxygen delivery. Thus these individuals are prone to problems created by the vascular insufficiency and inadequate tissue oxygen delivery. One of the consequences is diminished vascular supply to peripheral nerves via the vasa nervorum, creating peripheral neuropathies that are usually sensory although they can also be motor or mixed. These individuals are also prone to injury of the skin, invasive soft tissue infections, osteomyelitis, chronic ulceration, derangements of the skeletal architecture, and gangrene. The infections can be problematic owing to the insufficient blood supply needed for tissue repair. The chronic ischemia and sensory neuropathy place the skin and soft tissues at risk for destruction from even trivial injuries.[8] It is for these reasons that periodic foot examinations and aggressive foot care are so vital in the patient with diabetes. There are implications for the workplace in the patient with diabetes. Good shoes are important. Attention to issues such as prolonged walking and standing is important. Jobs that require foot immersion or ambulation without protection should be questioned for. Attention must be given to avoid situations placing the worker at risk for traumatic injuries to the feet, even trivial ones. These considerations and job modification recommendations are the responsibility of the disability evaluating or the primary attending physician. Off-work issues and job modifications need to be discussed with both the patient/examinee and the employer if the patient/examinee with diabetes develops signs of soft tissue infection or tissue ischemia.

THE UPPER EXTREMITY

Claudication in the upper extremities is not as common as in the lower extremities. It is estimated that only 5% of patients with limb ischemia as evidenced by muscle fatigue, claudication, ischemic rest pain, digital necrosis, or atheroembolization will have their disease in the upper extremities.[1] It is more common for the patient to complain of fatigue as opposed to true pain. Additionally, and importantly, the position of the arms may be very important. This must be addressed historically. Individuals with vascular disease in the subclavian or axillary arteries may be limited when performing muscular activities above their heads with no limitations at levels below the shoulders.

The subclavian steal syndrome is an important entity to discuss, not owing to its frequency, but rather owing to its frequency of mention and its confusion with the thoracic outlet syndrome. It is a very unusual situation wherein there is a reversal of flow in the ipsilateral vertebral artery distal to a proximal subclavian lesion. When the vascular demand of the upper extremity increases during exercise, the upper extremity increases its blood supply by "stealing" it from the vertebral artery. Symptoms include visual disturbances, vertigo, ataxia, syncope, dysphasia, dysarthria, sensory deficits of the face, and motor and sensory problems in the extremity. These patients will frequently have significant disease in other arteries of the upper torso, neck, and head.[7]

The thoracic outlet syndrome (TOS) presents with upper extremity symptoms owing to compression of the neurovascular bundle in the thoracic outlet area. The neurovascular bundle consists of nerves, arteries, and veins. Each of these elements can be compressed separately, usually against a cervical or rudimentary first rib, producing distinct symptom complexes. When using the term thoracic outlet syndrome, it should be designated by the structure that is compromised. Thus there is a neurogenic, arterial, and venous thoracic syndrome. Neurogenic TOS is the most common, accounting for up to 95% of cases. Venous TOS accounts for 2 to 3% of cases, with arterial TOS being the most rare, with 1% of all cases. It is a condition that is seen more commonly in female patients (70%) and in younger patients (20- to 45-year-olds). The symptoms of neurogenic TOS are the same as for any other type of compression neuropathy: pain, paresthesias, and weakness. These patients will often have a history of neck trauma preceding their symptoms. Cold hands, color changes, and swelling may be seen but these symptoms are usually the result of increased sympathetic activity in the lower brachial plexus and are more properly termed neurogenic TOS. These symptoms may also be seen with vascular TOS, but this syndrome usually presents with claudication, ischemic ulcers, and gangrenous fingertips (arterial TOS) or swelling (venous TOS). Physical examination findings include neurologic abnormalities with certain positions of the head or arms. The Adson sign (loss of the radial pulse in certain positions) occurs in 31% of patients with TOS, but also in 13 to 53% of normal individuals.[7] Individuals who engage in overextended shoulder motion activities are more likely to develop vascular TOS and this condition may limit a person's work activities.[9]

Raynaud's syndrome is a clinical condition that is characterized by episodic attacks of vasospasm in the most distal parts of the extremities. It is caused by a closure of the small arteries and arterioles in response to cold or emotional stress. The upper extremities are affected more commonly than the lower.

The classical description is one of intense pallor, followed by cyanosis, and then rubor on rewarming the extremity, although most patients only have the pallor or cyanosis during attacks. Most patients will have symptoms that last only 30 to 60 minutes although some individuals will have attacks that last until rewarming. Between 70% and 90% of patients are female. Random population surveys reveal variable presence with 3% to 30% of individuals having symptoms. Individuals living in cool, damp climates are more frequently affected. On the average, however, approximately 5% of the population will have this condition. It can be seen in certain occupations where the incidence may increase by as much as tenfold. These occupations include those dealing with vibrating tools and extreme changes in temperatures. Tools associated with this syndrome include pneumatic tools, chainsaws, chipping hammers, and others. The term "vibration-induced white finger" has been proposed for this subset of patients.[6(pp1170–1172)] Workers with early or mild cases may have their symptoms disappear on weekends or other times off work. Later, the symptoms may be more permanent. Paresthesias and neurosensory deficits are common but ischemic ulceration of the fingertips is rare. Spontaneous remission is seen only in early and mild cases.[3(p119)] The best treatment for occupational Raynaud's is to discontinue the activity that precipitates the problem. Other forms of treatment for Raynaud's can also be attempted. The cause of the injury is unknown.[9(pp1232–1234)] Other workers who are prone to the development of Raynaud's syndrome are those who are exposed to rapid and intense temperature changes such as individuals in food-processing industries where, again, the incidence has been reported to be 10 times higher than in controls.[6(p1172)] Finally, workers with Raynaud's syndrome should be evaluated for the temperature in which they work. Gloves and other types of clothing may provide sufficient protection; if not, a job change may be required.

Hypothenar hammer syndrome is another vascular occupational disease affecting the hand. At the ulnar base of the palm (the hypothenar eminence), the ulnar artery is fairly superficial. If this area is repeatedly traumatized, there can be ulnar or digital artery spasm, aneurysms, occlusions, or any combination of these entities. Embolization to the distal digital arteries can also occur. This condition is seen in individuals who engage in repetitive use of the palm with pushing, pounding, and twisting; for example, in carpenters and mechanics. Typical symptoms include Raynaud's syndrome symptoms, paresthesias, and stiffness.[9(pp1234–1236)] The most important element of treatment is a change in the occupation to allow for diminished use of the hand in this fashion.

Exposure to vinyl chloride monomer may lead to a condition that resembles scleroderma. It affects the hands of workers and presents with symptoms of Raynaud's syndrome. Additionally, it presents with acro-osteolysis or resorption of the distal tufts of the fingers. Digital artery occlusions and stenoses can be found. Again, cessation of exposure is the first goal of treatment.[2(pp1042–1043),9(p1236)]

VENOUS DISEASE

General Concepts

As noted in Chapter 27, venous diseases of the extremities are common. The lower extremity is affected much more commonly than the upper extremities. Chronic venous diseases and lymphedema cause impairment and disability due to their propensity to cause ulceration. They also create a need for the affected individual to treat the condition with intrusive measures such as frequent clinic visits or elevation of the extremity that can interfere with the patient's ability to be present in the workplace.

Ulceration can, of course, have many etiologies. Venous ulcers, however, can be recurrent and recalcitrant to treatment. Infected ulcers may also give rise to socially unacceptable odors that prevent a person from being present in the workplace. Moneta et al reviewed several studies and noted that of venous ulcer patients, 42% have a diminished ability to participate in leisure activities, 40% experience diminished earning capacities, and 5% lose their job because of this problem. They reference a 1988 study that stated that up to 2 million workdays are lost each year in the United States due to venous ulceration.[5(p1982)]

References

1. Cherry KJ: Arteriosclerotic occlusive disease of brachiocephalic arteries. In Rutherford RB (ed): Vascular Surgery, 5th ed. Philadelphia, WB Saunders, 2000, pp 1140–1162.
2. Cordasco EM, Kerkay J, Demeter SL, et al: Plasticizers, vinyl chloride, polyvinyls, and pyrolysis products: Biochemical and clinical aspects. In Zenz C (ed): Occupational Medicine, 2nd ed. Chicago, Year Book Medical Publishers, 1988, pp 1040–1048.
3. Mathias CGT: Occupational dermatoses. In Zenz C, Dickerson OB, Horvath EP (eds): Occupational Medicine, 3rd ed. St. Louis, Mosby, 1994, pp 93–131.
4. McDermott MM, Greenland P: Clinical significance and functional implications of peripheral arterial disease. In Hirsch AT (ed): Primary Care Series: Peripheral Arterial Disease and

Intermittent Claudication. Belle Mead, NJ, Excerpta Medica, 2001, pp 20–26.
5. Moneta GL, Nehler MR, Porter JM: Pathophysiology of chronic venous insufficiency. In Rutherford RB (ed): Vascular Surgery, 5th ed. Philadelphia, WB Saunders, 2000, pp 1982–1990.
6. Porter JM, Edwards JM: Occlusive and vasospastic diseases involving distal upper extremity arteries—Raynaud's syndrome. In Rutherford RB (ed): Vascular Surgery, 5th ed. Philadelphia, WB Saunders, 2000, pp 1170–1183.
7. Sanders RJ, Cooper MA, Hammond SL, Weinstein ES: Neurogenic thoracic outlet syndrome. In Rutherford RB (ed): Vascular Surgery, 5th ed. Philadelphia, WB Saunders, 2000, pp 1184–1200.
8. Seabrook GR, Towne JB: Management of foot lesions in the diabetic patient. In Rutherford RB (ed): Vascular Surgery, 5th ed. Philadelphia, WB Saunders, 2000, pp 1093–1011.
9. Yao JST: Occupational vascular problems. In Rutherford RB (ed): Vascular Surgery, 5th ed. Philadelphia, WB Saunders, 2000, pp 1232–1240.

CHAPTER

62

Dermatological Disability

JAMES S. TAYLOR, MD

Individuals with impairing and disabling dermatologic disorders require evaluation according to guidelines and criteria discussed in Chapter 28 (Dermatological Impairment). These include a complete medical and dermatologic evaluation—history, physical examination, ancillary diagnostic tests as required (e.g., cultures for microorganisms, skin biopsies, other laboratory tests, and allergy tests, such as epicutaneous patch and intracutaneous prick tests, etc.). An accurate diagnosis is imperative, and dermatologic consultation should be obtained when in doubt. Specialized referral is also indicated for determining whether a cause-and-effect-relation exists between a skin condition and an occupation (causation) in putative workers' compensation cases.

DISABLING SKIN CONDITIONS

Table 62–1 contains a list of skin conditions that may require time away from work; this information is based on personal experience. Studies by Finlay and colleagues[3,4] may be helpful in determining the extent of disability for psoriasis. In psoriasis, a sickness impact profile and psoriasis disability index have been studied and validated. The sickness impact profile allows comparison of the impairment of some of the activities of daily living experienced by patients with other systemic diseases; the disability index gives a rapid overall measure of psoriasis impairment based on responses to 15 questions about daily activities, work or school activities, personal relationships, leisure activities, and treatment. The responses were graded on a seven-point linear analogue scale. The same sickness impact profile of 136 questions has also been used to measure health-related dysfunction in atopic eczema and basal cell carcinoma. A much shorter and simpler 10-question instrument, the Dermatology Life Quality Index, has been validated for use in the general outpatient setting, in patients with severe eczema, in severe acne, in patients with basal cell carcinoma, in Bechét's disease, and in auditing the effectiveness of an inpatient service in improving the quality of life of patients with severe skin disease.[5]

TEMPORARY TOTAL IMPAIRMENT

If a worker has an occupationally related skin condition that significantly precludes working, then temporary total impairment may exist, and an appropriate amount

TABLE 62–1

Selected Dermatologic Conditions That May Require Time Away From Work

1. Localized involvement of the hands and/or feet: contact dermatitis, psoriasis, discoid lupus erythematosus, congenital or acquired bullous disorders, pressure urticaria, other dermatitis and other dermatoses
2. Disseminated dermatoses: contact dermatitis, psoriasis, bullous disorders, erythroderma, other dermatitis and other dermatoses
3. Burns: chemical or thermal
4. Cutaneous infections: viral, bacterial, fungal, and other micro-organisms; primary or secondary
5. Allergy: to a substance in the workplace; e.g., penicillin in a penicillin manufacturing plant; putative severe allergic contact dermatitis, urticaria, angioedema, etc., until allergen is identified.
6. Localized involvement of other body areas from disease or trauma: nails, scalp, arms, legs, trunk, etc.

of time away from work may be warranted under most workers' compensation laws. The treating physician usually makes this determination, and the disability may last a number of weeks and rarely several years. In my experience the most common skin disorders resulting in temporary total disability are severe cases of irritant and allergic contact hand eczema in workers such as machinists and hairdressers.

When Does Temporary Total Impairment End?

It is important for examining and treating physicians to know when temporary total impairment ceases. This occurs with one of the following events: 1) the patient has reached maximum medical improvement, or is "medically stationary"; 2) the condition has become permanent; 3) the patient has a valid job offer within his or her physical capabilities; 4) the patient states that he or she is capable of returning to work; or 5) the patient returns to work. Koral[8] states that temporary total benefits may be discontinued for any of three reasons: 1) "the employee is able or is released to return to work (either the employee's regular job or a light duty position)"; temporary partial disability benefits "may be paid if the job-related injury or disease results in a temporary physical impairment resulting in a decrease of the employee's earning capacity"; or 2) "the employee reaches maximum medical improvement (if the employee cannot return to work with the employer vocational rehabilitation benefits may become payable"; or 3) "the employee resists treatment or otherwise unnecessarily engages in behavior that hinders the employee's recovery." The burden of this decision-making is frequently left to the treating physician, except where employers or managed care oversight organizations are vigilant.

PROBLEMATIC DERMATOLOGIC DISABILITY CLAIMS

Some employers utilize third-party consulting firms to review all claims or "outlying" claims. Typical examples include workers with frequent recurrences of dermatitis, those with chronic hand eczema, or those whose dermatitis persists despite a job change. Permanent partial disability claims are often reviewed, with employers seeking the lowest possible percentage when rating impairment and employees the highest possible percentage. Other problematic cases are those with transient skin complaints and few objective findings, cases of chronic urticaria with a putative occupational connection, and cases of putative multiple chemical sensitivity syndrome, with symptoms involving the skin and multiple organ systems. In my experience most cases of chronic urticaria or recurrent acute urticaria are not occupationally related. The clear exception is those workers with latex urticaria, whose disease may range form contact and generalized urticaria to angioedema and anaphylaxis.

Workers' compensation cases become more difficult to resolve the longer the employee is off of work, and in some cases where "alternative and complementary" medical practitioners are consulted. In some cases workers develop excessive and unwarranted phobias after reading Material Safety Data Sheets (MSDSs). This is especially true if a primary care physician or specialist confirms those fears by certifying that the employees' complaints are work-related and recommends no return to work.

RETURN-TO-WORK GUIDELINES

Physicians should consult their own state's guidelines, if any, for temporary total disability or return to work. The state of Minnesota at one time published a permanent partial disability schedule and the Minnesota Medical Association previously published a temporary total impairment guide (Table 62–2).

At least three private disability guides provide information on diagnosis, therapy, and time away from work. The Medical Disability Advisor[10] lists a large number of medical diagnoses including information on diagnosis, differential diagnosis, outcome, complications, restrictions and accommodations, factors influencing disability, and expected length of disability. These estimates were often compiled by consensus and are diagnosis-dependent without specific guidelines for estimating time away based on factors such as disease severity, functional impairment, and extent or frequency of treatment. A number of dermatologic diagnoses are included in the

TABLE 62–2

Factors Determining Return to Work for Dermatologic Disorders

1. Severity of condition
2. Site and/or surface area of involvement
3. Effect of therapy, nonsurgical and surgical
4. Effect of comorbid conditions
5. Age
6. Recurrence or chronicity of disorder
7. Effect of adequate job description and availability and of alternative work
8. Results of ancillary diagnostic tests (culture, biopsy, laboratory tests, and allergy epicutaneous patch and intracutaneous prick testing) to make a more accurate diagnosis

Adapted from Denniston PL Jr (ed): ODG (Official Disability Guidelines), Special Edition: Top 100 Conditions. Corpus Christi, Tex, Work Loss Data Institute, 2001, pp 15, 20, 83–87.

Advisor, which seems useful to personnel departments and occasionally to physicians. The section on dermatitis appears to have been written by a non-dermatologist. The section Managing Medical Absences, which discusses the interaction of the Americans With Disabilities Act, the Family and Medical Leave Act, workers' compensation, and disability benefits laws, is a very helpful outline.

Milliman and Robertson[11] published Healthcare Management Guidelines for Workers' Compensation and Industrial Medicine in August 1998. Access is available on their Web site for a complimentary 30-day trial. Few if any dermatologic diagnoses are included in this edition.

The Official Disability Guidelines (ODG)[2] provide length-of-disability data from three U.S. government databases: The National Health Interview Study (NHIS) and the National Hospital Discharge Study (NHDS) from the National Center for Health Statistics of the Centers for Disease Control and Prevention, and the annual reports of Occupational Injuries and Illnesses (OII) from the Bureau of Labor Statistics (BLS), all listed according to ICD-9-CM code. Table 62–3 lists top dermatologic disability diagnoses sorted by occurrence from ODG. The ODG are meant to be used to identify cases that fall out of the norm. Work-related skin disorders generally cause more time lost from work than nonwork-related disorders. Guidelines for essentially the same ICD-9 code vary somewhat. For contact dermatitis and other eczema (ICD-9-CM code 692) limited surface area is rated 0 days return to work, but is not defined, and could be as disabling as extensive surface area involvement (15 days return to work), especially if the hands (limited surface area) were involved. Recurrence of a condition makes guideline determination more difficult. This is certainly true of hand eczema and acute intermittent problems, such as urticaria. It is also important to note that the ICD-9-CM codes are hierarchical. As an example, patch testing would allow more accurate coding to five digits and hence a better disability determination.

SPECIFIC EXAMPLES OF RETURN-TO-WORK ISSUES

■ Example 1: A 50-year-old automotive assembler had a 3-year history of recurrent hand eczema. Barrier cream given by the plant nurse did not help. Topical corticosteroids improved but did not clear condition. A severe flare required short course of systemic corticosteroids and 2 days off work. He was referred to a dermatologist for patch testing for a putative allergy to the anaerobic adhesives that he handled daily. He had positive patch test reaction to the neomycin present in the topical antibiotic prescribed by his primary care physician and to parachlorometaxylenol present in the barrier cream. His eczema cleared after stopping the topical antibiotic and barrier cream, as well as using a no-touch technique to handle the adhesive. The adhesive was thought to be a cause of irritant contact dermatitis.

Comment: Patch testing identified more than one allergen, which was not suspected by either the patient or his physician. The worker was told to stop direct skin contact with the adhesive, which was also contributing to the dermatitis through irritation. Thus allergen substitution and irritant avoidance resulted in a cure.[13]

■ Example 2: A 28-year-old cosmetologist with a history of childhood eczema had a 2-year history of severe dermatitis of the hands. She had seen her primary care physician for multiple episodes of recurrent

TABLE 62–3

Top Dermatologic Disability Diagnoses Sorted by Occurrence (From CDC-P Self-reported Data on All Disabilities): Hypertension Listed for Comparison

Percent of Total Occurrences	Percent of Total Disability Days	Mean Length of Disability	ICD-9-CM Code	Diagnosis/Disease Description
4.81%	2.34%	14.38	401	Hypertension
0.90%	0.10%	4.50	692	Contact dermatitis and other eczema
0.80%	0.71%	9.44	799	Other ill-defined and unknown cause conditions*
0.67%	0.05%	5.75	706	Diseases of sebaceous glands
0.57%	0.06%	7.46	703.0	Ingrown nail
0.45%	0.01%	7.13	698	Pruritus and related conditions

Adapted from Denniston PL Jr (ed): ODG (Official Disability Guidelines), Special Edition: Top 100 Conditions. Corpus Christi, Tex, Work Loss Data Institute, 2001, pp 15, 20, 83–87.

*Includes mostly nondermatologic conditions, but does include skin symptoms (ICD-9-CM Code 782) and rash and nonspecific skin eruption (ICD-9-CM Code 782.1).

dermatitis, which spread to her face and chest. She missed several weeks of work at a time, and required systemic antibiotics for secondary infections as well as continual corticosteroids. Her workers' compensation managed care organization referred her for dermatologic consultation. Patch testing was recommended and approved and she was allergic to glyceryl thioglycolate, present in acid permanent waves. It was recommended that she wear 4-H laminate gloves when giving permanent waves and to limit her exposure to perms. She was able to continue to work with only occasional flares of her dermatitis.

Comment: Accommodation in the workplace with the use of a protective glove, impervious to the permanent wave solution, controlled the dermatitis.[13]

■ Example 3: A 40-year-old phlebotomist had a 5-month history of hives when she wore latex gloves. Her atopic hand eczema was also aggravated by glove use and she experienced swelling of the vulva following a gynecologic examination. She attributed the problem to glove powder, but a switch to nonpowdered gloves did not clear her skin disorder. She had a positive radioallergosorbent test (RAST) to natural rubber latex and was given nonlatex gloves to wear, which cleared her hives and dermatitis.

Comment: This person, with natural rubber latex allergy, was accommodated by substituting nitrile gloves for the natural rubber latex gloves. She continued to work without further hives or dermatitis. She was given the following information on latex allergy: general information on allergen exposure and avoidance; a latex-safe protocol to give to her health care providers, for use during routine examinations and during medical procedures and surgery; a list of potentially cross reacting fruits and foods (the patient developed angioedema after eating bananas); and a list of occult sources of latex along with the Web site addresses for two latex allergy support groups.

Comment: The Occupational Safety and Health Administration Blood Borne Pathogen standard requires that allergic workers be provided with alternative gloves.[6,7,12,14,15]

■ Example 4: A 35-year-old surgeon had recurrent episodes of urticaria, angioedema, rhinitis, and asthma every time he operated. He had fewer symptoms in the outpatient clinic, but required frequent use of inhalers and antihistamines. Systemic steroids were prescribed on several occasions and he injected himself with an EpiPen on one occasion when he had difficulty breathing. Switching to nonlatex gloves helped his local skin reactions but did not improve his respiratory symptoms. He had a positive latex RAST and skin prick test to natural rubber latex gloves. The occupational physician recommended that he be given the information and substitute gloves as in Example 3. He also recommended that the hospital stop using powdered latex gloves for the other employees in the operating room, and give them substitute nonpowdered, nonlatex gloves.

Comment: This further accommodation allowed the surgeon to operate without cutaneous or respiratory symptoms. Hospitals and health care facilities must be aware of latex allergy and be able to provide a latex-safe environment for allergic patients.[6,7,12,14,15]

OTHER RETURN-TO-WORK ISSUES

Unduly restrictive limitations upon return to work, such as avoiding all contact with chemicals, may jeopardize a worker's job. Before writing such recommendations they must be discussed with the patient/employee and employer. This is especially important owing to the chronicity of some cases of occupational skin disease, in which a change of jobs does not always result in clearing of a worker's dermatitis. Some union-management contracts may also restrict worker placement.

Some skin diseases become chronic and do not clear with treatment and allergen and irritant avoidance. Possible reasons are listed in Table 62–4.

Table 62–5 discusses fitness to work with skin disease and lists selected conditions that may disqualify an individual for work.

Table 62–6 lists some work-aggravated skin disorders that may require accommodation by an employer.

Few instances of skin disease exclude a person from performing a given job, although a specific skin disorder may be considered a basis for exclusion in certain circumstances. Most individuals with chronic skin conditions can perform normal work activities, but in some instances require accommodations in the workplace.

TABLE 62–4
Causes of Prolonged and Recurrent Dermatoses

1.	Incorrect dermatologic diagnosis
2.	Proper diagnosis of occupational contact dermatitis but failure to establish cause
3.	Correct diagnosis and discovery of cause, but failure to eliminate the cause completely
4.	Improper medication
5.	Evolvement of secondary dermatoses
6.	Poor washing facilities and improper cleansing agents
7.	Placing dermatitis-prone individuals on hazardous new jobs
8.	Cross-sensitivity
9.	Multiple reactivities
10.	Malingering

Adapted from Birmingham DJ: Prolonged and recurrent occupational dermatitis. Occup Med 1:349–356, 1986.

TABLE 62–5

Selected Dermatologic Conditions That Under Some Circumstances May Exclude an Individual From Work

Disorder	Excluded Job
1. Herpes simplex virus whitlow of a finger, recurrent and not controllable	Health care work with direct patient contact
2. Dermatophyte infection of the palms, recurrent and not controllable	Massage therapy
3. Recurrent impetigo in chronic pyogenic *Staphylococcus aureus* infection	Health care work
4. Dermatoses of the feet	Police and fire work
5. Thermoregulatory skin disorders: anhidrotic ectodermal dysplasia	Extremely hot with potential for prolonged heat stress
6. Thermoregulatory skin disorders: patients with chronic erythroderma	Extremely cold indoor or outdoor jobs
7. Physical agent intolerance: lupus erythematosus	Extensive outdoor work
8. Physical agent intolerance: Raynaud's disease	Prolonged cold exposure
9. Physical agent intolerance: cold urticaria	Prolonged cold exposure; ocean or lake lifeguard
10. Hand dermatitis	May limit grip strength

Adapted from Nethercott JR: Fitness to work with skin disease and the Americans With Disability Act of 1990. Occup Med 9:11–18, 1994.

TABLE 62–6

Selected Dermatologic Conditions That May Require Accommodation

Disorder	Problem or Accommodation
1. **Dermatophyte infection of the palms**	Gloves, because a large innoculum is required to transmit the infection
2. **Psoriasis and lichen planus**	Frequent trauma that induces Koebner phenomenon; e.g., welder
3. **Vitiligo**	Disfiguring cosmetically, but does not impair work unless in strong sunlight
4. **Endogenous eczema or atopic dermatitis**	Avoid wet work as much as possible; inhalant allergens and heavy physical work may aggravate the condition
5. **Contact dermatitis**	Avoidance, allergen substitution, protective equipment
6. **Hyperhidrosis**	Certain tasks such as handling paper documents and working with cement and other chemicals
7. **Stasis ulcers recurrent in a setting of postphlebitic syndrome**	Prolonged standing may aggravate the condition
8. **Type 1 fair complexion (patient always sunburns and never tans)**	Prolonged outdoor work in sunlight may be a hazard even with sunscreen and protective clothing
9. **Hereditary or acquired bullous disorders**	Physical work involving friction and pressure

Adapted from Nethercott JR: Fitness to work with skin disease and the Americans With Disability Act of 1990. Occup Med 9:11–18, 1994.

References

1. Birmingham DJ: Prolonged and recurrent occupational dermatitis. Occup Med 1:349–356, 1986.
2. Denniston PL Jr (ed): ODG (Official Disability Guidelines), Special Edition: Top 100 Conditions. Corpus Christi, Tex, Work Loss Data Institute, 2001, pp 15, 20, 83–87.
3. Finlay AY, Kelly SE: Psoriasis: An index of disability. Clin Exp Dermatol 12:8–11, 1987.
4. Finlay AY, Khan GK, Luscombe DK, Salek MS: Validation of sickness impact profile and psoriasis disability index in psoriasis. Br J Dermatol 123:751–756, 1990.
5. Finlay AY, Ryan TJ: Disability and handicap in dermatology. Int J Dermatol 35:305–311, 1996.

6. Hamilton RG, Biagini RE, Krieg EF: Diagnostic performance of Food and Drug Administration–cleared serologic assays for natural rubber latex-specific IgE antibody. J Allergy Clin Immunol 103:925–930, 1999.
7. Holness DL, Mace SR: Results of evaluation of health care workers with prick and patch testing. Am J Contact Dermat 12:88–92, 2001.
8. Koral AM: Managing medical absences. In Reed P (ed): The Medical Disability Advisor, Workplace Guidelines for Disability Duration, 3rd ed. Boulder, Colo, Reed, 1997, p 1689.
9. Nethercott JR: Fitness to work with skin disease and the Americans With Disability Act of 1990. Occup Med 9:11–18, 1994.
10. Reed P (ed): The Medical Disability Advisor, Workplace Guidelines for Disability Duration, 3rd ed. Boulder, Colo, Reed, 1997.
11. Schibanoff JM (ed): Workers Compensation, Volume 7, Healthcare Management Guidelines. San Diego, Milliman and Robertson, 1998.
12. Smedley J, Jury A, Bendall H, et al: Prevalence and risk factors for latex allergy: A cross sectional study in a United Kingdom hospital. Occup Environ Med 56:833–836, 1999.
13. Taylor JS: Contact Dermatitis in Scientific American Medicine. New York, Web MD, 2001.
14. Taylor JS, Wattanakrai P, Charous BL, Ownby DR: Latex Allergy in Allergic Skin Disease: Causes and Treatment. New York, Marcel Dekker, 2000, pp 237–269.
15. Warshaw EM: Latex allergy. J Am Acad Dermatol 39:1–24, 1998.

CHAPTER

63

Endocrinological Disability

RICHARD P. LEVY, MD

Endocrine disorders are common, especially diabetes mellitus, thyroid disorders, and menopause, but the impairment they cause is usually minor enough not to cause major disability. Many endocrinopathies, however, including hypothalamic, pituitary, thyroid, parathyroid, gonadal endocrinopathies, and diabetes mellitus, may cause a feeling of malaise and depression that contributes to abnormalities specific to the endocrinopathy itself. In the everyday practice of adult endocrinology, the effects of diabetes and thyroid disease dominate the causes of impairment, disability, and handicap, and therefore are emphasized in the following.

DIABETES MELLITUS

Diabetes has undergone a large increase in prevalence in developed countries worldwide.[1] At the same time, there have been major advances in treatment that have changed the character of impairment and disability due to diabetes so that these are now mostly due to the late complications of diabetes: visual impairment, peripheral and autonomic neuropathy, renal failure, and accelerated atherosclerosis. The assessment and management of these complications is discussed in other chapters and is similar regardless of whether the individual is diabetic or not. On the other hand, hyperglycemia and hypoglycemia are common in diabetes and can cause disability and impairment.

Hyperglycemia

Elevated blood glucose concentrations below the renal threshold for glucose (about 180 mg/dL) do not cause impairment although even this degree of hyperglycemia is an important cause of the late complications of diabetes listed previously. As the blood glucose increases further, impairment both at home and at work may result from generalized weakness, weight loss, blurred vision, polyuria, and various infections. Insulin treatment must be begun in patients with Type 1 diabetes. A variety of oral agents are available for management of Type 2 diabetes either as monotherapy or as a combination of agents. Hypoglycemia can occur with any of these agents, but the risk is much lower with the oral agents than with insulin. Exercise, a prudent diet, and blood glucose monitoring are appropriate for all patients with diabetes. When blood glucose control is good without insulin treatment, impairment and disability are minimal.

On the other hand, insulin treatment causes impairment and disability to a greater or lesser extent. The standard of care requires self-measurement of blood glucose, ideally at least four times daily. With current devices this can be done almost painlessly in less than 1 minute with the result immediately visible and stored automatically. This can be done in all but the dirtiest and most hostile environments. Insulin needs to be given one to six times daily but there are automatic and semiautomatic devices to simplify insulin administration. For automatic insulin injection, insulin pumps are costly devices that the individual can wear continuously. They deliver insulin under the person's control either continuously (basal doses) or intermittently (bolus doses), selected to cover a feeding or to correct hyperglycemia.

Less complicated and less expensive devices are insulin "pens," whereby a person can dial in the dose and inject it immediately. Both quick-acting and intermediate-acting insulin cartridges are available.

In use in Europe and being investigated in the United States are implantable insulin pumps, which can contain 6000 units of a unique quick-acting insulin that is stable at body temperature for up to 6 months. Basal and bolus insulin doses are programmed using a small radio transmitter. The pump is implanted subcutaneously and the delivery catheter is directed into the peritoneal cavity. Premarketing experience is encouraging, demonstrating excellent blood glucose control with a reduced incidence of hypoglycemia.

Earlier in development is a subcutaneous glucose sensor that automatically measures and records glucose concentrations at frequent intervals. With the proper algorithms, data from the monitor could be able to adjust the insulin output from a pump to provide regulation of blood glucose at near normal concentrations.

With currently available devices diabetes can be controlled well enough to minimize impairment and disability and prevent or delay the complications of diabetes.

Hypoglycemia

Hypoglycemia can be a spontaneous event but it is rare and usually correctable. Hypoglycemia from insulin treatment is relatively common. Hypoglycemia from oral antidiabetic agents can occur but is unusual in an ambulatory patient eating regular meals and monitoring blood glucose. Early in the course of diabetes there are warning signs of hypoglycemia before marked changes in mental function begin, permitting timely self-administration of a rapidly absorbed hexose such as sugar tablets. Hormonal counter-regulatory secretion also occurs with release of epinephrine, glucagon, and growth hormone. As the diabetes progresses, the warning symptoms and hormonal counter-regulation diminish. At that time the first symptom of hypoglycemia may be neurologic, with alteration of mental function including loss of consciousness. Impairment and disability can be major. Living alone, driving a car, and operating dangerous machinery have become important problems. With the instruction of significant others, supervisors, and coworkers, most insulin takers function well in nonhazardous situations. This can include driving a car if the blood glucose is self-measured before starting and periodically thereafter. Driving commercial trucks and flying aircraft is generally forbidden (see Chapters 49 and 50).

THYROID DISEASE

Goiters (thyroid enlargement) are common even in iodine-replete areas such as the United States but they seldom become large enough to alter the quality of life. Hyperthyroidism and hypothyroidism are relatively common. The former can occur at any age; the latter has an increasing prevalence with increasing age.

Hyperthyroidism

Hyperthyroidism affects about 1 in 1000 persons—more women than men. Its onset may be gradual or sudden; its severity can be mild or severe. In the mild form, atrial fibrillation may be the presenting symptom. In more severe cases, weight loss, decreased ability to exercise, proximal muscle weakness, palpitations, heat intolerance, diarrhea, and ophthalmopathy can occur in any combination. If untreated, major impairment and disability will result. Treatment with either antithyroid drugs or 131-iodine usually results in prompt remission. Hypothyroidism is a frequent complication of radioiodine treatment. Laboratory confirmation of the diagnosis is readily available and relatively inexpensive. The ophthalmopathy is not correlated with the degree of thyrotoxicosis. It can be cosmetically disfiguring. It can cause diplopia, excess blinking and tearing, severely decreased visual acuity, and blindness. Treatment is generally unsatisfactory. Considerable irreversible impairment and disability can be expected in severe cases.

Hypothyroidism

Hypothyroidism is more common than hyperthyroidism, with the same preponderance of women. Its prevalence increases with age, affecting as many as 10% of women over 60. Onset may be subtle and symptoms overlap those of depression. Symptoms vary from patient to patient. They include slowed mentation, cold intolerance, hoarseness, constipation, modest weight gain, dry skin, and edema. Impairment is usually gradual. A well-known pediatrician with severe hypothyroidism continued to work full time until a routine electrocardiogram revealed the characteristic changes of severe hypothyroidism, which led to its diagnosis. In retrospect, the patient recalled having some symptoms of the disorder at least 2 years previously. Laboratory confirmation of the diagnosis is straightforward with an elevated serum thyroid stimulating hormone and decreased serum thyroxine concentration. Treatment is also straightforward with oral tablets of levothyroxine. Symptoms begin to abate in about 10 days and remission is complete in 4 to 6 weeks. Hypothyroidism is not an important cause of disability.

OTHER ENDOCRINOPATHIES

Menopause, which can cause altered mood and hot flashes, may cause some impairment. Replacement estrogen generally provides quick relief.

Hypothalamic-pituitary Disorders

Antidiuretic hormone (ADH) is made in the hypothalamus and transported to the posterior pituitary.

Deficiency in this system produces diabetes insipidus with polyuria and polydipsia. Impairment is minimal because treatment with an inhaled or injectable ADH analog is very successful.

Abnormalities in the anterior pituitary may cause visual impairment due to pressure on the optic chiasm. When there is hypersecretion or hyposecretion of one or more of the pituitary trophic hormones a variety of syndromes may result. From the standpoint of impairment and disability, Cushing's syndrome, acromegaly, and panhypopituitarism are the most important.

Pituitary disorders generally cause nonspecific symptoms such as weakness, depression, and easy fatigability. Treatment outcomes are variable, ranging from prompt and complete remission to severe and persistent disability. Parathyroid malfunction is generally mild and treatment results are usually good. Adrenal disease is rare. Cushing syndrome, already discussed, can cause considerable impairment; it is usually completely correctable. Adrenal insufficiency is readily correctable. Gonadal disorders other than menopause can cause infertility, impotence, hirsutism, and decreased sense of well-being.

SUMMARY

Within the endocrine system, diabetes mellitus is the principal cause of impairment, disability, and handicap. The so-called late complications are the major factors. Hyperglycemia can cause impairment until corrected. Hypoglycemia as a consequence of insulin treatment can preclude some activities. Thyroid disease can cause temporary disability. Other endocrinopathies are unusual causes of long-term disability.

CHAPTER

64

Gastrointestinal Disability

JAMES R. McPHERSON, MD, MSc, FACP

There is great variability in an individual's capacity to meet personal, social, and occupational demands when he or she has an impairment of the gastrointestinal tract. Changes in capacity occur with age of the patient, different stages of a disease, and the development of new therapies. Unfortunately, a return to the normal state is rare as a result of chronic gastrointestinal diseases.

A variety of mechanisms cause disability in gastrointestinal disease and some or all may play a role and should be considered. Some mechanisms are as follows:

1. Malnutrition secondary to dysphagia, inadequate digestion, malabsorption, or anorexia
2. Generalized fatigue and loss of stamina such as in chronic liver disease or inflammatory bowel disease
3. Anemia secondary to frequent bleeding or chronic disease
4. Debility associated with chronic unremitting pain
5. Massive fluid retention with peripheral edema and ascites
6. Necessity for special diets, regimens, and medical visits
7. Generalized intractable pruritus in cholestatic liver disease and ductal obstruction
8. Persistent viral carrier states such as hepatitis B and C
9. Intestinal stomas and fistulae or internal anastomoses requiring special attention
10. Intractable diarrhea and/or anal incontinence

OROPHARYNX

The inability to move food particles from the mouth to the esophagus secondary to radiation injury or neuromuscular dysfunction may be severe enough to prompt a feeding gastrostomy. Pooled saliva may be frequently aspirated. Owing to the necessity of a feeding tube or medical complications such as aspiration and malnutrition, disability is frequent and frequently total.

ESOPHAGUS

Strictures often require repeated dilatations with inherent risks.[7] A dilated proximal esophagus in achalasia can create permanent disability even after successful myotomy or pneumatic dilatation of the gastroesophageal sphincter.[6] Primary disease such as scleroderma may be complicated by a stricture caused by recurrent reflux. These individuals are frequently completely disabled for reasons similar to those listed under the oropharynx.

STOMACH

Disability after distal gastric resections is usually mild to moderate. Proximal gastrectomy has more potential for increased disability. Postgastrectomy dumping syndrome and reactive hypoglycemia usually are amenable to treatment but may add to the disability. The proximity of and ability to use washroom facilities often dictates specific jobs that a person may be capable of performing. Reactive hypoglycemia can also affect the nature of jobs, that a person can engage in. This will be dictated by the frequency, severity, and duration of the symptomatic period.

SMALL INTESTINE

Massive resection with 200 cm or less remaining of the small intestine will require parenteral nutrition for survival and a home program for the long term. The latter has allowed some patients to feel that they are able to do what they wish to do; however, the requirements of 8 hours of parenteral infusion, usually at night while sleeping, require great adaptation and attendant care. The risk of catheter-associated infection, metabolic disease of the liver, and bone disease are significant.[8]

Limited resections of small intestine are usually reasonably tolerated and unlikely to be disabling, although one may require dietary adjustment.

Motility disorders with pseudo-obstruction and refractory celiac sprue can be devastating and medications may not provide much relief. Untreated celiac sprue can cause retarded growth and spinal deformity.

PANCREAS

Chronic relapsing pancreatitis may be disabling owing to the unpredictable timing of attacks, chronic pain, and exocrine and endocrine deficiency. If pancreatectomy is required for pain relief, the complex nature of the various anastomoses is an additional disability factor.[2]

LIVER AND BILIARY TRACT[1,3,4]

Chronic hepatitis with its systemic effects and a viral carrier state are major factors preventing active involvement in health care industries and in the food service industry.

The development of complications such as bleeding, fluid retention, and renal disease in all forms of cirrhosis creates a major disability. Patients are usually restricted to sedentary jobs, depending on the degree of medical complications associated with the cirrhosis and/or results of treatment. Job placement becomes more problematic as the degree of complications and/or incomplete response to treatment progresses. Early treatment of hereditary hemochromatosis may lessen impairment and hence disability to frequent rechecks and phlebotomies four to six times per year. The same would apply to Wilson's disease with treatment.

Primary biliary cirrhosis progresses from minimal to complete disability in most cases. The sequence may be the same in primary sclerosing cholangitis.

Survival rates following liver transplant are more than 85% at 1 year and 70% at 5 years. Problems related to immunosuppressive therapy and complications such as fever, infection, depression, hypertension, diabetes mellitus, hyperlipidemia, and renal dysfunction add significant risk of disability. Despite this, the vast majority of recipients report a remarkable improvement in quality of life and some report a normal lifestyle. Frequent medical visits are required.

COLON

Ulcerative colitis and Crohn's disease cause varying degrees of disability due to systemic effects and diarrhea, abdominal pain, and bleeding. Colectomy offers a cure in the case of ulcerative colitis and a major benefit in Crohn's disease of the colon. The Brooke ileostomy is well tolerated in most patients. An ileal pouch–anal anastomosis is attractive to many, particularly young adults, but requires considerable attention.[1,5]

Partial resection and end-to-end anastomosis for isolated colon diseases such as tumors and angiomata have excellent results with only minimal change in a patient's bowel habits.

Severe irritable bowel may interfere with and even prevent employment in some fields requiring continuous attention.

Anal incontinence may be severe and intractable to treatment. A diverting descending colostomy to provide greater security may be of value and should be considered.

Most individuals with a colostomy will be capable of doing most jobs, although this decision is best made on a case-by-case basis with a knowledge of the job description.

ABDOMINAL WALL HERNIAS

If repair of a symptomatic hernia is not possible or feasible, then a disability exists for heavy manual labor.

References

1. Balan V, Scolapio JS, Harrison J, et al: Survival in Wilson's disease. Gastroenterology 106:A863, 1994.
2. Brandhagen D, Fairbanks V, Batts K: Update on hereditary hemochromatosis. Mayo Clin Proc 74:917–921, 1999.
3. Cooper MJ, Williamson RCN, Benjamin IS, et al: Total pancreatectomy for chronic pancreatitis. Br J Surg 74:912–915, 1987.
4. Desmet VJ: Current problems in diagnosis of biliary disease and cholestases. Semin Liver Dis 6:233–245, 1986.
5. Kohler LW, Pemberton JH, Zinsmeister AR, et al: A comparison of Brooke ileostomy, koch pouch and ileal pouch—anal anastomosis. Gastroenterology 101:679–684, 1991.
6. McCord GS, Staiano A, Clouse RE, et al: Achalasia, diffuse spasm and nonspecific disorders. Baillieres Clin Gastroenterol 5:307–335, 1991.
7. Pope CE II: Acid reflux disorders. N Engl J Med; 331:656–660, 1994.
8. Scolapio JS, Fleming CR, Kelly DG, et al: Survival of home parenteral nutrition–treated patients: 20 years experience at the Mayo Clinic. Mayo Clin Proc 74:217–222, 1999.

Bibliography

Sleisinger MH, Fordtran JS (eds): Gastrointestinal Disease, 6th ed., Philadelphia, WB Saunders, 1998.

CHAPTER

65

Renal Disability

KARL D. SCHWARZE, MD, MS

The intent of the federally funded end stage renal disease (ESRD) program, initiated in 1972, was to provide life-sustaining dialysis to patients suffering from terminal chronic renal failure.[13] As a consequence of this act, more patients with ESRD lived longer. Patients suffering from terminal renal failure found it financially feasible to stay alive and, hopefully, remain productive members of society.

Advances in ESRD management have altered many of the dialysis complications and expected survival time. Patients reaching end stage renal failure die within weeks if not placed on dialysis. Once renal replacement therapy has been initiated, the remaining life expectancy for a 40- to 44-year-old is 7 to 10 years according to the United States Renal Data System 1998 report, although this varies with race and other comorbid factors.[26]

Unfortunately, society has not kept up with these advancements. Patients are still perceived as unemployable. Only 13% of chronic dialysis patients under age 65, and without obvious disability, are employed outside the home.[12]

DISABILITY CAUSED BY RENAL FAILURE

When considering the work capabilities of a person with renal disease, the first two issues that need to be discussed are the etiology and the severity of the renal disease. By and large, the only types of primary renal disease leading to work restrictions (other than cancer) are those that lead to altered renal physiology. Generally, few activity restrictions are found until the creatinine clearance falls below 25 to 30 mL/min.

Once placed on some form of renal replacement therapy, it takes approximately 30 days to reach a steady state. Prior to this the patient still may have uremic signs and symptoms present to varying degrees, volume status may not be optimized, and the target weight (weight used in ultrafiltration calculations) may not have been established. After this period there are four areas of concern in determining functionality and possible employment: cognition, cardiovascular, neuropathy, and endurance.

Cognition is a concern when considering any occupation. Cognition is typically spared in ESRD patients and should not provide an occupational barrier. However, there is an entity, dialysis dementia, which can be seen in patients who have been dialyzed for many years. This neurologic syndrome is characterized by myoclonus, mental changes, speech disturbances, hallucinations, and seizures. Patients affected by this malady have been found to have high aluminum levels in brain tissue.[1] Aluminum containing phosphate binders were frequently used in the past. Because aluminum toxicity was seen with greater regularity in the ERSD population, the use of these binders has dropped and agents not containing aluminum are now used.

Cardiovascular involvement is frequent in ESRD patients, with 70% dying from cardiovascular disease due to enhanced atherogenesis leading to coronary artery disease, hypertension, and anemia that can cause a cardiomyopathy. The anemia increases cardiac work during exertion leading to restrictions on jobs that require significant physical exertion.

Neuropathies (peripheral and autonomic; see following) may accompany ESRD. The peripheral neuropathy is an asymmetric, distal, mixed sensorimotor polyneuropathy. This ailment is common in the ESRD patient. Sensory symptoms predominate, particularly dysesthesias with prickling or burning sensations. Motor symptoms are less common. "Restless legs," more common at night, are a nuisance but usually do not lead to physical impairments, although one may see sleep deprivation in these patients. Jobs requiring fine manual dexterity conceivably could be hampered if the polyneuropathy is severe. Autonomic neuropathy can also be seen. When present, it primarily affects the cardiovascular reflexes. This could lead to orthostatic hypotension. Jobs requiring bending and stooping may be hampered by this complication. However, this is seldom clinically significant. Most typically, symptoms of orthostasis are found immediately following dialysis before volume redistribution has a chance to occur.

Endurance is also affected in the ESRD patient. To a certain extent, the decreased endurance varies with the type of renal replacement therapy with the transplant patient's endurance being affected the least.[20,22] There are several causes of this decreased endurance, including cardiovascular dysfunction, anemia, acidosis-related muscle wasting, hyperparathyroidism, neuropathies, reduced bone density, and glucose intolerance.[14] Additionally, it is common for ESRD patients to be placed on a low-protein diet. This has a significant potential to further reduce muscle mass.[4] Also, as the renal failure patient approaches the need for dialysis, activity levels typically decrease due to fatigue and malaise. This leads to deconditioning, which further reduces the muscle mass. Typically, this lack of endurance will be manifest as a diminished exercise capacity with an inability to perform many of the activities of daily living. It has been documented that the exercise capacity of nondialyzed ESRD patients is well below values expected for sedentary, nondiseased individuals.[9,20–22,25] Unfortunately, studies have shown that physicians typically underestimate or fail to recognize the functional disability of these patients.[2]

There are numerous tests, both objective and subjective, used to assess the exercise capacity and endurance of this population. The definitive tests to assess the exercise capacity are the complete cardiopulmonary exercise stress test and the functional capacity assessment (see Chapters 24 and 51). There is increasing evidence that self-report instruments, such as the Medical Outcomes Study Short-Form 36 (SF-36), may be sufficient to detect the deterioration in functional capabilities.[5,6,18,24,27] The SF-36 consists of eight health constructs or scales. These scales are further divided into those representing the physical and the mental aspects of function. The physical component scale has been shown by Lowrie et al to correlate better with the risk of death than sex, race, or diabetes mellitus. Low mental component scores also have been shown to correlate with mortality when age and other clinical measures were controlled.[17]

Once the diminished endurance has been assessed, it may be possible to break the pattern of disability by early referral to physical therapy. According to the Life Options Rehabilitation Advisory Council, the ideal rehabilitation program for dialysis patients consists not only of medical treatment, education, counseling, and dietary regimens, but also exercise in order to improve the physical function in these patients.[3] Most exercise training studies of dialysis patients document significant improvements in cardiorespiratory fitness. Only by making physical therapy and exercise integral parts of the treatment will the ESRD patient be able to reach his or her full potential for a long and productive life. The importance of ongoing monitoring in this population cannot be overstated. It is well documented that this population has a large propensity for progressive deconditioning and eventual death.

Despite this downward spiraling cascade, motivated patients are able to perform quite physically demanding tasks. Further, this lack of endurance does not necessarily correlate with the vocational capabilities of the patient. Prudence would dictate that in patients pursuing physically demanding occupations, stress testing and tests designed to measure specific physical performance be performed prior to release for work.[23]

DISABILITY DUE TO THE EFFECTS OF RENAL FAILURE ON OTHER ORGAN SYSTEMS

Chronic renal failure can secondarily affect most, if not all, organ systems. During this progression from renal insufficiency to renal failure, each of the other organ systems becomes more compromised with the progressive deterioration of renal function. It is beyond the scope of this chapter to specifically detail all the nuances involved in this and only a brief discussion follows.

As noted before, the cardiovascular system is particularly vulnerable and the majority of chronic renal failure patients die from cardiovascular causes. The majority of patients are hypertensive, which leads to further renal compromise as well as cardiac damage.

Many patients have anemia further stressing the cardiac system, leading to high cardiac output states and left ventricular hypertrophy. Anemia of renal failure in addition to the cardiac manifestations probably accounts for many of the general symptoms attributed to uremia, including diminished exercise capacity, diminished cognitive function and mental acuity, decreased immune responsiveness, altered sleep patterns, poor nutrition, and sexual dysfunction.[7]

Dyslipidemias occur early in the course of renal failure, further compromising the cardiovascular system. Additionally, all of the above mentioned problems are amplified by smoking.

Renal bone disease is particularly bothersome owing to its clinically asymptomatic nature until very late in its course. There is now broad agreement that, in order to prevent the complications of secondary hyperparathyroidism, attention to this disorder must be paid very early in the course of renal insufficiency, well before the patient starts renal replacement therapy.

Metabolic acidoses ensue owing to the inability of the kidney in chronic renal failure to excrete excess hydrogen ions. This may lead to exertional breathlessness, which at times has been mistakenly attributed to the affects of anemia or pulmonary edema.

Malnutrition is common owing to anorexia, acidosis, and insulin resistance. The loss of muscle mass is commonly overlooked owing to a stable weight caused by fluid retention. Laboratory values useful in assessing this issue are the serum albumin, prealbumin, transferrin, and cholesterol. Under these circumstances a fall in serum creatinine is often misinterpreted as an improvement in renal function.

ESRD patients also have a bleeding diathesis, partially as a consequence of abnormal platelet function. This is particularly important owing to its silent manifestations of gastrointestinal blood loss.

The dermatologic manifestations can be a source of significant discomfort. Common manifestations are diffuse brown pigmentation, xerosis, and pruritus. The pruritus is variable and unpredictable but can be extremely debilitating. It usually is a late manifestation.

Neurologic manifestations are divided into central, peripheral, and autonomic neuropathies, as discussed previously. The extreme central neurologic manifestations are coma and seizures, although these are rarely seen. More commonly, the patient will experience cognitive impairment, but again this is a late finding and is usually an indication of the need to start dialysis. Opiate toxicity due to retention of active metabolites is additive and may aggravate or mimic uremic encephalopathy. This must be kept in mind when prescribing analgesics to this population. Symptoms related to peripheral and autonomic neuropathies are unusual in patients prior to needing dialysis.

Endocrinologic abnormalities causing symptoms have already been touched on and include hyperparathyroidism, decreased erythropoietin levels, and insulin resistance.

Psychological manifestations such as depression and anxiety are frequent. These are understandable and are seen more commonly in younger patients. Additionally, as the renal failure progresses, the patient becomes more fatigued and inactive, which only amplifies many of the debilitating conditions previously outlined.[14]

This is usually the time that the patient files for and is granted disability. Further inactivity and compromise in the patient's overall condition is found. It is during this downward cascade that the patient needs a physician well versed with the process. The goal of this physician in the past has not been to maintain the patient at his or her current level of activity but rather to treat the specific abnormalities as they present in order to preserve the patient's life until dialysis is instituted. This falls far short in many cases of maintaining the patient as a productive member of society. Owing to this lack of insight, the patient progresses to end stage renal failure in a debilitated and deconditioned state. If one is to reverse this trend, the physician must not only treat the organic consequences early and aggressively but also pay particular attention to deconditioning, balance, muscle weakness, range of motion, and nutritional status. Physical therapy should play a significant role in this process.

DISABILITY CAUSED BY THE TREATMENT OF RENAL FAILURE

Although few theoretical occupational limitations are placed on the ESRD patient, each treatment modality has specific hindrances. These are described in the following sections according to the specific modality. Limitations placed on the patient owing to hemodialysis are further classified in terms of access type—natural fistula, polytetrafluoroethylene (PTFE) graft, or tunnel catheter.

The hemodialysis patient should be qualified to perform either a sedentary or physical occupation providing that he or she is properly conditioned. Despite this, the patient may be severely impaired immediately following dialysis. Nausea, fatigue, headaches, and orthostatic symptoms are quite common during the immediate postdialysis time. In properly dialyzed patients, these symptoms should only last for several hours. Employment opportunities may be limited by the dialysis center schedules. Typically hemodialysis is performed three times a week with average run times of 4 hours. This can preclude meaningful participation at work when the traveling time is added to the recovery time.

Limitations can be placed on the patient by the presence of arterial-venous (AV) fistulas or PTFE grafts. There should be no situation in which the patient has to wear constricting bands or clothing around the access area because of the potential for thrombosis of the access. It would also be prudent to avoid occupations that would place the AV access in areas where it is at risk of being cut or punctured. In many instances the AV access has blood flows in excess of 1 liter per minute. A laceration of the access could lead to rapid exsanguination.

Tunneled catheters are used until an AV fistula can be created and mature. They usually contain a Dacron cuff circumscribing the catheter just prior to its exit from the skin. Ingrowth of fibrous tissue occurs at the cuff site providing a barrier to infection and an anchor for the catheter. Once the catheter has been placed and is well healed, the dialysis staff routinely performs examinations and cleaning of the exit site at the time of dialysis. It is imperative that the catheter be immobilized to prevent tension and trauma. Following satisfactory healing, showering and swimming are permitted. Exit site infections are a major problem related to this type of access. Thus occupations requiring significant exposures to dirt, grime, and dust are best avoided.

The peritoneal dialysis patient has other restrictions created by either the catheter or by the physical constraints related to the procedure itself. As with the hemodialysis-tunneled catheters, the peritoneal catheter usually contains a Dacron cuff circumscribing the catheter just prior to its exit from the skin. Ingrowth of fibrous tissue occurs at this cuff site, providing for a barrier to infection and an anchor for the catheter. Once the catheter has been placed and is well healed, frequent examinations by the patient are required to inspect for exit site and for tunnel infections. Daily or alternate day cleaning of the exit site are performed to remove dirt. It is imperative that the catheter be immobilized to prevent tension and trauma. Following satisfactory healing, showering and swimming are permitted.[16]

There are two basic forms of peritoneal dialysis in practice today: continuous ambulatory peritoneal dialysis (CAPD) and continuous cyclic peritoneal dialysis (CCPD). CAPD treatment is given continuously. Each exchange consists of two liters of dialysate solution. The two liters are infused into the peritoneal cavity via the peritoneal catheter. The solution is left in the peritoneal cavity for roughly 6 hours (this is referred to as a 6-hour dwell time) and then drained out through the same catheter. Three exchanges are done during the day and one at night. The night exchange usually has a little longer dwell time so that the patient is allowed to sleep throughout the night. These exchanges are manually performed and require a clean area to perform an exchange of peritoneal fluid. CCPD treatment is also continuous. Three to five exchanges are performed at night with aid of cycler. Typically there is one long exchange throughout the day with a dwell time of 14 to 16 hours. The average exchange volume is again two liters.

Peritoneal dialysis may allow more activity in patients as it does not require frequent visits to a dialysis center. However, it does require a clean environment to perform the actual exchanges. Because this technique requires operator participation and cleanliness, it would not be advantageous for a person employed in a dirty environment.

Finally, the continuous presence of a large volume of dialysis solution in the peritoneal cavity increases intra-abdominal pressure, which can further increase physical activity restrictions such as walking, jogging, and lifting. Continuous elevations of intra-abdominal pressures predispose to abdominal hernias (incisional, inguinal, diaphragmatic, or umbilical) and dialysate leaks, especially in older debilitated patients with or without previous surgical scars. Dialysis leaks occur when the dialysate solution leaks through soft tissue planes from incision sites or from soft tissue defects in a hernia. They present as edema of the abdominal wall, labia, scrotum, and penis. These frequently have been attributed to heavy lifting or straining causing excess intra-abdominal pressure. Equally important would be the overall condition of the abdominal musculature and fitness of the individual. If he or she has normally performed heavy lifting and exertion throughout his or her employment and has remained in good physical condition, then there would be little reason to suspect that he or she would not be able to continue with his or her occupation once the peritoneal catheter has been properly placed and healed. One may also consider CCPD over CAPD with smaller volumes during the daytime cycle to ensure no excess intra-abdominal pressure buildup.

The last modality considered is renal transplantation. Exercise capacities are higher in transplant recipients than in dialysis patients.[20,22] The average increase in exercise capacity in pre- to post-transplantation patients has been shown to be 28%. This increase was independent of increases in the hematocrit or physical activity.[20] Kempeneers et al point out that transplant recipients remained limited in exercise capacity by musculoskeletal factors.[15] Muscle wasting effects due to glucocorticoid treatment are well known. It has also been documented that quadriceps muscle strength in renal transplant recipients is only 70% of normal.[10,11] This side effect may be counteracted by resistance exercise training.[10,11] Two studies reported that cardiovascular training in renal transplant recipients resulted in significant improvements in exercise capacity.[15,19] Unfortunately, despite significant improvements in exercise capacity and feeling better after kidney transplantation, daily activity did not significantly improve at 6 months in one study. The reason given was that many recipients were fearful of doing anything that would harm their new organ.[8] The physical capacity to improve cardiovascular fitness, muscle strength, and health is present in this population. Even vigorous exercise training for competition is not contraindicated in the renal transplant recipient. However, these patients must gradually increase their cardiorespiratory fitness and strength before proceeding with a vigorous training program.

Thus it would seem that the average transplant recipient should be able to participate in both sedentary as well as physically challenging occupations with little difficulty. There are two potential exceptions. The first is transplant recipients who are medicated with immunosuppressive medications. Higher doses are used just after transplantation or during a rejection episode. During these times the individual should not be exposed to contagious illnesses. Once the immunosuppressives are tapered, he or she may resume normal activities. Further, there are other side effects of these medications: some are patient specific (e.g., nausea), on other organ systems (e.g., liver), or on other components of the blood (e.g., anemia or thrombocytopenia), which may limit work, depending on the nature of the work and the deficit that the individual experiences. The second exception occurs when the person develops significant renal failure from a recurrence of the primary renal disease or from chronic rejection.

CONCLUSION AND SUMMARY

Theoretically, individuals with chronic renal failure should be able to maintain their occupations with very few exceptions. Unfortunately, society has found it easier to label these people as totally disabled. The medical profession has also allowed this to happen by setting its goal at keeping these individuals alive but not necessarily maintaining their occupational capability. In the future more emphasis must be placed on returning these people to their respective occupations. There is little reason to expect less of these individuals with the progress that has been made in treating this affliction.

References

1. Alfrey AC, Le Gendre GR, Kaehny WD: The dialysis encephalopathy syndrome. Possible aluminum intoxication. N Engl J Med 294:184, 1976.
2. Calkins DR, Rubenstein LV, Cleary PD, et al: Failure of physicians to recognize functional disability in ambulatory patients. Ann Intern Med 114:451–454, 1991.
3. Carlson L, Carey S: Staff responsibility to exercise. Advances in Renal Replacement Therapy 6:172–180, 1999.
4. Castaneda C, Gordon PL, Uhlin KL, et al: Resistance training to counteract the catabolism of a low protein diet in patients with chronic renal insufficiency. Ann Intern Med 135:965–976, 2001.
5. Curtin RB, Lowrie EG, DeOreo PB: Self reported functional status: An important predictor of health outcomes among end-stage renal disease patients. Advances in Renal Replacement Therapy 6:133–140, 1999.
6. Edgell ET, Cooons SJ, Carter WB, et al: A review of health related quality of life measures used in end stage renal disease. Clin Ther 18:887–938, 1996.
7. Eschbach JW: Anemia in chronic renal failure. In Johnson RJ, Feehally J (eds): Comprehensive Clinical Nephrology. St Louis: Mosby, 2000.
8. Gallagher-Lepak S: Functional capacity and activity levels before and after renal transplantation. Am Nephrol Nurs Assoc J 18:378–382, 1991.
9. Goldberg AP, Geltman EM, Hagberg JM, et al: Therapeutic benefits of exercise training for hemodialysis patients. Kidney Int S16:S303–S309, 1983.
10. Horber FF, Scheidegger FR, Grunig BE, et al: Evidence that prednisone-induced myopathy is reversed by physical training. J Clin Endocrinol Metab 61:83–88, 1985.
11. Horber FF, Scheidegger JR, Grunig BE, et al: Thigh muscle mass and function in patients treated with glucocorticoids. Eur J Clin Invest 15:302–307, 1985.
12. Ifudu O, Paul H, Mayers J, et al: Pervasive failed rehabilitation in center based maintenance hemodialysis patients. Am J Kidney Dis 23:394–400, 1994.
13. Johansen KL: Physical functioning and exercise capacity in patients on dialysis. Advances in Renal Replacement Therapy 6:141–148, 1999.
14. Karasnoff J, Patricia P: The physiological consequences of bed rest and inactivity. Advances in Renal Replacement Therapy 6:124–132, 1999.
15. Kempeneers G, Myburgh KH, Wiggins T, et al: Skeletal muscle factors limiting exercise tolerance of renal transplant patients: Effects of a graded exercise training program. Am J Kidney Dis 14:57–65, 1990.
16. Khanna R, Nolph KD, Oreopoulos DG: The Essentials of Peritoneal Dialysis. New York, Kluwer Academic Publishers, 1993, pp 30–33.
17. Lowrie EG, Zhang H, LePain N, et al: SF-36 and Mortality. CQI Memorandum (Reference No. 98-01-16). Boston, Mass, Fresenius Medical Care North America, 1998.
18. Meyer KB, Espindle DM, DeGiacomo JM, et al: Monitoring dialysis patients' health status. Am J Kidney Dis 24:267–279, 1994.
19. Miller TD, Squires RW, Gau GT, et al: Graded exercise testing and training after renal transplantation: A preliminary study. Mayo Clin Proc 62:773–777, 1987.
20. Painter P, Hanson P Messer-Rehak D, et al: Exercise tolerance changes following renal transplantation. Am J Kidney Dis 10:452–456, 1987.
21. Painter P, Johansen K: Introduction: a call to activity. Advances in Renal Replacement Therapy 6:107–109, 1999.
22. Painter PL, Messer-Rehak D, Hanson P, et al: Exercise capacity in hemodialysis, CAPD, and renal transplant patients. Nephron 42:47–51, 1986.
23. Painter P, Stewart AL, Carey S: Physical functioning: Definitions, measurement, and expectations. Advances in Renal Replacement Therapy 6:110–123, 1999.
24. Rettig RA, Sadler JH, Meyer KB, et al: Assessing health and quality of life outcomes in dialysis: A report on an Institute of Medicine workshop. Am J Kidney Dis 30:140–155,1997.
25. Shalom R, Blumenthal JA, Williams RS, et al: Feasibility and benefits of exercise training in patients on maintenance dialysis. Kidney Int 25:958–963,1984.
26. U.S. Department of Health and Human Services: United States Renal Data System: USRDS 1998 Annual Data Report. Bethesda, Md, The National Institutes of Health, National Institute of Diabetes and Digestive and Kidney Diseases, U.S. Department of Health and Human Services, 1998.
27. Wilson IB, Cleary PD: Linking clinical variables with health related quality of life. JAMA 273:59–65,1995.

CHAPTER

66

Hematological and Oncological Disability

ALVIN MARKOVITZ, MD, FACP, FACOEM, FAADEP

Evaluating disability in hematologic disorders is more complex than in other organ systems. The evaluation of cardiac disorders utilizes objective testing such as exercise testing. Pulmonary function tests are the cornerstone of pulmonary disability evaluation. However, hematologic disabilities may result in diverse abnormalities in body functions that interfere with one's ability to work and compete in the open labor market. As always, disability assessments should be made only when the disease process is reasonably stable.

Rather than dealing with a specific hematologic disease on its own, it is more reasonable to group various hematologic entities into categories according to how they affect body function and their impact on activities of daily living (ADLs). These categories are as follows: red blood cell (RBC) diseases, white blood cell (WBC) diseases, coagulation defects, thrombosis, and acquired immunodeficiency syndrome (AIDS).

RBC DISEASES

Hematologic disorders may produce anemia, which decreases oxygen carrying capacity, resulting in exercise intolerance and fatigue. Mechanisms include interference with bone marrow production (as in leukemias), increased RBC destruction (as in hemolytic anemias), or bleeding (caused by clotting disorders). Hemoglobinopathies, including sickle cell disease, are associated with alterations of the erythrocyte that cause anemia. Myelofibrosis produces anemia by interfering with bone marrow production and is associated with fibrosis of the marrow. Whatever the mechanism, the development of anemia will cause impairment and subsequent disability. Erythrocytosis, on the other hand, rarely produces impairment/disability unless it is severe enough to produce vascular occlusion. (See the section on thrombosis.)

The complete cardiopulmonary exercise stress test (CPEST) (see Chapter 24) is of value when assessing disability due to anemia. A person's maximum exercise capabilities can be quantitated and these capabilities can be compared with job descriptions and the energy costs of various activities. Of concern in impairment evaluation, the CPEST only provides global assessments of exercise capabilities without discriminating between the effects of the anemia and possible coexistent diseases such as cardiac or pulmonary problems. For the disability assessment, that is only of minor concern, as the goal of the assessment is to arrive at work or activity capabilities/incapacitation.

Another method is to utilize the ADLs to determine a claimant's ability to work. Anemia occurs regularly in acute leukemia and frequently in chronic leukemia. The level of hemoglobin generally correlates with the level of fatigue, although there can be individual differences in two people's work capabilities even with the same level of anemia. If the development of the anemia is more rapid, such as in acute leukemia or in acute bleeding, then a person is more likely to be symptomatic earlier and more profoundly. If the anemia develops slowly, such as in chronic leukemia, then a worker will tolerate lower levels of hemoglobin with little reduction in work capabilities due to compensatory mechanisms. This is due to compensatory RBC (increase in the 2,3-diphosphoglycerate [DPG]) on this and other organ systems. In general terms, if the hemoglobin remains greater than 9 gm%, in the person with chronic anemia, a worker should be able to maintain reasonably normal job duties. Once the hemoglobin approaches 7 gm%, a reduction in work capacity is obvious, although an occasional worker will report normal work habits at levels at or below 7 gm%. Heavy labor, of course, will mitigate this general rule.

A suggested classification for the disturbances in ADLs for hematologic disorders appears in Table 66–1. This functional classification is in effect a description of the ADL. In taking a patient's history, the examiner determines the level that a worker was capable of prior to the illness and compares it to the activities tolerated at the time of evaluation with the reduced hemoglobin. One can estimate the percentage of work efforts lost (see following example).

■ A construction worker who regularly did heavy work, including lifting of 100 pounds or more, developed chronic myelocytic leukemia (CML). The disease process was controlled with therapy and hemoglobin levels were stable between 8 and 9 gm%. He was unable to tolerate his previous heavy job but was able to tolerate light work. He was transferred successfully to the position of inspector where he would spend 8 hours per day walking, standing, or sitting, with minimal demands for physical activity. One could estimate therefore that he lost approximately 50% of his preinjury capacity to work as a result of this hematologic disease.

A similar worker with CML and more advanced disease maintained a hemoglobin of only 7 gm% and suffered from chronic fatigue. He was only capable of working in a modified position in an office setting. The disability recommendations would restrict him to a more sedentary job only.

The AMA Guides, fifth edition,[1] also uses transfusion requirements when assessing rating impairment (see Table 9–2, p 193). Such transfusion requirements vary by the nature or cause of the anemia. Hemolytic anemias and acute bleeding will require blood transfusions more frequently, whereas relatively stable anemias such as sickle cell anemia and other hemoglobinopathies require less. The frequency of blood transfusions can interfere with ADLs, and one should correlate this with the disability (see following example).

■ A patient with CML is stable with a hemoglobin at 9 gm%. He is asymptomatic and works as a mechanic. The examiner would assign a descriptive term such as "no very heavy work," which would translate to a percentage disability in certain jurisdictions.

Another person with chronic hemolytic anemia fatigues with activities beyond sedentary. His hemoglobin is approximately 7 gm% despite transfusions every 6 to 8 weeks. He is restricted to sedentary work. Additionally, because of his frequent transfusion-requirements, he would likely have frequent periods of temporary disability.

Therefore, whatever the mechanism of the anemia, once the hematologic condition is stable, and by utilizing the CPEST, the frequency of transfusion requirements, and Table 66–1, the examiner can make a disability assessment.

TABLE 66–1

Functional Classification of Hematologic System Disease

Class	Description
I (None)	No signs or symptoms of disease despite laboratory abnormalities; individual performs the usual activities of daily living.
III (Minimal)	Some signs or symptoms of disease; individual performs the usual activities of daily living with some difficulty.
II (Moderate)	Signs and symptoms of disease; individual requires varying amounts of assistance from others to perform the usual activities of daily living.
IV (Marked)	Signs and symptoms of disease; individual requires assistance to perform most or all activities of daily living.

From Cocchiarella L, Andersson GBJ (eds): Guides to the Evaluation of Permanent Impairment, 5th ed. Chicago, American Medical Association, 2001, p 192, with permission.

WBC DISEASES

Hematologic conditions may increase a person's risk of infections. Leukemias reduce the WBC count and conditions like multiple myeloma interfere with the production of gamma globulin by producing clones of WBCs that produce abnormal globulins.

Leukemias are a group of diseases caused by the development of abnormal clones of WBCs. Acute leukemia develops rapidly and if unsuccessfully treated can be fatal within months. Chronic leukemia is more insidious and individuals may live for years and continue to work. Unless complete remission occurs in workers with acute leukemia, they generally remain totally disabled. The effects of the disease process itself and the toxic effects of chemotherapy generally preclude employment. Chronic leukemias, on the other hand, may last for years and are compatible with employment depending on the RBC count.

The WBC count usually does not increase the risk for infection by itself until the count falls well below 5000/cc. Decreases in WBC occur in hematologic malignancies (such as leukemia), drug reactions (such as agranulocytosis), and aplastic anemias (whether idiopathic or chemically induced). Low WBC counts can also occur in systemic diseases (such as systemic lupus erythematosus) or viral infections (such as human immunodeficiency virus [HIV]). The AMA Guides, fifth

TABLE 66–2

Criteria for Rating Permanent Impairment Due to White Blood Cell Disease

Class 1: 0% to 15% Impairment of the Whole Person	Class 2: 16% to 30% Impairment of the Whole Person	Class 3: 31% to 55% Impairment of the Whole Person	Class 4: 56% to 100% Impairment of the Whole Person
Symptoms or signs of leukocyte abnormality **and** needs no or infrequent treatment **and** performs all or most daily activities	Symptoms and signs of leukocyte abnormality **and** performs most daily activities, although requires continuous treatment	Requires continuous treatment **and** interference with the ability to perform daily activities; requires occasional assistance from others	Symptoms and signs of leukocyte abnormality **and** requires continuous treatment **and** experiences difficulty in performing activities of daily living; requires continuous care from others

From Cocchiarella L, Andersson GBJ (eds): Guides to the Evaluation of Permanent Impairment, 5th ed. Chicago, American Medical Association, 2001, p 200, with permission.

edition[1] utilizes the ADL as a major determinant of the severity of impairment to determine impairment in WBC disease (Table 66–2).

The criteria do not rely on the actual WBC count itself but rather on the effects on the ADLs and the need for treatment. Therefore, when discussing impairment and disability caused by WBC disorders, it is more reasonable to discuss the resulting complications such as infection and the need for treatment and discussing their interferences in the ADLs (see following example).

■ An individual with aplastic anemia has WBC counts of 1500 and below, has frequent skin and respiratory infections, and requires frequent courses of antibiotics that interfere with his duties as a clerk. Based on Table 66–2 and the interferences in his ADL, he has a disability limiting him to light work.

Hematologic malignancies, such as macroglobulinemia or multiple myeloma, also predispose to infections. When one considers disability due to WBC disease, factors other than the actual WBC count often determine the disability rating.

COAGULATION DISORDERS

"Coagulation disorders" refers to any disease process that interferes with the various blood elements that maintain hemostasis. The interference with these blood elements causes coagulation defects and, thus, a bleeding disorder. Examples include platelet abnormalities (either quantitative or qualitative), deficiency of plasma clotting factors, or production of anticlotting factors (such as in lupus anticoagulant or fibrinolysins). Coagulation defects are a result of a variety of hematologic disorders. In leukemia, the bone marrow infiltration reduces the numbers of megakaryocytes, which are the precursors for platelets. Immune reactions (such as in drug reactions or in lupus) reduce platelets by interfering with the release of platelets from megakaryocytes in the marrow. Immune processes can cause increased peripheral destruction of platelets (such as in idiopathic thrombocytopenic purpura [ITP]).

In general, platelet counts above 50,000/cc should not cause bleeding and therefore do not cause a work restriction. Between 10,000 and 50,000, bleeding can occur with surgery or trauma but spontaneous bleeding is not likely to occur. At platelet counts below 10,000, even minor trauma can cause bleeding and spontaneous bleeding may occur. At platelet counts below 5000, there is high risk for spontaneous bleeding, including intracranial hemorrhage. Therapy with platelet transfusions, steroids, and splenectomy (if appropriate) is needed, as well as specific treatment for the disease process causing this disorder. At platelet counts below 5000, impairment may not be evident if bleeding has not occurred, but because of the high likelihood of spontaneous bleeding, the evaluator must consider the actual platelet count and estimate the risk of spontaneous, atraumatic bleeding. One should consider the nature of the job and the prophylactic restrictions that should be given based on the job description and whether that job description contains a significant risk for trauma and subsequent bleeding, as in the following example:

■ A machine worker sustains frequent cuts on the job. He has ITP and his platelet counts, after therapy, are approximately 20,000/cc or below. This worker requires a change of occupation and the need for vocational rehabilitation to lessen the chance for traumatic bleeding.

Other coagulation disorders restrict a person's ability to work depending on the level of the abnormality and the nature of the work. A worker may be found to have a plasma clotting factor deficiency, either congenital or acquired, which is mild enough not to be detected in early life. Mild hemophiliacs, with an antihemophilic globulin of greater than 1%, are unlikely to have spontaneous bleeding but are at high risk for bleeding with trauma. A lupus patient developing a lupus anticoagulant may be at risk for bleeding even though there is no spontaneous bleeding at rest. Von Willenbrand's disorder, the most common hereditary hemorrhagic disorder, results in increased bleeding time with a slight reduction of the antihemophilic globulin, generally causing bleeding only after surgery or trauma. These individuals may have no impairment but would need to have prophylactic work restrictions to prevent trauma.

Workers with an antihemophilic globulin of less than 0.1% or with a platelet count of less than 5000 are at high risk of spontaneous bleeding and therefore have limited safe employment opportunities. Here again, one must evaluate the clinical picture and estimate the ability to continue work without significant risk and, if appropriate, give descriptive prophylactic work restrictions as the disability rating.

Additionally, impairment and disability ratings in these individuals will also reflect the damage to other organ systems due to the coagulation disorder (see following example).

■ A hemophiliac with repetitive, spontaneous, or traumatic bleeds into the joints will develop hemarthrosis that interferes with joint function. His disability also needs to take into account the joint damage and loss of function.

THROMBOTIC DISORDERS

Thrombotic disorders are hematologic conditions that predispose a person to develop blood clots in arteries and/or veins, thus interfering with the blood supply to or from a part of the body. Such disorders can be inherited; examples include protein C, protein S, or antithrombin III deficiencies and Factor V Leiden mutation. Blood factors such as antiphospholipids produce thrombosis and some malignancies produce blood clotting factors that in turn may result in multiple venous thromboses. Physical factors such as postsurgical states, immobility, and pregnancy can predispose to thrombosis. Drugs such as oral contraceptives may create a hypercoagulable state. Other causes include metabolic disorders (such as hyperhomocystenemia) and primary blood disorders (such as polycythemia vera or hereditary thrombocythemia).

The impairment evaluation reflects the damage and severity of the damage of the various organs whose blood supply is interfered with. The disability depends on this damage and its interference with one's work. Examples include the effects of strokes, myocardial infarction, mesenteric insufficiency, amputations of limbs, and chronic venous insufficiency. Those individuals with thrombotic disorders may have no abnormalities at the time of evaluation. For these individuals prophylactic restrictions for certain activities causing trauma or stasis may be necessary.

AIDS

AIDS impairment and disability depend on the clinical state of the disease. A positive HIV antibody test with no clinical disease and relatively normal CD4 counts implies functioning cellular immunity and/or response to treatment. When the disease progresses, damage to various organ systems can be assessed. For example, Pneumocystis pneumonia can cause lung impairment, which, when stable, can be rated on a pulmonary basis. HIV neuropathies can be rated on a neurologic basis. When the CD4 count falls below 200 cells/mm, a high risk of infection may prevent a person from working at a job due to the risk of infection even though the AIDS may not be clinically active (see following example).

■ A health care worker or a schoolteacher with HIV who comes in contact with individuals who may transmit respiratory or gastrointestinal infections would be at higher risk for acquiring these infections when his or her CD4 count is below 200 cells/mm. Therefore, prophylactic work restrictions for these individuals are appropriate.

One must also consider the treatment of AIDS. With multiple drug therapy, particularly with the protease inhibitors, there has been a dramatic reversal in short-term mortality and quality of life. These drugs have potential toxicities, including abnormal fat deposits, cardiac problems, and diabetes. One must therefore consider the impairment of any organ system damaged, not only by AIDS but also by its treatment, and determine work restrictions by these impairments.

Reference

1. Cocchiarella L, Andersson GBJ (eds): Guides to the Evaluation of Permanent Impairment, 5th ed. Chicago, American Medical Association, 2001.

SECTION

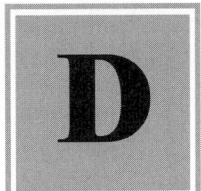

Neurological Disability

CHAPTER

67

Central Nervous System Disability

EDWIN H. KLIMEK, MD, FRCPC, FAADEP

Advances in general health have increased the lifespan and long-term survival of individuals with central nervous system (CNS) disorders. Although the magnitude of the societal effect is dependent on the definition of a CNS disorder, 1.4% of all deaths but 28% of all years of life lived with a disability result from CNS disorders.[45] The unrecognized demographic effect of pediatric CNS disability can be compared to the iceberg that shows only a fraction of its full mass. In the United States, 10% of children aged birth to 18 years have a chronic illness or disability.[35] The World Health Organization has ranked the disabling global effects of conditions. The Global Burden of Disease Study documents international statistics on the burden of diseases combining mortality and disability. For this study, a universal disability weighting was established for evaluation and priority setting in a wide range of health disorders.[71] According to the Global Burden of Disease Study, cerebrovascular accidents are the second leading cause of mortality worldwide, with 3 million of 4.4 million deaths arising in developing countries.[49] Leading causes of disability-adjusted life years (DALYs) predicted by the baseline model were (in descending order) ischemic heart disease, unipolar major depression, road-traffic accidents, cerebrovascular disease, chronic obstructive pulmonary disease, lower respiratory infections, tuberculosis, war injuries, diarrheal diseases, and human immunodeficiency virus (HIV).[48] The two major forces propelling the impact of disability globally are the demographic transition of aging and an increased burden of noncommunicable diseases.[9] By 2020, stroke will become the second most common cause of DALYs (Table 67–1).

TABLE 67–1
Disorders Ranked by Disability Adjusted Life Years

Health Condition	Rank	Median	Mean (SD)
Quadriplegia	1	2	3.3 (3.2)
Dementia	2	4	4.9 (3.6)
Active psychosis	3	4	5.3 (3.6)
Paraplegia	4	5	5.9 (3.3)
Blindness	5	6	6.8 (4.0)
Major depression	6	6	6.8 (4.0)
Drug dependence	7	8	7.8 (3.9)
HIV infection	8	9	8.8 (5.2)
Alcoholism	9	9	9.2 (3.6)
Total deafness	10	10	9.4 (3.7)
Mild mental retardation	11	10	9.9 (3.6)
Incontinence	12	10	10.2 (4.1)

HIV, human immunodeficiency virus.

These data suggest that research into neurodisability and rehabilitation is urgently required. Valid clinical evaluations from medical professionals trained in neurologic disease and well versed in impairment and disability will be a growth industry. To a great extent these individuals are currently largely self-taught. In part this is because medical training does not recognize disability medicine as an area of specialty pursuit or academic interest. As a result, practical instruction in evaluation is limited or nonexistent. Students are typically not given even rudimentary instruction, such as avoiding conflicting attending care duties when evaluating disability. This conflict of interest compromises the patient care relationship by casting doubt on the advocacy role of the doctor when functioning as the evaluating physician. Simultaneously rating impairment within a therapeutic ongoing patient-physician relationship permits allegations of medical negligence, professional misconduct, and collusion with the third party requesting a disability evaluation.

WORKPLACE INJURY AND DISABILITY

Motivation for study of impairment and disability arose from concern about workplace safety and compensation for injured workers. This social conscience emerged out of the industrial revolution in the 1800s and a new employer-worker relationship. In England, safeguards legislated in the 19th century enabled injured workers to claim guaranteed benefits, or to bring a case to the courts under the common law. In 19th century Germany a system was based on collective responsibility and administered by the state to ensure that the cost of industrial accidents was shared among society, industry, and government. In North America, labor movements gained strength and a worker's injury became compensable beyond his or her wage. That this may not always coincide with the dominant economic interest of any region or state can be seen from the resistance of employers today. North American workers' compensation legislation responded to the changes demanded by the industrial revolution and the rise of trade unionism, although Canada and the United States had slightly different responses to this challenge.

OUTCOME ASSESSMENT SCALES

The neurodisability evaluator is required to produce a numeric or scaled estimate of disability or impairment. These estimates should be based on a thorough understanding of the disease process or injury. Documentation of the manifestations of the injury or disease requires consideration of outcome measures and investigations that have been excerpted from their original setting. As a result the evaluator must be familiar with the origin and intent of outcomes measurement before any interpretation is possible. Often the clinician is familiar with mortality, laboratory values, symptoms, and signs as endpoints, but function in terms of motor, psychological, social, cognitive, and vocational performance and quality of life are foreign concepts.

In training, medical doctors are exposed to the Glasgow Coma Scale (GCS) (Fig. 67–1), which serves as a useful example of the utility and misuse of a scale. Clinicians studying the course of brain-injured patients developed the GCS. Coma was defined on the GCS as a score of 8 or less. The patient who showed no eye opening (1), did not obey commands (5), or give any comprehensible verbal response (2) was considered comatose. The clinical profile of the original case published by the authors follows (Fig. 67–2). The best GCS score predicts the potential of patients to recover from coma, providing complications do not develop. The GCS was designed to evaluate individual patients and distinguish clinically meaningful changes in consciousness. However it has been appropriated to characterize extent of brain injury outside of this clinical context.

The GCS is an examination-based global outcome scale. There are two types of outcome scales commonly encountered in the practice of disability evaluation: global outcome scales and activity of daily living (ADL) measurements. Global outcome scales measure severity of illness using defined criteria and ADL measurements estimate the burden imposed by the illness on patients or caregivers. Outcomes scales can be either specific for a disease of interest or nonspecific. Outcome scales are used in two mutually excusive ways. Discriminative scales measure differences between people and evaluative scales measure changes in the same individual. For example, height and intelligence tests compare individuals and are therefore discriminative, but pain questionnaires estimate change in the same individual and are therefore evaluative.

Outcome scales are also developed to monitor outcomes in large groups of patients when detailed studies of functions are not needed or impossible given time constraints. Most are not sufficiently sensitive to monitor individuals. The presumption of unbiased cooperation of the patient is inherent in the design of most clinical trials by virtue of double blinded assessment. The utility of these scales in the unblended clinical setting is not always clear.

All scales allocate specific outcomes to ordinal or linear representations of nondimensional phenomenae amalgamating diverse features.[42] Scales can be either single state scales measuring disease severity at a point in time or transition scales indicating change in severity of a disease process. The hierarchical progression suggests rankings are discrete, nonoverlapping and reasonable in the allocation of order, responsive to change, and of proven reliability and validity. This aura of mathematical authority may exceed the clinical importance of the scale scores or score differences.

VALIDITY OF OUTCOME SCALES

Validity refers to the extent something actually accomplishes whatever it purports to do. A valid outcome scale used to estimate neurodisability must actually measure neurodisability. Valid measurements that also precisely reflect changes in severity of an underlying condition are responsive measurements. A valid measurement is free of systematic and random error. Measurements must be reliable to be valid, but reliable, precise measurements, without random or systematic error, still may not be valid. For example, measurement of height and weight is not a valid estimate of athletic ability. Reliability is an index of reproducibility of results from repeated trials. Reliability presumes understanding the effects of random error and can also be considered an estimate of precision.

Validity is subdivided into content validity, criterion-related validity, construct validity, and others. Content validity is an index of how well the instrument reflects the components of what is being measured. If the scale

Pupil scale (mm)				TIME
1	COMA SCALE	EYES OPEN	4 SPONTANEOUSLY	
2			3 TO SPEECH	
3			2 TO PAIN	
4			1 NONE	
5		BEST VERBAL RESPONSE	5 ORIENTED	
6			4 CONFUSED	
7			3 INAPPROPRIATE WORDS	
8			2 INCOMPREHENSIVE	
			1 NONE	
		BEST MOTOR RESPONSE	6 OBEY COMMANDS	
			5 LOCALIZES TO PAIN	
			4 FLEXION WITHDRAWAL	
			3 ABNORMAL FLEXION	
			2 EXTENSION	
			1 FLACCID	
	TOTAL →			
	PUPIL	RIGHT	SIZE	
			REACTION	
		LEFT	SIZE	
			REACTION	

Figure 67–1. Glasgow Coma Scale.

demonstrates that outcomes are clustered at one part the scale is difficult to interpret. Criterion validity is a comparison of the instrument to another measurement scale or, ideally, the gold standard. Concurrent validity is best demonstrated if the gold standard and the instrument correlate closely. Predictive validity relates scores of the instrument to the future changes of the system under examination. Discriminant validity refers to the ability of the scale to differentiate among observations. Convergent validity refers to the close correlation with other instruments of measurement.

Construct validity is a measure of compatibility with a theoretical framework without regard to the merits of the theory. The theoretical framework itself may be erroneous even if a measurement demonstrates excellent construct validity. Valid and reliable measurements may be meaningless if casuality is unproven. A delightful example[2] (acknowledgement is made to Dr. Phil Osbourne) relates to the construct validity of the sunrise's relationship to the rooster and the alarm clock. Convergent validity is demonstrated each and every day that the rooster crows and the alarm sounds upon

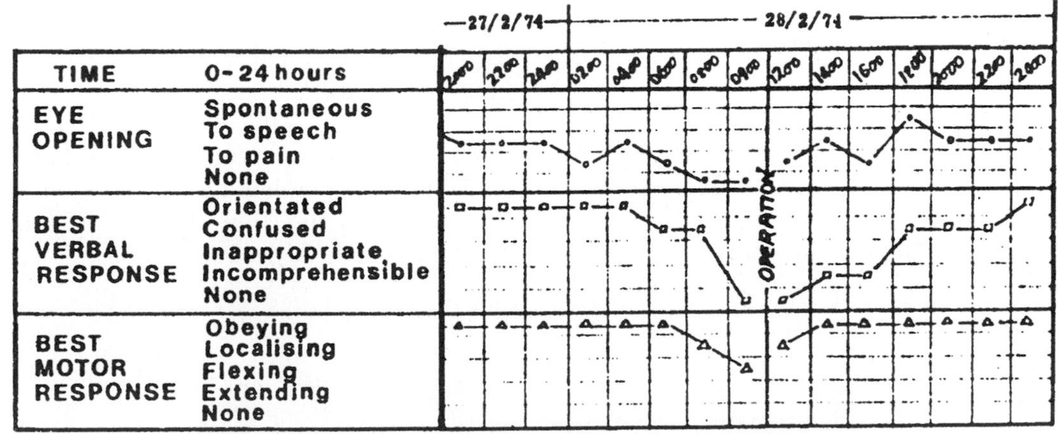

Figure 67–2. Glasgow Coma Scale clinical course. (From Teasdale G, Jennet B: Assessment of coma and impaired consciousness: A practical scale. Lancet 2:81–84, 1974.)

sunrise. Discriminant validity is untested until the sun fails to rise or the rooster fails to crow or the alarm fails to ring. Note the theoretical notion that the rooster or the alarm causes the sun to rise is neither supported nor refuted by the most reliable and precise measurements. In other words, causality is not established by valid and reliable measurements. Outcome scales may be validated in specific disorders but one must ensure that validation is relevant to the disability evaluation.

Even if a scale is valid and reliable, it may still be incapable of application in a specific circumstance because it is insensitive at the extremes. Scales usually have a "ceiling" or a "basement" effect inherent in their design intent. For example, Grade 8 on the Rancho Los Amigos Scale could be further subdivided readily. Nevertheless, the patient cannot be graded above Grade 8, yet a patient with a Grade 8 on the Rancho Los Amigos Scale may not be "normal."

Rancho Los Amigos Scale

1. No response
2. Generalized response
3. Localized response
4. Confused agitated
5. Confused inappropriate
6. Confused appropriate
7. Automatic appropriate
8. Purposeful appropriate

Some scales are intended only for institutionalized patients and used in forecasting death rates.[72] For example, a Barthel Index[43] score greater than 60 correlates with return home and greater than 95 score indicates independent self care. The Barthel Index lacks evaluation of cognitive and language function. This shortcoming of this scale has encouraged enhanced scales with expanded subcategories. One such scale is the Functional Independence Measure.[28] This adds communication (expression and comprehension) and social cognition (social interaction, problem solving, and memory).

Barthel Index

Feeding
Moving from wheelchair to bed and return
Personal toilet
Getting on and off toilet
Bathing self
Walking on level surface
Ascending and descending stairs
Dressing
Controlling bowels
Controlling bladder

The Rankin Disability Scale[54] is another example of a validated ordinal scale in wide use in outcome assessment.

Rankin Disability Scale

Grade 1—No significant disability; able to carry out all usual duties of daily living
Grade 2—Slight disability; unable to carry out some previous activities but able to look after own affairs without assistance
Grade 3—Moderate disability; requires some help but able to walk without assistance
Grade 4—Moderately severe disability; unable to walk or attend to own bodily needs without assistance
Grade 5—Severe disability; bedridden, incontinent, and requiring constant nursing care and attention

QUALITY OF LIFE, SELF PERCEPTION, AND FAMILY PERCEPTION SCALES

Outcome scales tend to rely on an examiner to undertake direct observation or examination, but there is also a case for including self-reported quality of life measurements into outcome assessment.[14,19] Often the disability evaluator is given a self-report of perceived impairment (e.g., Oswestry Low Back Pain Disability Questionnaire[23]). The Oswestry is a valid measure of a person's perceived disability. Experienced evaluators usually compare their own understanding of the case with the examinee's self-perception as an insight into the possibility of symptom magnification.

In some studies it has been felt that observations made by family members may contribute to more accurate assessment as clinicians may miss subtle changes. For example, the Geriatric Evaluation by Relatives Rating Instrument (GERRI) scale[63] used 49 items of interest to evaluate the at-home functioning of geriatric patients that were considered to be areas of cognitive functioning, social functioning, and mood. It is noteworthy that raters estimated the mood component to be the least reliable as mood must be verbalized to be evaluated. Items dependent on verbalization of symptoms—i.e., self-reporting that did not obtain acceptable reliability—include the following:

Wakes up at night
Daytime drowsiness
Awakens in the early morning and unable to go back to sleep
Poor appetite
Reports feeling faint and dizzy
Reports muscular aches and light backaches

Reports feeling tired and lacking energy
Sexually inappropriate
Reports feeling nervous
Reports pain in chest or heart
Reports heart irregularities (beating faster or pounding)
Reports nausea
Reports stomach upset

DISEASE-SPECIFIC SCALES

The abovementioned scales are nonspecific and may be used to measure outcome regardless of etiology. For example, the GCS estimates brain injury severity without regard to etiology. This contrasts with disease-specific outcome measurements that have the desirable feature of inclusion of all manifestations of the disease of interest. The significance of these manifestations in terms of functional impairment may not be independently weighted. An example of this type of scale is the Expanded Disability Status Scale (EDSS).[38] In 1983, the EDSS considered eight functional systems intended to be independent of each other and, in combination, reflecting all manifestations of neurologic impairment in multiple sclerosis. These subsections were pyramidal, cerebellar, brainstem, sensory, bowel and bladder, visual, cerebral or mental, and other. The first four refer to impairment of body parts below the head; brainstem refers to cranial nerves 3 through 12. The EDSS, shown in Table 67–2, is clearly an examination-based scale.

Although the EDSS contains steps 1.0 to 10.0, the arithmetic linearity of the scale is deceptive. An EDSS score of 4 is not "twice as bad" as 2. The lowest grades (up to step 4.0) presume the ability to ambulate fully for 500 meters and carry out full daily activities, and are determined by impairment of functional systems. The principle of objective abnormality without impairment of function is accepted with step 3.0, being "mild impairment without impeding normal functions except in rare individuals (steeplejacks or concert pianists)." Graphing the EDSS gives the appearance of a Gaussian distribution, wrongly suggesting that estimates of central tendencies such as means and standard deviations might be meaningful. The EDSS correlates with the magnetic resonance imaging–defined volume of plaque burden closely for pyramidal subscores. This probably indicates that factors other than volumetrically determined lesion load are important determinants for disability.[56]

STROKE

Data on stroke survival and outcome are available to permit planning of health and social policy. Stroke outcome scales are useful in comparing effects of treatment outcome. The difficulty in such a scale is to select clinical endpoints that are reasonably straightforward and still reflect the consequences of stroke on physical, psychological, and social performance. For example, the Scandinavian Stroke Study published in 1985 was designed to observe the effect of hemodilution in ischemic stroke during the first 24 hours. The Scandinavian Stroke Scale (SSS) was devised to assess medical impairment due to stroke and monitor outcome of treatment.[60] The SSS was subdivided into nine sections comprising consciousness, eye movements, arm power, hand power, leg power, orientation, speech, facial palsy, and gait. Although the study failed to define a benefit to treatment it prompted a series of other stroke-specific impairment scales and thoughtful review of outcome measures in stroke.[74]

Subsequent stroke scales were as notable due to the success or failure of the clinical trial with which they were associated, as much as to their inherent value. These include the Canadian Neurologic Scale,[16] the European Stroke Scale (ESS),[30] and the National Institute of Neurologic Disorders and Stroke Scale (NINDS),[50] among others. As a practical choice at the author's institution, the ESS was chosen by nursing staff after considering the nursing time required in training and administering the various scales (about 3 minutes); neurology staff use the NINDS for specific protocols of acute treatment. In all of these scales, the depression that follows stroke is not recognized as an outcome or in its contribution to disability. This is one of the unmet needs in neurodisability, more common in patients with left frontal lobe infaractions than in right hemisphere or brainstem stroke.[57]

DEMENTIA

The Mini-Mental State Examination (MMSE)[17] is in common use for screening patients with cognitive disorders. The score of the MMSE is age- and education-dependent in the normal population, suggesting that the threshold to be considered abnormal must be adjusted.[29] The median MMSE score is 29 for individuals with at least 9 years of schooling, 26 for those with 5 to 8 years of schooling, and 22 for those with 0 to 4 years of schooling. The score of the MMSE fluctuates and is of limited value in individual patients for periods less than 3 years because of a large measurement error.[15] This scale has a window suitable for only a narrow segment of the spectrum of neurodisability due to dementia. Using a score of 23 as a cutoff, the sensitivity and specificity for the MMSE is 87% and 82%, respectively, for detecting delirium in hospitalized patients. The score of the MMSE does not provide a specific diagnosis: patients with dementia, delirium, retardation, schizophrenia, or depression obtain low scores.

Other scales specifically designed for dementia trials include the Global Deterioration Scale, which identifies seven stages of cognitive decline,[55] and the Alzheimer's Disease Assessment Scale, with 21 cognitive items of

TABLE 67-2

Kurtzke Expanded Disability Status Scale (EDSS)

0.0—Normal neurologic examination (all grade 0 in all functional system [FS] scores).

1.0—No disability, minimal signs in one FS (i.e., grade 1).

1.5—No disability, minimal signs in more than one FS (more than one grade 1).

2.0—Minimal disability in one FS (one FS grade 2, others 0 or 1).

2.5—Minimal disability in two FS (two FS grade 2, others 0 or 1).

3.0—Moderate disability in one FS (one FS grade 3, others 0 or 1) or mild disability in three or four FS (three or four FS grade 2, others 0 or 1) although fully ambulatory.

3.5—Fully ambulatory but with moderate disability in one FS (one grade 3) and one or two FS grade 2; or two grade 3 (others 0 or 1) or 5 grade 2 (others 0 or 1).

4.0—Fully ambulatory without aid, self-sufficient, up and about some 12 hours a day despite relatively severe disability consisting of one FS grade 4 (others 0 or 1), or combination of lesser grades exceeding limits of previous steps and the patient should be able to walk >500 meters without assist or rest.

4.5—Fully ambulatory without aid, up and about much of the day, may otherwise require minimal assistance; characterized by relatively severe disability usually consisting of one FS grade 4 (others 0 or 1) or combinations of lesser grades exceeding limits of previous steps and walks >300 meters without assist or rest.

5.0—Ambulatory without aid for at least 50 meters; disability severe enough to impair full daily activities (e.g., to work a full day without special provision). (Usual FS equivalents are one grade 5 alone, others 0 or 1; or combinations of lesser grades.) Patient walks >200 meters without aid or rest.

5.5—Ambulatory without aid for at least 100 meters; disability severe enough to preclude full daily activities. (Usual FS equivalents are one grade 5 alone, others 0 or 1; or combinations of lesser grades.) Enough to preclude full daily activities. (Usual FS equivalents are one grade 5 alone, others 0 or 1; or combinations of lesser grades.)

6.0—Intermittent or unilateral constant assistance (cane, crutch, brace) required to walk at least 100 meters. (Usual FS equivalents are combinations with more than one FS grade 3.)

6.5—Constant bilateral assistance (canes, crutches, braces) required to walk at least 20 meters. (Usual FS equivalents are combinations with more than one FS grade 3.)

7.0—Unable to walk at least 5 meters even with aid, essentially restricted to wheelchair; wheels self and transfers alone; up and about in wheelchair some 12 hours a day. (Usual FS equivalents are combinations with more than one FS grade 4+; very rarely pyramidal grade 5 alone.)

7.5—Unable to take more than a few steps; restricted to wheelchair; may need aid in transfer; wheels self but cannot carry on in wheelchair a full day. (Usual FS equivalents are combinations with more than one FS grade 4+; very rarely pyramidal grade 5 alone.)

8.0—Essentially restricted to chair or perambulated in wheelchair, but out of bed most of day; retains many self-care functions; generally has effective use of arms. (Usual FS equivalents are combinations, generally grade 4+ in several systems.)

8.5—Essentially restricted to bed most of day; has some effective use of arm(s); retains some self-care functions. (Usual FS equivalents are combinations, generally 4 in several systems.)

9.0—Helpless bed patient; can communicate and eat. (Usual FS equivalents are combinations, mostly grade 4+.)

9.5—Totally helpless bed patient; unable to communicate effectively or eat or swallow. (Usual FS equivalents are combinations, almost all grade 4+.)

10.0—Death due to MS.

which 60% are weighted toward cognitive and memory tasks.[58] The latter was tested on patients who were screened for mild to moderate dementia. Patients with severe behavioral dysfunction were not included.

EPILEPSY

The causes of sudden loss of consciousness are extensive, but are broadly either neurologic or cardiovascular in origin. The most important differentiation is that of convulsive syncope from epilepsy, the main neurologic deficit.[75] Epilepsy is distinct among diseases for fleeting yet severe impact on employment, social life, and sense of well-being. Epilepsy studies of recurrence after a first tonic-clonic seizure give conflicting predictions of recurrence, with a meta-analysis suggesting a 2-year risk of recurrence greater than 40%.[5] Epilepsy is also unique as a potential cause of paroxysmal behavioral change that has on rare occasion been raised as a defense for violent crime.[70]

A difficulty commonly encountered in neurodisability evaluations involving epilepsy ensues after the evaluation is completed. Employers are hesitant to recognize that their employees, despite having epilepsy, are not disabled if reasonable accommodations can be made. The employer is often reluctant to allow these individuals to continue at the workplace, fearing workplace disruption or repercussion of potential workplace injury. Objections from employers or other partisan advocates become adversarial. The "reasonableness" of the accommodation is not a medical issue.

The other issue generating antagonism concerns the privilege to drive. The Epilepsy Foundation of America states: "While the Epilepsy Foundation of America opposes mandatory physician reporting laws, it does support state laws which give physicians 'good faith' immunity for participating in the driver licensing process, and for voluntarily reporting those patients, who pose an imminent threat to public safety because they are driving against medical advice. 'Good faith' should be defined as acting in accordance with a reasonable standard of care."[20]

All jurisdictions regulate eligibility of persons with certain medical conditions to possess a driver's license. The most common requirement for people with epilepsy is that they be seizure free for a specified period of time and submit a physician's evaluation of their ability to drive safely. Some jurisdictions require a 1-year seizure-free period and allow exceptions under which a license may be issued after a shorter period. Spudis et al[66] reviewed episodic brain dysfunction and suggested that idiopathic isolated attacks should be treated more favorably than recurrent attacks with abnormal investigations. Examples of possible exceptions include a breakthrough seizure due to physician-directed medication change, an isolated seizure where the medical examination indicates that another episode appears unlikely, a seizure related to a temporary illness, a seizure due to an isolated incident of not taking medication, an established pattern of nocturnal seizures, an established pattern of seizures that do not impair driving ability, or an established pattern of an extended warning aura.

Patients who should not be driving or who should be driving only under certain circumstances should be so advised. Most physicians have a standard letter (or a form providing for specific variations) and many provide the patient with a copy. Whereas the confidential nature of the physician-patient relationship is of the utmost importance, some jurisdictions have an explicit reporting requirement the physician should call to the patient's attention. Six states (California, Delaware, Nevada, New Jersey, Oregon, and Pennsylvania) currently have mandatory physician reporting requirements. The exact requirements vary in Canada.[11,25,52] They generally state that any physician who diagnoses or treats a person with epilepsy must report that person's name, age, and address to a central state agency, usually the Department of Motor Vehicles or Department of Public Safety. Some statutes give physicians immunity for their opinions and recommendations to the state DMV.

In refractory epilepsy, the role of the physician becomes more involved and additional sources of guidance are available in part developed as pharmaceutical instruments. Clinically significant changes in seizure frequency, type, and severity are outcome measurements of interest in clinical trials. As a result, validated patient-based seizure severity scales[3] were developed to reflect interventional effects. One should review these features when addressing impairment and disability issues in epilepsy.

TRAUMATIC BRAIN INJURY

The understanding of mild traumatic brain injury (MTBI) is evolving and sometimes confusing because the terms describing the study population have changed and are casually used and not carefully defined. Severe traumatic brain injury is obvious to the layperson and is infrequently mistaken. MTBI is less apparent. Disability following head injury varies depending on injury mechanism, neuropathology, and other factors, including medical complications.[41] The neuropathologic hallmark of severe brain injury is traumatically induced axonal injury.[53] It may result in partial or complete paralysis, speech problems, impaired cognitive functioning, disability from employment, long periods of coma, long-term care requirements, and CT, MRI, and other brain imaging changes.

Classification of head injury by the GCS[68] assesses motor and verbal responses along with eye opening on command to evaluate gross levels of consciousness after head injury. A score of 13 or above (out of 15 possible) places patients in the "mild" category for head trauma. In 1986, Jenkins et al studied 50 patients by MRI within 1 week of a head injury and found intracerebral lesions only in patients who had lost consciousness. These were present in most (29 of 42) but not all patients whose consciousness was still impaired on arrival at hospital.[33] Possibly the use of GCS scores 13 to 15 to define mild head injury permits excessive heterogeneity in injury severity and contributes to the variability in neurobehavioral outcome.[18] Some authors suggest that mild head injury should be redefined as a GCS score of 15 without acute radiographic abnormalities, whereas high-risk mild head injury should be defined as either GCS scores of 13 or 14 or a GCS score of 15 with acute radiographic abnormalities.[31]

MTBI may result from a head injury that is unaccompanied by a loss of consciousness.[6,21,39] The traumatic events that can cause an MTBI include the following:

- The head being struck
- The head striking an object
- Acceleration/deceleration movement without direct external trauma to the head

Symptoms may include headaches,[44] dizziness, lethargy, memory loss, irritability, personality changes, cognitive deficits, and/or perceptual changes. These symptoms have been characterized under various names, including minor head injury,[37] mild head injury,[4] closed head injury,[12] postconcussive syndrome,[8] postconcussional syndrome,[32] postconcussional disorder,[2] minor traumatic brain injury,[36] traumatic cephalgia, post brain injury syndrome, and post-traumatic syndrome.

A review by Andary et al of TBI refers to MTBI, noting that no single test is adequate to confirm the diagnosis. It indicates that the amount of trauma required to cause MTBI is unknown and that cumulative trauma from seemingly insignificant insults can cause abnormalities on neuropsychological testing, EEG, and CT scanning.[1] Treatment of these patients is geared toward the bias of each particular practitioner or clinic and the benefits of cognitive therapy are unproven.

Contrary to a popular perception, most patients with litigation or compensation claims are not cured by a verdict.[22] At least one study predating current terminology also suggested that litigation has a negligible effect on symptoms of post-concussion syndrome (PCS).[24] Others note that compensation claims were not associated with the rate of psychiatric illness,[64] suggesting that at least some individuals do not delay progress by either consciously or subconsciously "producing" MTBI symptoms. Analyses have revealed evidence of neuropsychological impairment in "minor head injury" patients suggesting that minor head injuries are not always innocuous, fully reversible conditions that resolve within days or a few weeks of injury. Rather, some patients appear to suffer enduring neuropsychological impairments.[39]

Depression is found after traumatic brain injury (TBI) and can impede the achievement of optimal functional outcome, whether in the acute or chronic stage of recovery. Symptoms may be temporary. After TBI with localized intracranial abnormalities the median duration for nonanxious depression was 1.5 months (7.5 months for anxious depressions, and 1.5 months for concurrent global anxiety disorder).[34] At least one article suggests that a combination of neuroanatomic, neurochemical, and psychosocial factors may be responsible for the onset and maintenance of depression.[46] It cannot be definitively concluded that the underlying substrates of depression seen after MTBI and clinical depression are the same.[10]

Contrary to this, others suggest that the symptoms of PCS may simply be attributable to the anticipation, widely held by individuals who have had no opportunity to observe or experience postconcussive symptoms, that PCS will occur following mild head injury.[47] Similarly, another study suggests the psychological reaction of preoccupation with symptoms and emotional distress is not unique to concussion. It also occurs after severe head injury and back injury and relates more to the personal interpretation of the effect of the trauma than to objective indicators of brain injury severity.[27] One group concluded there is no strong evidence for a specific effect of mild head injury on cognitive functioning.[59]

One review of individuals with mild closed head injury (CHI) indicates:

> . . . [T]he consensus is that minor head injuries are sufficient to produce cognitive deficit and postconcussional symptoms which have a characteristic time course of at least 2 to 6 weeks and possibly a residual decrement in cognitive capacity which is evident only under stressful conditions. Although individual differences in recovery are impressive, most persons experience at least a transient phase of reduced cognitive efficiency and emotional malaise during which they are vulnerable to secondary disturbances which often arise because of premature resumption of stressful activities. The converging lines of evidence support a neurogenic etiology for postconcussional symptoms and congitive sequelae during the early stage of recovery, whereas other factors probably account for the delayed onset and marked prolongation of these problems.[40]

DELAYED DIAGNOSIS OF MTBI

What if an individual involved in an accidental motor vehicle collision states that he or she did not see the car or did not recall telephoning from the emergency room (ER)? Was he or she confused, dazed, or disoriented? Were the emergency medical technicians, ER nurses, and ER doctors remiss in assessing the presentation? The Ontario Brain Injury Association advocates on behalf of the brain injured. It indicates the following about the use of the GCS in determining the presence of TBI at the time of the trauma:

> The best measures of GCS are those taken at the scene of the trauma (provided by trained Emergency Medical Technicians– EMTs) or upon admission to the Emergency Room of most hospitals in Ontario. These GCS assessments are generally expertly conducted although it is not unusual for an injured individual to have some variability in responsiveness from the time of the trauma to admission to the ER. For example, an individual can have limited alertness at the scene, and have a GCS say of 10, but deteriorate substantially on route to the hospital. The variability of response can continue within the ER. Emergency room staff (nurses, attending physicians, etc.) generally conducts a GCS assessment on a regular basis, perhaps even as often as every fifteen minutes. Again, these assessments are expertly done and usually quite accurate. However, the GCS can be affected by the use of sedating drugs or by intubation.[51]

If an altered state of consciousness is present with a brain injury, then a criterion of the American Congress of Rehabilitation Medicine (ACRM) for MTBI is met. However, meeting a criterion of the ACRM does not confirm a brain injury. Diagnostic errors may occur, in part because evidence for actual injury is hard to obtain in minor cases and most symptoms tend to be subjective and have high base rates in the normal, uninjured population.[73] It is a logical fallacy to permit membership in a category to substitute for confirmation of underlying cause. The ACRM classification becomes trivial if misused with absurd results.

WHIPLASH

"Whiplash" is a form of acceleration/deceleration injury sometimes seen with MTBI. The pathologic lesions accounting for chronically symptomatic whiplash injuries are by no means certain.[69] A complete review of the topic might suggest that divergent opinions exist about the significance and existence of whiplash injuries and the role of compensation for pain and suffering.[13] Some investigators found no evidence of a significant relation between detectable morphologic or functional brain damage and impaired cognitive performance in the late whiplash syndrome. Results indicate triggering of emotional and cognitive symptoms on the basis of initial injury of the cervical spine.[7] The theory of neuronal degeneration in the etiology of whiplash-related cognitive complaints is not supported, nor is the specificity of neuropsychological tests in detecting the subtle effects of brain trauma.[67] Some have stated that "the cognitive complaints of non-malingering post-whiplash patients are more likely a result of chronic pain, chronic fatigue or depression."[61]

However, it can be argued that a definitive understanding of this condition does not exist in part because selection bias has not permitted a truly representative cohort of accident victims to be followed prospectively.[26] Retrospective studies such as the Quebec Task Force Cohort Study[65] and the Lithuanian study[62] have suggested a high spontaneous recovery rate but could not answer fundamental questions based on accumulated data.

References

1. Andary MT, Vincent F, Esselman PC: Chronic pain following head injury. Office Management of Pain 4:141–150, 1993.
2. Anderson SD: Postconcussional disorder and loss of consciousness. Bull Am Acad Psychiatry Law 24:493–504, 1996.
3. Baker G, Smith D, Dewey M, et al: The development of Seizure Severity Scale as an outcome measure in epilepsy. Epilepsy Res 8:245–251, 1991.
4. Beers SR: Cognitive effects of mild head injury in children and adolescents. Neuropsychol Rev 3:281–320, 1992.
5. Berg AT, Shinnar S: The risk of seizure recurrance following a first unprovoked seizure: A quantitative review. Neurology 41:965–972, 1991.
6. Binder LM: Persisting symptoms after mild head injury: A review of the post-concussive syndrome. J Clin Exp Neuropsychol 8:323–346, 1986.
7. Bogdan RP, Bicik I, Dvorak J, et al: Relation between neuropsychological and neuroimaging findings in patients with late whiplash syndrome. J Neurol Neurosurg Psychiatry 66:485–489, 1999.
8. Bohnen N, Jolles J: Neurobehavioral aspects of postconcussive symptoms after mild head injury. J Nerv Ment Dis 180:683–692, 1992.
9. Bonita R: Epidemiology and diagnosis. Plenary: The coming epidemic (abstract). BMJ 352(S4):4, 1998.
10. Busch CR, Alpern HP: Depression after mild traumatic brain injury: A review of current research. Neuropsychol Rev 8:95–108, 1998.
11. Canadian Guidelines for the Assessment of Neurological Fitness in Pilots, Flight Engineers and Air Traffic Controllers (1995). Civil Aviation Medicine Division, Medical Services Branch, Health Canada, 6th Floor, Tower C, Place de Ville, Ottawa, Ontario K1A ON5, Canada.
12. Capruso DX, Levin HS: Cognitive impairment following closed head injury. Neurol Clin 10:879–893, 1992.
13. Cassidy JD, Carrol LJ, Cote P, et al: Effect of eliminating compensation for pain and suffering on the outcome of insurance claims for whiplash injury. N Engl J Med 342:1179–1186, 2000.
14. Chadwick D: Measuring antiepileptic therapies: The patient vs. the physician viewpoint. Neurology 44(S8):S24–S28, 1994.
15. Clark CM, Sheppard L, Fillenbaum GG, et al: Variability in annual Mini-Mental State Examination score in patients with probable Alzheimer disease. A clinical perspective of data from the Consortium to Establish a Registry for Alzheimer's Disease. Arch Neurol 56:857–862, 1999.
16. Cote R, Battista RN, Wolson C, et al: The Canadian Neurologic Scale: Validation and reliability assessment. Neurology 5:638–643, 1989.
17. Crum RM, Anthony JC, Bassett SS, Folstein MF: Population-based norms for the Mini-Mental State Examination by age and educational level. JAMA 269:2386–2391, 1993.
18. Culotta VP, Sementilli ME, Gerold K, Watts CC: Clinicopathological heterogeneity in the classification of mild head injury. Neurosurgery 38:245–250, 1996.
19. Deyo RA, Andersson G, Bombardieer C, et al: Outcome measures for studying patients with low back pain. Spine 19:2032s–2036s, 1994.
20. Epilepsy Foundation Position Statements: On Driver Licensing. http://www.efa.org/advocacy/drivelaw/efaposition.html. Accessed June 23, 2002.
21. Esselman PC, Uomoto JM: Classification of the spectrum of mild traumatic brain injury. Brain Injury 9:417–424, 1995.
22. Evans RW: The postconcussion syndrome and the sequelae of mild head injury. Neurol Clin 10:815–847, 1992.
23. Fairbank JCT, Couper J, Davies JB, O'Brien JP: The Oswestry Low Back Pain Disability Questionnaire. Physiotherapy 66:271–273, 1960.
24. Fee CR, Rutherford WH: A study of the effect of legal settlement on post-concussion symptoms. Arch Emerg Med 5:12–17, 1988.
25. Fit for Flying? A Guide for Mandatory Medical Reporting. Canadian Medical Association Department of Communication, P.O. Box 8650, Ottawa, Ontario K1G 0G8, Canada, 1992.
26. Freeman MD, Croft AC, Rossignol AM: Whiplash associated disorders: Redefining whiplash and its management, by the Quebec Task Force. A critical evaluation. Spine 23:1043–1049, 1998.
27. Gasquoine PG: Postconcussion symptoms. Neuropsychol Rev 7:77–85, 1997.
28. Guide for the Uniform Data Set for Medical Rehabilitation. State University of New York at Buffalo, 1996.
29. Grigoletto F, Zappala G, Anderson DW, Lebowitz BD: Norms for the Mini-Mental State Examination in a healthy population. Neurology 53:315–320, 1999.
30. Hantson L, De Weerdt W, De Keyser J, et al: The European Stroke Scale. Stroke 25:2215–2219, 1994.
31. Hsiang JN, Yeung T, Yu AL, Poon WS: High-risk mild head injury. J Neurosurg 87:234–238, 1997.
32. Jacobson RR: The post-concussional syndrome: Physiogenesis, psychogenesis and malingering. An integrative model. J Psychosom Res 39:675–693, 1995.
33. Jenkins A, Teasdale G, Hadley MD, et al: Brain lesions detected by magnetic resonance imaging in mild and severe head injuries. Lancet 23:445–446, 1986.
34. Jorge RE, Robinson RG, Starkstein SE, et al: Depression and anxiety following traumatic brain injury J Neuropsychiatry Clin Neurosci 5:369–374, 1993.

35. Kaplan LC: Community-based disability services in the USA: A paediatric perspective. Lancet 354:761–762, 1999.
36. Katz RT, DeLuca J: Sequelae of minor traumatic brain injury. Am Fam Physician 46:1491–1498, 1992.
37. King N: Mild head injury: Neuropathology, sequelae, measurement and recovery. Br J Clin Psychol 36(Pt 2):161–184, 1997.
38. Kurztke JF: Rating neurologic impairment in multiple sclerosis: An Expanded Disability Status Scale (EDSS). Neurology 33:144–152, 1983.
39. Leininger BE, Gramling SE, Farrell AD, et al: Neuropsychological deficits in symptomatic minor head injury patients after concussion and mild concussion. J Neurol Neurosurg Psychiatry 53:293–296, 1990.
40. Levin HS: Outcome after head injury: Part II: Neurobehavioral recovery. In Becker DP, Povlishock JT (eds): Status Report on Central Nervous System Trauma Research. Bethesda, Md, National Institute of Neurological and Communicative Disease and Stroke, 1985, p 294.
41. Macciocchi SN, Reid DB, Barth JT: Disability following head injury. Curr Opin Neurol 6:773–777, 1993.
42. MacKenzie CR, Charlson ME: Standards for the use of ordinal scales in clinical trials. BMJ 292:40–43, 1986.
43. Mahoney FI, Barthel DW: Functional evaluation: The Barthel Index. Md State Med J 14:61–65, 1965.
44. Martelli MF, Grayson RL, Zasler ND: Posttraumatic headache: Neuropsychological and psychological effects and treatment implications. J Head Trauma Rehabil 14:49–69, 1999.
45. Menken M, Munsat TL, Toole JF: The Global Burden of Disease Study: Implications for neurology. Arch Neurol 57:418–420, 2000.
46. Mitchell R, Christensen BK, Ross TP: Review article—Depression following traumatic brain injury. Arch Phys Med Rehabil 79:90–103, 1998.
47. Mittenberg W, DiGiulio DV, Perrin S, Bass AE: Symptoms following mild head injury: Expectation as aetiology. J Neurol Neurosurg Psychiatry 55:200–204, 1992.
48. Murray CJL, Lopez AD: Alternative projections of mortality and disability by cause 1990–2020: Global Burden of Disease Study. Lancet 349:1498–1504, 1997.
49. Murray CJL, Lopez AD: Mortality by cause for eight regions of the world: Global Burden of Disease Study. Lancet 349:1269–1276, 1997.
50. National Institute of Neurologic Disorders and Stroke r-TPA Stroke Study Group: Tissue plasminogen activator for acute ischemic stroke. N Engl J Med 333:1581–1587, 1995.
51. Ontario Brain Injury Association: http://www.obia.on.ca/definit.html. Accessed April 3, 2000 (no longer available).
52. Physicians Guide to Driver Examination (revised 1986). Canadian Medical Association, 1867 promenade Alta Vista, Ottawa, Ontario K1G 3Y6, Canada.
53. Povlishock JT, Christman CW: The pathobiology of traumatically induced axonal injury in animals and humans: A review of current thoughts. J Neurotrauma 12:555–564, 1995.
54. Rankin J: Cerebrovascular accidents in patients over the age of 60. Scott Med J 2:200–215, 1957.
55. Reisberg B, Ferris SH, DeLeon MJ, Crook T: The Global Deterioration Scale for assessment of primary degenerative dementia. Am J Psychiatry 139:1136–1139, 1982.
56. Riahi F, Zijdenbos A, Narayanan S, et al: Improved correlation between scores on the Expanded Disability Status Scale and the cerebral lesion load in relapsing-remitting multiple sclerosis. Results of the application of new imaging methods. Brain 121:1305–1312, 1998.
57. Robinson AG, Price TR: Post-stroke depressive disorders: A followup study of 103 patients. Stroke 13:635–641, 1982.
58. Rosen WG, Mohs RC, Davis KI: A new rating scale for Alzheimer's disease. Am J Psychiatry 141:1356–1364, 1984.
59. Satz PS, Alfano MS, Light RF, et al: Persistent post-concussive syndrome: A proposed methodology and literature review to determine the effects, if any, of mild head and other bodily injury. J Clin Exp Neuropsychol 21:620–628, 1999.
60. Scandinavian Stroke Study Group: Multicenter trial of hemodilution in ischemic stroke—Background and study protocol. Stroke 16:885–890, 1985.
61. Schmand B, Lindeboom J, Schagen S, et al: Cognitive complaints in patients after whiplash injury: The impact of malingering. J Neurol Neurosurg Psychiatry 64:339–343, 1998.
62. Schrader H, Obeliemene D, Bovim G, et al: Natural evolution of late whiplash syndrome outside the medicolegal context. Lancet 347:1207–1211, 1996.
63. Schwartz GE: Development and validation of the Geriatric Evaluation by Relatives Rating Instrument (GERRI). Psychological Reports 53:479–488, 1983.
64. Shoumitro D, Lyons I, Koutzoukis C, McCarthy G: Rate of psychiatric hlness 1 year after traumatic brain injury. Am J Psychiatry 156:374–378, 1999.
65. Spitzer WO, Skovron ML, Salmi LR: Scientific monograph of the Quebec Task Force on Whiplash Associated Disorders: Redefining "whiplash" and its management. Spine 20(Suppl.):1S–73S, 1995.
66. Spudis EV, Penry JK, Gibson P: Driving impairment caused by episodic brain dysfunction. Arch Neurol 43:558–564, 1986.
67. Taylor AE, Cox CE, Mailis A: Persistent neuropsychological deficits following whiplash: Evidence for chronic mild traumatic brain injury? Arch Phys Med Rehabil 77:529–535, 1996.
68. Teasdale G, Jennet B: Assessment of coma and impaired consciousness: A practical scale. Lancet 2:81–84, 1974.
69. Teasell RW, Shapiro AP: Whiplash injuries: An update. Pain Res Management 3:81–90, 1998.
70. Treiman DM: Epilepsy and violence: Medical and legal issues. Epilepsia 27(Suppl 2):S77–S104, 1986.
71. Üstün TB, Rehm J, Chatterji S, et al: Multiple-informant ranking of the disabling effects of different health conditions in 14 countries. Lancet 354:111–115, 1999.
72. Wagner DP, Knaus WA, Draper EA: Statistical validation of a severity of illness measure. Am J Publ Health 73:878–884, 1983.
73. Weight DG: Minor head trauma. Psychiatr Clin North Am 21:609–624, 1998.
74. Wood-Dauphinee SL, Willaims JI, Shapiro SH: Examining outcome measures in a clinical study of stroke. Stroke 21:731–739, 1990.
75. Zaidi A, Clough P, Scheepers B, Fitzpatrick A: Treatment resistant epilepsy or convulsive syncope? BMJ 317:869–870, 1998.

CHAPTER

68

Peripheral Nervous System Disability

MARC T. TAYLOR, MD

DISABILITY AND RETURN TO WORK ISSUES IN PERIPHERAL NERVOUS SYSTEM DISORDERS

Returning the patient with a history of a peripheral nervous system (PNS) disorder to the prior position in the workplace is frequently a challenging and frustrating event for all those involved in the process. The return to work process is affected by many factors. There are tremendous legal and vocational differences in the different workers' compensation systems from state to state and jurisdiction to jurisdiction. Other factors that can have a major effect on the return to work process are the type of work performed by an individual, the required essentials of a particular workplace position, and the flexibility of the employer. Even without all these nonmedical factors, it is a challenge for any physician to understand and manage the medical issues in a patient who presents to the office with what is thought to be a work-related musculoskeletal disorder or a PNS disorder. This chapter discusses the medical, disability, and return to work issues concerning patients with temporary musculoskeletal inflammatory conditions and PNS disorders.

DEFINING A MEDICAL DISORDER AND SEPARATING OUT WORKPLACE ISSUES

As pointed out in the chapter on PNS impairment (Chapter 35), the temporary loss of function and complaints of pain seen with muscle fatigue and the soft tissue inflammation associated with repetitive activities using the extremities that resolve with conservative medical treatment or rest are not PNS disorders. These exertional myalgias, muscle imbalances, and muscle weakness problems create a clinical picture in the physician's office of complaints of pain, weakness, and muscle fatigue, and they can occur at any point in the employment history of an individual. Frequently, the underlying muscle weakness and the physical inability of an individual to perform an essential task required of a position in the workplace are not created or the result of the workplace position. Whether there is a work-related injury and the cause of injury aspect can be confusing to a treating or examining physician, especially when the clinical picture develops in an individual after he or she performs some type of repetitive task using the extremities as part of the required essentials for a workplace position.

Although in some situations these individuals may have a recurrent clinical picture of the development of musculoskeletal pain in an area from exertional myalgias and musculoskeletal inflammation after performing certain types of repetitive activities required for the position within the workplace, there is frequently no ongoing medical condition or underlying disease process. These temporary musculoskeletal inflammatory clinical conditions can be work related, because they develop after performing work-related tasks. They respond to medical evaluation and short-term conservative treatment, but they are not permanent.

Imbalances in muscle strength, muscle weakness, and other physical attributes play a large role as to when and how often a physician might see this recurrent inflammatory clinical picture of complaints of pain, weakness, and muscle fatigue in a patient. The evaluating physician must separate out the workplace functional ability issues from any underlying medical disease or a pathologic process involving the PNS that would benefit from further active medical care or surgery. Following the clinical response of an individual to any treatment and documenting the specific factors surrounding any recurrence of symptoms are important points to consider in managing the person. In addition to the response to treatment of any temporary musculoskeletal inflammatory process, at some point and in some clinical situations the results of tests, such as needle electrodiagnostic testing, the two-point discrimination test, the Semmes-Weinstein touch pressure threshold monofilament test, and imaging studies, can provide additional objective data that can help define any underlying medical pathology.

The development of pain in areas of the body after performing a physical activity in the workplace does not mean that the workplace created a permanent pathologic process or an active medical condition. A frequent cause of this clinical situation is that the worker might not be capable of carrying out a specific required repetitive activity in the workplace on a prolonged or daily basis. As pointed out in Chapters 55 and 56, it is difficult to determine some of these functional ability limitations through any type of standard or even job-specific testing process.

For instance, during a job-specific functional ability testing procedure done on an individual prior to being hired or being returned to the workplace following successful treatment, an individual might be capable of sewing a single button on a shirt. That same individual might not be capable of sewing 50 buttons a day on shirts or sewing 50 buttons a day on shirts day in and day out without developing muscle soreness and pain in the upper extremities. If the workplace position requires sewing 50 buttons a day on shirts day in and day out, then in this case the individual cannot meet the essentials of the workplace position. Unfortunately, the physical limitations in terms of the person's capabilities in the workplace are frequently not found or do not develop until long after he or she has been hired or after a prolonged period of employment.

RELEASE FROM MEDICAL CARE AND RETURNING THE INDIVIDUAL TO THE WORKPLACE

If there is no objective evidence in the medical records, the patient history, or diagnostic studies that there is an active ongoing pathologic condition or medical condition that developed from an activity in the workplace, the individual should be returned to the workplace as soon as the temporary inflammatory musculoskeletal condition resolves. When there is no active underlying work-related medical condition that would preclude an individual from returning to the workforce, he or she should not be taken or kept out of the workforce just because he or she is not capable of meeting the essentials of his or her position in the workplace. Even in people who have a history of treatment or surgery for a peripheral nerve disorder, without objective documentation of an ongoing underlying pathology, there is no medical indication to continue to certify that an individual has a work-related medical condition preventing him or her from returning to the workplace. The fear of developing pain, the complaint of pain, or the inability to perform the essentials of a job without the development of pain are not indications to remove an individual from the workforce or to maintain an individual out of the workplace.

The definition of maximum medical improvement in the AMA Guides is based on the concepts that the medical condition is stable and not amendable to further active medical treatment and that the employability and the impairment in an individual will not change significantly. This definition is a medically sound one that can be used in a clinical situation. It allows for the individual to have the opportunity to receive any needed active medical care or surgical procedure, but also provides to the physician a medical basis for making a decision concerning the release from medical care. If there has not been any normal medical progression or change in the overall clinical state, in spite of normal diagnostic tests, medical treatment, or remaining out of work, then the person is stable and at maximum medical improvement and should be released from medical care.

These clinical situations can be difficult to address with the examinee and the employer when this recurrent temporary inflammatory clinical picture is associated with repetitive activities that are a part of the required essentials of a position within the workplace of that employer. Frequently in this situation, the inability to perform the essentials of the position in the workplace without developing a temporary inflammatory condition or the complaint of pain means that the person cannot physically perform on a regular basis the essentials of the job. A new position in the workplace has to be found, which is usually not easy, especially in an older individual with limited education who can no longer perform the physical essential tasks required for a workplace position.

In spite of the difficulty of dealing with these situations, when there is no active medical condition that can be demonstrated on diagnostic testing or physical examination that will benefit from further active medical care or surgery, the medical literature demonstrates that removing an individual from the workforce without objective evidence of a medical condition or pathologic condition is contraindicated. This is a workplace issue. Although at times it might seem to a physician that he or she is helping a person by certifying him or her off work when no medical condition exists, the examining physician and treating physician must be careful not to help create or reward dysfunctional behavior in that individual.

Discussed in Chapter 39, the rewarding of dysfunctional or chronic pain behavior intentionally or unintentionally can lead to a chronic pain syndrome. This is not a diagnosis, but a description of a constellation of symptoms and behavior, including persistent complaints of pain, poor coping, dysfunctional pain behaviors, impoverished activities of daily living, major life disruptions, persistent complaints of pain, persistent attempts at trying to find an organic cause, and repeated visits to physicians. Chronic pain syndrome is further characterized by symptoms of depression, anxiety, physical deconditioning, family discord, and financial distress. There is a belief that because of the chronic pain, one is unable to meet not only occupational demands, but also domestic, family, and social responsibilities, and unable to engage in vocational and recreational activities. Unfortunately, at times this disability conviction may be reinforced by external variables such as family, friends, or health care providers.

In this situation, the peer-reviewed medical literature demonstrates that surgery, invasive procedures, and active medical treatment are contraindicated. Surgery and active medical treatment will lead to iatrogenic disability and impairment. Numerous studies have shown that, on a statistical basis, the longer an individual remains out of the workplace, regardless of the cause or medical condition, the less likely it is that he or she will ever return to the workplace. A workplace issue cannot be cured with a knife, needle, or additional periods of time away from the workplace, and returning the individual to the workplace and addressing the workplace issues will be in the best interest of the worker from a physical, mental, and financial point of view, based on the peer-reviewed medical literature.

RETURN TO THE WORKPLACE PROGRAMS AND STANDARDS

Whether an individual has been unable to work because of a peripheral nerve disorder or a temporary inflammatory musculoskeletal condition, it is important that the return to work process be discussed and begin as soon as possible. A first time visit to a physician's office for a musculoskeletal disorder that is work related might not seem to be much of a problem at first, but as pointed out previously, the physician should be aware of the potential for the development of very complex issues, many of which may not be medically related. The physician should inquire about the requirements and physical essentials of the position in the workplace. The documentation of certain risk factors in terms of the required physical tasks of a workplace position, such as the need for repetition, awkward postures, contact stress, and vibration, is important. Even when it is known that the patient will require a surgical procedure followed by a period of physical rehabilitation, the physician and patient should discuss as early as possible these workplace factors and address the workplace issues.

There is considerable variation from one state to the next in the nature of return to work programs. It is important for the treating or evaluating physician to be aware of how the return to work issues and programs are handled in his or her state or jurisdiction. Some states provide only minimal support with limited physical therapy or work hardening following any medical treatment or surgery for a work-related musculoskeletal disorder or PNS disorder. In some states there may not be any payment or financial assistance for occupational rehabilitation, vocational rehabilitation, or vocational retraining. If a return to work program is available from the employer, the patient and physician might have access to additional resources in the return to work process. It is important to begin the return to work, the vocational retraining, or repositioning process as soon as possible, as it can make an enormous financial difference to the patient in the long run.

Whenever possible, the physician should contact trained occupational therapists, vocational rehabilitation specialists, and ergonomic specialists to evaluate the position in the workplace and to assist the patient in the return to work process. Many states have excellent programs where these specialists work with the patient and the physician directly in the return to work process. It is important to determine and to recommend to the employer any necessary modifications of the workplace. Formal testing of the overall functional ability of the patient and the ability to perform job-specific tasks can help provide important information in terms of the ability of the patient to perform certain essentials in the workplace. Many employers have ergonomic specialists available who can work with the patient and the worksite. At times relatively minor changes in the height or position of objects in the workplace can decrease or eliminate the development of symptoms.

The Occupational Safety and Health Administration issued rules on November 14, 2000, concerning an ergonomics program standard. There are stringent requirements for most nonconstruction employers to identify and to abate musculoskeletal disorders. The requirement for the full implementation of an entire ergonomics program by the employer now depends entirely on the report of the signs and symptoms of a musculoskeletal disorder by the employee. Until such an occurrence, the final rule only requires employers to give employees basic information addressing recognition and reporting of a musculoskeletal disorder. The employer must address and investigate any reports, and if necessary, develop a complete ergonomics program.

It is important for the physician to begin the investigation of the workplace issues and the return to work process as early as possible. Once the medical treatment has been completed and the patient has reached maximum medical improvement, it is in the best interest of the patient to be released from medical care, regardless of the medical condition or peripheral nerve disorder, so that the workplace issues can be addressed.

Bibliography

American Board of Electrodiagnostic Medicine, American Association of Electrodiagnostic Medicine, 21 Second Street SW, Rochester, MN 55902.

Aronoff G, Feldman J: Preventing iatrogenic disability from chronic pain. Curr Rev Pain 3:67–77, 1999.

Cocchiarella L, Andersson GBJ (eds): Guides to the Evaluation of Permanent Impairment, 5th ed. Chicago, American Medical Association, 2001.

Matheson LN: Symptom magnification syndrome structured interview: Rationale and procedure. J Occup Rehab 1:43–56, 1991.

Nathan PA, Keniston RC, Myers LD, et al: Natural history of median nerve sensory conduction in industry: Relationship to symptoms and carpal tunnel syndrome in 588 hands over 11 years. Muscle Nerve 21:711–721, 1998.

Redmond DM, Rivner MH: False positive electrodiagnostic tests in carpal tunnel syndrome. Muscle Nerve 11:511–517, 1988.

Salerno DF, Franzblau A, Werner RA, et al: Median and ulnar nerve conduction studies among workers: Normative values. Muscle Nerve 21:999–1005, 1998.

SECTION

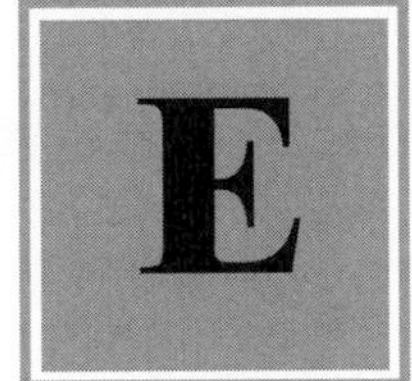

Psychiatric Disability

CHAPTER

69

Psychiatric Disability

MOSHE S. TOREM, MD

In this chapter, the term psychiatric disability is defined, and methods of assessing psychiatric disability and reporting the findings of psychiatric disability are covered.

DEFINITIONS

The World Health Organization (WHO)[8] defines impairment as a limitation due to a defect in a person's level of functioning. Handicap is defined as a limitation in social functioning creating a disadvantage for the individual with a handicap. Disability is defined as a specific limitation in one's activity (behavior and functioning) that is produced as a result of a person's interaction with the social or work environment. WHO classifies disabilities into three subgroups: 1) disability in personal self-care, such as eating, keeping oneself clean, dressing, grooming, and getting proper sleep and rest; 2) disability in social interaction, relating to a limitation that is manifested in the ability to properly interact in a social setting in an adaptive way; and 3) occupational disability, relating to a limitation in functioning adaptively in the work setting (see also Chapter 1).

ASSESSMENT

The assessment of psychiatric disability involves the assessment of several areas. First, it is important to assess the person's psychiatric diagnoses according to the Diagnostic and Statistical Manual of Mental Disorders, fourth edition (DSM-IV).[9] A five point axis system is used that includes the person's major psychiatric diagnosis (Axis I); the existence of a personality disorder (Axis II); the existence of a medical diagnosis that is significantly affected by the individual's psychiatric conditions or that affects the impairment of the psychiatric diagnoses (Axis III); the person's source of stresses such as the lack of a primary support group or work stress (Axis IV); and the individual's level of functioning with activities of daily living as measured by the Global Assessment of Functioning Scale (GAF) (Axis V).[2]

The assessment of social functioning is also extremely valuable and is done by using the social and occupational functioning scale described in DSM-IV[9] and based on work by Goldman and colleagues.[3]

In addition, the person's job must be assessed, including the job description and job history (work history), including notation of criticisms, praises, promotions, demotions, transfers, and the quality of his or her interactions with people at the workplace. In general, as pointed out by Kennedy and Gruenberg,[4] there are several aspects of psychiatric (mental) disability that are important to consider before one engages in such an assessment:

1. Each person is unique and the same degree of psychiatric impairment may produce different levels of disability in different persons. For example, a person with the diagnosis of attention deficit hyperactivity disorder (ADHD) may have a lifelong history of difficulties holding on to one job, may frequently fight with his supervisor, and may be described as rebellious and unreliable, whereas another person with the same diagnosis of ADHD and impairment may be a successful self-motivated consultant and entrepreneur.
2. The same person with the same psychiatric impairment may be disabled in one work environment and function without any disability in another work environment. For example, Mr. Z, a 35-year-old man, was diagnosed with a dependent personality

disorder. He worked as an assistant manager under a boss who was confident, secure, and in control, giving clear and regular task assignments with frequent feedback. In this environment, an individual with a dependent personality disorder may do reasonably well with little to no obvious work disability. When Mr. Z was promoted to a management position with several people reporting to him, he became very anxious, was unsure of himself, and could not adjust to the lack of daily and frequent feedback from a kind, confident, and reassuring boss. When Mr. Z was transferred back to his previous position, he quickly adjusted and the disability was gone. This example also illustrates the third point in assessing psychiatric disability.

3. A disability can be eliminated or reduced in severity by helping a specific individual to adjust to a specific job and by accommodating and changing the environment to fit the needs of the individual.
4. A specific disability may originate from impairments in more than one organ system, and the combination of two impairments may produce a disability greater than their sum. For example, Mr. A.S. was a 45-year-old engineer with a lifelong paranoid personality who functioned well enough to maintain his job and even get promotions in an office setting where there was a great emphasis on security and confidentiality. Files were always locked away. No document was ever left exposed. When the company was merged with another firm, the new CEO and President instituted a policy of greater openness. Mr. A.S. had a hard time adjusting, his paranoid tendencies became more severe and conspicuously abnormal in this new culture of openness, and he became dysfunctional on the job and eventually disabled.
5. Psychiatric disorders have a high degree of variability. For example, in the case of major depression, one individual with this diagnosis may respond well to a combination of psychotherapy with antidepressant pharmacotherapy, quickly recover into full remission, and return to work with little or no impairment. On the other hand, another individual of the same age, race, and sex may not respond to any known treatment for major depression and thus be diagnosed with chronic treatment-resistant major depression with poor progress, leading to severe impairment and disability.

STEPS IN ASSESSING PSYCHIATRIC DISABILITY

It is helpful to undertake the assessment of psychiatric disability in several consecutive steps.

Determine the Psychiatric Diagnosis

This is done based on the DSM-IV five-Axis system; for further detail, see Chapters 38 and 41.

Determine the Severity of the Psychiatric Impairment

Not every psychiatric diagnosis leads to an impairment in function. Many psychiatric ailments are chronic in nature with a history of relapses and remissions. When the psychiatric condition is in remission, there may be no impairment in function; however, when there is a relapse, functional impairment is clearly manifested. Good examples of such conditions are the diagnoses of bipolar mood disorder (manic depressive illness) or major depression, recurrent episodic type. However, some psychiatric conditions are progressive in nature and the person's functioning continues to deteriorate over time. Schizophrenia may fit into this category. On the other end of the spectrum, adjustment disorder is usually self-limiting and if no other condition is present the individual with the diagnosis of adjustment disorder may reach a full recovery once the stressful situation is resolved. The worker's psychiatric impairment may also change based on the place and circumstance of the assessment. For example, Mr. N.D., a 33-year-old man diagnosed with acute paranoid delusional disorder, decompensated at the workplace, requiring hospitalization. Following a 7-day hospital treatment with psychotherapy in a highly structured environment and in combination with proper psychotropic medications, his condition significantly improved and the impairment was barely evident. However, the same person assessed in an outpatient office visit with a highly open-ended unstructured interview may show significant impairment in thinking, feeling, reality judgement, and making decisions.

Activities of Daily Living (ADLs)

These activities include such functions as self-care, personal hygiene, ability to clearly communicate one's needs and requests and respond appropriately to communication from others, ambulation, travel, sleep, and caring for one's basic needs such as safety and nutritional needs. These activities are assessed based on the person's ability to perform them independently, with appropriate judgment, effectiveness, and sustainability. In addition, psychiatric impairment is assessed based on social functioning using the social functioning scale.[3]

The fifth edition of the AMA Guides to the Evaluation of Permanent Impairment,[1] p 363, includes a table that delineates five classes of impairment due to mental and behavioral disorders. These five classes are based on assessing the disturbances in the ADLs: social functioning; concentration, persistence in task completion, and pace in performing such functions; and the individual's ability to adapt to change in the workplace. The classes of impairment are as follows: Class 1, no impairment; Class 2, mild impairment, reflecting an impairment that is compatible with most useful functioning; Class 3, moderate impairment, reflecting an impairment that is compatible with some but not all useful functioning; Class 4, marked impairment, reflecting a level of impairment that significantly impedes useful functioning; and Class 5, extreme impairment, reflecting a level of impairment that precludes useful functioning.

Maximum Level of Improvement

Once the level of impairment has been determined the next step is to determine whether there can be an improvement in the assessed person's functioning by a different (yet untried) form of treatment or a higher level of treatment intensity. If there is a chance this may happen the assessed worker should be given the opportunity to receive the best available treatment and then reassessed 3 to 6 months later. If the assessed person is determined to have reached the maximum level of improvement, the next step can be undertaken.

Ability to Perform Previous Job

In spite of having an impairment a worker may still be able to perform his or her previous job. This must be carefully assessed by analyzing the worker's job description and requirements and comparing these requirements as well as the work setting with the specific worker's impairment. Sometimes this can only be assessed by a trial of returning to work associated with specific observations of how the impaired worker performs in his or her work environment. These observations are generated in writing specifying the worker's difficulties or impairments. Such observations can be organized into four different categories as suggested by the fifth edition of the AMA Guides.[1(p365)].
These categories are as follows:

1. Understanding and memory—The worker's ability to comprehend and remember work procedures as well as verbal and written instructions regarding work tasks and work assignments
2. Sustained concentration and persistence—The worker's ability to carry out both short and simple and more detailed and complex instructions; moreover, the worker's ability to maintain attention and concentration for extended periods of time and persist in performing required work activities with a given schedule
3. Social interaction—The worker's ability to properly interact with other people at work (including supervisors, from whom a worker must be able to take instructions and criticism) and maintain socially appropriate behavior in one's personal neatness, cleanliness, and attire
4. Adaptation—The worker's ability to adjust to changes in the workplace in a healthy, adaptive way that will preserve one's safety and the safety of one's coworkers; moreover, the ability to adjust to changing weather and traffic conditions in traveling to and from work

Workplace Accommodations

This is the next step to be determined in the process in a psychiatric disability assessment. Here the psychiatrist has to assess what type of workplace accommodations will improve the chances of a successful return to work. The options to be considered are the following:

1. Return to work full-time or part-time.
2. Return to work on a gradual increase of hours per day (from 2 hours a day gradually up to 8 hours a day as tolerated).
3. Return to the same shift or change to a different shift; for example, night shift to day shift, when there is usually more structure and supervision, or vice-versa.
4. Change the type of work, from heavy machinery to clerical work or vice-versa.
5. Change from a highly unstructured setting to a highly structured one, or vice-versa, based on the worker's needs.

Once the psychiatrist who performs the disability assessment determines what will be best for a specific worker, a recommendation is made in writing to try out in the workplace. If the company is unable to make the necessary accommodations, the worker may be assessed as disabled for his or her previous job with a specific company. However, the process is still not complete, and the question to be assessed is whether the worker is temporarily disabled or is permanently disabled and whether it is for all jobs or only for the specific job held before the disability started. This is a rather complex issue and involves the issue of motivation to return to work.

Motivation to Return to Work

A person's motivation to resume gainful employment is a very complex issue and depends not only on the level of disability and impairment but also on one's culture, personality, the presence of depression, personal values, and to what extent a person's self-esteem is connected to being gainfully employed. Moreover, the issue of secondary gain must be assessed as well. Secondary gain refers to the disabled worker's receiving of a monetary, financial, or other reward (gain) as a result of the disability and how much higher or lower it is compared to the worker's regular salary. In addition, the issue of primary gain should be assessed as well, concerning the worker's possible gain in personal standing in his or her family, village, etc., as a result of the impairment and disability. For example; being disabled due to a war injury and returning home as a hero is quite a different status from that of being disabled as a result of an infectious or contagious disease.

SPECIFIC ISSUES AND CONDITIONS

Diagnoses That Preclude Return to Work

Are there any psychiatric diagnoses that would preclude a return to work for a specific employee? The answer to this question is the result of an assessment of the type of work an employee had been engaged in and his or her specific diagnosis. The following are examples of when a worker should not return to his or her previous line of work.

1. *Paranoid schizophrenia and delusional disorder*: Persons diagnosed with active paranoid schizophrenia or delusional disorder or other types of schizophrenia should not return to previous jobs involving the use of firearms, such as police work or security.
2. *Panic attacks and agoraphobia*: Persons diagnosed with this condition who have active episodes of anxiety and panic in spite of treatment cannot return to work as an airplane pilot or in the operation of equipment in a closed and small place.
3. *Pedophilia and sociopathy*: Persons diagnosed with these conditions should be precluded from returning to work as teachers, guidance counselors, coaches, or any position involving children.

Threat of Violence to Self or Others

Workers who threaten violence to self or others in the workplace constitute a special safety hazard. Once a threat has been reported and identified, the company should not just remove the suspected employee from the workplace, but take him or her for an immediate assessment in the emergency room of a hospital where an emergency psychiatric examination can be thoroughly performed. Such an assessment should rule out the presence of alcohol and substance abuse, a previous history of violence and poor impulse control, and the presence of psychosis and severe depression or mania. If the presence of an acute psychiatric condition is identified the worker is offered intensive psychiatric treatment, many times involving hospitalization in an inpatient psychiatric unit for further evaluation and treatment. Once the patient has recovered from the acute state, if an act of violence took place, most companies are reluctant to accept the employee back. If only a threat occurred, the assessment must be done on a case by case basis and involve a thorough risk/reward assessment for the disabled worker as well as the employer as to whether to choose a return to the previous work setting, a change to another setting, or preclude a return to work all together.

Disability Assessment: Writing a Meaningful Report

The examining psychiatrist should receive a letter from the referring entity/agency requesting the disability assessment. The individual to be assessed should give written consent before the process and be aware that the assessment and examination is not for treatment purposes but for the purpose of a disability assessment and that a written report will be generated and sent to the referring agency giving the doctor's medical opinion and answering the specific questions asked in the referral letter. The following is an outline for writing a meaningful report of the disability assessment and examination.

Disability Assessment Report (Sample Outline)

Basic data
- Name of assessed worker (claimant)
- Social Security number
- Date of birth
- Date of injury
- Date illness began
- Last day of work
- Name of employer
- Name of examining psychiatrist
- Status of Board certification
- Date(s) of examination(s)
- Place of examination(s)
- Methods of assessment
  - Review of all available records
  - Interview of claimant
  - Interview of others (name them and their relationship to the claimant)
  - Mental status and psychiatric examination of the claimant
  - Psychological tests and screening scales used (name all tools)
  - Other sources of information

Family members
Employer
Treating physicians
Treating nonphysicians
(Specify how the information was obtained)

Relevant data from the medical history and the psychiatric interview

Chief complaint and current symptoms
Detailed history of illness or injury leading to impairment and disability
Data on attempts to return to work and their outcome
Family health history

Relevant data of personal, social, and family history

History of education and study habits
Ability to set educational goals and achieve them
Legal history; comment on any involvement with the police and court system
Military service; comment on ability to adjust to military discipline and handle authority
Enduring friendship and social ties
Comment on ability to function as spouse and parent

Relevant work history

Review previous jobs and what led the claimant to change places of work
Review promotions, bonuses, work evaluations, and any work terminations and reasons for them
Comment on the meaning of work in this claimant's value system
Comment on motivation to work (intrinsic versus necessity)
Comment on claimant's history of getting along with supervisors, peers, and subordinates

Relevant data from the mental status examination

For a detailed outline, see Chapters 38 and 41.

Psychological tests and screening scales

Comment on the results of any psychological tests and screening scales that were used and on the meaning of the results/scores.

Psychiatric diagnosis

Provide a diagnosis using the DSM-IV five-Axis system.[9]

Medical Opinion on Disability

This opinion can be formulated by answering the specific questions asked in the formal letter of referral. If the referral letter does not include a list of specific questions to be answered, the medical opinion regarding the worker's psychiatric disability status should include the following items:

The psychiatric diagnosis.
A statement about the relationship of the psychiatric condition to the workplace—this has high significance in cases of work injury. The statement should include information on the prognosis of the worker's condition and the level of impairment. The statement should also include information and recommendations regarding the present level of disability and the chances for vocational rehabilitation. Moreover, if the medical opinion includes a recommendation of returning to work, it should specify the following details:

When should the first day of return to work be?
Should any accommodations be made regarding return to work?
How many hours a day should the employee work the first week?
If a gradual increase in hours worked per day is recommended, the psychiatrist should be specific as to the rate of increase per day and how soon to begin increasing hours.
If the recommendation of return to work is on a trial basis, the psychiatrist should be specific as to how long, under what conditions, and what observations should be made and by whom regarding the employee's adjustment in returning to work.
If a reassessment is needed with the new data from the return to work on a trial basis, the examining psychiatrist should be specific as to when the reassessment is to be done and by whom.
The report should be signed by the examining psychiatrist and ideally completed within 7 to 14 days following the examination.

References

1. Cocchiarella L, Andersson GBJ (eds): Guides to the Evaluation of Permanent Impairment, 5th ed. Chicago, American Medical Association, 2001.
2. Endicott J, Spitzer RL, Fleiss JL, Cohen J: The Global Assessment Scale: A procedure for measuring overall severity of psychiatric disturbance. Arch Gen Psychiatry 33:766–771, 1976.
3. Goldman HH, Skodol AE, Lave TR: Revising Axis V for DSM-IV: A review of measures of social functioning. Am J Psychiatry 149:1148–1156, 1992.
4. Kennedy C, Gruenberg EM: A lexicology for the consequences of mental disorders. In Myerson AT, Fine T (ed): Psychiatric Disability: Clinical Legal and Administrative Dimensions. Washington, DC, American Psychiatric Press, 1987.
5. Massel KH, Liberman RP, Mintz J, et al: Evaluating the capacity to work of the mentally ill. Psychiatry 53:31–43, 1990.
6. Mischoulon D: An approach to the patient seeking psychiatric disability benefits. Academic Psychiatry 23:128–136, 1999.
7. Princess H, Kennedy C, Simmens S, et al: Determining disability due to mental impairment: APA's evaluation of Social Security Administration guidelines. Am J Psychiatry 148:1037–1043, 1991.
8. World Health Organization Psychiatric Disability Assessment Schedule (WHO/DAS). Geneva, WHO, 1988.
9. American Psychiatric Association: Diagnostic and Statistical Manual of Mental Disorders, 4th ed. Washington, DC, American Psychiatric Association, 1994.

PART

IV

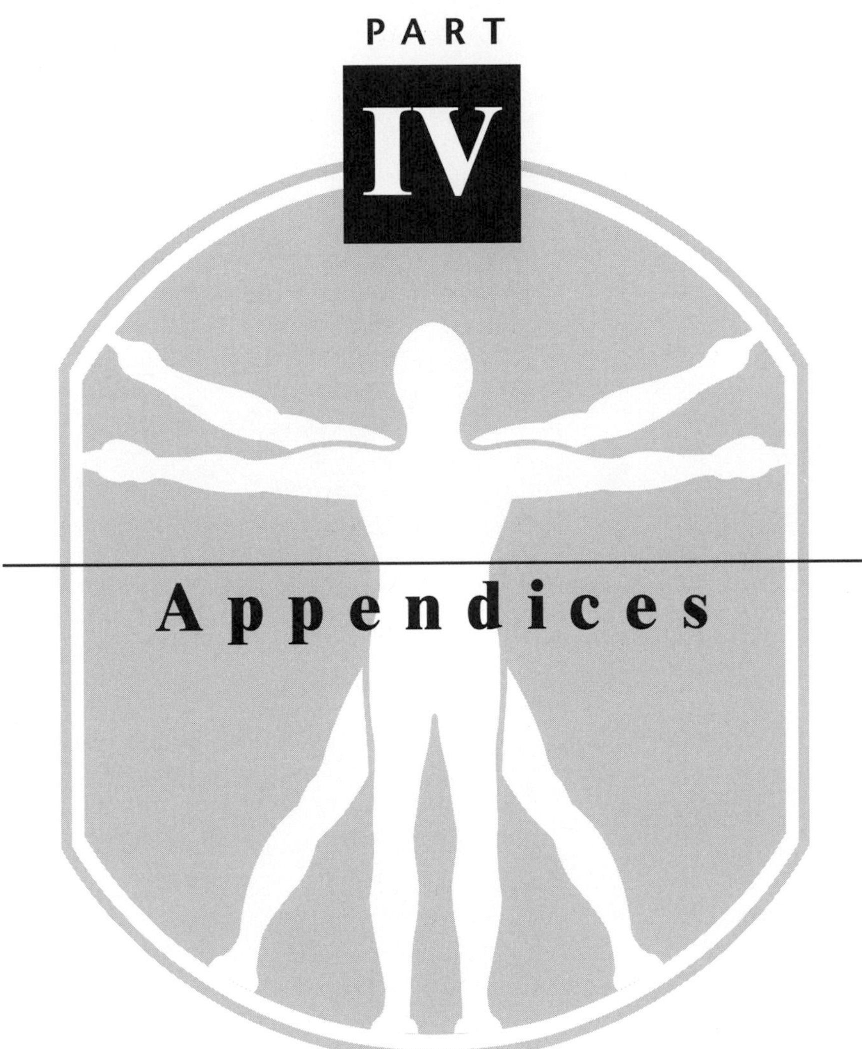

Appendices

A P P E N D I X   A

Biostatistics and Epidemiology: A Review of Topics Found in this Book

STEPHEN L. DEMETER, MD, MPH

This Appendix briefly reviews some concepts and terms used in biostatistics and epidemiology applicable to this book. Many of the terms defined in this Appendix are used throughout the book and it is presented as a convenience for those readers who have forgotten what these terms define and are used for.

Biostatistics

Correlation Coefficient (r and r^2)

When two variables are being studied for any correlation between them (covariance), the results of the relationship between the two variables can be graphed. For example, if systolic blood pressure was being measured as a function of age, a data set would be produced that could be graphed. The tighter the relationship, the more the data points will approximate a straight line. The looser the relationship, the more the graph appears as a scatterplot (Fig. 1, Table 1).

The r value addresses the issue of validity and is used in developing a predictive model. The r value is the slope of the line resulting when one value is compared with another (or comparing x and y). For example, when comparing weight gain with caloric intake, the study results could be plotted as shown in Figure 2. The slope of the line gives the r value, ranging from +1.0 (perfect correlation) to −1.0 (perfect inverse correlation), with a value of 0 showing absolutely no correla-

TABLE 1

r Values

Absolute Value of *r*	Degree of Association
0.8–1.0	Strong
0.5–0.8	Moderate
0.2–0.5	Weak
0–0.2	Negligible

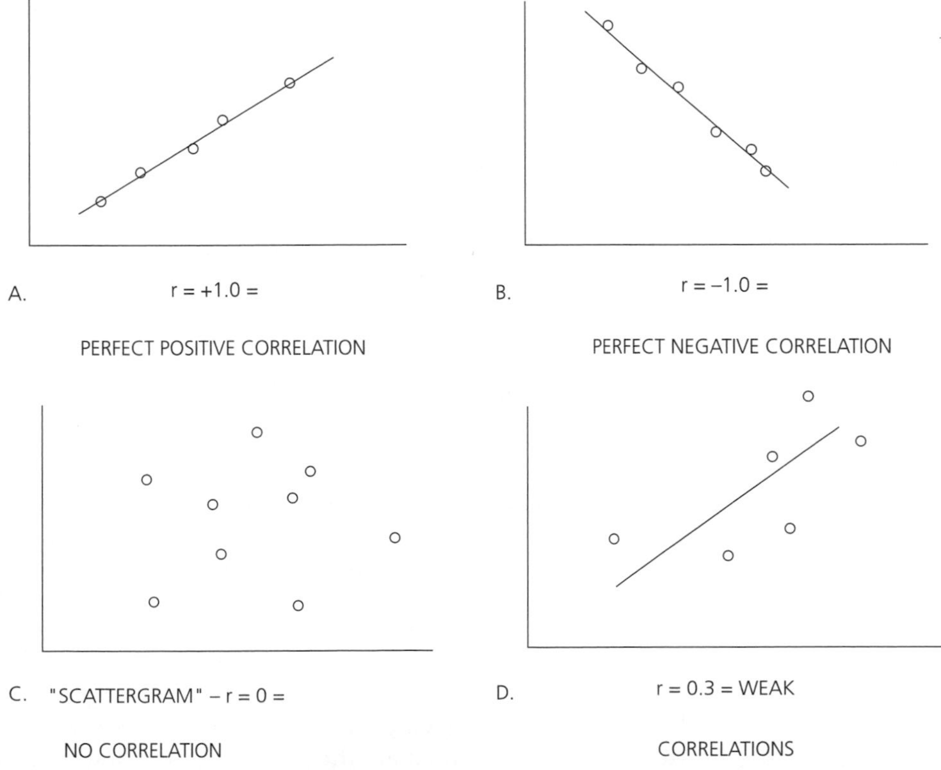

Figure 1. Correlation coefficients.

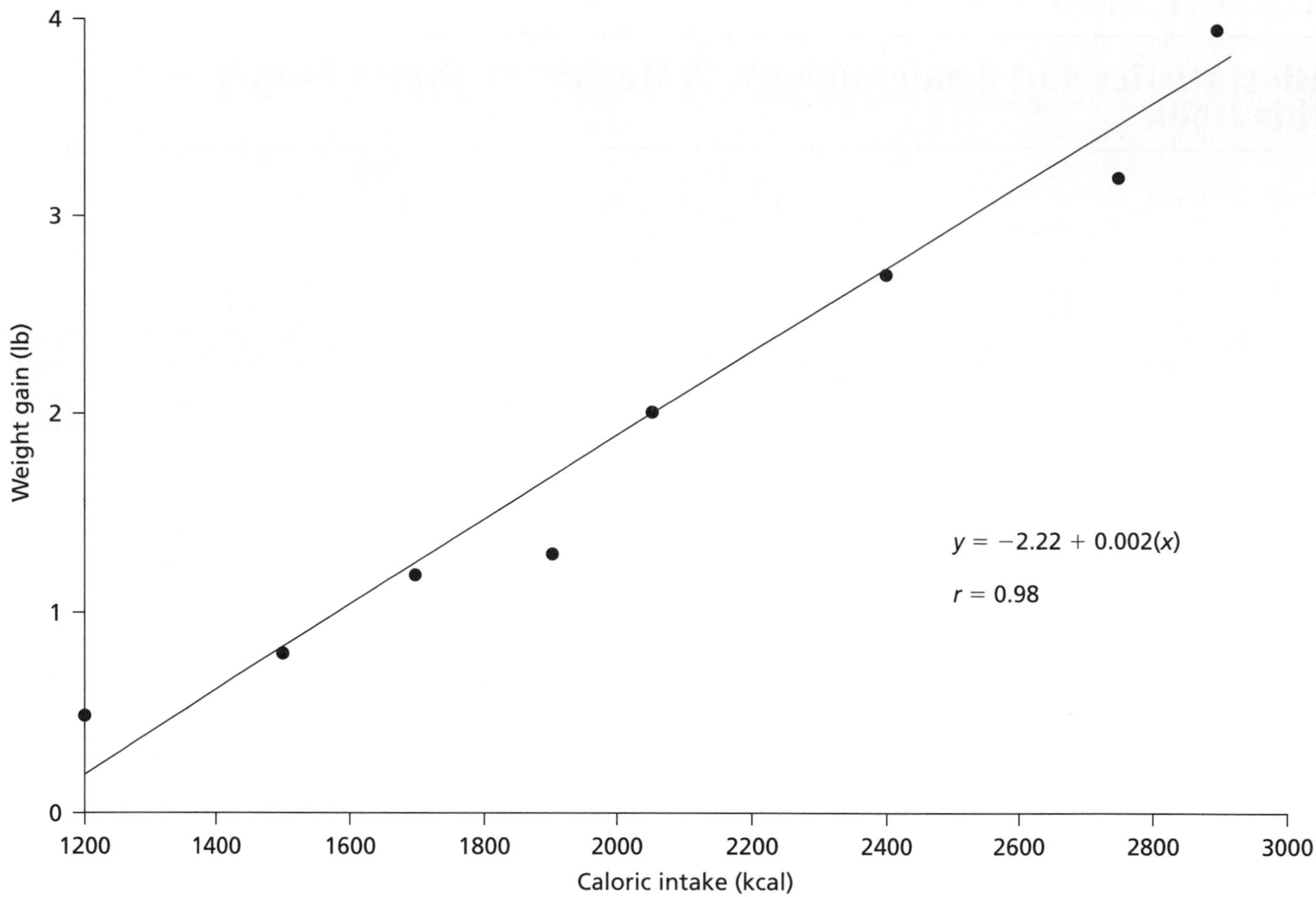

Figure 2. Regression line.

tion. Table 1 translates the slopes or r values into usable terms of statistical association.

The r^2 refers to the coefficient of determination. If it is multiplied by 100%, it reflects the percentage of variation in the dependent variable that is explained by the value of the independent variable.

Mean, Median, and Mode

Mean, median, mode, and standard deviation are terms applied to the distribution of results.

The mean is the average of a range of values and is denoted by the symbol yn; Sy is the sum of values in a sample containing n values. Mathematically, yn equals the sum of the values (Sy) divided by the number of values (n). Assume a study yields 19 observations (n = 19) and the observed values (y) are as follows:

1 2 2 2 3 3 3 4 4 6 6 6 7 7 7 7 8 8 9

The sum of these values, or Sy, is 95. To find yn (the mean), the sum (Sy or 95) must be divided by the number of values (n or 19), yielding a value of 5 (the yn) (Fig. 3).

The median is the value that lies in the middle of the sample. It is calculated by multiplying the number of values (n) plus one by 0.5. If n is odd, the median is the (0.5) (n + 1) value; if n is even, the median lies between the two middle values. For example, if n = 19, the median lies at the (0.5) (19 + 1) value, or the 10th y, which is 6. If n = 20, the median lies at the (0.5) (20 + 1) value, which would be at the 10.5 value. Since there is no 10.5 value, the median is determined as the average between the y value at position 10 and the y value at position 11.

The mode is the most frequently occurring value in the sample. In Figure 3, the mode is 7.

The mean, median, and mode do not necessarily equal each other. When they do equal each other, the distribution is said to form a normal curve (Fig. 4*A*). When the mean, median, and mode are not equal, the curve is skewed to the left or right (Fig. 4*B* and *C*). The greater the difference between the mean and the median, the greater the skewing of the curve.

Normal Distribution

In many biological studies, the correlations between two variables are studied. If we choose to have frequency as one of the variables, then we will derive graphs similar to those seen in Figure 4. In medicine, when we refer to the "normal range" or "within normal limits," we are generally referring to the central 95% of the variables studied with 2.5% on each side of the curve excluded as outliers (Fig. 5). These outliers are referred to as being outside of 2 standard deviations (SD) (see following).

Null Hypothesis and P Value

The null hypothesis states that any differences between two groups result from random variation or chance rather than a statistically meaningful association. When a study is performed, the null hypothesis must be stated and then either accepted or rejected on statistical grounds. The expressions used for either acceptance or rejection are the significance level and the probability (*P*) value.

We may develop the hypothesis that a computed tomography (CT) scan is a useful test for diagnosing a herniated disc. A study is performed and the results analyzed. The null hypothesis states that there is no association between the CT scan findings and the proven presence of a herniated disc. There can only be one of three results:

1. The CT scan correctly identifies a herniated disc in all (or almost all) circumstances.
2. It correctly identifies it in only some circumstances, but not enough to make it a worthwhile or valid test.
3. There is no correlation between the two (the null hypothesis).

To be able to make these descriptive statements, one must turn to a statistical analysis. This statistical analysis also addresses three issues:

1. Is the correlation correct?

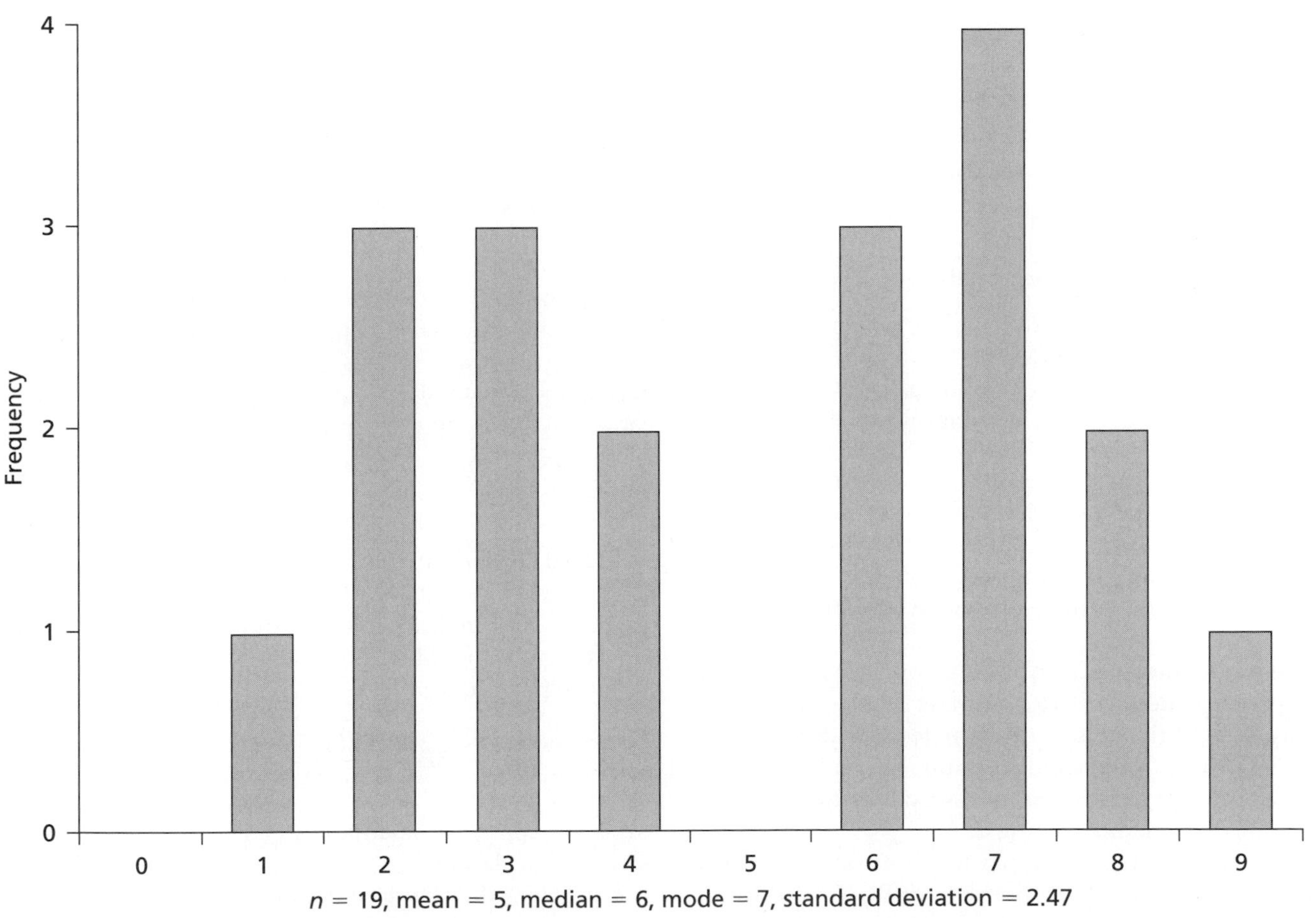

Figure 3. Frequency distribution (n = 19, mean = 5, median = 6, mode = 7, standard deviation = 2.47).

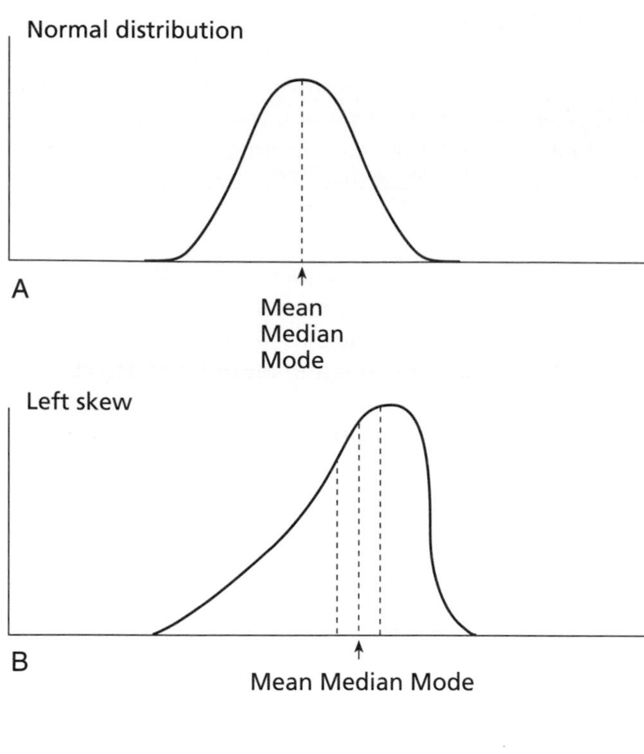

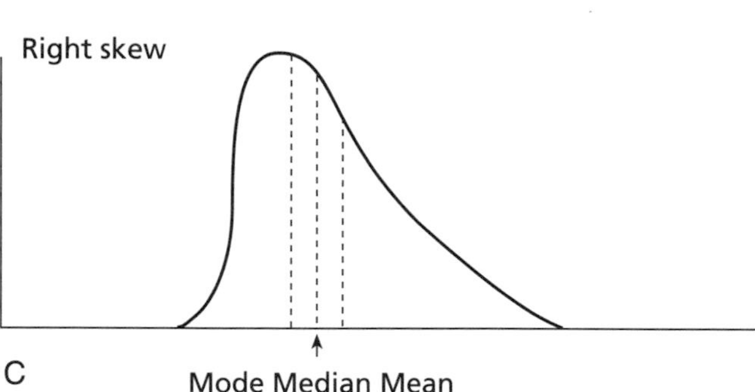

Figure 4. Normal and skewed distributions. *A*, Normal distribution; *B*, Left skew; *C*, Right skew.

2. Was there any confounding factor or bias that resulted in the apparently positive or negative relationship?
3. Was there any random variation that could have produced the positive or negative relationship?

The second issue should not be a concern if the study were properly designed to eliminate all known sources of bias. Also, if the results of many tests, addressing the same hypothesis, yield similar results, the chance of bias is (theoretically) eliminated unless exactly the same bias is present in each and every test.

Statistical analysis attempts to eliminate the third issue as a cause for the observed result. To do this, a test statistic (derived from Student t-test or from the chi-square test) is computed and compared with a predetermined value that provides a tangible meaning to the statistical values derived from the test (termed the critical value). When the test statistic exceeds the critical value, then the null hypothesis is rejected and the test results are accepted as showing a true relationship. The critical value is arbitrarily placed, usually at 5% (that is, all the results fall within 2 SD of expected values). Repeated testing of the same hypothesis is used to accept or reject the association. If repeated testing has not been or cannot be performed, the significance level is examined to determine if the test results should be accepted or rejected. If the significance level is 10%, 25%, or 50%, we should be wary of accepting the results. (When using the t-test or the chi-square test, the higher the number, the lower the probability.)

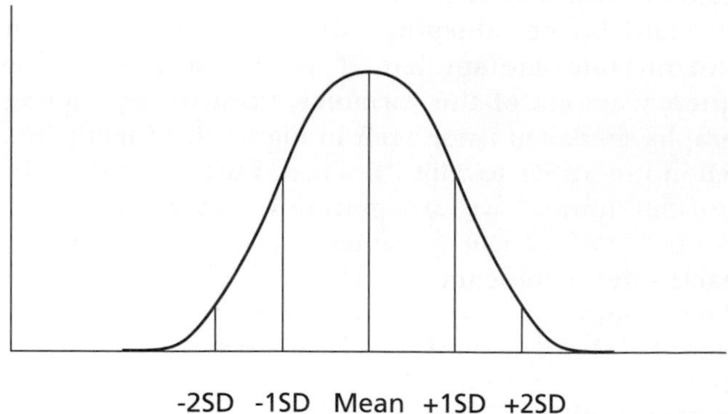

Figure 5. Standard deviations of a normal distribution.

Probability

The probability or *P* value expresses the probability that a difference as large as that observed would happen by chance. A *P* value of 0.05 (or 5%) is usually chosen in most clinical studies. The validity of the test increases as the *P* value decreases (for example, to 0.01 or 0.001).

Standard Deviation

The standard deviation, designated s or SD, reflects how much each value in the sample deviates from the mean, or average, value. Mathematically, it is derived using the following formula:

$$SD = \sqrt{\frac{\sum(y - \bar{y})^2}{n - 1}}$$

Most inexpensive calculators can easily calculate the standard deviation.

What does the standard deviation reveal about the distribution of values in a sample? Why is the standard deviation commonly identified in biological and medical studies? The standard deviation reveals the "spread" of the values, which leads to an analysis of whether the findings have statistical significance or result from chance. For a normal distribution curve, 68% of the observations fall within 1 SD of the mean, 95% within 2 SD, and 99.7% within 3 SD (Fig. 5).

Statistical Significance

In a normal curve, all the y values within 2 SD are found in an area comprising 95% of the total area (see Fig. 5). If a population study of height versus sex yielded a histogram resembling a normal curve, any given result could be expressed as being within or outside 2 SD. These findings would then have statistical significance depending on where they fell.

Epidemiology

Epidemiology is defined as the study of disease occurrence in a given population. This discussion focuses on the terms needed to understand the ideas presented in this text. These terms include, most importantly, sensitivity, specificity, incidence, and prevalence; other terms and their definitional formulae are listed in Table 2. The concepts represented by these terms allow the application of statistical values to population groups and are derived from a standard 2 × 2 table (Table 3).

Incidence and Prevalence

Incidence rates reflect the occurrence of an event happening in a given time period. Incidence can be calculated as the number of new cases in a given time period divided by the population at risk during that time period. Prevalence rates reflect the cumulative number of these events at any given time. Prevalence is found by dividing the total number of events at a given time by the population at risk during that time period.

As an example of how prevalence and incidence are used, if factory workers with herniated discs in a specific factory were studied, the denominator for both incidence and prevalence would be the total number of workers in that factory at risk for developing a herniated disc. If this number is 100, and 10 workers had pre-existent disc disease and an additional 10 developed disc disease during the study period, then the incidence rate (or the number of new cases during the period of study) would be 10/100, which is 10%, whereas the prevalence (or total number of cases at any given time) would be (10 + 10)/100, or 20%.

TABLE 2

Epidemiologic Terms and Formulas*

Name	Formula
Total positive tests	$a + b$
Total negative tests	$c + d$
True positives	a
True negatives	d
False positives	b
False negatives	c
Sensitivity	$a/(a + c)$
Specificity	$d/(b + d)$
Positive predictive value	$a/(a + b)$
Negative predictive value	$d/(c + d)$

*See Table 3 for *a*, *b*, *c*, *d*.

TABLE 3

2 × 2 Table

Screening Test	Final diagnosis: Disease Present	Final diagnosis: Disease Absent	Total
Positive	a	b	$a + b$
Negative	c	d	$c + d$
Total	$a + c$	$b + d$	$a + b + c + d$

Relative Risk

This concept is defined as the incidence rate among the exposed divided by the incidence rate in the nonexposed populations. This is not a measure of probability. For example, it addresses the concept of the number of lung cancers in smokers vs nonsmokers, not the probability or rate that a smoker will develop lung cancer.

Reliability/Validity

Reliability refers to the ability to reproduce the same results when a test is done over. It is a measure of the degree of stability when the measurements are performed under identical conditions.

Validity refers to the accuracy of a test. It is a reflection of the ability to trust the inferences of a study, especially when generalizations are extended beyond the study sample (extrapolation).

The two terms are not synonymous nor should they be used interchangeably. A study may be reliable but not valid, valid but not reliable, both, or neither. For example, a boy scout is out in the woods. His compass is off by 10 degrees. No matter where in the woods he is, the compass is always off by 10 degrees. It is therefore reliable but not valid (or reproducible vs accurate). If he holds the compass too close to his steel canteen, it may not be reliable as it will give a slightly different reading depending on the proximity of the canteen. Thus, the reliability and validity of a test depends on the construct of the test (i.e., free or not free from bias), the working state of the test machinery, and other factors.

Sensitivity and Specificity

Sensitivity is the proportion of disease-positive individuals correctly identified by a positive test. Specificity is the proportion of disease-negative individuals correctly identified by a negative test. How reliable and valid a test is relates to its sensitivity and specificity. Decisions regarding whether to accept the data gathered in testing rest on epidemiologic studies comparing the events expected with the observed outcomes. (The following mnemonic is useful: Se*n*sitivity [NIH] refers to positive in disease; s*p*ecificity [PID] refers to negative in health; to use the mnemonic, cross the P with NIH and N with PID). Positive predictive values refer to the number or proportion of disease-positive individuals with a positive test and negative predictive values refer to the frequency of no disease in test-negative individuals.

General Principles in Applying Statistics and Epidemiologic Concepts

The following points should be noted:

- The greater the number of experimental observations made, the greater is the reliance on the statistical expression; for example, if a study comprises only three results, the fact that all three are positive (100%) is less conclusive than if 97 of 100 were positive (97%).
- A p value of 0.051 (greater than the "accepted cutoff" of 0.05) in a large study differs little from a p value of 0.049.
- Because a study shows statistical significance does not automatically mean that this should or would be accepted clinically; for example, a benign but imperfect treatment for a benign disease can be compared with a new treatment that causes death at a p value less than 0.05 but results in a cure for that benign condition. Clinically, the former may be more acceptable because we are dealing with a benign disease.

A P P E N D I X B

How to Fill Out Disability and Return-to-Work Forms

STEPHEN L. DEMETER, MD, MPH

Social Security

As explained in Chapter 6, the purpose of the Social Security disability forms sent to health care providers (which only cover the medical evidence of a patient's case) is to determine whether a person is capable of performing sustained remunerative work activities. The physician filling out these forms is not "granting" disability, nor is he or she making a determination whether his or her patient qualifies for Social Security Disability. Administrators within the Social Security Administration (SSA), not the treating physician, make the decision whether a person qualifies for Social Security Disability. This team is employed by the Department of Disability Services (DDS) (a State agency that is fully funded by the federal government. It is termed the "adjudicative team" and consists of a medical or psychological consultant [a physician or psychologist] and a layperson called a "disability examiner"). The decision is based not only on the medical facts of the case but also on other issues including the patient's age, educational background, special skills and training, and other facts and issues. These forms are sent to all physicians who the patient has identified as being ones that he or she has seen and been treated by in the past few years (usually limited to the past 12 months).

In general, the SSA is looking for a variety of items of information when compiling the evidence for review of a case. These items include a compilation of the medical or psychological diagnoses; the laboratory evidence of these diagnoses and the information supporting the severity of each illness; and the impact of these medical or psychological conditions on the performance of the activities of daily living, especially their impact on the performance of work-related activities (as this is a disability program). The SSA takes into account the subjective symptoms of a person's health status and tries to make an assessment based on the following criteria (from page 16 of Disability Evaluation under Social Security, SSA Publication No. 64-039, Social Security Administration, Office of Disability, 1998—also referred to as the "Blue Book"):

- The claimant's daily activities
- The location, duration, frequency, and intensity of the pain or other symptoms
- Precipitating and aggravating factors
- The type, dosage, effectiveness, and side effects of any medications
- Treatments, other than medications, for the relief of pain or other symptoms
- Any measures the claimant uses or has used to relieve pain or other symptoms
- Other factors concerning the claimant's functional limitations due to pain or other symptoms

Figures 1 through 3 are an example of a form for a patient whom I was treating. She had severe asthma, arthritis, and a history of peptic ulcer disease. The form was sent to me as her treating pulmonary specialist. Forms were also sent to other physicians who she identified as treating physicians. In fact, she gave a list of physicians to the SSA who had treated her over the past 4 years; a total of eight physicians received forms from the SSA. The forms that the other physicians received were different from mine based on their specialty. Thus, her rheumatologist and orthopedist received forms that focused on joint mobility and strength in addition to the location and amount of arthritis. Her gastroenterologist received forms that focused on her peptic ulcer disease. Her primary care physicians (there were four who got forms) received forms that focused on her general state of health.

Many of these forms that these other physicians received contained questions that overlapped questions found on my forms. For example, in the forms I received, there were questions regarding her ability to think and reason and her ability to care for herself. It would seem more logical for the primary care

Rehabilitation Services Commission Bureau of Disability Determination

Please comment on asthmatic condition to include:

A. What usually precipitates asthma attacks for this patient?

B. Dates of visits to your office for treatment of asthma attacks:

C. Was parenteral or inhaled treatment administered in your office? _______ If so, please provide dates and type of treatment provided:

D. Have attacks required a visit to the ER or inpatient stays greater than 24 hours? _______ If so, please specify including dates and length of stay:

E. Has patient required oral steroid treatment in the past 12–24 months? _______ If so, give the frequency of use and the duration of treatment of each time:

- Please describe the current treatment prescribed to your patient: (including oral bronchodilators, steroids (inhaled or oral), inhaled bronchodilators—hand held or home nebulisation).

Type of Treatment	Medication	Dosage	How Administered	Frequency

- Do you feel this patient is compliant with prescribed therapy? _______ If no, please explain:

Figure 1. Sample of form sent by a state DDS to a physician from the SSA for a disability determination (DDS, Department of Disability Services; SSA, Social Security Administration).

provider to address those issues rather than her pulmonary specialist. These overlap questions were placed in these forms intentionally by the SSA. Again, the purpose of these forms is for the administrative team to be able to document whether a person qualifies for SSA disability. The duplication of questions allows the reviewers to better assess the applicant. Additionally, the DDS does not know which medical professional can best address these types of questions; hence the duplication.

The state agencies of the SSA have some degree of autonomy, especially with respect to the forms that are sent to medical providers. Therefore, the forms found in Figure 1 may not look like the forms that a physician practicing in a state other than Ohio may receive.

The forms are, again, one sent to a pulmonary specialist. They are reprinted to provide an example of the type of information that is requested by the SSA. They are intended to provide an example of how to fill out these forms. A copy of the Social Security rules can be found in the book "Disability Evaluation Under Social Security," which can be obtained from the local SSA office. It may also be downloaded from the SSA Web site at http://www.ssa.gov from the "forms" section (request SSA Pub. #64-039 or merely the "Blue Book"). Another useful form is the form that the SSA will send the patient (SSA-3368—Disability Report Adult) for the information that an applicant must fill out. Other useful information sites are found at the end of Chapter 6.

The general rule with these, or any other forms found in this section, is that no health care provider should attempt to answer or opine regarding any question unless he or she feels comfortable and qualified to answer it, especially for questions outside one's own specialty.

Health care providers, as a rule, may answer the SSA in one of four ways: by sending copies of their progress notes, laboratory tests, and hospitalization summaries; by filling in the forms; by dictating their responses (available in most localities); or by any combination of the above.

- On clinical examination of the chest does the patient have the following signs *between acute exacerbations* (if yes, please describe and characterize wherever possible):

  Rales: ______________________ Wheezing: ______________________

  Rhonchi: ______________________ Prolonged expiration: ______________________

  Increased A-P diameter: ______________________

  Cyanosis and other pertinent observations: ______________________
- Please send copies of any Emergency Room reports or discharge summaries, if available.
- Have pulmonary function studies been done? If yes, please report all of the following if available and send copies of the actual SPIROMETRIC TRACINGS.
- Height ____________ Weight ____________ Date obtained ____________

  Are these measurements without shoes on?

  Date testing done ____________

  Before bronchodilators After bronchodilators

  FVC ______________________ ______________________

  FEV_1 ______________________ ______________________
- Please send a copy of the most recent chest x-ray report.
- Please describe manifestations of patient's emotional problem that you have noted:
- Please estimate level of intellectual function:
- Please describe:
  - patient's ability to relate to others
  - ability to care for personal needs, personal appearance
  - any recent changes in interests or habits
  - any impairment in recent or remote memory
  - any restrictions of daily activities

Figure 2. SSA form. *Continued*

As noted, this form (Figs. 1 through 3) was sent to a pulmonary specialist, regarding a person who has many different diseases. However, the pulmonary specialist is only responsible for a limited part of the patient's medical problems; that part may or may not be sufficient to meet the SSA's criteria for disability.

The purpose of questions B through E in the forms is to obtain a history of the severity of her pulmonary disease by using the frequency of exacerbations as a surrogate for the severity of her illness. Additionally, the issue regarding the precipitating events for the asthmatic attacks (A) is important to the evaluating team as it may indicate certain jobs or conditions that the applicant may not be able to tolerate. After all, these are disability determinations, not impairment evaluations.

Again, the severity of the illness is judged by the frequency of exacerbations, especially those requiring steroid rescues, emergency room (ER) visits, or hospital admissions. It is also rated, or judged, by the types of medications administered, the frequency of those medications, and whether these medications are used as a metered dose inhaler versus aerosol, parenteral versus enteral, etc. Questions are also asked concerning whether the patient, in the physician's opinion, is compliant with the medications prescribed. This assists the evaluating team in assessing the severity of the patient's asthma.

- Diagnosis
- What is current therapy and response (including medication(s) and dosage)?

We would like to have a statement (you may respond at the bottom of this page or on the back), based on your opinion about; the patient's ability, despite the functional limitations imposed by the impairment(s), to do work-related activities or if a child, age appropriate daily activities and to behave in an age appropriate manner such as:

Physical activities:	Mental activities:
sitting	understanding and memory
standing	sustained concentration and persistence
walking	social interaction and adaptation
bending	
lifting	
carrying	
handling objects	
hearing	
speaking	
traveling	

Please provide any other relevant information that you may have.

- Should we need to contact you for additional information, what hours would be most convenient to call?

Date first examined ____________________ Date last examined ____________________

Signature ______________________________ Date ____________________

- If we decide that a consultative examination is needed and if you have an ongoing doctor/patient relationship with this individual, would you be willing to perform a new exam or special testing?

If you do not respond to this question we will assume you do not wish to perform an exam and it will be scheduled with another doctor.

Your medical specialty: ______________________________

Figure 3. SSA form. *Continued*

The next part of the form (Fig. 2) contains questions concerning the clinical examination between exacerbations. Remember that an administrative team is looking for information that will allow for a disability determination based on SSA rules. If the patient is compliant with medication (established in the previous set of questions) and still has unremitting asthma, then there may well be grounds for determining that this person is disabled. The ER (emergency room) sheets and discharge summaries are requested. If there are frequent exacerbations, despite adequate usage of medications, and if these exacerbations are documented by office records, pulmonary function tests (PFTs), ER visits, and/or hospitalizations, then the evaluating team can make an intelligent determination of whether a disability exists (remember that under SSA, this means that the person is not capable of sustained employment).

Questions are next asked about the patient's PFTs. These requests from the SSA are for pre-existent information only. The medical provider is not being asked to schedule a new examination or new tests. If the provided information is incomplete, the SSA will make that determination and purchase the needed test.

TIP: "Doctor, Do I Qualify?"

Often, a patient will ask his or her physician whether he or she would qualify for SSA disability. As mentioned previously, this is a decision made by analyzing both medical and nonmedical criteria. However, sometimes the physician can give his or her patient a reasonable estimate by examining the medical evidence and referring to the "Blue Book."

For example, if this patient were 66 inches tall (without shoes; the SS listings request a height without shoes on) and the measured forced vital capacity (FVC) were 1.40 L, then the administrative team would generally find that this patient was eligible for SS disability based on the medical criterion (as long as the nonmedical criteria were also met; see Table 1, reprinted from the "Blue Book," p 43). The physician could then respond to his or her patient appropriately.

If the FVC were 1.90 L, but the FEV_1 were 1.20 L, then the patient would still meet the medical criteria. However, if the FVC were 1.90 L and the FEV_1 were 1.60 L, then the patient would not (see the values listed in Table 2, from page 43 of the "Blue Book"). At this point, the administrative team would look at other medical conditions that the applicant had to see if there were other qualifying medical conditions. If not, then the fact that the spirometric criteria were close to the disability cutoffs would be taken into consideration. If the patient had other criteria, which by themselves were close but not qualifying, then the totality of the medical conditions and how close they were would be taken as a whole to determine eligibility. This is what the SSA refers to as a "medical equivalent." The team considers the numbers and severities of the patient's illnesses and forms a Gestalt opinion as to whether the totality of the illnesses would equal the criteria for a single illness. With increasing numbers and with increasing severities of these illnesses, the greater the likelihood that the patient will qualify as being medically disabled.

Another alternative is that the team would look at other criteria to make the determination. For the asthmatic, this might include factors such as the precipitating factors of the asthma. It might include whether the person has the background skills, education, or intellectual capability to perform work other than manual labor. Thus one cannot always give a reliable answer to a patient when that person does not meet the strict eligibility criteria found in the SSA manual.

Also at this point, the physician filling out the forms might state that he or she does not use the tests requested by the SSA. Thus a spirometry or full PFT was performed but not in accordance with the rules stated in the "Blue Book." The physician might feel that the tests performed are more state-of-the-art than those requested by the SSA. As discussed in Chapter 25, the rules created by the SSA are unique to that system. Each system assessing impairment or disability formulates rules and regulations that are unique to that system. Each disability or impairment system has its own way of doing things. Each has its own method of analysis. Each has its own lists of tests that are acceptable, accepted, and required. It is the physician's job to adhere to these requirements rather than trying to impose his or her desires upon the "system."

This difficulty is handled in one of two ways. First, fill out the form as if the information were obtained in the "correct" fashion and provide a copy of the test. The physician reviewers in the SSA may be familiar with alternative tests and will make the determination that the test provided meets their criteria as an alternative method of obtaining the desired information. This is another example of a "medical equivalency." For example, if the physician reviewers see that a flow-volume loop was used to obtain the FVC and FEV_1 rather than a volume-time curve, they will most likely accept the results even though it is not the specified test.

The physician may also state on the form that the information was not obtained. That part of the form will then be left blank or (better) the physician writes "N/A" or "not available" or "not done." There will be space provided at the end of the form (usually) for additional comments. The physician may make use of that part of the form to discuss the results of the alternative or "better" tests. For example, if a test of airway resistance was obtained rather than a FEV_1, but the information is equivalent in the opinion of the medical provider, then he or she should provide that information at that point and in this fashion.

TABLE 1

FVC Requirements for Disability Under the SSA (Social Security Administration)

Height Without Shoes (cm)	Height Without Shoes (in)	FVC Equal to or Less Than (L, BTPS)
154 or less	60 or less	1.25
155–160	61–63	1.35
161–165	64–65	1.45
166–170	66–67	1.55
171–175	68–69	1.65
176–180	70–71	1.75
181 or more	72 or more	1.85

FVC = forced vital capacity; L = liter; BTPS = body temperature and pressure saturated with water vapor.
From Disability Evaluation under Social Security, SSA Publication No. 64–039, Social Security Administration, Office of Disability, 1998, p 43, with permission.

TABLE 2

FEV_1 Requirements for Disability Under the SSA

Height Without Shoes (cm)	Height Without Shoes (in)	FEV_1 Equal to or Less Than (L, BTPS)
154 or less	60 or less	1.05
155–160	61–63	1.15
161–165	64–65	1.25
166–170	66–67	1.35
171–175	68–69	1.45
176–180	70–71	1.55
181 or more	72 or more	1.65

FEV_1, forced expiratory volume in 1 second; L = liter; BTPS = body temperature and pressure saturated with water vapor.
From Disability Evaluation under Social Security, SSA Publication No. 64–039, Social Security Administration, Office of Disability, 1998, p 43, with permission.

In the form shown in Figure 2, the SSA is requesting objective documentation by its request for the x-ray reports. This section also asks some of the "overlap" questions, discussed previously, such as the patient's intellectual, emotional, and behavioral levels. Again, other physicians whom the patient has seen will also provide this information. What may be noted or apparent to one physician may be ignored, not examined, or not assessed by another. The degree of emotional/intellectual repercussions of a disease process created by a problem in one organ system may not be necessarily the same as those observed by another specialist or by the generalist. The same holds true for restrictions in activities of daily living (ADLs). Thus the pulmonary specialist may have a more accurate idea of the emotional issues created by the chronic obstructive pulmonary disease (COPD) than the patient's primary care physician. He or she may also be in a better position to assess the restrictions in ADLs than will the primary care physician based on his or her expertise in a particular specialty.

Included in Figure 3 is a request for an opinion about the patient's general physical and mental capabilities in specific areas. This part of the form is, again, asking for an opinion as opposed to an assessment, unless the responding physician is a psychologist or psychiatrist. It is not a request for a functional capacity assessment. If one is needed, the SSA will purchase it. However, if the physician possesses that information, he or she should not hesitate to fill out this form, while making sure that he or she makes some notification that the results are derived from a formal study as opposed to being opinions.

Also, if the physician has not performed an assessment that would allow him or her to fill out this part of the form, there is nothing compelling him or her to do so. Just placing a comment stating that this was not examined and will be sufficient for the SSA. Finally, the physician should not rely solely on the patient's assessment of his or her abilities. The SSA is looking for factual information or for an educated opinion, based on knowledge of the patient. Again, if the physician does not feel comfortable filling out this part of the form, he or she should not do so. Placing a N/A or N/E (not available or not examined) or crossing out an item to indicate that it is not being filled out is sufficient.

It is also at this point that the physician may add other information that he or she feels is important. This is the area in which the physician can provide information concerning testing that falls outside the realm of those accepted by the SSA (see "Tip"). For example, although dobutamine stress testing is not addressed in the "Blue Book" (the Social Security Listings), it can be an acceptable test if the physician elaborates on the utility of the test and describes the equivalency with accepted tests. Conversely, the physician may make comment on the home circumstances of the patient or his or her inability to obtain training that would allow him or her to seek alternative employment. The patient may have open wounds caused by peripheral vascular disease that are resistant to treatment, require frequent visits to a wound center, and are expected to last for a year or greater. The form might detail how a patient, who is otherwise compliant with treatments, has been unable to lose weight, despite concentrated efforts by the patient and the physician. In other words, describe anything that you, the physician, feel may allow the reviewer to better understand the circumstances behind a patient's medical conditions that would potentially make the difference between a positive versus a negative response by the SSA. These circumstances will generally be revealed during an appeal and there is no reason to withhold them at this stage.

At this point, the SSA makes a determination whether the applicant qualifies for SS disability. If the submitted material by all the physicians of record is insufficient for a determination, then the SSA will purchase a separate independent medical evaluation and use that for the medical component of its determination (this is called a consultative examination; it may be done by the treating physician if desired and approved by the SSA—see the last "*" on the form).

Points to Remember

1. You are filling out a form only.
2. You are not making a determination whether your patient does or does not qualify for SS disability.
3. You need to fill out the form to the best of your ability and in an honest and ethical manner. The information that you provide should be within the realm of your personal knowledge based on your relationship with and knowledge of your patient and based on your prior histories, physical examinations, laboratory investigations, and observations.
4. You are not being asked to schedule an appointment for your patient or to perform a complete history and physical examination to fill out this form. Also, you are not being asked to perform any new tests. The requested information is only the material that is found in your existing medical records.
5. The more complete the document, the better the administrators in the SSA can do their job.
6. If data are crucial and missing or not performed, the SSA will make an independent judgment whether they should be obtained. If they are, the SSA will independently make arrangements for those tests.
7. Finally, and most importantly, although you may be the primary physician for this claimant and may feel that your role is that of a patient advocate, your only responsibility with respect to this form and with respect to your patient's claim is to fill out this form accurately, ethically, and as completely as your information will allow.

Department of Labor Style of Forms

These forms all take on a similar appearance. They relate to the Department of Labor (DOL) criteria for manual work. Unfortunately, they rarely, if ever, spell out the meaning of the terms used on the forms. Even when they do, these explanations are usually incomplete or misleading. See Chapter 48 for a complete discussion of these issues. A type of form that you might be asked to fill out for one of your patients might look like Figures 4 through 8.

As discussed in Chapter 1, the purpose of an impairment or disability examination/evaluation is to be able to communicate the findings, recommendations, and ratings with someone else. That "someone else" is usually a layperson. When filling out return-to-work (RTW) forms, that person is usually an administrator of an insurance program, a person in the human resources division of a company, a government agent, etc. Therefore, the purpose of filling out the forms is to make RTW recommendations available and usable to a person who may only possess rudimentary medical knowledge. More importantly, and even more dangerously, it may be a person who, while only possessing a modicum of medical information and background, may think that he or she possesses more information and expertise than he or she actually has.

The other side of the coin is equally true. Although these forms appear to be written in plain English and ask simple questions, the verbiage used is actually quite technical and conveys special information to the receiver. Therefore, the physician who fills out these forms must understand what is being asked. Further, he or she must understand the meaning of the terms used in these forms. Unfortunately, although the terms used in these forms appear to be simple ones, written in plain English, this is far from the truth. For example, the meaning of the term "sedentary work" appears obvious. For a person who is not knowledgeable in these terms, it seems to mean that a person has a desk job and is responsible for no manual labor. In actuality, it can mean something quite different. It can mean that a person will be expected to stand or walk up to 2 hours per an 8-hour workday. It can also mean that this person will also be expected to perform some minimal activities involving manual labor. This person might also be expected to lift up to 3 hours per an 8-hour working day with objects weighing up to 10 pounds, to perform repetitious activities up to 100 times per an 8-hour working day, and/or to carry objects weighing up to 10 pounds up to 3 hours per an 8-hour working day. All these activities are included under the umbrella term "sedentary activities" by the Department of Labor.

Therefore, the physician filling out these forms must understand what the terms found on this or any other form actually mean or refer to rather than relying on his or her understanding of the English language. Communication, as described in Chapter 1, is essential. Therefore, all parties must speak in a common language. This tenet is no more important for the recipient of the communication as it is for the sender of the information.

It cannot be overemphasized that the physician who fills out these forms bears liability for potential malpractice if his or her patient is returned to the work-

Name ______________________ S. S. No. ____________ Date ________
First Initial Last

The above person has been under my care or evaluated for the following illness / injury: List diagnoses - not symptoms.
(Please regard patient / physician confidentiality for non-work related conditions.)

Date of illness / injury

1) ____________________ ________
2) ____________________ ________
3) ____________________ ________

He / She has been under my care from ____________ until ____________ ☐ INITIAL CARE ☐ SUBSEQUENT CARE ☐ NOT APPLICABLE (If emergency care or evaluation.)

EMPLOYEE DISABLED FROM WORK?
☐ No ☐ Yes
First Day Off ____________

DATE ABLE TO RETURN TO WORK:
Full Duty ____________ ☐ Estimate ☐ Actual
Modified Duty ____________ ☐ Estimate ☐ Actual

OTHER INSTRUCTIONS (Describe work modifications, or list additional information.)
If work limitations have been recommended previously and are unchanged, mark this box ☐

____
____
____

Signed ______________________ M.D., D.C. Next appointment date ____________
(Physician's Signature Mandatory)

Print Last Name ____________ Phone (   ) ____________ Federal ID No. ____________

Address ______________________
Street City State Zip

IF EMPLOYEE CAN RETURN TO MODIFIED DUTY WORK, MARK APPROPRIATE WORK LIMITATIONS BELOW.

☐ SEDENTARY WORK. Lifting 10 pounds maximum and occasionally lifting and carrying such articles as dockets, ledgers, and small tools. Jobs are sedentary if walking and standing are required only occasionally and other sedentary criteria are met.

☐ LIGHT WORK. Lifting 20 pounds maximum with frequent lifting and / or carrying of objects weighing up to 10 pounds. Requires walking or standing to a significant degree, or sitting with a degree of pushing and pulling of arm and / or leg controls.

☐ LIGHT MEDIUM WORK. Lifting 30 pounds maximum with frequent lifting and / or carrying of objects weighing up to 20 pounds.

☐ MEDIUM WORK. Lifting 50 pounds maximum with frequent lifting and / or carrying of objects weighing up to 25 pounds.

☐ LIGHT HEAVY WORK. Lifting 75 pounds maximum with frequent lifting and / or carrying of objects weighing up to 40 pounds.

☐ HEAVY WORK. Lifting 100 pounds maximum with frequent lifting and / or carrying of objects weighing up to 50 pounds.

1. IN AN 8 HOUR WORK DAY EMPLOYEE MAY:

STAND/WALK	SIT	DRIVE
☐ None	☐ None	☐ None
☐ 1-4 Hrs	☐ 1-3 Hrs.	☐ 1-3 Hrs.
☐ 4-6 Hrs.	☐ 3-5 Hrs.	☐ 3-5 Hrs.
☐ 6-8 Hrs.	☐ 5-8 Hrs.	☐ 5-8 Hrs.

2. EMPLOYEE MAY:

	BEND	TWIST	SQUAT	CLIMB	REACH
Not at all	☐	☐	☐	☐	☐
Occasionally	☐	☐	☐	☐	☐
Frequently	☐	☐	☐	☐	☐

3. EMPLOYEE ☐ MAY ☐ MAY NOT USE HAND(S) ARM(S) FOR:

GRASPING ☐ MANIPULATION ☐ PUSHING & PULLING ☐

Figure 4. An example of a Department of Labor Style of form.

OPINION OF PHYSICAL CAPACITIES

INSTRUCTIONS:

- Complete the following items based on your clinical evaluation and other testing results of the claimant per an eight-hour workday.
- Any item that you do not believe you can answer should be marked N/A (not answerable).
- Check appropriate boxes as you are completing this form.

Name of claimant	Claim number

Give the full capacity for each activity the claimant is able to perform in an eight-hour workday

TOTAL AT ONE TIME

	0	1	2	3	4	5	6	7	8
Sit	☐	☐	☐	☐	☐	☐	☐	☐	☐
Stand	☐	☐	☐	☐	☐	☐	☐	☐	☐
Walk	☐	☐	☐	☐	☐	☐	☐	☐	☐

TOTAL DURING AN ENTIRE 8 HOUR DAY

	0	1	2	3	4	5	6	7	8
Sit	☐	☐	☐	☐	☐	☐	☐	☐	☐
Stand	☐	☐	☐	☐	☐	☐	☐	☐	☐
Walk	☐	☐	☐	☐	☐	☐	☐	☐	☐

Occasionally—1%-33%, Frequently—34%-66%, Continuously—67%-100%

LIFTING

	Never	Occasionally	Frequently	Continuously
Up to 5 lbs	☐	☐	☐	☐
6-10 lbs	☐	☐	☐	☐
11-20 lbs	☐	☐	☐	☐
21-25 lbs	☐	☐	☐	☐
26-50 lbs	☐	☐	☐	☐
51-100 lbs	☐	☐	☐	☐

CARRYING

	Never	Occasionally	Frequently	Continuously
Up to 5 lbs	☐	☐	☐	☐
6-10 lbs	☐	☐	☐	☐
11-20 lbs	☐	☐	☐	☐
21-25 lbs	☐	☐	☐	☐
26-50 lbs	☐	☐	☐	☐
51-100 lbs	☐	☐	☐	☐

CLAIMANT IS ABLE TO:

	Never	Occasionally	Frequently	Continuously
Bend	☐	☐	☐	☐
Squat	☐	☐	☐	☐
Crawl	☐	☐	☐	☐
Climb	☐	☐	☐	☐
Reach	☐	☐	☐	☐

RESTRICTION OF ACTIVITIES INVOLVING:

	Never	Mild	Moderate	Total
Unprotected heights	☐	☐	☐	☐
Being around moving machinery	☐	☐	☐	☐
Exposure to marked changes in temperature & humidity	☐	☐	☐	☐
Driving automotive equipment	☐	☐	☐	☐
Exposure to dust, fumes & gases	☐	☐	☐	☐

USE OF HANDS IN REPETITIVE ACTION SUCH AS:

	Simple Grasping	Pushing & Pulling Arm Controls	Fine Manipulation
Right	☐ Yes ☐ No	☐ Yes ☐ No	☐ Yes ☐ No
Left	☐ Yes ☐ No	☐ Yes ☐ No	☐ Yes ☐ No

USE OF FEET IN REPETITIVE MOVEMENTS OF LEG CONTROLS

Right	☐ Yes	☐ No
Left	☐ Yes	☐ No
Both	☐ Yes	☐ No

REMARKS ON ABOVE, OR OTHER FUNCTIONAL LIMITATIONS:

____

____

____

____

____

____

Physician's signature	Date

BWC-2977 (Rev. 4/91)

RH-27 Page 2 (Formerly OIC-6077/ICRD-27)

23-S

Figure 5. An example of a Department of Labor Style of form.

OPINION OF PHYSICAL CAPACITIES

INSTRUCTIONS:
- Complete the following items based on your clinical evaluation and other testing results of the claimant per an eight-hour workday
- Any item that you do not believe you can answer should be marked N/A (not answerable).
- Check appropriate boxes as you are completing this form.

Name of claimant	Claim number

Give the full capacity for each activity the claimant is able to perform in an eight-hour workday

TOTAL AT ONE TIME	0	1	2	3	4	5	6	7	8	TOTAL DURING AN ENTIRE 8 HOUR DAY	0	1	2	3	4	5	6	7	8
Sit	☐	☐	☐	☐	☐	☐	☐	☐	☐	Sit	☐	☐	☐	☐	☐	☐	☐	☐	☐
Stand	☐	☐	☐	☐	☐	☐	☐	☐	☐	Stand	☐	☐	☐	☐	☐	☐	☐	☐	☐
Walk	☐	☐	☐	☐	☐	☐	☐	☐	☐	Walk	☐	☐	☐	☐	☐	☐	☐	☐	☐

Occasionally—1%-33%, Frequently—34%-66%, Continuously—67%-100%

Figure 6. Department of Labor Style of form—section on sitting, standing, and walking.

LIFTING	Never	Occasionally	Frequently	Continuously	CARRYING	Never	Occasionally	Frequently	Continuously
Up to 5 lbs	☐	☐	☐	☐	Up to 5 lbs	☐	☐	☐	☐
6-10 lbs	☐	☐	☐	☐	6-10 lbs	☐	☐	☐	☐
11-20 lbs	☐	☐	☐	☐	11-20 lbs	☐	☐	☐	☐
21-25 lbs	☐	☐	☐	☐	21-25 lbs	☐	☐	☐	☐
26-50 lbs	☐	☐	☐	☐	26-50 lbs	☐	☐	☐	☐
51-100 lbs	☐	☐	☐	☐	51-100 lbs	☐	☐	☐	☐

CLAIMANT IS ABLE TO:	Never	Occasionally	Frequently	Continuously
Bend	☐	☐	☐	☐
Squat	☐	☐	☐	☐
Crawl	☐	☐	☐	☐
Climb	☐	☐	☐	☐
Reach	☐	☐	☐	☐

RESTRICTION OF ACTIVITIES INVOLVING:	Never	Mild	Moderate	Total
Unprotected heights	☐	☐	☐	☐
Being around moving machinery	☐	☐	☐	☐
Exposure to marked changes in temperature & humidity	☐	☐	☐	☐
Driving automotive equipment	☐	☐	☐	☐
Exposure to dust, fumes & gases	☐	☐	☐	☐

USE OF HANDS IN REPETITIVE ACTION SUCH AS:

USE OF FEET IN REPETITIVE MOVEMENTS OF LEG CONTROLS

Figure 7. Department of Labor Style of form—section on lifting, carrying, and other activities.

USE OF HANDS IN REPETITIVE ACTION SUCH AS:

	Simple Grasping	Pushing & Pulling Arm Controls	Fine Manipulation
Right	☐ Yes ☐ No	☐ Yes ☐ No	☐ Yes ☐ No
Left	☐ Yes ☐ No	☐ Yes ☐ No	☐ Yes ☐ No

USE OF FEET IN REPETITIVE MOVEMENTS OF LEG CONTROLS

Right	☐ Yes	☐ No
Left	☐ Yes	☐ No
Both	☐ Yes	☐ No

REMARKS ON ABOVE, OR OTHER FUNCTIONAL LIMITATIONS:

Figure 8. Department of Labor Style of form—section on use of hands and feet.

TABLE 3

DOL Divisions of Hours Per Day (DOL, Department of Labor)

%	Hours Per Day
1–33%	0–3
34–66%	3–6
67–100%	6–8

TABLE 5

Work Demands of the Job Categorized by Activity Type and METS

Term	Activity	Amount	Approximate Amount of Work
Sedentary	Lift	0–10 Pounds	
	Carry	None	1.5 METS
	Sit	6–8 Hours	
	Stand	0–2 Hours	
	Walk	0–2 Hours	
Light	Lift	20 Pounds	
	Carry	10 Pounds	3.0 METS
	Stand	4–8 Hours	
	Walk	0–4 Hours	
Medium	Lift	50 Pounds	
	Carry	25 Pounds	4.5 METS
	Stand	8 Hours	
	Walk	8 Hours	
Heavy	Lift	100 Pounds	
	Carry	50 Pounds	6.0 METS
	Stand	8 Hours	
	Walk	8 Hours	
Very Heavy	Lift	>100 Pounds	
	Carry	>50 Pounds	>7.5 METS
	Stand	8 Hours	
	Walk	8 Hours	

place, is placed in an inappropriate job (on the basis of the physician's recommendation), and reinjures himself or herself while appropriately performing the specified activities of his or her job. These forms can be misleading and a physician, by not understanding the words used in these forms, may find himself or herself placing his or her patient into a work situation that is not the situation that was intended. Be careful and know what you are authorizing/recommending.

For analysis, the forms shown in Figures 4 through 8 will be split into several areas with comments on each. Although the forms in Figures 4 through 8 appear more "user friendly" than most, they still require a bit of explanation.

For example, the concepts of 1% to 33% found in Figure 5 refer to the numbers of hours per day. In the case of 1% to 33%, it refers to 3 hours per day. It is difficult to divide an 8-hour workday by three. Why these forms do not use 1% to 25%, 26% to 50%, etc. is unclear but this is standard. Therefore, Table 3 should be used for this part.

The concepts of sit, stand, drive, and walk are self-explanatory. Again, see Chapter 48 for a more complete explanation.

The form in Figure 7 is more easily understood when two tables (Tables 4 and 5) are examined. They are adapted from Table 48–1. Notice the words never, occasionally, frequently, and continuously. What, exactly, do they mean? As discussed, the person filling out these forms must adhere to the definitions used by the requestor. For these terms, the definitions in Table 4 are recommended.

Thus, when asked whether the patient/examinee can lift, carry, bend, squat, crawl, climb, or reach or when there is a restriction of activities involving unprotected heights, being around moving machinery, being exposed to marked changes in temperature and humidity, driving automotive equipment, or being exposed to dust, fumes, and gases, the words never, occasionally, frequently, and continuously can be placed into proper context. Never translates into 0 time or 0 hours per 8-hour day (note that all subsequent times are meant to be a reflection of an 8-hour day), occasionally is up to 3 hours per day, frequently is 3 to 6 hours per day, and continuously is 6 to 8 hours per day. Therefore, the asthmatic patient might be placed into a never category for exposure to dust and fumes. The patient with a bad back might be placed into a category wherein he or she may lift occasionally. However, although this restriction is placed on the patient/examinee and/or company, there is nothing to state that the 3 hours may not be continuous. The physician may have meant that the patient/examinee can lift only once in a while. This is not what the form states. It states that the patient/examinee may lift up to 3 hours but does not specify whether these 3 hours are to be on a continuous or a noncontinuous basis.

TABLE 4

Lifting Demands of Work by Frequency

Physical Demand	Occasionally	Frequently	Continuously
% of time	0–33% of day	34–66% of day	67–100% of day
Approximate repititions	1–100 per 8-hour day	101–500 per 8-hour day	500+ per 8-hour day

TABLE 6

Activity Types in Work

- SEDENTARY WORK. Lifting 10 pounds maximum and occasionally using and carrying such articles as dockets, ledgers, and small tools. Jobs are sedentary as walking and standing are required only occasionally and other sedentary criteria are met
- LIGHT WORK. Lifting 20 pounds maximum with frequent using and/or carrying of objects weighing 10 pounds. Require walking of standing to a significant degree, or sitting with a degree of pushing and pulling of and/or leg controls.
- LIGHT MEDIUM WORK. Lifting 30 pounds maximum with frequent lifting and/or carrying of objects weighing up to 20 pounds.
- MEDIUM WORK. Lifting 50 pounds maximum with frequent lifting and/or carrying of objects weighing up to 25 pounds.
- LIGHT HEAVY WORK. Lifting 75 pounds maximum with frequent lifting and/or carrying of objects weighing up to 40 pounds.
- HEAVY WORK. Lifting 100 pounds maximum with frequent lifting and/or carrying of objects weighing up to 50 pounds.

The same holds true for the various activity levels. To check off that the patient/examinee may frequently carry or lift 21 to 25 pounds states that this activity can be done 4 to 6 hours per day and that these 4 to 6 hours may or may not be continuous.

Other parts of the form use terms such as sedentary, light, medium, heavy, or very heavy. Again, exactly what do these terms mean? Table 6 (derived from various Department of Labor style forms; see also Fig. 4) gives a description of what is meant.

Therefore, if you wish to state that a person with a bad back is incapable for sitting for more that 2 hours at a time, merely stating that he or she can do sedentary work is insufficient. The amount of time that that patient/examinee may sit must be spelled out. This table should also be used in conjunction with the table listing the amount of time that a person can do these types of activities. The number of repetitions must be specified as well.

As noted, sometimes the forms can be confusing or even misleading. Also, as noted, the purpose of filling out the forms is to communicate work capabilities/incapabilities to another person. An example of how the forms can be misleading is seen in the first form in this section. The pertinent part is reprinted in Table 4.

Note that the concepts of sedentary, light, etc. are described in easily understood English. However, this form is following the DOL style and there are actually subtle differences between simple English and what is actually implied. For example, the concept of sedentary work described perviously does not detail the frequency of repetitions nor does it indicate the amount of time that a person would be permitted to perform these activities. The same comments can be made for the other classifications.

For purposes of convenience, Tables 3 through 5 have been combined into one (Table 7). It would be very useful when filling out these forms to have a copy of this table next to the form so that the physician filling out the form knows exactly what he or she is committing his or her patient/examinee to in terms of job activities.

Table 7 is very busy, but, by its completeness, it should help the physician fill out the forms correctly based on his or her intent for his or her patient/examinee. If, in the opinion of the physician who fills out the forms, a particular cell in the table does not adequately describe the activities that he or she wishes to describe for his or her patient/examinee, then the alternative is to state that the terms used do not adequately describe the patient's/examinee's limitations or capabilities and prepare a handwritten prescription that explains these issues better.

Figure 8 shows the last part of the form. Note the new issues to be resolved involving the hands and feet. Note, also, the opportunity to be creative regarding the functional limitations. When these limitations are creatively described, these remarks will be similar to the handwritten notes discussed in the next section.

Handwritten Return-to-work Forms

As described in the previous section, forms may be filled out using the DOL criteria. If the physician does not feel that this system adequately describes the restrictions or work capabilities, then the alternative is to write a RTW prescription. However, the physician should be aware of two major concerns when composing these forms: liability and work description.

Liability—A physician is responsible for the content of the RTW form. The physician can be sued in two ways if the RTW form is filled out incorrectly. The physician can be sued for malpractice if the allowed activities/restrictions are inappropriate. For example, if the physician states that the patient/examinee can return to a given job, and if that patient/examinee injures him- or herself on the job while correctly performing the job, then the physician may be liable for malpractice. For example, if the physician states that the patient/examinee may return to work and places an activity restriction on the patient of lifting 100+ pounds on a frequent but not continuous basis and if that patient/examinee then suffers further harm to his or her lower back while working within these parameters, then the patient/examinee might sue the physician for placing him or her in a position where further injury was the likely foreseeable result. The physician may also be sued for breach of doctor-patient confidentiality if the RTW form contains information that is superfluous or irrelevant to the scope of the RTW opinion. Additionally, there are special issues involving the Americans With Disabilities Act (ADA) regarding liability and the patient's/employee's ability to retain his or her

TABLE 7

Activities Per 8-Hour Work Day Using Department of Labor Categorizations

Activity	% Of Day (Occasionally)	% Of Day (Frequently)	% Of Day (Continuously)	Amount	Approximate Amount of Work
Lift	0–3 Hours per day	4–6 Hours per day	6–8 Hours per day	0–10 Pounds	
Number of repetitions	1–100 per day	101–500 per day	500+ per day		
Carry	0–3 Hours per day	4–6 Hours per day	6–8 Hours per day	None	1.5 METS
Sit				6–8 Hours	
Stand				0–2 Hours	
Walk				0–2 Hours	
Lift	0–3 Hours per day	4–6 Hours per day	6–8 Hours per day	20 Pounds	
Number of repetitions	1–100 per day	101–500 per day	500+ per day		
Carry	0–3 Hours per day	4–6 Hours per day	6–8 Hours per day	10 Pounds	3.0 METS
Stand				4–8 Hours	
Walk				0–4 Hours	
Lift	0–3 Hours per day	4–6 Hours per day	6–8 Hours per day	50 Pounds	
Number of repetitions	1–100 per day	101–500 per day	500+ per day		
Carry	0–3 Hours per day	4–6 Hours per day	6–8 Hours per day	25 Pounds	4.5 METS
Stand				8 Hours	
Walk				8 Hours	
Lift	0–3 Hours per day	4–6 Hours per day	6–8 Hours per day	100 Pounds	
Number of repetitions	1–100 per day	101–500 per day	500+ per day		
Carry	0–3 Hours per day	4–6 Hours per day	6–8 Hours per day	50 Pounds	6.0 METS
Stand				8 Hours	
Walk				8 Hours	
Lift	0–3 Hours per day	4–6 Hours per day	6–8 Hours per day	>100 Pounds	
Number of repetitions	1–100 per day	101–500 per day	500+ per day		
Carry	0–3 Hours per day	4–6 Hours per day	6–8 Hours per day	>50 Pounds	>7.5 METS
Stand				8 Hours	
Walk				8 Hours	

job. A careful reading of the ADA section of Chapter 47 is highly recommended.

Work description—A good rule to remember is to be proactive rather than restrictive when writing a RTW prescription. In other words, it is far better to describe what the patient/examinee can do than describe what the patient/examinee cannot do. It is critical to remember that a person may lose his or her job based on a RTW prescription. It is also easier for the company's human resources department to place a person in a job if the physician clearly describes the person's capabilities rather than restrictions.

Several examples of handwritten RTW prescriptions are provided in the following with commentary on each.

Example 1: Off-work slip for a patient with acute bronchitis:

> John Doe
> Dx: acute bronchitis
> Off work × 2 wks.
> Next appt.—2 wks.

The problem with this RTW form is the diagnosis. This can be construed as a breach of the doctor-patient privilege. Some individuals have stated that, by giving this slip to the patient, there is no breach, as the patient willingly gives it to the employer with this information on it, thereby giving implied consent to the release of the information. It is also suggested that if the slip is given to the patient in a sealed envelope, then the patient no longer can be aware of the release of information and, therefore, the breach now exists. For this matter, and for all the technicalities associated with legal matters, one should seek legal advice. This same comment applies for all examples not only in this section, but all sections in Appendix B.

Another problem with this slip is the time duration for off-work for a diagnosis of acute bronchitis. Putting in the diagnosis thus creates problems for the physician in two ways. The employer or the human resources representative will want to know why the employee had to be off work for 2 weeks for this type of diagnosis. Now the physician will have to detail the condition, complications, treatment, and past medical history justifying such an extended leave.

Example 2: Off-work slip for patient with acute bronchitis:

> John Doe
> Off work × 2 wks.
> Next appt.—1 wk.

This form is better in that it does not give the diagnosis. However, it omits certain elements of important information for the employer. It does not give a date. It is unclear whether the off-work for 2 weeks is for the previous 2 weeks or whether it is for the past week, 1 additional week, and a re-evaluation at that time.

Example 3: RTW for a patient who had acute bronchitis:

> John Doe
> May return to work 6/18
> Dx: acute bronchitis
> No restrictions

The problems with this form are as follows:

- No date
- The diagnosis is given
- No signature
- No duration of off-work

Example 4: RTW for a patient who had acute bronchitis:

> John Doe
> May return to work 6/18
> No restrictions
>
> S. Demeter, M.D.
> 5/30

This form is quite well done. It does not breach confidentiality, gives a RTW date, and states that there are no restrictions. It could be done a bit better by being proactive rather than restrictive (even though there are no restrictions) by stating that John can return to his regular duties.

However, there are problems with this form as well. It does not give a total duration of time off work. More importantly, it lists the date as 5/30 and states that the employee is to be off until 6/18. The employer or the employer's representative may question the additional 2 weeks off work without a re-examination or other reason for the extra time off work.

Example 5: RTW for a patient who had an asthma exacerbation:

> John Doe
> May return to work 6/18
> No exposure to fumes, dust, or extremes of temperature

The problems with this form are as follows:

- No date
- No signature
- No duration of time off-work
- No date of re-evaluation (depending on the date of examination and the date of RTW)
- Most importantly, a very vague list of restrictions. Exactly what does it mean that the person cannot be exposed to "fumes, dust, or extremes of temperature"? How does an employer keep an employee away from dust? It would be better for the RTW form to specify vague amounts than to ignore the issue. Exact amounts should be given whenever possible. It is easier to do this for certain types of restrictions than for others. In the asthmatic, for example, it may impossible to quantify exactly the amount of dust or fumes that the patient may be exposed to although the temperature ranges may be more possible. For the patient with low back pain, it may be easier to quantify the amount of pounds that that person may lift or carry (even though it is an educated estimate).

TIP: Educated Guesses

All physicians creating RTW forms need to be aware of an important issue at this point. A lot of the information that will be placed on these slips will be estimates. However, they are intelligent or educated estimates. There is little chance of physician liability attached to an educated estimate or opinion if the physician does this in good faith and within the limits of his or her professional judgment. Remember, educated opinions/estimates/recommendations are far superior to noneducated guesses, which is what the employer's representative will make unless guided by the physician.

Example 6: RTW for a patient with asthma

John Doe
May return to work 6/18
Restricted from exposures to medium to high levels of dust, smoke, and fumes
Restricted from temperatures below 30 degrees F
These restrictions are to be considered permanent

This example is very well done. The only things missing are the date and signature.

Family and Medical Leave Act Forms

These forms usually come with an explanation attached to the last page. Thus, they are self-explanatory. Samples of these explanations are included at the ends of the forms reprinted in Figure 11. Also see Chapters 46 and 47 for details regarding this Act, who it covers, which companies are to be in compliance with this law, and other details. Remember that it covers individuals who are off work for either personal or for family-related health matters. The employee will not receive pay during this time but his or her job will be held and his or her benefits will continue as if he or she were continuously employed. Some important points that are covered in Chapters 46 and 47 are reviewed in the following.

1. This Act requires that the health care provider (and there are many individuals who are defined as health care providers, not just allopathic or osteopathic physicians) certify that his or her patient is unable to work based on a serious health condition.
2. Another justification for a leave covered in this Act is when the spouse, child, or parent of the employee has a serious health condition and the employee/patient must be off work in order to take care of that individual. Thus the physician may be filling out this form for the employee who is not his or her patient, but the spouse, parent, or child of his or her patient.
3. The law anticipates that the employer will submit a list of the essential job functions to the certifier.
4. There are provisions for intermittent or reduced leave.
5. The description of the medical illness and treatment(s) is a valid request by the employer upon the certifier. There is no breach of confidentiality when complying with these requests, as it is understood by the employee that this is part of the certification process.
6. If the employer is dissatisfied with the written material provided by the certifier, there are provisions for second and third opinions.
7. The employer may require that the physician provide a certification of fitness for duty and a RTW slip when the absence is created by a serious health problem, prior to returning to work.
8. Substance abuse programs for the patient or the family member are covered under this act as a health issue.

Request For Leave of Absence

I, ______________________________, [Social Security Number ______ - ______ - ______] am requesting a Leave Of Absence beginning on ______________ ending on ______________ for the following reason(s):

HR ______ Approved
- O Birth of a child
- O Adoption of a child
- O Serious health condition of spouse, child, or parent
- O My serious health condition (including Workers' Compensation)
- O Medical Leave of Absence (only available after all benefit and FMLA time exhausted)

Director ______ Approved
- O Military — Approved Denied Date: ______________
- O Departmental (non-qualifying FMLA issues)
- O Personal (non-qualifying FMLA issues) — **Director Signature**: ______________________

Status:(Please circle one) FT SFT PT OC (Please circle one) Nonbargaining ONA USWA

Please initial the item(s), which apply to you:

________ I wish to continue participating in my Flexible Resources benefits plans. During a paid leave, all benefit plans continue at the same premium. A paid leave includes payment from sick, vacation, or holiday time paid through the payroll system it does not include Workers' Compensation, LTD, Social Security, etc. During an unpaid leave, I understand that I am responsible for submitting payment to Human Resources on a monthly basis. I understand late or unpaid premiums will result in cancellation of coverage. Please refer to the Human Resource policy manual or call the benefits helpline at for details on what benefits may be continued, how long they may be continued, and the cost of each.

________ I wish to cancel my benefit coverage while on leave. I understand that I may reinstate my coverage after an FMLA leave if I enroll within 30 days of returning to work in a benefits eligible position. No waiting period or Evidence of Insurability will apply. If I return to a benefits eligible position following an LOA other than FMLA, I will have the opportunity to enroll for benefits coverage immediately upon return to work at the conclusion of my LOA or during the next open enrollment period.

________ I am not participating in any benefits programs (medical, long-term disability, life or reimbursement accounts).

I realize that approval of any leave is contingent upon notice of proper medical verification and/or supportive evidence of the necessity for the leave. A completed Certification of Health Care Provider form for any FMLA must be supplied. Furthermore, I understand that I am required by hospital policy to inform my department director prior to the end of the approved leave period if my return will be delayed in any manner and to submit any additional documentation to support an extension to any leave. Failure to do so may result in disciplinary action up to and including discharge.

Employee Signature: ______________________________ Date: __________ Department: ____________.

Request for a Medical Leave of Absence has been approved for the requested period.
Request for a Medical Leave of Absence has been approved for the following date(s) only ______________________.
Request for a Medical Leave of Absence has been denied for the following reason(s):
- O Insufficient medical documentation
- O Other ______________________________

Request for leave has been approved as FMLA qualifying leave for the requested period.
Request for leave has been approved as FMLA qualifying leave for the following date(s) only ______________________.
Request for leave has been approved as FMLA qualifying reduced schedule. It is your responsibility to work out an acceptable schedule with your department in order to accommodate your need for leave.
Request for leave has been denied as FMLA qualifying leave for the following reason(s):
- O You have not met the 12 months of service and/or the 1250 hours worked in the past 12 months
- O The Certification of Health Care Provider form was received greater than 30 days after the request for such certification
- O Condition does not qualify under FMLA guidelines
- O Insufficient medical documentation
- O Other ______________________________

LOA Specialist: ______________________________ Date: ______________________

Figure 9. FMLA style form.

Certification of Health Care Provider

(Family and Medical Leave Act of 1993)

To the Physician or Practitioner: Our employee has requested time off pursuant to the Family Medical Leave Act. In order to consider this request, we require the information requested below to make a determination. Please complete all questions.

1. Employee's Name: ______________________________

2. Patient's Name (if different from employee): ______________________________

3. Please note that a "serious health condition" under the Family and Medical Leave Act is defined on page 4. Does the patient's condition[1] qualify under any of the categories described? If so, please check the applicable category.

   (1)____ (2)____ (3)____ (4)____ (5)____ (6)____, or None of the above ____

4. Describe the medical facts which support your certification, including a brief statement as to how the medical facts meet the criteria of one of these categories:

5.a. State the approximate date the condition commenced, and the probable duration of the condition (and also the probable duration of the patient's present incapacity[2] if different):

b. Will it be necessary for the employee to take work only intermittently or to work on a less than full schedule as a result of the condition (including for treatment described in Item 6 below)? ____

If yes, give the probable duration:

---

1 Here and elsewhere on this form, the information sought relates only to the condition for which the employee is taking FMLA leave.

2 "Incapacity," for purposes of FMLA, is defined to mean inability to work, attend school or perform other regular daily activities due to the serious health condition, treatment therefore, or recovery therefrom.

Figure 9. *Continued*

c. If the condition is a chronic condition (condition #4) or pregnancy, state whether the patient is presently incapacitated[2] and the likely duration and frequency of episodes of incapacity[2]:

6.a. If additional treatments will be required for the condition, provide an estimate of the probable number of such treatments.

b. If the patient will be absent from work or other daily activities because of treatment on an intermittent or part-time basis, also provide an estimate of the probable number and interval between such treatments, actual or estimated dates of treatment if known, and period required for recovery if any.

c. If any of these treatments will be provided by another provider of health services (*e.g.*, physical therapist) please state the nature of the treatments.

d. If a regimen of continuing treatment by the patient is required under your supervision, provide a general description of such regimen (*e.g.*, prescription drugs, physical therapy requiring special equipment):

7.a. If medical leave is required for the employee's absence from work because of the employee's own condition (including absences due to pregnancy or a chronic condition), is the employee unable to perform work of any kind? ____

b. If able to perform some work, is the employee unable to perform any one or more of the essential functions of the employee's job (the employee or the employer should supply you with information about the essential job functions)? ____ If yes, please list the essential functions the employee is unable to perform:

2

Figure 9. *Continued*

c. If neither a. nor b. applies, is it necessary for the employee to be absent from work for treatment? ____

8.a. If leave is required to care for a family member of the employee with a serious health condition, does the patient require assistance for basic medical or personal needs or safety or for transportation? ____

b. If no , would the employee's presence to provide psychological comfort be beneficial to the patient or assist in the patient's recovery? ____

c. If the patient will need care only intermittently or on a part-time basis, please indicate the probable duration of this need:

(Signature of Health Care Provider) (Type of Practice)

(Address) (Telephone Number)

To be completed by the employee needing family leave to care for a family member:

State the care you will provide and an estimate of the period during which care will be provided, including a schedule if leave is to be taken intermittently or if it will be necessary for you to work less than a full schedule.

(Employee Signature) (Date)

3

Figure 9. *Continued*

A "Serious Health Condition" means an illness, injury, impairment, or physical or mental condition that involves one of the following:

1. Hospital Care
Inpatient care (*i.e.*, an overnight stay) in a hospital, hospice, or residential medical care facility, including any period of incapacity[2] or subsequent treatment in connection with or consequent to such inpatient care.

2. Absence Plus Treatment
(a) A period of incapacity[2] of more than three consecutive calendar days (including any subsequent treatment or period of incapacity[2] relating to the same condition) that also involves:
(1) Treatment[3] two or more times by a health care provider, by a nurse or physician's assistant under direct supervision of a health care provider, or by a provider of health care services (*e.g.*, physical therapist) under orders of, or on referral by, a health care provider; *or*
(2) Treatment by a health care provider on at least one occasion with results in a regimen of continuing treatment[4] under the supervision of the health care provider.

3. Pregnancy
Any period of incapacity due to pregnancy, or for prenatal care.

4. Chronic Conditions Requiring Treatments
A chronic condition which:
(1) Requires periodic visits for treatment by a health care provider, or by a nurse or physician's assistant under direct supervision of a health care provider;
(2) Continues over an extended period of time (including recurring episodes of a single underlying condition); and
(3) May cause episodic rather than a continuing period of incapacity[2] (*e.g.*, asthma, diabetes, epilepsy, etc.).

5. Permanent / Long-term Conditions Requiring Supervision
A period of incapacity[2] which is permanent or long-term due to a condition for which treatment may not be effective. The employee or family member must be under the continuing supervision of, but need not be receiving active treatment by, a health care provider. Examples include Alzheimer's, a severe stroke, or the terminal stages of a disease.

6. Multiple Treatments (Non-Chronic Conditions)
Any period of absence to receive multiple treatments (including any period of recovery therefrom) by a health care provider or by a provider of health care services under orders of, or on referral by, a health care provider, either for restorative surgery after an accident or other injury, or for a condition that would likely result in a period of incapacity[2] of more than three consecutive calendar days in the absence of medical intervention or treatment such as cancer (chemotherapy, radiation, etc.), severe arthritis (physical therapy), kidney disease (dialysis).

---

3 Treatment includes examinations to determine if a serious health condition exits and evaluations of the condition. Treatment does not include routine physical examinations, eye examinations, or dental examinations.

4 A regimen of continuing treatment includes, for example, a course of prescription medication (*e.g.*, an antibiotic) or therapy requiring special equipment to resolve or alleviate the health condition. A regimen of treatment does not include the taking of over-the-counter medications such as aspirin, antihistamines, or salves, or bed-rest, drinking fluids, exercise, and other similar activities that can be initiated without a visit to a health care provider.

Figure 9. *Continued*

9. Also covered is the time required for the birth or care of the newborn (or adopted child) for both the mother and the father.
10. The employer may request recertification after 30 days.
11. There are other legal provisions restricting the circumstances and material that the employer may request as well as whether modified duty exists and is to be performed by the employee/patient. See Chapter 47 for details.

As noted, these forms are self-explanatory but a careful reading is recommended, as all forms will be slightly different. The language and explanations given in forms 10 and 11 are taken directly from the Act itself.

The author expresses his gratitude to the following individuals who helped with Appendix B: Charles Atkins, Esq., Barry Eigen, Esq., of the SSA, and the people in the Social Security Division of Medical and Vocational Policy: Karen Erzine, MD, Carolyn Kiefer, and William Anderson.

APPENDIX C

Resource Lists

BARBARA JUDY, RN, MA

"Reasonable accommodation" for a qualified individual with a disability refers to a modification of the work situation or environment that enables the individual to meet the same job demands and conditions of employment as any other individual in the same job or similar job.

In a recent survey conducted by the Job Accommodation Network, 78% of all accommodations cost less than $1000. In addition, employers, in response to another survey, reported that they believed the return on investment in an accommodation was more than 30 to 1.

The following list identifies resources at community, state, and national levels that provide both information and support regarding the Americans With Disabilities Act (ADA) and reasonable accommodation.

These resources span the spectrum of information and services and are available to individuals who are in need of information and assistance; to executives, staff, managers, and workers in the business and industrial communities; to claims adjusters and managers in the insurance industry; to professionals and consultants in all fields; and to any other interested parties.

They may be used when there is a particular problem to solve or to obtain general information. There are resources to help with all aspects of accommodation from analyzing the capabilities of a person with a disability to on-site job analysis and designing the accommodation in a particular case.

Federal Agencies That Provide ADA Assistance

Title I
U.S. Equal Employment Opportunity Commission
1801 L Street, NW, Washington, DC 20507
(202) 663-4900 (Voice); (202) 663-4494 (TTY)
Local Field Office (800) 669-4000 (Voice);
(800) 669-6820 (TTY)
www.eeoc.gov

Title II and III
U.S. Department of Justice—Office of the Americans With Disabilities Act Civil Rights Division
PO Box 66738, Washington, DC 20035-6738
(202) 307-0663 (Voice/TTD); (202) 307-1198 (Fax)
ADA (800) 514-0301 (Voice); (800) 514-0383 (TTY)
http://www.usdoj.gov/crt/ada/adahom1.htm

Department of Transportation
400 Seventh Street, SW, Washington, DC 20590
(202) 366-4000 (Voice); (202) 755-7687 (TTY)
www.fta.dot.gov/office/civ.htm

Title IV
Federal Communication Commission
445 Twelfth Street, SW, Washington, DC 20554
(888) 225-5322 (Voice); (888) 835-5322 (TTY)
www.fcc.gov/cib/dro

ADA Accessibility Guidelines
Architectural and Transportation Barriers Compliance Board
The Access Board, 1331 F Street, NW, Suite 1000,
Washington, DC 20004-1111
(800) 872-2253 (Voice); (800) 993-2822 (TTY)
www.access-board.gov

Office of Disability Employment Policy (ODEP)
Job Accommodation Network (JAN)
West Virginia University, 918 Chestnut Ridge Road,
Suite 1, PO Box 6080, Morgantown, WV 26506-6080
(800) 526-7234 (Voice/TDD)
www.jan.wvu.edu

Regional Disability and Business Technical Assistance Centers (DBTACs)

(800) 949-4232 (Voice/TDD)
A free call will ring through to the NIDRR DBTAC responsible for the region that contains your area code.

Region	Address/Phone/Fax/TDD
I-New England DBTAC CT, ME, MA, NH, RI, VT	Adaptive Environments Center, Inc. 374 Congress Street, Suite 301, Boston, MA 02210 (617) 695-0085 (V/TTY); (617) 482-8099 (Fax) http://www.adaptenv.org
II-Northeast DBTAC NJ, NY, PR, VI	United Cerebral Palsy Associations of New Jersey 354 South Broad Street, Trenton, NJ 08608 (609) 392-4004 (V); (609) 392-7044 (TTY); (609) 392-3505 (Fax)
III-Mid-Atlantic DBTAC DE, DC, MD, PA, VA, WV	TransCen, Inc. 451 Hungerford Drive, Suite 607, Rockville, MD 20850 (301) 217-0124 (V/TTY); (301) 217-0754 (Fax) http://www.adainfo.org
IV-Southeast DBTAC AL, FL, GA, KY, NC, SC, MS, TN	UCP National Center for Rehab Technology at Georgia Tech 490 Tenth Street, Atlanta, GA 30318 (404) 385-0636 (V/TTY); (404) 385-0641 (Fax) http://www.sedbtac.org
V-Great Lakes DBTAC IL, IN, MI, MN, OH, WI	University of Illinois/Chicago Dept on Disability & Human Development 1640 West Roosevelt Road, Chicago, IL 60608 (312) 413-1407 (V/TTY); (312) 413-1856 (Fax)
VI-Southwest DBTAC AR, LA, NM, OK, TX	http://www.adagreatlakes.org Independent Living Research Utilization 2323 South Shepherd Boulevard, Suite 1000, Houston, TX 77019 (713) 520-0232 (V/TTY); (713) 520-5785 (Fax) http://www.ilru.org/dbtac
VII-Great Plains DBTAC IA, KS, NE, MO	ADA Project, University of Missouri/Columbia 100 Corporate Lake Drive, Columbia, MO 65203 (573) 882-3600 (V/TTY); (573) 884-4925 (Fax) http://www.adaproject.org
VIII-Rocky Mountain DBTAC CO, MT, ND, SD, UT, WY	Meeting the Challenge, Inc. 3630 Sinton Road, Suite 103, Colorado Springs, CO 80907 (719) 444-0268 (V/TTY); (719) 444-0269 (Fax) http://www.ada-infonet.org
IX-Pacific DBTAC AZ, CA, HI, NV, Pacific Basin	California Public Health Institute 2168 Shattuck Avenue, Suite 301, Berkeley, CA 94704-1307 (510) 848-2980 (V); (510) 848-1840 (TTY); (510) 848-1981 (Fax) http://www.pacdbtac.org
X-Northwest DBTAC AK, ID, OR, WA	Washington State Gov. Com. on Disability Issues & Employment PO Box 9046, MS 6000, Olympia, WA 98507-9046 (360) 438-4116 (V/TTY); (360) 438-3208 (Fax) http://www.wata.org/NWD

State Rehabilitation Agencies

Alabama (AL)
Alabama Department of Rehabilitation Services
2129 East South Boulevard
PO Box 11586
Montgomery, AL 36116
(334) 281-8780/(800) 441-7607
(334) 613-2249 (TDD)
(334) 281-1973 (Fax)
http://www.rehab.state.al.us

Alaska (AK)
Alaska Division of Vocational Rehabilitation
801 West 10th Street, Suite 200
Juneau, AK 99801
(907) 465-2814/(800) 478-2815
(907) 465-2856 (Fax)
http://www.educ.state.ak.us/vocrehab/home.html

Arizona (AZ)
Arizona Rehabilitation Services Administration
1789 West Jefferson 2, NW
Phoenix, AZ 85007
(602) 542-3332/(800) 563-1221
(602) 542-3778 (Fax)
http://www.azrsa.org

Arkansas (AR)
Arkansas Rehabilitation Services
1616 Brookwood Drive
PO Box 3781
Little Rock, AR 72203
(501) 296-1600/(800) 330-0632
(501) 296-1669 (TDD)
(501) 296-1655 (Fax)

California (CA)
California Health and Human Service Agency
Department of Rehabilitation
2000 Evergreen Street
Sacramento, CA 95815
(916) 263-8981 (Voice)
(916) 263-7477 (TTY)
http://www.rehab.cahwnet.gov

Colorado (CO)
Colorado Department of Human Services
2211 West Evans, Building B
Denver, CO 80223
(720) 884-1234 (Voice & TDD)
(720) 884-1213 (Fax)
http://www.cdhs.state.co.us/ods/dvr/index.html

Connecticut (CT)
Bureau of Rehabilitation Services
Department of Social Services
25 Sigourney Street 11th Floor
Hartford, CT 06106
(800) 842-1508
(800) 842-4542 (TTY)
http://www.dss.state.ct.us/divs/brs.htm

Board of Education and Services for the Blind
Vocational Rehabilitation Division
184 Windsor Avenue
Windsor, CT 06095
(860) 602-4000/(800) 842-4510
(860) 602-4002 (TTY)

Delaware (DE)
Delaware Division of Vocational Rehabilitation
4425 North Market Street
PO Box 9969
Wilmington, DE 19809-0969
(302) 761-8275 (Voice/TTY)
(302) 761-6611 (Fax)

District of Columbia (DC)
D.C. Rehabilitation Services Administration
800 9th Street, SW, Fourth Floor
Washington, DC 20024-2487
(202) 645-5883
(202) 645-5847 (TDD)
(202) 645-3857 (Fax)
(202) 645-5798 (Chinese Speaking)
(202) 645-5875 (Spanish Speaking)
http://dhs.Washington.dc.us/

Florida (FL)
Division of Vocational Rehabilitation
2002-A Old Saint Augustine Road
Tallahassee, FL 32399-0696
(850) 488-6210/(800) 451-4327
(850) 488-8062 (Fax)
http://www.state.fl.us/vocrehab

Florida Division of Blind Services
2551 Executive Center Circle West
Tallahassee, FL 32399
(850) 488-1330/(800) 342-1828
(850) 487-1804 (Fax)

Georgia (GA)
Division of Rehabilitation Services
Georgia Department of Human Resources
2 Peachtree Street, NW
35th Floor
Atlanta, GA 30303-3142
(404) 657-3000
(404) 657-3086 (Fax)
http://www.state.ga.us/departments/dhr/

Hawaii (HI)
Hawaii Vocational Rehabilitation & Services for the Blind
The State Kakuhihewa Building
601 Kamokila Boulevard, Room 515
Kapolei, HI 96707
(808) 692-7722
http://www.state.hi.us

Idaho (ID)
Idaho Division of Vocational Rehabilitation
Agency of the State Board of Education
650 West State Street, Room 150
PO Box 83720
Boise, ID 83720-0096
(208) 334-3390/(800) 856-2720
(208) 334-5305 (Fax)
http://www.state.id.us/idvr/idvrhome.htm

Illinois (IL)
Department of Human Services
Office of Rehabilitation Services
623 East Adams Street, PO Box 19429
Springfield, IL 62794
(800) 843-6154 (customers)
(800) 804-3833 (providers)
(800) 447-6404 (TTY)

Indiana (IN)
Division of Disability, Aging & Rehabilitative Services
402 W. Washington Street C-453
PO Box 7083
Indianapolis, IN 46207-7083
(317) 232-1252 (customers)
(317) 232-6478 (Fax)
http://www.state.in.us/fssa

Iowa (IA)
Iowa Division of Vocational Rehabilitation Services
510 East 12th Street
Des Moines, IA 50319
(515) 281-6731/(800) 532-4703 (Iowa only)
(515) 281-4703 (Fax)
http://www.dvrs.state.ia.us

The Iowa Department for the Blind
524 Fourth Street
Des Moines, IA 50309
(515) 281-1333/(800) 362-2587
(515) 281-1263 (Fax)
http://www.blind.state.ia.us

Kansas (KS)
Department of Social and Rehabilitation Services
915 Harrison Street Office Building
Topeka, KS 66612
(785) 296-3959
(785) 296-2173 (Fax)
http://www.ink.org/public/srs/ISD.htm

Kentucky (KY)
Kentucky Department of Vocational Rehabilitation
209 St. Clair Street
Frankfort, KY 40601
(800) 372-7172 (Voice/TDD)
http://www.ihdi.uky.edu/projects/dvr/dvrhome.htm

Kentucky Department for the Blind
209 St. Clair Street
PO Box 757
Frankfort, KY 40602
(502) 564-4754/(800) 321-6668
(502) 564-2929 (TDD)
(502) 564-2951 (Fax)

Louisiana (LA)
Louisiana Rehabilitation Services
8225 Florida Boulevard
Baton Rouge, LA 70806
(504) 925-4131/(800) 737-2958
(504) 925-4184 (Fax)
http://www.dss.state.la.us

Maine (ME)
Maine Bureau of Rehabilitation Services
150 State House Station
Augusta, ME 04333-0150
(207) 624-5950/(207) 624-5955
(800) 698-4440 (TTY)
(207) 624-5980 (Fax)

Division for the Blind and Visually Impaired
150 State House Station
Augusta, ME 04333-0150
(207) 624-5959/(207) 624-5955
(800) 698-4440 (TTY)
(207) 624-5980 (Fax)
http://janus.state.me.us/labor/brs/vr.htm

Maryland (MD)
Maryland State Department of Education
Division of Rehabilitation Services
2301 Argonne Drive
Baltimore, MD 21218-1696
(410) 554-9388/(888) 554-0334
(800) 735-2258 (TDD)
(410) 554-9412 (Fax)
www.dors.state.md.us

Massachusetts (MA)
Massachusetts Rehabilitation Commission
Fort Point Place
27-43 Wormwood Street
Boston, MA 02210-1616

(617) 204-3600/(800) 245-6543
(617) 204-3868 (TTY or Voice)
(617) 727-1354 (Fax)
www.state.ma.us/mrc

Massachusetts Commission for the Blind
88 Kingston Street
Boston, MA 02111-2227
(617) 727-5550/(800) 392-6450
(800) 392-6556 (TDD)
(617) 727-5960 (Fax)
www.state.ma.us/mcb

Michigan (MI)
Michigan Department of Career Development
Rehabilitation Services
608 Allegan, PO Box 30010
Lansing, MI 48909
(800) 605-6722
(888) 605-6722 (TTY)
(517) 373-0565 (Fax)
http://www.mrs.state.mi.us

FIA, Michigan Commission for the Blind
PO Box 30652
Lansing, MI 48909
(517) 373-2062/(800) 292-4200
(517) 373-4025 (TDD)
(517) 335-5140 (Fax)

Minnesota (MN)
Department of Economic Security
Rehabilitation Services Branch
390 North Robert Street
Saint Paul, MN 55101
(612) 296-5616/(800) 328-9095
(612) 296-3900 (TTY)/(800) 657-3973
(612) 296-5159 (Fax)
www.des.state.mn.us/burgendy/rehab.htm

Mississippi (MS)
Mississippi Department of Rehabilitation Services
PO Box 1698
Jackson, MS 39215-1698
(601) 853-5321
(601) 853-5325 (TTY)
(601) 853-5310 (Fax)

Missouri (MO)
Missouri Division of Vocational Rehabilitation
3024 West Truman Boulevard
Jefferson City, MO 65109
(573) 751-3251/(800) 735-2466
(573) 751-0881 (TTY)/(800) 735-2966 (TTY)
http://services.dese.state.mo.us/divvocrehab

Missouri Rehabilitation Services for the Blind
PO Box 88
Jefferson City, MO 65103-0088
(573) 751-4249/(800) 592-6004
(573) 751-4984 (Fax)

Montana (MT)
Montana Vocational Rehabilitation
111 Sanders
PO Box 4210
Helena, MT 59604-4210
(406) 444-2590 (Voice/TDD)
(406) 444-3632 (Fax)
http://www.dphhs.mt.gov

Nebraska (NE)
Nebraska Department of Education
Vocational Rehabilitation
PO Box 94987
301 Centennial Mall, South
Lincoln, NE 68509-4987
(402) 471-3644/(800) 742-7594
(402) 471-0788 (Fax)
http://nde4.nde.state.ne.us/VR/VocRe.html

Nevada (NV)
Bureau of Vocational Rehabilitation
505 East King Street, Room 501
Carson City, NV 89701-3704
(775) 684-4070 (Voice/TDD)
(775) 684-4186 (Fax)
http://detr.state.nv.us/rehab/reh_vorh.htm

New Hampshire (NH)
Department of Education
Division of Vocational Rehabilitation
78 Regional Drive
Concord, New Hampshire
(603) 271-3471/(800) 299-1647
(800) 735-2964 (TDD)
(603) 271-7095 (Fax)
http://www.state.nh.us/doe/

Department of Education
Services for the Blind and Visually Impaired
78 Regional Drive
Concord, NH 03301-3537
(603) 271-3537/(800) 339-9900
(800) 735-2964 (TDD)
(603) 271-7095 (Fax)
http://www.state.nh.us/doe/

New Jersey (NJ)
New Jersey Division of Vocational Rehabilitation
Services
135 East State Street, PO Box 398

Trenton, NJ 08625-0398
(609) 292-5987/(609) 292-8347
(609) 292-2919 (TDD)

New Jersey Department of Human Services
Commission for the Blind and Visually Impaired
153 Halsey Street, 6th Floor
PO Box 47017
Newark, NJ 07101
(973) 648-3333
(973) 648-7364 (Fax)

New Mexico (NM)
New Mexico Division of Vocational Rehabilitation
435 St. Michael's Drive, Building D
Santa Fe, NM 87505
(505) 954-8500/(800) 224-7005
(505) 954-8562 (Fax)
http://www.state.nm.us/dvr

New Mexico Commission for The Blind
P.E.R.A. Building, Room 553
Santa Fe, NM 87503
(505) 827-4479/(888) 513-7968
(505) 827-4475 (Fax)
http://www.state.nm.us/cftb/

New York (NY)
Vocational and Educational Services for Individuals with Disabilities
99 Washington Avenue
Albany, NY 12234
(800) 222-JOBS
(518) 486-4154 (Fax)
http://web.nysed.gov/vesid

Commission for the Blind and Visually Handicapped
40 North Pearl Street
Albany, NY 11243-0001
(518) 474-7079 (Voice)
(518) 474-7501 (TTY)
(518) 486-5819 (Fax)
www.dfa.state.ny.us/cbvh/

North Carolina (NC)
North Carolina Division of Vocational Rehabilitation Services
805 Ruggles
Raleigh, NC 27603
(919) 733-3364
(919) 733-7968 (Fax)
http://www.dhhs.state.nc.us

North Carolina Division of Services for the Blind
2601 Mail Service Center
Raleigh, NC 27699
(919) 733-9700
(919) 733-9700 (TDD)
(919) 715-8771 (Fax)
http://www.dhhs.state.nc.us/dsb/

North Dakota (ND)
N.D. Disability Services Division
Vocational Rehabilitation
600 South 2nd Street, Suite 1B
Bismark, ND 58504
(701) 328-8950/(800) 755-2745
(701) 328-8968 (TDD)
(701) 328-8969 (Fax)

Ohio (OH)
Ohio Rehabilitation Services Commission
400 East Campus View Boulevard
Columbus, OH 43235-4604
(614) 438-1200 (Voice/TYY)/(800) 282-4536 (Ohio only)
(614) 438-1257 (Fax)
http://www.state.oh.us/rsc/

Oklahoma (OK)
Department of Rehabilitation Services
3535 NW 58th, Suite 500
Oklahoma City, OK 73112
(405) 951-3400
(405) 951-3529 (Fax)

Oregon (OR)
Disability Determination Services
500 Summer Street, NE
Salem, OR 97310-1020
(503) 945-5878/(800) 452-2147
(503) 945-6273 (TTY)
(503) 378-3439 (Fax)

Vocational Rehabilitation Division
Administration Office
500 Summer Street, NE
Salem, OR 97310-1018
(503) 945-5880
(503) 945-5894 (TTY)
(503) 945-8991 (Fax)

Pennsylvania (PA)
Office of Vocational Rehabilitation
Attn: Social Security Administration/Vocational Rehabilitation State Coordinator
Room 1300
Labor and Industry Building
7th and Forster Street
Harrisburg, PA 17120
(800) 442-6351

Rhode Island (RI)
Department of Human Services
Office of Rehabilitation Services

40 Fountain Street
Providence, RI 02903-1898
(401) 421-7005
(401) 421-4016 (TDD)
(401) 421-9259 (Fax)
http://www.ors.state.ri.us

Services for the Blind and Visually Impaired
40 Fountain Street
Providence, RI 02093-1898
(401) 222-2300/(800) 752-8088 ext 2300
(401) 222-3010 (TDD)
(401) 222-1328 (Fax)
http:www.ors.state.ri.us/sbvipage.htm

South Carolina (SC)
South Carolina Vocational Rehabilitation Department
State Office Building, 1410 Boston Ave
PO Box 15
West Columbia, SC 29171-0015
(803) 896-6500
http://www.scvrd.net/scvrinfo.htm

South Carolina Commission for the Blind
PO Box 79
1430 Confederate Avenue
Columbia, SC 29202-0079
(803) 898-8700/(800) 922-2222
(803) 898-8800 (Fax)
www.sccb.state.sc.us

South Dakota (SD)
Division of Rehabilitation Services
East Highway 34, Hillsview Plaza
c/o 500 East Capitol
Pierre, SD 57501-5070
(605) 773-3195
(605) 773-5483 (Fax)
www.state.sd.us/state/executive/dhs/drs/drs.htm

Tennessee (TN)
Department of Human Services
Division of Rehabilitation Services
Citizens Plaza Building, Room 1100
400 Deaderick Street
Nashville, TN 37248-6100
(615) 313-4902
(615) 741-6508 (Fax)

Texas (TX)
Texas Rehabilitation Commission
4900 North Lamar
Austin, TX 78751
(512) 424-4063/(800) 628-5115
(512) 424-4730 (Fax)

Texas Commission for the Blind
4800 North Lamar
Austin, TX 78756
(512) 459-2608/(800) 252-5204
(512) 467-6462 (TTY)
(512) 459-2685 (Fax)
http://www.tcb.state.tx.us

Utah (UT)
Utah State Office of Rehabilitation
250 East 500 South
Salt Lake City, UT 84111
(801) 538-7530/(800) 473-7530
(801) 538-7522 (Fax)
http://www.usor.state.ut.us

Vermont (VT)
Division of Vocational Rehabilitation
Department of Aging and Disabilities
Agency of Human Services
Osgood Building, 103 Main Street
Waterbury, VT 05671-2303
(800) 361-1239
(802) 241-2186 (TTY)
(802) 241-3359 (Fax)
http://www.dad.state.vt.us/dvr/

Division for the Blind and Visually Impaired
Department of Aging and Disabilities
Agency of Human Services
Osgood Building, 103 Main Street
Waterbury, VT 05671-2303
(802) 241-2210
(802) 241-3359 (Fax)
http://www.dad.state.vt.us/dbvi/main.htm

Virginia (VA)
Virginia Department of Rehabilitation Services
8004 Franklin Farms Drive
Richmond, VA 23288
(800) 552-5019
(800) 464-9950 (TTY)
(804) 662-9533 (Fax)
www.state.va.us/hhr/drs

Virginia Department for the Visually Handicapped
397 Azalea Avenue
Richmond, VA 23227-3697
(804) 371-3140/(800) 622-2155
(804) 371-3351 (Fax)
http://dit1.state.va.us/hhr/dvh

Washington (WA)
Department of Services for the Blind
1400 South Evergreen Park Drive, SW
Suite 100
PO Box 40933
Olympia, WA 98504-0933
(206) 721-4056/(360) 586-1224/(800) 552-7103

(206) 721-4056 (TDD)
(360) 586-7627 (Fax)

State of Washington, Division of Vocational Rehabilitation
Mailing Address: PO Box 45340
Olympia, WA 98504
Street Address: 612 Woodland Square Loop SE
Lacey, WA 98503-1044
(800) 637-5627/(360) 438-8000 (Voice/TTY)
(360) 438-8007 (Fax)
http://www.wa.gov/dshs/dvr

West Virginia (WV)
The West Virginia Division of Rehabilitation Services
PO Box 50890, State Capitol
Charleston, WV 25305-0890
(304) 766-4600/(800) 642-8207
(304) 766-4690 (Fax)

Wisconsin (WI)
Wisconsin Division of Vocational Rehabilitation
2917 International Lane
Suite 300, PO Box 7852
Madison, WI 53707-7852
(608) 243-5600/(800) 442-3477
(608) 243-5601 (TTY)
(608) 243-5680 (Fax)
http://www.dwd.state.wi.us/dvr

Wyoming (WY)
Wyoming Division of Vocational Rehabilitation
1100 Herschler Building
1st Floor East Wing
Cheyenne, WY 82002
(307) 777-7389
(307) 777-5939 (Fax)

Additional Resources

The following information may not be an all-inclusive list.

AIDS/HIV

AIDS Action
1906 Sunderland Place, NW
Washington, DC 20036
(202) 530-8030
(202) 530-8031 (Fax)
http://www.aidsaction.org

American Red Cross
Workplace HIV/AIDS Program
50 E. 42nd Street, 19th Floor
Falls Church, VA 22042-1203
(800) 375-2040
http://www.redcross.org/

Centers for Disease Control and Prevention (CDC)
Business and Labor Resource Service
PO Box 6003
Rockville, MD 20849-6003
(800) 458-5231
(800) 243-7012 (TTY)
(301) 562-1098 (international)
http://www.brta-lrta.org/

Centers for Disease Control and Prevention (CDC)
National AIDS Hotline
American Social Health Association
PO Box 13827
Research Triangle Park, NC 27709
(800) 342-AIDS/(800) 342-2437
(800) 243-7889 (TTY)
http://www.ashastd.org/nah/index.html

Centers for Disease Control and Prevention (CDC)
National Center for HIV, STD and TB Prevention (NCHSTP)
1108 Corporate Square
Atlanta, GA 30329
(404) 639-8040
http://www.cdc.gov/nchstp/od/nchstp.html

The AIDS Memorial Quilt
PO Box 5552
Atlanta, GA 31107
(404) 688-5500
(404) 688-5552 (Fax)
http://www.aidsquilt.org

National Association of People with AIDS (NAPWA)
1413 K Street, NW, 7th Floor
Washington, DC 20005
(202) 898-0414
(202) 898-0435 (Fax)
http://www.napwa.org/

National Minority AIDS Council (NMAC)
1931 13th Street, NW
Washington, DC 20009-4432
(202) 483-6622
(202) 483-1135 (Fax)
http://www.nmac.org

National Native American AIDS Prevention Center (NNAAPC)
134 Linden Street
Oakland, CA 94607
(510) 444-2051
http://www.nnaapc.org

Alcoholism

Addiction Resource Guide
PO Box 8612

Tarrytown, NY 10591
(914) 725-5151
(914) 631-8077 (Fax)
http://www.addictionresourceguide.com

Alcoholics Anonymous World Services, Inc. (AA)
PO Box 459, Grand Central Station
New York, NY 10163
(212) 870-3400
(212) 870-3003 (Fax)
http://www.alcoholics-anonymous.org

American Society of Addiction Medicine (ASAM)
4601 North Park Avenue, Arcade Suite 101
Chevy Chase, MD 20815
(301) 656-3920
(301) 656-3815 (Fax)
http://www.asam.org

Canadian Centre on Substance Abuse (CCSA)
75 Albert Street, Suite 300
Ottawa, ON, Canada K1P 5E7
(613) 235-4048
(613) 235-8101 (Fax)
http://www.ccsa.ca

Equal Employment Opportunity Commission (EEOC)
1801 L Street, NW
Washington, DC 20507
(800) 669-4000/(202) 663-4900
(202) 663-4494 (TTY)
(800) 669-6820 (TDD)
http://www.eeoc.gov

National Association on Alcohol, Drugs & Disability (NAADD)
2165 Bunker Hill Drive
San Mateo, CA 94402-3801
(650) 578-8047 (Voice/TTY)
(650) 286-9205 (Fax)
http://www.naadd.org

The National Center on Addiction and Substance Abuse at Columbia University (CASA)
633 Third Avenue, 19th Floor
New York, NY 10017-6706
(212) 841-5200
(212) 956-8020 (Fax)
http://www.casacolumbia.org

The National Clearinghouse for Alcohol and Drug Information (NCADI)
PO Box 2345
Rockville, MD 20847-2345
(800) 729-6686/(301) 468-2600
(800) 487-4889 (TTY)
(301) 468-6433 (Fax)
http://www.health.org

National Council on Alcoholism and Drug Dependence (NCADD)
20 Exchange Place, Suite 2902
New York, NY 10005
(800) NCA-CALL/(212) 269-7797
(212) 269-7(510) (Fax)
http://www.ncadd.org

National Institute on Alcohol Abuse and Alcoholism (NIAAA)
6000 Executive Boulevard, Willco Building
Bethesda, MD 20892-7003
(301) 443-3885
http://www.niaaa.nih.gov

Office of Disability Employment Policy
Job Accommodation Network
West Virginia University, PO Box 6080
Morgantown, WV 26506-6080
(800) 526-7234/(800) ADA-WORK (Voice/TTY)
(304) 293-7186
(304) 293-5407 (Fax)
http://www.jan.wvu.edu

The Research Institute on Addictions (RIA)
1021 Main Street
Buffalo, NY 14203-1016
(716) 887-2566
http://www.ria.org

The Substance Abuse and Mental Health Services Administration (SAMHSA)
Room 12-105 Parklawn Building
5600 Fishers Lane
Rockville, MD 20857
(301) 443-4795
(800) 729-6686 (clearinghouse)
http://www.samhsa@dhhs.gov

Arthritis Resources

American Autoimmune Related Diseases Association, Inc.
Washington Office
750 17th Street, NW, Suite 1100
Washington, DC 20006
(202) 466-8511
http://www.aarda.org

The Arthritis Foundation
PO Box 7669
Atlanta, GA 30357-0669
(800) 283-7800
http://www.arthritis.org

Missouri Arthritis Rehabilitation Research and Training Center
130 AP Green, DC 330.00
One Hospital Drive
Columbia, MO 65212
http://www.hsc.missouri.edu/~arthritis

National Institute of Arthritis and Musculoskeletal and Skin Diseases (NIAMS)
National Institutes of Health (NIH)
1 AMS Circle
Bethesda, MD 20892-3675
(301) 495-4484
http://www.nih.gov/niams

National Osteoporosis Foundation
1232 22nd Street NW
Washington, DC 20037-1292
(202) 223-2226
http://www.nof.org

Office of Disability Employment Policy
Job Accommodation Network
West Virginia University, PO Box 6080
Morgantown, WV 26506-6080
(800) 526-7234/(800) ADA-WORK (Voice/TTY)
(304) 293-7186
(304) 293-5407 (Fax)
http://www.jan.wvu.edu

The Road Back Foundation
PO Box 447
Orleans, MA 02653
(614) 227-1556

Attention Deficit Disorder and Learning Disabilities Resources

American Association for Higher Education
(Equal Access to Software & Information)
1 Dupont Circle, Suite 360
Washington, DC 20036
(202) 293-6440
(202) 293-0073 (Fax)
http://www.rit.edu/~easi

Association on Higher Education and Disability (AHEAD)
University of Mass. of Boston
100 Morrissey Boulevard
Boston, MA 02125-3393
(617) 287-3880
(617) 287-3882 (TTY)
(617) 287-3881 (Fax)
http://www.ahead.org

Children and Adults with Attention Deficit Disorder (CH.A.D.D.)
8181 Professional Place, Suite 201
Landover, MD 20785
(800) 233-4050/(301) 306-7070
(301) 306-7090 (Fax)
http://chadd.org

HEATH (Higher Education and Adult Training for People with Handicaps)
Resource Center
One Dupont Circle, Suite 800
Washington, DC 20036
(800) 544-3284/(202) 939-9300
http://www.Heath-Resource-Center.org

International Dyslexia Association (formerly the Orton Dyslexia Society)
8600 LaSalle Road, Chester Building, Suite 382
Baltimore, MD 21286-2044
(410) 296-0232
(410) 321-5069 (Fax)
(800) ABC-D123 (messages)
http://www.interdys.org

Learning Disabilities Center
The University of Georgia
331 Milledge Hall
Athens, GA 30602-5875
(706) 542-4589
(706) 542-0001 (Fax)
http://www.coe.uga.edu/ldcenter

Mainstream, Inc.
6930 Carroll Avenue, Suite 240
Takoma Park, MD 20912
(301) 891-8777
(301) 891-8778 (Fax)
e-mail: Info@Mainstreaminc.org

National Attention Deficit Disorder Association (ADDA)
1788 Second Street, Suite 200
Highland Park, IL 60035
(847) 432-ADDA
(847) 432-5874 (Fax)
http://www.add.org

National Center for Law and Learning Disabilities
PO Box 368
Cabin John, MD 20818
(301) 469-8308

National Center for Learning Disabilities (NCLD)
381 Park Avenue South, Suite 1401
New York, NY 10016

(212) 545-7510
(212) 545-9665 (Fax)
(888) 575-7373 (referral number)
http://www.ncld.org

National Council of Independent Living Programs (NCIL)
1916 Wilson Boulevard, Suite 209
Arlington, VA 22201
(703) 525-3406
(703) 525-4153 (TTY)
(703) 525-3409 (Fax)
www.ncil.org

National Information Center for Children & Youth with Disabilities (NICHCD)
PO Box 1492
Washington, DC 20013-1492
(800) 695-0285 (Voice/TTY)
(202) 884-8200 (Voice/TTY)
(202) 884-8441 (Fax)
http://www.nichcy.org

National Institute for Literacy
1775 I Street, NW, Suite 703
Washington, DC 20006-2401
(202) 233-2025
(202) 233-2050 (Fax)
http://novel.nifl.gov/nalldtop.htm

National Rehabilitation Information Center (NARIC)
1010 Wayne Avenue, Suite 800
Silver Spring, MD 20910
(301) 562-2400
(301) 562- 2401 (Fax)
(301) 495-5626 (TTY)
(800) 346-2742
(800) 34NARIC
http://www.naric.com/

Office of Disability Employment Policy
Job Accommodation Network
West Virginia University, PO Box 6080
Morgantown, WV 26506-6080
(800) 526-7234/(800) ADA-WORK (Voice/TTY)
(304) 293-7186
(304) 293-5407 (Fax)
http://www.jan.wvu.edu

Recording for the Blind and Dyslexic (RFB)
20 Roszel Road
Princeton NJ 08540
(609) 452-0606/(800) 221-4792
(609) 987-8116 (Fax)
http://www.rfbd.org

Rehabilitation Engineering and Assistive Technology Society of N. America (RESNA)
Technical Assistance Project, 1700 North Moore Street, Suite 1540
Arlington, VA 22209-1903
(703) 524-6686
(703) 524-6639 (TTY)
(703) 524-6630 (Fax)
http://www.resna.org

Trace Research & Development Center
University of Wisconsin–Madison
5901 Research Park Boulevard
Madison, WI 53719
(608) 262-6966
(608) 2632-5408 (TTY)
(608) 262-8848 (Fax)
http://trace.wisc.edu

WebABLE, Inc.
50 Franklin Street
Boston, MA 02110
(866) 932-2253 (Fax)
http://www.webable.com/

Back

American National Standards Institute
Washington, DC Headquarters
1819 L Street, NW, 6th Floor
Washington, DC 20036
(202) 293-8020
(202) 293-9287 (Fax)
http://www.ansi.org/

ANSI/HFS 100
Obtained from American National Standards Institute
11 West 42nd Street
New York, NY, 10036
(212) 642-4900

ErgoWeb Inc.
PO Box 1089, 93 West Main
Midway, UT 84049
(888) ER-GOWeb
(888) 374-6932
(435) 654-4284
(435) 654-5433 (Fax)
http://www.ergoweb.com/

National Institute for Occupational Safety and Health
NIOSH Publications
4676 Columbia Parkway, Mailstop C-13
Cincinnati, OH 45226-1998
http://www.cdc.gov/niosh/homepage.html/

National Institute for Occupational Safety and Health
Clearinghouse for Occupational Safety and Health Information
4676 Columbia Parkway
Cincinnati, OH 45226
(800) 35-NIOSH

Occupational Safety and Health Administration
(800) 35-NIOSH
(513) 533-8573 (Fax)
http://osha.gov/govsites.html/

Office of Disability Employment Policy
Job Accommodation Network
West Virginia University, PO Box 6080
Morgantown, WV 26506-6080
(800) 526-7234/(800) ADA-WORK (Voice/TTY)
(304) 293-7186
(304) 293-5407 (Fax)
http://www.jan.wvu.edu

Brain Injury

American Association for Higher Education
(Equal Access to Software & Information)
1 Dupont Circle, Suite 360
Washington, DC 20036
(202) 293-6440
(202) 293-0073 (Fax)
http://www.rit.edu/~easi

Association for the Advancement of Rehabilitation Technology (RESNA)
Technical Assistance Project
1700 North Moore Street, Suite 1540
Arlington, VA 22209-1903
(703) 524-6686
(703) 524-6639 (TTY)
(703) 524-6630 (Fax)
http://www.resna.org

The Brain Injury Association Inc.
105 North Alfred Street
Alexandria, VA 22314
(703) 236-6000
(703) 236-6001 (Fax)
http://www.biausa.org/national.htm

Brain Injury Association of Tennessee
699 W. Main Street, Suite 112
Hendersonville, TN 37075
(615) 264-3052/(877) 885-7511
(615) 264-1693 (Fax)

Centre for Neuro Skills
CNS–California
2658 Mt. Vernon Avenue
Bakersfield, CA 93306
(800) 922-4994/(805) 872-3408
(805) 872-5150 (Fax)
http://www.neuroskills.com

Closing the Gap, Inc.
PO Box 68, 526 Main Street
Henderson, MN 56044
(507) 248-3294
(507) 248-3810 (Fax)
http://www.closingthegap.com/

CNS–Texas
3501 N. MacArthur, Bldg. 200
Irving, TX 75062
(800) 554-5448/(972) 580-8500
(972) 255-3162 (Fax)
www.neuroskill.com

disAbility Resource Center
607-S.E. Everett Mall Way, Suite 9B
Everett, WA 98208
(425) 347-5768 (Voice/TTY)
(800) 315-3583 (Voice/TTY)
http://www.wa-ilsc.org/

HEATH Resource Center
National Clearinghouse Postsecondary Education for Individuals with Disabilities, American Coun. on Ed.
One Dupont Circle, Suite 800
Washington, DC 20036-1193
(800) 544-3284 (Voice/TTY)
http://www.heath-resource-center.org/

Independent Living Research Utilization Program
2323 South Shepherd, Suite 1000
Houston, TX 77019
(713) 520-0232
(713) 520-5136 (TDD)
(713) 520-5785 (Fax)
http://www.ilru.org/ilru-overview.html

Dr. Glen Johnson, Clinical Neuropsychologist
Clinical Director Neuro-Recovery Head Injury Program
5123 North Royal Drive
Traverse City, MI 49684
(231) 929-1313
http://www.tbiguide.com

Mainstream, Inc.
3 Bethesda Metro Center, Suite 830
Bethesda, MD 20814
(301) 654-2400
(301) 654-2403 (Fax)
http://www.mainstream-mag.com/

National Council of Independent Living Programs (NCIL)
1916 Wilson Boulevard, Suite 209
Arlington, VA 22201
(877) 525-3400
(703) 525.3409 (Fax)
www.ncil.org

National Information Center for Children & Youth with Handicaps (NICHY)
PO Box 1492
Washington, DC 20013-1492
(800) 695-0285/(202) 884-8200
(202) 884-8441 (Fax)
http://www.nichy.org

National Center for Injury Prevention
Mailstop K65
4770 Buford Highway NE
Atlanta, GA 30341-3724
(770) 488-1506
(770) 488-1667 (Fax)
http://www.cdc.gov/ncipc/dacrrdp/tbi.htm

National Rehabilitation Information Center (NARIC)
1010 Wayne Avenue, Suite 800
Silver Spring, MD 20910
(301) 562-2400/(800) 346-2742
(301) 562-2401 (Fax)
(301) 495-5626 (TTY)
http://www.naric.com./

The National Resource Center for Traumatic Brain Injury
PO Box 980542
Richmond, VA 23298-0542
(804) 828-9055
(804) 828-2378 (Fax)
http://www.neuro.pmr.vcu.edu/material/material.htm

Office of Disability Employment Policy
Job Accommodation Network
West Virginia University, PO Box 6080
Morgantown, WV 26506-6080
(800) 526-7234/(800) ADA-WORK (Voice/TTY)
(304) 293-7186
(304) 293-5407 (Fax)
http://www.jan.wvu.edu

Ohio Valley Center for Brain Injury Prevention and Rehabilitation
480 W. 9th Avenue, 1166 Dodd Hill
Columbus, OH 43215
(614) 293-3802
(614) 293-8886 (Fax)
http://www.osu.edu/virtual/OhioValley/

The Perspectives Network, Inc.
PO Box 1859
Cumming, GA 30028-1859
(770) 844.6898 (Voice/Fax)
(800) 685-6302 / (334) 639-5037
e-mail: TPN@tbi.org
http://www.tbi.org

Santa Clara Valley Medical Center/The Traumatic Brain Injury Project
950 S. Bascom Avenue, Suite 2011
San Jose, CA 95128
(408) 295-9896
(408) 295-9913 (Fax)
http://www.tbi-sci.org/

Trace Research & Development Center
University of Wisconsin–Madison
5901 Research Park Boulevard
Madison, WI 53719-1252
(608) 262-6966
(608) 263-5408 (TTY)
(608) 262-8848 (Fax)
http://trace.wisc.edu/

Traumatic Brain Injury Fact Sheet
http://www.tnbiat.org/TBIFACT2.htm

Traumatic Brain Injury Web Resources
http://busboy.sped.ukans.edu/~music/resources/tbi/tbi.shtml

World Institute on Disability
510 16th Street
Oakland, CA 94612-1500
(510) 763-4100
(510) 208-9493 (TTY)
(510) 763-4109 (Fax)

Cancer Resources

American Cancer Society
1599 Clifton Road, NE
Atlanta, GA 30329
(800) ACS-2345
http://www.cancer.org

American Institute for Cancer Research
1759 R Street, NW
Washington, DC 20009
(800) 843-8114
http://www.aicr.org

Cancer Care, Inc.
275 7th Avenue
New York, NY 10001

(800) 813-HOPE/(212) 302-2400/(212) 221-3300
(212) 719-0263 (Fax)
http://www.cancercare.org

Cancer Information Service
Building 31, Room 10A16
31 Center Drive, MSC 2580
Bethesda, MD 20892-2580
(800) 4-CANCER/(301) 435-3848
http://www.nci.nih.gov/info/what.htm

Centers for Disease Control and Prevention (CDC)
1600 Clifton Road
Atlanta, GA 30333
(404) 639-3311
http://www.cdc.gov

Cancer Help Network
Two North Road, Suite A
Chester, NJ 07930-2308
(877) Hope-Net
www.cancerhelpnet.org

National Bone Marrow Transplant Link
20411 W. 12 Mill Road, Suite 108
Southfield, MI 48076
(800) LINK-BMT
http://comnet.org/nbmtlink

National Cancer Institute
31 Center Drive, MSC 2580
Bethesda, MD 20892-2580
(800) 4-CANCER/(301) 435-3848
http://www.nci.nih.gov

National Coalition for Cancer Survivorship
1010 Wayne Avenue, Suite 770
Silver Spring, MD 20910-5600
(877) NCCS-YES/(301) 650-9127
(301) 565-9670 (Fax)
http://www.cansearch.org

National Marrow Donor Program
3001 Broadway Street, NE, Suite 500
Minneapolis, MN 55413-1753
(800) MARROW-2
http://www.marrow.org

National Organization for Rare Disorders, Inc
PO Box 8923
New Fairfield, CT 06812-8923
(800) 999-6673/(203) 746-6518
(203) 746-6481 (Fax)
http://www.rarediseases.org

Office of Disability Employment Policy
Job Accommodation Network
West Virginia University, PO Box 6080
Morgantown, WV 26506-6080
(800) 526-7234/(800) ADA-WORK (Voice/TTY)
(304) 293-7186
(304) 293-5407 (Fax)
http://www.jan.wvu.edu

Cardiovascular Resources

American Heart Association
7272 Greenville Avenue
Dallas, TX 75231

Customer Heart and Stroke Information
(800) AHA-USA1/(800) 242-8721

Women's Health Information: (888) MY-HEART
http://www.americanheart.org

Centers for Disease Control and Prevention (CDC)
1600 Clifton Road
Atlanta, GA 30333
(404) 639-3534 or 3311/(800) 311-3435
http://www.cdc.gov

Heart and Stroke Foundation of Canada
160 George Street, Suite 200
Ottawa, ON, Canada K1N 9M2
(613) 241-4361
www.heartandstroke.ca

National Heart, Lung, and Blood Institute (NHLBI)
National Institutes of Health (NIH)
Bethesda, MD 20892-2580
http://www.nhlbi.nih.gov/index.htm

National Organization for Rare Disorders, Inc. (NORD)
PO Box 8923
New Fairfield, CT 06812-8923
(800) 999-6673/(203) 746-6518
(203) 746-6481 (Fax)
http://www.rarediseases.org

Office of Disability Employment Policy
Job Accommodation Network
West Virginia University, PO Box 6080
Morgantown, WV 26506-6080
(800) 526-7234/(800) ADA-WORK (Voice/TTY)
(304) 293-7186
(304) 293-5407 (Fax)
http://www.jan.wvu.edu

Texas Heart Institute
1101 Bates Avenue
Houston, TX 77030
(800) 292-2221/(713) 791-4011
www.TexasHeartInstitute.org

Chemical Sensitivity

American Industrial Hygiene Association (AIHA)
2700 Prosperity Avenue, Suite 250
Fairfax, VA 22031
(703) 849-8888
(703) 207-3561 (Fax)
http://www.aiha.org/

Anderson Laboratories, Inc.
PO Box 323
West Hartford, VT 05084
(802) 295-7344
http://www.andersonlaboratories.com

Chemical Injury Information Network (CIIN)
PO Box 301
White Sulphur Springs, MT 59645
(406) 547-2255
(406) 547-2455 (Fax)
http://www.ciin.org/

Environmental Health Network (EHN)
PO Box 1155
Larkspur, CA 94977-1155
(415) 541-5075
http://www.ehnca.org

Fragranced Products Information Network
(801) 340-3578 (Fax)
http://www.ameliaww.com/fpin/fpin.htm

Human Ecology Action League, Inc. (HEAL)
PO Box 29629
Atlanta, GA 30359-0629
(404) 248-1898
(404) 248-0162 Fax
http://members.aol.com/HEALNatnl/index.html

MCS Referral & Resources, Inc.
508 Westgate Road
Baltimore, MD 21229
(410) 362-6400/(410) 362-6401
http://www.mcsrr.org/whoweare.html

The National Air Filtration Association (NAFA)
1518 K Street, NW, Suite 503
Washington, DC 20005
(202) 628-5328
(202) 638-4833 (Fax)
http://www.nafahq.org/

National Center for Environmental Health Strategies, Inc.
1100 Rural Avenue
Voorhees, NJ 08043
(856) 429-5358
http://www.ncehs.org/

National Coalition Against the Misuse of Pesticides
701 E Street, SE, #200
Washington, DC 20003
(202) 543-5450
(202) 543-4791
http://www.beyondpesticides.org/

National Foundation for the Chemically Hypersensitive
4407 Swinson Road
Rhodes, MI 48652
(517) 689-6369
(517) 689-6877 (Fax)
http://www.mcsrelief.com

National Pesticide Telecommunications Network
Oregon State University
333 Weniger Hall
Corvallis, OR 97331-6502
(800) 858-7378
(541) 737-0761 (Fax)
http://ace.ace.orst.edu/info/nptn/

Office of Disability Employment Policy
Job Accommodation Network
West Virginia University, PO Box 6080
Morgantown, WV 26506-6080
(800) 526-7234/(800) ADA-WORK (Voice/TTY)
(304) 293-7186
(304) 293-5407 (Fax)
http://www.jan.wvu.edu

Chronic Fatigue Resources

American Association for Chronic Fatigue Syndrome
c/o Harborview Medical Center
PO Box 359780, 325 Ninth Avenue
Seattle, WA 98104
(206) 521-1932
(206) 521-1930 (Fax)
http://www.aacfs.org

Chronic Fatigue and Immune Dysfunction Syndrome Association of America
PO Box 220398
Charlotte, NC 28222-0398
(800) 442-3437
(704) 365-9755 (Fax)
http://www.cfids.org

National Chronic Fatigue and Fibromyalgia Syndrome Association (NCFFSA)
PO Box 18426
Kansas City, MO 64133
(816) 931-4777

National Organization for Rare Disorders (NORD)
PO Box 8923
New Fairfield, CT 06812-8923
(800) 999-6673/(203) 746-6518
http://www.rarediseases.org

Office of Disability Employment Policy
Job Accommodation Network
West Virginia University, PO Box 6080
Morgantown, WV 26506-6080
(800) 526-7234/(800) ADA-WORK (Voice/TTY)
(304) 293-7186
(304) 293-5407 (Fax)
http://www.jan.wvu.edu

Chronic Pain Resources

American Academy of Pain Management
13947 Mono Way, #A
Sonora, CA 95370
(209) 533-9744
http://www.aapainmanage.org

American Chronic Pain Association
PO Box 850
Rocklin, CA 95677-0850
(916) 632-0922
(916) 632-3208 (Fax)
http://www.theacpa.org

American Pain Foundation
201 N. Charles Street, Suite 710
Baltimore, MD 21201-4111
http://www.painfoundation.org

American Pain Society
4700 West Lake Avenue
Glenview, IL 60025
(847) 375-4715
(877) 734-8758 (Fax)
http://www.ampainsoc.org

Centers for Disease Control and Prevention (CDC)
1600 Clifton Road
Atlanta, GA 30333
(404) 639-3534/(800) 311-3435
http://www.cdc.gov

International Association for the Study of Pain (IASP)
909 NE 43rd Street, Suite 306
Seattle, WA 98105-6020
(206) 547-6409
(206) 547-1703 (Fax)
http://dasnet02.dokkyomed.ac.jp/IASPM/IASP.html

National Chronic Pain Outreach Association (NCPOA)
7979 Old Georgetown Road, Suite 100
Bethesda, MD 20814
(301) 652-4948
(301) 907-0745 (Fax)
http://neurosurgery.mgh.harvard.edu/ncpainoa.htm

National Organization for Rare Disorders (NORD)
PO Box 8923
New Fairfield, CT 06812-8923
(800) 999-6673/(203) 746-6518
http://www.rarediseases.org

North American Chronic Pain Association of Canada (NACPAC)
150 Central Park Drive, Unit 105
Brampton, ON, Canada L6T 2T9
(800) 616-PAIN/(905) 793-5230
(905) 793-8781 (Fax)
http://www.chronicpaincanada.org

Office of Disability Employment Policy
Job Accommodation Network
West Virginia University, PO Box 6080
Morgantown, WV 26506-6080
(800) 526-7234/(800) ADA-WORK (Voice/TTY)
(304) 293-7186
(304) 293-5407 (Fax)
http://www.jan.wvu.edu

Diabetes Resources

American Association of Diabetes Educators
100 West Monroe, Suite 400
Chicago, IL 60603-1901
(312) 424-2426
(312) 424-2427 (Fax)
http://www.aadenet.org

American Diabetes Association
1701 North Beauregard Street
Alexandria, VA 22311
(800) 342-2383
http://www.diabetes.org/

American Dietetic Association
National Center for Nutrition and Dietetics
216 West Jackson Boulevard
Chicago, IL 60606-6995
(800) 366-1655 (Consumer Nutrition Hotline)
(800) 745-0775/(312) 899-0040
http://www.eatright.org

American Heart Association National Center
7272 Greenville Avenue
Dallas, TX 75231
(800) AHA-USA1/(214) 373-6300
http://www.americanheart.org/

Diabetes Exercise and Sports Association DESA
PO Box 1935
Litchfield Park, AZ 85340
(800) 898-4322/(623) 535-4593
(623) 535-4741 (Fax)
http://www.diabetes-exercise.org

Indian Health Service
Diabetes Program
5300 Homestead Road, NE
Albuquerque, NM 87110
(505) 248-4101

Juvenile Diabetes Foundation International
120 Wall Street
New York, NY 10005-4001
(800) JDF-CURE/(212) 785-9500
(212) 785-9595 (Fax)
http://www.jdf.org

National Diabetes Information Clearinghouse
One Information Way
Bethesda, MD 20892-3560
(800) 860-8747/(301) 654-3327
(301) 907-8906 (Fax)
http://www.niddk.nih.gov/health/diabetes/ndic.htm

National Eye Institute
National Eye Health Education Program
2020 Vision Place
Bethesda, MD 20892-3655
(800) 869-2020 (for health professionals only)
(301) 496-5248
http://www.nei.nih.gov

National Kidney Foundation, Inc. (NKF)
30 East 33rd Street, Suite 1100
New York, NY 10016
(800) 622-9010/(212) 889-2210
(212) 689-9261 (Fax)
http://www.kidney.org/

Office of Public Health and Science
U.S. Department of Health and Human Services
Office of Minority Health Resource Center
PO Box 37337
Washington, DC 20013-7337
(800) 444-MHRC/(800) 444-6472
(301) 230-7198 (Fax)
http://www.omhrc.gov/

Veterans Health Administration (VHA)
Program Chief, Diabetes
Veterans Health Affairs
810 Vermont Avenue, NW
Washington, DC 20420
(202) 273-5400
http://www.va.gov/health/diabetes/

Fibromyalgia Resources

American Fibromyalgia Syndrome Association, Inc.
6380 E. Tanque Verde, Suite D
Tucson, AZ 85715
(520) 733-1570
http://www.afsafund.org

The Arthritis Foundation
PO Box 7669
Atlanta, GA 30357-0669
(800) 283-7800
http://www.arthritis.org

Centers for Disease Control and Prevention (CDC)
1600 Clifton Road
Atlanta, GA 30333
(800) 311-3435/(404) 639-3311
http://www.cdc.gov

Chemical Injury Information Network (CIIN)
PO Box 301
White Sulphur Springs, MT 59645
(406) 547-2255
(406) 547-2455 (Fax)
http://www.ciin.org/

Environmental Health Network (EHN)
Working Fragrance Free
PO Box 460461
San Francisco, CA 94146-0461

Death by Perfume?
By A. Marsh
http://users.lanminds.com/~wilworks/WFF/watsntes.htm

Environmental Health Network (EHN)
PO Box 1155
Larkspur, CA 94977-1155
(415) 541-5075
http://users.lanminds.com/~wilworks/ehnindex.htm

Fibromyalgia Network
PO Box 31750
Tucson, AZ 85751
(800) 853-2929
http://www.fmnetnews.com/main.html

Fragranced Products Information Network
(This site is financed, owned and maintained by Betty Bridges, RN)
http://www.ameliaww.com/fpin/fpin.htm
e-fax: (801) 340-3578

Human Ecology Action League, Inc. (HEAL)
PO Box 29629
Atlanta, GA 30359-0629
(404) 248-1898
(404) 248-0162 (Fax)
http://members.aol.com/HEALNatnl/index.html

National Center for Environmental Health Strategies, Inc.
1100 Rural Avenue
Voorhees, NJ 08043
(856) 429-5358
http://www.ncehs.org/ (under construction)

National Chronic Fatigue and Fibromyalgia Syndrome Association (NCFFSA)
PO Box 18426
Kansas City, MO 64133
(816) 931-4777

National Fibromyalgia Partnership, Inc. (NFP)
140 Zinn Way
Linden, VA 22642-5609
(866) 725-4404
(540) 622-2998 (Fax)
http://www.fmpartnership.org

National Foundation for the Chemically Hypersensitive
4407 Swinson Road
Rhodes, MI 48652
(517) 689-6369
(517) 689-6877 (Fax)
http://www.mcsrelief.com (under construction)

National Institute of Arthritis and Musculoskeletal and Skin Diseases (NIAMS)
National Institutes of Health (NIH)
Bethesda, MD 20892-2350
(301) 495-4484
http://www.nih.gov/niams

National Organization for Rare Disorders (NORD)
PO Box 8923
New Fairfield, CT 06812-8923
(800) 999-6673/(203) 746-6518
(203) 746-6481 (Fax)
http://www.rarediseases.org

MCS Referral & Resources, Inc.
508 Westgate Road
Baltimore, MD 21229
(410) 362-6400
(410) 362-6401 (Fax)
http://www.mcsrr.org/whoweare.html

Miningco.com
Miningco guide to Fragrance Sensitivity
1440 Broadway
New York, NY 10018
(212) 204-4000
http://allergies.miningco.com/library/weekly/aa022299.htm

Office of Disability Employment Policy
Job Accommodation Network
West Virginia University, PO Box 6080
Morgantown, WV 26506-6080
(800) 526-7234/(800) ADA-WORK (Voice/TTY)
(304) 293-7186
(304) 293-5407 (Fax)
http://www.jan.wvu.edu

Oregon Fibromyalgia Foundation (OFF)
1211 SW Yamhill, Suite 303
Portland, OR 97205
http://www.myalgia.com

Research Institute for Fragrance Materials
Two University Plaza, Suite 406
Hackensack, NJ 07601

Selected Abstracts on the Health Effects of Perfume
http://members.aol.com/chemxpose/abstracts.html

Sweet Poison: What Your Nose Can't Tell You About The Dangers of Perfume
By Andrea Des Jardins
http://members.aol.com/chemxpose/perfume.html

Hearing Related Resources

Alexander Graham Bell Association for the Deaf & Hard of Hearing
3417 Volta Place, NW
Washington, DC 20007-2778
(202) 337-5220 (Voice/TTY)
(202) 337-8314 (Fax)
http://www.agbell.org/

American Academy of Audiology
8300 Greensboro Drive, Suite 750
McLean, VA 22102
(703) 790-8466/(800) AAA-2336
(703) 790-8631 (Fax)
http://www.audiology.com/

American Speech Language Hearing Association (ASHA)
10801 Rockville Pike

Rockville, MD 20852
(800) 638-8255 (Voice/TTY)
http://www.asha.org/

American Tinnitus Association (ATA)
PO Box 5
Portland, OR 97207-0005
(800) 634-8978/(503) 248-9985
(503) 248-0024 (Fax)
http://www.ata.org/

Better Hearing Institute
515 King Street, Suite 420
Alexandria, VA 22314
(703) 684-3391
http://www.betterhearing.org/

National Association of the Deaf (NAD)
814 Thayer Avenue
Silver Spring, MD 20910-4500
(301) 587-1788
(301) 587-1789 (TTY)
(301) 587-1791 (Fax)
http://www.nad.org/

National Institute on Deafness and Other Communication Disorders (NIDCD)
National Institutes of Health
31 Center Drive, MSC 2320
Bethesda, MD 20892-2320
(301) 496-7243
(301) 402-0252 (TTY)
(301) 402-0018 (Fax)
http://www.nidcd.nih.gov/

Office of Disability Employment Policy
Job Accommodation Network
West Virginia University, PO Box 6080
Morgantown, WV 26506-6080
(800) 526-7234/(800) ADA-WORK (Voice/TTY)
(304) 293-7186
(304) 293-5407 (Fax)
http://www.jan.wvu.edu

Hepatitis Resources

American Liver Foundation
75 Maiden Lane, Suite 603
New York, NY 10038
(800) 465-4837
(888) 443-7222
http://www.liverfoundation.org/

CDC, Hepatitis Branch
Mailstop G37
Division of Viral and Rickettsial Diseases
National Center for Infectious Diseases
Centers for Disease Control and Prevention
Atlanta, GA 30333
Hepatitis Hotline: (888) 4HEPCDC/(888) 443-7232
http://www.cdc.gov/ncidod/diseases/hepatitis/index.htm

Hepatitis C Education and Support Network
PO Box 1231
Locust Grove, VA 22508
(888) 437-2376
http://www.hepcesn.net/index.html

The Hepatitis C Foundation
National Headquarters
1502 Russett Drive
Warminster, PA 18974
(215) 672-2606
http://www.hepcfoundation.net/

Hepatitis Education Project
4603 Aurora Avenue, N.
Seattle, WA 98103
(206) 732-0311
(206) 732-0312 (Fax)
http://www.scn.org/health/hepatitis/

Hepatitis Foundation International
30 Sunrise Terrace
Cedar Grove, NJ 07009-1423
(800) 891-0707/(973) 239-1035
(973) 857-5044 (Fax)
http://www.hepfi.org/

The Hepatitis Information Network
3535 Trans-Canada Highway
Pointe Claire, Quebec, Canada H9R 1B4
http://www.hepnet.com/

National Digestive Diseases Information Clearinghouse
2 Information Way
Bethesda, MD 20892-3570
(301) 654-3810
http://www.niddk.nih.gov

Latex Allergy Resources

American Academy of Allergy, Asthma & Immunology
611 East Wells Street
Milwaukee, WI 53202
(800) 822-2762/(414) 272-6071
(414) 272-6070 (Fax)
http://www.aaaai.org/

American College of Allergy, Asthma & Immunology
85 West Algonquin Road, Suite 550
Arlington Heights, IL 60005
(800) 842-7777 (Allergist Referral Service)
(847) 427-1200
(847) 427-1294 (Fax)
http://allergy.mcg.edu/

American Latex Allergy Association (A.L.E.R.T., Inc.)
PO Box 13930
Milwaukee, WI 53213
(888) 97ALERT (972-5378)
(262) 677-2808 (Fax)
http://www.latexallergyresources.org/

Canadian Latex Allergy Association
96 Cavan Street
Port Hope, ON, Canada L1A 3B7
(905) 885-9708
http://members.tripod.com/claa/

ELASTIC (Education for Latex Allergy/Support-Team and Information-Coalition)
Lise C. Borel, DMD, National Director
PO Box 2228
West Chester, PA 19380
(610) 436-4801
(610) 436-1198 (Fax)
http://www.latex-allergy.org/

(NIOSH) Latex Allergy: A Prevention Guide
http://www.cdc.gov/niosh/98-113.html

(NIOSH) Preventing Allergic Reactions to Natural Rubber Latex in the Workplace
4676 Columbia Parkway
Cincinnati, OH 45226-1998
(800) 356-4674
(513) 533-8573 (Fax)

Rubber Latex in the Workplace
http://www.cdc.gov/niosh/latexalt.html

National Institute of Occupational Safety & Health (NIOSH)
Technical Information and Assistance
(800) 35-NIOSH (356-4674)
(513) 533-8328
(888) 232-3299 (Fax-on-demand)
(513) 533-8573 (Fax)
http://www.cdc.gov/niosh/homepage.html

Occupational Safety and Health Administration (OSHA)
U.S. Department of Labor
Occupational Safety & Health Administration
Office of Public Affairs–Room N3647
200 Constitution Avenue
Washington, DC 20210
(202) 693-1999/(800) 321-6742
http://www.osha.gov/

Office of Disability Employment Policy
Job Accommodation Network
West Virginia University, PO Box 6080
Morgantown, WV 26506-6080
(800) 526-7234/(800) ADA-WORK (Voice/TTY)
(304) 293-7186
(304) 293-5407 (Fax)
http://www.jan.wvu.edu

On-line Discussion Group
Natural Rubber Latex Allergy Discussion Group
http://www.Immune.com/rubber/index.html

OSHA Technical Bulletin—Potential for Allergy to Natural Rubber Latex Gloves and other Natural Rubber Products (May 1999)
http://www.osha-slc.gov/html/hotfoias/tib/TIB19990412.html

Lupus Resources

American Autoimmune Related Diseases Association, Inc.
Washington Office
750 17th Street, NW, Suite 1100
Washington, DC 20006
(202) 466-8511
Literature Requests: (800) 598-4668
http://www.aarda.org

The American Lupus Society
23751 Madison Street
Torrance, CA 90505
(800) 558-0121/(301) 670-9292

The Arthritis Foundation
PO Box 7669
Atlanta, GA 30357-0669
(800) 283-7800
http://www.arthritis.org

Lung Line
National Jewish Medical and Research Center
1400 Jackson Street
Denver, CO 80206
(800) 222-LUNG (5864)/303-388-4461
http://www.njc.org

Lupus Canada
Box 64034 5512–4 ST NW
Calgary, AB, Canada T2K 6J1
(403) 274-5599
Toll free (in Canada): (800) 661-1468
http://www.lupuscanada.org

Lupus Foundation of America
1300 Piccard Drive, Suite 200
Rockville, MD 20850-4303
(800) 558-0121/(301) 670-9292
http://www.lupus.org

National Institute of Arthritis and Musculoskeletal and Skin Diseases (NIAMS)
National Institutes of Health (NIH)
1 AMS Circle
Bethesda, MD 20892-3675.
(301) 495-4484/(877) 22-NIAMS
(301) 565-2966 (TTY)
(301) 718-6366 (Fax)
http://www.nih.gov/niams

National Organization for Rare Disorders, Inc.
PO Box 8923
New Fairfield, CT 06812-8923
(800) 999-6673/(203) 746-6518
(203) 746-6481 (Fax)
http://www.rarediseases.org

Office of Disability Employment Policy
Job Accommodation Network
West Virginia University, PO Box 6080
Morgantown, WV 26506-6080
(800) 526-7234/(800) ADA-WORK (Voice/TTY)
(304) 293-7186
(304) 293-5407 (Fax)
http://www.jan.wvu.edu

Mental Retardation Resources

American Association on Mental Retardation
444 North Capitol Street, NW, Suite 846
Washington, DC 20001-1512
(800) 424-3688
http://www.aamr.org

The ARC of the United States
1010 Wayne Avenue, Suite 650
Silver Spring, MD 20910
(301) 565-3842
(301) 565-3843 (Fax)
http://www.thearc.org

Asperger Syndrome Coaltion of the US
PO Box 351268
Jacksonville, FL 32235-1268
(866) 4-ASPRGR
http://www.asperger.org

Association for Persons in Supported Employment
1627 Monument Avenue, Room 301
Richmond, VA 23220
(804) 278-9187
http://www.apse.org

Autism Society of America (ASA)
7910 Woodmont Avenue, Suite 300
Bethesda, MD 20814-3015
(800) 3-AUTISM/(301) 657-0881
(301) 657-0869 (Fax)
http://www.autism-society.org

Center for the Study of Autism
PO Box 4538
Salem, OR 97302
http://www.autism.org

National Down Syndrome Society
666 Broadway, 8th Floor
New York, NY 10012-2317
(800) 221-4602
http://www.ndss.org

National Organization on Fetal Alcohol Syndrome
216 G Street, NE
Washington, DC 20002
(202) 785-4585
(202) 466-6456 (Fax)
http://www.nofas.org

Office of Disability Employment Policy
Job Accommodation Network
West Virginia University, PO Box 6080
Morgantown, WV 26506-6080
(800) 526-7234/(800) ADA-WORK (Voice/TTY)
(304) 293-7186
(304) 293-5407 (Fax)
http://www.jan.wvu.edu

President's Committee on Mental Retardation
352 G Hubert Humphrey Building, 200 Independence Avenue
Washington, DC 20201
(202) 619-0634

President's Task Force on Employment of Adults with Disabilities
U.S. Department of Labor
200 Constitution Avenue, NW, Suite S-2220
Washington, DC 20210
(202) 693-4939
(202) 693-4920 (TT)

United Cerebral Palsy Association (UCPA)
1660 L Street, NW, Suite 700
Washington, DC 20036-5602
(800) USA-5-UCP/(800) 872-5827 (Voice/TT)
http://www.ucpa.org/

Migraine Resources

American Academy of Neurology
1080 Montreal Avenue
St. Paul, MN 55116
(651) 695-1940
http://www.aan.com

American Council for Headache Education (ACHE)
19 Mantua Road
Mt. Royal, NJ 08061
(856) 423-0258

(856) 423-0082 (Fax)
http://www.achenet.org/

Australian Brain Foundation
National/Victoria Branch
746 Burke Rd. Camberwell
Victoria, Australia 3124
(800) 677-579/ 03 9882 2203
03 9882 5737 (Fax)
http://www.brainfunction.org.au/

"The Excedrin Headache Relief Update" newsletter
The Excedrin Headache Resource Center
1350 Liberty Avenue
Hillside, NJ 07205
(800) 580-4455
http://www.excedrin.com

"Headache" newsletter
ACHE (American Council for Headache Education)
19 Mantua Road
Mt. Royal, NJ 08061
(800) 255-ACHE, extension 2243
(856) 423-0082 (Fax)
http://www.achenet.org

"HeadWay" newsletter
Glaxo Wellcome Migraine Information Center
(888) 825-5249
http://www.migrainehelp.com/resources.html

Irish Migraine Association
Carmichael House
4 North Brunswick Street
Dublin 7, Ireland
353 01 8724137
353 01 8724157 (Fax)

JAMA (Journal of the American Medical Association)
http://www.ama-assn.org/special/migraine/migraine.htm

M.A.G.N.U.M., Inc. (Migraine Awareness Group: A National Understanding for Migraineurs)
Washington, DC Office
113 South Saint Asaph Street, Suite 300
Alexandria, VA 22314
(703) 739-9384
(703) 739-2432 (Fax)
http://www.migraines.org

Migraine Action Association (formerly the British Migraine Association)
Unite 6, Oakley Hay Lodge Business Park
Great Folds Road
Great Oakley, Northants NN189AS, UK
01536 46133
01536 46144 (Fax)
http://www.migraine.org.uk/

The Migraine Association of Canada
356 Bloor Street East, Suite 1912
Toronto, ON, Ontario M4W 3L4
(416) 920-4916
(416) 920-3677 (Fax)
(800) 663-3557 (to order information)
(416) 920-4917 (24-hour Information on Line)
http://www.migraine.ca

Migraine Trust
45 Great Ormond Street
London, England WC1N 3HZ
020 7831 4818
020 7831 5174 (Fax)

National Headache Foundation
428 W. St. James Place, 2nd Floor
Chicago, IL 60614-2750
(888) NHF-5552
(773) 525-7357 (Fax)
http://www.headaches.org

National Institute of Neurological Disorders and Stroke
National Institutes of Health
31 Center Drive, Bldg 31, Rm 8A-06
Bethesda, MD 20892-254
(800) 352-9424
http://www.ninds.nih.gov/

Neurological Foundation of New Zealand
PO Box 110022
Auckland 1030, New Zealand
09 309 7749
09 377 0614 (Fax)

Office of Disability Employment Policy
Job Accommodation Network
West Virginia University, PO Box 6080
Morgantown, WV 26506-6080
(800) 526-7234/(800) ADA-WORK (Voice/TTY)
(304) 293-7186
(304) 293-5407 (Fax)
http://www.jan.wvu.edu

Swiss Migraine Trust Foundation/Migraine Action
Postfach 4037
4002 Basel, Switzerland
41-61-423 10 80
41-61-423 10 82 (Fax)

Multiple Sclerosis Resources

The Center for Universal Design
North Carolina State University
PO Box 8613
219 Oberlin Road
Raleigh, NC 27695-8613
(800) 647-6777/(919) 515-3082
(919) 515-3023 (Fax)
http://www.design.ncsu.edu/cud

Delta Society National Service Dog Center (NSDC)
289 Perimeter Road East
Renton, WA 98055-1329
(800) 869-6898
(425) 226-7357
http://petsforum.com/deltasociety/dsb000.htm

Independent Living Research Utilization Program (ILRU)
2323 S Shepherd, Suite 100
Houston, TX 77019
(713) 520-0232
(713) 520-5136 (TDD)
(713) 520-5785 (Fax)
http://www.bcm.tmc.edu/ilru

International MS Support Foundation (IMSSF)
PMB# 291
9420 E. Golf Links Road, #291
Tucson, AZ 85730-1340
http://www.msnews.org

Multiple Sclerosis Association of America (MSAA)
706 Haddonfield Road
Cherry Hill, NJ 08002
(800) LEARN-MS
http://www.msaa.com

Multiple Sclerosis Foundation, Inc. (MSF)
6350 N. Andrews Avenue
Fort Lauderdale, FL 33309
(800) 441-7055/(954) 776-6805
http://www.msfacts.org
http://www.msfocus.org

Multiple Sclerosis Society of Canada (MSSOC)
250 Bloor Street East, Suite 1000
Toronto, ON, Canada M4W 3P9
(800) 268-7582/(416) 922-6065
(416) 922-7538 (Fax)
http://www.mssociety.ca

National Multiple Sclerosis Society (NMSS)
733 3rd Ave, 6th Floor
New York, NY 10017
(800) 344-4867/(212) 986-3240
http://www.nmss.org

Office of Disability Employment Policy
Job Accommodation Network
West Virginia University, PO Box 6080
Morgantown, WV 26506-6080
(800) 526-7234/(800) ADA-WORK (Voice/TTY)
(304) 293-7186
(304) 293-5407 (Fax)
http://www.jan.wvu.edu

Muscular Dystrophy Resources

Centers for Disease Control and Prevention (CDC)
1600 Clifton Road
Atlanta, GA 30333
(404) 639-3534
http://www.cdc.gov

Facioscapulohumeral Dystrophy (FSHD) Society
3 Westwood Road
Lexington, MA 02420
(781) 860-0501
(781) 860-0599 (Fax)
http://www.fshsociety.org

International Myotonic Dystrophy Organization
PO Box 1121
Sunland, CA 91041-1121
(866) 679-7954 (toll free in the USA)/(815) 951-2311
http://www.myotonicdystrophy.org

Muscular Dystrophy Association (MDA)
3300 E. Sunrise Drive
Tucson, AZ 85718
(800) 572-1717
http://www.mdausa.org

Muscular Dystrophy Association of Canada
2345 Yonge Street, Suite 900
Toronto, ON, Canada M4P 2E5
(800) 567-2873/(416) 488-0030/(416) 488-0033
416-488-7523 (Fax)
http://www.mdac.ca

The Muscular Dystrophy Family Foundation, Inc.
2330 North Meridian Street
Indianapolis, IN 46208-5730
(800) 544-1213/(317) 923-6333
http://www.mdff.org/

National Institute of Arthritis and Musculoskeletal and Skin Diseases (NIAMS)
National Institutes of Health (NIH)
1 AMS Circle
Bethesda, MD 20892-3675
(877) 22-NIAMS/(301) 565-2966 (TTY)
(301) 718-6366 (Fax)
http://www.nih.gov/niams

National Organization for Rare Disorders (NORD)
PO Box 8923
New Fairfield, CT 06812-8923
(800) 999-6673/(203)746-6518
http://www.rarediseases.org

Office of Disability Employment Policy
Job Accommodation Network
West Virginia University, PO Box 6080

Morgantown, WV 26506-6080
(800) 526-7234/(800) ADA-WORK (Voice/TTY)
(304) 293-7186
(304) 293-5407 (Fax)
http://www.jan.wvu.edu

Parent Project for Muscular Dystrophy Research
1012 N University Boulevard
Middletown, OH 45044
(800) 714-KIDS (-5437)/(513) 424-0696
(513) 425-9907 (Fax)
http://www.parentprojectmd.org

Myasthenia Gravis Resources:

Myasthenia Gravis Foundation of America
5841 Cedar Lake Road, Suite 204
Minneapolis, MI 55416
(952) 545-9438/(800) 541-5454
(952) 545-6073 (Fax)
http://www.myasthenia.org

Myasthenia Gravis-A Summary http://www.myasthe-nia.org/information/summary.htm
Authored by Dr. James F. Howard, Dpt of Neurology, The University of North Carolina at Chapel Hill.

National Organization for Rare Disorders
PO Box 8923
New Fairfield, CT 06812-8923
(800) 999-6673/(203) 746-6518
http://www.rarediseases.org

Office of Disability Employment Policy
Job Accommodation Network
West Virginia University, PO Box 6080
Morgantown, WV 26506-6080
(800) 526-7234/(800) ADA-WORK (Voice/TTY)
(304) 293-7186
(304) 293-5407 (Fax)
http://www.jan.wvu.edu

Neurological (Miscellaneous) Resources:

AACPDM—Site of the American Academy for Cerebral Palsy & Developmental Medicine
6300 North River Road, Suite 727
Rosemont, IL 60018-4226
(847) 658-1635
(847) 823-0536 (Fax)
http://www.aacpdm.org

Access Board—Federal Agency Responsible for Accessibility Specifications of Buildings
U.S. Architectural & Transportation
Barriers Compliance Board (The Access Board)
1331 F Street, NW, Suite 1000
Washington, DC 20004-1111
(202) 272-5434
http://www.access-board.gov

American Academy of Neurology
1080 Montreal Avenue
St. Paul, MN 55116
(800) 879-1960
http://www.aan.com

The Family Village
Waisman Center, University of Wisconsin Madison
1500 Highland Avenue
Madison, WI 53705-2280
http://www.familyvillage.wisc.edu

Office of Disability Employment Policy
Job Accommodation Network
West Virginia University, PO Box 6080
Morgantown, WV 26506-6080
(800) 526-7234/(800) ADA-WORK (Voice/TTY)
(304) 293-7186
(304) 293-5407 (Fax)
http://www.jan.wvu.edu

RESNA—(Rehabilitation Engineering and Assistive Technology Society of North America)
1700 North Moore Street, Suite 1540
Arlington, VA 22209-1903
(703) 524-6686/(703) 524-6639 (TTY)
(703) 524-6630 (Fax)
http://www.resna.org

TASH
29 W. Susquehanna Avenue, Suite 210
Baltimore, MD 21204
(410) 828-8274
(410) 828-6706 (Fax)
http://www.tash.org

Trace Research and Development Center
University of Wisconsin – Madison
5901 Research Park Boulevard
Madison, WI 53719 -1252
(608) 262-6966/(608) 263-5408 (TTY)
(608) 262-8848 (Fax)
http://www.trace.wisc.edu

UCP National
1660 L Street, NW, Suite 700
Washington, DC 20036
(202) 776-0406/(202) 973-7197 (TTY)
(202) 776-0414 (Fax)
http://www.ucpa.org

Parkinson's Resources

American Parkinson Disease Association, Inc.
1250 Hylan Boulevard, Suite 4B
Staten Island, NY 10305
(800) 223-2732/(718) 981-8001
(718) 981-4399 (Fax)
http://www.apdaparkinson.org

Centers for Disease Control and Prevention (CDC)
1600 Clifton Road
Atlanta, GA 30333
(404) 639-3534
http://www.cdc.gov

Michael J. Fox Foundation for Parkinson's Research
381 Park Avenue S., Suite 820
New York, NY 10016
(212) 213-3525
(212) 213-3523 (Fax)
http://www.michaeljfox.org

National Parkinson's Foundation (NPF)
Bob Hope Parkinson Research Center
1501 N.W. 9th Avenue, Bob Hope Road
Miami, FL 33136-1494
(800) 327-4545/(305) 547-6666
(305) 243-4403 (Fax)
http://www.parkinson.org

Office of Disability Employment Policy
Job Accommodation Network
West Virginia University, PO Box 6080
Morgantown, WV 26506-6080
(800) 526-7234/(800) ADA-WORK (Voice/TTY)
(304) 293-7186
(304) 293-5407 (Fax)
http://www.jan.wvu.edu

Parkinson Act Network
300 N. Lee Street, Suite 500
Alexandria, VA 22314
(800) 850-4726
(730) 518-8877
(730) 518-0673 (Fax)
http://www.parkinsonaction.org

Parkinson's Disease Foundation, Inc. (PDF)
710 West 168th Street
New York, NY 10032-9982
(800) 457-6676/(212) 923-4700
(212) 923-4778 (Fax)
http://www.pdf.org

Parkinson's Foundation of Canada
4211 Yonge Street, Suite 316
Toronto, ON, Canada M2P 2A9
(800) 565-3000/(416) 227-9700
http://www.parkinson.ca

The Parkinson's Institute
1170 Morse Avenue
Sunnyvale, CA 94089-1605
(800) 786-2958/(408) 734-2800
http://www.parkinsonsinstitute.org

Psychiatric Disabilities Resources

Anxiety Disorders Association of America
11900 Parklawn Drive, Suite 100
Rockville, MD 20852-2624
(301) 231-9350
http://www.adaa.org

Center for Psychiatric Rehabilitation, Boston University
940 Commonwealth Avenue
Boston, MA 02215
(617) 353-3549
(617) 353-7700 (Fax)
http://www.bu.edu/sarpsych/

Judge David L. Bazelon Center for Mental Health Law
1101 15th Street, NW, Suite 1212
Washington, DC 20005
(202) 467-5730
(202) 467-4232 (TTY)
(202) 223-0409 (Fax)
http://www.bazelon.org

Knowledge Exchange Network (KEN)
PO Box 42490
Washington, DC 20015
(800) 789-CMHS/(800) 789-2647
(301) 443-9006 (TTY)
(301) 984-8796 (Fax)
http://www.mentalhealth.org

National Alliance for the Mentally Ill (NAMI)
Colonial Place 3
2107 Wilson Boulevard, Suite 300
Arlington, VA 22201
(800) 950-NAMI/(800) 950-6264/(703) 524-7600
(703) 524-9094 (Fax)
(703) 516-7227 (TTY)
http://www.nami.org

National Depressive/Manic Depressive Association
730 North Franklin, Suite 510
Chicago, IL 60610
(312) 642-0049
(312) 642-7243 (Fax)
(800) 82-NDMDA/(800) 826-3632
http://www.ndmda.org

National Foundation for Depressive Illness, Inc.
PO Box 2257
New York, NY 10116

(800) 239-1265 (Fax)
http://www.depression.org

National Mental Health Association
1021 Prince Street
Alexandria, VA 22314
(703) 684-7722/(800) 969-6642
(703) 684-5968 (Fax)
(800) 433-5969 (TTY)
http://www.nmha.org

National Mental Health Consumer Self-Help Clearinghouse
1211 Chestnut Street, Suite 1207
Philadelphia, PA 19107
(800) 553-4KEY/(800) 555-4539
(215) 751-1810
(215) 636-6312 (Fax)
http://www.mhselfhelp.org

Obsessive Compulsive Foundation Inc
337 Notch Hill Road
North Branford, CT 06471
(203) 315-2190
(203) 315-2196 (Fax)
http://www.ocfoundation.org

Office of Disability Employment Policy
Job Accommodation Network
West Virginia University, PO Box 6080
Morgantown, WV 26506-6080
(800) 526-7234/(800) ADA-WORK (Voice/TTY)
(304) 293-7186
(304) 293-5407 (Fax)
http://www.jan.wvu.edu

Washington Business Group on Health
Employers' Resource Center on the ADA and Workers with Psychiatric Disabilities
50 F Street, NW, Suite 600
Washington, DC 20001
(202) 628-9320
(202) 628-9244 (Fax)
http://www.wbgh.com

Sleep Disorder Resources

American Academy of Sleep Medicine
6301 Bandel Road, Suite 101
Rochester, MN 55901
http://www.aasmnet.org

The American Sleep Apnea Association
1424 K Street, NW, Suite 302
Washington, DC 20005
(202) 293-3650
(202) 293-3656 (Fax)
http://www.sleepapnea.org

Equal Employment Opportunity Commission (EEOC)
(800) 669-4000
(800) 669-6820 (TDD)
http://www.eeoc.gov

Narcolepsy Network
10921 Reed Hartman Highway
Cincinnati, OH 45241
(513) 891-3522/(513) 891-3836
http://www.websciences.org/narnet/

National Institute on Disability and Rehabilitative Research
400 Maryland Avenue, SW
Washington, DC 20202-2572
(202) 205-8134/(202) 205-4475
http://www.ed.gov/offices/OSERS/NIDRR/

National Institutes of Health
Bethesda, MD 20892
http://search.info.nih.gov

National Institute of Neurological Disorders and Stroke
PO Box 5801
Bethesda, MD 20824
(301) 352-9424
http://www.ninds.nih.gov/index.htm

National Sleep Foundation
729 Fifteenth Street, NW, Fourth Floor
Washington, DC 20005
http://www.sleepfoundation.org

Office of Disability Employment Policy
Job Accommodation Network
West Virginia University, PO Box 6080
Morgantown, WV 26506-6080
(800) 526-7234/(800) ADA-WORK (Voice/TTY)
(304) 293-7186
(304) 293-5407 (Fax)
http://www.jan.wvu.edu

Sleep Medicine Associates of Texas, P.A.
8140 Walnut Hill Lane, Suite 100
Dallas, TX 75231
(214) 750-7776
(214) 750-4621 (Fax)
http://www.sleepmed.com/sleepdisorders.html#Narcolepsy

Social Security Administration (SSA)
6401 Security Boulevard, Room 4-C-5 Annex
Baltimore, MD 21235
(800) 772-1213
(800) 325-0778 (TDD)
http://www.ssa.gov

U.S. Department of Justice
Civil Rights Division
PO Box 66738
Washington, DC 20035-6738
(800) 514-0301
(800) 514-0383 (TDD)
(202) 307-1198 (Fax)
http://www.usdoj.gov/crt/ada/adahom1.htm

U.S. Small Business Administration (SBA)
Office of Advocacy/Office of Economic Research
409 Third Street, SW, Suite 7600
Washington, DC 20416
(800) 8-ASK-SBA/(202) 376-6200
(202) 205-7064 (Fax)
(202) 205-7333 (TDD)
http://www.sbaonline.sba.gov

Trauma Resources

American Industrial Hygiene Association (AIHA)
2700 Prosperity Avenue, Suite 250
Fairfax, VA 22031
(703) 849-8888
(703) 207-3561 (Fax)
http://www.aiha.org

American National Standards Institute (ANSI)
1430 Broadway
New York, NY 10018
(212) 642-4900
http://web.ansi.org

American Society of Safety Engineers (ASSE)
1800 E. Oakton Street
Des Plaines, IL 60018
(847) 699-2929
(847) 768-3434 (Fax)
http://www.asse.org

The Association for Repetitive Motion Syndromes (A.R.M.S.)
PO Box 471973
Aurora CO 80047-1973
(303) 369-0803
http://www.certifiedpst.com/arms

Canadian Centre for Occupational Health and Safety (CCOHS)
250 Main Street East
Hamilton, ON, Canada L8N 1H6
(905) 572-4400/(800) 267-0441
(905) 572-4500 (Fax)
http://www.ccohs.ca

CTD Resource Network (CTDRN)
2013 Princeton Court
Los Banos, CA 93635
(209) 827-0801
http://www.ctdrn.org

Human Factors and Ergonomics Society
PO Box 1369
Santa Monica, CA 90406-1369
(310) 394-1811
(310) 394-2410 (Fax)
http://hfes.org

National Institute for Occupational Safety and Health (NIOSH)
4676 Columbia Parkway, Mail Stop C-13
Cincinnati, OH 45226-1998
(800) 35-NIOSH/(513) 533-8326
http://www.cdc.gov/niosh/homepage.html

National Safety Council
1121 Spring Lake Drive
Itasca, IL 60143-3201
(630) 285-1121
(630) 285-1315 (Fax)
http://www.nsc.org

Occupational Safety & Health Administration (OSHA)
US Department of Labor, Public Affairs Office
Room 3647, 200 Constitution Avenue
Washington, DC 20210
(202) 693-1999/(800) 321-OSHA
http://www.osha.gov

Office of Disability Employment Policy
Job Accommodation Network
West Virginia University, PO Box 6080
Morgantown, WV 26506-6080
(800) 526-7234/(800) ADA-WORK (Voice/TTY)
(304) 293-7186
(304) 293-5407 (Fax)
http://www.jan.wvu.edu

Rehabilitation Engineering Society of North America (RESNA)
1700 North Moore Street, Suite 1540
Arlington, VA 22209-1903
(703) 524-6686
(703) 524-6630 (Fax)
(703) 524-6639 TTY
http://www.resna.org

Vision Impairments Resources

American Council of the Blind (ACB)
1155 15th Street, NW, Suite 1004
Washington, DC 20005
(202) 467-5081/(800) 424-8666
(202) 467-5085 (Fax)
http://www.acb.org

American Foundation for the Blind (AFB)
11 Penn Plaza, Suite 300
New York, NY 10001
(212) 502-7600/(800) AFB-LINE (232-5463)
http://www.afb.org

The Foundation Fighting Blindness
11435 Cronhill Drive
Owings Mills, MD 21117-2220
(888) 394-3937/(800) 683-5551 TDD
(410) 568-0150/(410) 363-7139 TDD
http://www.blindness.org

National Braille Press
88 St. Stephen Street
Boston, MA 02115
(617) 266-6160
(617) 437-0456 (Fax)
http://www.nbp.org

National Federation of the Blind (NFB)
1800 Johnson Street
Baltimore, MD 21230
(410) 659-9314
(410) 685-5653 (Fax)
http://www.nfb.org
http://www.nfb.org/states/newjob.htm

DB-LINK: The National Information Clearinghouse on Children Who Are Deaf-Blind
345 N. Monmouth Avenue
Monmouth, OR 97361
(800) 438-9376
(800) 854-7013 (TTY)
(503) 838-8150 (Fax)
http://www.tr.wou.edu/dblink

Recordings for the Blind & Dyslexic
20 Roszel Road
Princeton, NJ 08540
(609) 452-0606
(609) 987-8116 (Fax)
(800) 803-7201 (customer service)
http://www.rfbd.org

Rehabilitation Research and Training Center on Blindness and Low Vision
PO Drawer 6189, Mississippi State University
Mississippi State, MS 39762
(662) 325-2001
(662) 325-8989 (Fax)
(662) 325-8693 TDD
http://www.blind.msstate.edu

Trace Research & Development Center
University of Wisconsin–Madison
5901 Research Park Boulevard
Madison, WI 53719-1252
(608) 262-6966
(608) 262-8848 (Fax)
(608) 263-5408 (TTY)
http://trace.wisc.edu

Wheelchair Users Resources

AgrAbility
1146 Agricultural Engineering Building
West Lafayette, IN 47907-1146
(800) 825-4264
(765) 494-5088 (Voice/TT)
(765) 496-1356 (Fax)
http://abe.www.ecn.purdue.edu/ABE/Extension/BNG/agrabilityproject.html

The ALS Association
27001 Agoura Road, Suite 150
Calabasas Hills, CA 91301-5104
(800) 782-4747/(818) 880-9007
(818) 880-9006 (Fax)
http://www.alsa.org

American National Standards Institute (ANSI)
25 West 43rd Street, 4th Floor
New York, NY 10036
(212) 642-4900
(212) 398-0023 (Fax)
http://web.ansi.org

Arthritis Foundation
PO Box 7669
Atlanta, GA 30357-0669
(800) 283-7800/(404) 872-7100
http://www.arthritis.org

The Center for Universal Design
North Carolina State University
PO Box 8613
Raleigh, NC 27695-8613
(800) 647-6777/(919) 515-3082
(919) 515-3082 (Voice/TTY)
http://www.design.ncsu.edu/cud

Christopher Reeve Paralysis Foundation
500 Morris Avenue
Springfield, NJ 07081
(800) 225-0292
http://paralysis.org

Computer/Electronic Accommodations Program (CAP)
US Department of Defense
TRICARE Management Activity
5111 Leesburg Pike, Suite 810
Falls Church, VA 22041
(703) 681-3976 (Voice/TTY)

(703) 681-9075 (Fax)
http://www.tricare.osd.mil/cap

Delta Society National Service Dog Center (NSDC)
289 Perimeter Road East
Renton, WA 98055-1329
(425) 235-1076 (Fax)
www.deltasociety.org/

Independent Living Research Utilization Program (ILRU)
2323 S Shepherd, Suite 100
Houston, TX 77019
(713) 520-0232
(713) 520-5136 (TDD)
(713) 520-5785 (Fax)
http://www.bcm.tmc.edu/ilru

The Muscular Dystrophy Association (MDA)
3300 East Sunrise Drive
Tucson, AZ 85718
(800) 572-1717
http://www.mdausa.org/about.html

National Center on Accessibility (NCA)
Indiana University
2805 East 10th Street, Suite 190
Bloomington, IN 47408-2698
(812) 856-4422
(812) 856-4421 (TTY)
(812) 856-4480 (Fax)
http://www.indiana.edu/~nca

National Institute for Occupational Safety and Health (NIOSH)
4676 Columbia Parkway
Cincinnati, OH 45226-1998
(800) 35-NIOSH
(513) 533-8573 (Fax)
http://www.cdc.gov/niosh/homepage.html

The National MS Society (NMSS)
733 Third Avenue
New York, NY 10017
(800) Fight-MS (344-4867)
http://nmss.org

National Spinal Cord Injury Association (NSCIA)
6701 Democracy Boulevard, Suite 300-9
Bethesda, MD 20817
(800) 962-9629/(301) 588-6959
http://www.spinalcord.org

National Spinal Cord Injury Statistical Center
UAB Spain Rehabilitation Center
Room 544, 1717 6th Avenue, S.
Birmingham, AL 35233-7330
(205) 934-3320

National Stroke Association (NSA)
9707 E. Easter Lane
Englewood, CO 80112
(800) STROKES/(303) 649-9299
http://www.stroke.org

Occupational Safety & Health Administration (OSHA)
US Department of Labor
200 Constitution Avenue, NW
Washington, DC 20210
(202) 693-1999
http://www.osha.gov

Office of Disability Employment Policy
Job Accommodation Network
West Virginia University, PO Box 6080
Morgantown, WV 26506-6080
(800) 526-7234/(800) ADA-WORK (Voice/TTY)
(304) 293-7186
(304) 293-5407 (Fax)
http://www.jan.wvu.edu

Paralyzed Veterans of America (PVA)
801 Eighteenth Street, NW
Washington, DC 20006-3517
(800) 424-8200
http://www.pva.org

Index

Note: Page numbers followed by f refer to figures; page numbers followed by t refer to tables.